Orthodontics in the Vertical Dimension

A Case-Based Review

Orthodontics in the Vertical Dimension

A Case-Based Review

Thomas E. Southard, DDS, MS

Steven D. Marshall, DDS, MS

Laura L. Bonner, DDS, MS

University of Iowa
Iowa City, Iowa
USA

WILEY Blackwell

Published by John Wiley & Sons, Inc., Hoboken, New Jersey
Published simultaneously in Canada

Library of Congress Cataloging-in-Publication Data:

Southard, Thomas E., author.
Orthodontics in the vertical dimension : a case-based review / Thomas E. Southard, Steven D. Marshall, Laura L. Bonner.
p. ; cm.
Includes index.
ISBN 978-1-118-87021-1 (cloth)
I. Marshall, Steven D., author. II. Bonner, Laura L., author. III. Title.
[DNLM: 1. Malocclusion–Case Reports. 2. Malocclusion–Problems and Exercises. 3. Orthodontics–methods–Case Reports. 4. Orthodontics–methods–Problems and Exercises. 5. Vertical Dimension–Case Reports. 6. Vertical Dimension–Problems and Exercises. WU 18.2]
RK521
617.6′43–dc23

2015004424

Set in 9/11pt Minion by SPi Global, Pondicherry, India

10 9 8 7 6 5 4 3 2 1

Contents

Preface

The goal of this book is to teach—to provide students with a solid foundation in diagnosis, treatment planning, and "in-treatment" decision-making when managing malocclusions—with special emphasis on the vertical dimension. Problems in the vertical dimension can be especially challenging to manage, and a clinician must achieve a high level of proficiency in addressing these challenges. Careful study of our book will provide the foundation for achieving this proficiency.

The practice of orthodontics and dentofacial orthopedics is a cognitive discipline. Over 90% of what an orthodontist does is observe, reason, and make decisions. Treatment planning and treatment delivery for each patient essentially consist of your ability to correctly answer a seemingly infinite series of questions related to that patient's care. During orthodontic residency, when you examine a patient, the attending faculty asks what problems you observe, and you answer. The attending faculty asks how you would treat these problems, you answer, and the faculty provides you with positive and constructive feedback. Whether in the classroom or clinic, we have found orthodontic residents mature fastest and best using this method of question–answer teaching.

The format of our book is similarly based on this question–answer style of teaching, as we view our book as an orthodontic miniresidency. We use the question–answer format in order to keep you intellectually involved, to encourage critical thinking, to offer you the opportunity to reflect on our questions and your answers, and to gauge the progress of your understanding. Using this format, we will coach you to address a very broad range of challenging clinical problems and to formulate appropriate decisions. To grasp the principles upon which we focus, we recommend that you study each case from beginning to end at one sitting. Carefully think through answers to the questions we present (ideally, by writing down your answers), and make the best decisions you can. You should do this <u>before</u> you refer to the answers we have provided. Answer each question as thoughtfully as you would if the patient was sitting in front of you, and you had to make the right decision to care for him or her. Your orthodontic diagnostic, treatment planning, and in-treatment decision abilities will strengthen in direct proportion to your efforts to work through each problem presented—before making your decision and reading our answers.

You will find certain principles are emphasized and applied repeatedly throughout this text. This is our objective—to instill patterns of analysis and habits of rational decision making by repetition and by presenting many different patients with a multitude of problems. Problems in the vertical dimension are inextricably related to problems in the anteroposterior and transverse dimensions. The principles and cases presented comprehensively illustrate these interrelationships and will strengthen your ability to treat patients in all three dimensions. Also, as occurs with every patient you will treat in your practice, each patient presented in this text has diverse problems apart from the primary problems in the vertical, anteroposterior, and transverse dimensions. Many of the problems that you will likely encounter in private practice will be examined and addressed in this text.

The answers we provide for the cases presented are based on our many years of teaching, literature review, and clinical experience at the University of Iowa and in private practice. It does not mean, however, that our answers are necessarily "correct." Everything taught in our specialty must be challenged and questioned. If our ideas cannot withstand the rigor of scrutiny and the test of time, then we must modify our position. If you disagree with concepts in this text, please discuss them with your colleagues, attending faculty, or us. Constructive dialogue makes us better orthodontists, results in better care for our patients, and strengthens our specialty. Our book contains important references for many clinical and scientific concepts, but was not written as a systematic review reference source. The treatment principles contained in this text will be valid for your lifetime of clinical practice, but the specific scientific and clinical study references may change over the years.

The spectrum of vertical problems encompasses deep bites and open bites of both skeletal and dental origin, and our book is organized accordingly into the following chapters: Foundations, Dental Deep Bites, Skeletal Deep Bites, Dental Anterior Open Bites, Skeletal Anterior Open Bites, Posterior Open Bites, and Appendix. In Chapter 1, we provide an overview of the spectrum of vertical dimension problems, important craniofacial growth concepts, and fundamental principles of diagnosis and treatment planning. These principles are applied repeatedly with every case throughout the text. In Chapter 2, an introduction provides overall concepts of dental deep bite diagnosis and treatment. The cases that follow encompass comprehensive dental deep bite cases, which you will work through from initial patient presentation to debond/deband and retention. The same chapter organization is repeated for subsequent chapters. The Appendix presents a cephalometric analysis primer, the Iowa AP Classification Primer, useful tables, and abbreviations. We wish to note that every case we present in the book was painstakingly chosen from a cumulative clinical practice of over one-half century, with the intent of providing a broad range of problems. Our ultimate goal is your goal: to help you become a superb orthodontist. As teachers, Steve, Laura, and I will always strive to help you become a better orthodontist than we are. We experience no greater professional joy than when our students rise above us. If you learn from this book, then our years of teaching will have been worthwhile.

You will find no mention of specific orthodontic bracket types or specific orthodontic bracket manufacturers in this text. Why? Excellent orthodontic care depends on the orthodontist's intelligence, education, experience, skill, and desire. The specific appliance used by each doctor is a matter of personal preference. When you first enter practice, you will be exposed to new brackets, wires, appliances, and biomechanics that are purported to be "the answer" to orthodontic treatment. Be skeptical. When someone announces they have the answer, or a panacea for treatment, demand that they provide you with evidence (independently confirmed from different university studies in high impact, peer-reviewed journals), that clearly documents the efficacy of their claims of treatment superiority.

We wish to acknowledge the diagnostic skill, treatment outcomes, and patient care provided by Dr. Karin A. Southard who kindly allowed us to include many of her cases in this book. Karin is a clinician's clinician and an educator's educator. We thank her for her teaching and her many contributions to excellent patient care. We also wish to thank Dr. Michael L. Swartz for his permission to use orthodontic clipart in developing many of the illustrations in this text, and Drs. Nathan E. Holton, Veerasathpurush Allareddy, and Ms. Chris White for their thorough review and many insightful suggestions. Finally, we wish to thank Dr. James Vaden for providing us with material from the Charles H. Tweed International Foundation for Orthodontic Research and Education.

This book is dedicated to every man or woman who strives daily to become proficient in the art and science of orthodontics and dentofacial orthopedics, and who endeavors, uncompromisingly, to provide outstanding care to his or her patients. Doctor, we salute you.

CHAPTER 1

Foundations

The Spectrum of Vertical

Q: Emily is a 20-year-old who presents to you for treatment (Figure 1.1). Compare her soft tissue midface height to her soft tissue lower anterior facial height (LAFH). What do you observe?

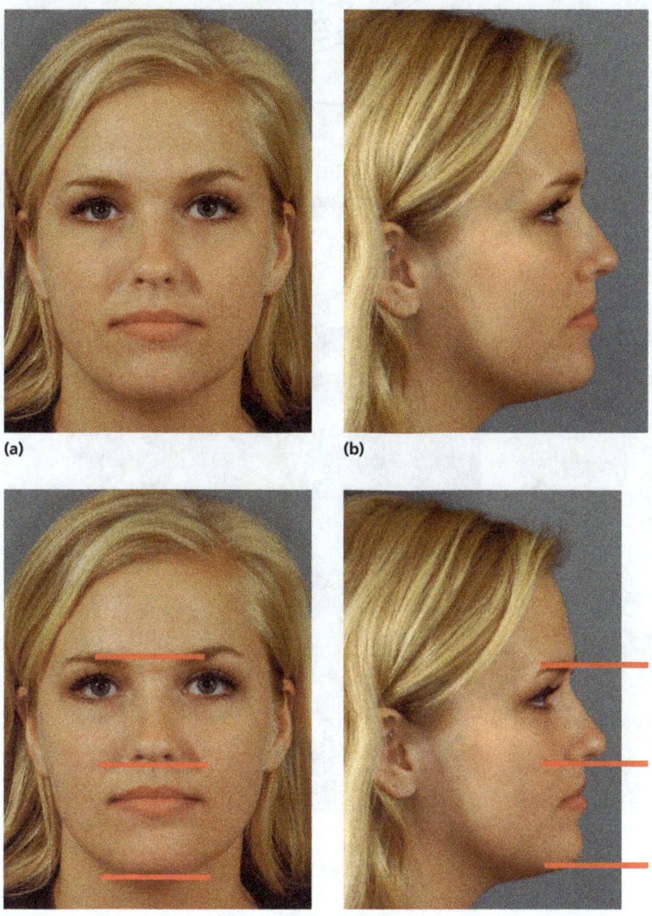

Figure 1.1 (a, b) Emily's facial photographs. (c, d) Soft tissue midface height (vertical distance from supraorbital ridges/soft tissue Glabella to Subnasale) is compared to LAFH (vertical distance from Subnasale to soft tissue Menton). Abbreviations used in this book are defined in the Appendix.

A: Emily's soft tissue proportions are nearly ideal. Her soft tissue midface height is equal to her soft tissue LAFH. [1, 2] Also, the distance from Subnasale to Stomion is approximately one-half of the distance from Stomion to soft tissue Menton. She exhibits lip competence without either an interlabial gap (ILG) or an overclosed appearance.

Q: Next, evaluate her vertical skeletal and dental features using her cephalometric tracing (Figure 1.2). What do you observe?

A: The (percentage) skeletal LAFH is expressed as a proportion of (linear) skeletal LAFH to (linear) skeletal TAFH (total anterior facial height). TAFH is the distance Nasion–Menton. LAFH is the distance measured from Menton along a Nasion–Menton line to a point where ANS projects perpendicularly to the Nasion–Menton line. For Emily, the LAFH/TAFH ratio (expressed as a percentage) is 54%. Ideal LAFH/TAFH is 55%, and one standard deviation difference from ideal is approximately 2% [3]. So, Emily's LAFH/TAFH is normal. In terms of mandibular plane (MP) angles, her FMA is normal (26°; ideal is 25°) and SNMP is normal (30°; ideal is 32°). Her maxillary first molar root apices are located below the palatal plane, a feature generally found in patients with vertical maxillary excess. Finally, the maxillary central incisor tip extends below the upper lip by approximately 4 mm (ideal 2–4 mm) [4]. A primer on the determination of facial height and other cephalometric parameters used in this book can be found in the Appendix.

Q: A number of Emily's skeletal and dental features were described as normal, but not ideal. Should not the terms normal and ideal be synonymous? In other words, if the ideal (average) FMA is 25°, should not this exact value be considered normal and all other FMA values considered abnormal?

A: No. *"Normal" constitutes a range of values and not one specific number*. That is why we say, "within the range of normal," or WRN. In other words, an FMA of 25° is normal but so can FMAs of 26°, 27°, 28°, 24°, 23°, and 22° be considered WRN. The same can be said for LAFH/TAFH proportions, ANB values, FMIA values, and so forth. Ideal can be considered one specific value, for instance, the average value measured from a population, but normal is a range—not a number. Think of it this way, there exists a broad range of what we consider beautiful human faces, and normal human faces cover an even broader range. A discussion of "normal" cephalometric values can be found in the Appendix.

Q: Evaluate Emily's vertical dental features, as seen intraorally (Figure 1.3a). What do you observe?

A: Overall, she presents with normal overbite (10–20% vertical overlap of her mandibular incisors by her maxillary central incisors measured in centric occlusion, Figure 1.3b). Variation

Orthodontics in the Vertical Dimension: A Case-Based Review, First Edition. Thomas E. Southard, Steven D. Marshall and Laura L. Bonner.

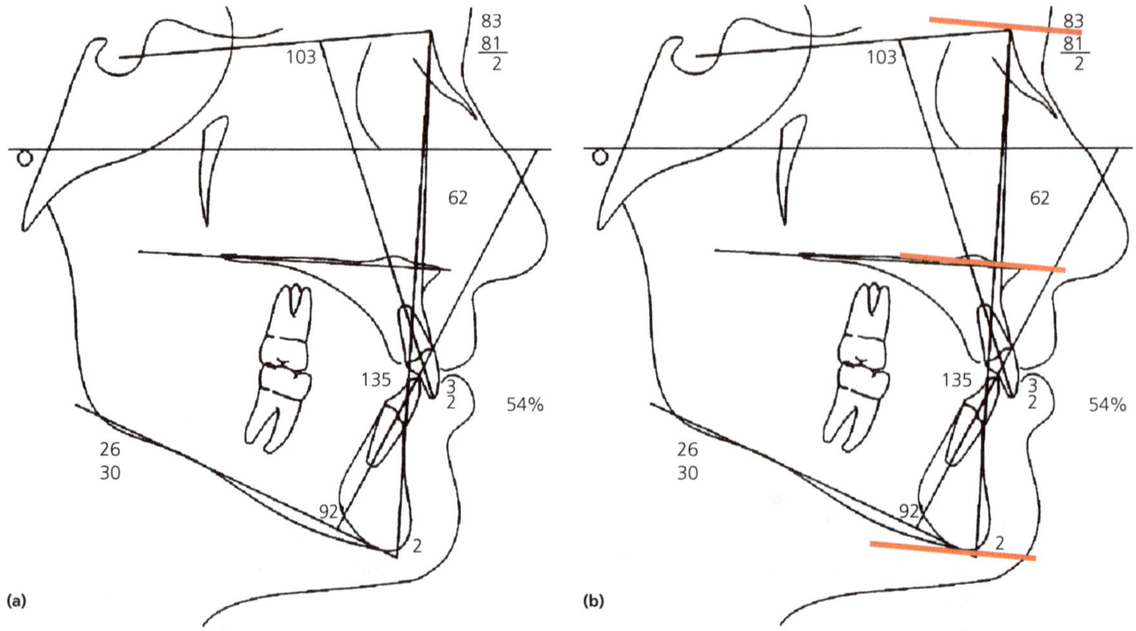

Figure 1.2 (a) Emily's lateral cephalometric tracing. (b) Skeletal TAFH is the distance Nasion–Menton. Skeletal LAFH is the distance measured from Menton along a Nasion–Menton line to a point where ANS projects perpendicularly to the Nasion–Menton line. A primer on the determination of facial height and other cephalometric measurements used in this book can be found in the Appendix.

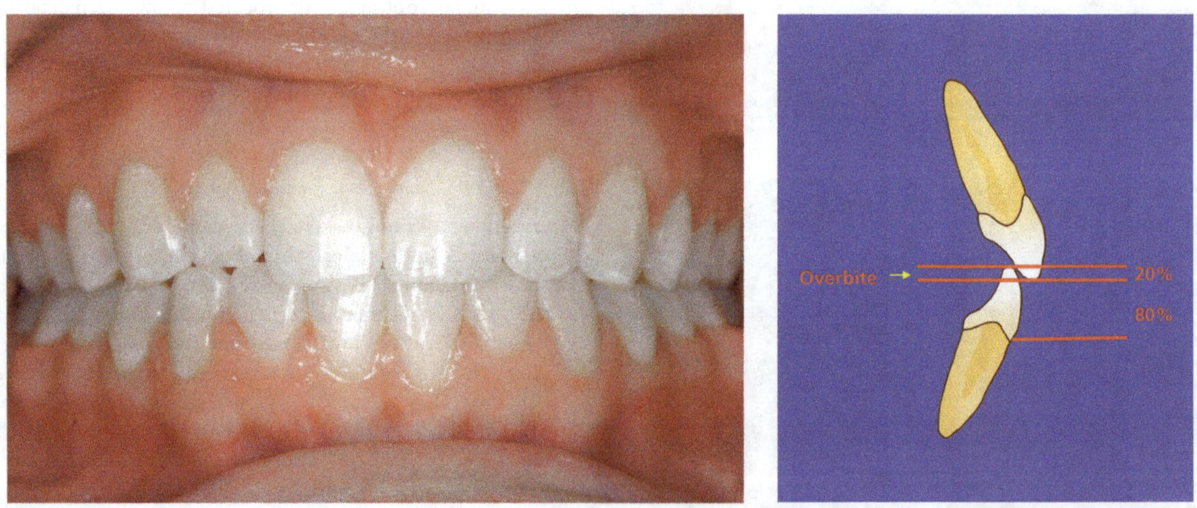

Figure 1.3 (a) Frontal intraoral view of Emily with (b) approximately 20% central incisor overbite measured relative to mandibular central incisor crown length.

in overbite is illustrated in Figure 1.4, which ranges from excessive vertical overlap (deep OB, Figure 1.4 left) to an absence of vertical overlap (open bite, Figure 1.4 right). Emily's maxillary right lateral incisor (Figure 1.3a) exhibits inadequate vertical overlap with her mandibular right lateral incisor—resulting in dark incisal embrasures. Her maxillary central incisor gingival margins are at the same level (ideal), her right and left maxillary lateral incisor gingival margins are about even but stepped down slightly compared to the centrals (ideal), and her right canine gingival margin is stepped up slightly compared to the right lateral (ideal, central–lateral–canine gingival heights are "high–low–high"). Her left canine gingival margin is even with her left lateral gingival margin (less ideal). Finally, her midlines are coincident (ideal), and the height of the gingival papilla between the maxillary central incisors is about one-half the vertical crown length of the central incisors (ideal) [5].

Combining Emily's soft tissue (clinical), skeletal (cephalometric), and dental (intraoral) features, we conclude that she is vertically normal. If we imagine a spectrum of patients presenting with varying degrees of vertical facial development (Figure 1.5), then we can imagine plotting Emily as normal.

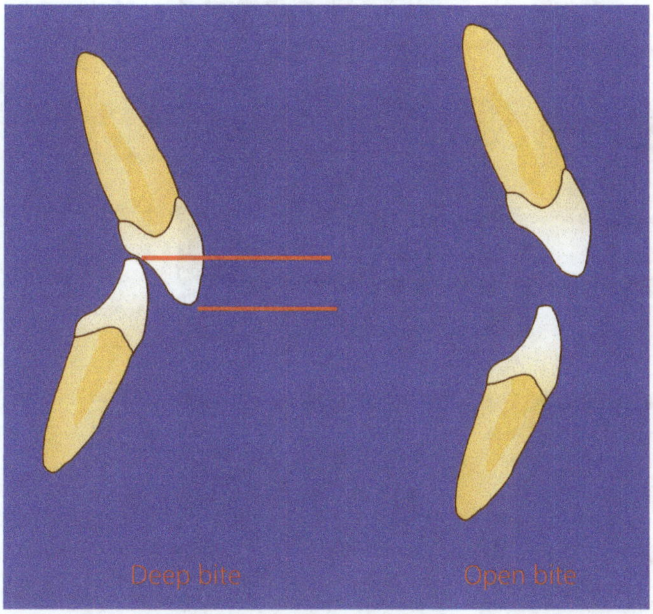

Figure 1.4 Illustration of maxillary and mandibular central incisors in the sagittal view depicting incisor overbite, ranging from deep (left) to open (right).

Q: Let's use our spectrum to compare subjects who vary considerably in vertical facial development. Three more patients present for examination (Figure 1.6, left to right Kelly, Ashley, and Alexis). Compare their soft tissue midface heights to their soft tissue LAFHs. Compare other facial features. What do you observe?

A: A stark contrast in vertical soft tissue proportions exists between Kelly, Ashley, and Alexis. Kelly's LAFH is shorter than her midface height, Ashley's LAFH is equal to her midface height, and Alexis's LAFH is longer than her midface height. Kelly and Ashley are facially symmetric, while Alexis has a slight chin deviation to her right. Kelly appears overclosed. Kelly and Ashley demonstrate lip competence with the distance from Subnasale to Stomion approximately one-half the distance from Stomion to soft tissue Menton (ideal). Alexis presents with lip incompetence (ILG), so Stomion (the midpoint of the oral fissure when the lips are closed) does not exist. Alexis presents with an ILG of 8 mm. An ILG of up to 2 mm may be considered normal [6].

Q: Evaluate and contrast their respective vertical skeletal and dental features using cephalometric tracings (Figure 1.7). What do you observe?

A: Kelly's skeletal LAFH/TAFH is 50%, more than two standard deviations less than ideal (55%) (Figure 1.7d). Ashley's LAFH/TAFH is 56%, normal (Figure 1.7e). Alexis's LAFH/TAFH is

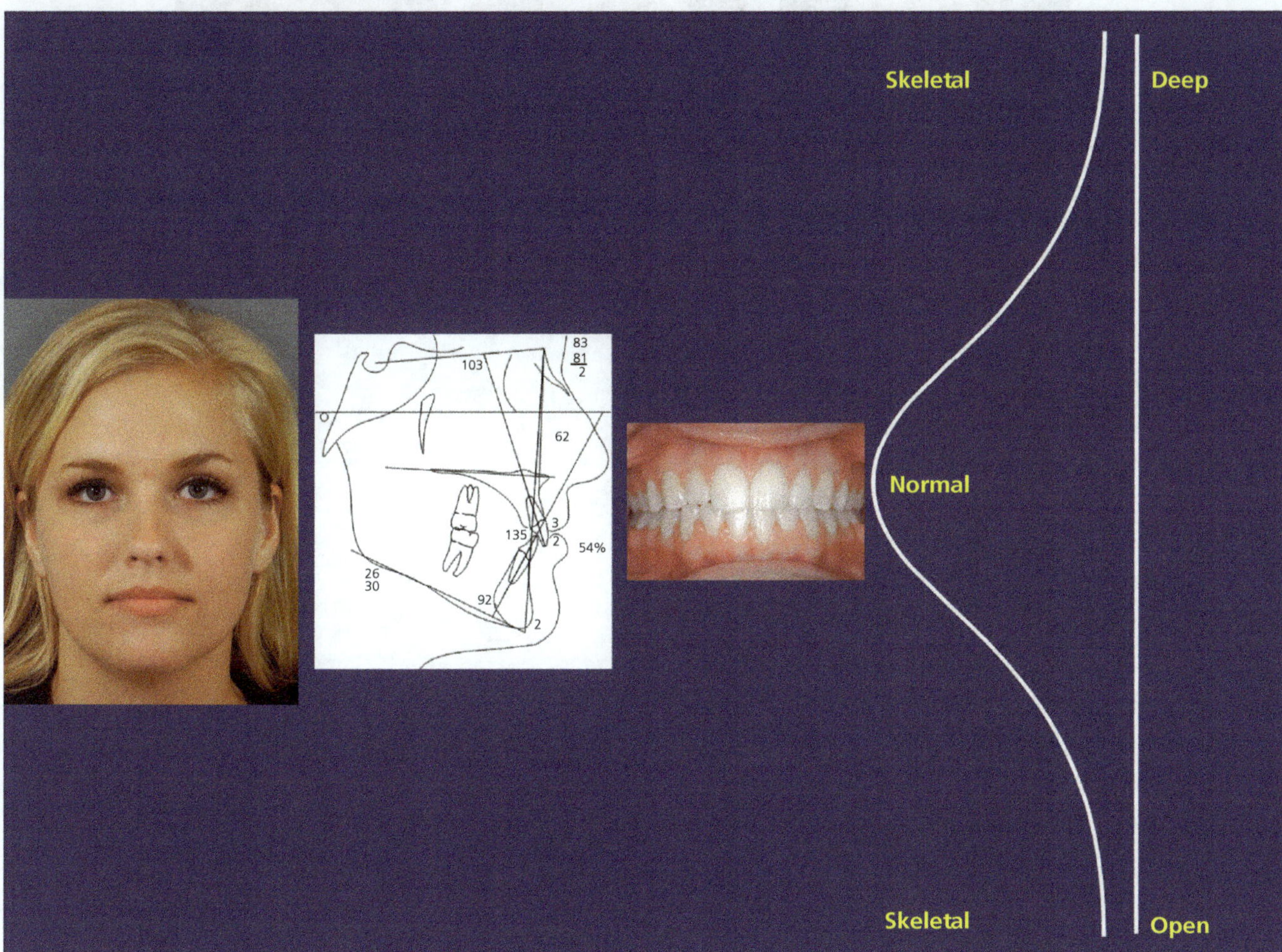

Figure 1.5 The spectrum of vertical facial development depicted on the right ranges from deficient (top, usually associated with deep bite) to excessive (bottom, usually associated with open bite). Emily is located in the center of this range and exhibits normal vertical facial development.

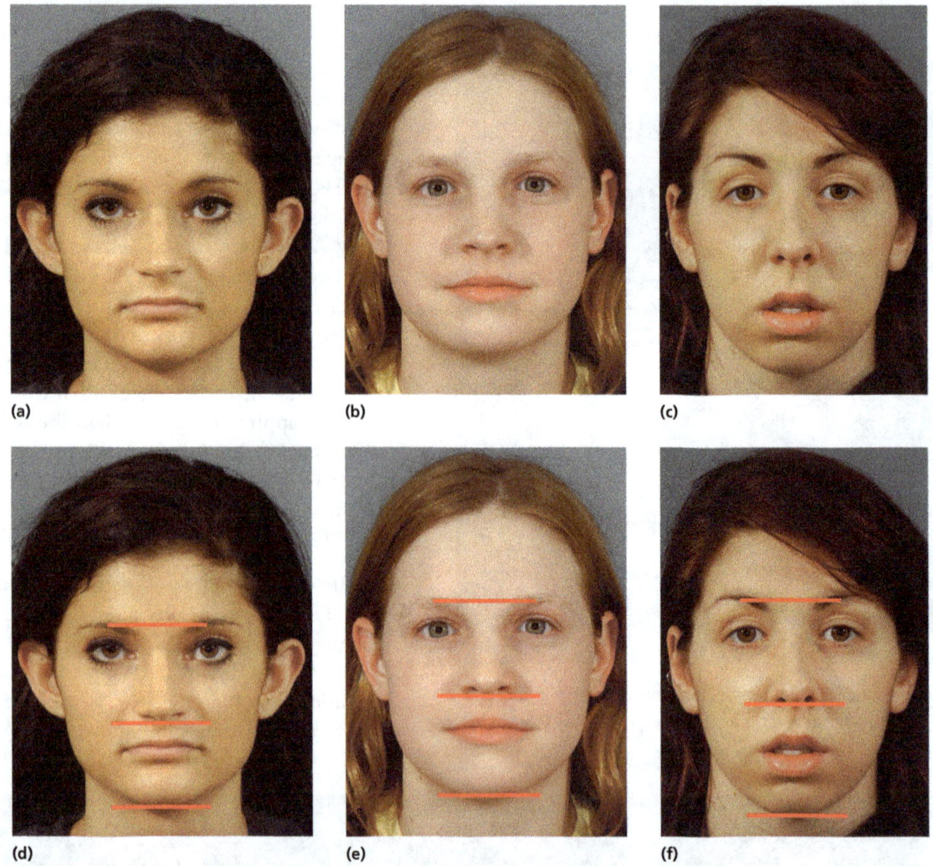

Figure 1.6 Variation of vertical soft tissue proportions: (a, d) Kelly, (b, e) Ashley, and (c, f) Alexis.

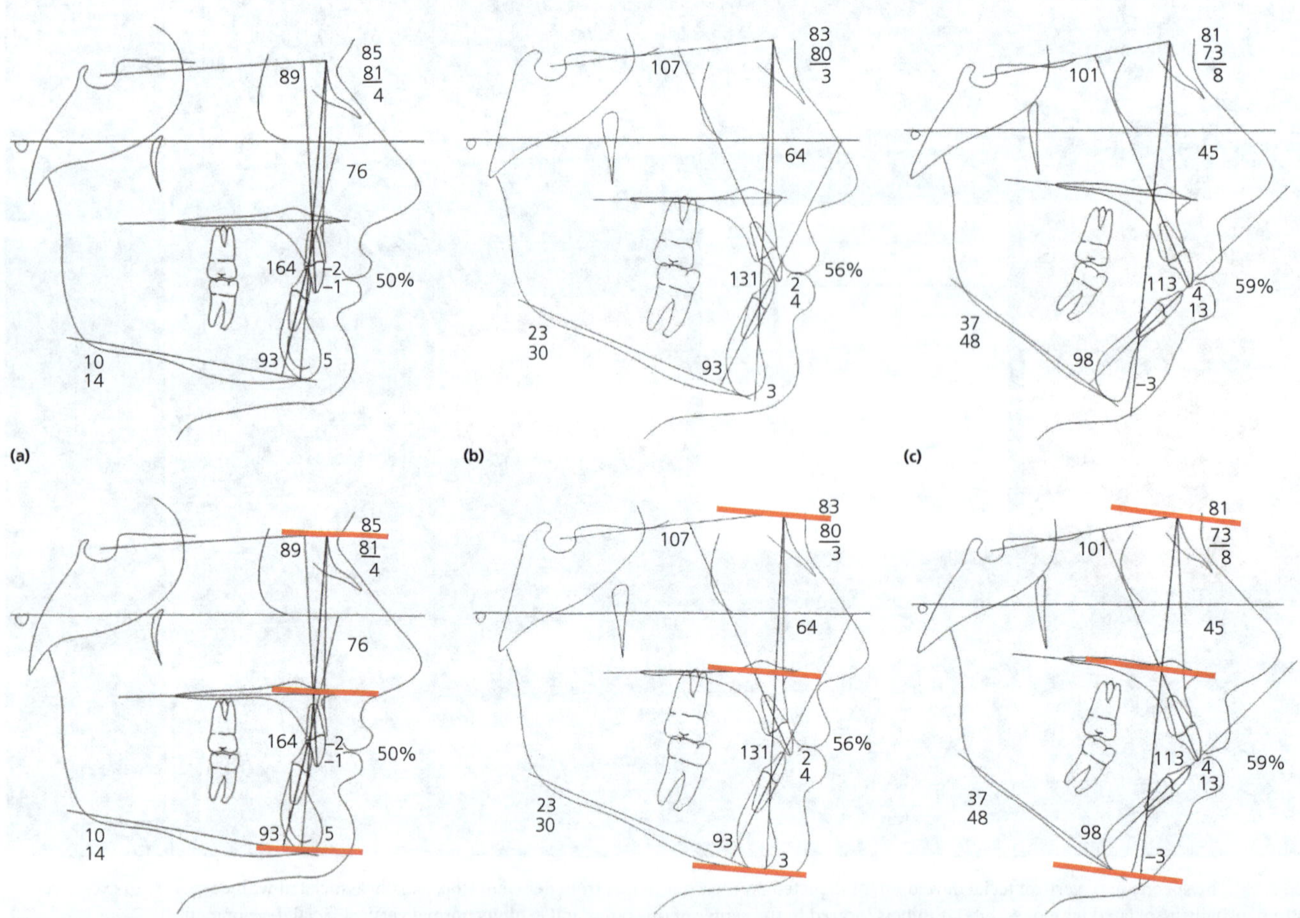

Figure 1.7 Variation of vertical skeletal and dental features: (a, d) Kelly, (b, e) Ashley, and (c, f) Alexis.

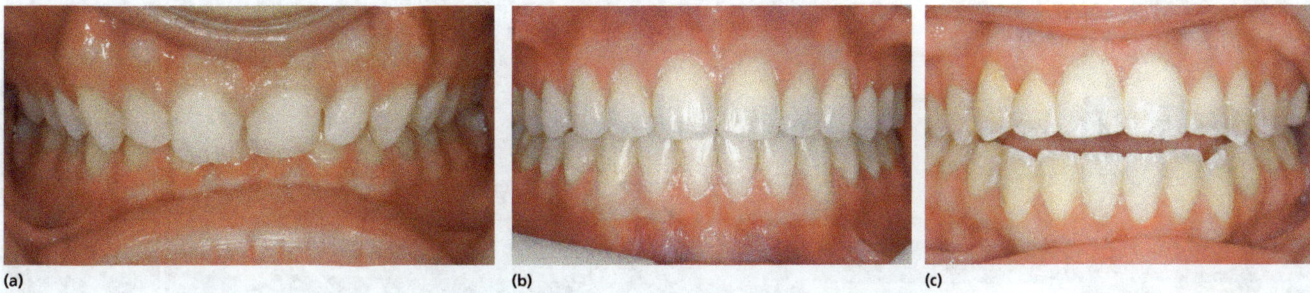

Figure 1.8 Variation of intraoral vertical dental features for the subjects shown in Figure 1.6: (a) Kelly, (b) Ashley, and (c) Alexis.

59%, two standard deviations greater than ideal (Figure 1.7f). Kelly's MPAs are flat (FMA = 10°, SNMP = 14°) compared to ideal (FMA = 25°, SNMP = 32°), and her MP, FH, and SN (Sella–Nasion) lines are roughly parallel. Ashley's MPAs are normal (FMA = 23°, SNMP = 30°). But Alexis's MPAs are steep (FMA = 37°, SNMP = 48°), and her MP, FH, and SN lines diverge significantly. Kelly and Ashley's maxillary first molar apices are located at their respective palatal planes (ideal), while Alexis's maxillary first molar apices have erupted well below her palatal plane. Kelly's maxillary central incisor tip extends below her maxillary lip by about 4 mm (ideal 2–4 mm), but this maxillary lip coverage could change if she were to separate her jaws slightly and let her maxillary lip relax. Ashley's and Alexis's maxillary incisor tip extends below their maxillary lips by 1–2 mm.

Q: Finally, evaluate their vertical dental features, as seen intraorally (Figure 1.8). What do you observe?

A: Kelly presents with 100% OB (Figure 1.8a, 100% overlap of her mandibular incisors by her maxillary incisors). Her maxillary incisors are "stepped down" relative to her maxillary posterior teeth. Ashley has an ideal OB of 10–20% (Figure 1.8b). Alexis has a 2–3 mm anterior open bite with maxillary incisors stepped up relative to the maxillary posterior teeth and mandibular incisors stepped down relative to the mandibular posterior teeth (Figure 1.8c). In terms of gingival levels, all Kelly's maxillary incisors have gingival margins at the same level (due to central incisor overeruption). Ashley's central incisor gingival margins are slightly uneven, but she demonstrates reasonably normal high–low–high gingival margin relationships proceeding from maxillary central incisors to canines. Alexis's maxillary central incisor gingival margins are even, and she demonstrates a reasonable high–low–high gingival margin relationship proceeding from central incisors to canines. Coincidence of maxillary and mandibular midlines cannot be ascertained in Kelly's frontal view, Ashley's midlines are coincident, and Alexis's midlines appear to be reasonably coincident. Kelly demonstrates a short gingival papilla between her supraerupted maxillary central incisor crowns. Ashley's and Alexis's maxillary incisor gingival papilla heights are approximately ideal (one-half of their respective central incisor crown lengths).

Q: Based on soft tissue (clinical), skeletal (cephalometric), and dental (intraoral) features, where would you place Kelly, Ashley, and Alexis on the spectrum of vertical facial development?

A: Kelly's features place her at one end of the vertical spectrum—skeletal deep bite. Alexis has features placing her at the other end of the vertical spectrum—skeletal open bite. Ashley is normal, similar to Emily in Figure 1.1. Kelly and Alexis are plotted with Emily along the vertical spectrum in Figure 1.9.

Q: Let's complete our vertical spectrum. Three additional patients present for examination (Figure 1.10, Cassie (a), Grace (b), and Adair (c)). Compare their soft tissue midface heights to their soft tissue LAFHs. Compare other facial features. What do you observe?

A: All three are reasonably similar and normal. Cassie, Grace, and Adair have LAFHs equal to their midface heights (ideal). All three are symmetric and demonstrate lip competence, do not appear overclosed, and present with Subnasale to Stomion heights approximately one-half their Stomion to soft tissue Menton heights.

Q: Evaluate and contrast their respective vertical skeletal and dental features using cephalometric tracings (Figure 1.11). What do you observe?

A: In terms of vertical skeletal relationships, all three are quite similar and WRN. Cassie's LAFH/TAFH is ideal (55%), Grace's is normal (54%), and Adair's is normal (56%). All three have MPAs that range widely but are still WRN: Cassie's FMA is 27° and her SNMP is 35°, Grace's FMA is 20° and her SNMP is 30°, and Adair's FMA is 27° and his SNMP is 38°. Cassie's and Grace's maxillary first molar apices are erupted away from the palatal plane, while Adair's maxillary first molar apices are level with his palatal plane (ideal). Finally, Cassie's maxillary central incisor tip extends below the upper lip by about 2–4 mm (ideal), Grace's maxillary incisor tip extends below the upper lip by about 2 mm (normal), and Adair's maxillary incisor tip is about at the level of the upper lip (less than normal).

Q: Evaluate their vertical dental features, as viewed intraorally (Figure 1.12).

A: This is where significant differences exist between the three patients. Cassie has a 50–60% OB with overerupted maxillary central incisors, Grace has an OB WRN (10–20%) with stepped up maxillary incisors, and Adair has an open bite of 1–2 mm with stepped up maxillary incisors. In terms of gingival levels, Cassie's central incisor gingival margins are uneven—her right maxillary central incisor gingival margin is low due to its supraeruption. All four of Grace's maxillary incisor gingival margins are approximately even and sit above her maxillary canine gingival margins. Adair's central incisor gingival margins are approximately even and are situated much higher than either his lateral incisor or his canine gingival margins. Cassie, Grace, and Adair did not exhibit ideal high–low–high gingival margin relationships (proceeding from maxillary central incisors to maxillary canines). All three have approximate coincidence of maxillary and mandibular midlines. Cassie demonstrates a short gingival papilla height between her supraerupted maxillary central incisor crowns; Grace's and Adair's gingival papilla heights between the central incisors are ideal (about one-half of her and his central incisor crown lengths).

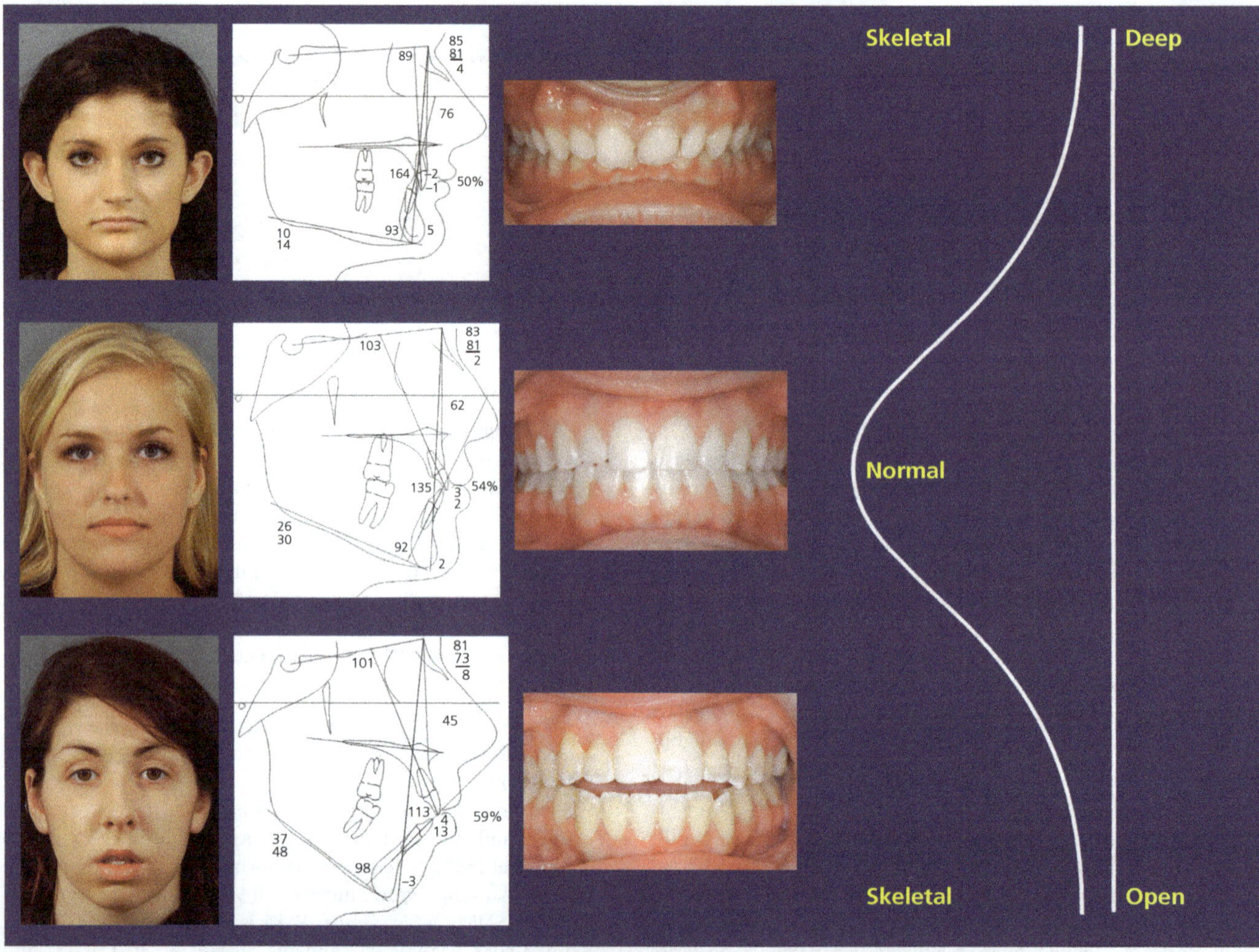

Figure 1.9 Kelly, Emily, and Alexis plotted on the spectrum of vertical facial development.

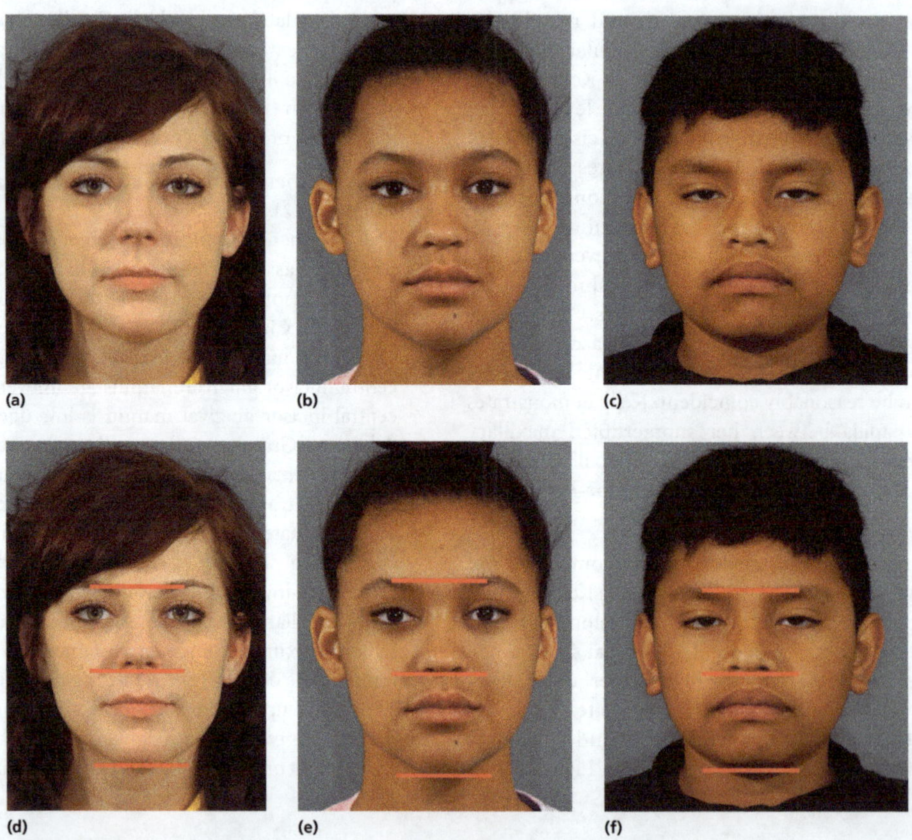

Figure 1.10 Variation of vertical soft tissue proportions: (a, d) Cassie, (b, e) Grace, and (c, f) Adair.

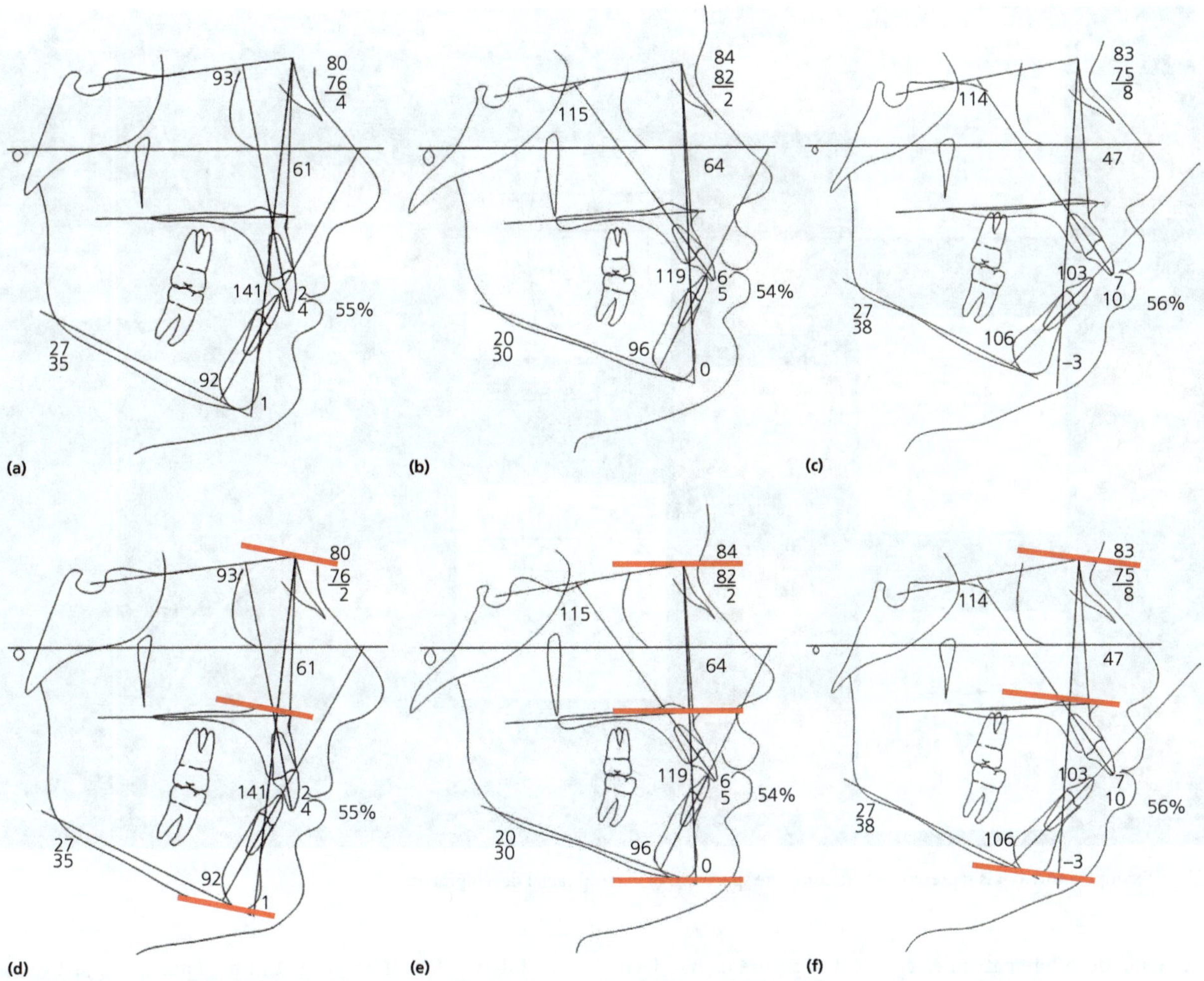

Figure 1.11 Variation of vertical skeletal and dental features: (a, d) Cassie, (b, e) Grace, and (c, f) Adair.

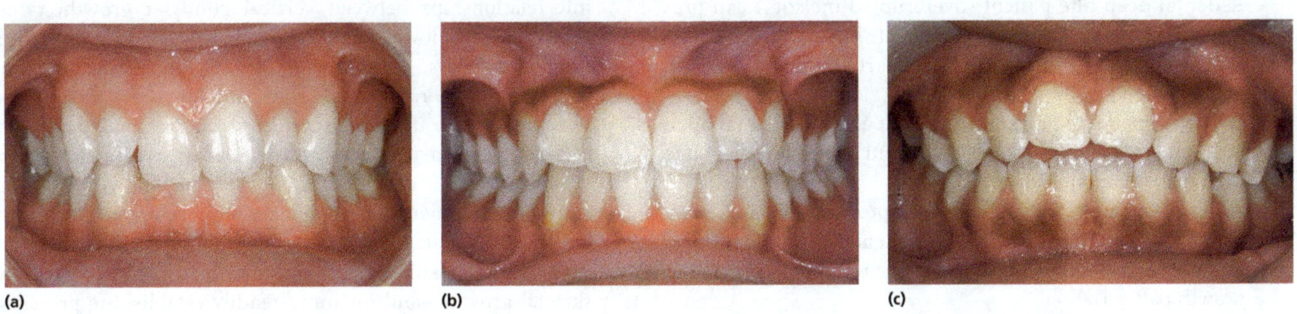

Figure 1.12 Variation of intraoral vertical dental features for the subjects shown in Figure 1.10: (a) Cassie, (b) Grace, and (c) Adair.

Q: If Cassie, Grace, and Adair are normal in terms of their vertical soft tissue (clinical) and vertical skeletal (cephalometric) features but differ in terms of their vertical dental (intraoral) features, where would you plot them on the spectrum of vertical facial development?

A: Since Cassie has normal vertical soft tissue/skeletal development but 50–60% OB, she should be plotted as a *dental* deep bite patient (Figure 1.13). Grace is normal in terms of vertical soft tissue/skeletal development and OB—similar to Emily in Figure 1.5. Since Adair has normal vertical soft tissue/skeletal development but an open bite, he should be plotted as a *dental* open bite patient. Figure 1.13 now illustrates examples of patients covering the complete range of anterior vertical problems: skeletal deep bite, dental deep bite, normal, dental open bite, and skeletal open bite.

Q: Can every patient be classified into one of these five, discrete, vertical spectrum categories—without overlap of features from another category?

A: No. *Many (most) patients present with some overlap of features between categories.* But, the greater the preponderance of features a patient presents with from any one of the categories, the more unambiguously the patient may be classified in that category. For example:

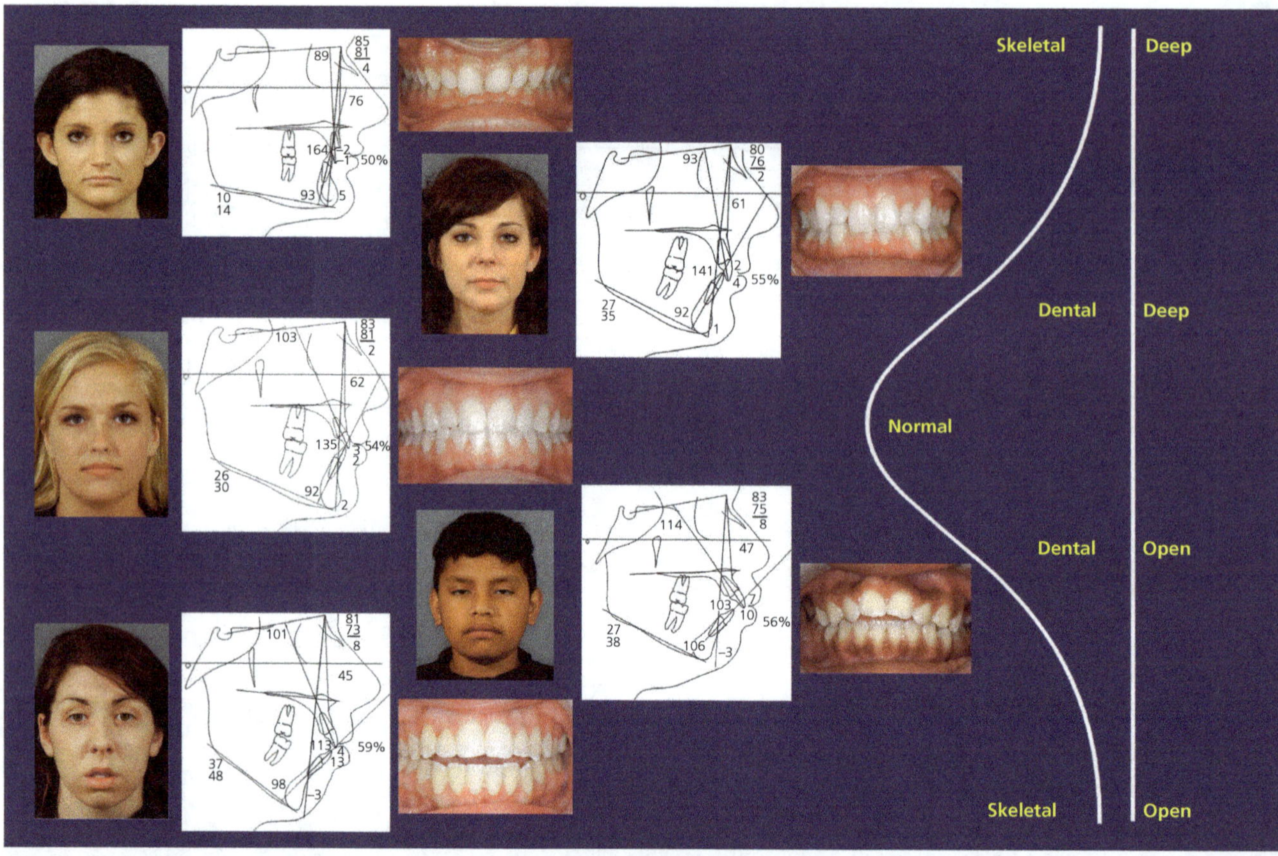

Figure 1.13 Example individuals representing the complete spectrum of vertical facial development.

- A dental deep bite patient can present as a pure dental deep bite—normal vertical facial growth and excess OB due solely to overerupted incisors.
- A dental deep bite patient (overerupted incisors) can present not only as a pure dental deep bite but also as a borderline skeletal deep bite (excess OB partially due to growth pattern).
- A dental open bite patient can present as a pure dental open bite—normal vertical facial growth and open bite solely due to undererupted incisors.
- A dental open bite patient (undererupted incisors caused by habit) can present not only as a pure dental open bite but also as a borderline skeletal open bite (open bite partially due to growth pattern).
- A severe skeletal deep bite patient can present as a pure skeletal deep bite—short LAFH with excess OB due entirely to the growth pattern and not excess incisor eruption.
- A severe skeletal deep bite patient (growth pattern, short LAFH) can also present with a dental deep bite (overerupted incisors) or even a dental open bite (undererupted incisors due to a habit).
- A severe skeletal open bite patient can present as a pure skeletal open bite—long LAFH with open bite due entirely to the growth pattern and not inadequate incisor eruption.
- A severe skeletal open bite patient (growth pattern, long LAFH) can also present with a dental open bite (undererupted incisors caused by habit), a normal OB, or even a dental deep bite (overerupted incisors). Of course, an open bite would not be present in the latter case, just the skeletal open bite growth pattern (LLAFH).

The point is that vertical dimension problems result from interrelationships between vertical condylar growth, ramus growth, sutural lowering of the maxillary corpus, growth rotation of the jaws, dentoalveolar growth, muscle growth, jaw function, and oral habits. The complex three-dimensional interplay of the developing facial structures and developing muscle function produces considerable variation in vertical dimension abnormalities of the facial complex. We've considered vertical dimension problems as a discrete spectrum for the purpose of education, portraying variation from normal vertical relationships due to aberrations in dentoalveolar and skeletal growth—and for more readily establishing principles of treatment.

Q: Mitchell presents to you for treatment (Figure 1.14). What vertical features do you observe? How would you classify Mitchell?

A: Examination in the frontal and profile views reveals an increased soft tissue LAFH (the distance Subnasale to soft tissue Menton is much greater than the distance soft tissue Glabella to Subnasale). There is also noticeable lip strain with the lips closed (Figure 1.14a), but a large ILG exists (Figure 1.14d) with lips at rest. These features are suggestive of a skeletal open bite. Looking at the cephalometric radiograph and tracing (Figure 1.14f, g), several diagnostic features also suggest a skeletal open bite: SN-MP is extremely high at 48°; skeletal LAFH/TAFH ratio, 60%, is over two standard deviations above normal; posterior facial height is short; gonial angle is very shallow at 140°; significant

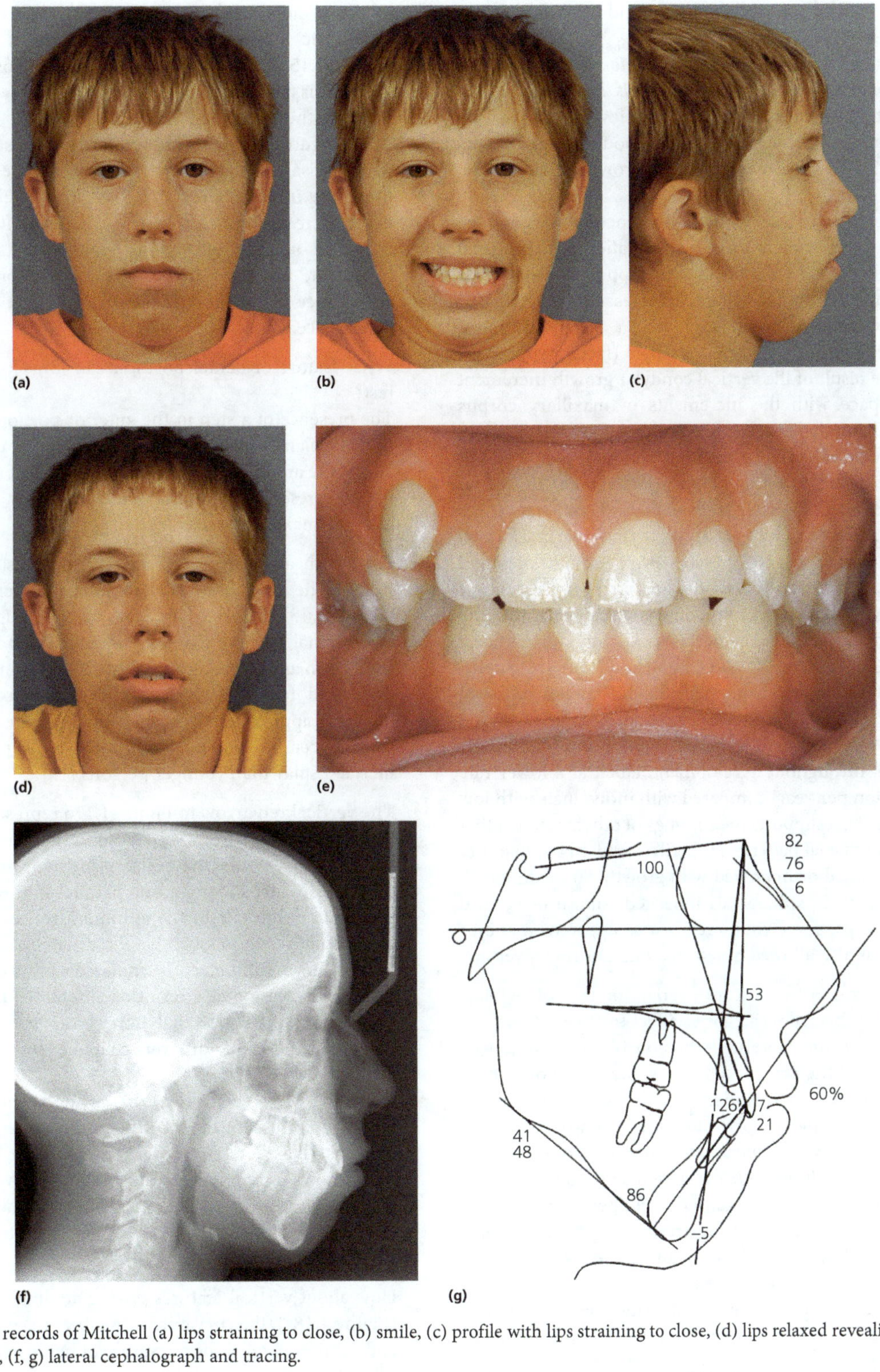

Figure 1.14 Initial records of Mitchell (a) lips straining to close, (b) smile, (c) profile with lips straining to close, (d) lips relaxed revealing an ILG, (e) intraoral photo, (f, g) lateral cephalograph and tracing.

antegonial notching is present; and maxillary first molar apices lie below the palatal plane, suggestive of excessive vertical descent of the posterior maxillary alveolar process and the maxillary molar teeth. Now look at Mitchell's intraoral photograph (Figure 1.14e). With the exception of the ectopic maxillary right canine, anterior overbite appears WRN (20% OB). In other words, *Mitchell has a skeletal open bite development pattern but with normal dental overbite.*

Q: In terms of the vertical spectrum of development, what is Mitchell an example of?

A: Mitchell is an example of overlapping features between categories. He has a preponderance of skeletal open bite features but with normal dental OB. Our point in presenting Mitchell is to emphasize the spectrum of vertical as continuous, with overlapping features between categories, and not discrete.

Q: With the extreme steepness of his LAFH and SN-MP, how did Mitchell achieve 20% OB during growth?

A: The most probable explanation is that *additional eruption of his mandibular anterior teeth compensated for his developing skeletal open bite*. Note how much more Mitchell's lower incisors have erupted (Figure 1.14g) compared to the amount lower incisors erupt in individuals with normal vertical growth (Figures 1.2a, 1.7b, and 1.11a–c).

We can also assume that Mitchell experienced some counterclockwise (forward) mandibular growth rotation, which helped his OB. Bjork [7, 8] showed that clockwise apparent mandibular rotation during growth (SN-MP angle increasing) is associated with increased anterior facial height and a steep MP angle. Schudy [9, 10] reasoned a steep MP angle (facial hyperdivergence) was the result of the vertical condylar growth increment not keeping pace with the increments of maxillary corpus vertical descent and the vertical eruption of posterior teeth, causing backward mandibular rotation and increasing SN-MP angle. However, the majority of *individuals characterized as "skeletal open bite" by their cephalometric and soft tissue characteristics, do not exhibit a net apparent clockwise (backward) mandibular rotation during growth. Most exhibit apparent counterclockwise (forward) mandibular rotation*. For most individuals, even those with hyperdivergent patterns, the SN-MP angle remains the same or decreases slightly during facial growth [11–13]. Karlsen [14] and Chung and Wong [15] demonstrated that individuals with high SN-MP angles followed longitudinally during childhood and adolescence displayed apparent forward (counterclockwise) rotation and decreasing SN-MP angles throughout development, albeit at a lower rate (degrees rotation per year) compared with individuals with low SN-MP angles. This supports the findings of others [16, 17] that a hyperdivergent facial pattern is inherited, and, in the majority of cases, maintained or improved with growth. So for Mitchell, it is plausible that, in spite of his inherited pattern of vertical facial relationships, some counterclockwise apparent mandibular rotation has also allowed him to maintain normal overbite.

Q: How does the concept of feature overlap, or lack of overlap, between vertical spectrum categories affect treatment?

A: On the one hand, the more unambiguously a patient can be classified in one of the vertical categories, the more you should follow the principles of treatment for that category. On the other hand, *the more overlap of features between two categories a patient presents with, the more your care should encompass treatment principles from both categories*. For example, if an open bite patient presents as a pure dental open bite, then you should care for that patient using treatment principles for a dental open bite. But, if a dental open bite patient also presents with borderline skeletal open bite features—then the care you provide should encompass treatment principles for a dental open bite *plus* treatment principles for a skeletal open bite.

Q: Mitchell has overlap of features between categories. How will this overlap affect your treatment decisions?

A: In spite of the fact that he has a normal overbite—you must address the skeletal open bite pattern during treatment—you must control vertical dentoalveolar growth and eruption of posterior teeth. If you do not, then backward mandibular rotation, increase in LAFH, and an anterior open bite may occur.

Q: Let's now turn to consider other aspects of the vertical dimension (and other features impacting facial esthetics as seen in the frontal view). In Figure 1.15a, b, we see two facially symmetric patients with normal vertical proportions. In Figures 1.15c and 1.15d, the amount of incisor display is visible when their teeth are slightly separated and their lips are relaxed. What do these figures illustrate?

A: These figures illustrate the amount of incisal display at rest. Ideal incisal display at rest varies with age and gender [4]. *Maxillary incisal display at rest decreases with age as philtrum length increases (even after age 30), and maxillary incisal display is less in males compared to females* [18, 19]. In terms of treatment, increased incisal display can project a youthful appearance. Decreased incisal display can project an aged appearance.

Q: What feature of dental position can impact incisal display at rest?

A: The presence of a step in the anterior portion of the maxillary occlusal plane, either down (Figure 1.16a) or up (Figure 1.16b), affects the amount of incisal display at rest. If an anterior step is initially present, the amount of incisal display at rest will change after the maxillary arch is leveled.

Q: Lip length also affects the amount of incisal display at rest. What is the range of normal adolescent lip lengths in girls and boys ages 13–15 years? How does age affect lip length?

A: The normal range of maxillary lip length for adolescent girls is 17–23 mm and for adolescent boys 22–26 mm [20]. During the third and fourth decades of life, the maxillary lip length increases approximately 1 mm more than the maxillary incisor edge descends—which explains why older persons show less incisal display than younger persons [19].

Q: The vertical red arrow in Figure 1.17a represents the philtrum length (measured from Subnasale to the maxillary lip vermilion border), while the yellow line represents commissure height (measured along a line parallel to the philtrum length line from Subnasale to the commissure). In adults, the philtrum length–commissure height difference should be small, maybe a few millimeters. In adolescents, the difference may be greater (decreasing as a result of differential lip growth during maturation) [21–23]. What impact can the philtrum length–commissure height difference make on maxillary incisal display?

A: Compare Matt (Figure 1.17b), who has a small philtrum length–commissure height difference, to John (Figure 1.17c), who has a large philtrum length–commissure height difference. Matt shows 1 mm incisor display at rest, while John shows nearly 10 mm of maxillary incisor due to his short philtrum length. John has what is termed an "exaggerated cupid's bow" of his maxillary lip.

Q: How about vertical features during smiling? In a posed smile (Figure 1.18a), the curvature of Ashley's maxillary incisal edges and canines parallel the curvature of her lower lip. What is this called?

A: This relationship is termed an ideal smile arc [24].

Q: Compare Ashley's ideal smile arc (Figure 1.18a) with Eric's smile arc before (Figure 1.18b) and following (Figure 1.18c) treatment. What do you observe?

A: Whereas Ashley demonstrates an ideal smile arc, Eric initially presents with a *reverse* smile arc (Figure 1.18b). In other words, the edges of his maxillary incisors and canines curve upward, away from his lower lip, instead of curving downward

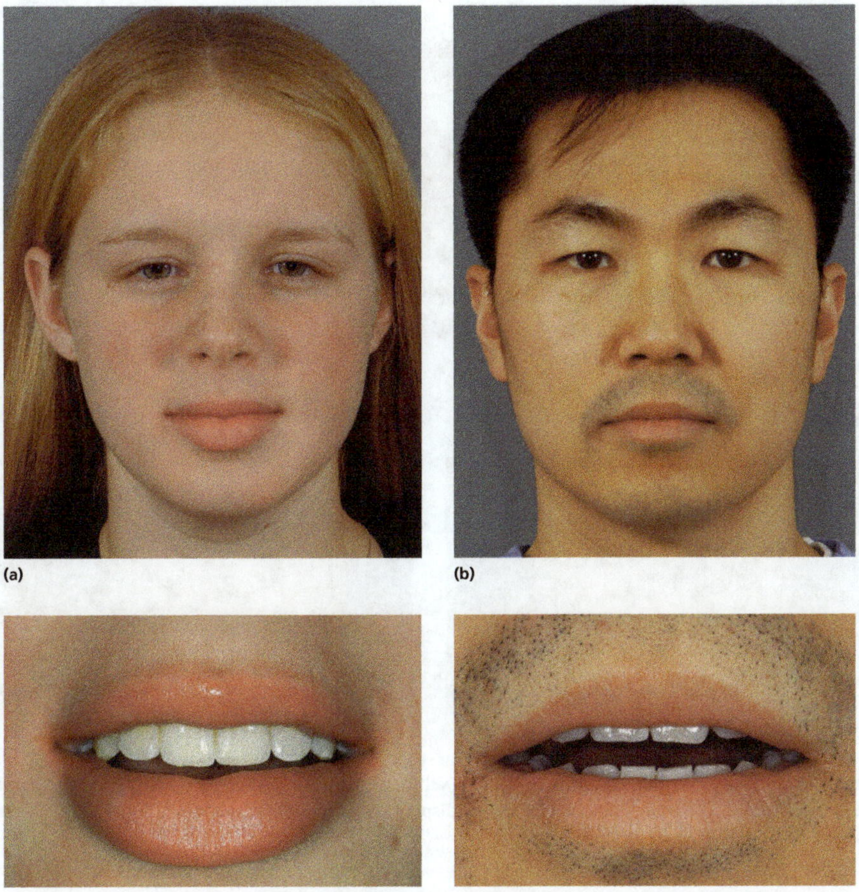

(a) (b) (c) (d)

Figure 1.15 Incisal display: (a, c) an adolescent girl, (b, d) a young man.

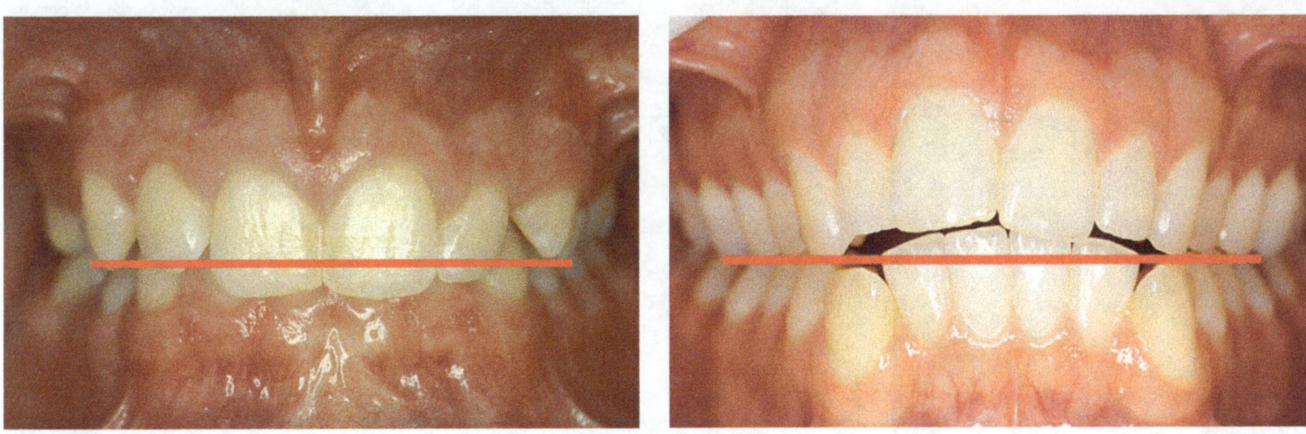

(a) (b)

Figure 1.16 Steps in the anterior portion of the maxillary occlusal plane affect the amount of incisal display at rest: (a) anterior teeth stepped down and (b) stepped up relative to the maxillary occlusal plane, which is defined by the occlusal surfaces of the posterior maxillary teeth bilaterally (red line).

following the curvature of his lower lip. Following treatment (Figure 1.18c), his smile arc is improved.

Q: What are the reasons for a patient presenting with *excessive* incisal and gingival display when smiling?

A: Excess incisal and gingival display can result from the following:

- Excess maxillary vertical growth
- Short maxillary lip (philtrum) length
- Stepped-down (overerupted) maxillary incisors
- Excessively long incisor crowns
- Delayed passive eruption (excess gingiva)
- Hyperactivity of (smiling) facial muscles

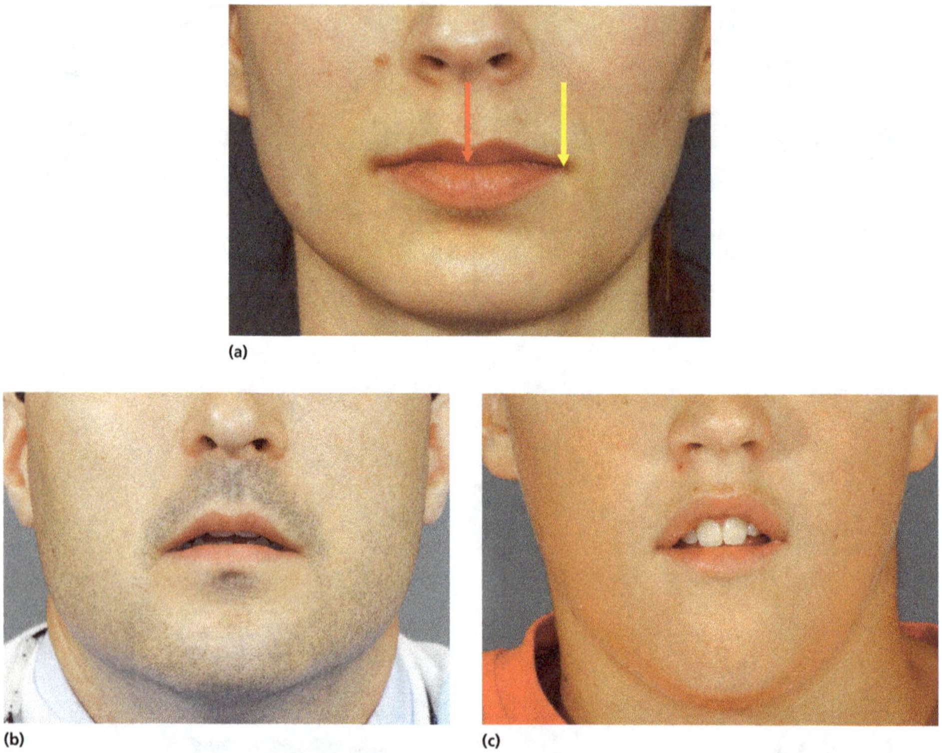

Figure 1.17 (a) Effect of philtrum length (red arrow)–commissure height (yellow arrow) difference on incisal display. (b) Matt has a small, 3–4 mm philtrum length–commissure height difference and exhibits 1 mm incisal display at rest. (c) John has a much larger philtrum length–commissure height difference and exhibits 10 mm of incisal display at rest.

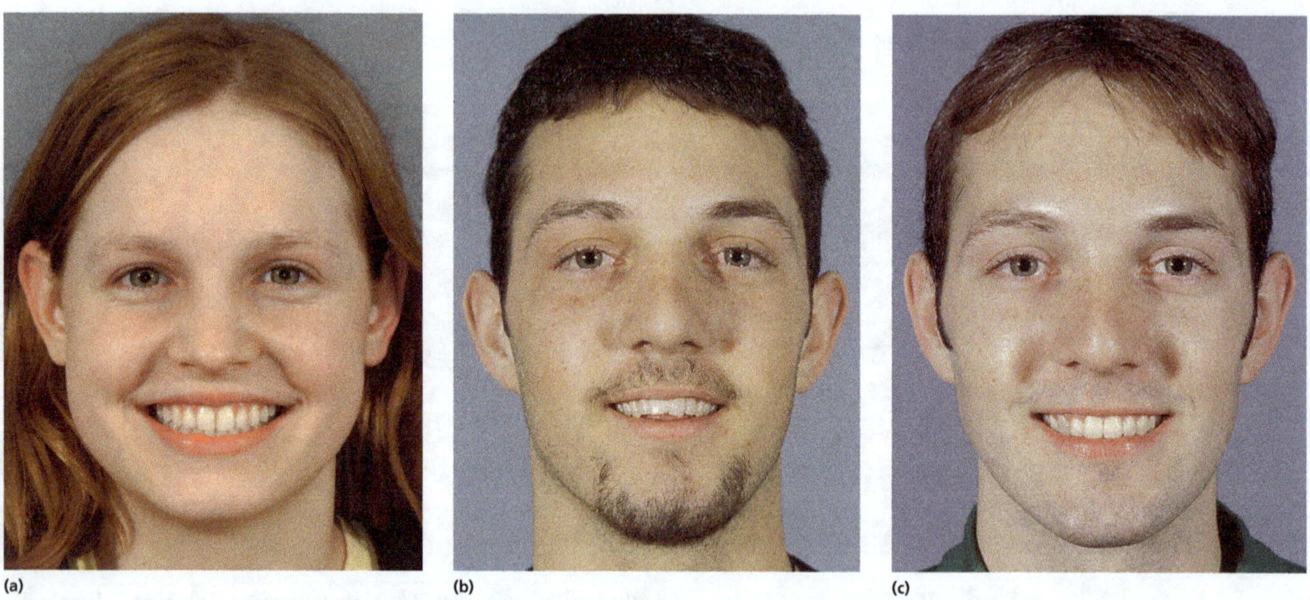

Figure 1.18 Smile arcs during a posed smile: (a) ideal smile arc, (b) reverse smile arc, (c) same patient, improved smile arc following treatment.

Q: What are the reasons for a patient presenting with *inadequate* incisal display when smiling?

A: Inadequate incisal and gingival display can result from the following:

- Inadequate maxillary vertical growth
- Long maxillary lip (philtrum) length
- Stepped-up (undererupted) maxillary incisors
- Worn or short incisor crowns
- Hypoactivity of (smiling) facial muscles

Q: Chris (Figure 1.19a) demonstrates facial symmetry and normal vertical proportions at rest. Compare the two photographs of him smiling (Figures 1.19b, c). What do you note?

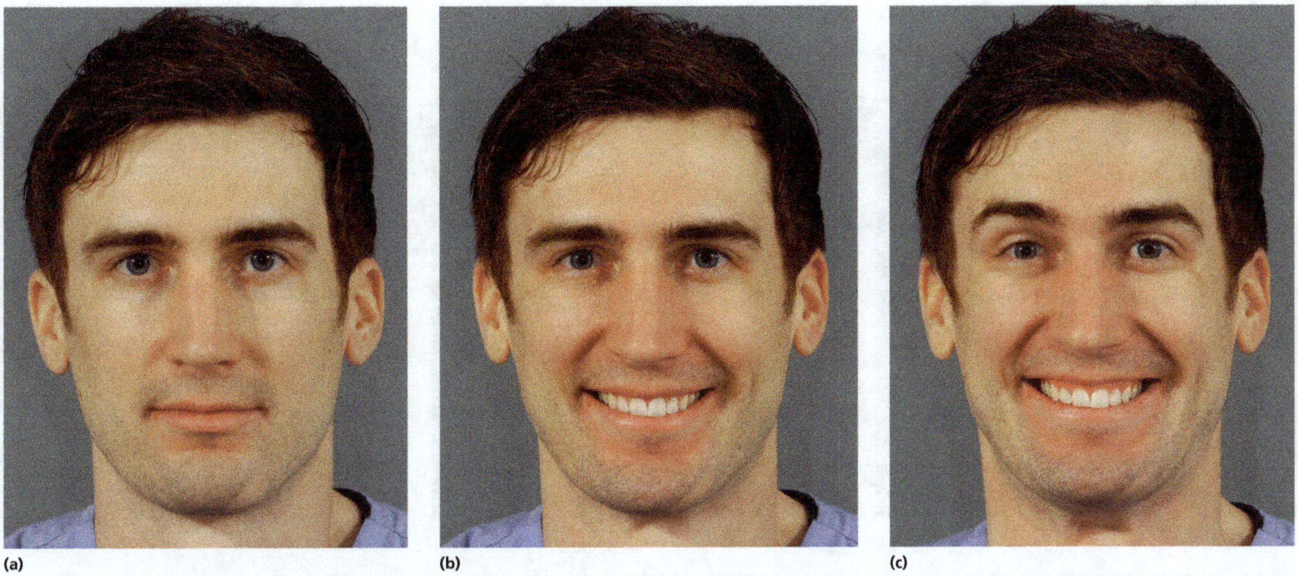

Figure 1.19 Chris: (a) at rest, (b) smiling in a posed smile, and (c) smiling in an unposed smile.

A: In Figure 1.19b, Chris is demonstrating a posed smile—a voluntary, repeatable, and sustainable smile typically made when posing for photographs (not elicited by emotion). In Figure 1.19c, he is demonstrating an unposed smile—a spontaneous smile elicited by joy or humor. We use the posed smile, not the unposed smile, to judge the position of the maxillary lip vermillion to the maxillary incisor gingiva.

Q: What is considered an attractive amount of gingival display in a posed smile?

A: In his posed smile (Figure 1.19b), the (vermillion) border of Chris's maxillary lip is at the same height as the gingival margins of his maxillary central incisors. This is considered ideal, the most attractive, vertical relationship [25–27]. However, it is not until the distance from the maxillary central incisor gingival margins to the maxillary lip is 3.0 mm or more that laypersons perceive a decrease in attractiveness. [28] This fact underscores the concept that attractiveness is a range, not a single value.

Q: Three patients (Figure 1.20; Tanner, Olivia, and Trevor) present to you with LAFHs (reasonably) WRN. As they smile (Figures 1.20d–f), compare their interpupillary lines to their respective right to left maxillary occlusal relationships. What do you observe?

A: They each present with an asymmetrical smile due to a *structural* maxillary occlusal cant. In other words, although each has their maxillary lip vermillion relatively parallel to their interpupillary line, Tanner's right maxilla/right dentition has descended more than his left—resulting in an occlusal cant. Olivia's and Trevor's left maxilla/left dentition has descended (slightly) more than their right.

Q: What percentage of the population has an asymmetrical smile due to a *structural* maxillary occlusal plane cant versus a functional (neuromuscular) canting of the upper lip?

A: Although this phenomenon has not been widely studied, one study (210 subjects) reported that 7% of their sample had an asymmetric smile due to an underlying maxillary (structural) occlusal cant, while 8% of their sample showed similar asymmetry due to a functional (neuromuscular) canting of the upper lip [29].

Q: How large of a right to left structural maxillary occlusal cant must exist to be noticed by laypersons?

A: A maxillary right canine to left canine cant of at least 3 mm is required for laypersons to rate it as noticeable. An occlusal plane cant can be an overwhelmingly displeasing smile characteristic to health professionals and laypeople, alike [30].

Q: Lynn (Figure 1.21) also has an asymmetrical smile. Is the asymmetrical smile due to a structural maxillary occlusal cant or a functional canting of the upper lip?

A: Closely compare her interpupillary line to her right to left occlusal plane. They are very nearly parallel. There has not been an uneven descent of her maxilla or teeth between left and right sides. Look at her maxillary lip vermillion at rest (Figure 1.21a). It runs right to left in a nearly parallel fashion with her interpupillary line. But, when she smiles (Figure 1.21b), her right maxillary vermillion is elevated higher by her facial musculature than her left. Also notice that her mandibular left lip vermillion is pulled down more than her mandibular right. Lynn's asymmetric smile is due to functional (neuromuscular) canting of her upper lip.

Q: Asymmetrical smiles result from structural or functional asymmetries. How does this impact treatment options?

A: If an asymmetrical smile results from structure (overgrowth of the maxilla on one side, overeruption of teeth on one side), then treatment to correct the asymmetrical structure may be appropriate. Treatment may include a differential Le Fort I maxillary osteotomy (combined with a mandibular osteotomy) to correct the occlusal cant in both jaws, or it may include orthodontic treatment only using TADs to intrude the maxillary or mandibular dentition on one side of the arch (with vertical elastics to correct the corresponding occlusal plane in the opposing jaw). On the other hand, if the asymmetrical smile results from function, then treatment that changes structure would be inappropriate. Treatments such as botulinum toxin injections can be considered to address excess hyperactivity of smiling musculature, but patients can experience unesthetic perioral animation effects with such treatments [31, 32]. Finally, remember that having an occlusal cant may not even be a

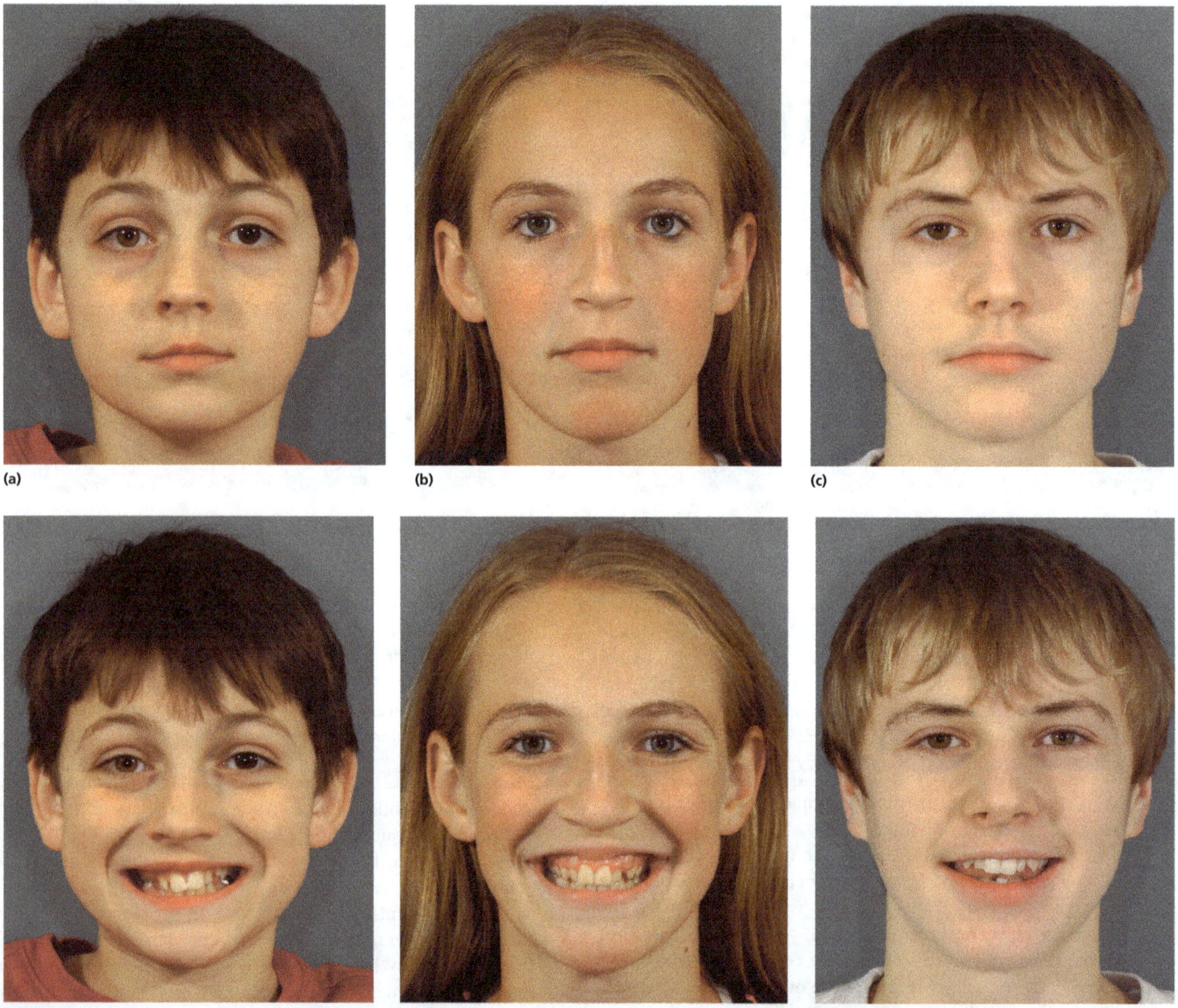

(a) (b) (c) (d) (e) (f)

Figures 1.20 Patients with asymmetrical smiles due to structural maxillary occlusal cants: (a, d) Tanner, (b, e) Olivia, and (c, f) Trevor.

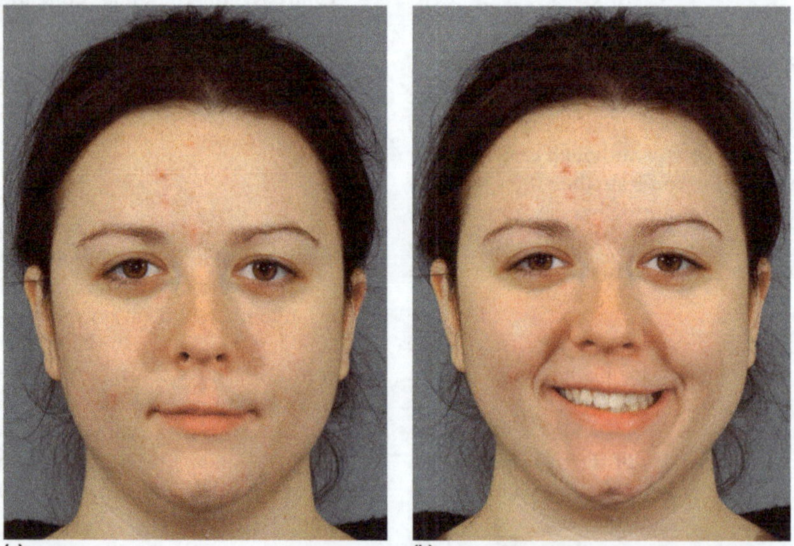

(a) (b)

Figure 1.21 (a, b) Patient with an asymmetrical smile due to unbalanced smile musculature function.

concern for a patient, and as the doctor you must be careful not to draw undue attention to problems that the patient may not be concerned with.

Q: Christina (Figure 1.22) presents with an asymmetrical smile. Is her asymmetry due to structure or function (trick question, look carefully)?

A: Her smile asymmetry is due to *both* structure and function. If you look carefully at her occlusal plane relative to her interpupillary line (Figure 1.22b), then you can see that she has a right to left maxillary occlusal cant (structure). Further, if you look very carefully at her maxillary lip vermillion at rest, you will also notice that it has a very slight right to left cant (structure, Figure 1.22a). Finally, if you look at her during a posed smile, you see that her maxillary lip is raised slightly more on her left than right (function, Figure 1.22b). Her smile asymmetry is due to both structure and function.

Q: What other features affect smile and lower facial esthetics?

A: Features that affect smile and lower facial esthetics include the following:

- Lip fullness: Scott et al. [33] reported that thicker vermillion (Figures 1.23a, b) are considered more attractive (and more feminine) than thinner vermillion (Figure 1.23c), which are considered less attractive (and more masculine).
- Central incisor midline position: The patient in Figure 1.24a demonstrates ideal central incisor midline positions: maxillary and mandibular central incisor midlines are coincident and in line with the facial midline. The patients in Figures 1.24b, c have midlines that are deviated to the right of their facial midlines by 2 mm and 3–4 mm, respectively. Whereas a recent systematic review reported a dental midline deviation of up to 2.2 mm as being acceptable to laypersons [34], other studies suggest that the majority of laypersons are unable to detect midline deviations up to 4 mm [30, 35].

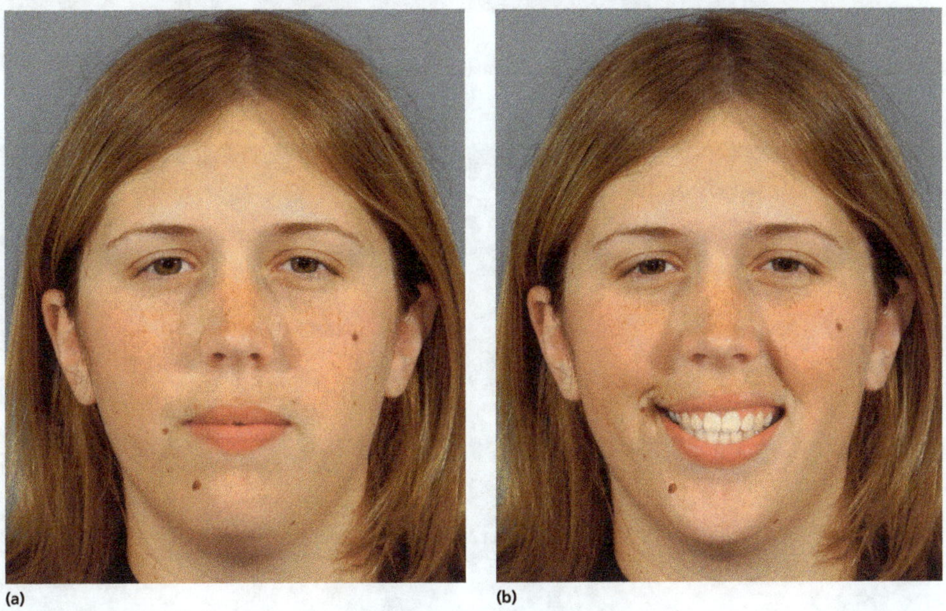

Figure 1.22 Christina presents with an asymmetrical smile.

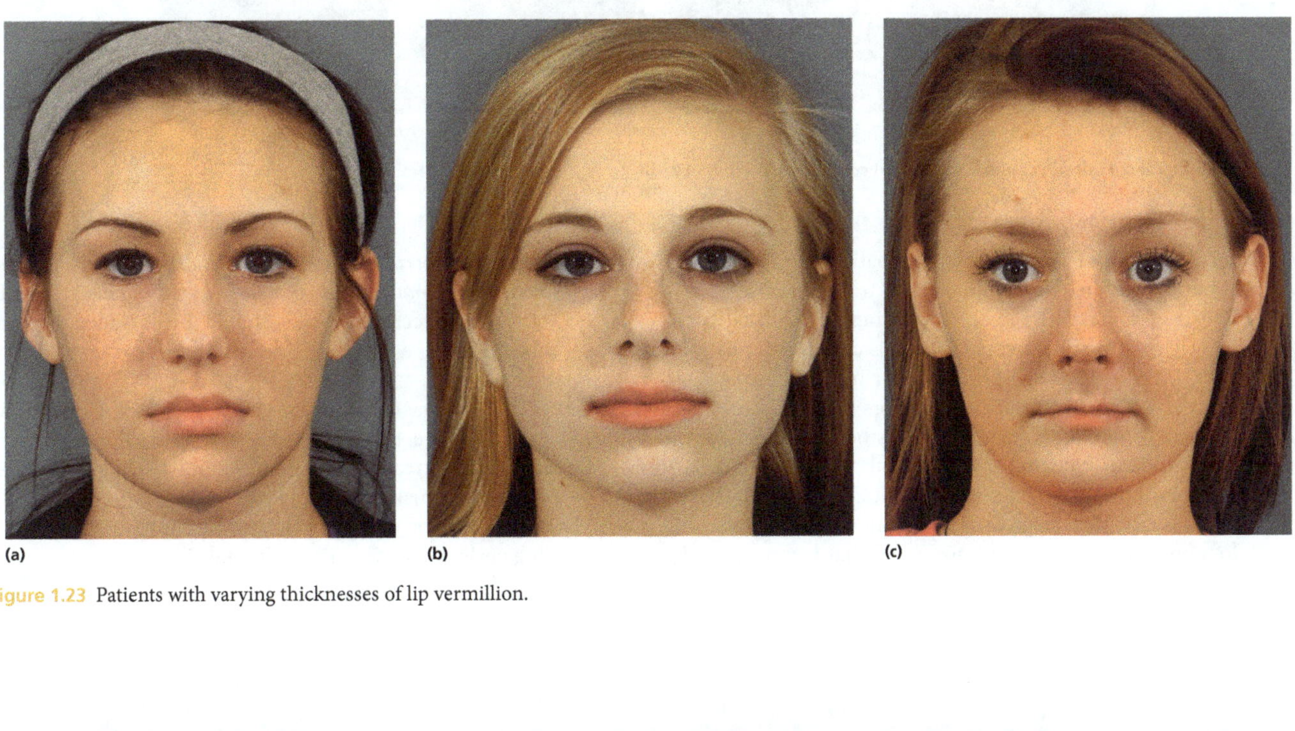

Figure 1.23 Patients with varying thicknesses of lip vermillion.

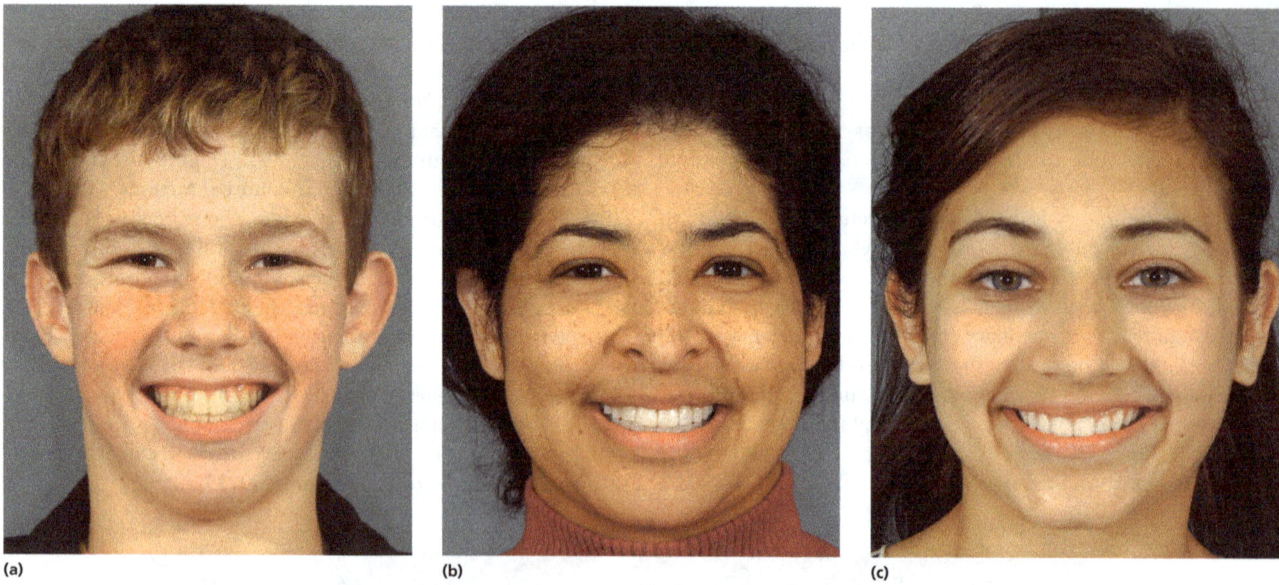

Figure 1.24 Incisor midline positions: (a) ideal, (b) 2 mm right deviation, (c) 3–4 mm right deviation.

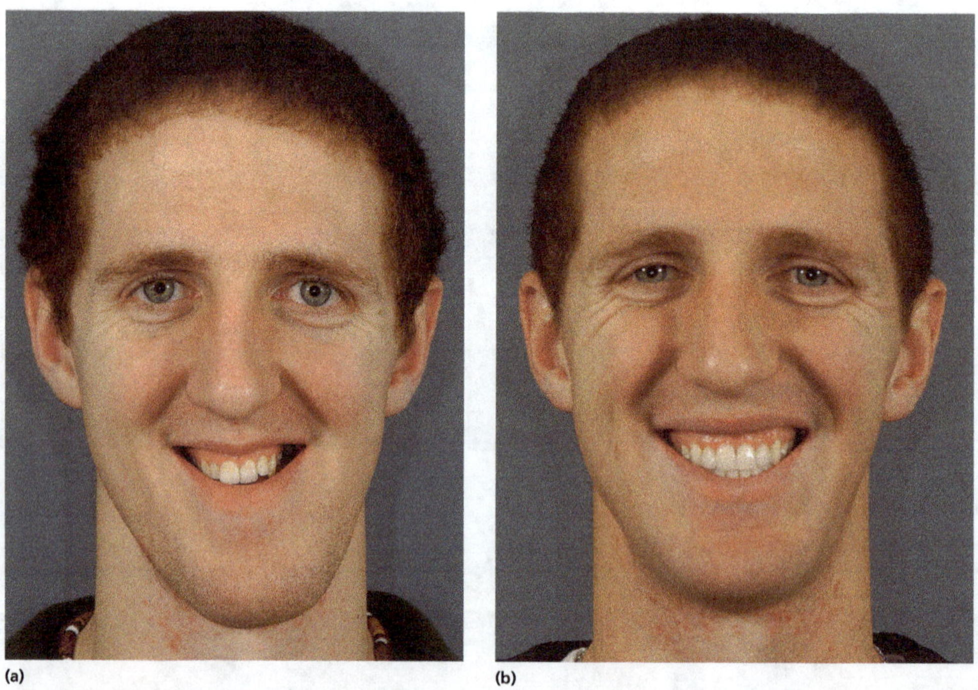

Figure 1.25 Buccal corridors: (a) initially large, (b) reduced following SARME

- Buccal corriodor size: Look at the patient in Figure 1.25. Initially (A), he had a maxillary transverse deficiency (constricted maxilla) and accompanying large buccal corridors (dark intraoral spaces between his cheeks and posterior teeth). Following SARME and orthodontic treatment (Figure 1.25b), his buccal corridors were dramatically reduced. In your opinion, is there an esthetic difference in his smile? Clearly, reduction in his buccal corridors (maxillary expansion) improved his smile esthetics. Although there has been disagreement regarding the influence of buccal corridors on smile esthetics [36], we found that *laypersons judge large buccal corridors (narrow maxillary arches) to be less esthetic than small buccal corridors (broad maxillary arches)* [37]. Large buccal corridors should be included in your problem list.

Q: Considering the fact that the two most important factors in an attractive face are the eyes and the smile [38], the esthetic impact of a well-treated occlusion (Figures 1.26a, b) compared to an untreated malocclusion (Figure 1.26c) is immeasurable. What are some of the factors contributing to an esthetically pleasing occlusion as seen in the frontal view?

A: Tooth shade (ideally, approaching the whiteness of the patient's orbital sclera), absence of crowding, alignment of incisal edges/cusp tips along arch of the occlusal plane, coincidence of maxillary and mandibular midlines, maxillary central incisor crowns having equal widths, maxillary central incisor crowns having ideal proportions (width/height ratio of 4/5) and a lack of wear/attrition, golden proportion of maxillary anterior teeth from anterior to posterior, proper long axis alignment of anterior teeth, absence of a reverse smile arc, ideal overbite and overjet, equal levels of maxillary central incisor gingival margins with canine gingival margins at about the same level and lateral incisor gingival margins slightly incisal, and absence of gingival embrasures (black triangles) or incisal embrasures [5, 30, 31, 35, 39, 40].

Q: Examine each occlusion in Figures 1.27a–o (frontal views). What unesthetic features can you identify in each image?

A: Unesthetic dental features include the following for each of Figure 1.27a–o:

- (a) Dark shade, significant generalized anterior tooth wear, edge-to-edge incisal relationship (lack of normal overbite and overjet), anterior crossbite of right central incisors.
- (b) Severe maxillary central incisor inclination, excessive OB with overerupted maxillary central incisors, gingival margins of maxillary central incisors are stepped down relative to the maxillary lateral incisor gingival margins, dark yellow shade, labial crown torque maxillary left canine, possible gingival recession/caries along the maxillary central incisor gingival margins.
- (c) Dark shade, uneven maxillary central incisor widths, maxillary central incisor crown widths equal to or greater than the incisor crown heights (width/height ratio of 4/5 violated) leading to a disruption in golden proportion of maxillary anterior teeth from anterior to posterior, midlines are not coincident, maxillary midline diastema, uneven maxillary central incisor gingival margins, maxillary left central incisor gingival margin lower than lateral incisor gingival margins, significant tip of maxillary right lateral incisor edge, significant cuspal wear of maxillary right canine.
- (d) Anterior open bite, reverse smile arc, excessive mesial crown tip of maxillary central incisors, malalignment of maxillary and mandibular anterior teeth, isolated white spot hypocalcified areas, excessive maxillary canine lingual crown torque (maxilla appears to be constricted).

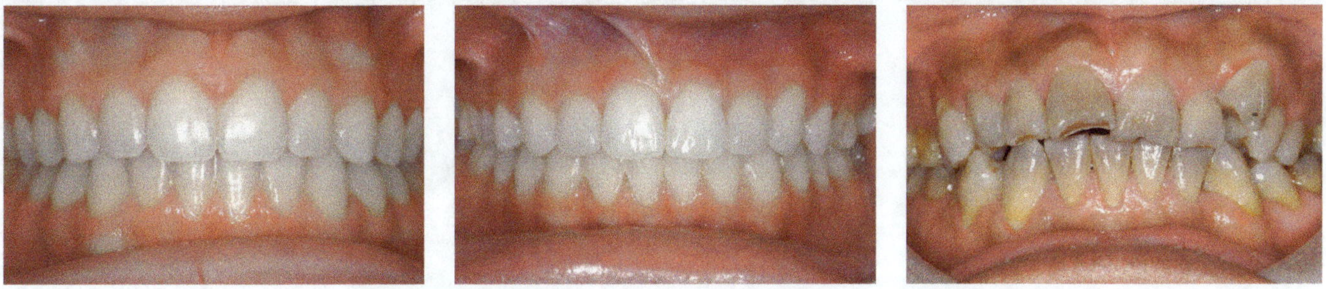

(a) (b) (c)

Figure 1.26 Dental features impacting esthetics: (a–b) well-finished occlusions, (c) a malocclusion possessing many unesthetic features.

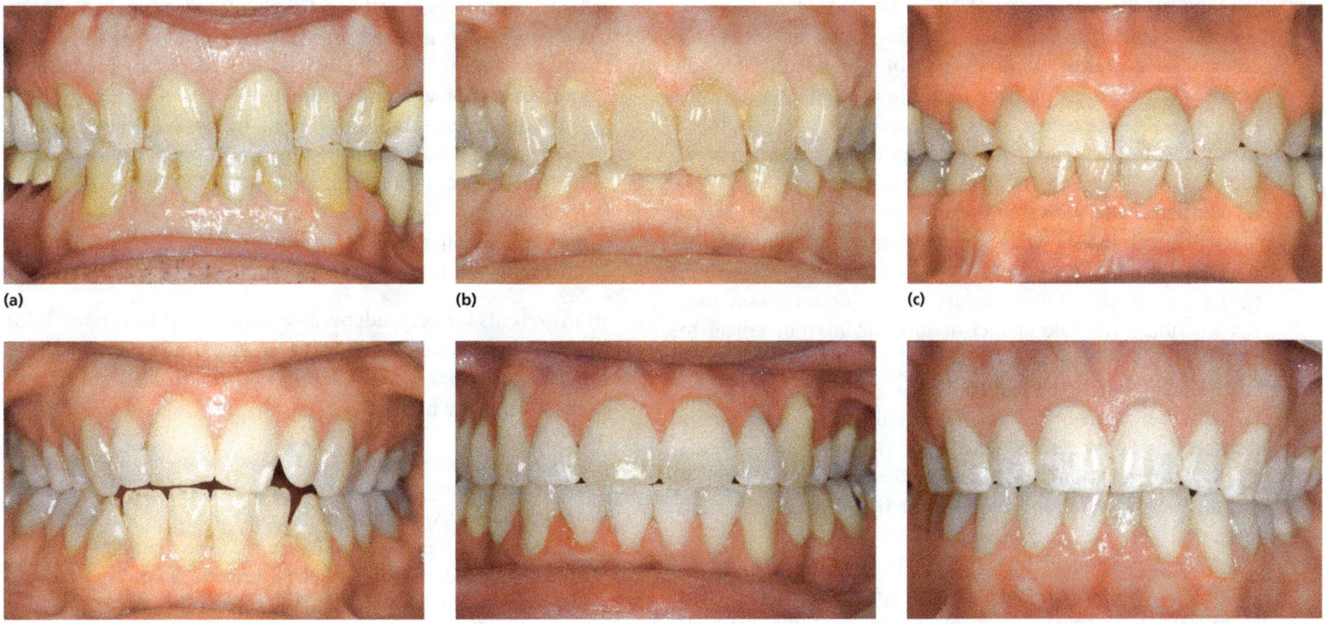

(a) (b) (c) (d) (e) (f)

Figure 1.27 (a–o) Unesthetic dental features.

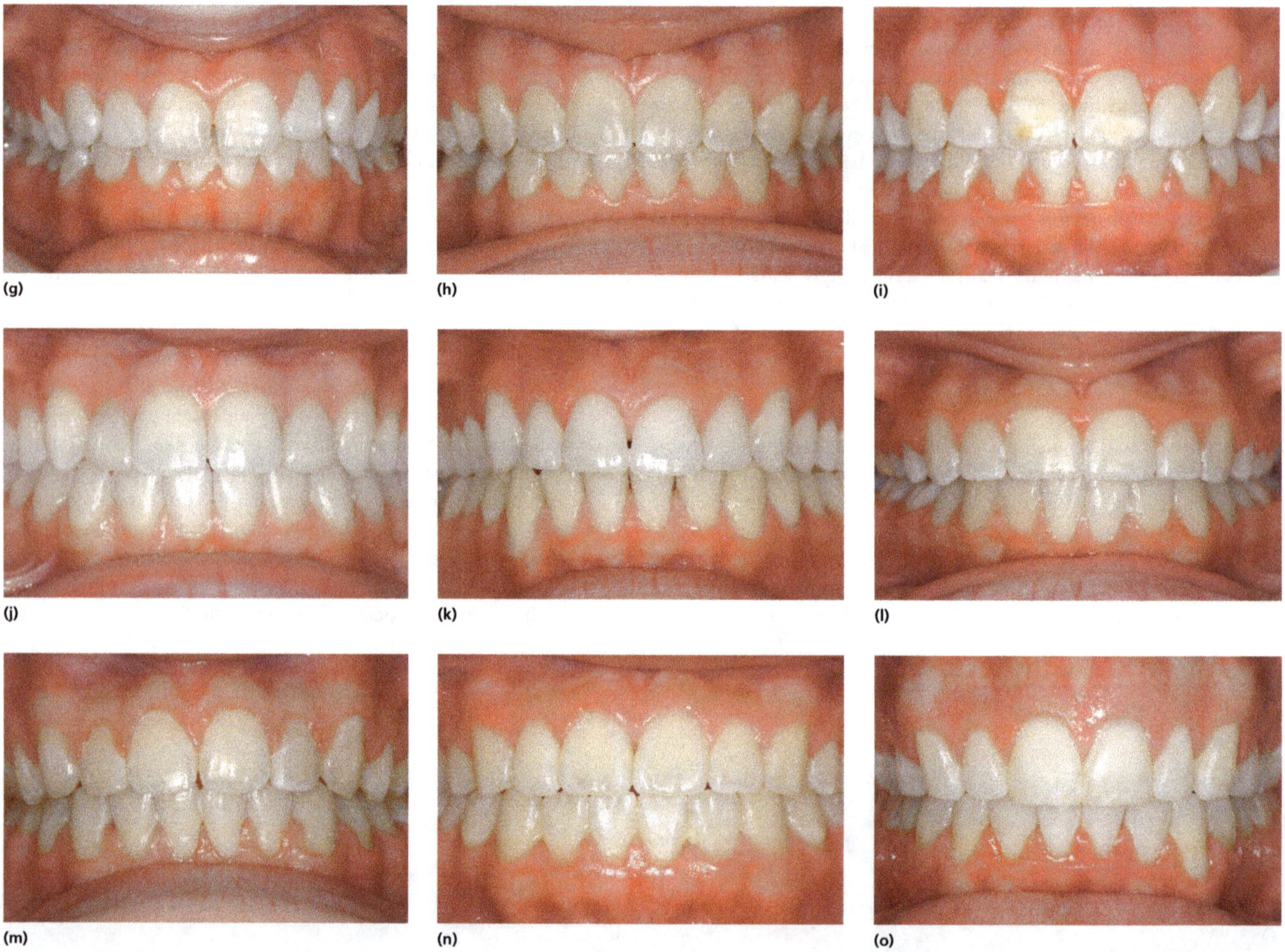

Figure 1.27 (Continued)

- (e) Maxillary central incisor crowns are nearly as wide as they are long (width/height ratio of 4/5 violated) leading to a disruption in golden proportion of maxillary anterior teeth from anterior to posterior, midlines are not coincident, edge-to-edge incisal relationship (lack of minimal overbite and overjet), incisal embrasures, gingival recession over roots of maxillary canines, shade (dark coloration of maxillary central incisors, white spots of maxillary lateral incisors).
- (f) Mottled shade, incisal embrasures, uneven and worn maxillary central incisal edges, malalignment of mandibular incisors.
- (g) Excessively deep OB, maxillary central incisor mesial root tip, maxillary left lateral incisor gingival margin apical to canine gingival margin.
- (h) Dark shade, uneven central incisor gingival margins.
- (i) Discolored central incisors, small incisal embrasure between maxillary central incisors.
- (j) Midlines not coincident, maxillary central incisor gingival margins slightly uneven, mesial root tip of maxillary right lateral incisor.
- (k) Maxillary central incisors gingival embrasure (black triangle), maxillary central incisor gingival margins uneven, maxillary left central incisor stepped down, incisal embrasure between maxillary right lateral incisor and mandibular right canine, gingival embrasures between mandibular incisors.
- (l) Maxillary central incisor crowns are wider than they are long (width/height ratio of 4/5 violated) leading to a disruption in golden proportion of maxillary anterior teeth from anterior to posterior, midlines are not coincident, right canines do not appear coordinated.
- (m) Mild reverse smile arc, central incisor incisal embrasure.
- (n) Excess mesial crown inclination of maxillary left central incisor, incisal embrasures, midlines not coincident.
- (o) A few white spots, maxillary right central incisor is wider than the maxillary left central incisor.

Let's complete this chapter by examining four patients.

Q: Brad presents for a consult because of his deep bite (Figure 1.28). What features would lead you to classify Brad as a dental deep bite patient? What features would lead you to classify Brad as a skeletal deep bite patient?

A: See Table 1.1

Q: Would you classify Brad as a dental deep bite patient, a skeletal deep bite patient, or a combination of both?

A: Dental deep bite. Brad's 80% OB resulted from mandibular incisor overeruption and not from skeletal growth. In the spectrum of vertical facial relationships, Brad lies in the normal skeletal range.

Q: What features would lead you to classify Robert (Figure 1.29) as a dental deep bite or a skeletal deep bite patient?

A: See Table 1.2

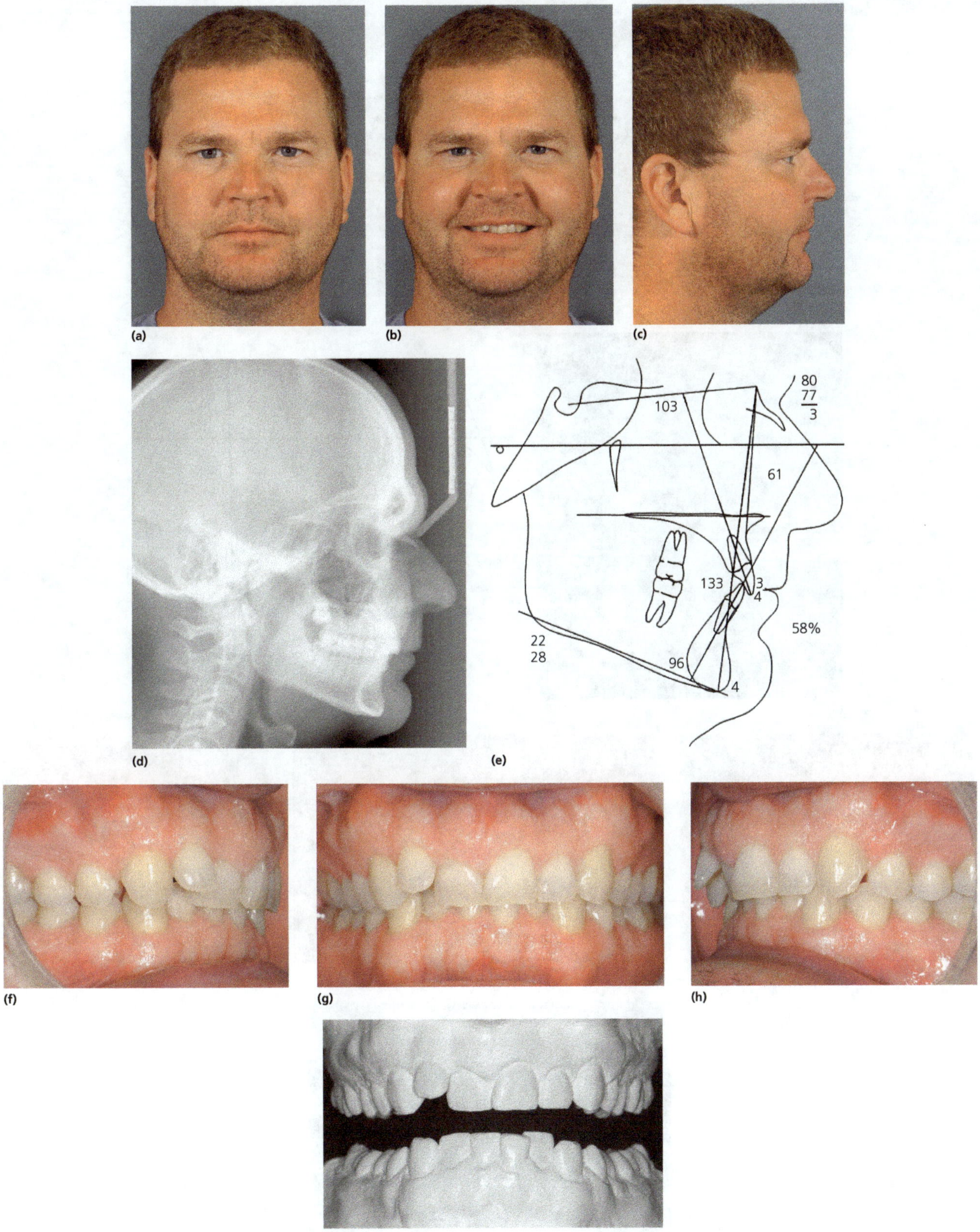

Figure 1.28 Initial records of Brad: (a–c) composite facial photographs, (d) lateral cephalograph, (e) cephalometric tracing, (f–h) intraoral photographs, and (i) models separated.

Table 1.1 Dental and skeletal features of Brad (Figure 1.28).

Skeletal deep bite features	Dental deep bite features
	• Soft tissue LAFH WRN • Skeletal LAFH mildly long (LAFH/TAFH 58%, > 1 standard deviation longer than ideal, 55%) • MPA WRN (FMA = 22° and SNMP = 28°) • Maxillary incisal display WRN (posed smile and as seen on his cephalograph) with maxillary central incisors neither stepped up nor stepped down (Figure 1.28i) • Mandibular incisors overerupted (deep curve of Spee)

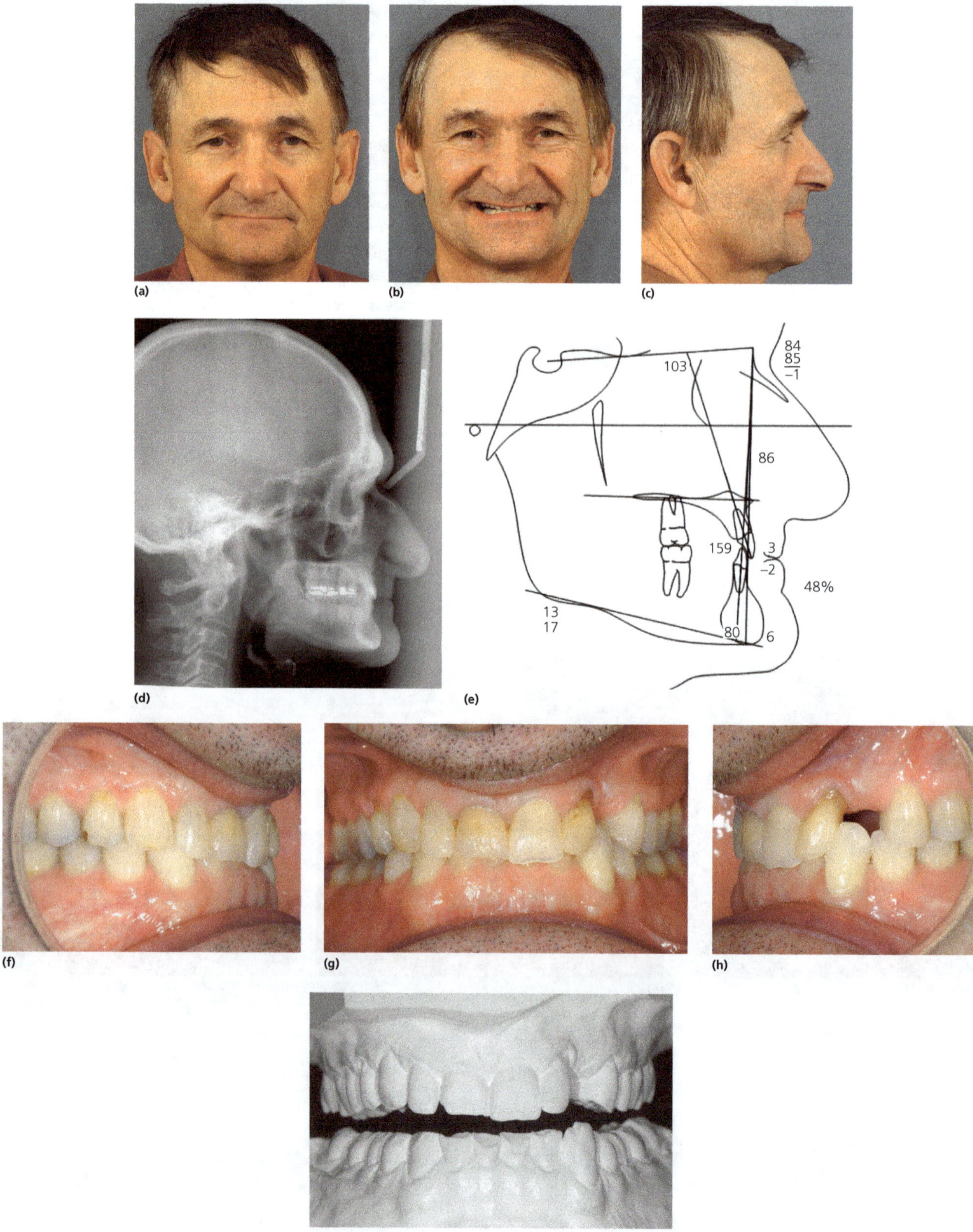

Figure 1.29 Initial records of Robert.

Table 1.2 Skeletal and dental features of Robert (Figure 1.29).

Skeletal deep bite features	Dental deep bite features
• Short soft tissue LAFH • Overclosed appearance • Short skeletal LAFH • Flat MPA • SN, FH, and MP nearly parallel • Maxillary incisal display inadequate (posed smile and cephalometrically) *with* maxillary incisors stepped down	• Overerupted maxillary incisors

Q: Would you classify Robert as a dental deep bite patient, a skeletal deep bite patient, or a combination of both?

A: Robert is a patient with a combination skeletal and dental deep bite. The fact that Robert's facial skeleton never developed vertically to keep pace with his facial soft tissue drape is clearly illustrated by Figures 1.30a–b. Figure 1.30a is, once again, Robert's initial frontal photo in maximal intercuspation. He looks overclosed. In Figure 1.30b, Robert was asked to separate his jaws until his lips were just touching. This is where his facial soft tissue drape is fully expressed (vertically). Do you see the difference in his appearance? In other words, *his facial skeletal vertical development was dramatically less than his facial soft tissue vertical development*. As Robert closes, his mandible rotates upward and forward until his teeth are in occlusion and his facial soft tissues are compressed, leaving him with an overclosed appearance.

This lack of vertical skeletal development also affects his smile (Figure 1.29b). Figure 1.30c illustrates his lack of incisal display at rest even though he has stepped-down maxillary incisors. In the spectrum of vertical facial development, Robert would be plotted in the extreme end of skeletal deep bite. But, he also has a dental deep bite due to overerupted maxillary incisors.

Q: What features would lead you to classify Kelly (Figure 1.31), a 17-year-old, as a dental open bite or a skeletal open bite patient?

A: See Table 1.3

Q: What questions should you ask Kelly? What should you check for?

A: You should check for the following:

- Although she exhibits lip competence, you should confirm that Kelly is not straining (mentalis strain) to achieve lip competence. This was not done. However, she also exhibits lip competence in her lateral cephalometric radiograph, which is a good sign. Many times, patients who strain to close their lips when photographs are taken will relax when the radiographs are being made. Even if she was straining to achieve lip competence, this could be due to the fact that her incisors are so proclined that her lips must strain to reach around them (and not due to the fact that her LAFH is long).
- Check for an anterior tongue interposition habit by asking Kelly to close her eyes. Then, ask her to open her eyes (to distract her) while you simultaneously draw her lower lip down and look for her tongue to be positioned between her anterior teeth. You find that she does not have an anterior tongue interposition habit. Ask her about a possible digit habit. She says she quit her thumb habit for a number of years but currently sucks her thumb when sleeping at night (the etiology of her dental open bite).

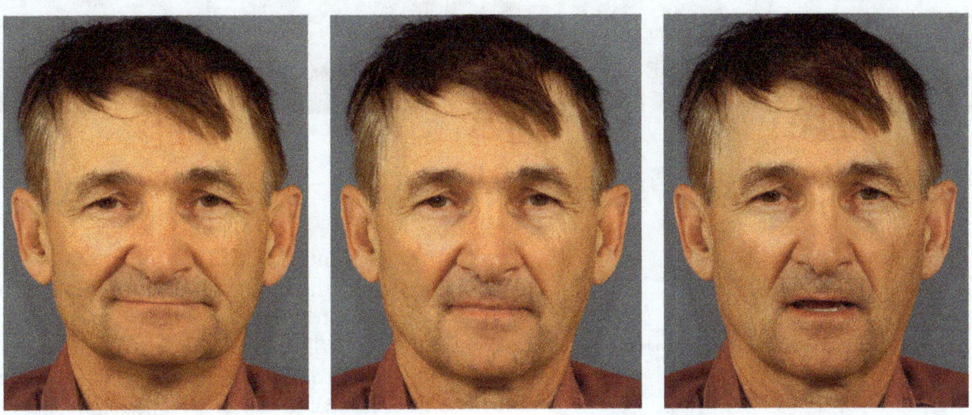

(a) (b) (c)

Figure 1.30 Robert: (a) initial photo again, in maximal intercuspation; (b) with jaws separated until lips relaxed and just touching; (c) opened until lips relaxed and parted to demonstrate degree of incisal display at rest.

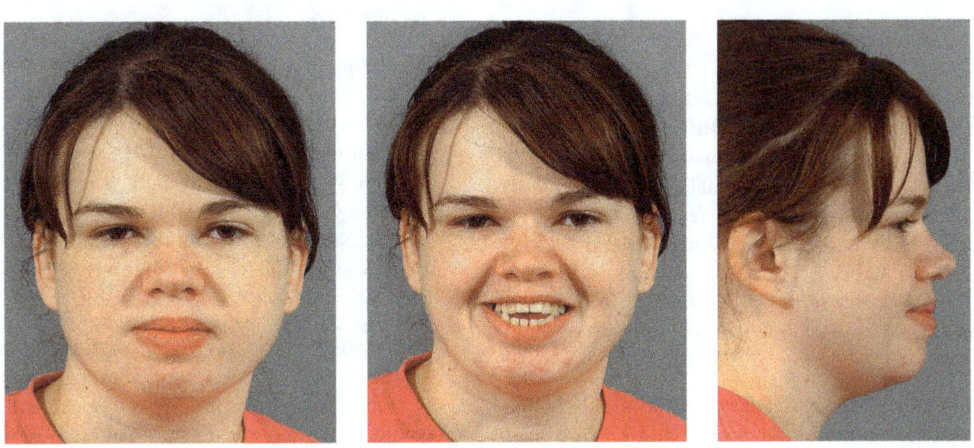

(a) (b) (c)

Figure 1.31 Initial records of Kelly.

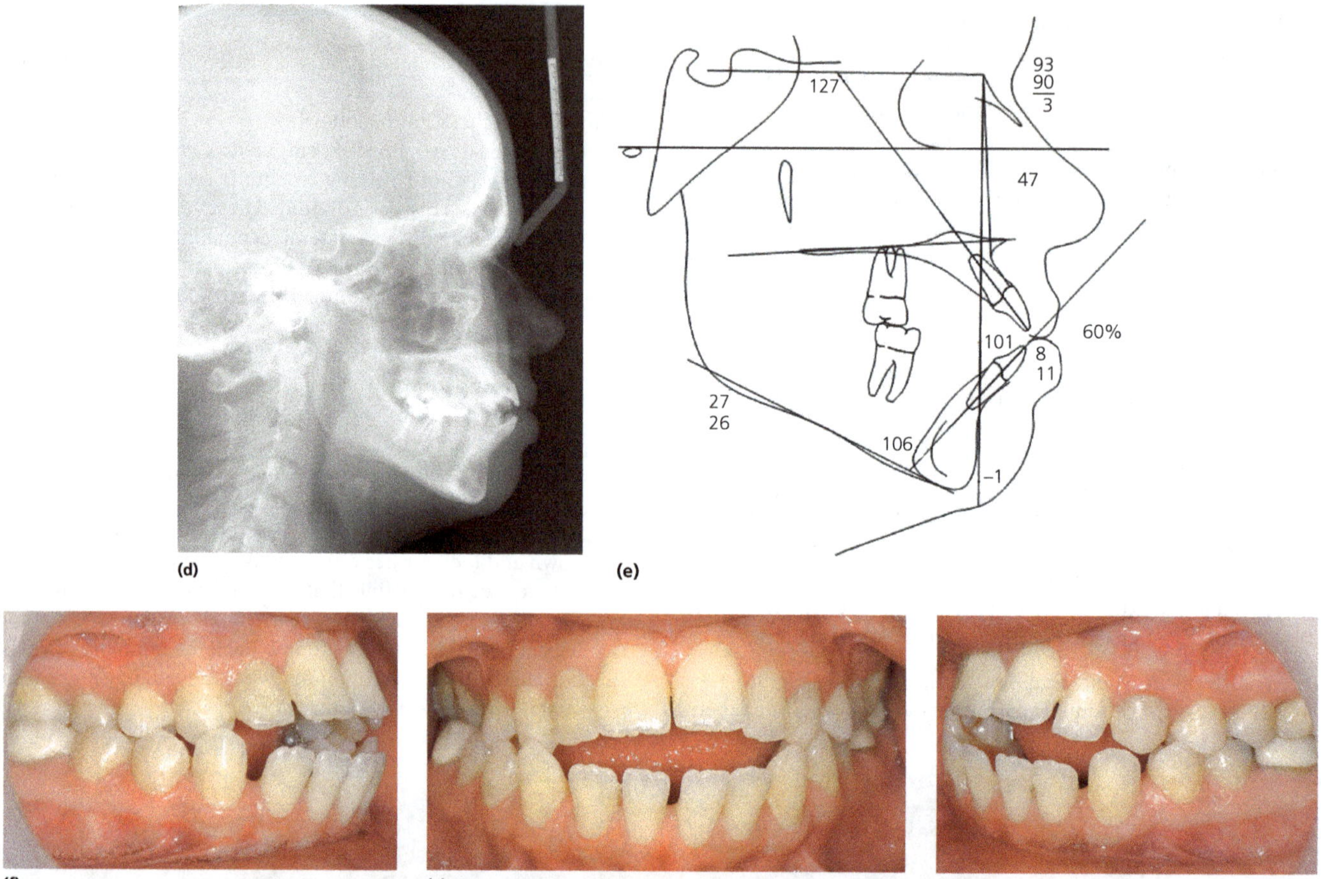

Figure 1.31 (Continued)

Table 1.3 Skeletal and dental features of Kelly (Figure 1.31).

Skeletal open bite features	Dental open bite features
• Long soft tissue LAFH • Long skeletal LAFH (LAFH/TAFH 60%)	• Lip competence (no ILG, mentalis strain?) • MPA WRN • Stepped-up maxillary incisors • Stepped-down mandibular incisors • Open bite limited to anterior teeth with the classic "football shape" indicative of an anterior functional habit

Q: Would you classify Kelly as a dental open bite patient, a skeletal open bite patient, or a combination of both?

A: Kelly should be considered a combination of both. She clearly presents with a dental (functional) open bite due to an active thumb habit. She also exhibits features of a skeletal open bite (long soft tissue LAFH and long skeletal LAFH) but has a normal MPA. In fact, *Kelly's midface appears short (Figure 1.31a), which contributes to the findings of long soft tissue LAFH and long skeletal LAFH even though she looks normal.*

Q: Do you recommend *treating* a patient like Kelly as a dental open bite, a skeletal open bite, or a combination of both?

A: This really comes down to questions of how far from normal do you feel Kelly's vertical development is, how much her vertical growth contributed to her open bite, and how much future growth she has left. We concluded that Kelly has a short midface, which contributes to her LLAFH features. In the spectrum of vertical, Kelly lies in the fairly normal skeletal range. Based upon this conclusion, we treated her as a dental open bite. This was reasonable, especially since she was a 17-year-old and had completed growth.

Q: What features would lead you to classify Owen (Figure 1.32) as a dental open bite or a skeletal open bite patient?

A: See Table 1.4

Q: What should you check for? What questions should you ask Owen?

A: First, discuss with Owen and his parents his breathing history. Is he an obligatory mouth breather? Does he snore at night? Does he stop breathing at night (sleep apnea)? He and his parents deny any history of breathing difficulty, and he breaths nasally. Next, check Owen for an anterior tongue interposition habit. You find he has one (Figure 1.33). He denies a history of a thumb or other digit-sucking habit.

Q: Would you classify Owen as a dental open bite patient, a skeletal open bite patient, or a combination of both?

A: A combination of both. In the spectrum of vertical, Owen would be plotted toward the extreme of skeletal open bite, but his dental (functional, tongue interposition habit) component must also be addressed during treatment.

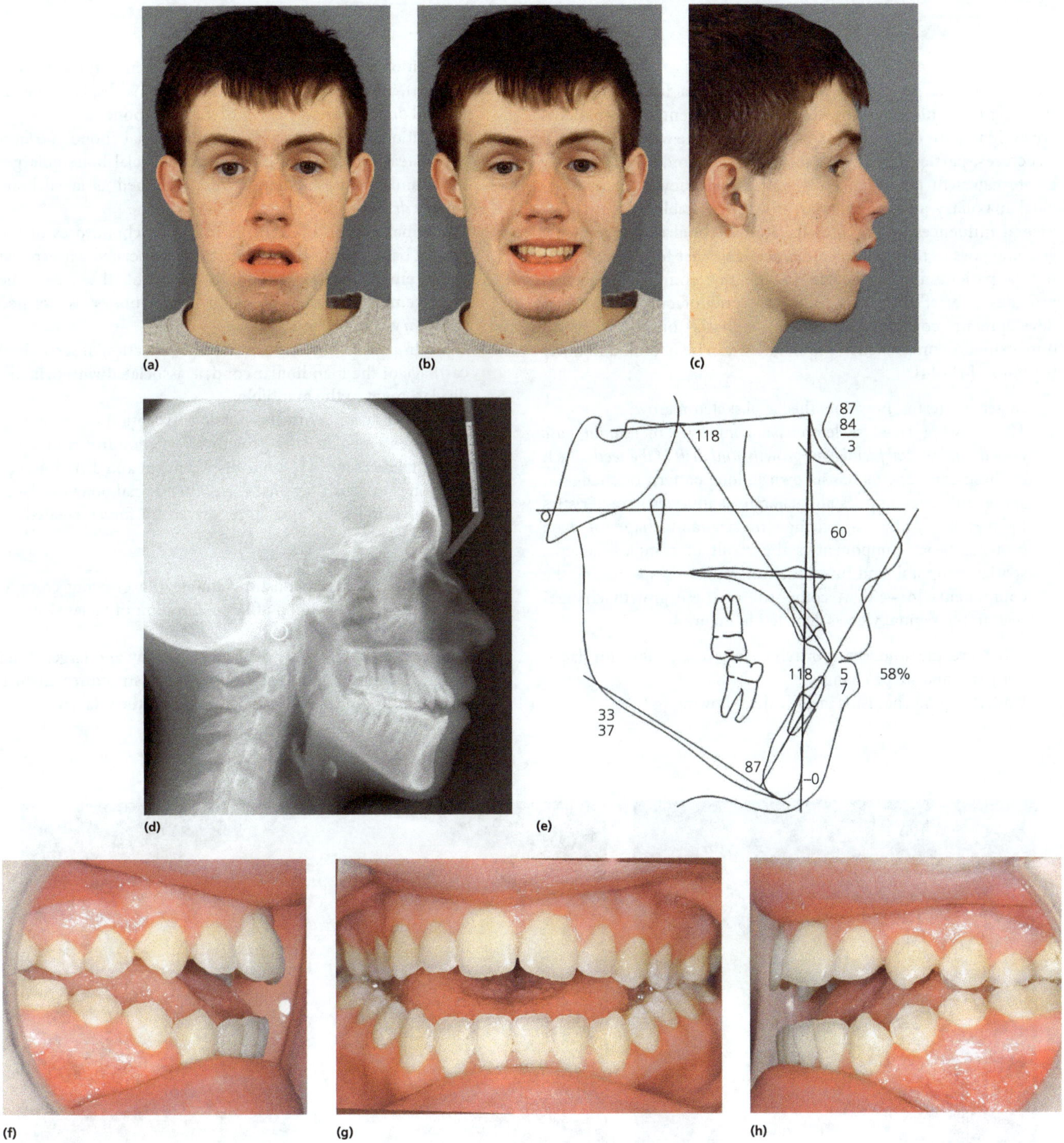

Figure 1.32 Initial records of Owen.

Table 1.4 Skeletal and dental features of Owen (Figure 1.32).

Skeletal open bite features	Dental open bite features
• Long soft tissue LAFH • Long skeletal LAFH • Large ILG • Steep MPA • Maxillary molar root apices erupted well below the palatal plane • Open bite extending to first molars	• Mandibular anterior teeth stepped down in an AP reverse curve (Figures 1.32f and 1.32h)

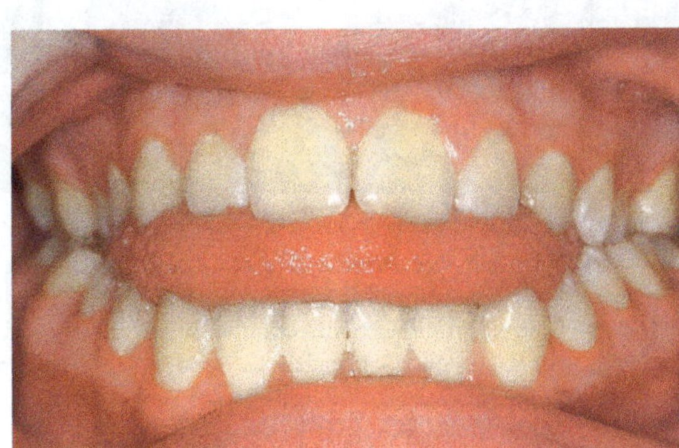

Figure 1.33 Tongue interposition habit of Owen.

Growth Foundations

Essential to the practice of our specialty is an in-depth understanding of craniofacial growth and development. Most patients are evaluated for orthodontic treatment at a time when their facial structures, particularly the maxilla and the mandible, have their greatest growth potential. Thus, exhaustive knowledge of postnatal maxillary and mandibular growth, heritable and environmental influences on jaw growth, and potential response of the growing jaws to intervention are crucial in order for the specialist to treat patients and to evaluate treatment outcomes. This section provides a brief review of important craniofacial growth and development concepts, with an emphasis on the vertical dimension. A comprehensive foundation can be obtained in other textbooks [41–44].

Q: In general terms, how does the facial skeleton grow?

A: The growing facial skeleton is a composite of *cranial base growth, individual facial bone growth, and drift of the teeth*. Each of these components has its own unique pattern of change in space and time but does not generate its unique characteristics independently. Instead, change in size and shape of each growing facial component is the result of complex genetic, spatial, temporal, and functional interrelationships among the components [41–43]. A composite of these growth changes seen in the sagittal view is depicted in Figure 1.34.

Q: What are the underlying mechanisms responsible for facial bone size and shape changes?

A: Underlying mechanisms include the following [42]:

- Appositional bone growth at the facial bone *sutures* (sutural growth) causing spatial displacement. This displacement is termed *primary displacement* of the facial bones.
- Appositional bone growth at the facial bone *surfaces* (periosteal growth) causing individual facial bone enlargement and change in shape. This is defined as facial bone *surface drift*.
- Interstitial growth of cartilage in the synchondroses of the cranial base and nasal septal cartilage associated with spatial displacement of the adjoining bones of the face. The displacement of the adjoining facial bones is termed *secondary displacement*.
- Chondrogenesis and endochondral ossification of secondary cartilage of the mandibular condyle associated with primary displacement of the mandible.

Important concept: With the possible exception of secondary displacement mediated by growth at synchondroses and the nasal septal cartilage [41], bone displacement and drift does not cause bones to "push" against each other. Facial bone displacement and drift is, by and large, driven by forces created by growth of the enveloping soft tissues.

Q: How do temporal relationships among the growing components of the facial skeleton affect maturation of facial size and shape?

A: Maturation of facial size and shape occurs, by and large, along a superior–inferior gradient [42]. Cranial structures mature first, followed by cranial base structures, then facial bones,

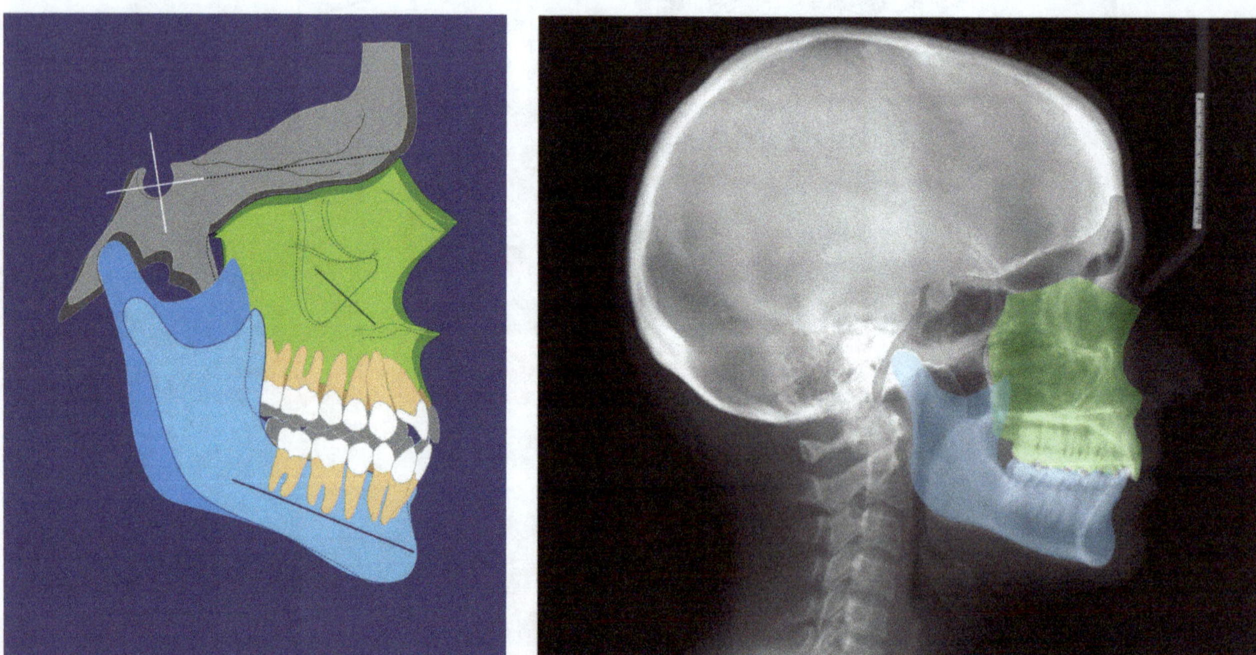

(a) (b)

Figure 1.34 (a) Changes in size, shape, and position of the major skeletal components contributing to the growth of the face as viewed in the sagittal. Approximate outline of the cranial base (gray), the maxilla (green), and the mandible (blue) as seen on a lateral cephalogram. Darker shades of color indicate the approximate location and direction of changes in size and shape due to drift and displacement of the cranial base, maxilla, mandible, and teeth during growth (Duterloo HS, Planche PG. Handbook of Cephalometric Superimposition. Hanover Park: Quintessence, 2001. Figure 3.23. Reprinted with permission from Quintessence Publishing Company Inc, Chicago.) (b) The location of the cranial base (gray), maxilla (green), and mandible (blue) on a lateral cephalogram.

and finally the mandible completes maturation after the maxilla. Aberrations in the temporal sequence result in significant craniofacial deformities. Some have characterized the gradient with distinct tiers (cranial, cranial base, facial), while others have argued for a continuous gradient with maturation of anatomic structures between tiers showing overlap [45]. Adding to the complexity of facial growth, the mediolateral structures of the cranial base do not mature in the same "tier," or at the same time, as those along the superior–inferior gradient. Midline cranial base structures, presumably influenced by maturation of the spheno-occipital synchondrosis, appear to mature well in advance of structures in the lateral cranial floor. Lateral cranial floor structures mature in a similar time frame to the mandible, suggesting a possible functional integration of the masticatory apparatus and the development of lateral cranial floor [45].

Q: How does the cranial base grow? How does cranial base growth contribute to facial growth? Provide a detailed review.

A: The cranial base provides the foundation for postnatal facial development. In the midline, the cranial base undergoes lengthening by primary displacement to accommodate the growing brain. Frontal and temporal lobe brain expansion corresponds with the endochondral bone replacement of cartilage in the sphenoethmoidal and spheno-occipital synchondroses. Frontal and temporal lobe expansion also drives anterior and middle cranial fossae anteroposterior, vertical, and lateral enlargement via sutural growth and drift. The resulting forward movement of the anterior cranial base has a forward displacement (secondary) effect on the nasomaxillary complex. The pterygoid processes move downward by drift and displacement. As frontal lobe expansion and sphenoethmoidal synchondrosis growth cease (approximately age 7), temporal lobe expansion continues, displacing the frontal lobe anteriorly with a continued secondary displacement effect on the anterior cranial base and the nasomaxillary complex. Temporal lobe expansion laterally and vertically also influences the position of the glenoid fossae, which are displaced posteriorly and inferiorly [46] until approximately age 15–16 years [45]—and to a greater degree during adolescence compared to childhood [47]. In general, a more obtuse cranial base angle (angle formed by Nasion–Sella and Sella–Basion) and/or a long anterior (relative to posterior) cranial base length is associated with a skeletal Class II relationship. A more acute cranial base angle and/or a short anterior cranial base length is associated with a skeletal Class III relationship [44]. A composite of these growth movements in the sagittal view is depicted in Figure 1.35.

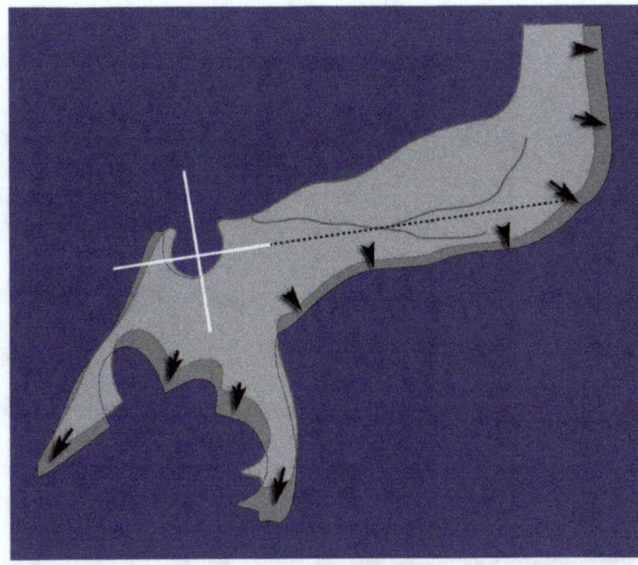

Figure 1.35 Changes in size, shape, and position of the cranial base during growth—as viewed in the sagittal. The intersection of the white lines indicates Sella point. Darker gray and dark arrows indicate approximate magnitude and direction of changes due to growth-driven drift and displacement. (Duterloo HS, Planche PG. Handbook of Cephalometric Superimposition. Hanover Park: Quintessence, 2001. Figure 3.25. Reprinted with permission from Quintessence Publishing Company Inc, Chicago.)

Q: How does the nasomaxillary complex grow?

A: Downward and forward growth of soft tissues creates tension that drives downward and forward nasomaxillary complex movement. That is, as a result of this tension, primary displacement occurs by growth at the sutures joining the maxilla with the frontal, zygomatic, sphenoid, ethmoid, nasal, lacrimal, and palatine bones. This is accompanied by backward downward drift at the posterior maxilla (tuberosity) with new bone available for eruption of permanent molar teeth and downward-directed drift of the hard palate. Nasomaxillary surface drift occurs in response to changing soft tissue and facial bone spatial relationships. Palatal inferior drift and development/vertical drift of permanent teeth contribute approximately 66% of the vertical height change in the maxilla [48, 49]. Vertical drift of maxillary teeth is controlled by forces of eruption (exact mechanism unknown) and forces opposing eruption (e.g., functional/parafunctional loading with mandibular teeth). The contribution of nasal cartilage interstitial growth to downward forward translation of the nasomaxillary complex (secondary displacement) remains equivocal and is thought to have early postnatal influence that diminishes as other displacement forces supersede in later postnatal development [42]. A composite of these growth movements in the sagittal view is depicted in Figure 1.36.

Q: How does the mandible grow?

A: The mandible is carried downward and forward by growth expansion of the enveloping soft tissues. In response, the mandible grows upward and backward largely by a combination of bone surface drift (membranous ossification) and primary displacement at the condyle (endochondral replacement of cartilage).

Q: The mandible consists of five developmentally important regions. What are they, and what role does each play?

A: The mandible consists of the condyle, coronoid process, ramus, corpus, and alveolar process (Figure 1.37). The role of each is as follows:

- Condyle: Along with the ramus, it is a major site of compensatory mandibular growth during downward and forward facial soft tissue expansion. It provides articulation with the temporal bone to mediate function between the maxillary and mandibular teeth. It performs these roles by virtue of the

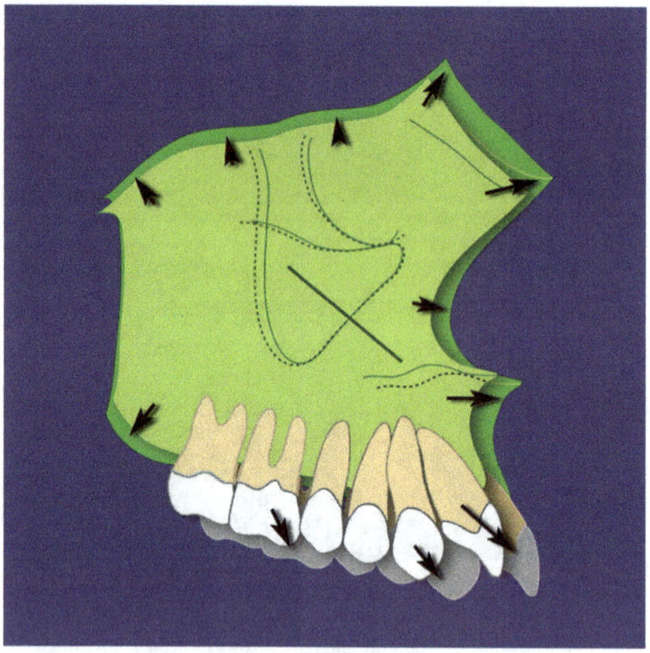

Figure 1.36 Changes in size, shape, and position of the maxilla and maxillary teeth during growth—as viewed in the sagittal. Darker color and dark arrows indicate approximate magnitude and direction of changes due to growth-driven drift and displacement. (Duterloo HS, Planche PG. Handbook of Cephalometric Superimposition. Hanover Park: Quintessence, 2001. Figure 3.29. Reprinted with permission from Quintessence Publishing Company Inc, Chicago.)

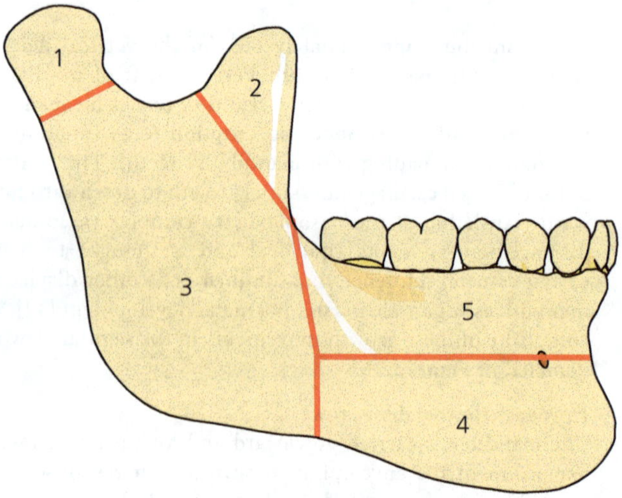

Figure 1.37 The mandible consists of five regions: 1, condyle; 2, coronoid process; 3, ramus; 4, corpus; 5, alveolar process.

condylar cartilage, a specialized secondary cartilage allowing endochondral bone growth to occur in the presence of masticatory compressive forces on the condylar head. The arrangement of secondary cartilage allows condylar growth to be adaptive, facilitating change in growth direction as pressure and tension on the condylar head change, and to maintain the relationship of the condyle and glenoid fossa as the mandible is carried downward and forward.

- Coronoid process: It provides attachment for the temporalis muscle, which supports the process of mastication. The coronoid process undergoes extensive drift upward, backward, and laterally during the downward and forward translation of the mandible.

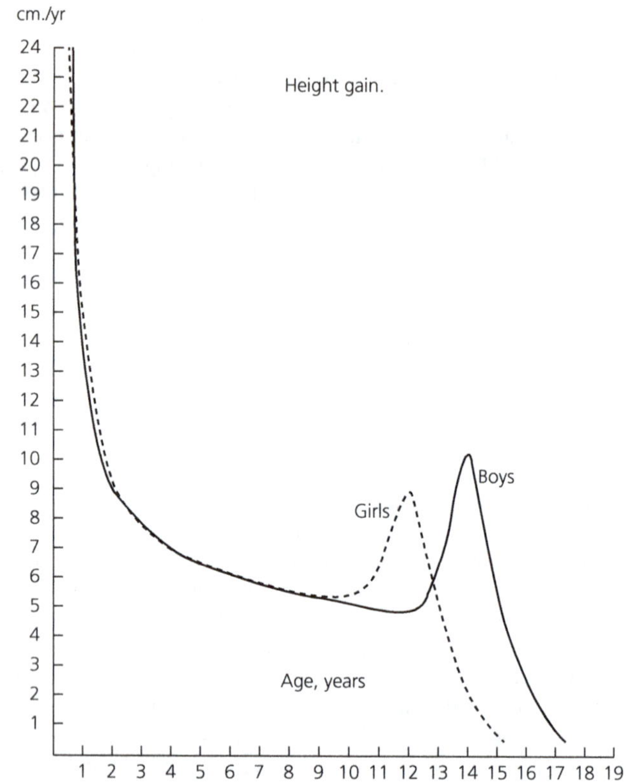

Figure 1.38 Plot of change in growth velocity with age. (Tanner JM, Whitehouse RH, Takaishi M. Standards from birth to maturity for height, weight, height velocity, and weight velocity: British children, 1965. Arch Dis Child. 1966 Oct;41(219):454–71. Reproduced with permission from BMJ Publishing Group Ltd.)

- Ramus: As a major site of adaptive growth and growth compensations, it is of equal importance to the condyle during downward and forward translation of the mandible. In order to maintain the appropriate spatial and functional relationship of the mandibular dentition with the maxillary dentition during growth, the ramus undergoes complex changes in width, breadth, height, and uprighting (gonial angle becoming more acute). Although it is common to encounter the term "condylar growth," signifying the condyle as the most important mandibular growth center, the importance of ramus growth is coequal in establishing balance or imbalance in mandibular position [42]. Also, the ramus provides attachment for the masseter and medial pterygoid muscles.
- Corpus: It supports the alveolar process and teeth during development and mastication. It provides attachment for many muscles, including the mentalis muscle.
- Alveolar process: It provides a bony housing for the eruption, drift, and function of teeth.

Q: Is facial growth coordinated with statural growth?

A: Yes. By and large, the temporal sequence of maturation is synchronized throughout the body. General body (somatic) growth, measured by change in stature with time (growth velocity), is an indicator of velocity changes in craniofacial dimensions during growth [50, 51]. This is in contrast to the neurocranium, which is more closely coordinated with neural growth.

Q: Do facial and statural growth proceed with constant velocity during development?

A: No. A typical plot of statural growth velocity (Figure 1.38) shows that change is not uniform. One-half of adult stature is attained within the first two years of life during a rapid deceleration of growth velocity. After which, a much slower deceleration of growth velocity occurs until the onset of puberty. The inflection point where deceleration of growth velocity changes to acceleration is the beginning of pubertal growth acceleration, often termed the "pubertal growth spurt." This pubertal growth acceleration increases growth velocity to a maximum, termed the peak height velocity (PHV), followed by a rapid deceleration in growth velocity [50, 52].

Q: What is the duration of pubertal growth acceleration?

A: Approximately 2–2.5 years [50].

Q: Does pubertal growth acceleration occur at the same age for males and females?

A: No. On average, females reach PHV at age 11.5–12 years and males reach PHV at age 14 years [50, 52, 53].

Q: Is peak facial growth velocity coordinated with PHV?

A: Yes. On average, females reach peak facial growth velocity at 10.9–12.3 years and males reach peak facial growth velocity at 14.1–14.3 years, [54–56] supporting the close association between change in stature and facial dimensions [50].

Q: How much growth occurs during pubertal growth acceleration?

A: On average, males add 20 cm in stature and females add 16 cm in stature. On average, the chin moves downward and forward, away from the cranial base (measured Sella to Gnathion), 1.8–2.0 cm in males and 1.1–1.2 cm in females [57].

Q: Are males and females similar in the downward and forward facial growth pattern during pubertal growth acceleration?

A: Possibly not. A recent longitudinal study of 111 untreated French-Canadian females demonstrated that during the period of pubertal growth acceleration, beginning at approximately 11.5 years of age, measures of vertical skeletal change showed acceleration, but measures of horizontal skeletal change did not. Moreover, in this sample, measures of horizontal skeletal change decelerated during adolescence. For this sample, female pubertal growth acceleration did not provide anteroposterior improvement in chin projection [58].

Q: Is the pattern and rate of forward and downward growth during pubertal growth acceleration the same as found prior to puberty?

A: No. Studies have shown that horizontal and vertical translation of the chin varies between prepubertal and pubertal growth periods. [16, 59–63] Growth-driven *anterior* movement of the chin has a greater velocity during childhood compared to the period of adolescence. In contrast, growth-driven *inferior* movement of the chin has less velocity during childhood compared to the period of adolescence. These findings suggest a tendency for facial height to increase more than facial depth during adolescence compared to childhood [63–65].

Q: Is there a measurable indicator of pubertal growth acceleration and PHV?

A: There is no one best indicator of pubertal growth acceleration and PHV. Maturation of hand–wrist and cervical spine bones has been studied as potential predictors of PHV but give unreliable estimates of PHV timing and peak facial growth velocity [54, 66–71]. Skeletal development of hand–wrist bones has been shown to be useful in estimating whether the pubertal growth acceleration has already occurred [54], but the method of assessing a patient's skeletal development by hand–wrist radiography against a radiographic atlas of normal hand–wrist skeletal development has low sensitivity in predicting whether the pubertal growth acceleration is impending or ongoing [50, 66]. That being said, measurement of growth acceleration itself, measured as *change in stature with time, may be considered the least invasive and most reliable predictor of pubertal growth acceleration and PHV* [54, 72].

Q: Can other periods of growth acceleration occur before puberty?

A: Yes. Statural growth acceleration has been reported to occur in the age range 6.5–8.5 years for some individuals (termed the midgrowth spurt) [73, 74]. Reports on the magnitude of change in statural growth velocity vary in characterization from "less deceleration" to mild acceleration, and are of considerably lower magnitude, compared to pubertal growth acceleration [73–76]. Midgrowth spurts in facial growth velocity have also been shown in some individuals. [54, 59, 77]

Q: How does "normal" vertical skeletal development occur?

A: "Normal" vertical skeletal relationships arise from a sequential coordination of the major elements of the craniofacial growth process:

- Cranial base growth
- Sutural lowering of the maxilla with drift of the palate/nasal floor
- Growth of the mandibular corpus, ramus, and condyle
- Maxillary and mandibular growth rotation
- Dentoalveolar development

These processes are directed by complex interrelationships between factors under genetic control and environmental (epigenetic) factors influencing this control.

Q: Is "normal" skeletal development a prerequisite for "normal" interocclusal dental relationships?

A: No. A Class I molar relationship is considered "normal," as is 1–2 mm of incisor overjet and 10–20% of incisor overbite. However, "normal" interocclusal dental relationships can occur in spite of abnormal skeletal relationships. For example, it is estimated that 50–55% of the US population have Class I malocclusion [78], meaning that they have Class I molars in spite of possible anteroposterior (AP), vertical, or transverse skeletal problems (in addition to dental problems, such as crowding). Among all human populations, there are individuals who vary significantly from others in vertical, AP, and transverse skeletal relationships yet have similar interocclusal relationships [42].

Q: The preceding answer raises the following question: what is the growth mechanism providing "normal" interocclusal molar relationships despite significant variation in skeletal relationships?

A: Simply put, it is the *compensatory growth potential* of each major element of the facial growth process. In other words, compensatory growth of one element can overcome unbalanced growth of another element, allowing for attainment and maintenance of normal interocclusal relationships [42]. For example, decreased cranial base flexure can be associated with skeletal mandibular retrusion; but, an individual with decreased cranial base flexure and increased ramus breadth growth will maintain a normal interocclusal relationship.

Q: By what one mechanism do skeletal problems develop?

A: This is a trick question. By and large, there is not one *single* causative mechanism for the development of skeletal problems. The development of skeletal problems is multifactorial, and "abnormal" skeletal relationships arise from aberrations in genetic and/or environmental influences. Aberrations produce altered growth intensity and/or altered temporal coordination of one or more major growth elements. Aberrations, sufficient in magnitude and/or duration to disrupt the interrelationships of these elements, result in adaptive growth movements of the maxilla and mandible that may lead to abnormal changes in the spatial relationship of the jaws [42, 79].

Q: With respect to craniofacial development in the vertical dimension, abnormal skeletal relationships are characterized using various cephalometric measures. Can you list, and describe, three of these measures?

A: Three cephalometric measures describing vertical development include the following:

- Ratio of posterior facial height (linear measurement from Sella to Gonion) to anterior facial height (linear measurement from Nasion to Menton) or PFH/AFH, viewed in the sagittal plane. A reduced PFH/AFH ratio is associated with greater divergence between the MP and cranial base, indicating a "skeletal open bite" facial pattern. Conversely, a large PFH/AFH ratio tends to indicate a "skeletal deep bite" facial pattern [80].
- Ratio of lower anterior facial height to total anterior facial height (linear measurement from Menton to ANS superimposed on the linear measurement of Menton to Nasion) or LAFH/TAFH. A reduced LAFH/TAFH ratio indicates a skeletal deep bite facial pattern, and a large ratio is associated with greater facial divergence and a skeletal open bite pattern.
- Angular measurement between the SN line and MP, or SN-MP angle. An elevated SN-MP angle indicates greater facial divergence and skeletal open bite facial pattern. A reduced SN-MP angle indicates a skeletal deep bite facial pattern.

Q: Extreme variations of craniofacial vertical growth appear to result from adaptive jaw displacement and remodeling. Skeletal open bites may result from adaptive jaw displacement and remodeling due to what?

A: Skeletal open bites may result from the following:

- Decreased cranial base flexure leading to superior spatial positioning of the temporomandibular fossae. However, this influence is not well understood and requires more study before it can be used reliably in diagnosis.
- Excessive sutural lowering (vertical growth/descent) of the maxilla
- Diminished vertical growth of the mandibular condyles (posterior-superior condylar growth)
- Backward mandibular (true/internal) rotation
- Excessive vertical posterior dentoalveolar development (excessive posterior tooth eruption)

Q: Conversely, skeletal deep bites may result from adaptive jaw displacement and remodeling due to what?

A: Skeletal deep bites may result from the following:

- Increased cranial base flexure leading to inferior spatial positioning of the temporomandibular fossae. However, this influence is not well understood and requires more study before it can be used reliably in diagnosis
- Deficient sutural lowering (vertical growth/descent) of the maxilla
- Excessive vertical growth of the mandibular condyles
- Forward mandibular (true/internal) rotation
- Deficient vertical posterior dentoalveolar development

Q: According to Schudy [9], how does vertical condylar growth relate to the sum of vertical maxillary descent *plus* maxillary/mandibular molar eruption during normal, hyperdivergent, and hypodivergent facial development?

A: Schudy suggests the following:

- When vertical condylar growth *matches* the sum of maxillary descent and posterior dentoalveolar development, *normal vertical development results.*
- With diminished vertical condylar growth relative to the sum of maxillary descent and posterior dentoalveolar development, facial hyperdivergence, decreased PFH/AFH, increased LAFH/TAFH, increased SN-MP, and a skeletal open bite pattern result.
- With excessive vertical condylar growth relative to the sum of maxillary descent and posterior dentoalveolar development, facial hypodivergence, increased PFH/AFH, decreased LAFH/TAFH, decreased SN-MP, and a skeletal deep bite pattern result.
- It is noteworthy that extreme patterns of vertical skeletal growth develop early and, by and large, remain relatively stable throughout craniofacial growth.

Q: Do we know the *exact* mechanisms by which aberrations in craniofacial growth processes create vertical skeletal abnormalities?

A: No. The exact mechanisms by which aberrations in craniofacial growth processes create vertical skeletal abnormalities remain unknown. Epigenetic (environmental) factors are thought to influence the interrelationship of these processes, but this influence is currently not well-defined. For example, structural and/or environmental conditions that restrict nasal breathing have long been associated with facial hyperdivergence (skeletal open bite). Enlarged adenoids being a conspicuous etiologic agent for restricted breathing, the term "adenoid facies" was widely used to describe the clinical picture of affected individuals. Extreme facial hyperdivergence, narrow maxillary arch, and lip incompetence are prominent clinical features. The theory of epigenetic influence proposed for the development of this skeletal pattern has been largely mechanistic: restricted nasal breathing demands mouth breathing and mouth breathing alters the tongue position, mandibular posture, and head posture. Altered postures lead to muscle imbalance, and muscle imbalance influences craniofacial growth—leading to decreased vertical condylar growth, increased sutural growth of the upper face, and increased posterior dentoalveolar development with negative (elongating) effects on vertical facial growth [81–85]. Although much study has been applied to this theory, a direct cause and effect relationship remains equivocal [86].

More recently, a new theory has been proposed that suggests restricted nasal breathing may be related to abnormal nocturnal secretion of growth hormone (GH) [87]. Children with obstructive sleep apnea share similar craniofacial characteristics to those earlier characterized with "adenoid facies" and also show abnormal nocturnal GH secretion. GH is known to have a positive mediating effect on mandibular ramus height during growth [88]. Further, recent information suggests that faulty GH receptors are a genetic marker for reduced ramus height during growth in certain populations [89–91]. Taken together, this information suggests that the mechanism by which restricted nasal breathing affects craniofacial form is due to a more complex sequence of epigenetic events than envisioned previously. Our point is that, even using one example, the *exact* mechanisms by which aberrations in craniofacial growth processes create vertical skeletal abnormalities are unknown.

Q: Is there a relationship between masticatory function and vertical facial dimensions?

A: Yes, variation in vertical facial dimensions is closely associated with masticatory performance. Studies have documented that an increase in the relative height of the anterior lower facial skeleton is predictably associated with a decrease in bite force magnitude, smaller cross-sectional area of the masticatory adductors (i.e., masseter, medial pterygoid, and temporalis), and reduced masticatory muscle activity. The precise influence of masticatory performance on facial form is not well understood, and there is debate regarding the causal nature of this relationship [92]. In a manner similar to habitual mouth breathing, reduced muscle function may alter the posture of the mandible and thus affect the pattern of mandibular rotation during development resulting in a long-face phenotype [93].

Q: What is meant by growth rotation of the jaws?

A: Viewed in the sagittal plane, the maxilla and mandible undergo patterns of rotation during facial growth and development. Björk [7, 94] identified three components of mandibular rotation and remodeling (matrix, intramatrix, and total rotation, Figure 1.39 illustrates an example) that have been more recently redefined [78]:

- Apparent rotation ("matrix" rotation) is a measure of angular changes of the mandibular inferior border relative to the anterior cranial base (usually measured as changes in SN-MP). It is the absolute change in MP angle during growth.
- Angular remodeling ("intramatrix" rotation) is a measure of change in the MP relative to the mandibular reference line representing the mandibular corpus (determined by mandibular structures stable during growth). It reflects remodeling along the mandibular lower border during growth.
- True rotation ("total" rotation, "internal" rotation) is a measure of change in the mandibular reference line (mandibular corpus) relative to cranial base reference line. True rotation is the sum of apparent rotation and angular remodeling. Apparent rotation is often less than true rotation due to the angular remodeling that minimizes SN-MP change during growth.

Q: How does growth rotation of the jaws influence the vertical dimension of the face?

A: Björk was the first to discover true growth rotation, defined as rotation of the maxillary or mandibular corpus relative to the cranial base, measured from stable references (implanted bone markers) in the sagittal view. [94, 95, 8] His studies demonstrated a relationship between true mandibular growth rotation and condylar growth:

- Greater true forward mandibular growth rotation is associated with vertical condylar growth of larger magnitude directed more anteriorly.

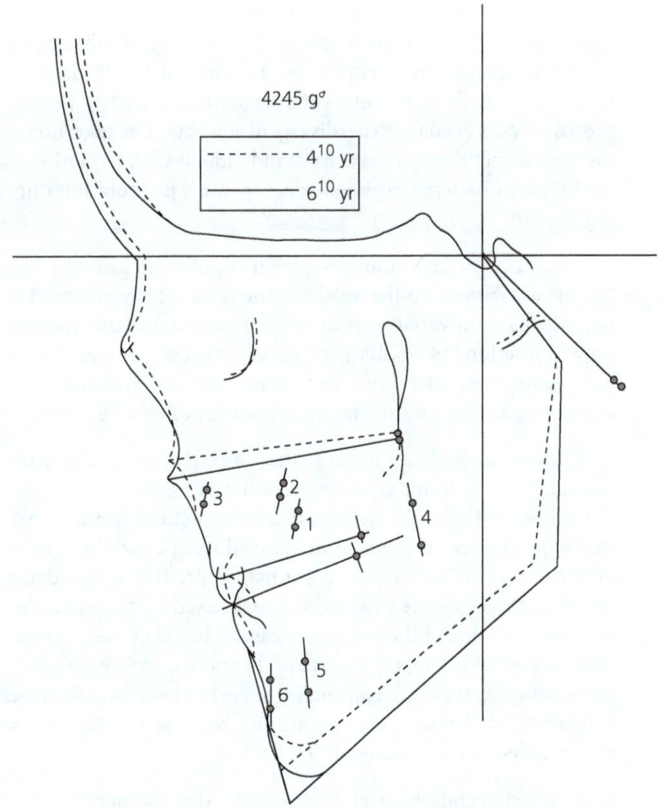

Figure 1.39 Overall superimposition of cephalometric tracings depicting 2 years of growth in a young male. Black dots indicate location of implant markers. Numbers 1, 2, and 3 indicate maxillary implant markers. Numbers 4, 5, and 6 indicate mandibular implant markers. Black lines bisecting dot pairs indicate the direction of implant marker displacement during growth. Note the equivalence in magnitude and direction of maxillary implant displacement indicating nominal true rotation. In contrast, the pattern of changes in magnitude and direction of the mandibular implants indicates true mandibular anterior rotation. The pattern of inferior mandibular border change suggests nominal apparent mandibular rotation due to angular remodeling. (Björk A. Facial growth in man, studied with the aid of metallic implants. Acta Odontol Scand. 1955;13:9–34. Reproduced with permission from Taylor & Francis Ltd.)

- Greater backward mandibular growth rotation is associated with vertical condylar growth of smaller magnitude directed more posteriorly.
- True forward mandibular rotation during growth is also associated with decreases in the gonial angle [96–99], decreases in MP angle [100], and increases in posterior facial height [95]. True forward rotation results in adaptive modeling of the mandible, including increased posterior ramus deposition, increased posterior lower border resorption, and increased anterior lower border deposition [101, 102].
- Extremes of true forward or backward mandibular rotation are associated with skeletal deep bite and skeletal open bite, respectively [80].

Q: What is the occurrence of forward or backward growth rotation of the jaws?

A: Measurement of selected populations longitudinally has suggested that *true mandibular growth rotation is, by and large, forward for most* individuals [14, 15, 103]. High-angle (increased SN-MP angle) subjects show less forward true rotation (degrees per year) and less condylar growth magnitude (mm per year) compared with low-angle (decreased SN-MP angle) subjects. In addition, these studies support the findings of Björk, namely, that apparent forward rotation (decreasing SN-MP) during growth occurs even for hyperdivergent subjects. The take-home message is that the vast majority of individuals with hyperdivergent skeletal patterns experience net forward jaw rotation during growth.

Q: Is rotation of the jaws uniform during craniofacial growth?
A: No. In a manner similar to the velocity of condylar growth, individuals show variation in amount, duration, and direction of growth rotation [14, 98, 100]. This means that some hyperdivergent individuals that experience a net forward rotation may experience backward rotation during some period of growth.

Q: Are there diagnostic indices that foretell an individual's maxillary or mandibular future growth rotation?
A: No. Björk [104] identified seven specific structural features that might develop as a result of remodeling during a particular type of growth rotation. His suggestions for predicting condylar rotation have, however, not been widely used by the specialty because (1) some of the indicators cannot be easily seen on the average cephalogram, (2) the use of the indicators is very time-consuming for the clinician, and (3) there has been no scientific validation of the suggested indicators because of difficulties encountered in study design [105, 106].

Q: Does growth rotation affect dentoalveolar development?
A: Yes. Greater mandibular incisor proclination, greater mandibular molar mesial drift, and relatively greater mandibular molar than incisor eruption have been related to greater true forward rotation [95, 107].

Q: Does dentoalveolar development and tooth eruption *cause*, or only adapt to, skeletal problems in the vertical dimension?
A: Dentoalveolar development and tooth eruption *adapt* to skeletal problems in the vertical dimension. Issacson [108] was the first to report on dentoalveolar development in three groups of subjects—those with short anterior facial height (hypodivergent), those with average anterior facial height, and those with excessive anterior facial height (hyperdivergent). Maxillary posterior alveolar development was found to decrease with decreasing SN-MP angle, with a difference of 5.1 mm of dentoalveolar development between hypodivergent and hyperdivergent individuals. This finding has subsequently been confirmed by others [109, 110]. Björk [95] suggested dentoalveolar development was coupled to vertical facial growth, a suggestion later verified in a longitudinal female sample. In this study, eruption of mandibular teeth followed vertical growth displacement of the mandible. Also, mandibular molar eruption showed greater plasticity than vertical mandibular growth, indicating that molar eruption *adapts* to vertical mandibular growth displacement [111].

Q: What causes abnormalities in vertical dentoalveolar development?
A: Vertical dentoalveolar development abnormalities manifest as supraeruption or infraeruption of teeth. Since vertical dentoalveolar development/tooth eruption is controlled by forces of eruption (exact mechanism unknown) and forces opposing eruption (e.g., functional/parafunctional occlusal loading), any disturbance of these forces may create abnormalities. Such disturbances may include the following:

- Diminished masticatory performance/diminished loading: This has been shown to be associated with increased posterior alveolar development, increased posterior tooth eruption, severe hyperdivergence, and skeletal open bite and may influence tooth eruption and jaw growth [92].
- Altered spatial relationship of the jaws: This can result in teeth left unopposed and absence of forces opposing eruption. For example, in a large Class II discrepancy patient (mandibular hypoplasia, large ANB angle), the mandibular incisors are unopposed by the maxillary incisors. The mandibular incisors can supraerupt creating an exaggerated curve of Spee.
- Tongue interposition, digit-sucking, and lip-biting habits: This can increase the duration/magnitude of forces opposing tooth eruption and result in anterior or posterior open bites.
- Ankylosis or tooth loss: This results in elimination of forces opposing eruption and supraeruption of teeth in the opposing arch.

Q: What is dentofacial orthopedics?
A: Orthopedic change can be defined as alteration in size, shape, growth velocity, or growth rotation of bones. Modifying craniofacial growth with orthodontic forces is termed dentofacial orthopedics.

Q: Which craniofacial elements are potentially alterable by dentofacial orthopedics?
A: Forces of significant magnitude and duration can potentially influence the following:

- Glenoid fossa portions of the cranial base
- Cranial base sutures adjoining the maxilla
- Corpus, dentoalveolar process, and teeth of the maxilla
- Condyle, ramus, dentoalveolar process, and teeth of the mandible

Q: Can you provide examples, or cite studies, of orthopedics influencing these elements?
A: One vivid example is the use of a "Milwaukee brace" to treat patients with scoliosis of the spinal column. Use of this device transmits significant force to the lower border of the mandible—producing changes in shape and growth direction for both the maxilla and mandible [112]. Various animal studies [113–116] have demonstrated that application of relatively high force over an extended period of time can produce measurable changes in the flexure of the cranial base, sutural growth of the maxilla, proliferation of condylar cartilage, shape and position of the glenoid fossae, growth rotation of the mandible, and position of teeth/dentoalveolar bone. Orthodontic treatment, with or without the extraction of permanent teeth, can redirect the drift of teeth and alveolar bone, providing treatment-induced adaptation or compensation of the maxillary and mandibular dentoalveolar processes [117].

Q: Can orthopedic treatment effects demonstrated in animal studies be extrapolated to humans?
A: Animal study findings, generally, cannot be directly extrapolated to humans. For example, differences in force magnitude are frequently found between animal studies and clinical application. Elder and Tuenge [113] used 1400 grams of force to produce measurable change in cranial base flexure in monkeys (small cranium), but typical clinical headgear force ranges from 200 to 400 grams per side and typical clinical maxillary protraction or mandibular chin cup forces range from 300 to 600 grams [118]. Also, differences in force duration are frequently found between animal studies and clinical application. For example, McNamara and Bryan studied the orthopedic effects of a mandibular protrusive appliance worn in monkeys from early

mixed dentition until maturity [119], but clinical application of protrusive appliances in persons is for much shorter periods (e.g., 6- to 9-month wear for a Herbst appliance [120, 121]).

Diagnosis and Treatment Planning Principles

Q: When evaluating a patient for orthodontic treatment, what steps are needed to obtain a comprehensive diagnosis and appropriate treatment plan?

A: We recommend a sequence of 10 steps in order to establish a final treatment plan:

1. Obtain a thorough history and establish the patient's chief complaint (CC).
2. Examine the patient clinically and with appropriate records.
3. Exhaustively list diagnostic findings/problems and make your diagnosis.
4. Define your treatment goals.
5. Focus on solving the *primary* problem in each dimension (plus other major problems).
6. Consider surgical options.
7. Establish unknowns you face—strive to reduce significant unknowns *before* presenting final treatment plan to the patient and before doing anything irreversible.
8. Consider benefits/costs of treating nonextraction.
9. Consider benefits/costs of treating with extraction of anterior teeth or posterior teeth.
10. Weigh benefits/costs of all viable treatment options.

Based upon all of the aforementioned steps, you should choose a recommended treatment plan (what you would do if you were the patient or if the patient was a member of your family).

These 10 steps will be used for all the cases presented in this text. Let's examine these steps in detail, using patients to exemplify how information is obtained and used in this process.

Step 1: Obtain a thorough history and establish the patient's CC.

Q: How do you establish the patient's CC?

A: By asking the direct question when discussing their history, "What is your chief concern?" and following with open-ended questions that elicit the patient's description of their concern and their feelings regarding why they are seeking change. For example, Monica (Figure 1.40) is a 41-year-old woman who presents to you with the CC, "I would like my crossbite corrected." Many patients are not so candid. When a patient first presents to you, it can be helpful to ask them questions that draw out their concerns, such as, "Hello Monica, thank you for

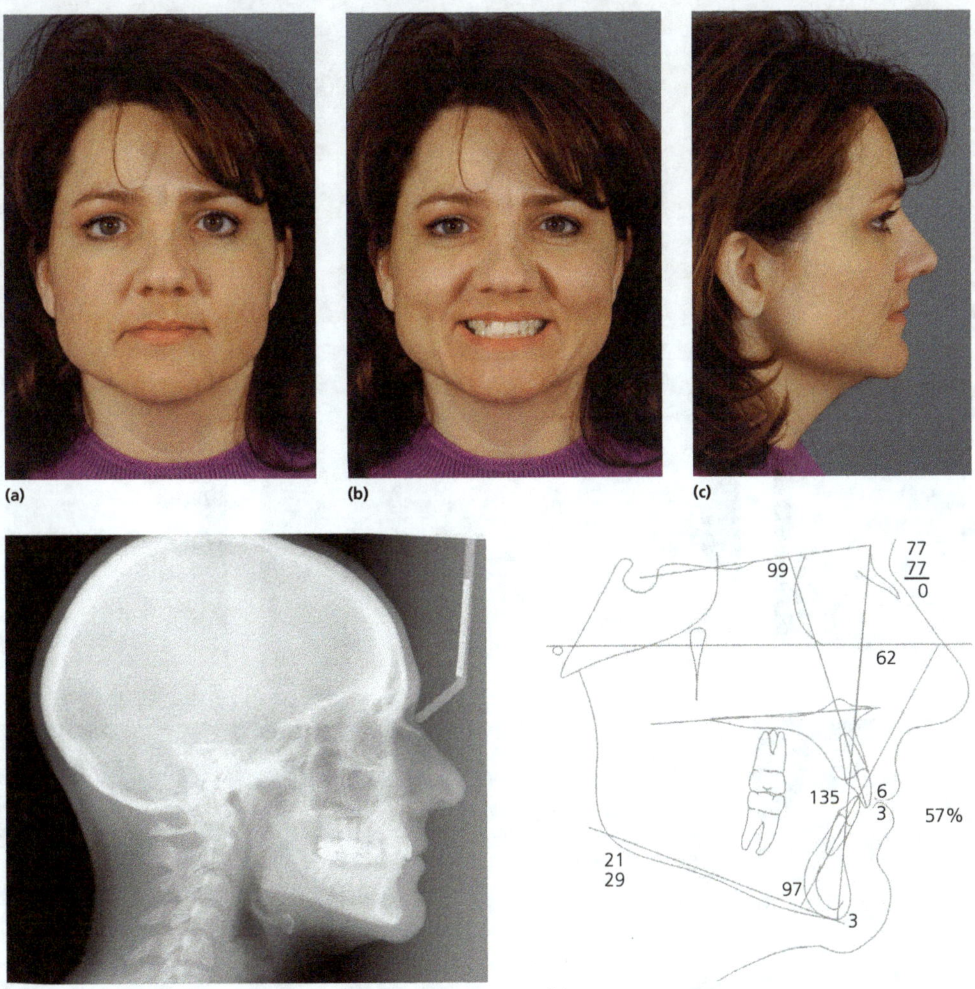

Figure 1.40 Initial records of Monica: (a–c) facial photographs, (d) lateral cephalograph, (e) cephalometric tracing, (f) pantomograph, (g–k) intraoral photographs, (l–q) model photographs.

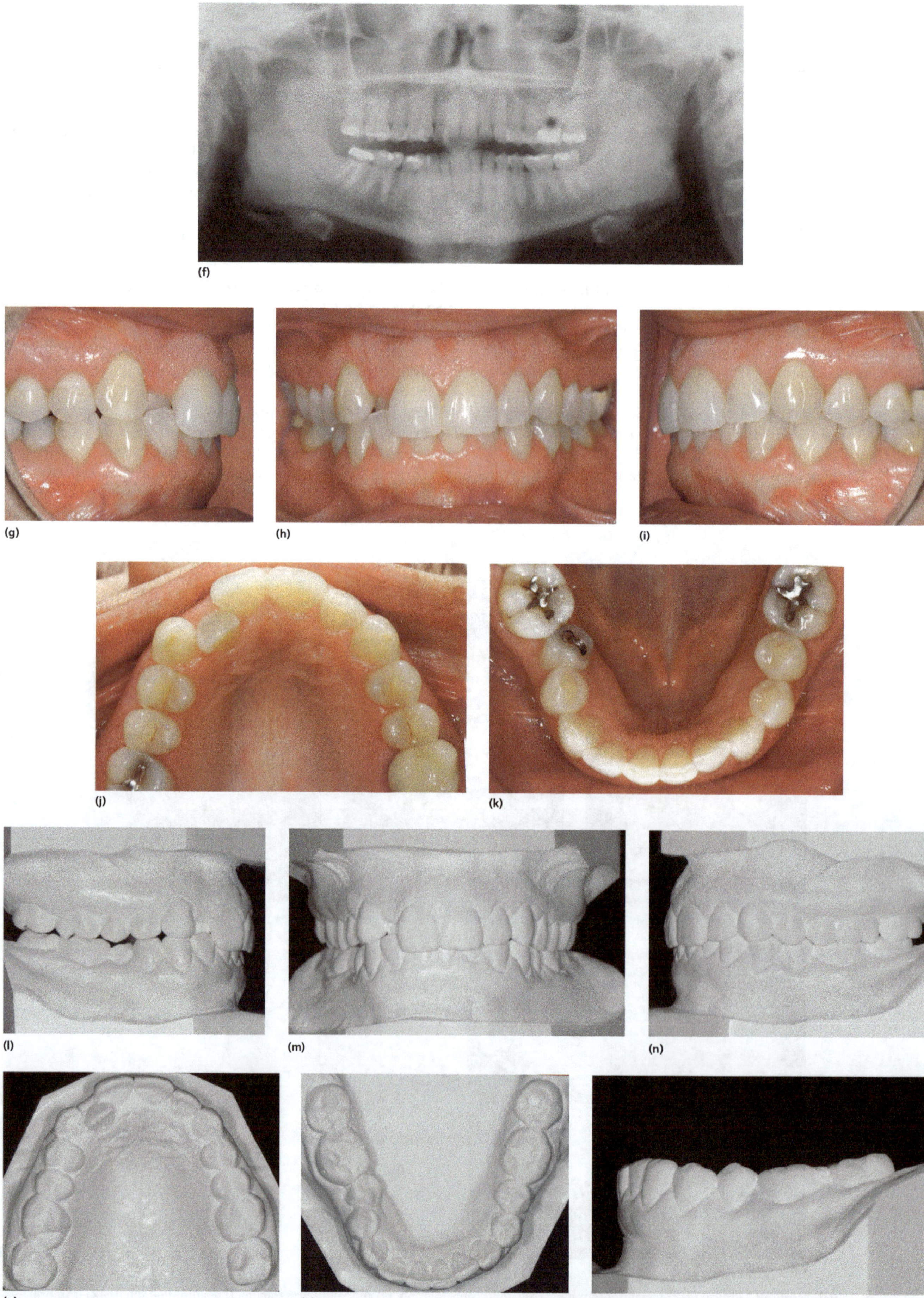

Figure 1.40 (Continued)

coming to see us. Is there any particular problem with your bite or your smile that has brought you here today?" The way you phrase such a question can make all the difference in helping to elicit their concerns. Many patients can benefit greatly from orthodontic treatment in terms of facial and smile esthetic improvement and self-image improvement but have difficulty communicating this. For example, a patient may present for an initial examination and ask you if they should have treatment. Providing the patient a hand-held mirror during the examination will facilitate a discussion about their concern regarding their bite or smile.

Step 2: Examine the patient clinically and with appropriate records.

Q: What should be included in your clinical examination, and what records are appropriate for diagnosis?

A: Your clinical examination should include the following: a review of the patient's past medical history (PMH) and past dental history (PDH), a temporomandibular joint (TMJ) examination, a complete head and neck examination, a periodontal/mucogingival examination, determination of their upper dental midline (UDML) position with respect to the midline of their face, evaluation of the incisal display and upper lip length in relaxed lip position, and a determination of any AP or lateral slide between centric relation and centric occlusion (CR–CO shift).

Appropriate records include facial and intraoral photographs, models or intraoral digital scans of the teeth and gingiva, and radiographic imaging of the facial bones and teeth. Radiographic imaging may include a cone-beam CT scan (CBCT), or separate lateral cephalometric and panoramic radiographs, and a complete mouth series of dental radiographs as you deem appropriate. Also, identify the patient's general dentist and physician and any dental specialists providing treatment, to allow you to communicate with other doctors involved in the patient's care.

For Monica, you perform a clinical examination and make a lateral cephalometric radiograph, panoramic radiograph, models, and photographs (Figure 1.40). Her PMH, PDH, and TMJs are WRN. You observe that CR=CO (there is no shift). Her periodontal examination is WRN.

Step 3: Exhaustively list diagnostic findings/problems and make your diagnosis.

Q: Do you have any suggestions to help make an exhaustive list of diagnostic findings and problems?

A: Yes, using a table to systematically list pertinent diagnostic data and problems that vary significantly from normal can help. An example is shown in Table 1.5.

Q: Looking at Monica's diagnostic records (Figure 1.40), what are her diagnostic findings and problems? (A blank Diagnostic Findings/Problem List table for you to copy is found in the Appendix.)

A: See Table 1.6

Q: Why is it important to view study models from the lingual aspect?

A: Some patients with mesially rotated maxillary first molars will appear Class II when viewed from the buccal but actually have their maxillary first molar lingual cusps properly seated in the mandibular first molar central fossa (Class I) when viewed from the lingual. As shown, Monica is clearly Class I when viewed from the lingual (Figure 1.41).

Table 1.5 Diagnostic findings and problem list with some common features to examine.

Full face and profile	**Frontal view**
	Facial symmetry
	Vertical facial balance
	Relaxed lip posture
	Buccal corridors
	Upper dental midline
	Incisal display during smile
	Gingival display during smile
	Profile view
	Overall profile curvature (convex, straight, concave)
	Nasal shape
	Nasolabial angle (NLA)
	Labiomental sulcus
	Chin position (retrusive, effective, protrusive)
	Lip–chin–throat angle
	Chin–throat length
Ceph analysis	**Skeletal**
	Maxillary position (anteroposterior (AP) and vertical)
	Mandibular position (AP and vertical)
	Bony chin position and form
	Vertical balance
	Dental
	Maxillary and mandibular incisor angulation
	Maxillary and mandibular incisor AP position
Radiographs	Dentition stage of development
	Root morphology
	Pathology
Intraoral Photos and Models	Angle classification
	Iowa classification
	Dental midlines
	Dental arch symmetry
	Dental arch crowding or spacing
	Absence of teeth
	Maxillary occlusal plane alignment
	Mandibular occlusal plane alignment
	Posterior tooth torque
	Transverse occlusal/skeletal discrepancies
	Gingiva and frena
Other	CR–CO shift, syndromes, systemic disease, impacted teeth, poor oral hygiene, etc.
Diagnosis	Angle classification of malocclusion
	Vertical and/or AP skeletal problems
	Vertical and/or AP dental arch problems

Q: How do you use study models to assess posterior tooth torque?

A: By looking at the models down the arch, from anterior to posterior (Figure 1.42).We see that Monica has slight buccal crown torque of the maxillary second molars and lingual crown torque of the mandibular molars. For Monica's treatment these torques may not be critical, but in many patients such torques will play a role in helping you to decide whether or not to expand the maxilla (providing overjet to later remove the torque).

Step 4: Define your treatment goals.

Q: What are "treatment goals"?

A: Treatment goals are the "big picture" objectives you have for a patient and should address the patient's CC and all problems that can feasibly be treated. Some problems, of concern to the patient or found during diagnosis, may not be amenable to treatment or require treatment for which the outcome is not certain. Therefore, compromises involving alternative treatment or no treatment for these problems should be discussed with the patient. Treatment goals are *not* the specific procedures used to achieve big picture objectives. For example, extraction of first premolars is not a treatment goal. It is a treatment procedure.

Table 1.6 Diagnostic findings and problem list for Monica (Figure 1.40).

Full face and profile	**Frontal view**
	Face is symmetric
	Vertical facial proportions appear WRN (Glabella–Subnasale ≈ Subnasale–soft tissue Menton)
	Deep paranasal folds
	Absence of an interlabial gap
	Upper dental midline is to the right of her facial midline ≈ 1 mm (UDML R ≈ 1 mm)
	Inadequate incisal display in a posed smile (central incisor gingival margins are hidden above vermillion border of maxillary lip)
	Profile view
	Upturned nose
	Obtuse NLA
	Straight profile
	Prominent chin
	Lip–chin–throat angle WRN
Ceph analysis	**Skeletal**
	Maxillary AP position is mildly deficient (A-Point lies behind Nasion-perpendicular line)
	Mandibular AP position appears WRN
	Effective bony Pogonion
	Vertical skeletal proportions WRN (FMA = 21°; SNMP = 29°; LAFH/TAFH = 57%)
	Dental
	Upright maxillary incisors (U1-SN = 99°)
	Mandibular incisors mildly proclined (FMIA = 62°)
Radiographs	Adult dentition
	Missing third molars
Intraoral photos and models	Angle Class I
	Iowa Classification: I II (2–3) I I
	OJ ≈ 1 mm
	OB ≈ 60%
	Curve of Spee (COS) depth ≈ 2 mm
	Midlines are not coincident (LDML to right of UDML by 1–2 mm)
	Mild mandibular and maxillary crowding
	Increased buccal crown torque maxillary second molars
	Increased lingual crown torque mandibular molars
Other	Anterior crossbite (single tooth)
Diagnosis	Angle Class I malocclusion
	Single tooth anterior crossbite

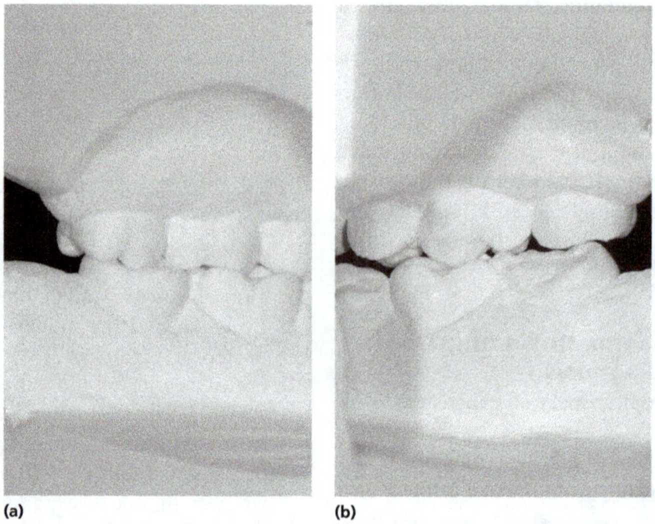

Figure 1.41 Lingual view of Monica's occlusion: (a) left, (b) right.

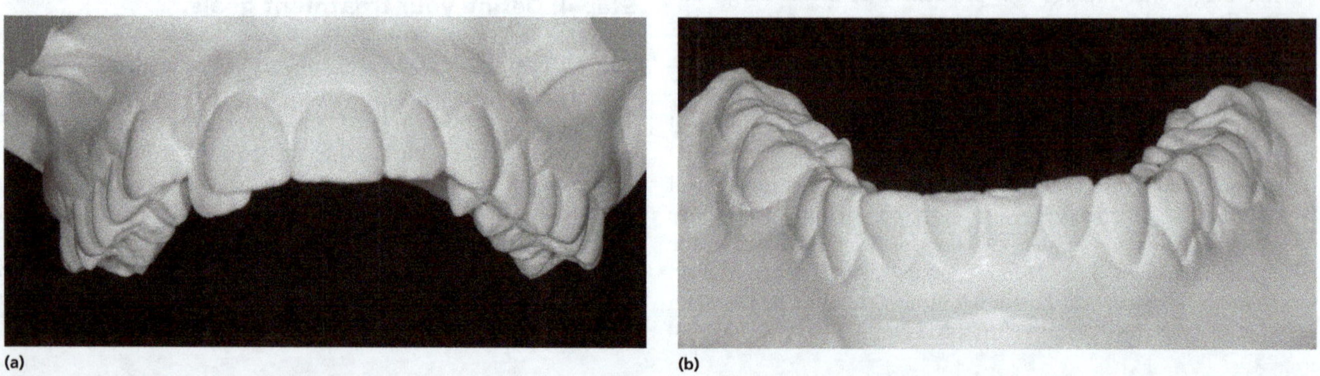

Figure 1.42 Separated models view of Monica.

Q: What would be appropriate goals for Monica? Do you anticipate any treatment compromises?

A: The most important goal is addressing her CC—correction of her crossbite. Other goals may include achieving a Class I AP relationship bilaterally (molars *and* canines since her right canines are initially Class II), deep bite correction (obtaining minimal overbite), and obtaining minimal OJ. No treatment compromises are anticipated.

Step 5: Focus on solving the *primary* problem in each dimension (plus other major problems).

Q: What is the importance of identifying the *major (primary)* problem in each dimension and other major problems?

A: Major problems having a direct impact on your treatment goals must be identified. This is one point we will emphasize throughout this text. If you learn only one thing from us this is it. You must never lose sight of the major problem you face in each dimension (plus other major problems). Avoid getting sidetracked during treatment on small issues (such as marginal ridge discrepancies between adjacent teeth) when you have larger AP, vertical, and transverse issues to deal with. Correct your major problems first, and then move on to addressing smaller problems. During your initial workup, *and as you examine the patient at each treatment appointment*, you should ask yourself: "What are the primary AP, vertical, and transverse problems in this patient (plus other major problems, such as impacted teeth)?" Then, focus on correcting these major problems.

Q: Why is this concept so important?

A: The following case is an example of why this concept is so important and why you can end up in trouble if you ignore this principle. Look at Corey (Figure 1.43), a 14-year-old boy who presents for treatment with the CC, "I have crowded teeth." His diagnostic findings and problem list are found in Table 1.7.

Q: Given your diagnostic findings and problem list, what are Corey's *primary* problems in the AP, vertical, and transverse dimensions? Are there other significant problems that will affect your treatment plan? (A blank Primary Problems table for you to copy is found in the Appendix.)

A: See Table 1.8

Q: Given your diagnostic findings and problem list, what are your treatment goals for Corey?

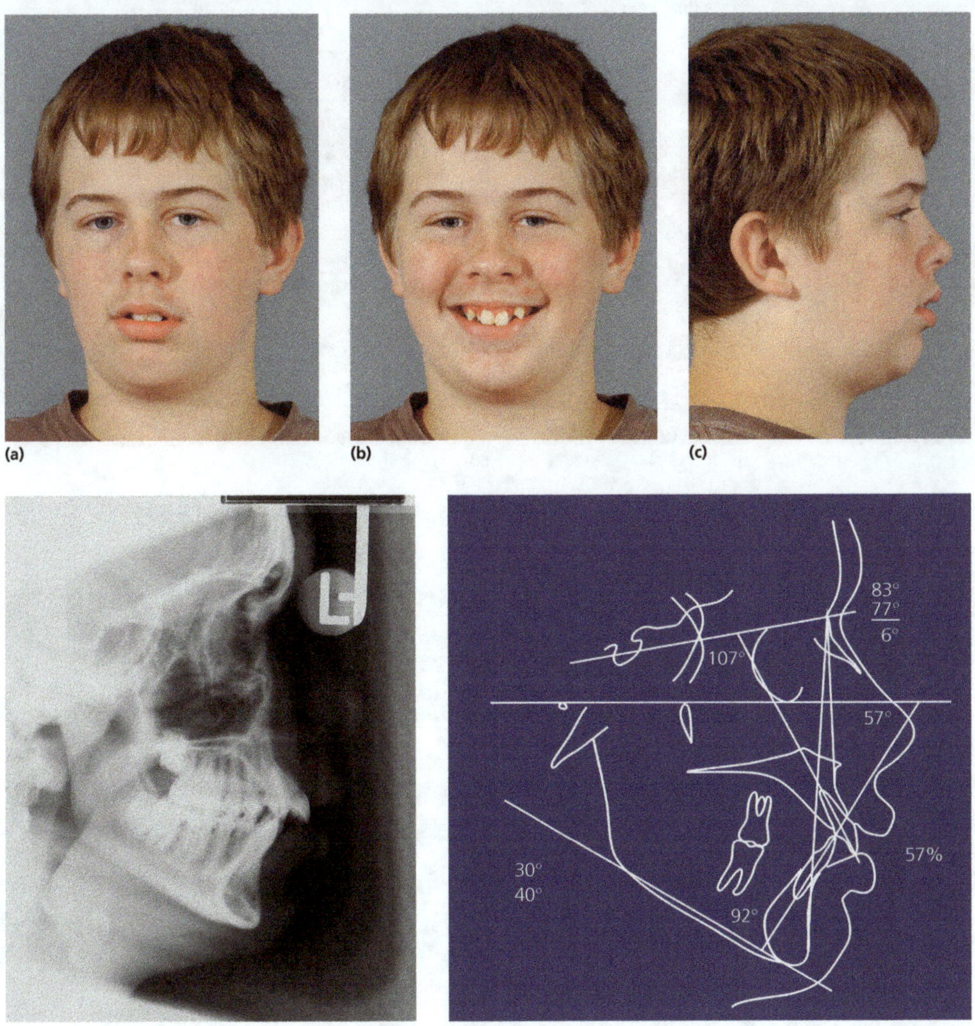

Figure 1.43 Initial records of Corey.

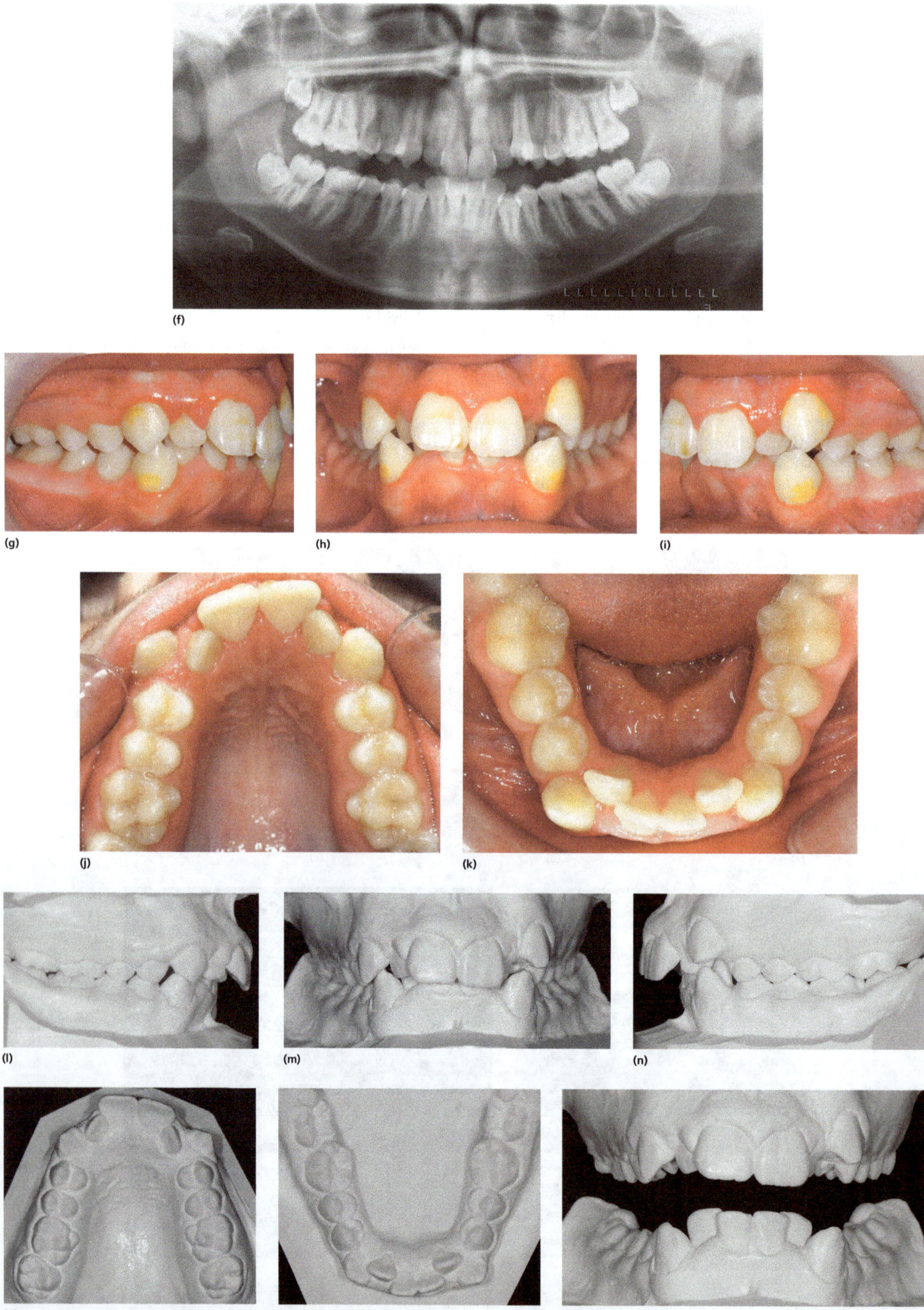

Figure 1.43 (Continued)

Table 1.7 Diagnostic findings and problem list for Corey (Figure 1.43).

Full face and profile	**Frontal view**
	Long lower anterior soft tissue height (LLAFH) (soft tissue Glabella–Subnasale < Subnasale–soft tissue Menton)
	Interlabial gap in relaxed lip position (ILG)
	Buccal corridors evident
	UDML to left of facial center
	Excessive incisal display at rest and during smile
	Excessive gingival display during smile
	Profile view
	Upturned nose
	NLA—WRN
	Convex profile
	Deep labiomental sulcus
Ceph analysis	**Skeletal**
	Maxillary AP position WRN
	Retrusive mandible with ineffective Pogonion
	Steep mandibular plane angle
	Short posterior facial height
	Dental
	Maxillary incisor proclination (U1-SN = 107°)
	Mandibular incisor proclination (FMIA = 57°)
Radiographs	Full permanent dentition
Intraoral photos and models	Angle Class II division 1
	Iowa Classification: II (6) II (6) II (6) II (6)
	Moderate maxillary and mandibular anterior crowding
	Mandibular incisors stepped up
	Narrow constricted maxillary arch
	Mandibular posterior lingual crown torque
Other	Poor oral hygiene
Diagnosis	Angle Class II division 1 malocclusion
	Mandibular skeletal retrusion
	Mildly excessive vertical anterior facial height
	Transverse maxillary skeletal deficiency with mandibular posterior transverse compensations

Table 1.8 Primary problems list for Corey *(apical base/skeletal discrepancies italicized).*

AP	II (6) II (6) II (6) II (6)
	Mandibular skeletal retrusion
Vertical	*Mildly excessive vertical anterior facial growth* (ILG, excess incisal display, steep MPA)
Transverse	*Constricted maxillary arch* with significant mandibular posterior lingual crown torque (mandibular posterior transverse dental compensations)
Other	Poor oral hygiene

A: Treatment goals include the following:

- Improve profile/chin projection.
- Obtain Class I canine relationship.
- Obtain normal overbite and overjet.
- Increase maxillary skeletal width/eliminate transverse posterior compensations.
- Relieve maxillary and mandibular dental arch crowding.
- Improve poor oral hygiene.

Q: Keeping his AP, vertical, transverse, and other major problems in mind (Table 1.8), how would you proceed with Corey's treatment?

A: Considering Corey's age, it would be wise to *begin orthopedic treatment immediately* in order to take advantage of any remaining growth. Further, it would be wise to delay orthodontic tooth movement until his major AP, vertical, and transverse problems have been addressed via dentofacial orthopedics. His maxilla should be skeletally expanded with an RME appliance, and he should be placed on a high-pull headgear (HPHG; to restrict his maxillary forward and downward growth) or a Herbst appliance (to restrict his maxillary growth and accelerate his mandibular growth). At the same time, every effort should be made to address his poor hygiene before he has orthodontic appliances placed and begins tooth movement. This would be the smart approach—focusing on his major problems.

However, this was not the approach taken. Yes, his maxilla was expanded with an RME appliance to begin, but he was then placed in fixed appliances to align his arches (Figure 1.44) for nearly a year (with the thought that he would be placed in a headgear or Herbst appliance sometime later).

Beginning with an RME appliance was prudent, but the lack of focus on his AP and vertical problems was not. By delaying headgear or Herbst treatment, any possible orthopedic benefits to improve Corey's AP and vertical problems were lost. Ignoring his primary AP and vertical problems could have necessitated a later need for orthognathic surgery to achieve treatment goals. Further, not immediately addressing his poor hygiene resulted in areas of decalcification (Figures 1.45d–f). In patients with high caries susceptibility, poor oral hygiene can force discontinuing treatment early leading to compromised results.

Q: It was at this time that Corey is transferred to you (Figure 1.44). How would you proceed?

A: Even at this late stage, you need to *focus on the primary problems in each dimension*. Corey still has skeletal problems in two dimensions (deficient mandibular AP growth and excess vertical maxillary growth). Since his skeletal problems are found in the basal bone of the jaws (in the bone apical to the alveolar process bone of the jaws), we can refer to Corey's primary problems as "apical base discrepancies" between the jaws. Apical base discrepancies are treated in three different ways: orthopedics, masking (camouflage), and surgery.

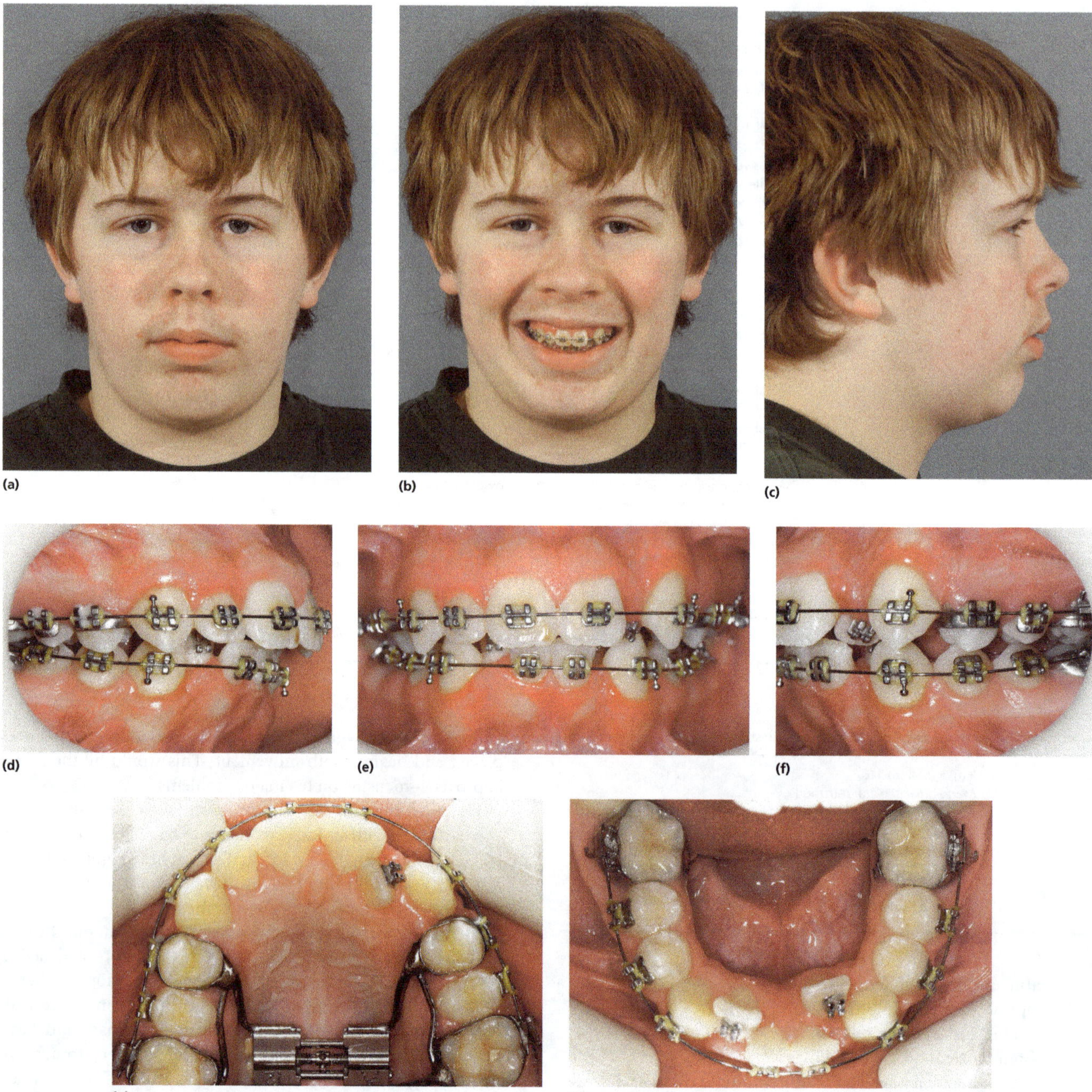

(a) (b) (c) (d) (e) (f) (g) (h)

Figure 1.44 Progress records of Corey.

Orthopedics is the modification of apical base discrepancies by modifying jaw growth. Two factors (in addition to patient compliance) determine your chances for success with orthopedics: the magnitude of the apical base discrepancy and the time remaining for growth to occur. If the patient has a mild apical base discrepancy with years of potential growth remaining, then you have a reasonable chance of correcting the problem. If the child has a severe apical base discrepancy with very little future growth potential, then you have a poor chance of correcting the problem (but with some growth you may achieve enough correction to be able to mask the problem).

Masking (camouflage) is orthodontic treatment directed at correcting the dental/occlusal relationships without addressing the underlying apical base discrepancies.

Surgery can correct moderate-to-severe apical base discrepancies when growth is considered complete.

In Corey's case, we lost the opportunity to use orthopedics to correct his Class II relationship (his parents state that he has now finished growing), and his parents are opposed to surgery. We are left with the possibility of masking (camouflage) if we think that a reasonable outcome can result. This is what was done. Corey's maxillary first premolars were extracted, and the extraction spaces were closed by retracting his maxillary canines and incisors distally. His deband photographs are shown in Figure 1.45.

Q: What do you think of Corey's outcome?

A: This was a compromised result. Notice his AP occlusion (Figures 1.45d–f). His canine relationship is slightly Class II

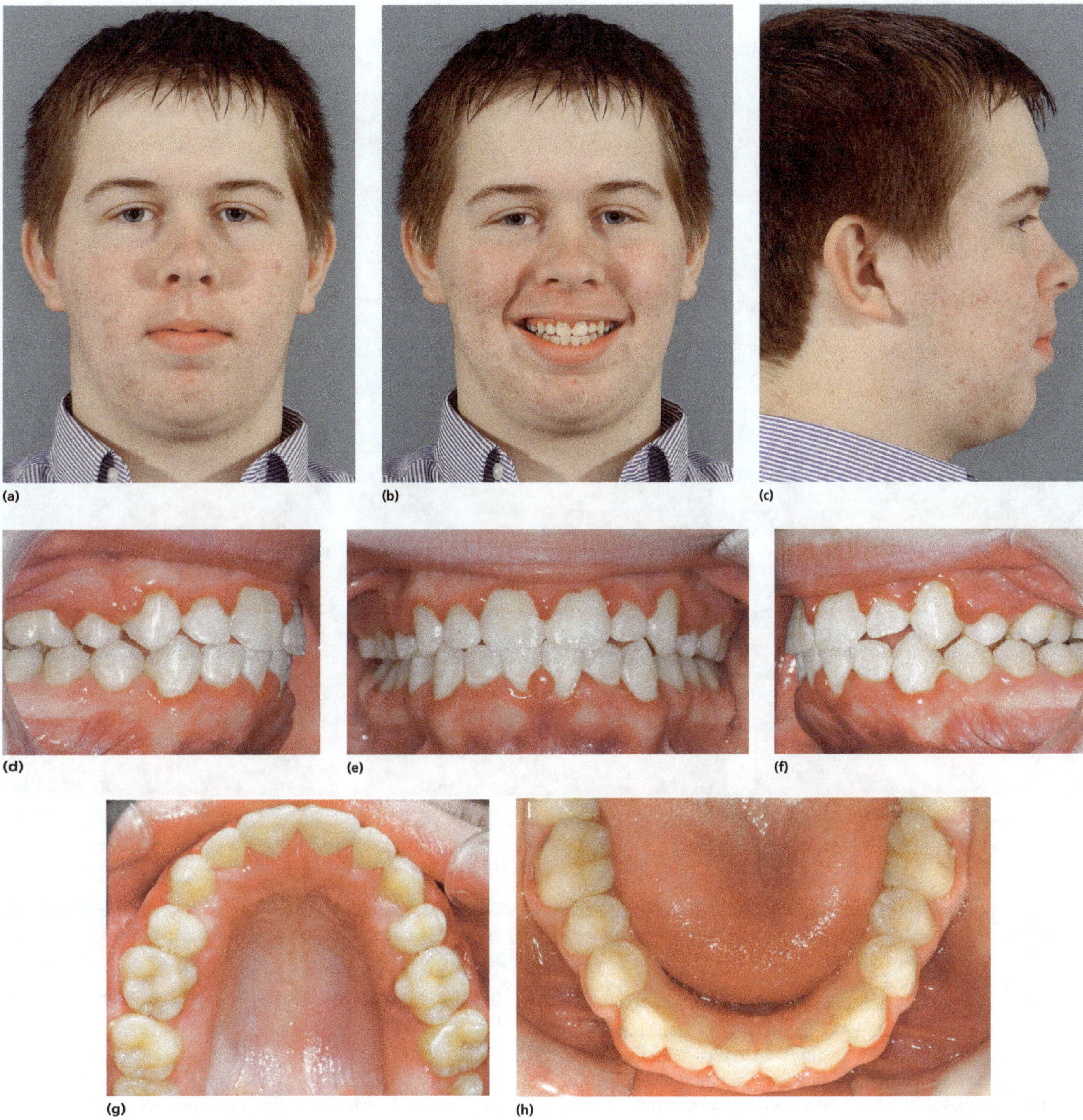

Figure 1.45 Deband records of Corey.

and his posterior teeth do not fit together in maximum intercuspation (he exhibits what is termed "Class II windows"). What could have been an excellent finish is now less than that—because *primary problems were not addressed initially and at every treatment visit.*

Q: Returning to Monica (Figure 1.40, Table 1.6), what are her primary problems in each dimension plus other problems relevant to your treatment plan?

A: Monica does not have overt apical base discrepancies. Her AP, vertical, and transverse skeletal relationships are reasonably normal. But, she does have primary problems in each dimension, as shown in Table 1.9. The correction of these problems should be considered at every appointment.

Table 1.9 Primary problems list for Monica.

AP	I II (2–3) I I
Vertical	60% deep bite (dental)
Transverse	–
Other	Anterior crossbite

Step 6: Consider surgical options.

Q: Why must you consider surgical options?

A: Many patients have severe apical base discrepancies and can benefit from orthognathic surgery. But *with every patient, you should always ask yourself whether orthognathic surgery would*

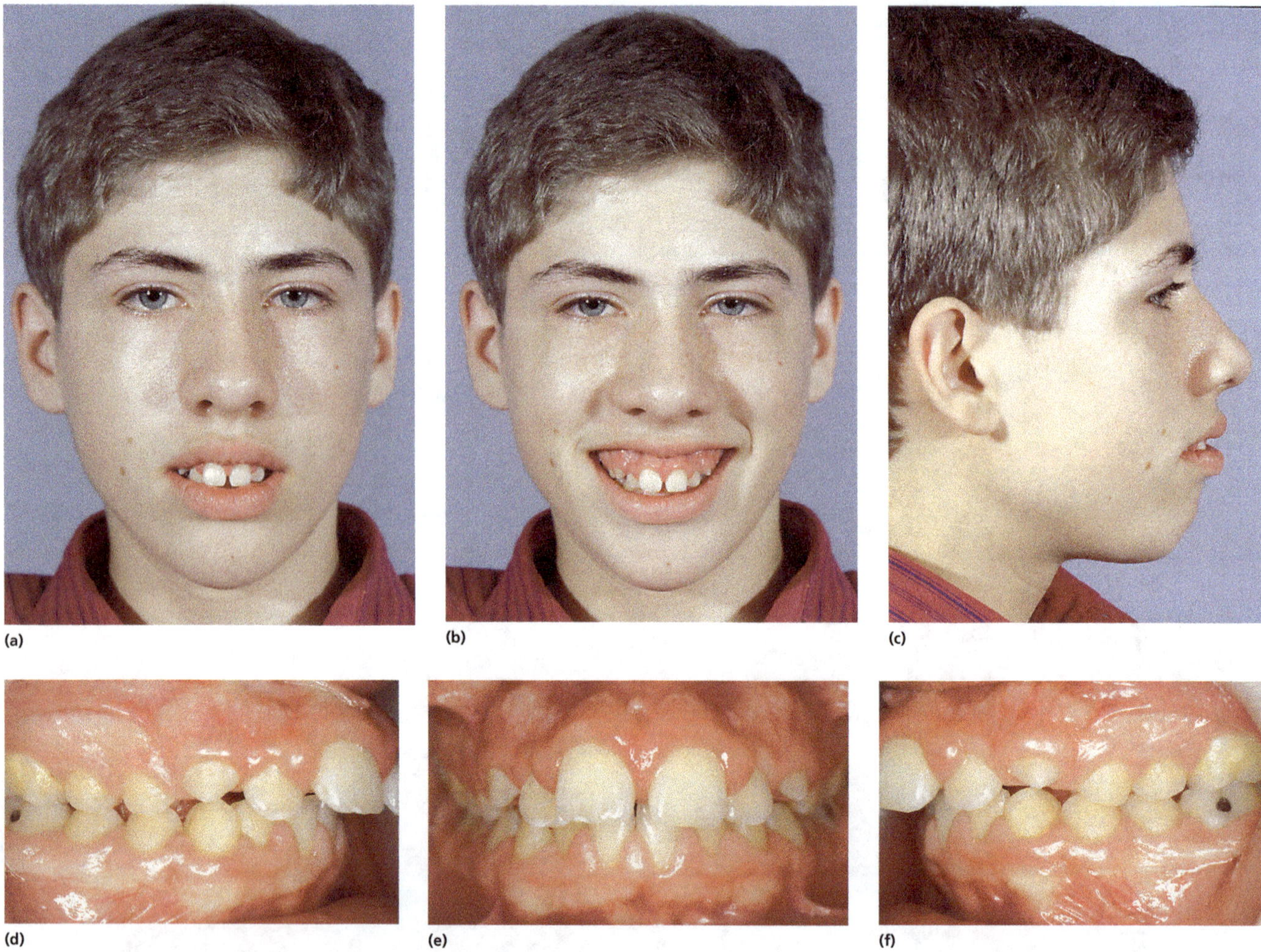

Figure 1.46 Initial records of Martin.

be a viable treatment option. With most patients you will quickly answer no, with some patients you will quickly answer yes, but with some borderline patients you will want to investigate the patient's concerns and desires further.

For example, look at Martin in Figure 1.46. He is a 19-year-old college student who is not happy with his appearance. It is quite apparent that he exhibits increased anterior facial growth. He shows too much maxillary incisor at rest (excessive incisal display), he shows too much gingiva when smiling (excessive gingival display), and he has a convex profile (inadequate chin projection/mandibular deficiency). After establishing a problem list and diagnosis, you must sensitively discuss his facial features that relate to his vertical and AP skeletal relationships and discuss the anticipated outcomes of orthodontic treatment alone versus treatment that includes jaw surgery.

This was done, and a surgical option was chosen by Martin. Surgery included a Le Fort I maxillary impaction osteotomy to move his maxilla superiorly and bilateral sagittal split mandibular advancement osteotomy to correct his Class II dental relationship and increase his chin projection. Figures 1.47a–h show his final result. Figures 1.47d–e show his initial and post-surgery lateral cephalometric radiographs, respectively. Note the significant improvement in his appearance and occlusion.

Another example is Jackie (Figure 1.48). Jackie is 15 years old and, according to her parents, has finished growing.

Q: What are Jackie's primary problems in the AP, vertical, and transverse dimensions, plus other problems relevant to your treatment plan?

A: See Table 1.10

Q: Jackie's mandibular skeletal deficiency is reflected in her convex profile. Should you discuss this problem with Jackie and her parents? If she would benefit from surgery, then what type of surgery would you recommend?

A: Yes, any time surgery is a viable alternative; you must discuss this option with the patient and parents. What you consider a minor concern, the patient may consider significant. Likewise, what you consider a significant concern may be unimportant to the patient. Jackie and her parents said they were not interested in surgery (mandibular advancement osteotomy), but you must document in her record that this option was presented and declined. Due to the fact that Jackie has finished growing, orthopedics was not an option in Jackie's treatment. The final option presented (masking) included extraction of the maxillary left first premolar with retraction of the maxillary anterior teeth into a Class I left canine relationship.

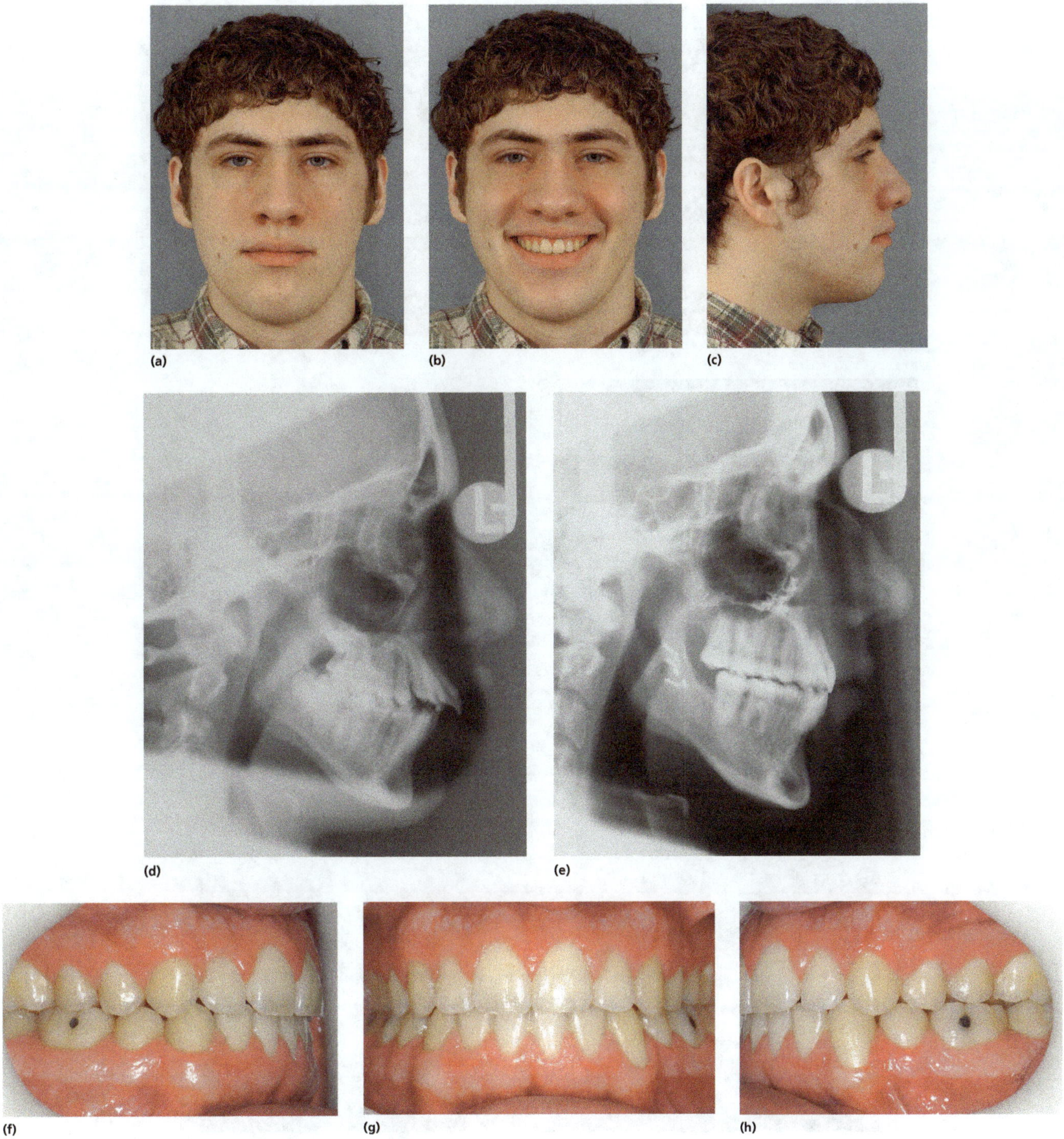

Figure 1.47 Deband records of Martin.

Note: You must discuss with the patient and parents treatment compromises that will occur if surgery is recommended but not chosen, that is, if masking the apical base discrepancy is chosen instead of surgery. If you are attempting to treat adolescent patients with orthopedics, it is usually wise to inform parents of potential future surgical needs if satisfactory growth, or satisfactory patient compliance, is not forthcoming during treatment. Be very considerate of the patient's feelings when bringing up potential surgical needs. In our eyes, every patient we have ever treated has been beautiful even before undergoing orthodontic/surgical care. As an orthodontist, you should inform the patient of structural discrepancies you observe that may limit correction without jaw surgery, but you should also phrase your comments in a thoughtful and sensitive manner.

Q: Returning to Monica (Figure 1.40, Table 1.6), should you discuss possible surgical options with her?

A: No, Monica is not a candidate for orthognathic surgery, and there is no need to discuss surgical options with her.

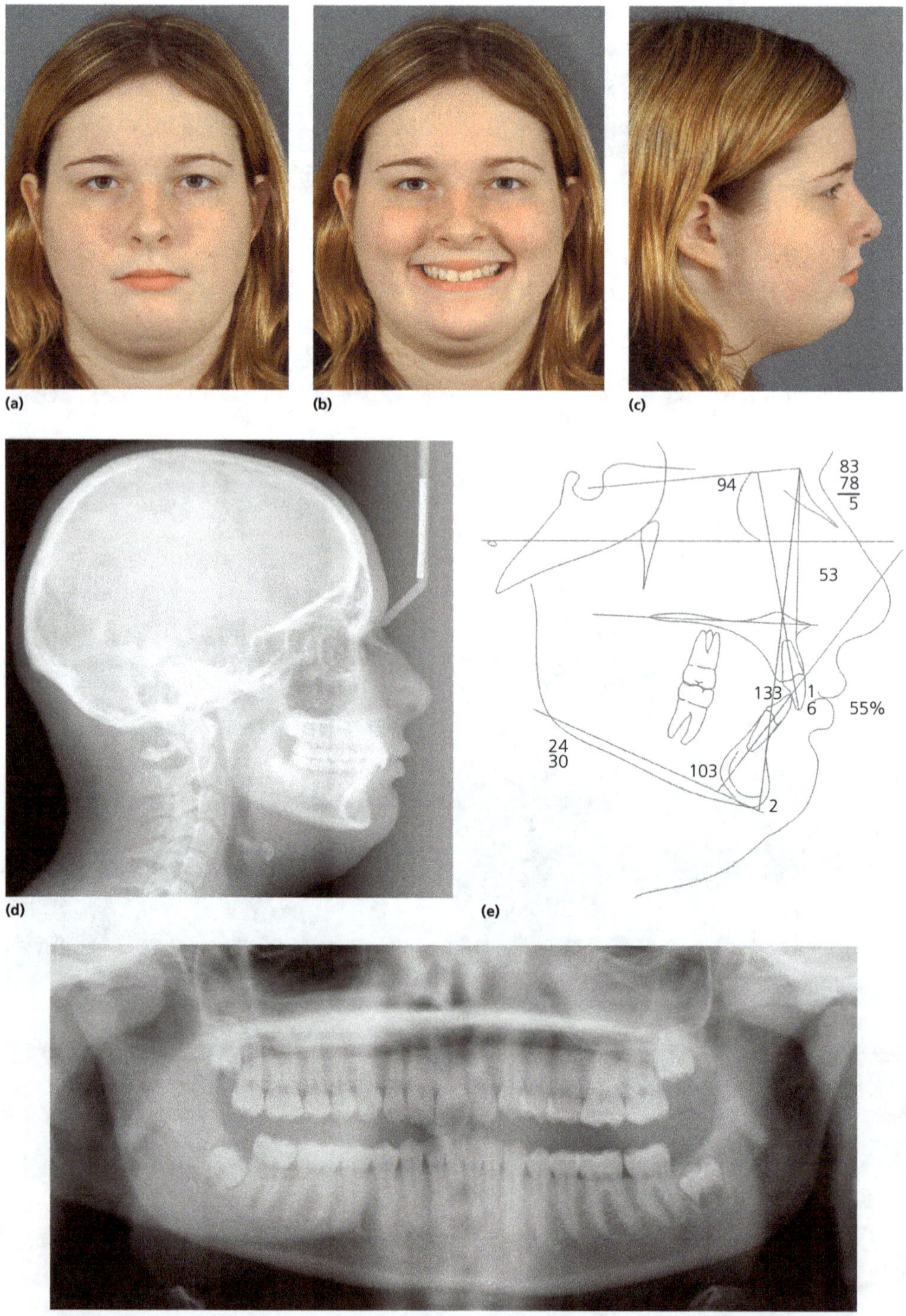

Figure 1.48 Initial records of Jackie.

Step 7: Establish unknowns you face—strive to reduce significant unknowns *before* presenting the final treatment plan to the patient and before doing anything irreversible.

Q: How do unknown conditions affect your treatment plan and the application of treatment?

A: If you only learn one thing from us—this is it: after you have defined the problems you will address with your treatment plan, always force yourself to answer this question, "what unknowns are present in treating this patient and what unknowns should I eliminate before I define my final treatment plan or do something irreversible?" Unknowns typically include variables such as magnitude and direction of jaw growth in adolescent patients, undetected CR–CO shifts, treatment cooperation, whether the midpalatal suture will split in late adolescence, possible tooth ankylosis, patient hygiene, and so forth. Explain to patients and parents the unknowns you face—they will be more understanding if you later need to modify

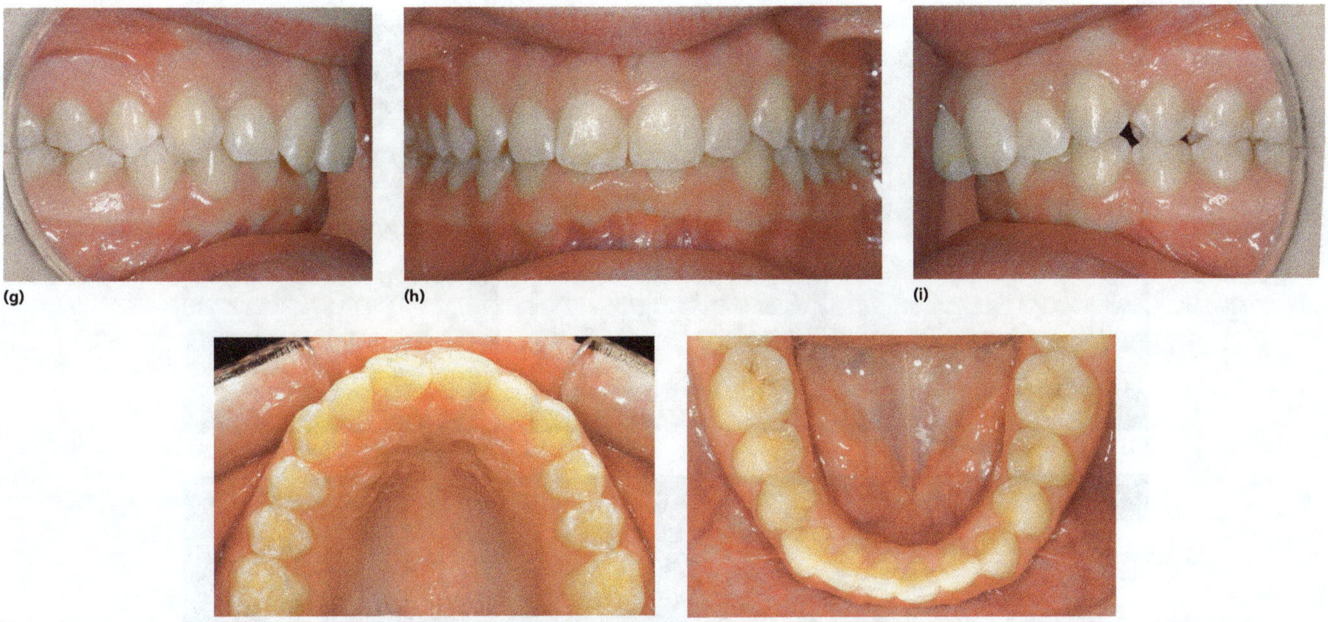

(g) (h) (i) (j) (k)

Figure 1.48 (Continued)

Table 1.10 Primary problems list for Jackie *(apical base/skeletal discrepancies italicized).*

AP	I II (3) II (3) *Mandibular skeletal retrusion*
Vertical	70–80% deep bite
Transverse	–
Other	–

your treatment plan as a result of these unknowns. Begin treatment by trying to reduce these unknowns before committing to irreversible treatment (e.g., extracting teeth).

As an example, what unknowns did you face earlier in treatment planning for Corey (Figure 1.43)?Unknowns include the following:

- If you could achieve maxillary midpalatal suture separation with his RME appliance
- How much mandibular (and maxillary) AP growth he had remaining
- How much vertical maxillary growth he had remaining (which might promote rotation of his mandible down and back—worsening his Class II relationship)
- How compliant Corey would be with treatment
- If he would improve his hygiene

Which of Corey's unknowns should have been eliminated before Corey and his parents were given a final treatment plan? Within a 9- to -12-month evaluation period, the unknowns of midpalatal suture opening, jaw growth, patient compliance, and hygiene should have been reduced/eliminated before a final, definitive treatment plan was established. As we discussed, Corey should have immediately been placed in an RME appliance and a HPHG or Herbst appliance while his hygiene was followed. Instead, the principle of reducing unknowns was ignored, resulting in compromised care for Corey.

As another example, Jesse (Figure 1.49) is 16 years, 6 months old. Because of his age, his significant mandibular retrusion (normal maxillary AP position, but ANB = 6°), and his profile concerns, Jesse's treatment plan included extraction of mandibular first premolars, mandibular space closure to upright his proclined mandibular incisors, and bilateral sagittal split osteotomy mandibular advancement. But his parents objected to extracting teeth and requested that a decision to extract teeth be made after Jesse's arches were leveled and aligned.

Q: What is the major unknown in Jesse's case?

A: His remaining facial growth potential. Even though Jesse is 16 years, 6 months old, he could still be growing. In fact, during the time that braces were put on Jesse, and his arches were being leveled and aligned, Jesse's mandible grew enough to where his profile was no longer a concern (Figure 1.50). The need for surgery was eliminated! Our point is this—unless Jesse's parents were absolutely sure that he had stopped growing for some time, orthopedic treatment should have at least been initially considered (maybe for a 6-month trial period while Jesse was being leveled and aligned) before a decision to commit to surgery was made. We would not have lost any time proceeding this way. Thankfully, nothing irreversible (e.g., mandibular premolar extractions) was done until the unknown (growth) was eliminated, even though no one planned it this way.

Q: Was the improvement in Jesse's profile really the result of growth or was it simply a posturing forward of his mandible once his bite was "unlocked" during leveling and aligning?

A: The improvement was due to growth. No CR–CO shift was noted before or after leveling and aligning of Jesse's arches. Interestingly, in a study of Class II division 2 children, proclination of upper incisors and deep bite correction (phase one of the treatment, unlocking the bite) did *not* result in mandibular anterior positioning [122].

Q: Regarding patients like Jesse, what is the current state of the art in predicting the amount and direction of facial growth in adolescents?

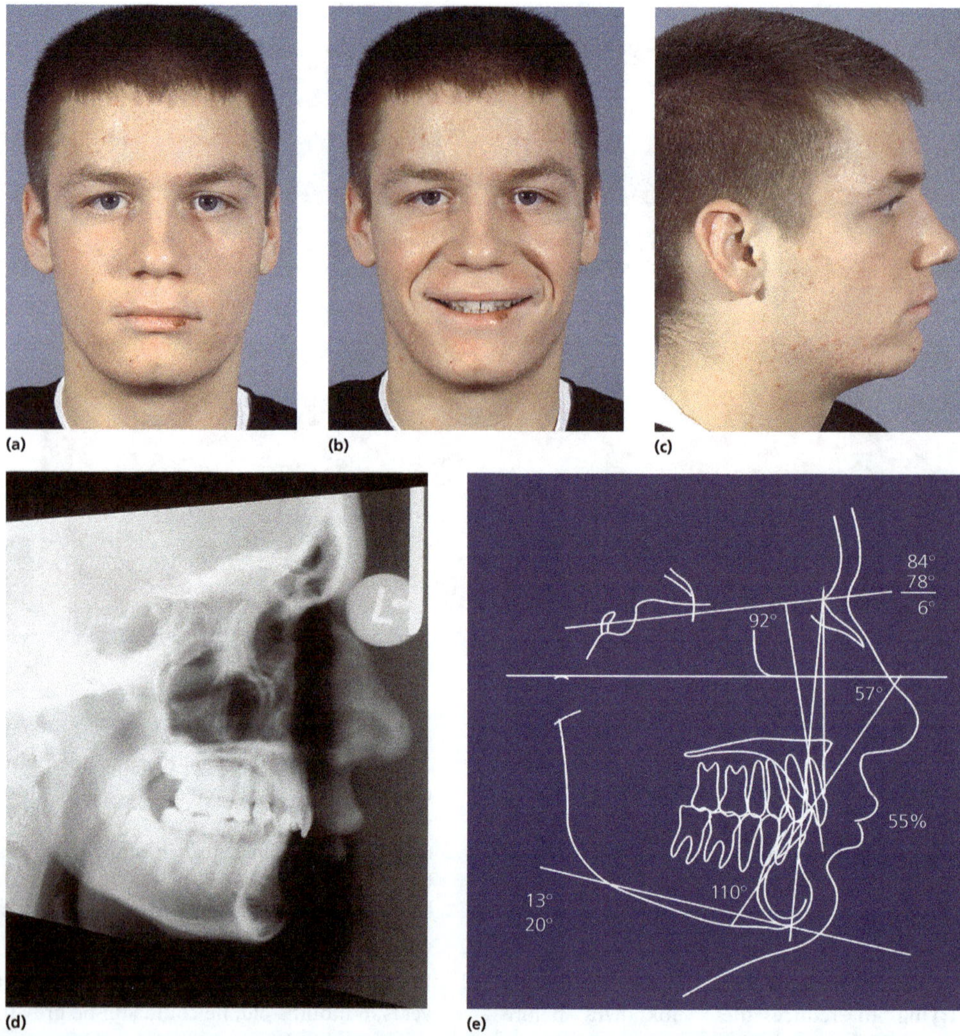

Figure 1.49 Initial records of Jesse.

A: In a recent systematic review [68], a number of salient points were made concerning facial growth prediction, which are as follows:

- Each individual's skeletal maturity is influenced by genetic and environmental factors.
- The same pattern of skeletal growth can be found in almost everyone, but the initiation, duration, and amount of growth varies considerably during the pubertal growth spurt. Some persons mature early with a relatively short pubertal growth spurt, whereas other persons mature late with a large pubertal growth spurt.
- Staging of skeletal development has been assessed using peak growth velocity in standing height, pubertal markers (voice changes in males, menarche in females, breast development, appearance of pubic hair, and appearance of axillary hair), radiographic assessment of bone maturation, and staging of dental development.
- Peak growth velocity in standing height forms a useful historic longitudinal measure of an individual's growth pattern but has little predictive value for future growth rate or percentage of total growth remaining.
- Ossification sequence and timing of skeletal maturity within the hand–wrist area show polymorphism and sexual dimorphism, which can limit their clinical predictive use.
- Skeletal maturity analysis of hand–wrist radiographs for use in predicting facial growth velocity should include bone staging as well as ossification events.
- Overall facial horizontal and vertical growth velocity is related to skeletal maturation indicators determined by analysis of hand–wrist radiographs.
- Maxillary and mandibular growth velocities are related to skeletal maturity, but the correlations are less robust than those for overall facial growth velocity.
- Dental development indicators are not reliable predictors of an individual's stage of skeletal development.
- The relationship between cranial base growth velocity and skeletal maturity has not been definitively established.

In perhaps the most extensive study of the pattern of facial growth and its relationship to maturity indicators [54] yet published, results demonstrated that

- The onset of average pubertal growth spurt in height was *9.3 years in girls and 11.9 years in boys.*
- Average stature (height) peaked *earlier* than facial skeletal growth (*girls 10.9 years, boys 14.0 years*).
- Hand–wrist stages provided the best indication that maturation had advanced to the peak.

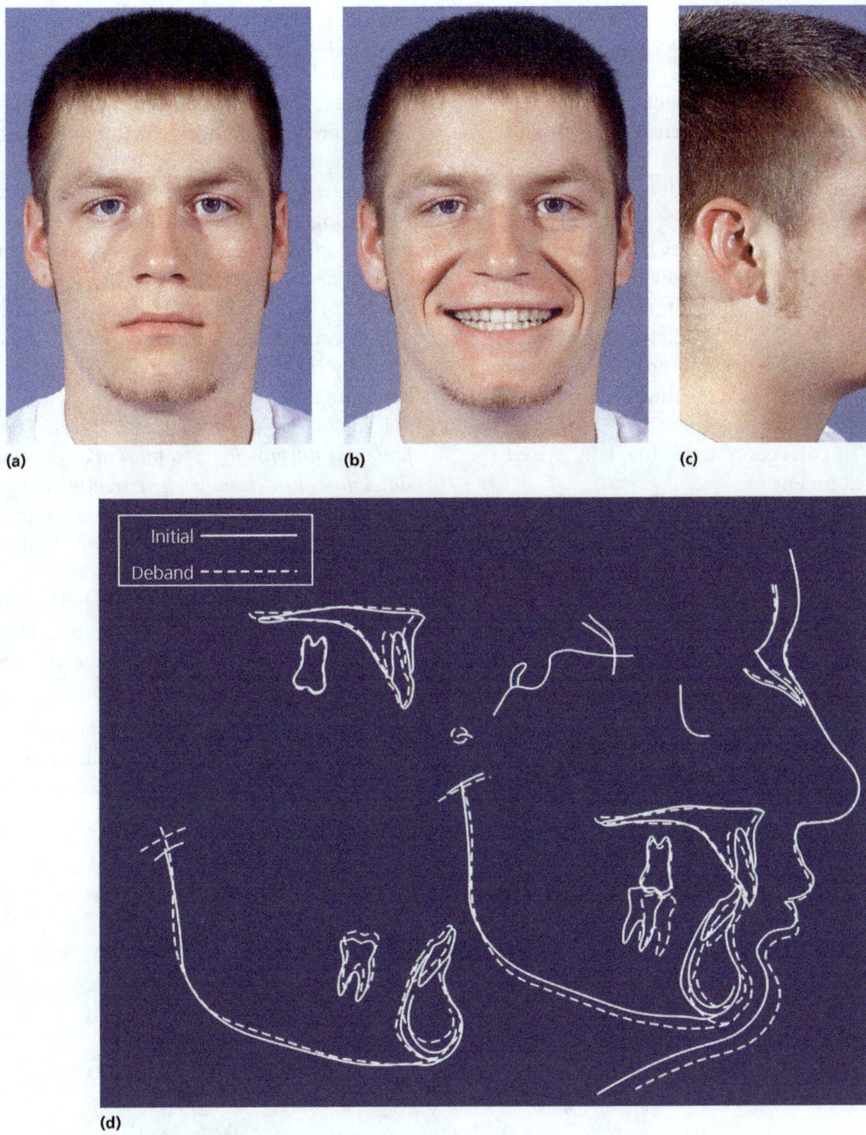

Figure 1.50 Deband records of Jesse. Note the additional growth he had.

- Vertebral stages were consistently the worst predictors (intrinsic lack of predictive ability). Recent evidence suggests that reliability of vertebral staging is questionable [70].
- Of the methods tested for the prediction of peak growth velocity, statural onset had the lowest errors.
- Chronologic age was nearly as good.
- Stature can be measured repeatedly—and may lead to improved prediction of the timing of the adolescent growth spurt.

The point is that the cervical vertebrae method has little clinical predictive value, but hand–wrist measurements do have value as indicators of maturation advancing to peak. Even hand–wrist measurements cannot predict the direction of future facial growth. Chronologic age, but especially repeated measures of stature, can be used clinically (and noninvasively) to improve indication of the adolescent growth spurt.

For girls:

- Peak rate of stature increase is reached prior to menarche [123].
- With the onset of menses, the rate of change in height drops to prepubertal levels and decreases sharply to an adult rate of change during the subsequent 2 years. Note: our clinical impression is that, for girls with hyperplastic mandibular growth, growth may continue far longer than this rule of thumb would suggest.

Q: Why is the prediction of remaining facial growth magnitude and direction so important in adolescents?

A: With a large amount of growth remaining (plus favorable growth direction plus excellent patient compliance), you have a better chance of orthopedically improving an apical base discrepancy (AP, vertical, or transverse) than with little growth remaining. Conversely, with a large amount of growth remaining following orthopedic treatment, it is more difficult to maintain a corrected occlusion afterwards (growth is not been normalized with orthopedic treatment).

Q: List "take-home pearls" in predicting the timing, amount, and direction of adolescent facial growth.

A: Take-home pearls include the following:

- We would like to predict the adolescent growth spurt so as to time orthopedic treatment and "bracket" or capture this growth period. Further, we would like to be able to predict the amount of remaining growth so that we can best judge when it is safe to discontinue orthopedic treatment (e.g., highpull chincup treatment in Class III patients) or when it is safe for a patient to undergo surgical correction—without fear of relapse from continued growth.

- The state of the art in predicting individual amount and direction of facial growth in adolescents is imprecise. For over 40 years, various radiographic schemes have purported the ability to predict *individual* facial growth. None have survived the test of time, and we are left with "rules of thumb" to guide us during treatment, such as the following:
  - For maximum orthopedic effect, apply an RPHG to an anteroposteriorly deficient maxilla at the time the maxillary incisors are erupting.
  - Wait to start Class II correction until the late mixed dentition stage of development.
  - Once a highpull chincup has corrected a Class III malocclusion, it should be worn until growth is complete.
  - To maximize transverse skeletal correction with RME appliance, apply it before or during puberty.
  - Surgery to correct excess jaw growth should be performed after growth is complete.
  - Surgery to correct a deficient mandible can be instituted earlier.
- Average onset of the statural growth spurt is a little more than 9 years for girls and a little less than 12 years for boys; peak of statural growth spurt is about 1½ to 2 years later; facial skeletal growth peaks later; but, there is considerable variation in these times among patients.
- At an adolescent's initial examination, ask the parents if they are measuring their child's height regularly and if the child has entered his or her growth spurt. Begin making height measurements. For girls, inquire about menarche—once menarche is reached you have about 2 years to capture any remaining growth. *As soon as you or the parents detect the growth spurt onset, consider beginning orthopedic Class II (headgear or functional appliance) or Class III (high-pull chin-cup) treatment*—regardless of whether the patient is still in early mixed dentition or not. It is generally better to error by beginning orthopedic treatment too early than by beginning too late.
- *For patients in late adolescence, if there is any chance that the patient is still growing, you must take this residual growth potential into consideration when treatment planning.* Otherwise, you may miss the chance either to improve the apical base discrepancy orthopedically or to maintain a correction, posttreatment.

Now back to our principle of establishing unknowns. As another example, look at the initial panoramic image and periapical radiographs of an 11-year-old girl shown in Figure 1.51.

Q: What do you see?

A: She is in the late mixed dentition stage of dental development, she is missing her maxillary lateral incisors and mandibular left second premolar, and the roots of her maxillary second premolars are very poorly developed.

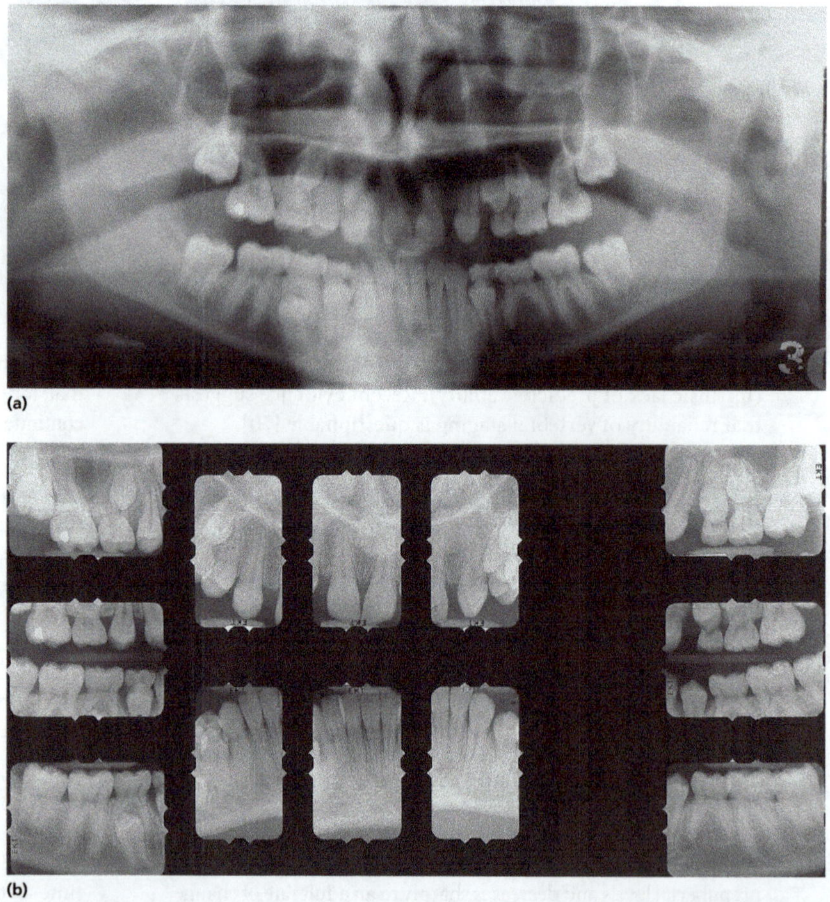

(a) (b)

Figure 1.51 Panoramic and complete mouth series radiographs for an 11-year-old female presenting for orthodontic evaluation.

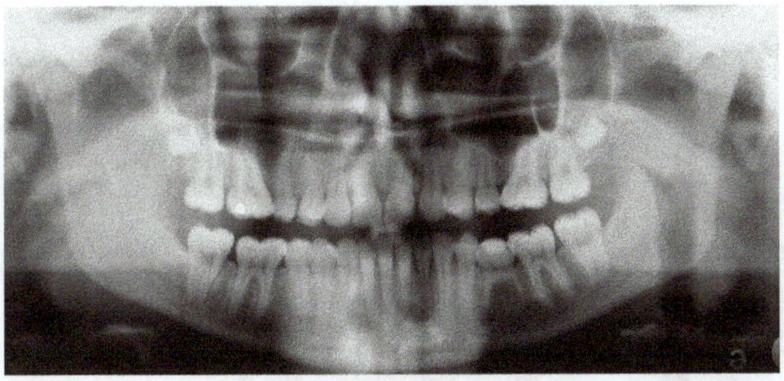

Figure 1.52 Posttreatment panoramic radiograph of the patient presented in Figure 1.51.

Q: So, in terms of these radiographs what are her unknowns?

A: Her unknowns include potential future ankylosis or loss of the retained mandibular left second primary molar and whether her maxillary second premolars will ever develop/erupt (whether they should be retained or extracted).

Q: How should you handle these unknowns?

A: *Wait and monitor*. Give the premolars some time to develop. Assuming there are no outstanding issues with facial growth that must be addressed, you should wait to begin treatment. Waiting is a very hard thing to do for most orthodontists, but waiting can potentially reduce this patient's unknowns to the point where you can finalize your treatment plan. This was done and the maxillary second premolars eventually developed and erupted and were aligned with orthodontic treatment (Figure 1.52). Given adequate time, if they had not developed complete roots, you could have considered extracting them. Note that the mandibular primary left second molar does appear to have ankylosed (slight step in the alveolar process bone between it and the adjacent teeth), and it has been covered with a composite buildup.

Q: Returning to our patient Monica, what are her unknowns?

A: Monica is an adult, so future growth is not a variable. However, her unknowns include the possibility of an undetected CR–CO AP or lateral shift. You must take the possibility of this shift into account and, if present, try to eliminate it before committing to a final treatment plan. In some patients, an undetected shift will not be discovered until habitual biting patterns are "broken up" during leveling and aligning with fixed appliances. Check for a CR–CO shift again at Monica's case presentation appointment and at every treatment appointment thereafter.

Step 8: Consider benefits/costs of treating nonextraction.

Step 9: Consider benefits/costs of treating with extraction of anterior teeth or posterior teeth.

Decisions to extract permanent teeth or not to extract permanent teeth depend on a myriad of factors, including magnitude of the AP apical base or dental discrepancy, amount and location of dental crowding, degree of proclination or uprightness of the anterior teeth, presence or absence of dental arch asymmetries, condition of the periodontium, condition of the teeth, frontal/profile soft tissue esthetics, and the decision to treat surgically or nonsurgically. A decision to extract teeth should never be taken lightly and should be made *only* after significant unknowns are eliminated and after considering the costs/benefits of treating the patient nonextraction, with extraction of different combinations of anterior teeth, with extractions of different combinations of anterior and posterior teeth, and with extraction of different combinations of posterior teeth.

Step 10: Weigh benefits/costs of all viable treatment options and establish the recommended plan and treatment objectives.

This is the time for "putting it all together." Consider every viable treatment option, exhaustively. If necessary, determine what preliminary treatment you must initiate in order to eliminate unknowns before you can decide on a final treatment plan. Many patients generally appreciate that you present a range of options to them at the case presentation, and they realize that you have taken the time to consider the costs/benefits of each. Be prepared to recommend which you consider to be the best treatment option.

The following two cases exemplify application of Steps 8, 9, and 10. Connie is a 33-year-old woman (Figure 1.53) who presents to you for treatment to eliminate her severe dental crowding. She is Class I with a deep bite and relatively straight profile.

Q: Should Connie be treated nonextraction, with extraction of anterior teeth only, with extraction of some combination of anterior and posterior teeth, or with extraction of some combination of posterior teeth only?

A: On the one hand, she has moderate-to-severe mandibular anterior crowding. As a general guideline, tooth extraction to alleviate anterior crowding is generally warranted when the amount of dental crowding is 10 mm or greater. Connie appears to meet this guideline. On the other hand, Connie's cephalometric tracing reveals that she has *very* upright incisors, and her lips are not protrusive. Moreover, she has a Class I dental relationship and a straight profile. These facts support a nonextraction treatment approach since space for her anterior teeth can be gained by proclining her incisors to a more normal inclination.

Proclination of anterior teeth to gain arch length is generally reasonable when the anterior teeth are initially upright. Look at Figure 1.54, top, where the mandibular incisors are upright. Proclining the incisors moves the crowns forward increasing arch length (Figure 1.54, bottom) and places the incisor long axes in a more ideal angulation. Of course, this assumes that the mandibular anterior periodontium can support forward root movement. In Connie's case (Figures 1.53g–i), there appears to be robust periodontium.

All things considered, Connie could benefit from nonextraction treatment, and there are no real costs to treating her nonextraction. But you should never get in the habit of considering only one treatment option. You should always force yourself to exhaustively consider all of your treatment options—including extraction of anterior and posterior teeth.

Q: So, exploring the cost/benefit of extractions, should Connie be treated with extractions?

A: Start by considering extraction of her anterior teeth. The only reasonable anterior tooth to extract would be a mandibular incisor. Extracting a mandibular incisor would help alleviate the anterior crowding and would not upright her anterior teeth more because the extraction space would be used entirely for dental alignment. However, because her maxillary anterior teeth are not small, extraction of a mandibular incisor would result in a mismatch in cumulative mesiodistal widths between maxillary anterior teeth and mandibular anterior teeth (anterior Bolton discrepancy). This mismatch would result in excess anterior overjet at the end of treatment.

Q: How about extracting posterior teeth?

A: Posterior extractions would alleviate her crowding, but you would need to extract symmetrically to keep her dental arches symmetric following space closure (since her arches are already symmetric). Extracting four first premolars would create over 14 mm of extraction space in each arch. Retracting anterior teeth through so much extraction space would result in further uprighting of her already upright incisors. The resulting incisor movement could retract the lips relative to her nose and chin causing a negative impact on her profile (a possible "dished in" profile).

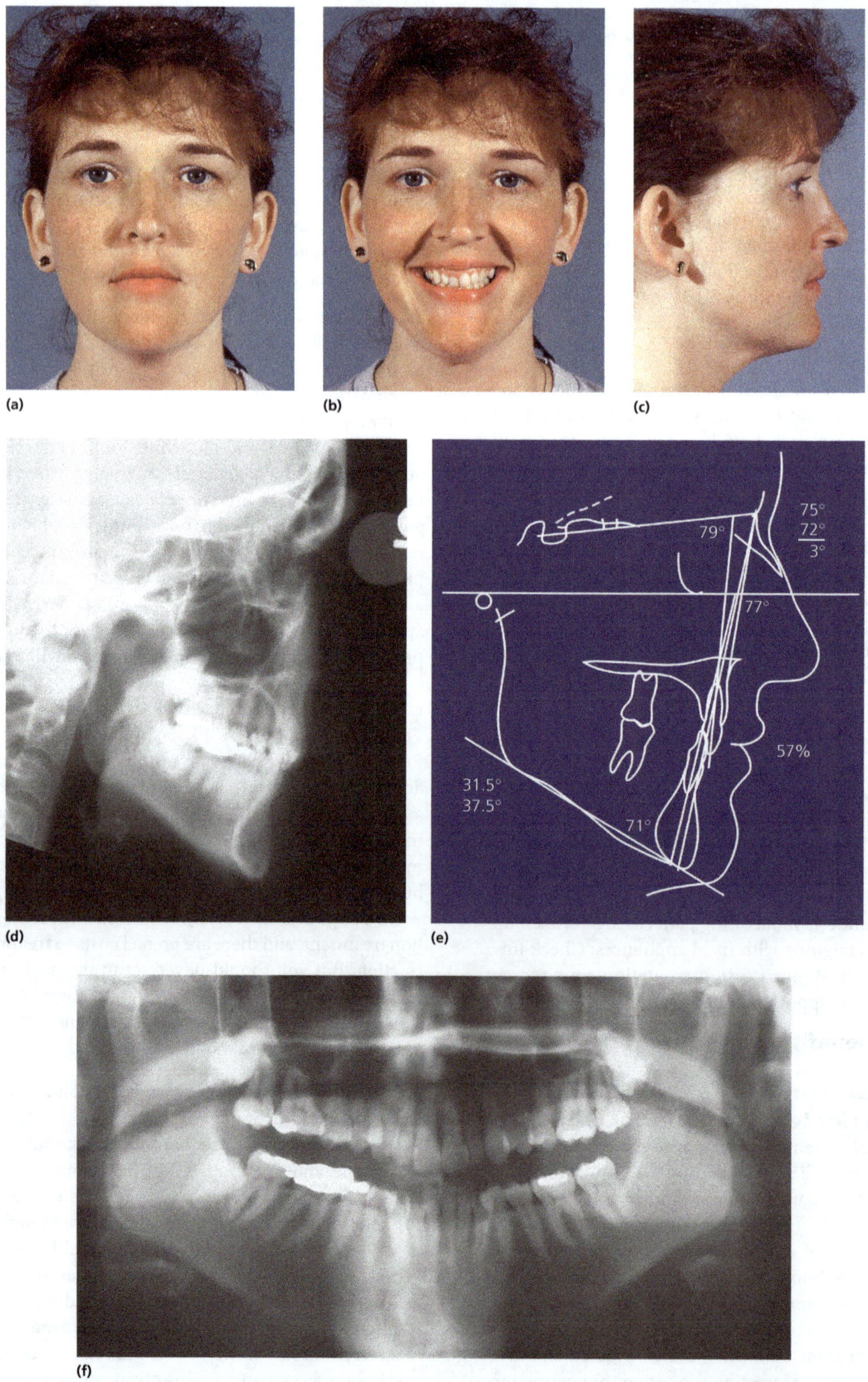

Figure 1.53 Initial records of Connie.

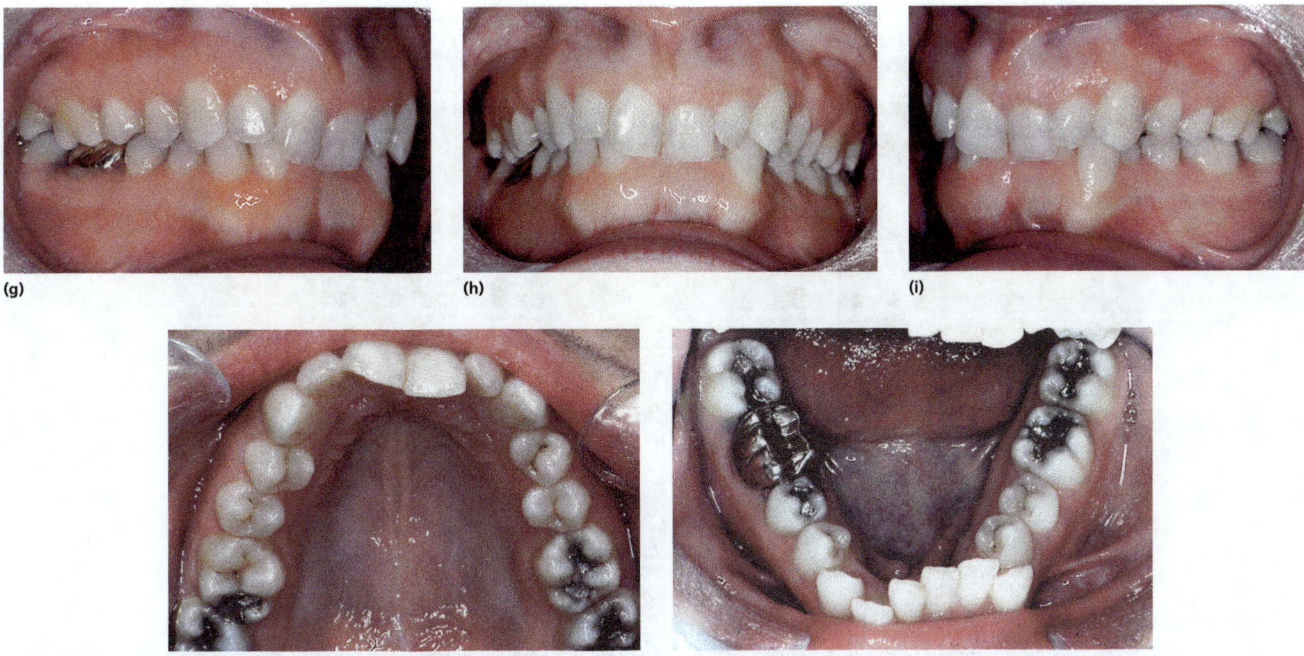

(g) (h) (i)

(j) (k)

Figure 1.53 (Continued)

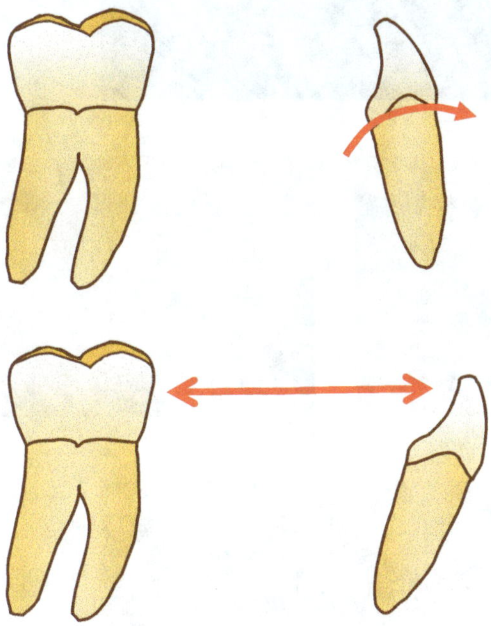

Figure 1.54 By proclining initially upright mandibular incisors (top) additional arch length can be gained (bottom).

Q: In cases where you are retracting maxillary incisors, what *ultimately* limits how far you can retract the maxillary incisors?

A: The position of the mandibular incisors limits the amount of maxillary incisor retraction (i.e. zero overjet). You cannot retract maxillary incisors beyond the mandibular incisors' edges, as you will put the patient in cross bite.

Connie was successfully treated nonextraction by aligning/proclining her incisors (Figure 1.55). The point we are trying to make is that these options must be considered in deciding whether to treat a patient nonextraction or with extractions. With every patient, you must weigh the benefits and costs of nonextraction treatment and different combinations of extraction treatment.

Pearl: With some borderline extraction patients, where you are having difficulty deciding whether to extract or not extract teeth, it makes sense to begin treatment nonextraction and reevaluate for extractions after leveling and aligning the arches. This is another example of reducing unknowns. However, in patients with extreme crowding, proclined incisors, lip protrusion, and steep MP angles, it may make sense to extract teeth (make space) at the very beginning of treatment.

Q: Your next patient is Phoebe (Figure 1.56) who is 11 years old. What are her primary problems in the AP, vertical, and transverse dimensions plus other problems relevant to your treatment plan?

A: See Table 1.11

Q: In terms of your decision to treat Phoebe nonextraction or with extraction of permanent teeth, can you list the factors that will play a role in your decision?

A: Factors to consider include Phoebe's

- Upturned nose (her nasolabial angle could become obtuse if maxillary incisors are retracted).
- Minimal overbite (which will tend to deepen if anterior teeth are retracted).
- AP relationship is normal (there is no need to extract teeth to achieve a Class I canine relationship).
- Moderate-to-severe crowding in the maxillary anterior (blocked-out maxillary permanent canines) and mild-to-moderate crowding in the mandibular anterior (mandibular primary second molars are still present).
- Bimaxillary dental protrusion with mild lip protrusion (both of which could improve if anterior teeth were retracted).

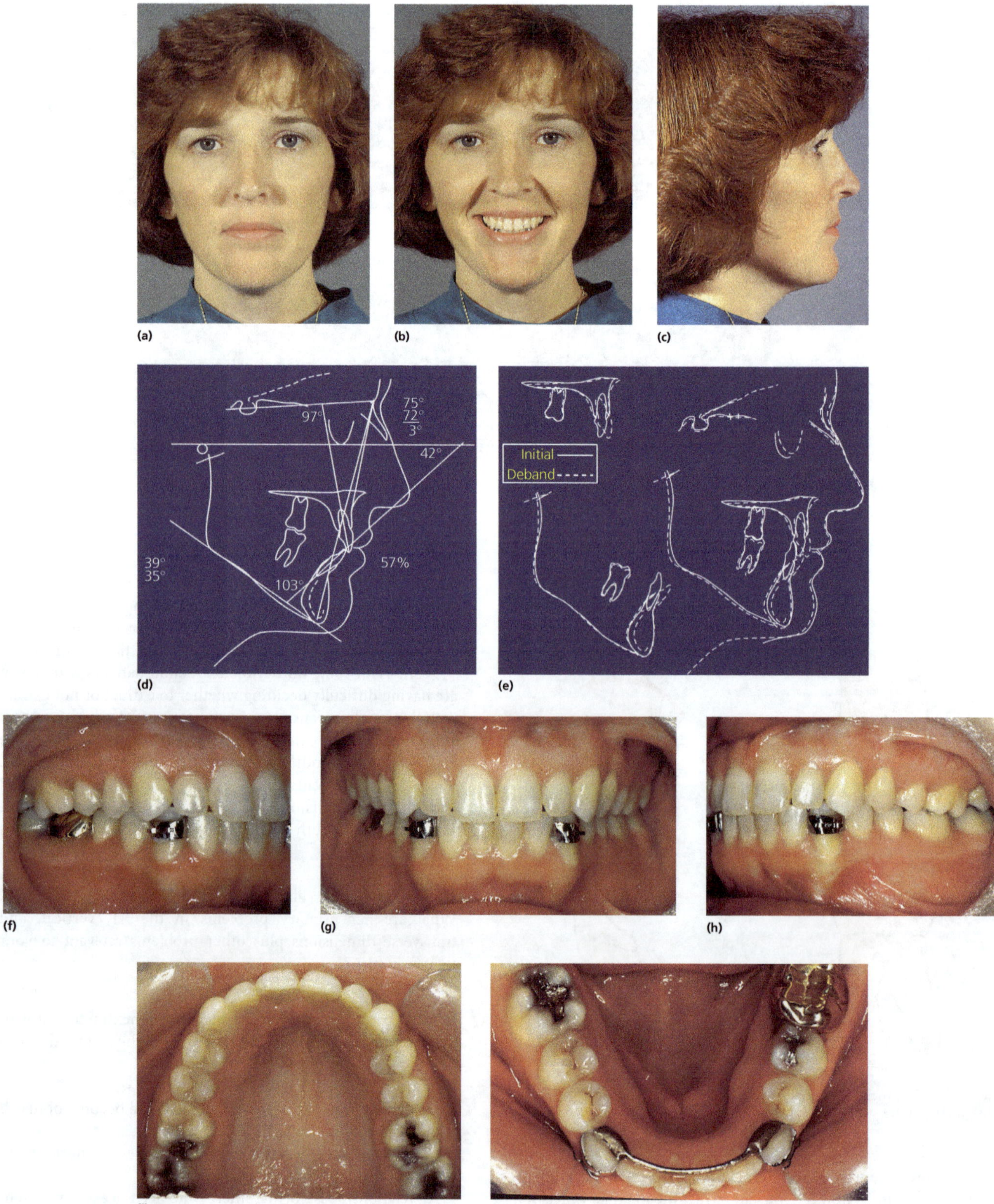

Figure 1.55 Deband records of Connie.

- Thin attached tissue covering roots of mandibular central incisors (will recession occur if the incisors are proclined?).

Q: Is Phoebe a good candidate for nonextraction treatment?

A: Although you can argue that every patient can be treated nonextraction, the cost of treating Phoebe without extractions could be high. Even if you expanded her maxillary arch to gain maxillary arch perimeter and make space for her canines, if she is treated nonextraction then her maxillary incisors could end up very proclined after they are aligned. Her lips could be very protrusive, and she could end up with mandibular anterior gingival recession. However, you could make a case for initially treating her nonextraction, placing a lower lingual holding arch (LLHA), expanding the maxillary arch, and reevaluating for extractions after all the permanent teeth erupt and you observe how much crowding you still have (reducing unknowns).

Q: Is Phoebe a good candidate for extracting anterior teeth?

A: Consider the following:

- If you initially placed an LLHA, allowed all her permanent teeth to erupt, then deemed mandibular tooth extraction still necessary, you could consider extracting a mandibular incisor to alleviate crowding. But, depending upon the cumulative mesiodistal widths of the remaining maxillary and mandibular anterior teeth, you could end up with excess anterior overjet (anterior Bolton discrepancy).
- In the maxilla, you could consider extracting the permanent canines (substituting the maxillary first premolars as canines) to alleviate crowding. If you did this, you would first need to confirm (CBCT scan) that the left lateral incisor root has not been resorbed by the canine crown.
- Or, you could consider extracting maxillary lateral incisors (substituting maxillary permanent canines as laterals and

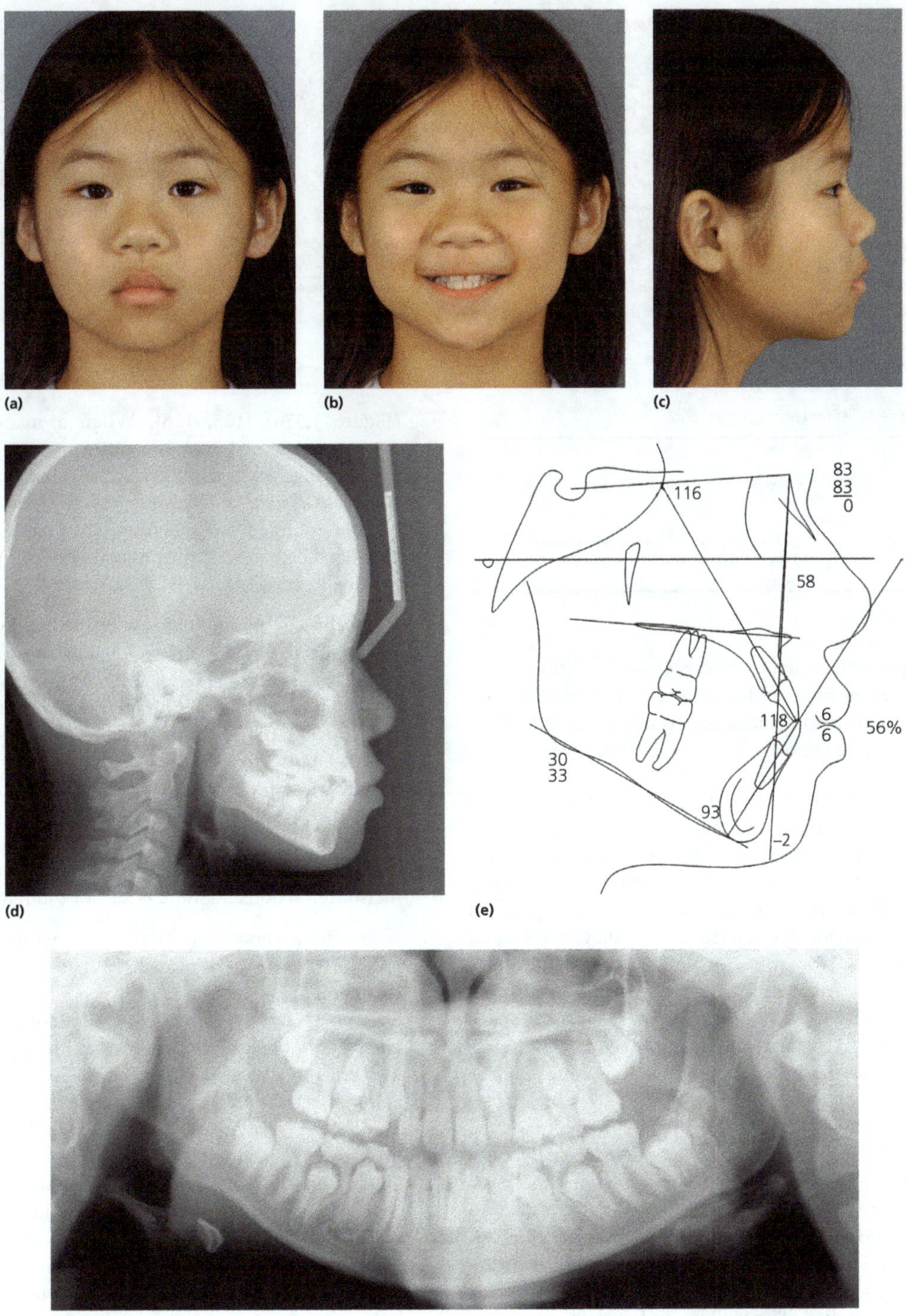

Figure 1.56 Initial records of Phoebe.

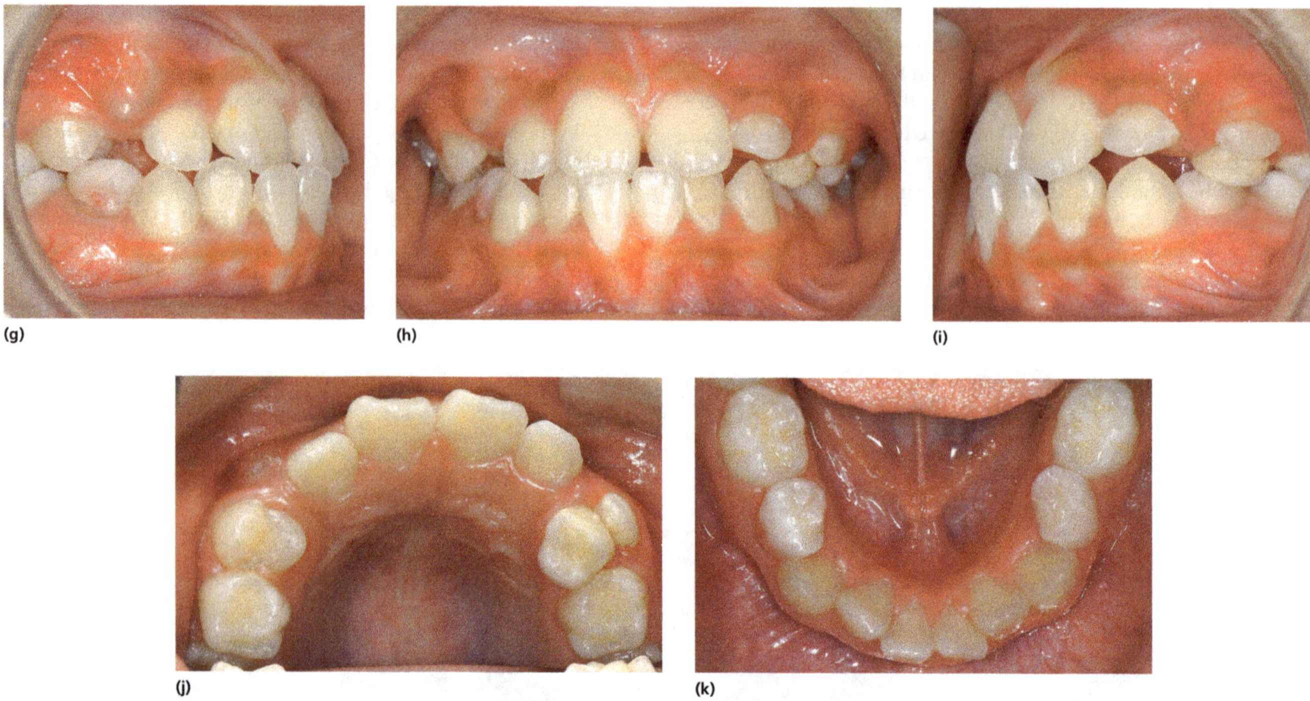

Figure 1.56 (Continued)

Table 1.11 Primary problems list for Phoebe (Figure 1.56).

AP	I I I I
Vertical	Minimal overbite
Transverse	–
Other	Anterior crossbite Blocked-out maxillary canines with the left canine overlapping the lateral incisor on panoramic image

substituting maxillary first premolars as canines). If you then ended up treating the mandibular arch nonextraction, you would need to protract the maxillary posterior teeth to place the maxillary first premolars in a Class I canine position.

Q: Patients with severe anterior crowding (incisor protrusion/lip protrusion) may be candidates for first premolar extractions, patients with moderate crowding (relatively acceptable profile) may be candidates for second premolar extractions [124], and patients with severe mandibular incisor crowding (with a corresponding anterior tooth–size discrepancy/peg-shaped maxillary lateral incisors) may be candidates for mandibular incisor extraction. Focusing on just the mandibular arch, what tooth movements are observed with reciprocal space closure (no use of TADs for anchorage) following second premolar extractions, first premolar extractions, and incisor extractions?

A: As a rule of thumb, when second premolars are extracted one can expect the posterior teeth to move mesially one-half the extraction space, leaving the remaining half for canine retraction, relief of crowding, and incisor retraction (Figure 1.57a). When first premolars are extracted, one can expect the posterior teeth to move mesially one-third of the space, leaving the remaining two-thirds of the space for canine retraction, relief of crowding, and incisor retraction (Figure 1.57b) [125, 126]. When a mandibular incisor is extracted (Figure 1.57c), the entire space is available for relief of crowding. *With incisor extraction, mesial movement of posterior teeth should not be anticipated.* Of course, when TADs are incorporated for anchorage, the entire tooth movement equation changes with the possibility of complete space closure in one direction.

Q: Is Phoebe a good candidate for extracting posterior teeth?

A: Extraction of all four first premolars would provide space to align (and upright) anterior teeth. However, before you extract all first premolars, you should examine the maxillary lateral incisor roots (CBCT scan) to confirm that the maxillary left lateral incisor root has not been severely resorbed by the permanent canine crown. Extraction of premolars may also necessitate surgical exposure of the maxillary left canine. Extraction of all four second premolars offers no advantage over extracting all four first premolars: space closure will result in less incisor retraction and more posterior tooth mesial movement.

Q: Is Phoebe a good candidate for extracting a combination of anterior and posterior teeth? What is your recommended treatment for Phoebe?

A: She was treated with extraction of a combination of anterior and posterior teeth. An LLHA was initially placed, but mandibular crowding was later deemed too severe to treat the lower arch nonextraction. Mandibular first premolars were removed. Due to the position of the maxillary left canine crown (and probable maxillary left lateral incisor root resorption), the maxillary lateral incisors were also extracted. All permanent teeth were allowed to erupt. Figure 1.58 illustrates Phoebe's final result after completion of fixed orthodontic treatment and canine composite veneers. As shown, she has a beautiful smile and profile. A small space exists distal to the mandibular left canine.

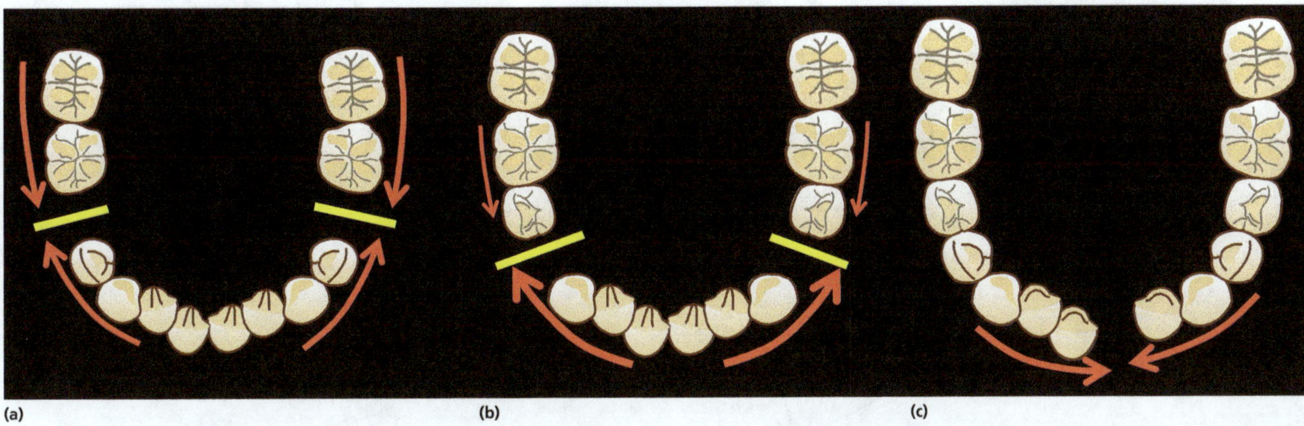

Figure 1.57 Illustration of the effect of (a) second premolar, (b) first premolar, or (c) incisor extraction on movement of teeth (red arrows) adjacent to mandibular extraction sites using conventional orthodontic mechanics without the aid of supplemental anchorage. Yellow lines in (a) and (b) indicate approximate location where translation of tooth segments will stop when extraction spaces are completely closed, reciprocally. Note in (c), protraction of posterior teeth is not seen.

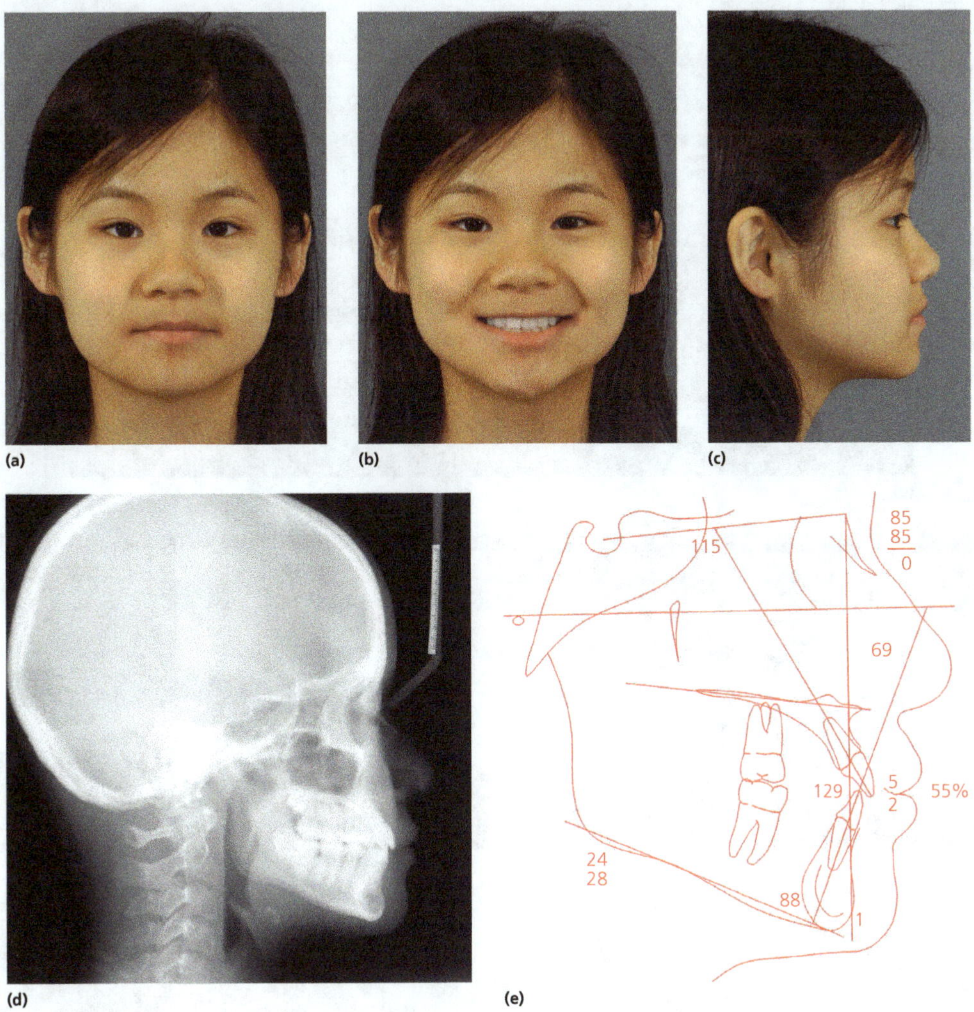

Figure 1.58 Deband records of Phoebe.

Once again, our point is to encourage you to consider all possible options in deciding whether to treat a patient nonextraction or with extractions. You must eliminate unknowns (e.g., placing an LLHA and evaluating space needs after the permanent teeth erupt), consider the costs/benefits of nonextraction treatment, and weigh the costs/benefits of every reasonable combination of anterior and posterior tooth extraction pattern.

Now let's look at a case by proceeding through all 10 steps of diagnosis and treatment planning. Lauris (Figure 1.59) presents to you for orthodontic treatment.

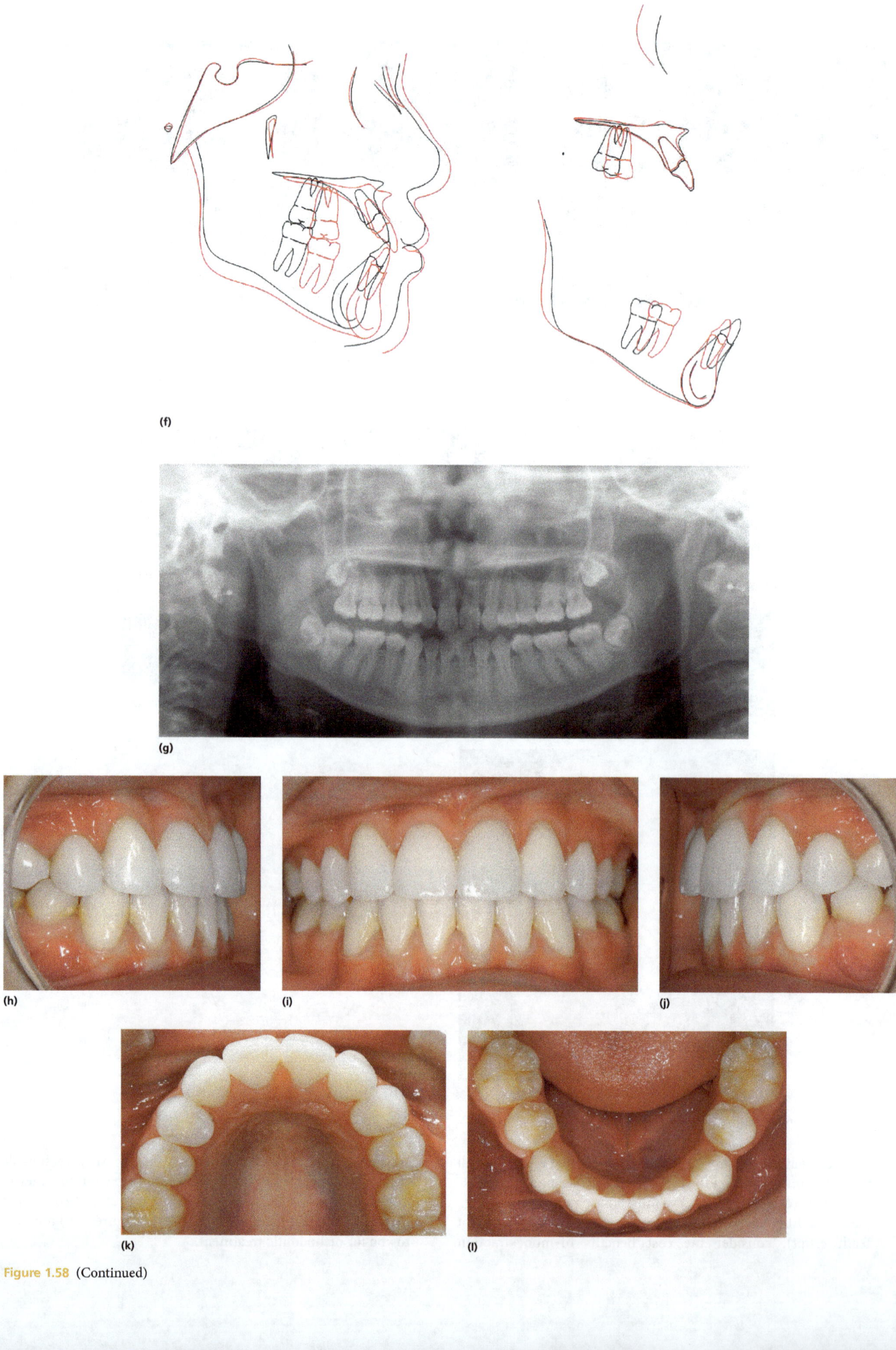

Figure 1.58 (Continued)

Q: Step 1: What is Lauris' history and CC?

A: Lauris is 42 years old with PMH WRN. PDH includes significant restorative dentistry experience. He states he wants his crossbite corrected.

Q: Step 2: What does your examination reveal? What records are required?

A: Periodontal and TMJ findings are WRN. UDML is centered with the face. No functional shifts are detected. Panoramic and cephalometric radiographs, a full photographic series, and study models are made (Figure 1.59, study models not shown).

Q: Step 3: After a thorough review of Lauris' history, examination, and records, what are his diagnostic findings and problems? Please prepare a list.

A: Lauris' diagnostic findings/problem list and diagnosis is shown in Table 1.12.

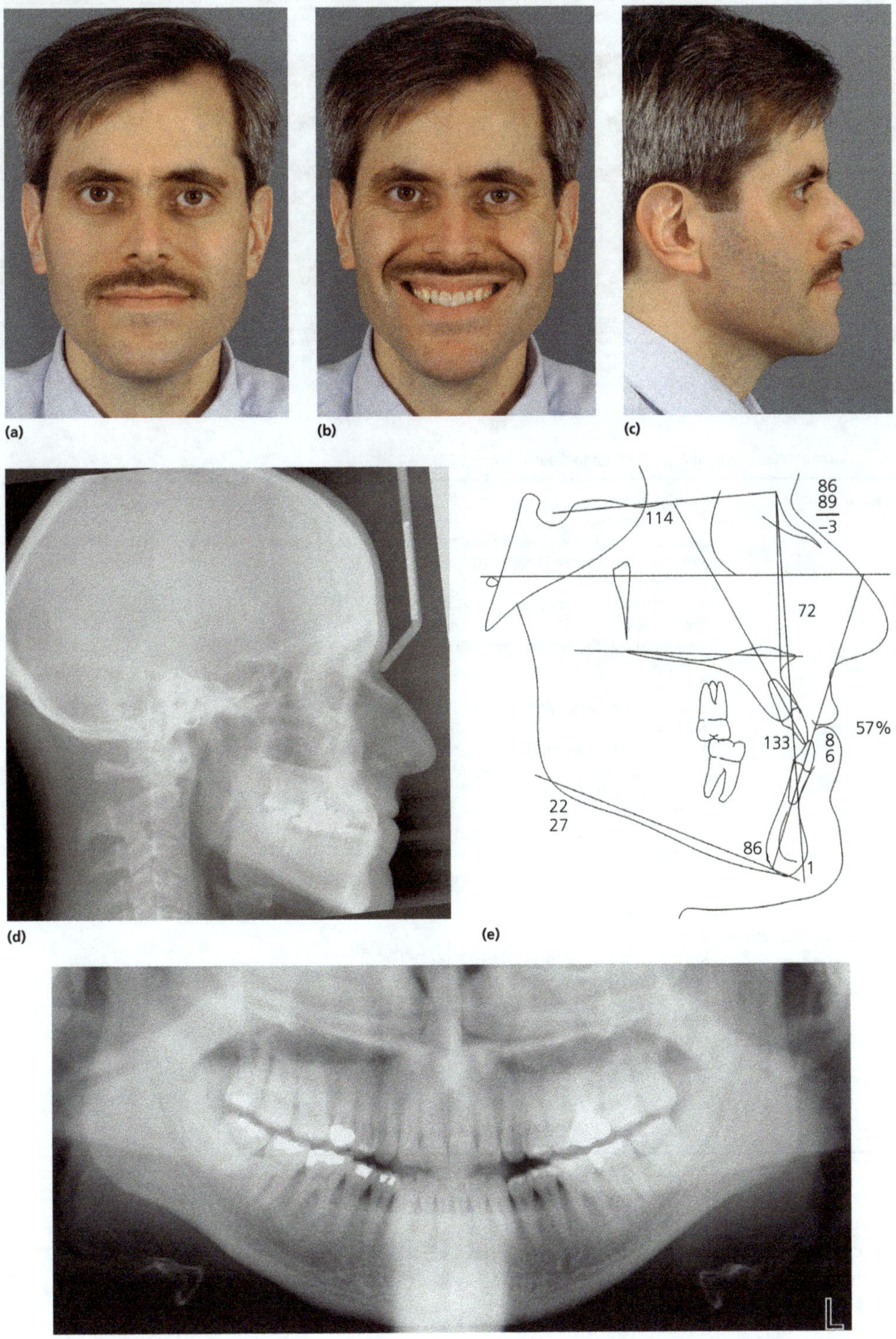

Figure 1.59 Initial records of Lauris.

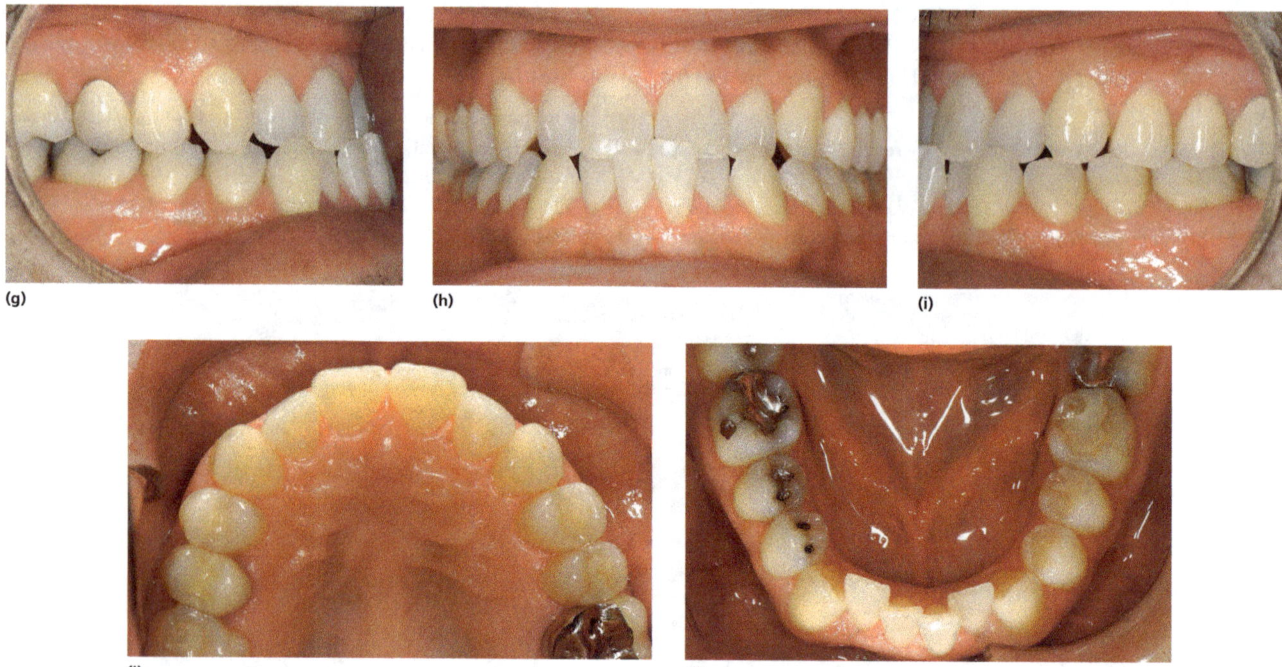

(g) (h) (i) (j) (k)

Figure 1.59 (Continued)

Table 1.12 Diagnostic findings and problem list for Lauris (Figure 1.59).

Full face and profile	**Frontal view** Face is symmetric Soft tissue long lower anterior facial height (soft tissue Glabella–Subnasale < Subnasale–soft tissue Menton) Absence of an interlabial gap (ILG) UDML WRN Incisal display during posed smile WRN **Profile view** Straight to slightly concave/anteriorly divergent profile NLA WRN Prominent chin Lip–chin–throat angle WRN
Ceph Analysis	**Skeletal** Maxillary AP position WRN Mandibular AP position protrusive (ANB = −3° with maxillary AP position WRN) Effective bony Pogonion Mildly increased skeletal lower anterior facial height: LAFH/TAFH = 57% FMA (22°) and SNMP (27°) mildly flat **Dental** Proclined maxillary incisors (U1-SN angle of 114°) Upright mandibular incisors (FMIA = 72°)
Radiographs	Adult dentition
Intraoral photos and models	Angle Class III Iowa Classification: III (4–5) III (4–5) III (4–5) III (4–5) Anterior crossbite occlusion OB 20% Midlines are not coincident (LDML to right of UDML by 1–2 mm) Moderate mandibular anterior crowding
Other	
Diagnosis	Angle Class III malocclusion Skeletal mandibular protrusion Anterior crossbite occlusion

Q: Step 4: What are your treatment goals?

A: Achieve Class I canines, achieve ideal overbite and overjet and correct his anterior crossbite.

Q: Step 5: What are Lauris' primary problems in the AP, vertical, and transverse dimensions (plus other significant problems)?

A: See Table 1.13

Table 1.13 Primary problems list for Lauris *(apical base/skeletal discrepancies italicized)*.

AP	III (4–5) III (4–5) III (4–5) III (4–5) *Mandibular skeletal protrusion*
Vertical	–
Transverse	–
Other	Anterior crossbite

Q: Step 6: Should you discuss surgical options with Lauris?

A: Yes. Lauris is a good example of the challenges you face in deciding treatment for patients with *moderate* apical base discrepancies. On the one hand, you could consider a mandibular setback osteotomy to address his mandibular protrusion and his dental Class III relationship. On the other hand, setting back his mandible could result in an unsatisfactory chin–throat length and profile convexity. It is important to discuss this with him, underscoring the limitations of treatment to ideal occlusion (treatment with surgery) versus treatment to acceptable occlusion with less dramatic effects on his profile (treatment without surgery). After your presentation and discussion, Lauris states that he does not want jaw surgery. Note: With any mandibular setback osteotomy, you must inquire whether the patient has a history of snoring or sleep apnea as the airway cross-section could be reduced with surgery [127]. A sleep study (polysomnography) may be warranted before beginning treatment in such a case.

Q: Step 7: What unknowns do you face? Specifically, what unknowns does he have that you should eliminate before doing anything irreversible (e.g., extracting permanent teeth)?

A: A previously *undetected CR–CO shift*. This underscores an important point regarding examination of patients with crossbites. Crossbite occlusions may occur as a result of a functional shift to avoid tooth interferences. In some instances, growth and dental drift may "convert" the shift to a stable mandibular position. However, in many instances, the shift is not stable and is due to neuromuscular control of the mandible to avoid interferences. Detecting a true path of closure may be difficult in such cases. Therefore, if you are uncertain whether Lauris has a shift, attempt to discover it at a later examination [128]. This was done and it was noted that Lauris has an anterior centric slide of 1 mm. This information will modify the cephalometric diagnosis, as the cephalometric radiograph is taken in maximum intercuspation. Note: As an aid in detecting CR–CO shifts, you can consider "deprogramming" the habitual occlusion by having the patient wear a bite plate or leveling the arches with fixed appliances.

Q: Steps 8 and 9: Because of his age, you cannot treat Lauris' apical base discrepancy with orthopedics. Further, he declined surgery. Therefore, your remaining option is masking. In terms of treating Lauris by masking his apical base discrepancy (either nonextraction or with extraction of permanent teeth), can you list the factors that will play a role in your decision?

A: Factors include the following:

- A 4–5 mm Class III AP dental relationship *but with a 1 mm anterior shift from CR to CO (which reduces the Class III relationship to only 3–4 mm)*
- Upright mandibular incisors and proclined maxillary incisors
- Mild-to-moderate crowding in the mandibular anterior
- Robust attached tissue covering roots of mandibular incisors

Q: Step 8: Is Lauris a good candidate for nonextraction treatment?

A: No. Achieving a Class I canine relationship without surgery or extractions may be heroic. Class III elastic wear can be effective in correcting a Class III patient a few millimeters but may be challenging with Lauris' 3–4 mm Class III discrepancy. The costs outweigh the benefits.

Q: Step 9: Is Lauris a good candidate for treatment with anterior tooth extractions?

A: No. Extracting anterior teeth (e.g., a lower incisor) has the benefit of relieving anterior crowding, but extracting an incisor will not help correct his Class III relationship. The cost is not finishing Lauris with a Class I canine relationship.

Q: Is Lauris a good candidate for treatment with posterior tooth extractions?

A: Yes. Extraction of mandibular premolars could provide space to retract the mandibular canines into a Class I relationship and unravel his mild mandibular anterior crowding. The cost is further uprighting his mandibular incisors.

Q: Step 10: Weighing the benefits/costs of these options, which is (are) best for Lauris? What is your recommended treatment plan?

A: The cost of treatment without extractions or with anterior tooth extractions outweighs their benefits. The cost of extracting mandibular premolars and retracting mandibular anterior teeth can be further uprighting of his mandibular incisors. However, the benefits of mandibular premolar extractions are correction of his anterior crossbite (his CC), improvement of his mandibular anterior tooth alignment, and finishing in Class I canine relationship. Extraction of mandibular first premolars was the option that was chosen.

Q: What are the specific objectives of treatment for the maxilla, mandible, maxillary dentition, and mandibular dentition in all three planes of space?

A: Specific objectives of treatment for Lauris are as follows:

Maxilla
- AP: Maintain.
- Vertical: Maintain.
- Transverse: Maintain.

Mandible
- AP: Maintain.
- Vertical: Maintain.
- Transverse: Maintain.

Maxillary dentition
- AP: Maintain molars. Maintain incisor position.
- Vertical: Maintain molars. Maintain incisor position.
- Intermolar width: Maintain.

Mandibular dentition
- AP: Protract molars. Retract canines. Upright incisors.
- Vertical: Maintain molars. Maintain incisor position.
- Intermolar/intercanine width: Maintain intermolar and intercanine widths.

Q: What was the outcome using this approach?

A: Progress and final records are shown in Figures 1.60 and 1.61. Note in Figure 1.60 how Lauris' first premolars have been extracted and his mandibular anterior teeth are being retracted, reciprocally, out of crossbite.Figure 1.61 illustrates Lauris at deband. Your treatment goals have been achieved. Lauris has a wonderful smile and bite, but his mandibular incisors have uprighted (superimposition, Figure 1.61f). Mandibular incisor crown retractions of this magnitude can result in reciprocal movement of mandibular incisor root apices forward through the alveolar process bone, although this does not appear to have happened here (Figure 1.61d). Extraction of lower premolars was an appropriate treatment for Lauris.

As the foregoing examples illustrate, much thought should go into considering whether you treat a patient nonextraction, with extraction of anterior teeth, with some combination of anterior and posterior teeth, or with some combination

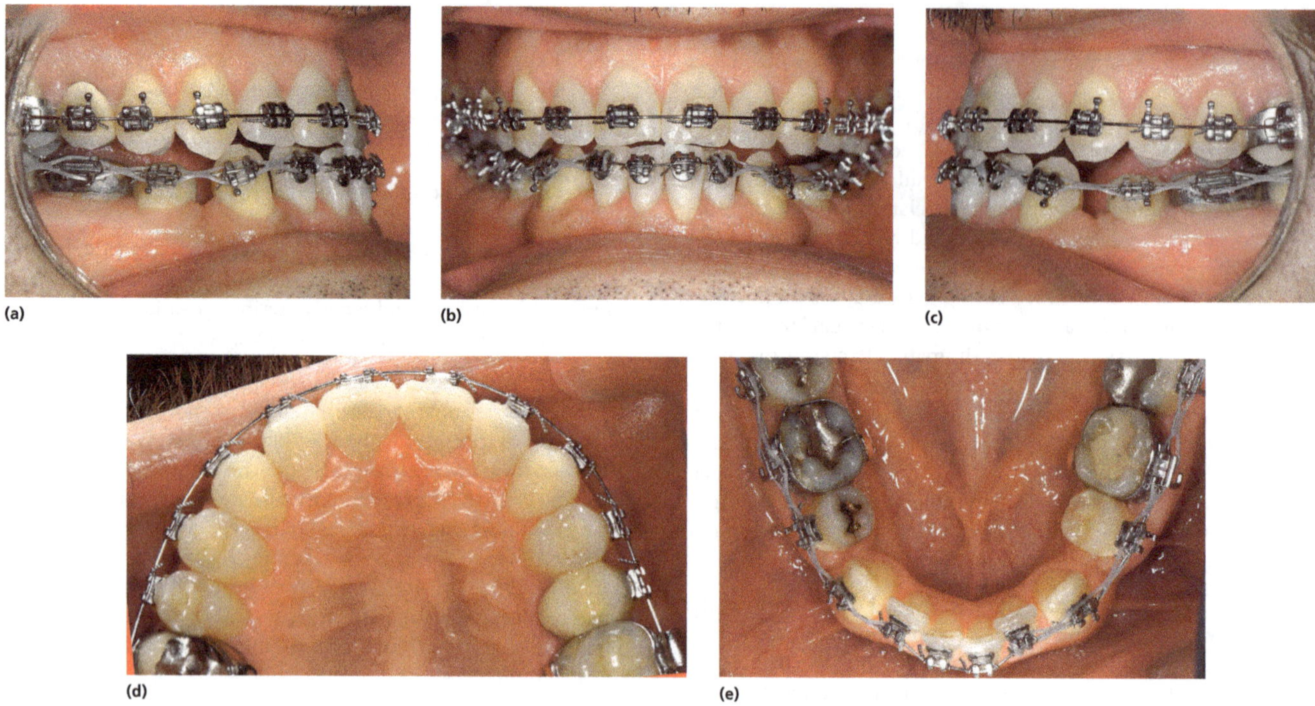

Figure 1.60 Progress records of Lauris.

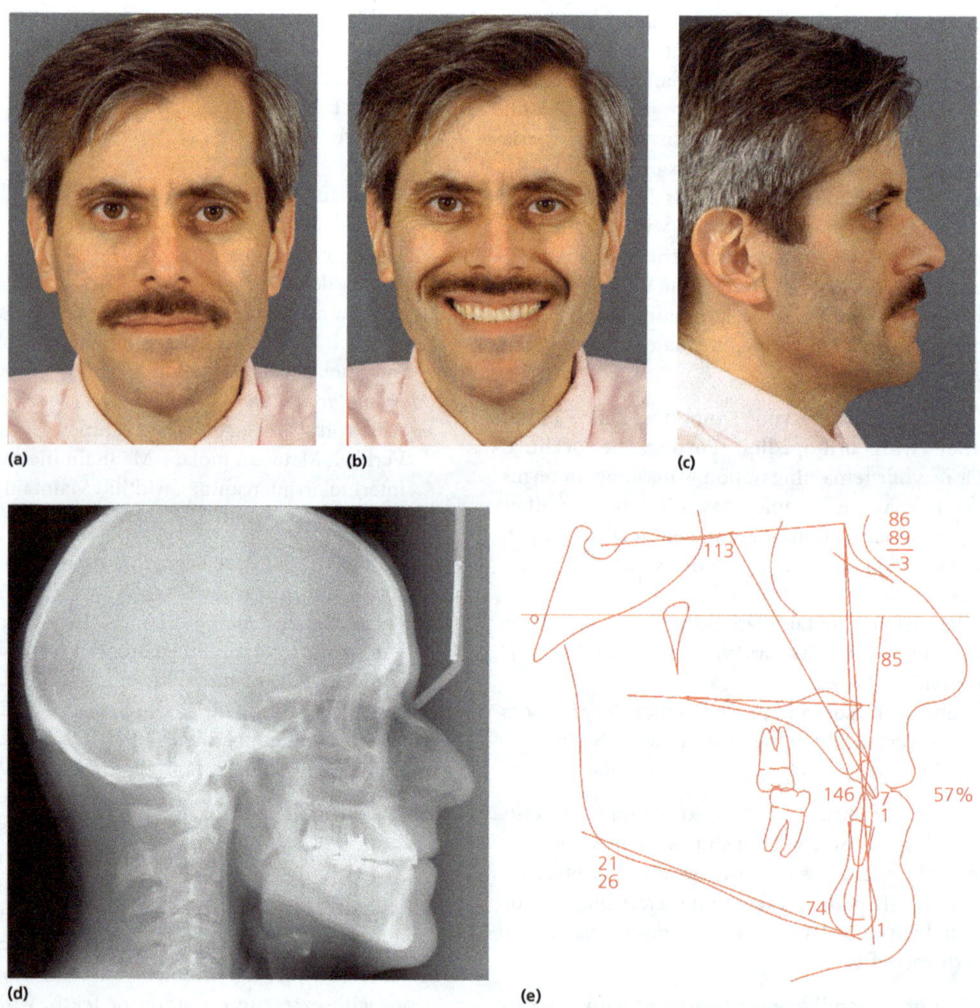

Figure 1.61 Deband records of Lauris.

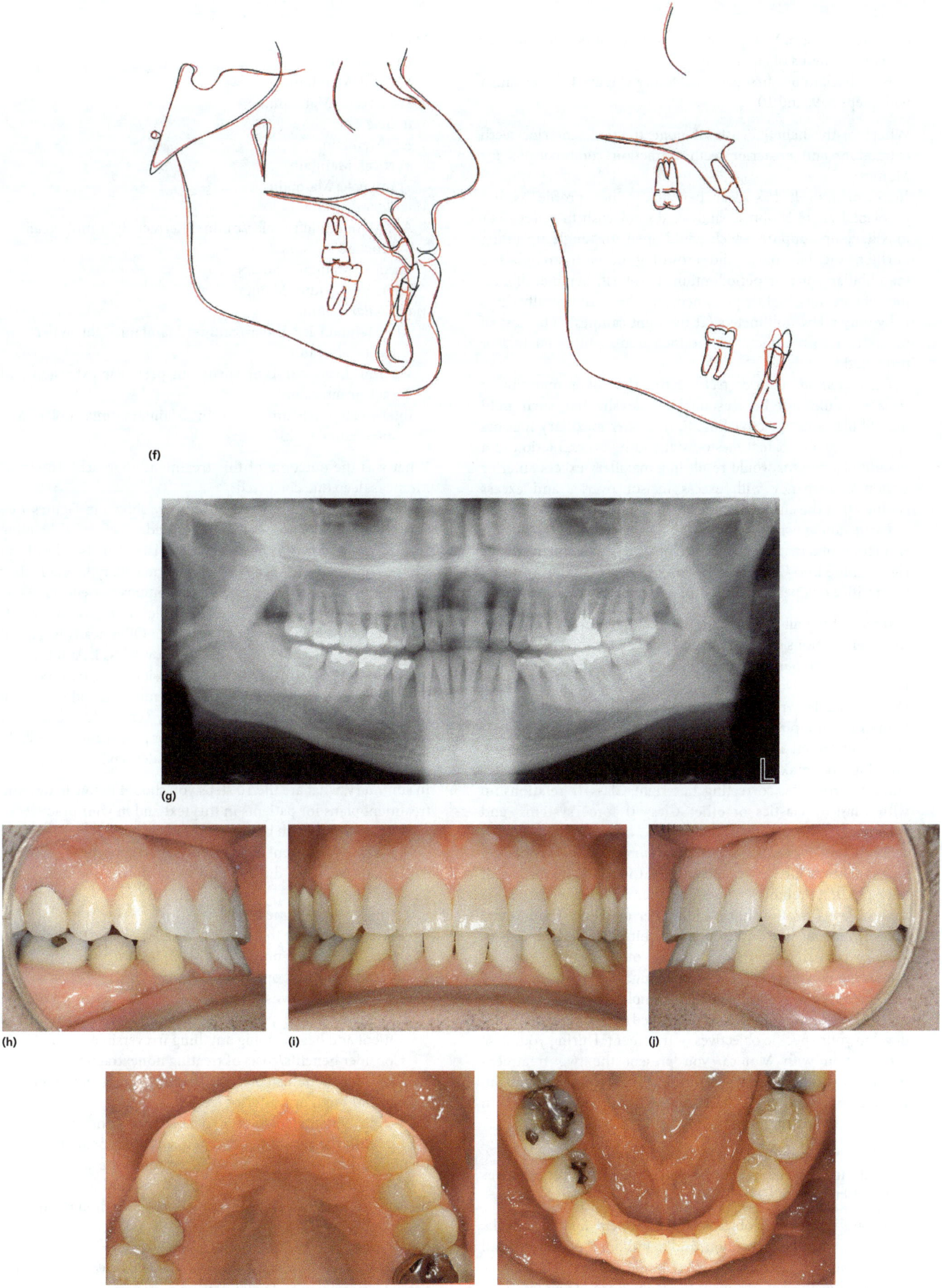

Figure 1.61 (Continued)

of posterior teeth. You should always force yourself to consider the costs/benefits of all options.

Now, back to our first patient, Monica (Figure 1.40) to finish with Steps 8, 9, and 10.

Q: What are the benefits/costs of nonextraction, anterior teeth extraction, and posterior teeth extraction combinations for Monica?

A: *Nonextraction*: It has clear benefits to her profile as her nasolabial angle is obtuse, and we do not wish to reduce her maxillary lip support, which could open this angle up more. Further, she has only mild crowding in both arches, her mandibular anterior periodontium is robust, her mandibular incisors are only slightly proclined, and she is unilaterally Class II by only a few millimeters (at the right canines). The cost of nonextraction treatment will be increased mandibular incisor proclination.

Extraction of anterior teeth: Extraction of a mandibular incisor would not be reasonable since she has such mild mandibular anterior crowding. Further, her maxillary incisors appear to be of normal mesiodistal width—so extraction of a mandibular incisor would result in a maxillary excess anterior Bolton discrepancy with excess incisor overjet and excess canine OJ at the end of treatment.

Extraction of posterior teeth: An argument could be made for extraction of a maxillary right premolar to move the maxillary right canine into Class I occlusion. The cost of doing so would be sacrifice of a permanent tooth.

Q: After weighing all nonextraction and extraction options, what treatment options do you recommend for Monica?

A: *Nonextraction:* banding/bonding arches (except for the maxillary lateral incisor), leveling/aligning arches, opening space for the maxillary right lateral incisor, placing the patient on a temporary bite plate (to open her bite and permit her maxillary right lateral incisor to swing forward out of crossbite), bonding the maxillary right lateral incisor, correcting her anterior crossbite, correcting her right Class II relationship with Class II elastics or other Class II force systems, and finishing.

Extraction of maxillary right first premolar: banding/bonding arches (except for her maxillary lateral incisor), extraction of her right first premolar, retraction of her maxillary right canine into a Class I relationship, bonding her maxillary right lateral incisor, placing her on a temporary bite plate, correction of anterior crossbite, leveling/aligning of arches, closure of remaining maxillary space, and finishing.

Remember, now that you have completed Steps 1–10, you must choose your final (recommended) treatment plan and develop your specific objectives of treatment. During your case presentation with Monica, you present the two treatment options. You determine that Monica will be a compliant patient. Patient compliance (e.g., elastic wear) will be an asset with either treatment approach.

Q: What is your recommended treatment plan for Monica?

A: Considering her compliance potential, Monica's final plan was nonextraction with Class II elastic wear on her right.

Q: What are the specific objectives of treatment for the maxilla, mandible, maxillary dentition, and mandibular dentition in all three planes of space?

A: Specific objectives of treatment for Monica are as follows:

Maxilla
AP: Maintain.
Vertical: Maintain.
Transverse: Maintain.

Mandible
AP: Maintain.
Vertical: Maintain.
Transverse: Maintain.

Maxillary dentition
AP: Maintain left molar/canine. Retract right molar/canine. Procline incisors.
Vertical: Maintain molars.
Intermolar width: Maintain.

Mandibular dentition
AP: Maintain left molar/canine. Maintain right molar/protract right canine.
Vertical: Level curve of Spee with premolar extrusion and incisor intrusion.
Intermolar/intercanine width: Maintain intermolar and intercanine widths.

Q: What was the outcome of this treatment approach? How was Monica's deep bite corrected?

A: Progress and final records for Monica are shown in Figures 1.62 and 1.63. Intraoral photographs made before debanding (Figure 1.62) show the maxillary right lateral incisor has been stepped up to balance her right and left maxillary lateral incisor gingival margins in preparation of composite veneers. Final images are shown in Figure 1.63. Her smile has improved dramatically, her crossbite has been corrected, her OB is nearly ideal, and her right Class II canine relationship is now Class I. As illustrated by her initial to posttreatment superimposition (Figure 1.63f), her deep bite was opened by mandibular molar eruption (which rotated her mandible down and back), very mild mandibular incisor proclination, and maxillary incisor proclination (the slight maxillary incisor eruption would tend to deepen her bite).

Q: In summary, what are the 10 steps you should follow to develop treatment plans for patients in this text and in your practice?.

A:
1 Obtain a thorough history and establish the patient's CC.
2 Examine the patient clinically and with appropriate records.
3 Exhaustively list diagnostic findings/problems and make your diagnosis.
4 Define your treatment goals.
5 Focus on solving the *primary* problem in each dimension (plus other major problems).
6 Consider surgical options.
7 Establish unknowns you face—strive to reduce significant unknowns *before* presenting final treatment plan to the patient and before doing anything irreversible.
8 Consider benefits/costs of treating nonextraction.
9 Consider benefits/costs of treating with extraction of anterior teeth or posterior teeth.
10 Weigh benefits/costs of all viable treatment options and establish the recommended plan and treatment objectives.

Remember, at every patient visit, examine the patient, force yourself to review your *primary problems*, and act to address these problems. Over time, the major problems should diminish and your attention can be drawn to smaller and smaller problems—until you finish treatment.

Finally, *at every patient visit do everything you can for the patient*. Even if you and your staff are very busy, do not procras-

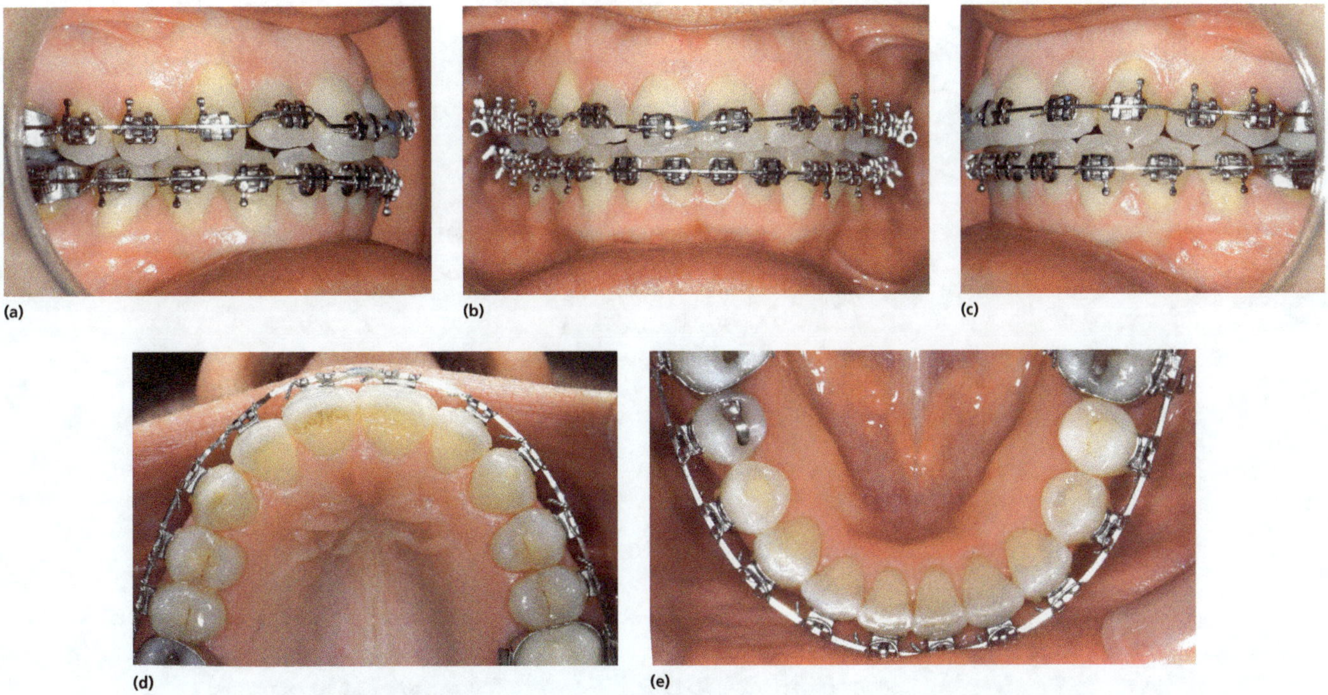

Figure 1.62 Progress records of Monica.

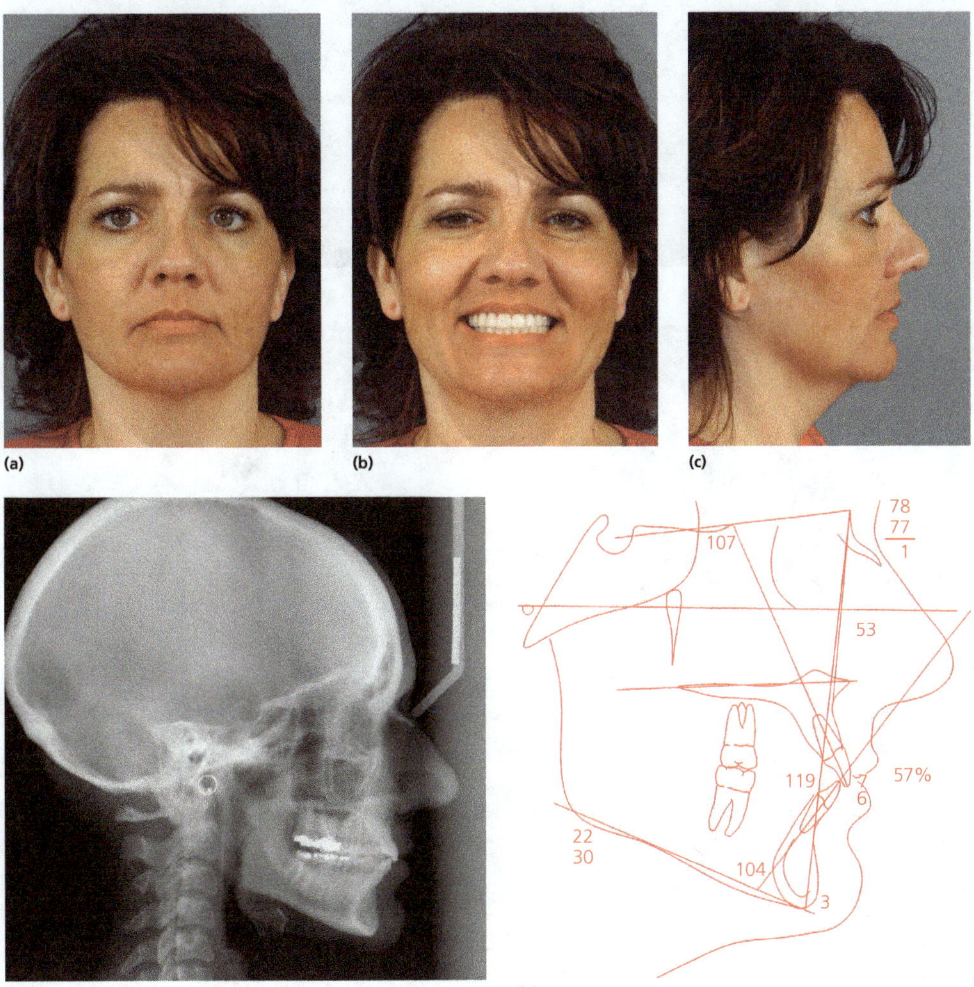

Figure 1.63 Deband records of Monica.

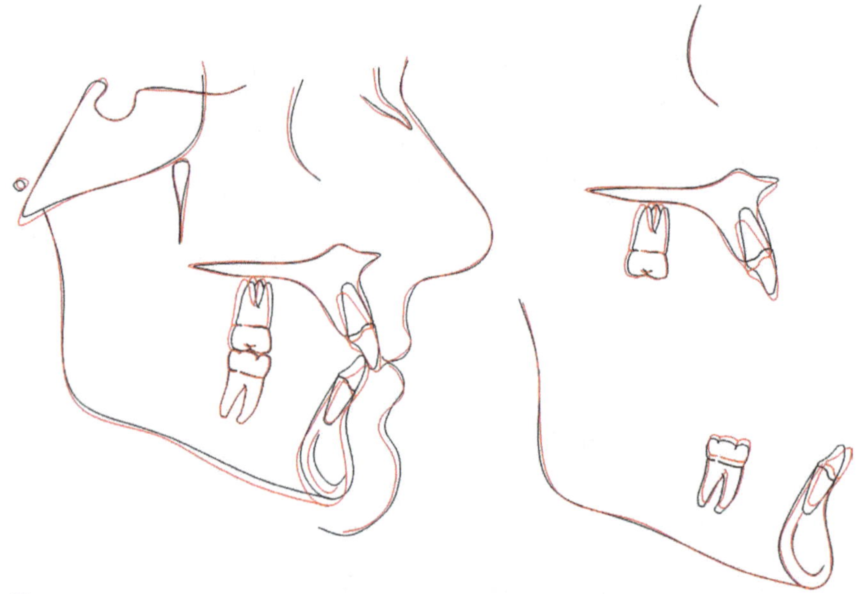

(f)

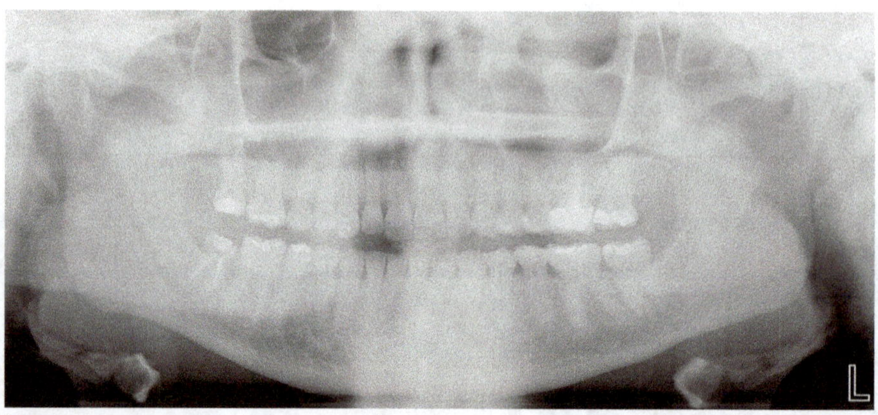

(g)

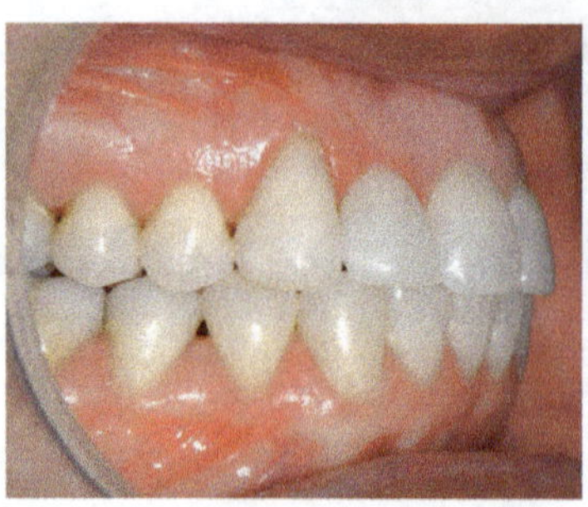

(h)

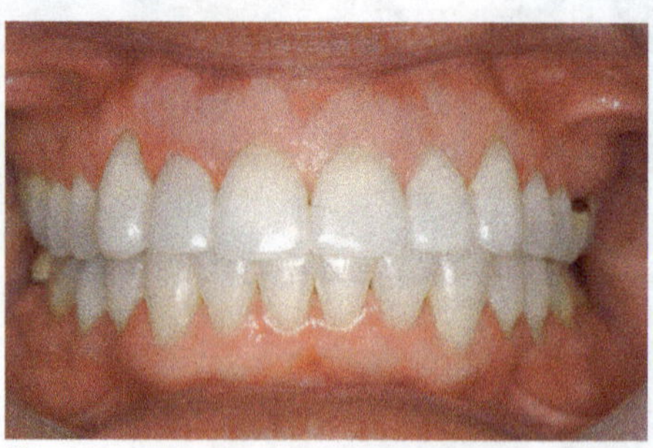

(i)

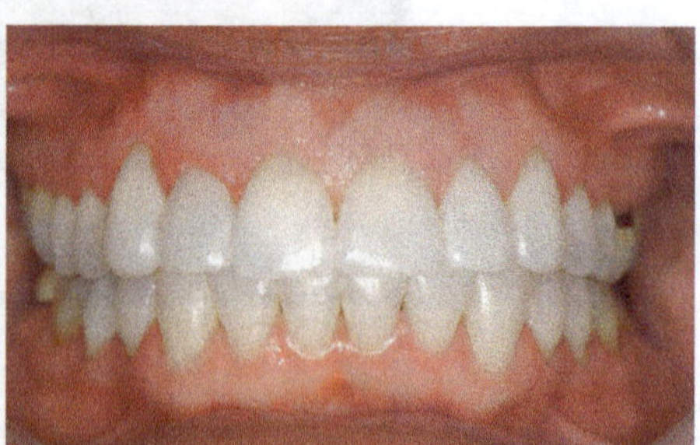

(j)

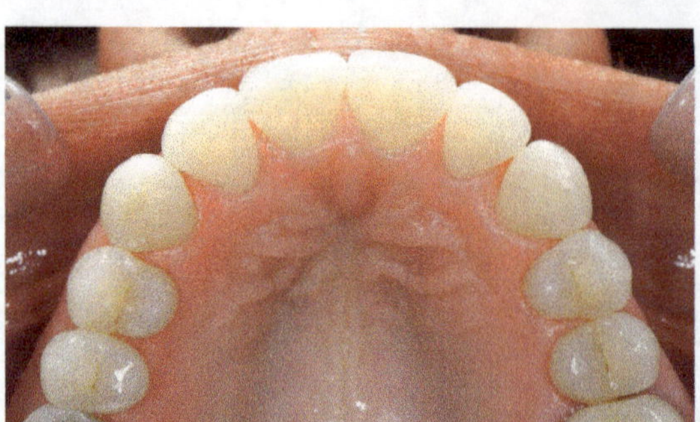

(k)

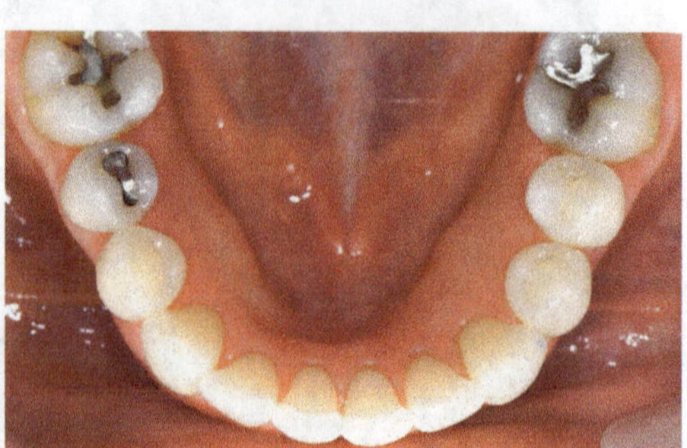

(l)

Figure 1.63 (Continued)

tinate until the next appointment to get as much done for that patient as possible. As a doctor you must follow the golden rule: Do for the patient what you would want done for yourself.

References

1 English JD, Do-Quang T-D, Salas-Lopez AM. Orthodontic records and case evaluation. In: English JD, Peltomaki T, Pham-Litschel K, editors. *Mosby's orthodontic review*. St. Louis: Mosby Elsevier; 2009. p. 39.

2 Proffit WR, Ackerman JL. Orthodontic diagnosis: the development of a problem list. In: Proffit WR, Fields HW, editors. *Contemporary Orthodontics*. 2nd ed. St. Louis: Mosby; 1993. p. 148.

3 Wylie WL, Johnson EL. Rapid evaluation of facial dysplasia in the vertical plane. *Angle Orthod*. 1952;**22**:165–81.

4 Vig RG, Brundo GC. The kinetics of anterior tooth display. *J Prosthet Dent*. 1978;**39**:502–5.

5 Kurth JR, Kokich VG. Open gingival embrasures after orthodontic treatment in adults: prevalence and etiology. *Am J Orthod Dentofac Orthop*. 2001;**120**:116–23.

6 Fridrich KL, Casko JS. Genioplasty strategies for anterior facial vertical dysplasias. *Int J Adult Orthodon Orthognath Surg*. 1997;**12**:35–41.

7 Bjork A. Facial growth in man, studied with the aid of metallic implants. *Acta Odontol Scand*. 1955;**13**:9–34.

8 Bjork A, Skieller V. Normal and abnormal growth of the mandible: a synthesis of longitudinal cephalometric implant studies over a period of 25 years. *Eur J Orthod*. 1983;**5**:1–46.

9 Schudy FF. Vertical growth versus anteroposterior growth as related to function and treatment. *Angle Orthod*. 1964;**34**:75–93.

10 Schudy FF. The rotation of the mandible resulting from growth: its implications in orthodontic treatment. *Angle Orthod*. 1965;**35**:36–50.

11 Skieller V, Bjork A, Linde-Hansen T. Prediction of mandibular growth rotation evaluated from a longitudinal implant sample. *Am J Orthod*. 1984;**86**:359–70.

12 Miller S, Kerr WJ. A new look at mandibular growth—a preliminary report. *Eur J Orthod*. 1992;**14**:95–8.

13 Spady M, Buschang PH, Demirjian A, LaPalme L. Mandibular rotation and angular remodeling during childhood and adolescence. *Am J Hum Biol*. 1992;**4**:683–9.

14 Karlsen AT. Craniofacial growth differences between low and high MP-SN angle males: a longitudinal study. *Angle Orthod*. 1995;**65**:341–50.

15 Chung CH, Wong WW. Craniofacial growth in untreated skeletal Class II subjects: a longitudinal study. *Am J Orthod Dentofacial Orthop*. 2002;**122**:619–26.

16 Bishara SE, Jakobsen JR. Longitudinal changes in three normal facial types. *Am J Orthod*. 1985;**88**:466–502.

17 Jacob HB, Buschang PH. Vertical craniofacial growth changes in French-Canadians between 10 and 15 years of age. *Am J Orthod Dentofacial Orthop*. 2011;**139**: 797–805.

18 Zankl A, Eberle L, Molinari L, Schinzel A. Growth charts for nose length, nasal protrusion, and philtrum length from birth to 97 years. *Am J Med Genet*. 2002;**111**:388–91.

19 Fundalej P. Long-term changes of the upper lip position relative to the incisor edge. *Am J Orthod Dentofacial Orthop*. 2008;**135**:204–9.

20 Burstone, C. Lip posture and its significance in treatment planning. *Am J Orthod*. 1967;**53**:262–84.

21 Vig PS, Cohen AM. Vertical growth of the lips a serial cephalometric study. *Am J Orthod*. 1979;**75**:405–15.

22 Sarver DM, Ackerman MB. Dynamic smile visualization and quantification: Part 1. Evolution of the concept and dynamic records for smile capture. *Am J Orthod Dentofacial Orthop*. 2003;**124**:4–12.

23 Mammandras AH. Linear changes of the maxillary and mandibular lips. *Am J Orthod Dentofacial Orthop*. 1988;**94**:405–10.

24 Sarver DM. The importance of incisor positioning in the esthetic smile: the smile arc. *Am J Orthod Dentofacial Orthop*. 2001;**120**:98–111.

25 Hulsey CM. An esthetic evaluation of lip-teeth relationships present in the smile. *Am J Orthod*. 1970;**57**:132–44.

26 Mackley RJ. An evaluation of smiles before and after orthodontic treatment. *Angle Orthod*. 1993;**63**:183–9; discussion 190.

27 Ackerman JL, Ackerman MB, Brensinger CM, Landis JR. A morphometric analysis of the posed smile. *Clin Orthod Res*. 1998;1:2–11.

28 Kokich VO, Kokich VG, Kiyak HA. Perceptions of dental professionals and laypersons to altered dental esthetics: asymmetric and symmetric situations. *Am J Orthod Dentofacial Orthop*. 2006;**130**:141–51.

29 Benson KJ, Laskin DM. Upper lip asymmetry in adults during smiling. *J Oral Maxillofac Surg*. 2001;**59**:396–8.

30 Kokich VO Jr, Kiyak HA, Shapiro PA. Comparing the perception of dentists and lay people to altered dental esthetics. *J Esthet Dent*. 1999:**11**;311–24.

31 Polo M. Botulinum toxin type A in the treatment of excessive gingival display. *Am J Orthod Dentofacial Orthop*. 2005;**127**:214–8.

32 Niamtu J 3rd. Botox injections for gummy smiles. *Am J Orthod Dentofacial Orthop*. 2008;**133**:782–3; author reply 783-4.

33 Scott CR, Goonewardene MS, Murray K. Influence of lips on the perception of malocclusion. *Am J Orthod Dentofacial Orthop*. 2006;**130**:152–62.

34 Janson G, Branco NC, Fernandes TM, Sathler R, Garib D, Lauris JR. Influence of orthodontic treatment, midline position, buccal corridor and smile arc on smile attractiveness. *Angle Orthod*. 2011;**81**:153–61.

35 Pinho S, Ciriaco C, Faber J, Lenza MA. Impact of dental asymmetries on the perception of smile esthetics. *Am J Orthod Dentofacial Orthop*. 2007;**132**:748–53.

36 Roden-Johnson D, Gallerano R, English J. The effects of buccal corridor spaces and arch form on smile esthetics. *Am J Orthod Dentofacial Orthop*. 2005;**127**:343–50.

37 Moore T, Southard KA, Casko JS, Qian F, Southard TE. Buccal corridors and smile esthetics. *Am J Orthod Dentofacial Orthop*. 2005;**127**:208–13.

38 Jornung J, Fardal O. Perceptions of patients' smiles: a comparison of patients' and dentists' opinions. *J Am Dent Assoc*. 2007;**138**:1544–53.

39 Dunn WJ, Murchison DF, Broome JC. Esthetics: patients' perceptions of dental attractiveness. *J Prosthodont*. 1996;**5**:166–71.

40 Correa BD, Viera Bittencourt MA, Machado AW. Influence of maxillary canine gingival margin asymmetries on the perception of smile esthetics among orthodontists and laypersons. *Am J Orthod Dentofacial Orthop*. 2014;**145**:55–63.

41 Dixon AD, Hoyte DA, Ronning O. *Fundamentals of craniofacial growth*. Boca Raton: CRC Press, 1997.

42 Enlow DH, Hans MG. *Essentials of facial growth*. 2nd ed. Ann Arbor: Needham Press; 2008.

43 Hartsfield JK Jr, Morford LA, Otero LM. In: Bourzgui F, editor. Genetic factors affecting facial growth, Orthodontics—basic aspects and clinical considerations. Rijeka, Croatia: InTech. [cited 2014 Aug 11]. Available from: http://www.intechopen.com/books/orthodontics-basic-aspects-and-clinical-considerations/genetic-factors-affecting-facial-growth. pp. 125–52.

44 Duterloo HS, Planché PG. *Handbook of cephalometric superimposition*. Hanover Park: Quintessence; 2011.

45 Bastir M, Rosas A, O'Higgins P. Craniofacial levels and the morphologic maturation of the human skull. *J Anat*. 2006;**209**:637–54.

46 Bjork A. Cranial base development. *Am J Orthod*. 1955;**41**:198–225.

47 Buschang PH, Santos-Pinto A. Condylar growth and glenoid fossa displacement during childhood and adolescence. *Am J Orthod Dentofacial Orthop*. 1998;**113**:437–42.

48 Bjork A, Skieller V. Growth of the maxilla in three dimensions as revealed radiographically by the implant method. *Br J Orthod*. 1977;**4**:53–64.

49 Baumrind S, Ben-Bassat Y, Bravo LA, Curry S, Korn EL. Partitioning the components of maxillary tooth displacement by the comparison of data from three cephalometric superimpositions. *Angle Orthod*. 1996;**66**:111–24.

50 Ranly DM. *A synopsis of craniofacial growth*. 2nd ed. Norwalk: Appleton and Lange; 1988.

51 Buschang PH. Craniofacial growth and development. In: English, JD, Peltomaki T, Litschel K, editors. *Mosby's orthodontic review*. St. Louis: Elsevier Mosby; 2009. pp. 1–12.

52 Tanner JM, Whitehouse RH, Takaishi M. Standards from birth to maturity for height, weight, height velocity, and weight velocity: British children, 1965. *Arch Dis Child*. 1966;**41**:454–71.

53 Malina RM, Bouchard C, Beunen G. Human growth: selected aspects of current research on well-nourished children. *Ann Rev Anthropol*. 1988;**17**:187–219.

54 Mellion ZJ, Behrents, RG, Johnston LE Jr. The pattern of facial skeletal growth and its relationship to various common indexes of maturation. *Am J Orthod Dentofacial Orthop*. 2013;**143**:845–54.

55 Bambha JK, Van Natta P. Longitudinal study of facial growth in relation to skeletal maturation during adolescence. *Am J Orthod*. 1963;**49**:481–93.

56 Hunter CJ. The correlation of facial growth with body height and skeletal maturation at adolescence. *Angle Orthod*. 1966;**36**:44–54.

57 Mitani H. Contributions of the posterior cranial base and mandibular condyles to facial depth and height during puberty. *Angle Orthod*. 1973;**43**:337–43.

58 Buschang PH, Jacob HB, Demirjian A. Female adolescent craniofacial growth spurts: real or fiction? *Eur J Orthod*. 2013;**35**:819–25.

59 Nanda RS. The rates of growth of several facial components measured from serial cephalometric roentgenograms. *Am J Orthod*. 1955;**41**:658–73.

60 Buschang PH, Tanguay R, Demirjian A, LaPalme L, Goldstein H. Modeling longitudinal mandibular growth: percentiles for gnathion from 6 to 15 years of age in girls. *Am J Orthod Dentofacial Orthop*. 1989;**95**:60–6.

61 van der Beek MC, Hoeksma JB, Prahl-Andersen B. Vertical facial growth and statural growth in girls: a longitudinal comparison. *Eur J Orthod*. 1996;**18**:549–55.

62 Buschang PH, Martins J. Childhood and adolescent changes of skeletal relationships. *Angle Orthod*. 1998;**68**:199–206; discussion 207-8.

63 Chvatal BA, Behrents RG, Ceen RF, Buschang PH. Development and testing of multilevel models for longitudinal craniofacial growth prediction. *Am J Orthod Dentofacial Orthop.* 2005;**128**:45–56.

64 Bishara SE, Peterson LC, Bishara EC. Changes in facial dimensions and relationships between the ages of 5 and 25 years. *Am J Orthod.* 1984;**85**:238–52.

65 van der Beek MC, Hoeksma JB, Prahl-Andersen B. Vertical facial growth: a longitudinal study from 7 to 14 years of age. *Eur J Orthod.* 1991;**13**:202-8.

66 Houston WJ. Relationships between skeletal maturity estimated from hand-wrist radiographs and the timing of the adolescent growth spurt. *Eur J Orthod.* 1980;**2**:81–93.

67 Hagg U, Taranger J. Maturation indicators and the pubertal growth spurt. *Am J Orthod.* 1982;**82**:299–309.

68 Flores-Mir C, Nebbe B, Major PW. Use of skeletal maturation based on hand-wrist radiographic analysis as a predictor of facial growth: a systematic review. *Angle Orthod.* 2004;**74**:118–24.

69 Hunter WS, Baumrind S, Popovich F, Jorgensen G. Forecasting the timing of peak mandibular growth in males by using skeletal age. *Am J Orthop Dentofacial Orthod.* 2007;**131**:327–33.

70 Gabriel DB, Southard KA, Qian F, Marshall SD, Franciscus RG, Southard TE. Cervical vertebrae maturation method: poor reproducibility. *Am J Orthod Dentofacial Orthop.* 2009;**136**:478.e1–7; discussion 478-80.

71 Nestman TS, Marshall SD, Qian F, Holton N, Franciscus RG, Southard TE. Cervical vertebrae maturation method morphologic criteria: poor reproducibility. *Am J Orthod Dentofacial Orthop.* 2011;**140**:182-8.

72 Baume RM, Buschang PH, Weinstein S. Stature, head height, and growth of the vertical face. *Am J Orthod.* 1983;**83**:477–84.

73 Tanner JM, Cameron N. Investigation of the mid-growth spurt in height, weight and limb circumferences in single-year velocity data from the London, 1966–67 growth survey. *Ann Hum Biol.* 1980;**7**:565–77.

74 Gasser T, Müller HG, Köhler W, Prader A, Largo R, Molinari L. An analysis of the mid-growth and adolescent spurts of height based on acceleration. *Ann Hum Biol.* 1985;**12**:129–48.

75 Molinari L, Largo RH, Prader A. Analysis of the growth spurt at age seven (mid-growth spurt). *Helv Paediatr Acta.* 1980;**35**:325–34.

76 Sheehy A, Gasser T, Molinari L, Largo RH. An analysis of variance of the pubertal and midgrowth spurts for length and width. *Ann Hum Biol.* 1999;**26**:309–31.

77 Buschang PH, Tanguay R, Demirjian A, LaPalme L, Turkewicz J. Mathematical models of longitudinal mandibular growth for children with normal and untreated Class II, division 1 malocclusion. *Eur J Orthod.* 1988;**10**:227–34.

78 Proffit WR, Fields HW Jr, Sarver DM, editors. *Contemporary orthodontics.* 4th ed. St. Louis: Mosby Elsevier Health Sciences; 2007.

79 Hartsfield, J.K., Jr. Genetics and orthodontics. In: Graber LW, Vanarsdall RL, Vig KWL, editors. *Orthodontics: current principles and techniques.* 5th ed. St. Louis: Elsevier Mosby; 2011. pp. 139–56.

80 Nielsen IL. Vertical malocclusions: etiology, development, diagnosis and some aspects of treatment. *Angle Orthod.* 1991;**61**:247–60.

81 Solow B, Kreiborg S. Soft-tissue stretching: a possible control factor in craniofacial morphogenesis. *Scand J Dent Res.* 1977;**85**:505–7.

82 Linder-Aronson S. Adenoids: their effect on mode of breathing and nasal airflow and their relationship to characteristics of the facial skeleton and the dentition. A biometric, rhino-manometric and cephalometro-radiographic study on children with and without adenoids. *Acta Otolaryngol Suppl.* 1970;**265**:1–132.

83 Linder-Aronson S Respiratory function in relation to facial morphology and the dentition. *Br J Orthod.* 1979;**6**:59–71.

84 Solow B, Siersbæk-Nielsen S, Greve E. Airway adequacy, head posture, and craniofacial morphology. *Am J Orthod.* 1984;**86**:214–23.

85 Behlfelt K, Linder-Aronson S, McWilliam J, Neander P, Laage-Hellman J. Craniofacial morphology in children with and without enlarged tonsils. *Eur J Orthod.* 1990;**12**:233–43.

86 Vig KW. Nasal obstruction and facial growth: the strength of evidence for clinical assumptions. *Am J Orthod Dentofacial Orthop.* 1998;**113**:603–11.

87 Peltomäki T. The effect of mode of breathing on craniofacial growth—revisited. *Eur J Orthod.* 2007;**29**:426–9.

88 Vogl C, Atchley WR, Cowley DE, Crenshaw P, Murray JD, Pomp D. The epigenetic influence of growth hormone on skeletal development. *Growth Dev Aging.* 1993;**57**:163–82.

89 Yamaguchi T, Maki K, Shibasaki Y. Growth hormone receptor gene variant and mandibular height in the normal Japanese population. *Am J Orthod Dentofacial Orthop.* 2001;**119**:650–3.

90 Zhou J, Lu Y, Gao XH, Chen YC, Lu JJ, Bai YX, et al. The growth hormone receptor gene is associated with mandibular height in a Chinese population. *J Dent Res.* 2005;**84**:1052–6.

91 Tomoyasu Y, Yamaguchi T, Tajima A, Nakajima T, Inoue I, Maki K. Further evidence for an association between mandibular height and the growth hormone receptor gene in a Japanese population. *Am J Orthod Dentofacial Orthop.* 2009;**136**:536–41.

92 van Spronsen PH. Long-face craniofacial morphology: cause or effect of weak masticatory musculature? *Semin Orthod.* 2010;**16**:99–117.

93 Buschang PH, Heider J, Carrillo R. The morphological characteristics, growth and etiology of the hyperdivergent phenotype. *Semin Orthod.* 2013;**19**:212–26.

94 Björk A. Variations in the growth pattern of the human mandible: longitudinal radiographic study by the implant method. *J Dent Res.* 1963;**42** Pt.2:400–11.

95 Björk A, Skieller V. Facial development and tooth eruption. An implant study at the age of puberty. *Am J Orthod.* 1972;**62**:339–83.

96 Odegaard J. Growth of the mandible studied with the aid of metal implant. *Am J Orthod.* 1970;**57**:145–57.

97 Odegaard J. Mandibular rotation studies with the aid of metal implants. *Am J Orthod.* 1970;**58**:448–54.

98 Lavergne J, Gasson N. Operational definitions of mandibular morphogenetic and positional rotations. *Scand J Dent Res.* 1977;**85**:185–92.

99 Sinclair PM, Little RM. Dentofacial maturation of untreated normals. *Am J Orthod.* 1985;**88**:146–56.

100 Lavergne J, Gasson N. Direction and intensity of mandibular rotation in the sagittal adjustment during growth of the jaws. *Scand J Dent Res.* 1977;**85**:193–6.

101 Buschang PH, Gandini Jr. LG. Mandibular skeletal growth and modelling between 10 and 15 years of age. *Eur J Orthod.* 2002;**24**:69–79.

102 Mojdehi M, Buschang PH, English JD, Wolford LM. Postsurgical growth changes in the mandible of adolescents with vertical maxillary excess growth pattern. *Am J Orthod Dentofacial Orthop.* 2001;**119**:106–16.

103 Kim J, Nielsen IL. A longitudinal study of condylar growth and mandibular rotation in untreated subjects with Class II malocclusion. *Angle Orthod.* 2002;**72**:105–11.

104 Björk A. Prediction of mandibular growth rotation. *Am J Orthod.* 1969;**55**:585–99.

105 Baumrind S, Korn EL, West EE. Prediction of mandibular rotation: an empirical test of clinician performance. *Am J Orthod.* 1984;**86**:371–85.

106 Leslie LR, Southard TE, Southard KA, Casko JS, Jakobsen JR, Tolley EA, et al. Prediction of mandibular growth rotation: assessment of the Skieller, Björk, and Linde-Hansen method. *Am J Orthod Dentofacial Orthop.* 1998;**114**:659–67.

107 Nanda SK. Growth patterns in subjects with long and short faces. *Am J Orthod Dentofacial Orthop.* 1990;**98**:247–58.

108 Isaacson JR, Isaacson RJ, Speidel TM, Worms FW. Extreme variation in vertical facial growth and associated variation in skeletal and dental relations. *Angle Orthod.* 1971;**41**:219–29.

109 Kuitert R, Beckmann S, van Loenen M, Tuinzing B, Zentner A. Dentoalveolar compensation in subjects with vertical skeletal dysplasia. *Am J Orthod Dentofacial Orthop.* 2006;**129**:649–57.

110 Janson GR, Metaxas A, Woodside DG. Variation in maxillary and mandibular molar and incisor vertical dimension in 12-year-old subjects with excess, normal, and short lower anterior face height. *Am J Orthod Dentofacial Orthop.* 1994;**106**:409–18.

111 Liu SS, Buschang PH. How does tooth eruption relate to vertical mandibular growth displacement? *Am J Orthod Dentofacial Orthop.* 2011;**139**:745–51.

112 Alexander RG. The effects on tooth position and maxillofacial vertical growth during treatment of scoliosis with the Milwaukee brace. *Am J Orthod.* 1966;**52**:161–89.

113 Elder, JR, Tuenge RH, Cephalometric and histologic changes produced by extra-oral high-pull traction to the maxilla in Macaca mulatta. *Am J Orthod.* 1974;**66**:599–616.

114 Stöckli PW, Willert HG. Tissue reactions in the temporomandibular joint resulting from anterior displacement of the mandible in the monkey. *Am J Orthod.* 1971;**60**:142–55.

115 Woodside DG., Metaxas A., Altuna G. The influence of functional appliance therapy on glenoid fossa remodeling. *Am J Orthod Dentofacial Orthop.* 1987;**92**:181–98.

116 Voudouris JC, Woodside DG, Altuna G, Angelopoulos G, Bourque PJ, Lacouture CY. Condyle-fossa modifications and muscle interactions during Herbst treatment, Part 2. Results and conclusions. *Am J Orthod Dentofacial Orthop.* 2003;**124**:13–29.

117 Bishara SE, Cummins DM, Zaher AR. Treatment and posttreatment changes in patients with Class II, Division 1 malocclusion after extraction and nonextraction treatment. *Am J Orthod Dentofacial Orthop.* 1997;**111**:18–27.

118 Ritucci R, Nanda R. The effect of chin cup therapy on the growth and development of the cranial base and midface. *Am J Orthod Dentofacial Orthop.* 1986;**90**:475–83.

119 McNamara JA Jr, Bryan FA. Long-term mandibular adaptations to protrusive function: an experimental study in Macaca mulatta. *Am J Orthod Dentofacial Orthop.* 1987;**92**:98–108.

120 Pancherz H. The effects, limitations, and long-term dentofacial adaptations to treatment with the Herbst appliance. *Semin Orthod.* 1997;**3**:232–43.

121 Konik M, Pancherz H, Hansen K. The mechanism of Class II correction in late Herbst treatment. *Am J Orthod Dentofacial Orthop.* 1997;**112**:87–91.

122 Demisch A, Ingervall B, Thüer U. Mandibular displacement in Angle Class II, division 2 malocclusion. *Am J Orthod Dentofacial Orthop.* 1992;**102**:509–18.

123 Marshall WA, Tanner JM: Puberty. In: Falkner F, Tanner J, editors. *Human growth: a comprehensive treatise. Vol. 2, Postnatal growth: neurobiology.* 2nd ed. New York: Plenum Publishing, 1986. pp. 171–203.

124 Brandt S, Safirstein GR. Different extractions for different malocclusions. *Am J Orthod.* 1975;**68**:15–41.

125 Creekmore TD. Where teeth should be positioned in the face and jaws and how to get them there. *J Clin Orthod.* 1997;**31**:586–608.

126 Kim TK, Kim JT, Mah J, Yang WS, Baek SH. First or second premolar extraction effects on facial vertical dimension. *Angle Orthod.* 2005;**75**:177–82.

127 Hwang S, Chung CJ, Choi YJ, Huh JK, Kim KH. Changes in hyoid, tongue and pharyngeal airway after mandibular setback surgery by intraoral vertical ramus osteotomy. *Angle Orthod.* 2010;**80**:302–8.

128 Okeson JP. *Management of temporomandibular disorders and occlusion.* 5th ed. St. Louis: Mosby; 2003.

CHAPTER 2

Dental Deep Bites

Introduction

Jane is a 43-year-old female (Figure 2.1) who presents to you with the chief complaint, "I am concerned with my deep bite and crowding." Her medical history (PMH) and temporomandibular joint (TMJ) evaluations are within the range of normal (WRN). Her periodontal evaluation is WRN and centric relation = centric occlusion (CR=CO). Her past dental history (PDH) includes previous comprehensive orthodontic treatment with extraction of four first premolars as an adolescent. She reports discontinuing orthodontic retainers "a long time ago."

Q: What are your diagnostic findings/problems (vertical dimension only)?

A: See Table 2.1

Q: What is the etiology of Jane's deep bite? How should you examine her to help answer this question?

A: Have her open with her lips slightly parted (Figure 2.2a) and then much wider with cheek retractors (Figure 2.2b).

Q: What do you see?

A: She has excess incisal display when relaxed (Figure 2.2a). She shows 5–6 mm of incisal display as opposed to an ideal of 2–4 mm of incisal display. Her maxillary central incisors are stepped down relative to her posterior occlusion (Figure 2.2b). This is true despite the fact that her maxillary anterior gingival margins (Figure 2.1h) are reasonably positioned relative to each other (central incisor-lateral incisor-canine gingival margins: high–low–high). Also, her mandibular anterior teeth are stepped up significantly relative to her posterior teeth (accentuated curve of Spee, COS).

Q: What other vertical measurement would be helpful?

A: We should measure maxillary lip length at the philtrum. You measure it and find her lip is 22 mm long.

Q: What is a normal range of maxillary lip length?

A: Lip length in a group of normal 13–15-year-old adolescents ranged from 17 to 23 mm (mean 20 mm) for females and 22–26 mm (mean 24 mm) for males [1]. Mean maxillary lip lengths in 18–19-year-old females and males, measured with a different measurement technique, were reported to be about 17 and 18 mm, respectively [2]. By age 30+, this same study reported that the mean female and male lip lengths had both increased to about 19 mm. So, based on either study, Jane's lip length is on the longer side of normal.

Q: What does Jane's lip length, coupled with her stepped down maxillary incisors, mean in terms of anticipated incisal display *after* you level her maxillary arch?

A: Since the maxillary incisors are stepped down relative to the maxillary posterior teeth, we can anticipate that the maxillary incisors will be *intruded* following leveling of the maxillary arch. Consequently, the amount of incisal display will diminish, which is a good thing.

Q: Taking all of these findings/problems together, is Jane's deep bite a *skeletal* deep bite, a *dental* deep bite, or a combination of both?

A: Dental deep bite. Her clinical lower anterior facial height (LAFH) is WRN (soft tissue Glabella—Subnasale=Subnasale–soft tissue Menton), and her cephalometric skeletal LAFH is WRN (LAFH/TAFH = 53%, FMA = 20° and SNMP = 32°). Her *skeleton is vertically normal.* On the other hand, her maxillary incisors are overerupted, as are her mandibular incisors (deep COS). The incisor overlap (deep bite) is due to incisor overeruption.

Q: Jane asks you why her deep bite developed. What explanation can you give her?

A: By and large, teeth continue to erupt throughout life until they meet resistance. We do not know Jane's occlusion when she was placed in retention after her orthodontic treatment. We know she did not wear retainers faithfully. Because Jane is Class II at her canines by 2–3 mm (Figure 2.1g and i), we can assume that her maxillary and mandibular incisors did not contact sometime after her previous orthodontic treatment, so they continued to erupt.

Q: Interestingly, as shown on her cephalometric radiograph (Figure 2.1d), Jane's maxillary incisors have erupted to the point where they are covered by her lower lip. What may this explain?

A: This fact may explain the "uprightness" of her maxillary incisors. The lower lip resting pressure (approximately 2.5 times greater than upper lip resting pressure) is linked to retroclination of the maxillary incisors [3, 4]. In other words, if eruption of the maxillary incisors places their incisal edges well below the lip line, the maxillary incisors will experience significantly more lingually directed pressure than maxillary incisors whose incisal edges are at the lip line. Consequently, her lower lip can push Jane's maxillary incisors to an upright position—and push the lower incisors to an upright position.

Q: How will the fact that Jane has a dental deep bite (versus a skeletal deep bite) affect your treatment plan?

A: *There are really only two ways to treat any deep bite. You can either (i) erupt the posterior teeth or (ii) intrude/procline the anterior teeth.* In Jane's treatment, there is no need to erupt her posterior teeth. In fact, such a movement would rotate her

Orthodontics in the Vertical Dimension: A Case-Based Review, First Edition. Thomas E. Southard, Steven D. Marshall and Laura L. Bonner.

mandible down and back, lengthening her LAFH, which is now normal. Instead, the ideal treatment is to intrude/procline her maxillary central incisors slightly and intrude/procline her mandibular anterior teeth.

Q: What are your vertical treatment goals?
A: To maintain Jane's skeletal vertical dimension, to reduce her labiomental sulcus depth slightly, and to decrease her overbite, OB (address her chief complaint).

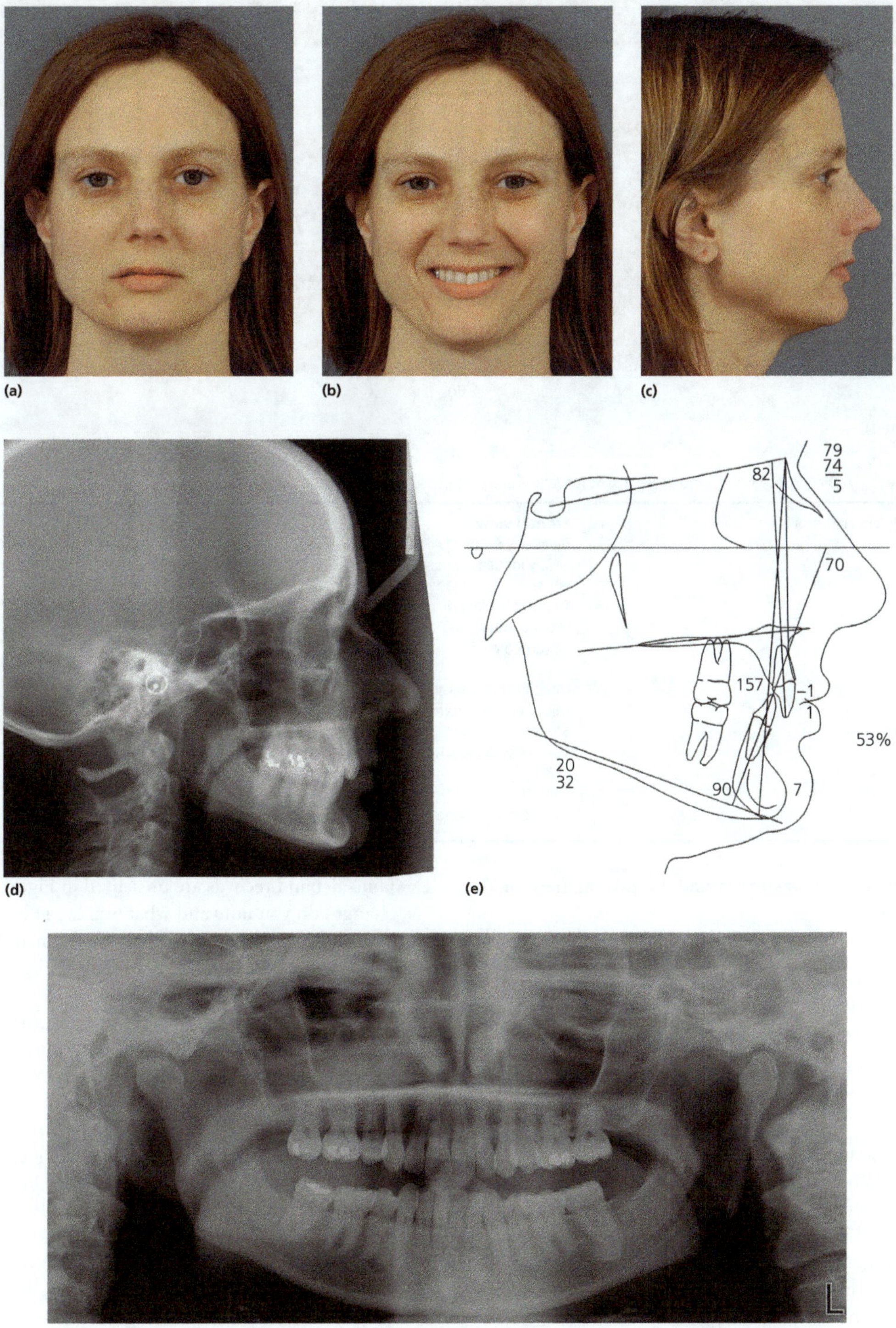

Figure 2.1 Initial records of Jane: (a–c) facial photographs, (d) lateral cephalograph, (e) cephalometric tracing, (f) pantomograph, and (g–k) intraoral photographs.

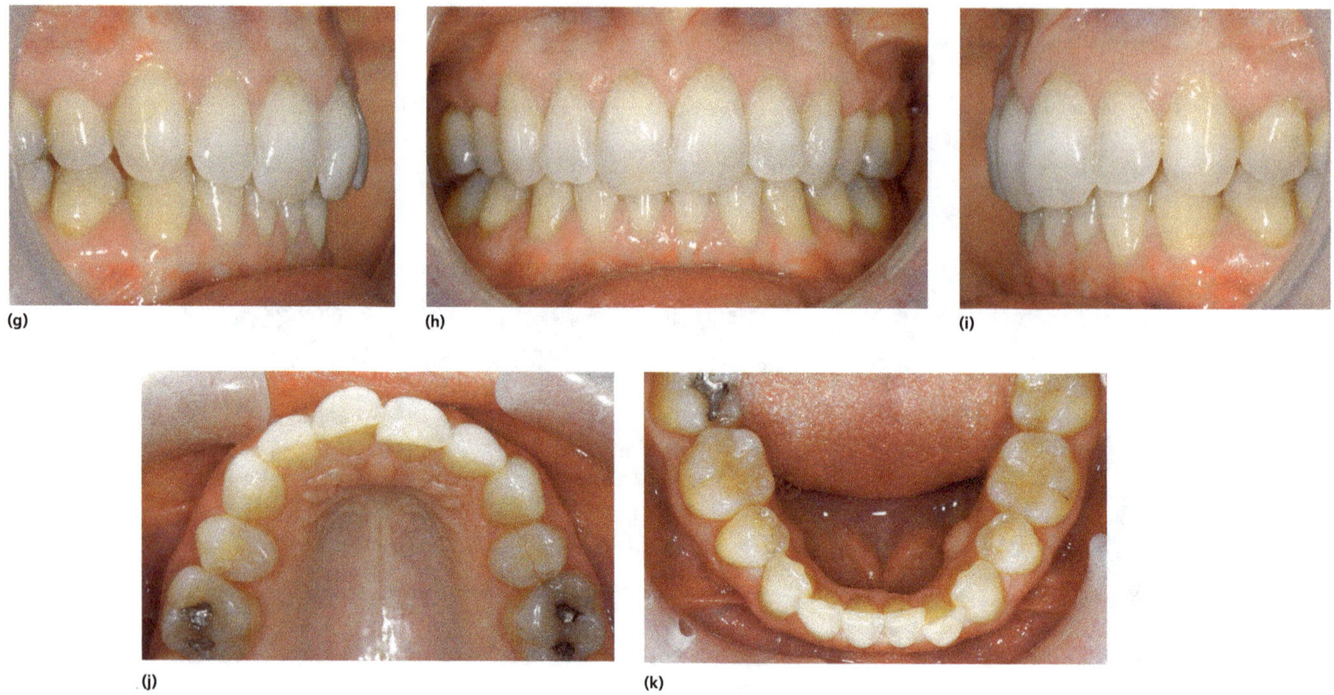

Figure 2.1 (Continued)

Table 2.1 Diagnostic findings and problems list for Jane (vertical dimension only).

Full face and profile	**Frontal view** Relatively normal LAFH (soft tissue Glabella–Subnasale = Subnasale–soft tissue Menton) Mildly inadequate display during posed smile (maxillary incisors not fully exposed) Lower lip vermillion covers the maxillary central incisor incisal edges Asymmetric lip pull during smile (left commissure slightly elevated) **Profile view** Upturned nose Obtuse NLA Deep labiomental sulcus Mildly everted lower lip
Ceph analysis	**Skeletal** Vertical skeletal WRN (LAFH/TAFH = 53%, FMA = 20°, SNMP = 32°)
Radiographs	WRN
Intraoral photos and models	OB: 60% Deep curve of Spee

Q: Is there a possible need for surgery and should you mention this possibility to Jane?
A: No.

Q: What unknowns do you face in treating Jane's vertical dimension? Specifically, are there any unknowns you should eliminate before irreversible treatment is initiated?
A: No. Her only unknowns are the presence of a (small) undetected vertical shift and compliance. However, these will not impact treatment.

Q: How do you wish to proceed with treatment?
A: Jane was treated non-extraction. Fixed appliances were placed in Jane's maxillary arch, and overjet, OJ (to provide space for bonding the mandibular incisors) was created by intrusion of the maxillary incisors (leveling the maxillary arch) and by trapping open-coil springs between the maxillary canines and maxillary lateral incisors. When OJ was adequate, the mandibular arch was banded/bonded. Both arches were leveled and aligned. Class II elastics were used to improve Jane's Class II relationship. Arches were coordinated and finished. Jane was debanded.

Q: Jane's deband records are presented in Figure 2.3. What vertical changes do you note and what was the effect of treatment?
A: Vertical changes and treatment effects include the following:
- Vertical dimension was maintained (Figure 2.3a and b versus Figure 2.1a and b).
- Mandibular plane has rotated down and back slightly (Figure 2.3f), following slight eruption of mandibular molars (with mandibular COS leveling, Figure 2.2b).
- Maxillary incisors intruded slightly (Figure 2.3f).
- Mandibular incisors intruded and proclined.
- Labiomental sulcus appears to have opened on the cephalometric superimposition (Figure 2.3f) but does not appear to have opened when viewed clinically (Figure 2.3c versus Figure 2.1c).
- OB reduced from 60 to 10% (Figure 2.1h versus Figure 2.3i).

Q: Were your vertical treatment goals achieved?
A: Yes and no. Although her vertical dimension was maintained and OB was decreased (her chief complaint), her labiomental sulcus depth did not improve clinically.

Q: How was Jane's deep bite corrected?

A: Her deep bite was corrected through the following:

- Slight posterior tooth eruption resulting in downward and backward rotation of her mandibular plane
- Maxillary incisor intrusion
- Mandibular incisor intrusion and proclination

Q: We anticipated that the amount of maxillary incisal display in a posed smile would diminish after leveling the maxillary arch. Did it diminish (Figure 2.3b versus Figure 2.1b)?

A: Not noticeably. The amount of incisor display and gingival display shown by a patient is dependent not only on structure (bone, teeth, and soft tissue) but also on function (facial muscle activity). On average, subjects can reproduce a natural smile at different sessions within 1 mm, with the upper lip showing more variation than the lower lip [5]. In Jane, these factors may have contributed to a change in incisal display not being noticeable after treatment (although the maxillary incisal edges do appear to have intruded by about 1 mm, Figure 2.3f).

Q: Jane asks you if you can tell her what will happen to her incisal display as she ages. What can you say?

A: You can tell her that during the third and fourth decades upper lip length increase exceeds skeletal length increase by approximately 1 mm [6]. So, she can expect less incisal display with age.

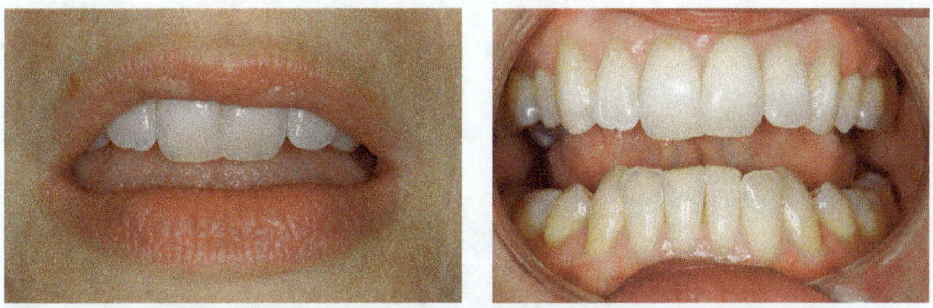

(a) (b)

Figure 2.2 Initial records of Jane: (a) incisal display with lips at rest and (b) intraoral view with teeth apart.

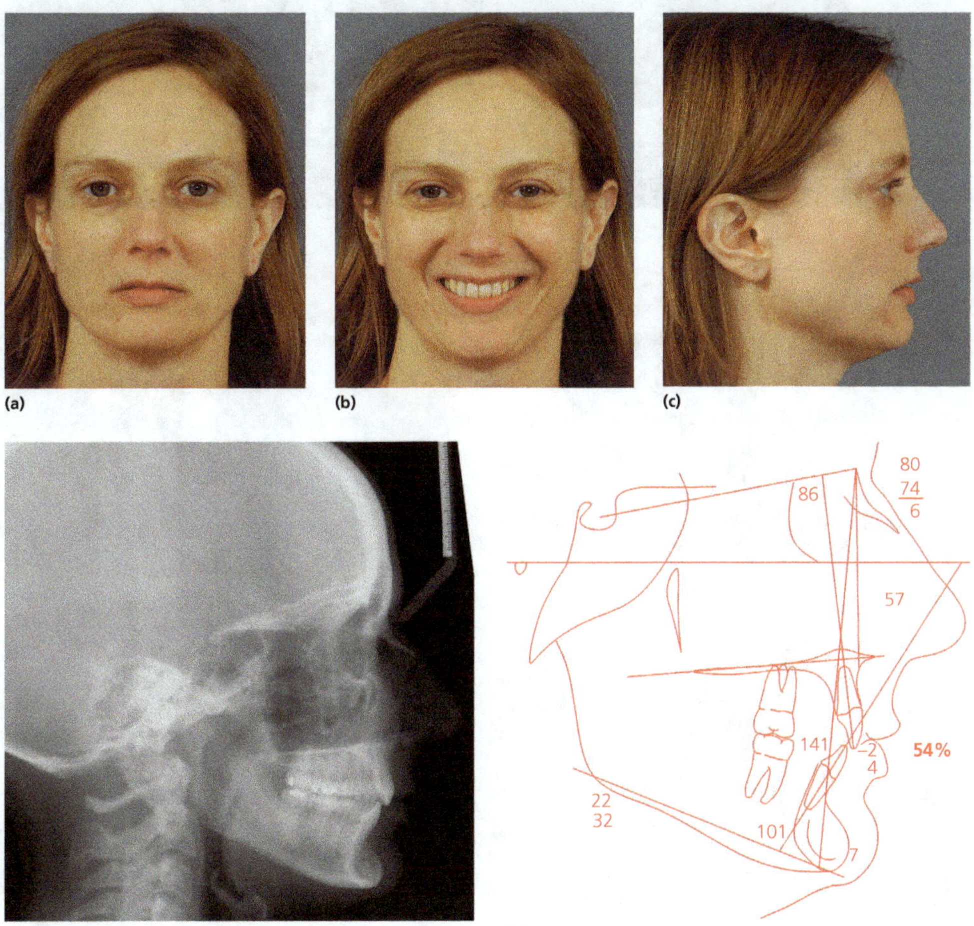

Figure 2.3 (a–l) Deband records of Jane.

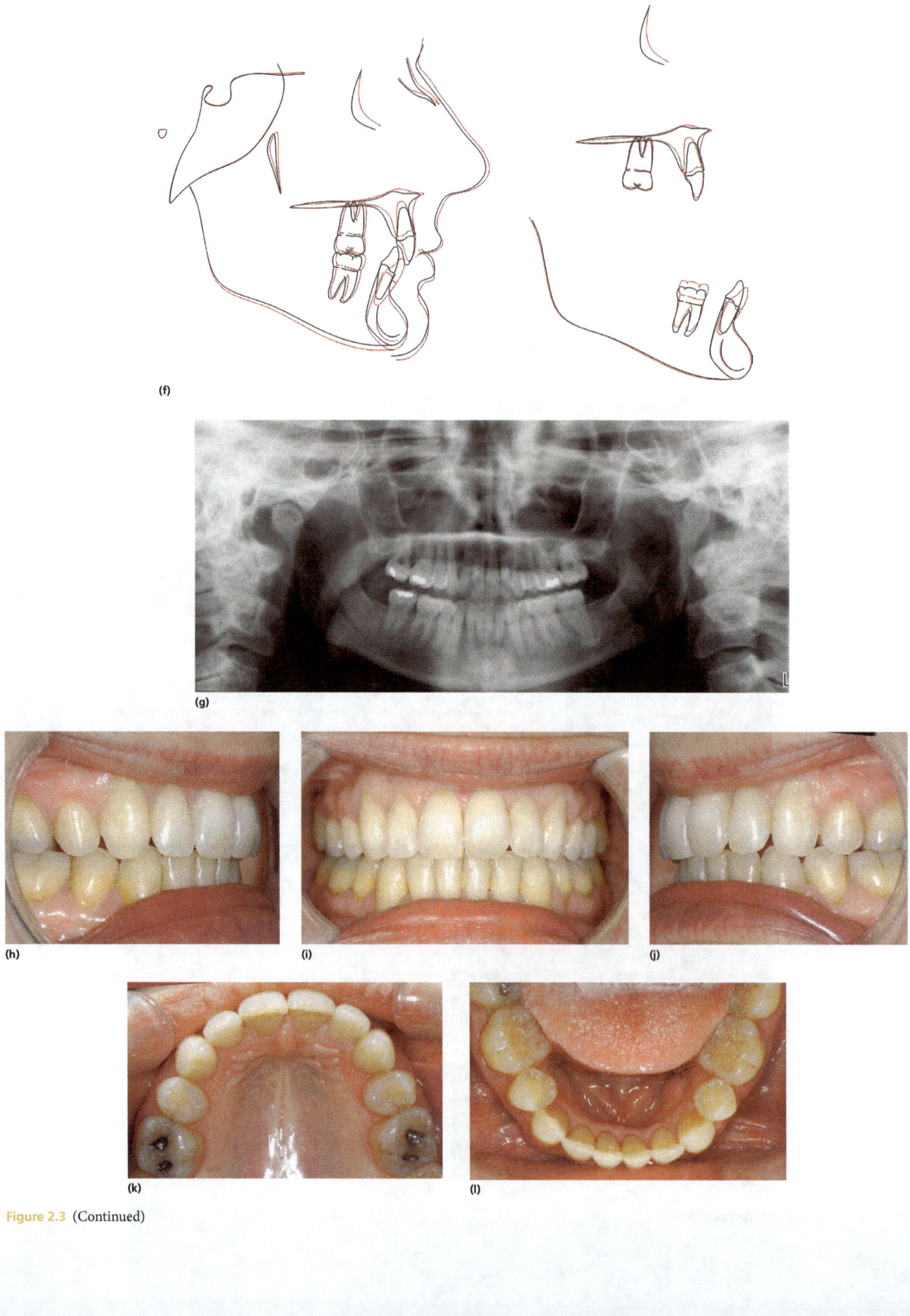

Figure 2.3 (Continued)

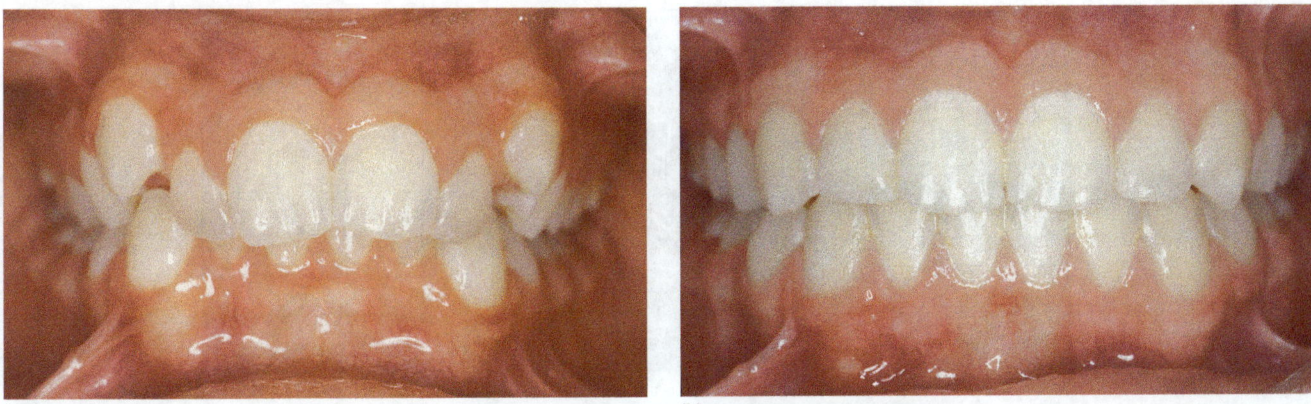

(a) (b)

Figure 2.4 Deep bite correction example: (a) initial OB of 70–80% and (b) following treatment OB of 10%.

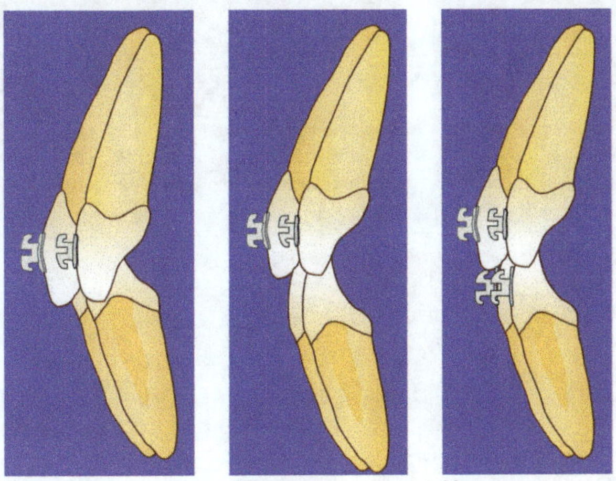

(a) (b) (c)

Figure 2.5 Opening a deep bite to permit bonding of mandibular anterior teeth: (a) initial deep bite with inadequate room for mandibular brackets, (b) deep bite corrected, and (c) mandibular brackets placed.

Q: Are there any "take-home" pearls from this case that you can carry into practice?

A: Yes, take-home pearls include the following:

- Pure dental deep bite patients have normal vertical skeletal relationships (normal vertical development).
- Dental deep bites result from overeruption (and uprighting) of maxillary and/or mandibular incisors.
- Dental deep bites are treated, ideally, by intruding overerupted anterior teeth and proclining upright anterior teeth.
- Intruding overerupted anterior teeth, with fixed orthodontic appliances and archwires, may be accompanied by reciprocal eruption of posterior teeth and changes in vertical dimension as the mandible rotates down and back (unless TADs are used intrude the anterior teeth, or TADs are used to prevent posterior tooth eruption).

Q: The deep bite in Figure 2.4a was opened as part of treatment (Figure 2.4b). List the reasons for correcting (opening) deep bites such as this.

A: Reasons for correcting (opening) deep bites:

- Create OJ to bond mandibular anterior teeth. In the presence of a deep bite (Figure 2.5a), inadequate OJ exists to place brackets on the mandibular incisors. The bite must be opened (Figure 2.5b) in order to bond the mandibular anterior teeth (Figure 2.5c).

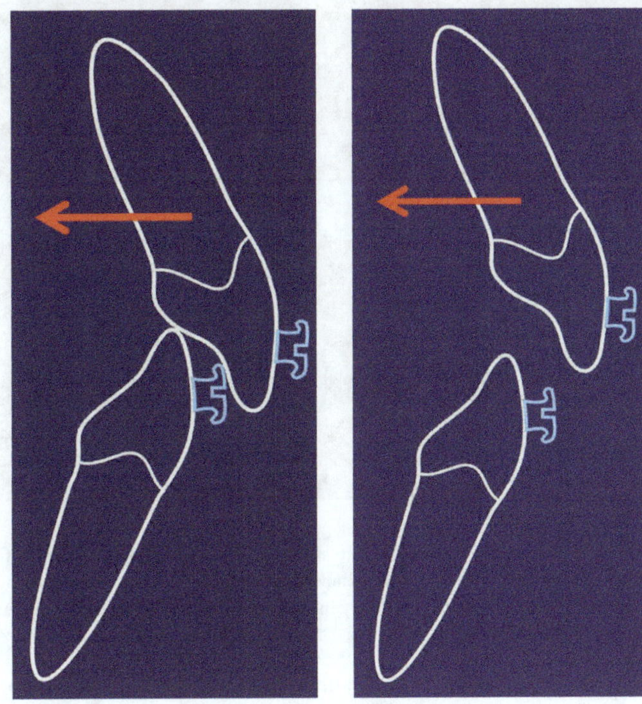

(a) (b)

Figure 2.6 Opening a deep bite to create OJ for maxillary incisor retraction: (a) deep bite with inadequate OJ to retract maxillary incisors and (b) deep bite correction creates OJ for maxillary incisor retraction.

- Create OJ to permit maxillary incisor retraction. In the presence of a deep bite (Figure 2.6a), the maxillary incisors hit the mandibular brackets during incisor retraction (maxillary space closure). The bite must be opened (Figure 2.6b) to create enough OJ to permit maxillary incisor retraction.
- Create space to permit restoration of teeth. Some patients exhibit significant bite deepening following maxillary incisor wear and compensatory maxillary incisor eruption (Figure 2.7a left to center). Opening the bite permits space for restorative material (Figure 2.7a, right). Figure 2.7b–d illustrate a deep bite patient with excessive wear and very thin enamel. The bite was opened with fixed appliances (Figure 2.7e) to provide OJ so that the teeth could be restored with composite veneers (Figure 2.7f).

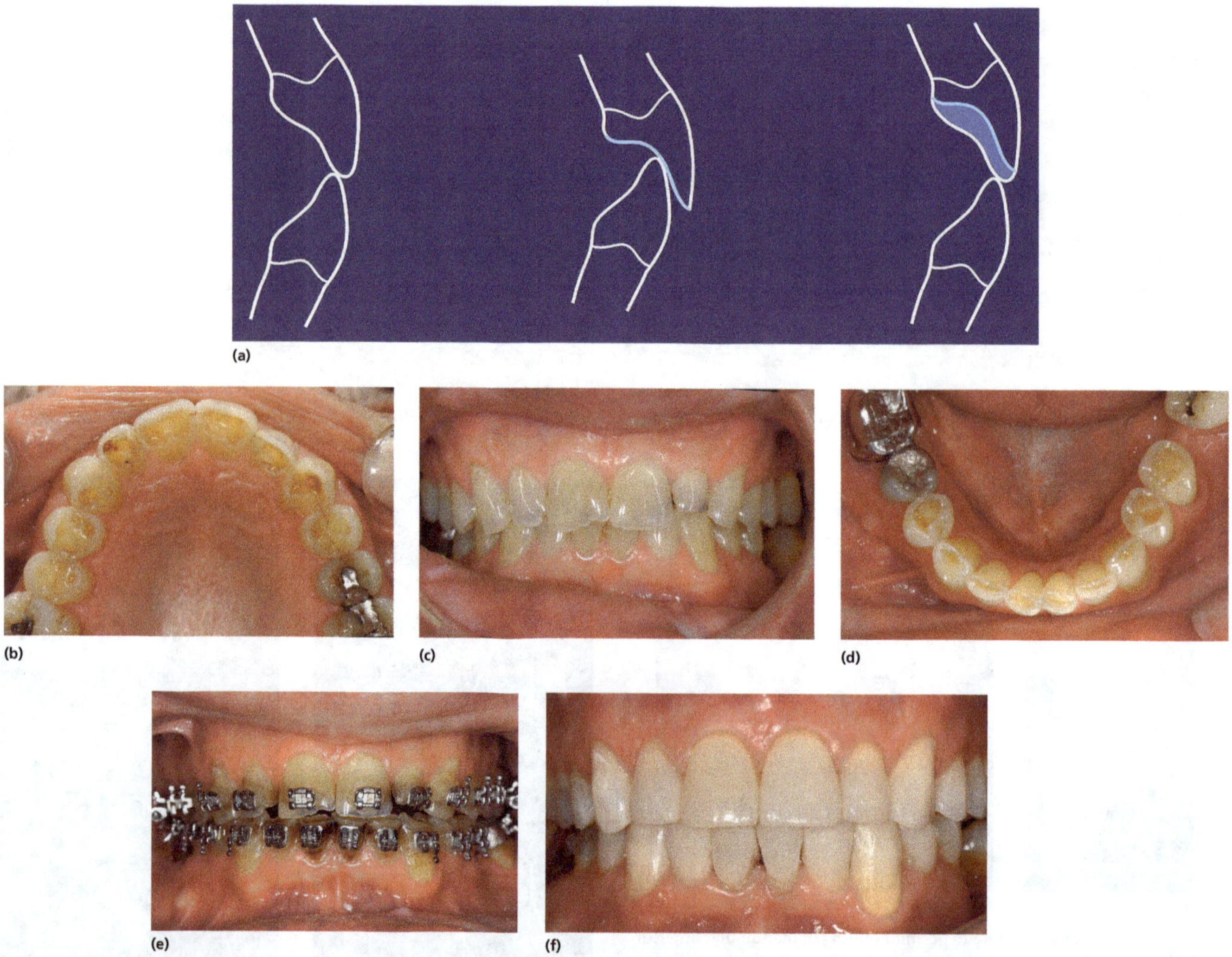

Figure 2.7 Opening a deep bite to create space for restoring badly worn teeth: (a) left-to-right normal OB, deep bite with badly worn maxillary incisors, deep bite corrected with maxillary incisor restored; (b–d) example of patient's initial intraoral photos showing severe wear and deep bite—there is no room on the lingual of the maxillary incisors to restore these teeth; (e) same patient following bite opening; and (f) and following deband/restoration.

- Prevent/reduce tissue trauma. In cases of excessively deep bites—mandibular incisors can impinge on the palate (Figure 2.8a–c) and strip soft tissues lingual to the maxillary incisors or labial to the mandibular incisors (Figure 2.8d and e).
- Resolve lip trapping. "Trapping" of the mandibular lip, with a resulting deep labiomental sulcus, can be seen in some patients with deep bites (Figure 2.9). Correcting the deep bite can resolve the lip trapping and open up the deep labiomental sulcus.

Q: COS depth (Figure 2.10a and b) is of significant interest during deep bite correction. Why?

A: Because *deep bites usually result, in part, from a deep COS (overeruption of mandibular incisors).* Leveling (flattening) of the COS helps open a deep bite by eruption of posterior teeth (rotating the mandible down and back), intruding anterior teeth, and proclining anterior teeth.

Q: How and when does the COS develop?

A: The COS develops from differential eruption of the teeth during growth. Specifically, Marshall et al. [7] reported that the COS is minimal in the primary dentition, increases to an average depth of 1.3 mm at the time permanent mandibular first molars and central incisors erupt (Figure 2.11, left red arrow), and increases again to 2.2 mm at the time permanent mandibular second molars erupt (Figure 2.11, right red arrow).

Q: Human beings naturally have a COS. So why does it make sense to level the COS during orthodontic treatment?

A: The COS found in deep bite patients is typically exaggerated. For example, the COS in Figure 2.12 is 3–4 mm deep, far deeper than a normal depth of 2 mm. It is reasonable to level such exaggerated curves if doing so can benefit treatment.

Q: Is the COS depth related to skeletal (cephalometric) factors?

A: Yes, an increase in the COS depth is related to a decrease in SNB angle [8]. This makes sense, since a decrease in SNB angle means the patient is more Class II—so there is a greater chance that the mandibular incisors are unopposed by the maxillary incisors (and free to erupt, deepening the COS).

Q: Does a deep bite "lock" the mandible back in Class II patients, preventing mandibular forward growth? In other words, does

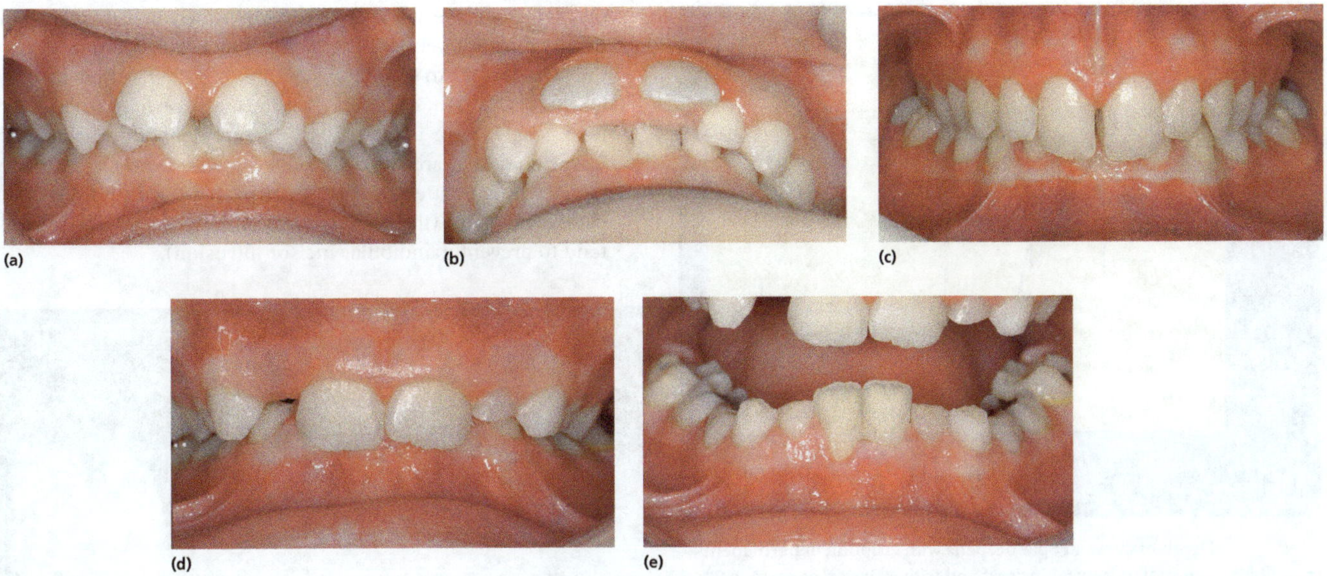

Figure 2.8 Deep bites can affect soft tissue: (a–c) mandibular incisors can bite into palate and (d and e) maxillary incisors can strip mandibular incisor labial gingiva.

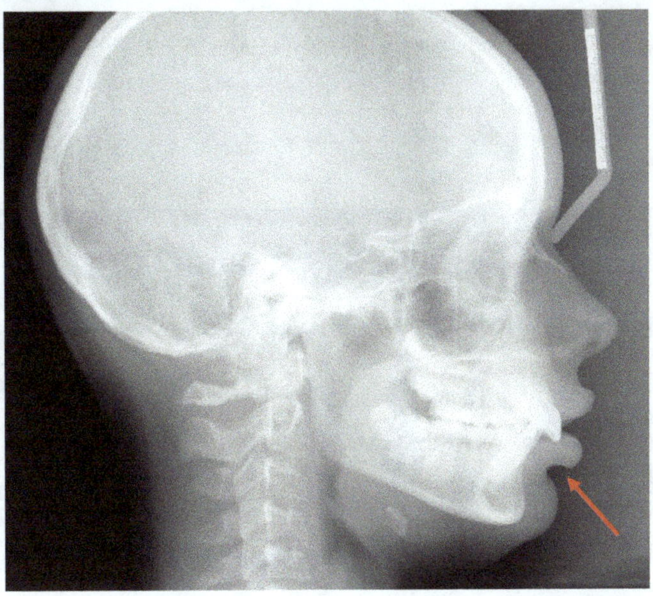

Figure 2.9 Deep bite resulting in lip "trapping" and a deep labiomental sulcus.

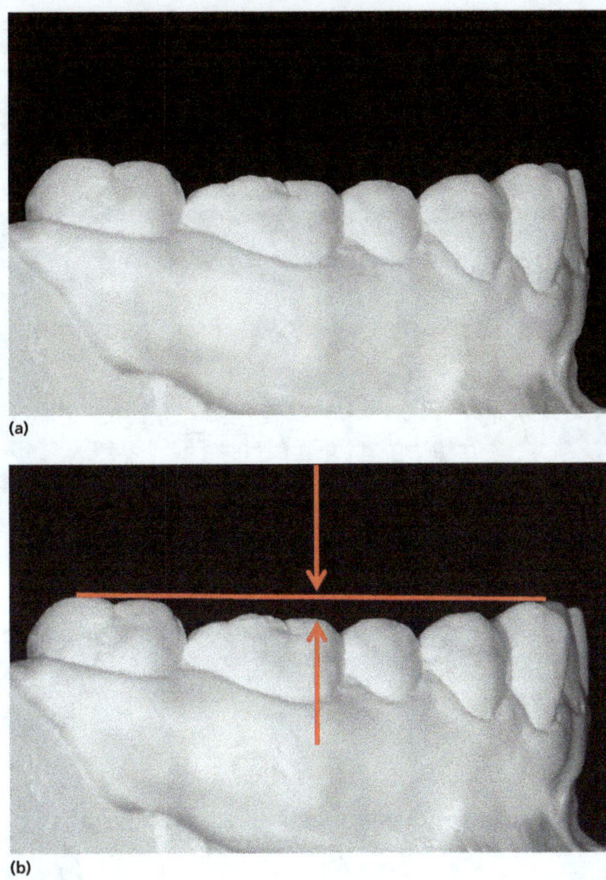

Figure 2.10 (a, b) Measurement of the curve of Spee depth.

unlocking (opening) a deep bite in Class II patients result in the mandible moving forward?

A: No. Demisch et al. [9] reported that incisor proclination (deep bite correction) did *not* result in mandibular anterior positioning to a more Class I relationship. In fact, Ingervall [10–12] reported that mandibular-deficient Class II division 2 children tended to already posture their mandibles forward compared to children with normal occlusions.

Q: How much incisor intrusion occurs during arch leveling?

A: This is a trick question. Incisors are not always intruded during arch leveling. Incisors may actually be extruded during leveling. Whether incisors are intruded or extruded during arch leveling with fixed orthodontic appliances and archwires is dependent on the incisor bracket slot positions relative to posterior tooth bracket slot positions. If the incisor bracket slots are *incisal* to the posterior tooth slots (Figure 2.13a and b), then the archwire is deflected incisally into the incisor brackets and the incisors will tend to be intruded. If the incisor bracket slots are *apical* to the posterior tooth slots (Figure 2.13c and d), then the archwire is deflected apically into the incisor brackets and the incisors will tend to be extruded.

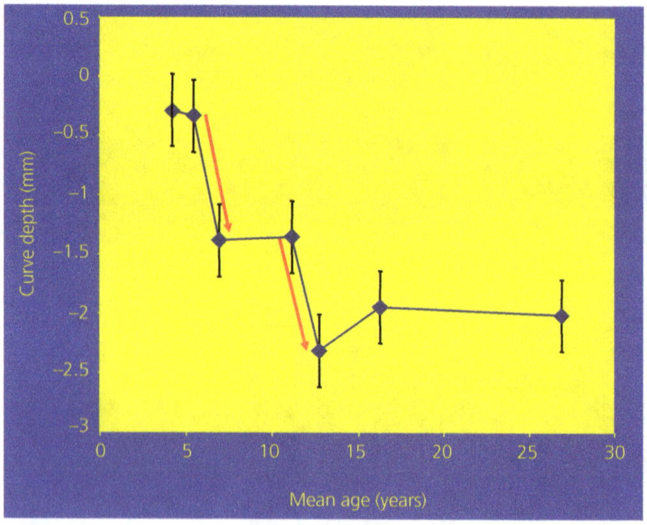

Figure 2.11 Depth of curve of Spee deepens with eruption of permanent mandibular first molars/central incisors and with eruption of permanent mandibular second molars [7]. (Marshall SD, Caspersen M, Hardinger RR, Franciscus RG, Aquilino SA, Southard TE. Development of the curve of Spee. Am J Orthod Dentofacial Orthop. 2008;134:344–52. Reprinted with permission from Elsevier.)

Q: Ok, let's rephrase the question. How much incisor intrusion occurs during leveling if the incisor bracket slots are incisal to the posterior tooth slots?

A: This is also a trick question. You must also specify what other biomechanics are in place. For example, mandibular incisor intrusion during arch leveling will be greater if only an archwire is placed—compared to if an archwire is placed plus Class III elastics are worn (the vertical force of the Class III elastics will tend to prevent mandibular incisor intrusion).

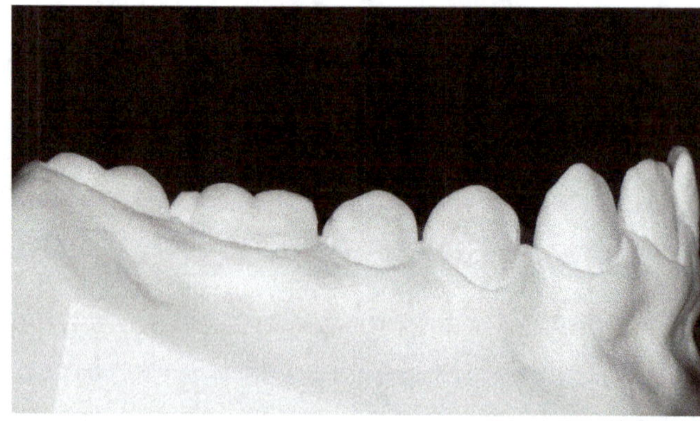

Figure 2.12 An exaggerated curve of Spee (3–4 mm deep).

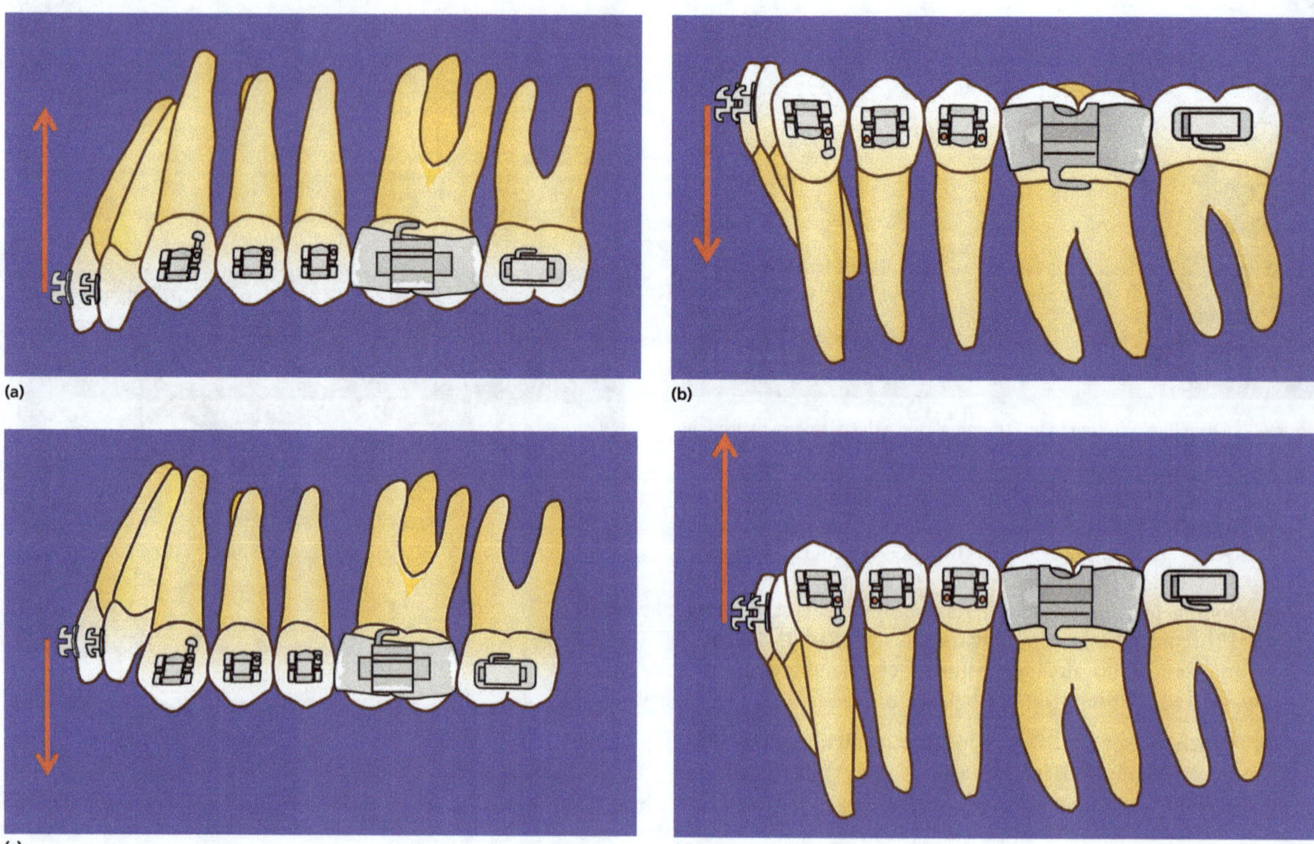

Figure 2.13 Incisor vertical movement during arch leveling: (a and b) if incisor brackets are positioned *incisal* to posterior brackets, then incisors will be intruded by the archwire; and (c and d) if incisor brackets are positioned apical to posterior brackets, then incisors will be extruded.

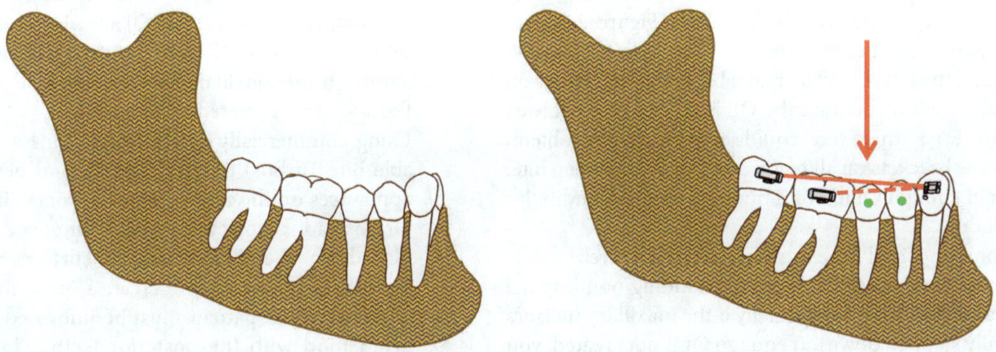

Figure 2.14 Second molars should be banded in deep bite patients: (a) mandibular second molars erupt higher on the ramus than first molars and (b) when second molars are banded, the archwire (solid line) must be deflected further to engage the premolars than if only the first molars are banded (dotted line archwire). So, a deep bite will open more readily if second molars are banded.

Q: Ok, let's rephrase this question one final time. What does the literature state will be the average amount of maxillary and mandibular incisor intrusion (with only archwires in place), if the incisors are stepped up (incisally) relative to the posterior teeth?

A: Maxillary incisor intrusion ranges from 0.26 to 1.88 mm. Mandibular incisor intrusion ranges from −0.19 to 2.84 mm [13].

Q: Although incisor intrusion and proclination tend to level the COS and open deep bites, how does *most* COS leveling occur when using a continuous AW?

A: When measured from the mandibular first molar as the terminal edgewise bracket, leveling the COS with a continuous archwire occurs by extrusion of mandibular premolars [14].

Q: Why would the fact that premolar extrusion plays such an important role in leveling the COS influence your decision to band mandibular second molars in deep bite patients?

A: As shown in Figure 2.14a, mandibular second molars erupt higher in the ramus than do the first molars. If the mandibular second molars are bonded (Figure 2.14b), then the archwire (solid red line) must deflect further to engage the premolar bracket slots (shown as green dots) than if the archwire (dashed red line) extends only to the mandibular first molars. If the second molars are bonded, then the COS flattens more and the deep bite opens more, than if only the first molars are bonded.

Q: What happens to the mandibular molars during COS leveling with an archwire?

A: You would think that deflection of the archwire from the molars apically to the premolar brackets would cause reciprocal intrusion of the molars. However, because the mandibular molars tip toward the mesial in the COS (Figure 2.14a), uprighting them will actually cause their mesial roots to extrude as the molars upright (Figure 2.15), rotating the mandibular plane down/back and opening the bite even more. This is precisely the reason why you should band/bond second molars in deep bite cases but avoid banding/bonding second molars in nonsurgery skeletal open bite cases.

The mandibular third molars erupt on the ramus even higher than the mandibular second molars. So, if the mandibular third molars are bonded, then the archwire is deflected down even more when the premolars are engaged. Figures 2.16a and b illustrate before and after leveling of a mandibular arch (first premolars extracted) when all molars (first, second, and third molars) were banded/bonded.

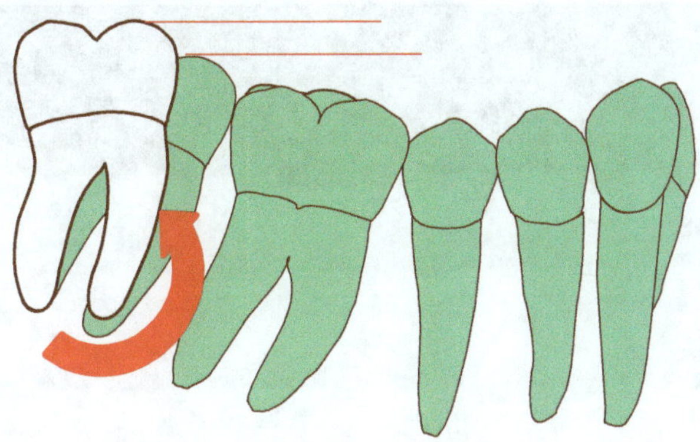

Figure 2.15 Uprighting mesially tipped mandibular molars results in their eruption.

Q: In summary, how is the COS leveled?

A: Premolar eruption, molar uprighting/eruption, incisor intrusion/proclination.

Q: Is leveling the COS (Figure 2.17a and b) stable or prone to relapse?

A: Leveling the COS is stable [15, 16]. Further, initial COS depth is not an indicator of COS relapse [16], and COS relapse has been reported to be greater using removable retainers rather than fixed [17].

Q: If leveling the COS occurs *primarily* by eruption of mandibular premolars, and if eruption of teeth is generally considered the least stable movement, then why is COS leveling stable?

A: Probably because leveling of the COS is one of the first things that is done with orthodontic treatment—and the leveled arch is held in that position for the remainder of treatment (1–1½ years). This apparently gives the tissues adequate time to remodel.

Q: Is there an outcome difference between deep bite treatment at puberty versus before puberty in the mixed dentition versus after growth is complete?

A: Yes, *deep bite treatment (biteplane followed by fixed appliances) results in significantly more favorable outcomes when treated at puberty* in the permanent dentition than when treated before puberty in the mixed dentition [18]. Deep bite correction by eruption of posterior teeth (which is what treatment with an anterior biteplate includes) is questionable in adults and contraindicated in patients with normal or long facial heights.

Q: A patient presents to you with a deep bite (Figure 2.18a–c) resulting, in part, from a deep COS. You wish to level the COS in order to open the bite, but you are unable to place brackets on the mandibular incisors because the OB is 70–80%. List at least five different ways that you could address this problem, eventually place brackets on all teeth, and correct the deep bite.

A: Ways to obtain enough OJ to bond brackets on the mandibular incisors include:

- Banding/bonding and leveling the maxillary arch alone, which may create enough OJ to permit banding/bonding the mandibular anterior teeth (especially if the maxillary incisors were initially stepped down). If enough OJ is not created, you could also trap compressed open coil springs between the maxillary canines and lateral incisors, and advance the incisors. This would create OJ allowing you to bond the mandibular incisors (Figure 2.19a–c). However, with this approach the maxillary incisors must be "round tripped" as the spaces you created are later closed.
- Using commercially available anterior biteplates (e.g., bondable Bite Turbos) to open the bite and permit placing fixed appliances on the mandibular incisors (Figure 2.20a and b). Or, instead, a small amount of composite material could be placed on the etched lingual surfaces of the maxillary incisors (Figure 2.20c) to create a "poor man's" bite plate. In either case, the patient must be informed of the inability to grind food with the posterior teeth. The patient must be advised to cut up food in small pieces and eat slowly and carefully.

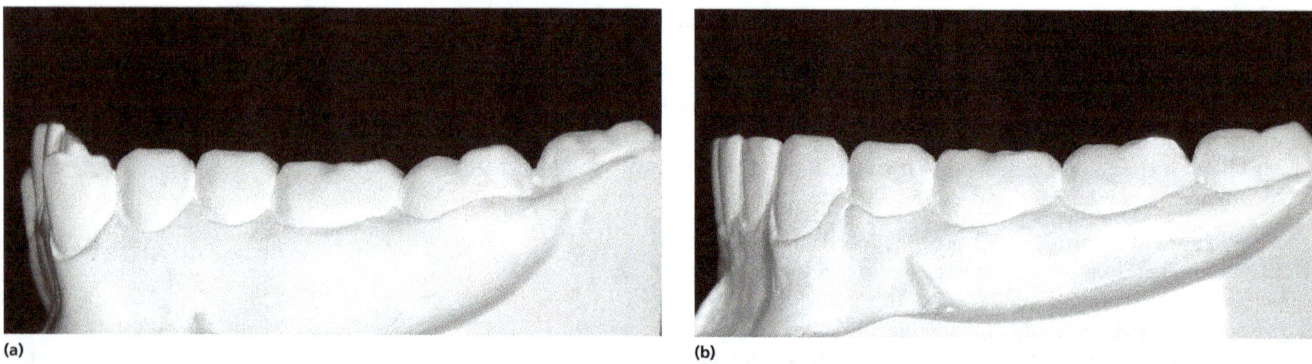

Figure 2.16 Leveling the curve of Spee using second *and* third molars: (a) before and (b) after.

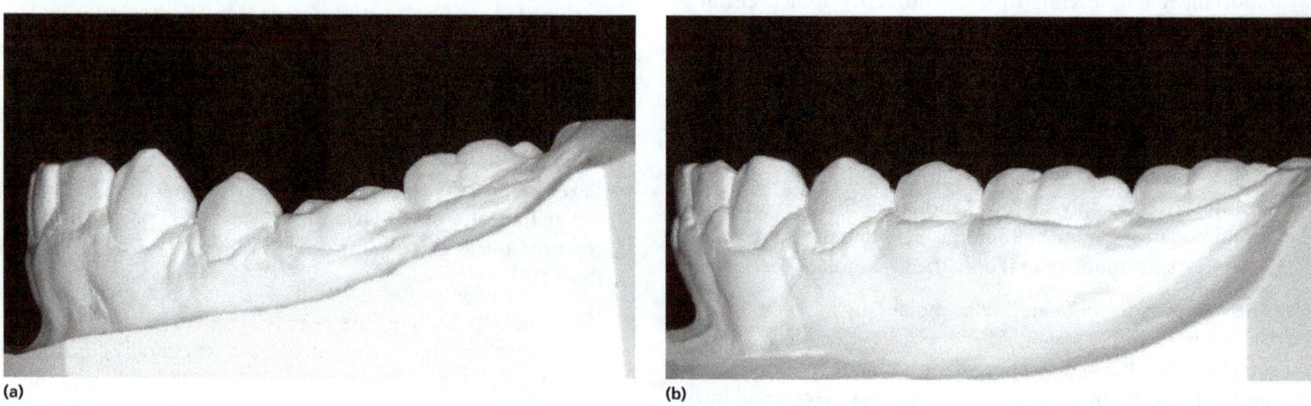

Figure 2.17 Another example of a curve of Spee that was leveled: (a) before and (b) after.

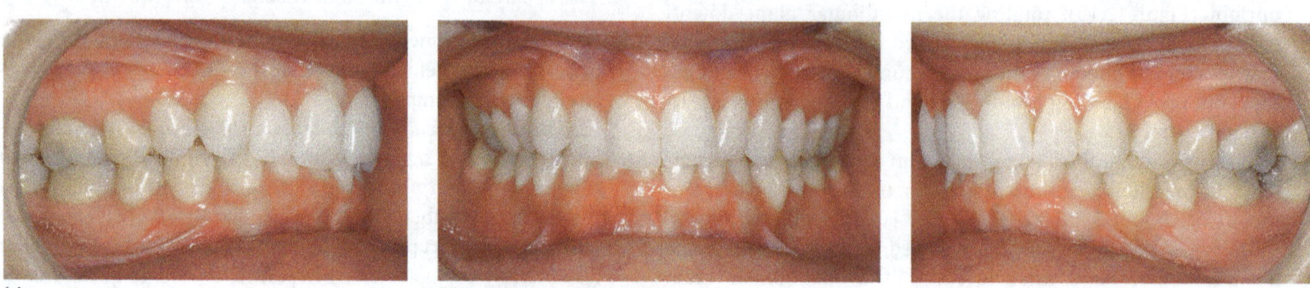

Figure 2.18 (a–c) Deep-bite patient with inadequate OJ to bond mandibular incisors.

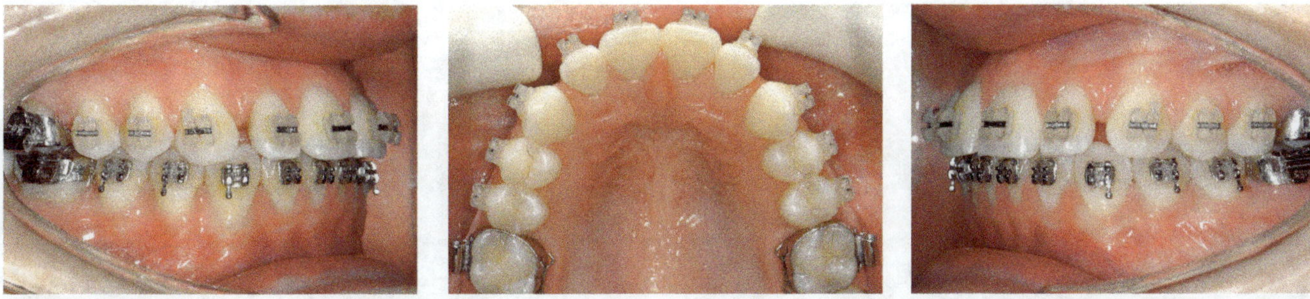

(a) (b) (c)

Figure 2.19 (a–c) Overjet created by proclining maxillary incisors (opening spaces distal to the maxillary lateral incisors), which then allows bonding of mandibular incisors.

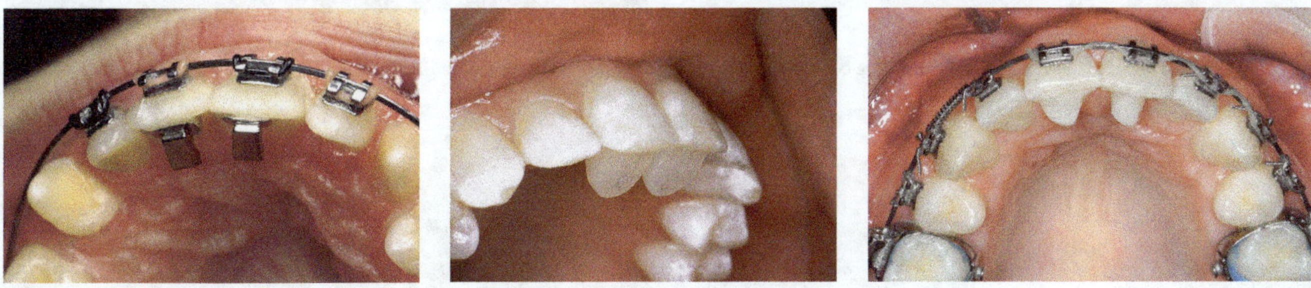

(a) (b) (c)

Figure 2.20 Overjet created by placement of anterior biteplates: (a and b) commercially available biteplates and (c) "poor man's" anterior biteplate formed using composite resin.

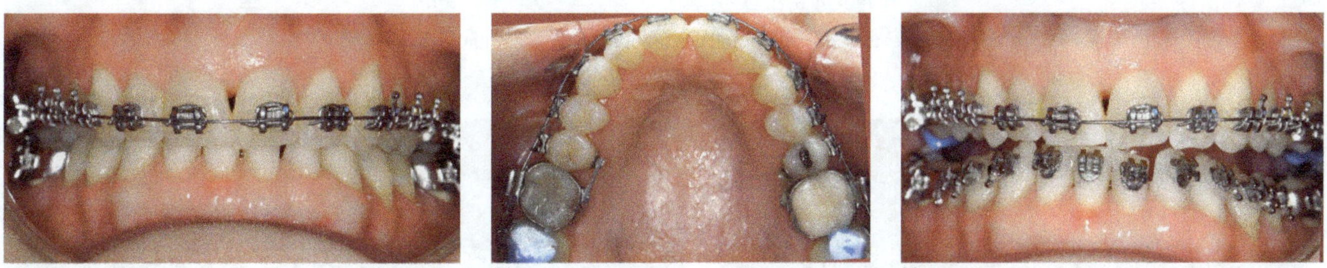

(a) (b) (c)

Figure 2.21 Overjet created by placement of orthodontic banding cement on posterior teeth: (a) inadequate OJ to bond mandibular incisors due to a deep bite, (b) banding cement placed on maxillary second molars to open bite, and (c) results in adequate OJ created to bond mandibular incisors.

- Using light-cured orthodontic banding cement placed on posterior teeth to open the bite and permit bonding of the mandibular incisors (Figure 2.21a–c). But, be sure to inform the patient that he/she will be chewing with only two molars.
- Using Ketac cement (or Triad gel/ropes) in place of orthodontic light-cured banding cement. But, regardless of which cement is used, please remember to place a lubricant on the opposing teeth and to have the patient bite/open into the material repeatedly while it is curing so that the upper and lower jaws do not lock together. In Figure 2.22a, an orthodontic resident placed an exceedingly thick "mandibular Ketac biteplate." Although the mandibular incisors can now be bonded, if this thick biteplate is left in place too long, the posterior teeth will be prevented from erupting and a posterior open bite can result (Figure 2.22b). In this particular growing patient, the posterior teeth should eventually erupt into occlusion—or vertical elastics can be used to help close the posterior open bite. Remember, the Ketac biteplate only needs to be thick enough to create enough OJ so that mandibular incisors can be bonded.
- Placing orthodontic cement on the maxillary canines, instead of on the molars, to open the bite (Figure 2.23a–c). Using this approach, the posterior teeth can erupt, helping to maintain the corrected deep bite when the cement is removed.
- Using a maxillary anterior removable biteplate to disclude the posterior teeth, open the bite, and permit the mandibular anterior teeth to be bonded. With the bite opened, and fixed appliances placed in the lower arch, vertical elastics can be used to erupt the posterior teeth (Figure 2.24a and b).
- Using Guray "bite raisers" (Figure 2.25a), which attach directly to the maxillary molar bands, immediately open the bite, separate the anterior teeth, and permit bonding of the mandibular incisors (Figure 2.25b).

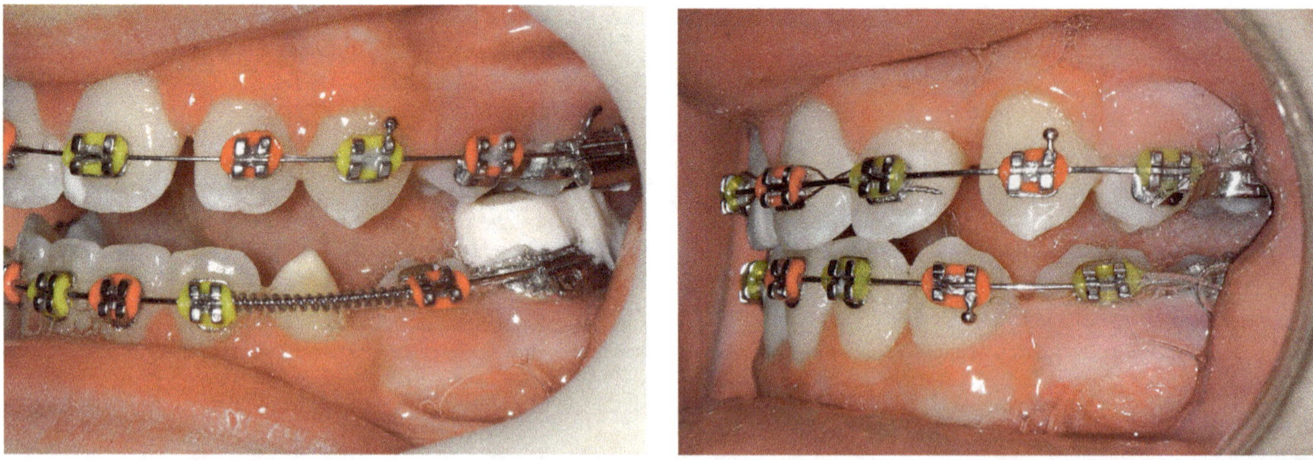

(a) (b)

Figure 2.22 (a) Placement of excessively thick banding cement on mandibular first molars permits bonding mandibular incisors but (b) resulted in a posterior open bite.

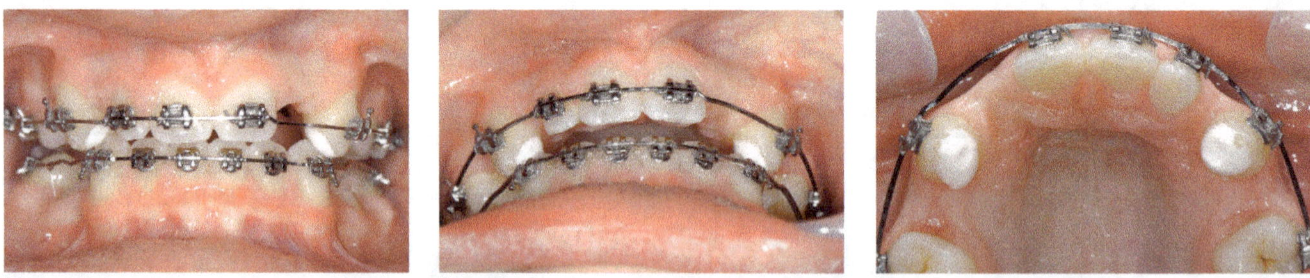

(a) (b) (c)

Figure 2.23 Orthodontic cement placed on canines to open the bite and permit bonding of mandibular incisors.

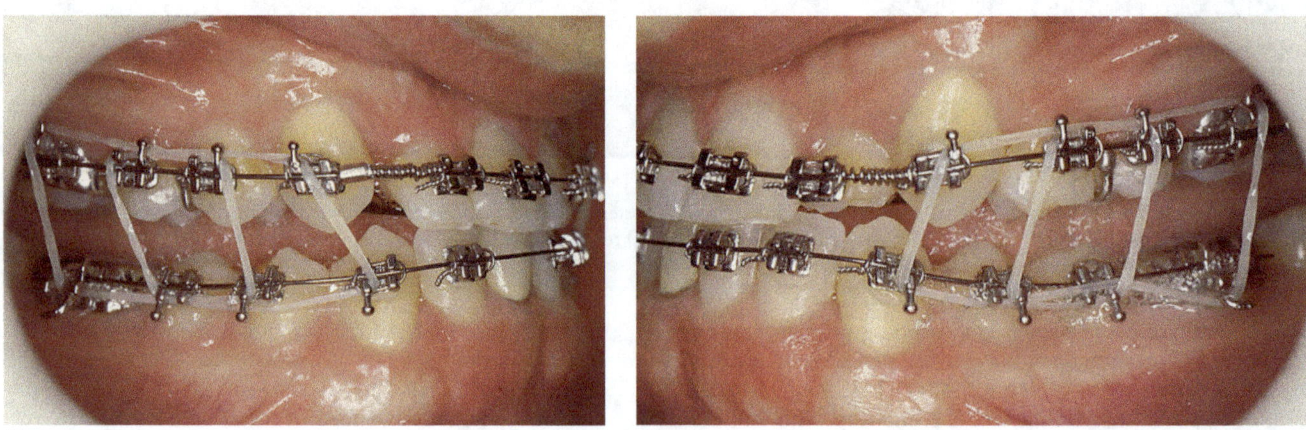

(a) (b)

Figure 2.24 Anterior biteplate used to open the bite for mandibular incisor bonding. Vertical elastics are being used to erupt the posterior teeth.

- Leveling the maxillary arch and the mandibular posterior arch from the mandibular canines to the mandibular second molars—using segmental archwires but without bonding the mandibular incisors (Figure 2.26a–c). Later, as the bite is opened (Figure 2.26d–f), the mandibular incisors are bonded, the arches leveled, and the occlusion finished (Figure 2.26g–i).

Q: What if you use none of the earlier mentioned techniques to create OJ to bond the mandibular incisors? What if you just bond the lower incisors when there is not enough OJ to bond them—so the patient ends up occluding on the lower incisor brackets as he/she bites? What will happen to the patient with this "bracket anterior biteplate"?

A: One of three outcomes will occur (two are bad): (i) the mandibular brackets will be popped off by the maxillary teeth, (ii) the mandibular brackets will wear off enamel from the maxillary teeth, or (iii) the mandibular brackets will indeed act as a biteplate—permitting the arch to be leveled. It is difficult to predict which outcome will occur.

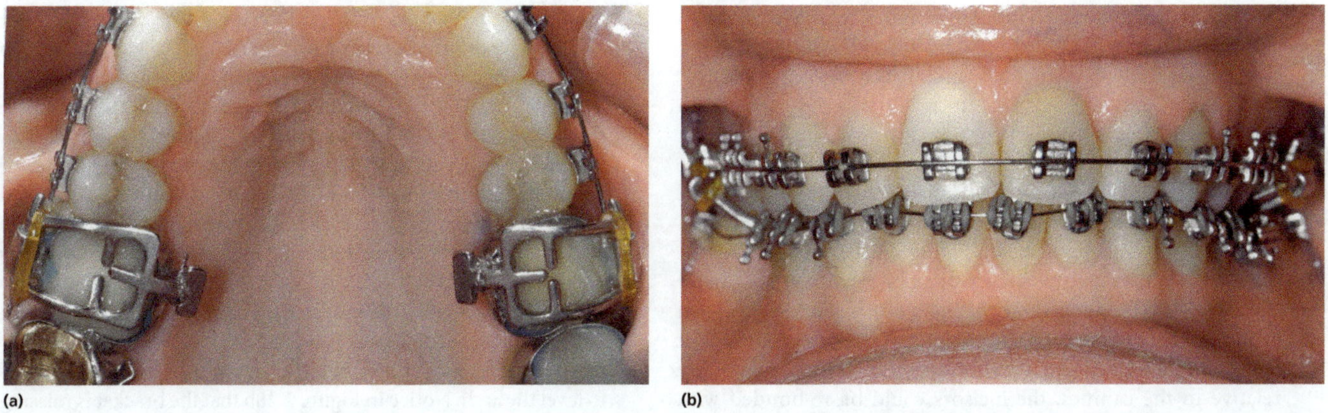

Figure 2.25 Guray "bite raisers": (a) placed on maxillary first molar bands and (b) patient biting on "bite raisers" that open the bite and allow bonding of mandibular incisors.

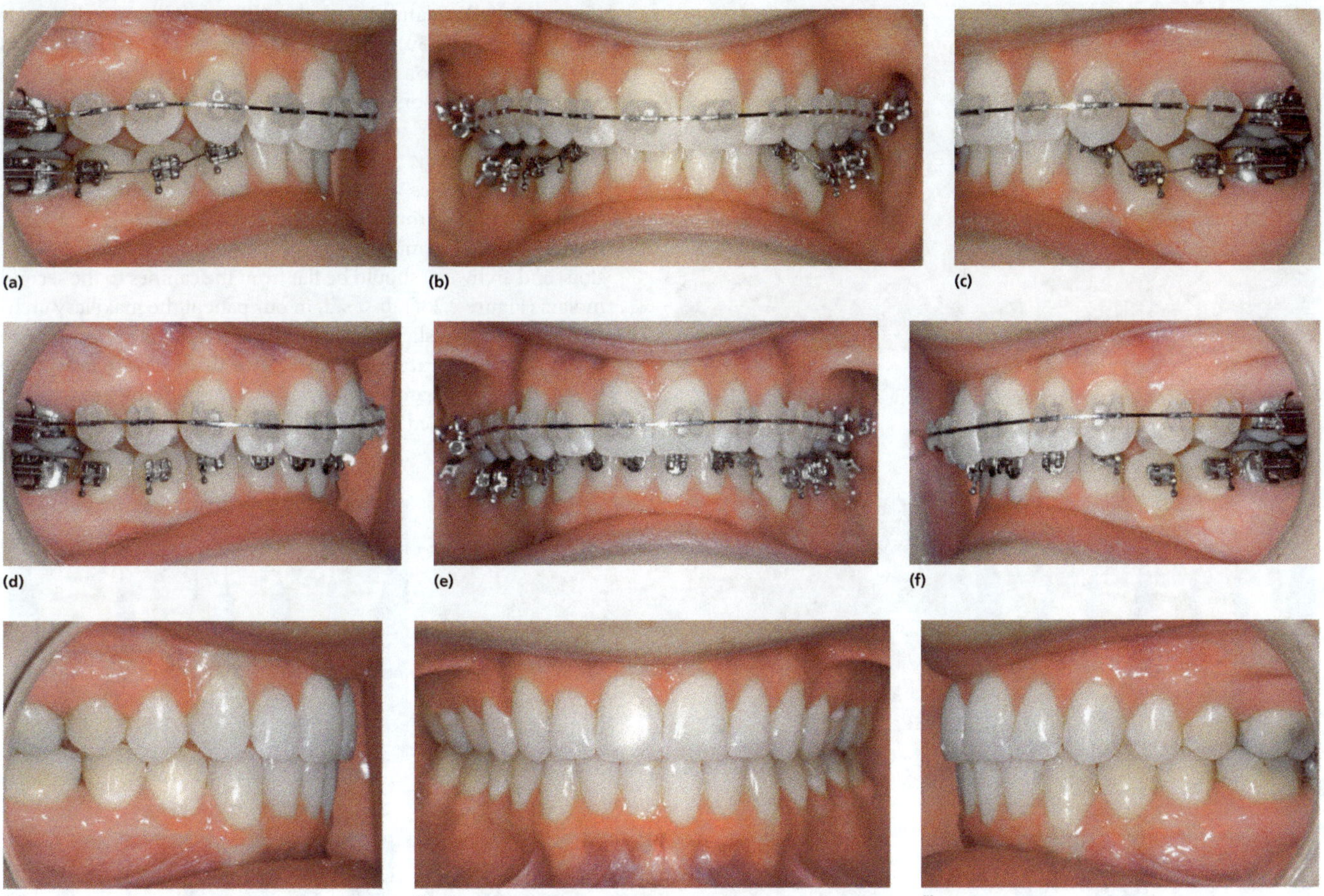

Figure 2.26 Leveling the mandibular arch using segmental archwires: (a–c) curve of Spee initially leveled using mandibular segmental wires from canines to molars, (d–f) as the bite is opened OJ is created permitting mandibular incisor bonding, and (g–i) final overbite and occlusion.

Q: Let's move on to some "in treatment" questions. A patient presents to you, already in fixed appliances, with a deep bite (Figure 2.27). The maxillary incisor edges are hitting the mandibular incisor brackets (note the wear spot where the mandibular left central incisor bracket is hitting the maxillary left central incisor edge). What do you look for, intraorally, to determine the cause of this deep bite? How could you proceed to correct (open) the deep bite?

A: Principle: when faced with this situation, always check the relationships between the following:

- Mandibular incisors relative to mandibular canines (Figure 2.28a)

- Mandibular canines relative to mandibular posterior teeth (Figure 2.28c)
- Maxillary incisors relative to maxillary canines (Figure 2.28d)
- Maxillary canines relative to maxillary posterior teeth (Figure 2.28f)

Mandibular incisors relative to mandibular canines: Have the patient open and check to see if the mandibular incisor teeth are stepped down slightly relative to the mandibular canines (Figure 2.28a). In our patient (Figure 2.28b), they are at the same level as the canines. To help open his bite, the mandibular incisors could be stepped down slightly by placing steps down in the archwire from distal of right lateral incisor to distal of left lateral incisor. Or, if the mandibular incisors were stepped up relative to the canines, the incisors could be re-bonded with brackets placed more incisally, and the arch leveled to intrude the incisors. In addition, as seen in Figure 2.28b, his mammelons are still present in the lower incisors. Slight enameloplasty could remove the mammelons, level out the incisal edges, and open the bite by the amount of incisal enamel removed.

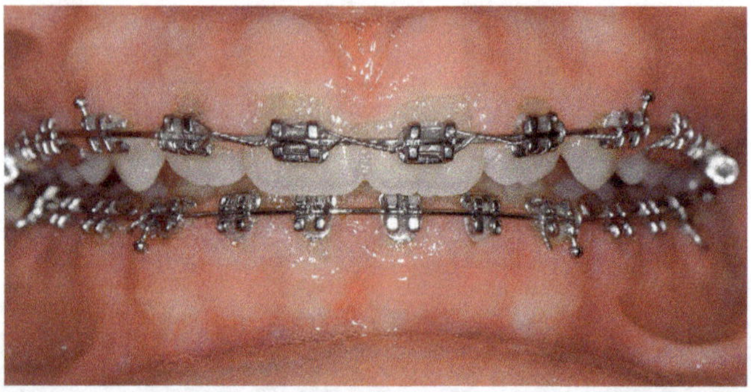

Figure 2.27 Patient presents in treatment with a deep bite and maxillary left central incisor edge hitting a lower bracket.

Mandibular canines relative to mandibular posterior teeth: Next, look posteriorly from the canines back (Figure 2.28b). To open the bite, you want the posterior occlusal surface to be perfectly flat (Figure 2.28c). The bracket slots and archwire should be flat, without curve or deflection. In our patient (Figure 2.28b), you can see a very mild curve in the posterior portion of the archwire. The archwire has not entirely eliminated the COS, leaving the mandibular anterior teeth higher than the posterior teeth. What should be done? Well, we can give this archwire more time to act; or we can remove the archwire to verify that the archwire is indeed flat and not distorted; or we can insert a heavier archwire to help extrude the premolars, upright/extrude the molars, and intrude/procline the mandibular incisors to level the arch. Notice in Figure 2.28b that the bracket is missing from the mandibular left second molar. To completely level the mandibular arch, both second molars should be bonded.

Maxillary incisors relative to maxillary canines: After examining the mandibular arch, check to see if the maxillary incisor teeth are stepped up slightly relative to the maxillary canines (Figure 2.28d). Examining the anterior maxillary arch of our patient (Figure 2.28e), notice that the maxillary central incisors (incisal edge attrition visible) are at the same level as the canines, or lower. The incisors should be stepped up slightly relative to the canines, either with archwire artistics or by re-bonding them more incisally, to open the bite.

Maxillary canines relative to maxillary posterior teeth: Next, look posteriorly from the maxillary canines to the molars (Figure 2.28e). The maxillary posterior (occlusal surfaces, bracket slots, and archwire) should be flat from the canines to the second molars (Figure 2.28f). Instead, in our patient the maxillary archwire curves down slightly toward the anterior teeth. How do you treat his maxillary arch? You could give this archwire more time to act, remove the archwire to verify that the archwire is indeed flat and not distorted, or insert a larger flat archwire.

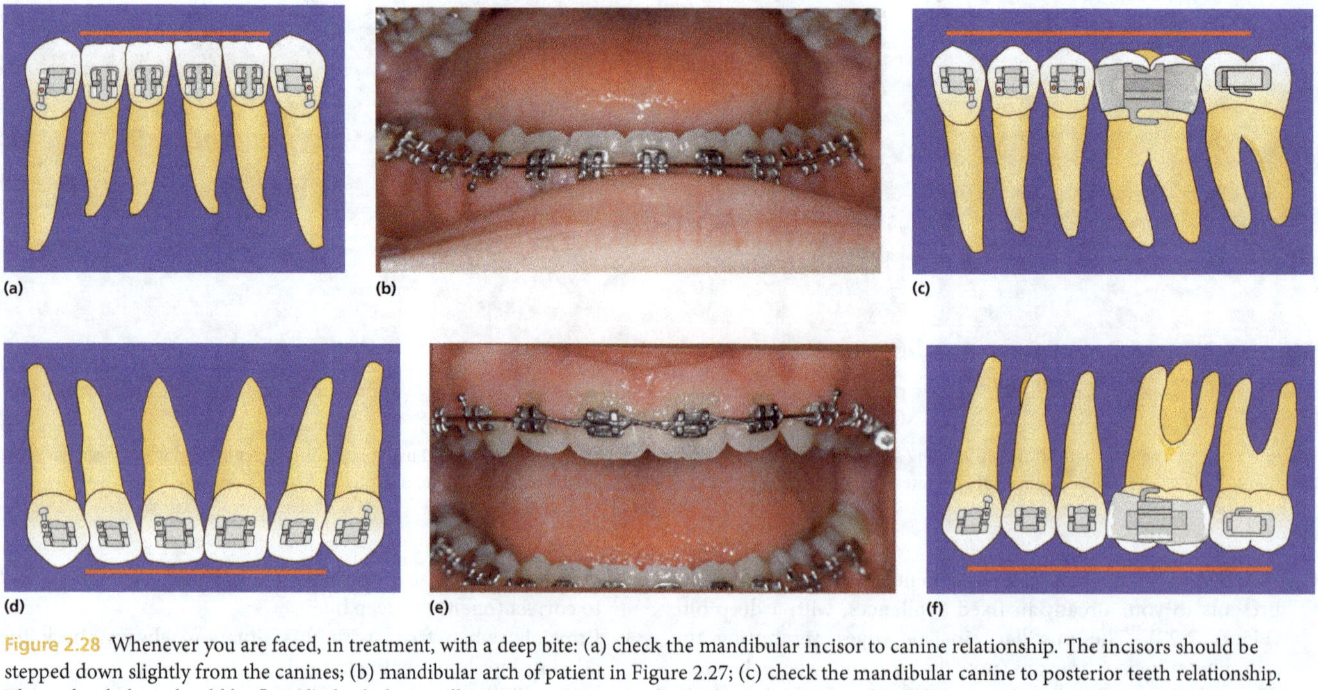

Figure 2.28 Whenever you are faced, in treatment, with a deep bite: (a) check the mandibular incisor to canine relationship. The incisors should be stepped down slightly from the canines; (b) mandibular arch of patient in Figure 2.27; (c) check the mandibular canine to posterior teeth relationship. The occlusal plane should be flat; (d) check the maxillary incisor to canine relationship. The incisors should be stepped up slightly from the canines; (e) maxillary arch of the patient in Figure 2.27; and (f) check the maxillary canine to posterior teeth relationship. The occlusal plane should be flat.

So, in summary, to open the deep bite of the patient in Figure 2.27:

- Bond the mandibular left second molar.
- Increase archwire sizes in both arches, making sure that the archwires are flat.
- Enameloplasty incisal edges (removing mammelons), as needed.
- Place steps in the anterior of the archwires to intrude the maxillary and mandibular incisors (or re-bond the incisors, prn).

Note: *Any decision to intrude (or extrude) maxillary incisors must include consideration of incisal display at rest and when smiling.* If you need to intrude incisors to open a deep bite in a patient with minimal maxillary incisal display, you may choose to intrude only the mandibular incisors.

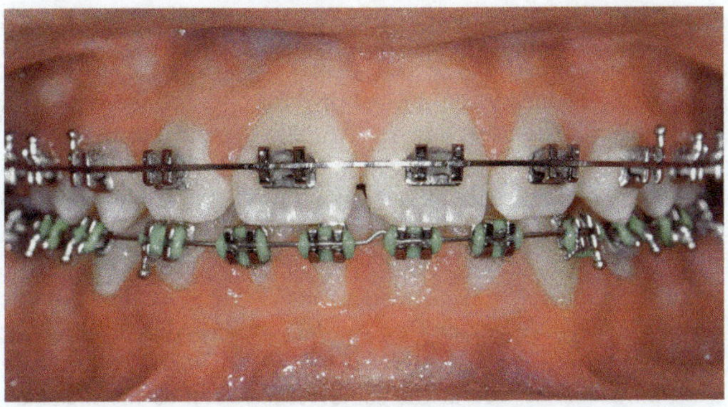

Figure 2.29 Patient presents with maxillary incisor edges hitting lower brackets.

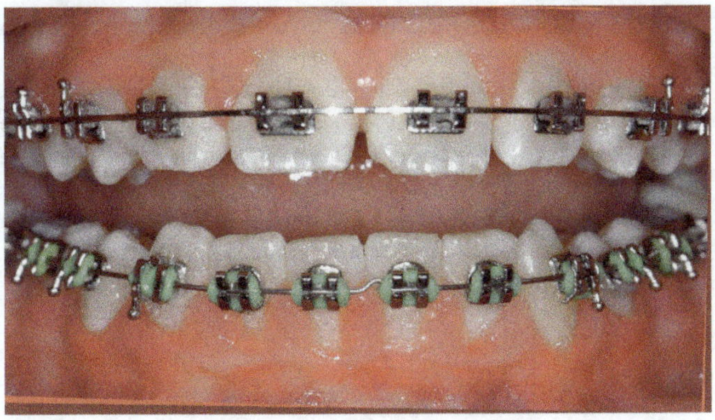

Figure 2.30 With the jaws separated, examine relationships between anterior teeth and between anterior and posterior teeth to help determine the cause of the deep bite (and how to correct it).

Q: Another patient presents to you, in treatment, with a deep bite. Her maxillary anterior teeth are hitting the mandibular anterior brackets (Figure 2.29). How do you proceed?

A: Ask the patient to open slightly (Figure 2.30). Look at relationships between the following:

- Mandibular incisors relative to mandibular canines
- Mandibular canines relative to mandibular posterior teeth
- Maxillary incisors relative to maxillary canines
- Maxillary canines relative to maxillary posterior teeth

Q: What do you observe?

A: Her mandibular incisors are stepped down slightly relative to the mandibular canines, which is good. However, there is a large, vertical step between the mandibular canines and the more posterior teeth. Also, if you look closely, you see that the mandibular left second molar is not bracketed. The maxillary incisors are stepped up slightly relative to the maxillary canines (good), and the maxillary posterior teeth appear to be level.

Q: What should you do to open the bite in the patient shown in Figures 2.29 and 2.30?

A: Bond the mandibular left second molar. Re-bond the mandibular premolars more apically and re-level to get rid of the step distal to the canines (you will need to decrease your archwire size anyway to insert an archwire into the re-bonded mandibular left second molar). Or, if all the mandibular spaces are closed, you could bend steps in the mandibular archwire distal to the mandibular canines to step down the canines (if you do this and keep the same mandibular archwire, you will need to insert a small "overlay" wire into the newly bonded left second molar to complete arch leveling). You do not need to do anything in the maxillary arch.

Q: A patient presents to you in treatment with a deep bite. The maxillary anterior teeth are touching the mandibular anterior brackets (Figure 2.31a). How do you proceed?

A: Ask the patient to open slightly (Figure 2.31b). Examine relationships between the following:

- Mandibular incisors relative to mandibular canines
- Mandibular canines relative to mandibular posterior teeth
- Maxillary incisors relative to maxillary canines
- Maxillary canines relative to maxillary posterior teeth

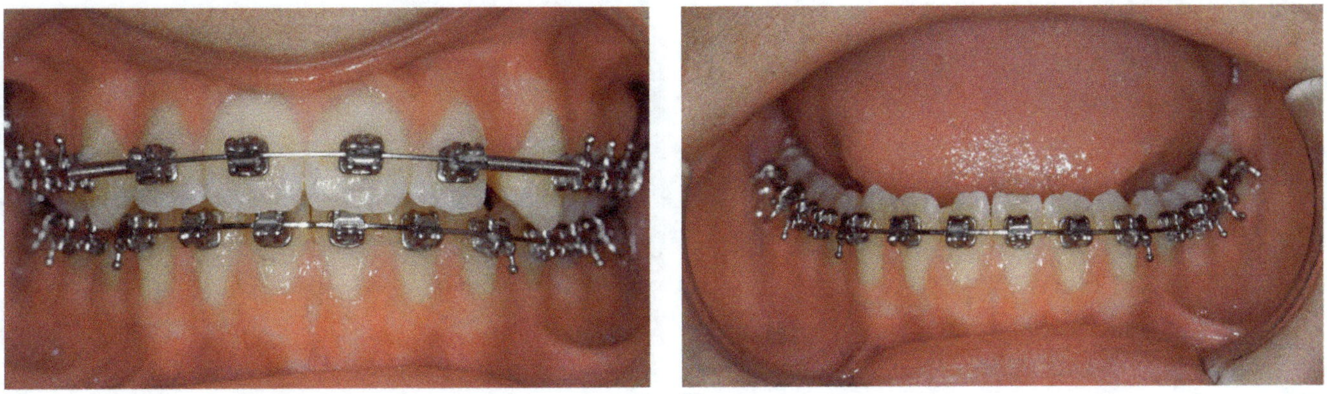

(a) (b)

Figure 2.31 Determining the cause of a dental deep bite: (a) Patient presents with maxillary incisors hitting the mandibular brackets and (b) examining the lower arch to look for factors contributing to the deep bite.

Q: What do you notice?

A: The mandibular incisors are chipped but look stepped up slightly relative to the mandibular canines. There is a step between the mandibular canines and the more posterior teeth. Also, there is a pronounced curve remaining in the mandibular archwire. The maxillary incisors (Figure 2.31a) are stepped up (excessively) relative to the maxillary canines, and the canine-to-posterior maxillary teeth look flat bilaterally, which is good. The maxillary arch is not contributing to the deep bite.

Q: How do you recommend opening the bite in the patient shown in Figure 2.31a?

A: Consider increasing the size of the mandibular archwire, or at least removing it to make sure that the archwire is flat—then re-inserting it to allow it to level the arch. Once the curve has been removed from the mandibular posterior arch, consider stepping down the mandibular incisors relative to the canines. Place a step in the archwire between the mandibular canines and first premolars to step down the anterior teeth from canine to canine. Or, re-bond the mandibular arch and re-level the arch.

Q: In the aforementioned situation, is it better to place steps in the archwire or to re-bond teeth (and re-level the arch)?

A: As a general rule, it is better to re-bond teeth/re-level the arch than it is to place (a lot of) steps in the archwire. The most frequent error when banding/bonding is not achieving vertical correspondence between teeth. When you first band a patient, and you see that a bracket is off vertically, replace it immediately. After you level the arches, check again for banding/bonding errors. When you see them, re-band/re-bond immediately. We advise that you save "artistic" steps for small bonding errors in the final archwire (so you do not need to replicate the artistic bend time and time again between increasing archwire sizes). Also, do not place bends in archwires if you still have spaces to close. Why? The archwire will bind when you try to close spaces. Other tips are to close all spaces before placing bends, place torques in the archwire before placing bends (it can be wicked to place torque in a wire if steps are present), and when placing artistic bends in wires, work from anterior to posterior.

Q: Why is there a bite deep in the patient shown in Figure 2.32?

A: Looking at the mandibular and maxillary posterior teeth bracket slots in Figure 2.32b, curves are seen along the posterior bracket slots. Also, the mandibular incisors' incisal edges are uneven and nearly at the level of the mandibular canines. The mandibular canines are stepped up relative to the mandibular first premolars, and the maxillary central incisors are at the same approximate level as the maxillary canines.

Q: How do you recommend opening the bite in the patient shown in Figure 2.32?

A: The curves along the posterior bracket slots need to be leveled (flattened). This would be accomplished by increasing the size and stiffness of the archwires. The mandibular incisors should be stepped down relative to the mandibular canines. The mandibular canines should be stepped down relative to the mandibular first premolars. Finally, the maxillary central incisors should be stepped up slightly.

Q: During maxillary central incisor retraction and space closure, the central incisors are seen to hit the mandibular incisor brackets in the patient shown in Figure 2.33a. You need to open the bite to continue incisor retraction. You ask the patient to open (Figure 2.33b) in order to determine why the bite is deep. What do you see?

A: The mandibular incisor edges are at the same level as the mandibular canine cusp tips. The slots of the mandibular posterior teeth form a gentle curve and follow the COS. The maxillary central incisors are at the same vertical level as the maxillary canine cusp tips, and the maxillary posterior arch appears flat.

Q: How do you recommend opening the bite in the patient shown in Figure 2.33?

A: A larger (stiffer) mandibular archwire should be placed to eliminate the remaining COS, artistic steps (down) placed in the mandibular archwire to intrude the mandibular incisors, and steps (up) placed in the maxillary archwire to intrude the maxillary central incisors (Figure 2.34a). These actions open the bite and permit continued maxillary space closure. Compare the bite depth in Figure 2.34b to the original bite depth in Figure 2.33a. Note that the bite has been opened through these actions by approximately 1–2 mm.

Q: An adult patient presents to you with a dental deep bite (Figure 2.35a and b). What *curves* could you place in the maxillary and mandibular archwires to assist in opening the bite?

A: You could place reverse COS in the mandibular archwire (Figure 2.35c, bottom) and compensating curve in the maxillary archwire (Figure 2.35c, top). The key to using these curves in this particular patient lies in the fact that his maxillary and

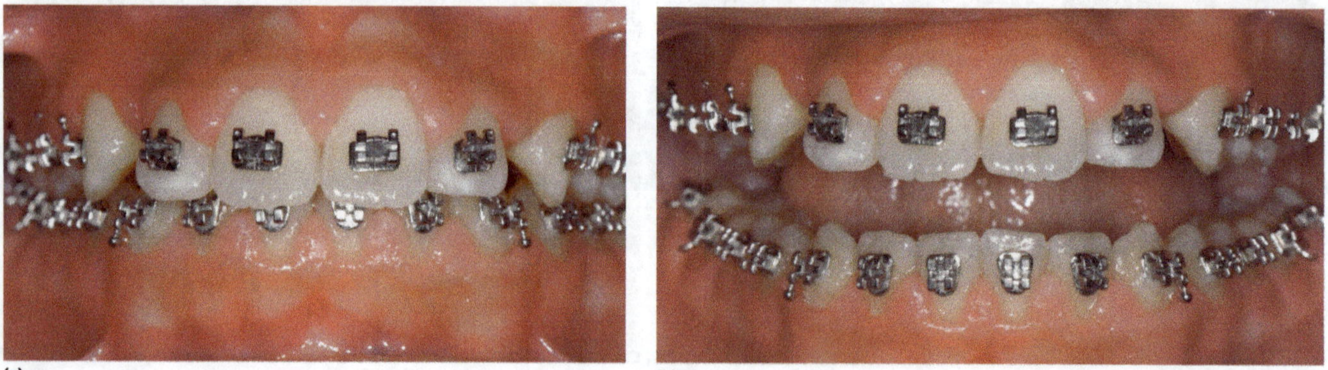

(a) (b)

Figure 2.32 Determining the causes of a dental deep bite: (a) patient presents with maxillary incisors overlapping lower brackets and (b) have the patient open to look for factors contributing to the deep bite.

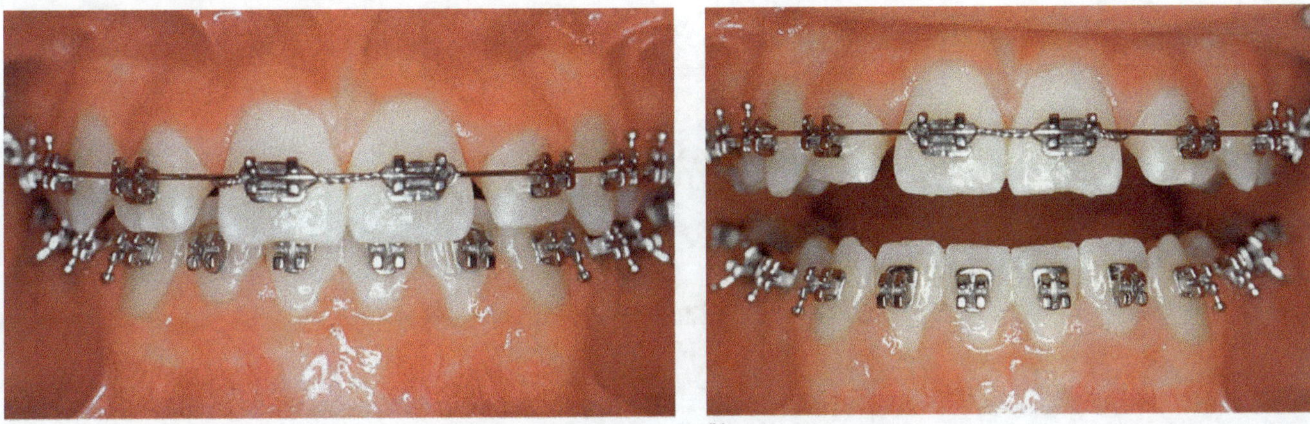

(a) (b)

Figure 2.33 Determining the cause of a deep bite: (a) the maxillary incisal edges contact the mandibular brackets during retraction/space closure and (b) the patient opens.

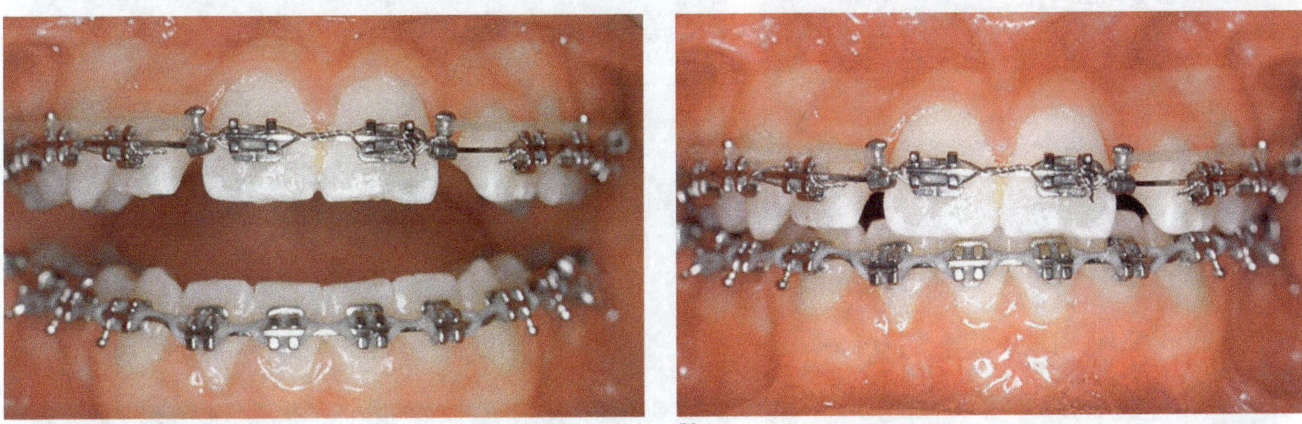

(a) (b)

Figure 2.34 Correcting the deep bite in Figure 2.33: (a) a larger/stiffer mandibular archwire was placed together with maxillary central incisor and mandibular incisor intrusion steps and (b) which opened the bite and create OJ. Central incisor retraction can now continue.

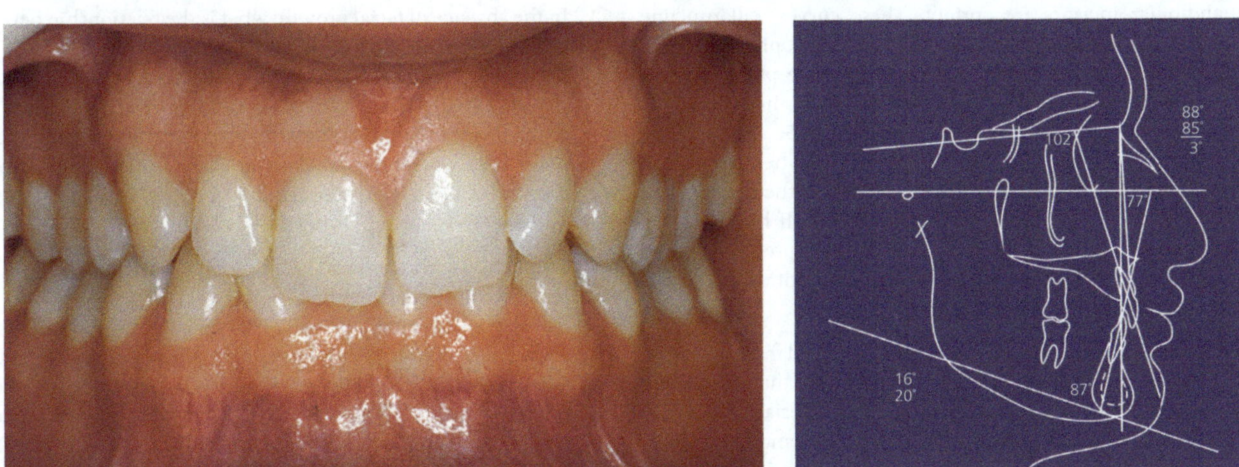

(a) (b)

Figure 2.35 Correction of a deep bite (and curve of Spee) by placement of *reverse* curve of Spee and compensating curve: (a and b) patient presents with a deep bite and upright incisors, (c) reverse curve of Spee is placed in the mandibular archwire and compensating curve is placed in the maxillary archwire, (d) the deep bite is corrected by, and (e and f) mandibular and maxillary incisor proclination/intrusion.

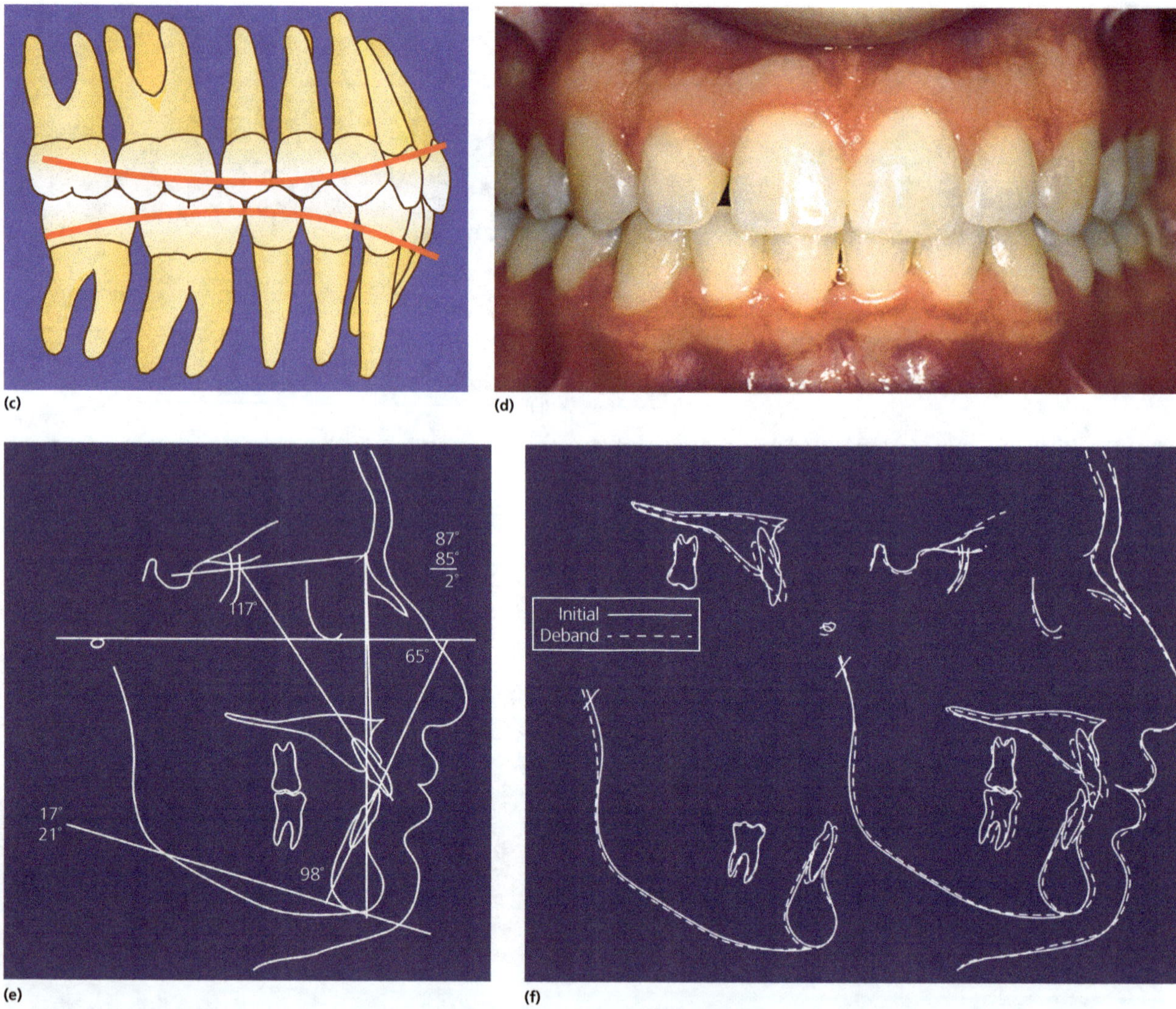

Figure 2.35 (Continued)

mandibular incisors are upright. These curves will procline anterior teeth readily, so you should start with upright incisors if you intend to use them. These curves were placed in this patient's archwires—rapidly proclining and intruding his maxillary and mandibular incisors (Figure 2.35e and f). If the incisors had initially been proclined (instead of being upright), then extra care would be needed to insure that the incisors had not become too proclined with these curves. If his maxillary and mandibular incisors had initially been proclined, then simply leveling with increasingly larger and stiffer, flat, archwires may have been prudent.

Q: You are trying to level a COS by erupting premolars in a patient, but the curve is proving to be intractable. Other than increasing the archwire size or using a stiffer archwire material, what could you do to increase the extrusive force on the premolars to erupt them?

A: One simple pearl: try inserting the archwire *under* the premolar brackets (Figure 2.36). However, remember that any extrusion of teeth can be prone to relapse—so the extruded teeth should be held in their extruded positions for many months.

Q: In the absence of facial growth, what is the relationship between vertical deep bite correction and AP change?

A: Molars and premolars are erupted during deep bite correction (leveling the COS). Whenever molars and premolars are erupted, the mandible tends to be rotated down and back—potentially worsening an existing Class II molar relationship, creating a Class II relationship where a Class I relationship initially exists, or improving a Class III relationship.

Q: Theoretically, how does LAFH affect horizontal change in B-point during bite opening?

A: Although bite opening occurs by a combination of molar/premolar eruption plus incisor intrusion/proclination, assume for a moment that bite opening occurs entirely by molar/premolar eruption—resulting in downward/backward mandibular rotation around the condyles. As illustrated in Figure 2.37, for a given amount of anterior OB reduction (vertical downward pointing yellow arrow) B-point/Menton/Pogonion will all rotate back less (horizontal arrow) with a short LAFH patient (left) than with a long LAFH patient (right). In both instances, the AP relationship becomes more Class II.

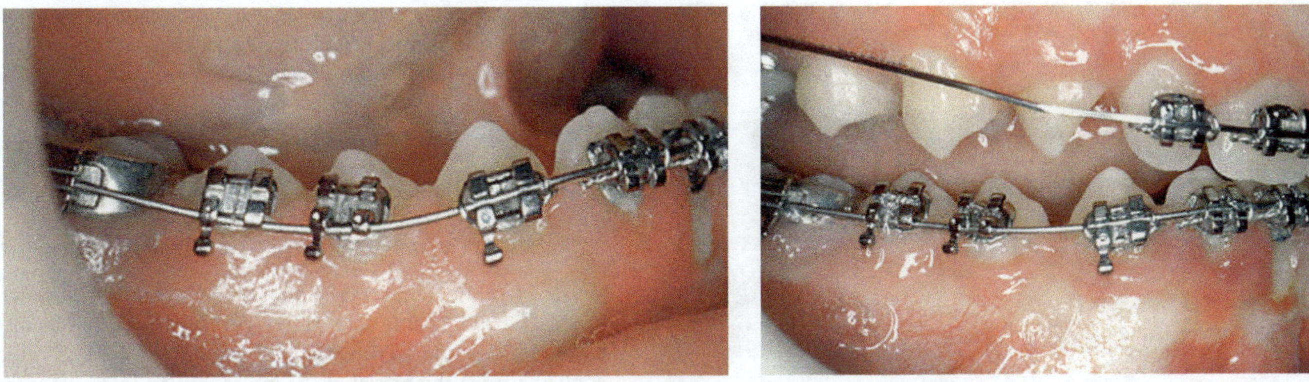

(a) (b)

Figure 2.36 Pearl to help level an intractable curve of Spee: (a) placing the archwire under brackets increases the wire deflection/eruptive force and (b) results in the mandibular occlusal plane leveling (at this time, the wire can be placed *in* the bracket slots).

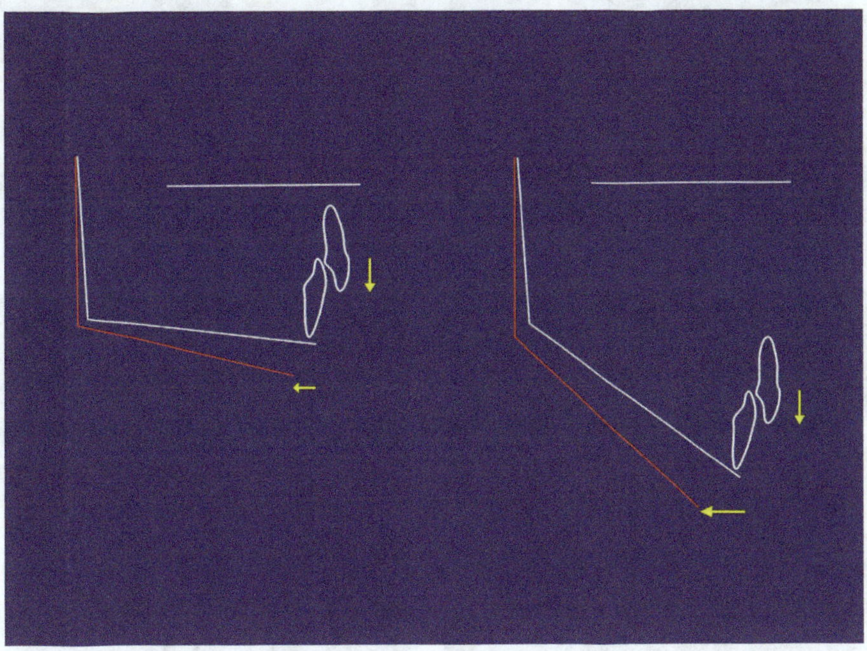

Figure 2.37 For the same amount of bite opening (vertical yellow arrow), B-point and Pogonion will move back less in a short LAFH patient (left, horizontal yellow arrow) than in a long LAFH patient (right).

Q: You wish to intrude overerupted mandibular incisors in a mixed dentition patient (Figure 2.38). How can you do this without bonding the entire arch?

A: One simple way is to bond/band the mandibular first molars and use them as anchorage with a utility arch to the incisors (a 2×4 appliance—a "two by four" appliance where two molars are banded plus four incisors bonded). The utility arch has a tip-back bend ("V bend," intrusion bend, or anchor bend) placed just mesial to the first molar (Figure 2.39a). Let's examine what happens as we lift the wire up to engage it in the incisor bracket (Figure 2.39b). Our intuition tells us that an intrusive force ($F1$) is placed at the incisor by this action and, if we take the cover off the molar bracket (Figure 2.39c), we find that an extrusive force is also applied against the mesial upper edge of the molar bracket ($F2$) and an intrusive force is applied against the distal lower edge of the molar bracket ($F3$). Now, assume that the distance between the distal edge of the molar bracket and the mesial edge of the molar bracket is "Y" and that the distance between the mesial edge of the molar bracket and the incisor bracket is "X."

For a static system, the sum of the moments around any point must equal zero. If we choose the mesial end of the molar bracket as this point, assign a positive value for a clockwise moment, and assign a negative value for a counterclockwise moment then,

$$\sum M_{\text{Mesial of bracket}} = 0 = F1 \cdot X - F3 \cdot Y + F2 \cdot 0$$

or,

$$F3 = F1 \cdot \frac{X}{Y}$$

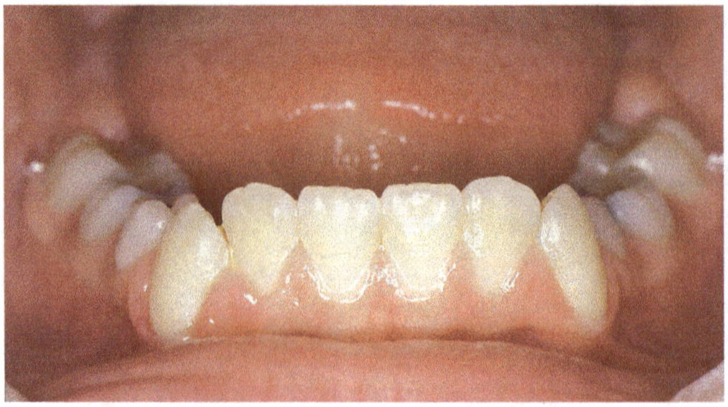

Figure 2.38 Overerupted incisors in a mixed dentition patient.

Also, the sum of the vertical forces in a static system must equal zero. If we assign a negative value to a downward force, and assign a positive value to an upward forces, then

$$\sum F_Y = 0 = F2 - F1 - F3$$

or,

$$F2 = F1 + F3 = F1 \cdot \left(1 + \frac{X}{Y}\right)$$

We find that the forces at each of our three points are as shown in Figure 2.39d. That is, an intrusive force ($F1$) is applied against the incisor, the sum of *two extrusive* forces ($F1$ plus $F1 \cdot X/Y$) are applied against the mesial of the molar, and an intrusive force

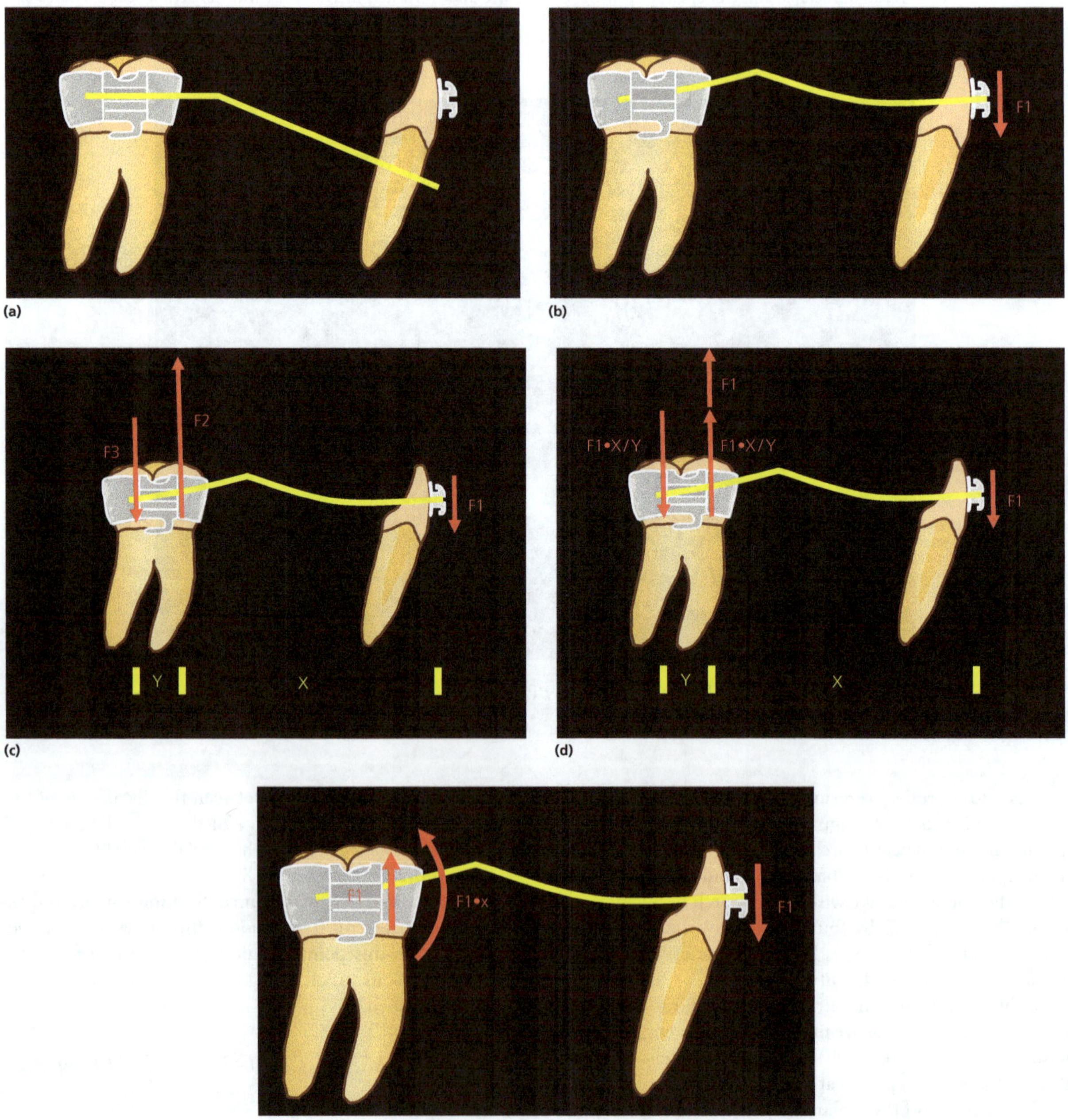

Figure 2.39 Effects of a "V bend" utility archwire: (a) bend placed just mesial to the first molar, (b–d) analysis of resulting forces acting on the molar and incisor, and (e) net result is a distal tipping moment on the molar, eruptive force on the molar, and intrusive force on the incisor.

$F1 \cdot X/Y$ is applied against the distal of the molar. The mesial and distal $F1 \cdot X/Y$ forces applied against the molar are equal but opposite forces and constitute a moment, or couple, of magnitude $F1 \cdot X$ (the value of one force multiplied by the distance Y between them), while the vertical effects of these two forces cancel out exactly. We are left (Figure 2.39e) with an intrusive force ($F1$) applied against the incisor, an extrusive force ($F1$) applied against the molar, plus a distal-tipping moment ($F1 \cdot X$) applied against the molar.

Q: Using these utility archwire mechanics (no TADs) in the mixed dentition patient shown in Figure 2.38, what would be a smart way to intrude the incisors *without* extruding or tipping back the mandibular first permanent molars?

A: Use the *primary second molars,* instead of the permanent first molars, for anchorage (Figure 2.40a and b). This way, you eliminate distal tipping/extrusion of the permanent first molars. Using this technique, notice the resulting mandibular incisor intrusion and distal tipping of the mandibular primary second molars (Figure 2.40c–e).

Q: Is it better to level the COS using a utility archwire or a continuous archwire?

A: Overall, the effects of both are very similar [19–21]:

- Both have similar reduction in OB.
- MPA may open slightly with both (molar extrusion). One study demonstrated 1.4° greater MPA increase using continuous archwires [20].
- Mandibular incisors intrude slightly (1–1.7 mm) with both. A study by Dake and Sinclair [19] demonstrated no incisor intrusion with continuous archwires, but Class III elastics were concurrently used when needed (which would tend to prevent intrusion of the lower incisors).
- Incisor proclination results are mixed. In the Dake and Sinclair study [19], the utility arch demonstrated more flaring of incisors. In the AlQabandi et al. study [21], the utility arch (wire cinched distal to the molar bracket) demonstrated incisor retroclination, while continuous wires produced incisor proclination.

Q: What can happen to the mandibular COS and maxillary compensating curve during space closure following premolar extractions (canine retraction and incisor retraction)? Why does this happen?

A: The mandibular COS can deepen, the maxillary compensating curve can reverse, OB can deepen, and the patient can develop a posterior open bite. Why? Look at Figure 2.41a. Here we see that maxillary and mandibular first premolars have been extracted, and the extraction spaces are being closed reciprocally. The anterior teeth are retracting, and the posterior teeth are protracting. As this happens, the anterior teeth tip distally and the posterior teeth tip mesially (rotating around their apicies). Consequently, the archwire deflects, the mandibular COS deepens, the maxillary compensating curve reverses, OB deepens, and a posterior open bite develops (Figure 2.41b). Figure 2.41c–h illustrates this situation, clinically, during canine retraction. As shown, as the canines are retracted in both arches through the first premolar extraction spaces, they tip distally while the molars tip mesially—deepening the mandibular COS, reversing the maxillary compensating curve, deepening the OB, and creating a posterior open bite. These effects result because space closure force is too heavy, archwires are too light (unable to generate adequate counter couples), and not enough time is allowed for tooth roots to translate through the alveolar process bone.

Q: Your associate comes to you concerned that this problem is developing in a patient. How would you correct it? How would you have prevented it?

A: Decrease the space closure force, increase the archwire size/stiffness in each arch, and give the patient more time between appointments for the teeth roots to move through bone. This was done for the previously shown patient (Figure 2.42a–f).

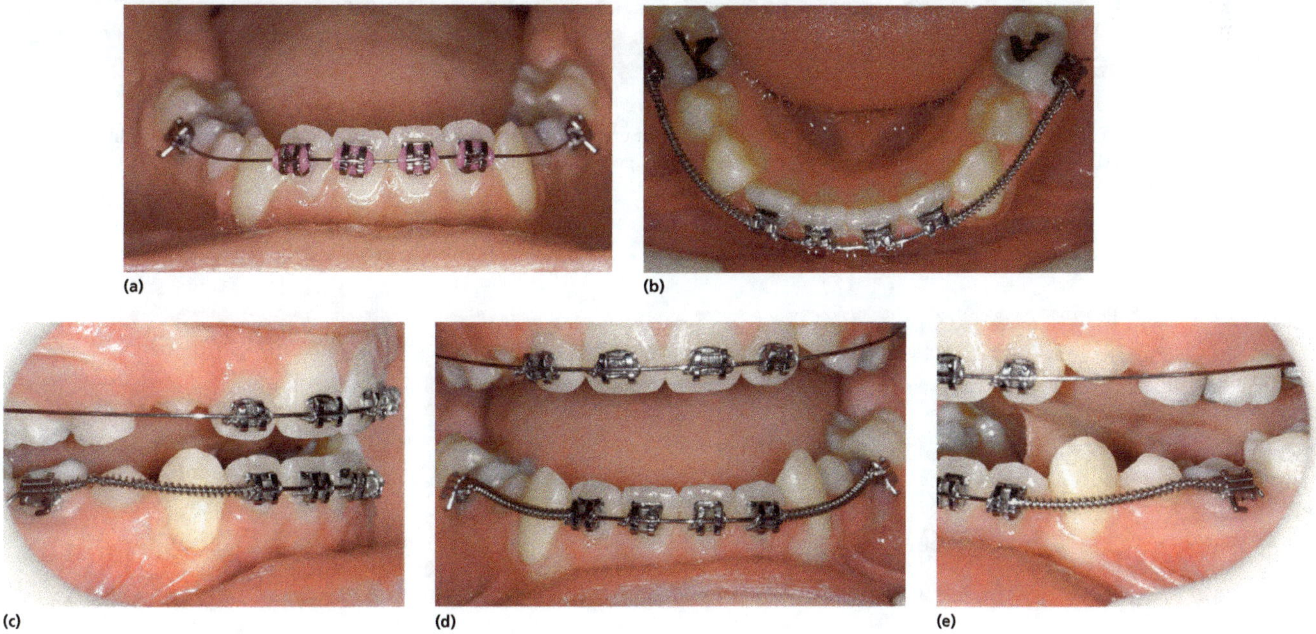

Figure 2.40 Effects of a "V bend" archwire: (a and b) incisors and *primary* second molars bonded and (c–e) incisors intruded, primary second molars tipped distally. Note "V bend" mesial to molars under the open-coil spring.

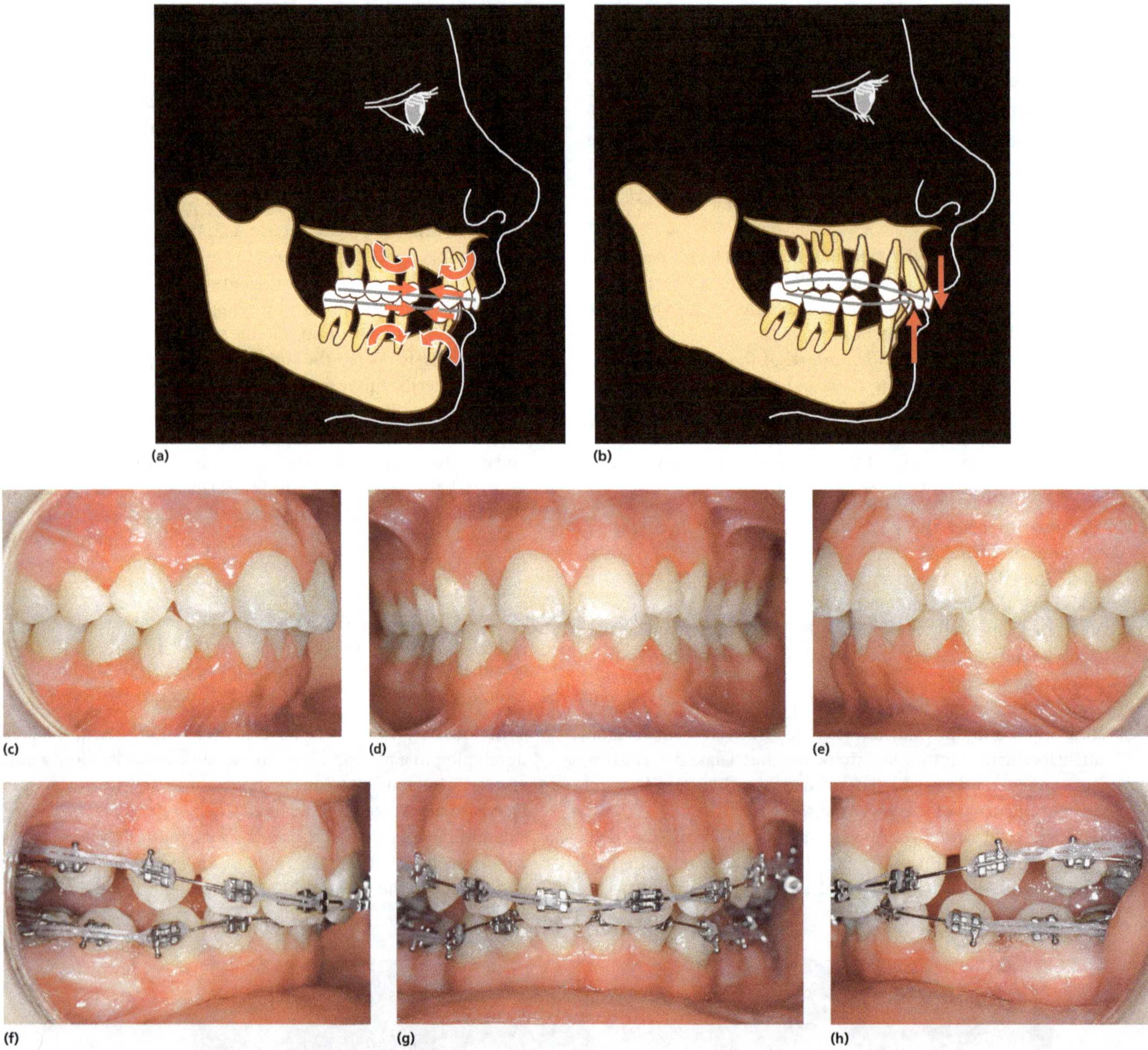

Figure 2.41 (a–h) Effects of reciprocal space closure following extraction of first premolars. As teeth tip into the extraction spaces, the mandibular curve of Spee deepens, the maxillary compensating curve reverses, OB deepens, and a posterior open bite can develop.

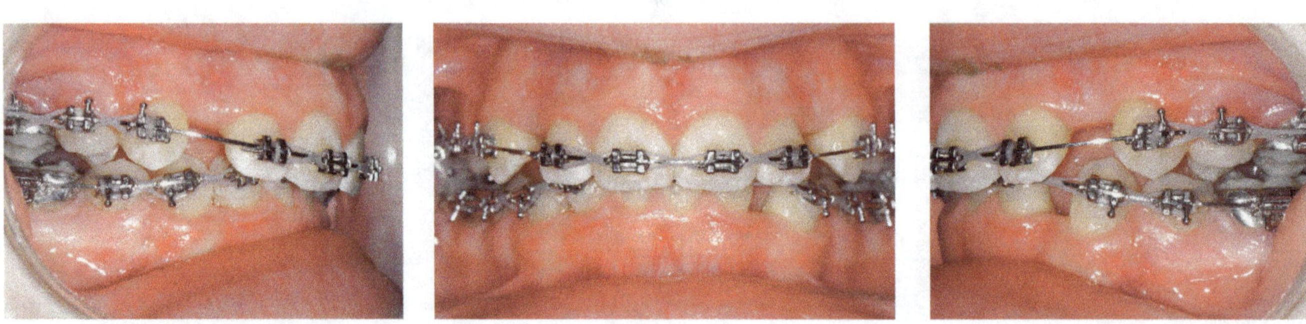

Figure 2.42 (a–i) The undesirable effects of space closure previously shown can be corrected by increasing archwire size, decreasing space closure force, and allowing adequate time for teeth roots to move through bone.

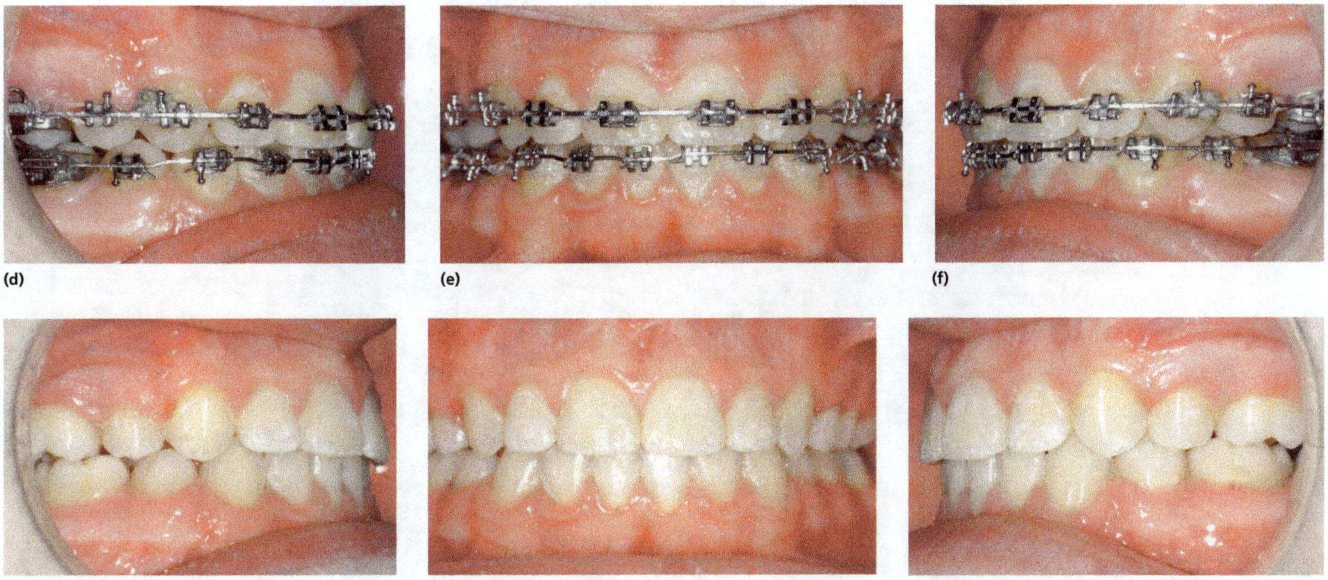

(d) (e) (f) (g) (h) (i)

Figure 2.42 (Continued)

The mandibular COS was eliminated, the maxillary reverse curve was eliminated, the OB was reduced, the posterior open bite was eliminated, and the spaces were closed (Figure 2.42g–i). The problem could have been prevented by leveling the COS before beginning space closure, decreasing the space closure force, using larger archwires capable of generating adequate counter couples during space closure, and allowing adequate time between appointments for tooth roots to move.

Q: What is an effective retention protocol for corrected deep bites?

A: At deband, immediately place the patient in vacuum-formed retainers during the day (maxillary vacuum-formed retainer shown in Figure 2.43a) and Hawley retainers at night (Figure 2.43b–f). The vacuum-formed retainers may be discontinued after 2–3 months. The Hawley retainers are worn, at night, forever. The maxillary Hawley retainer should include an anterior bite plate, which *slightly discludes the posterior occlusion* when the patient wears it at night. The patient should not wear the Hawley retainers full-time, because with the posterior teeth discluded, the posterior teeth will super-erupt. Such anterior "bite-raising" maxillary retainers are recommended to combat OB relapse [22, 23]. Note on the mandibular Hawley retainer the addition of acrylic labial to the anterior teeth which aids in maintaining incisor alignment. Such acrylic can also be placed labial to the maxillary anterior teeth. Fixed retainers (lingually bonded chains or wires across anterior teeth) can also be effective, but do not add a bite-raising effect.

Q: Is long-term deep bite correction stable?

A: Yes, reasonably stable. For example, look at the cephalometric superimposition of a dental deep bite patient treated in his early teen years (Figure 2.44a). As shown, his deep bite was opened through a combination of molar eruption, maxillary incisor intrusion, maxillary incisor proclination, and mandibular incisor proclination. His initial and deband intraoral frontal photographs are seen in Figure 2.44b and c, respectively, and illustrate a reduction in OB from 100 to 20%. Post treatment, he wore his Hawley retainers nightly. After 10 years (Figure 2.44d), his OB has increased to about 30–40%, mainly due to maxillary central incisor vertical eruption.

Follow-up of deep bite correction (initial OB of 4.5 mm or more) in children successfully treated nonextraction to a normal OB showed that, long-term, only minor relapse (mean 0.8 mm) occurred [24]. Interestingly, the control group of subjects in this study underwent a bite opening of 0.7 mm during the same period. In Class II division 2 patients specifically, OB correction appears to be reasonably stable with an average of 20% relapse at 2 years post retention [22] and doubling at 15 years follow-up [25]. In a sample of adults treated with utility arch mandibular incisor intrusion, long-term deep bite correction was found to be stable [26]. *Deep bite correction is reasonably stable* [27].

Q: Discuss possible etiologic factors that could influence deep bite relapse.

A: Possible etiologic factors:

- Riedel [28] suggested, and Ludwig [29] reported, a positive correlation between upright incisors (interincisal angle >140°) and OB relapse. However, Simons and Joondeph [30] found no such correlation.
- Protrusion of the mandibular incisors during orthodontic treatment to correct the OB was found to be correlated with OB relapse [30].
- Canut and Arias [31] reported a correlation between the number of years, which had elapsed after retention, OB relapse, and postretention mandibular irregularity. Overcorrection of OB was also seen to relapse.
- Removal of excess maxillary incisor overlap by the lower lip has been highlighted as an important treatment stability objective [32].
- High-angle patients show less deep bite relapse than normal or low-angle patients [33].
- Stability of deep bite correction by eruption of molars in adults (especially with low to average mandibular plane angles) is questionable [34, 35].

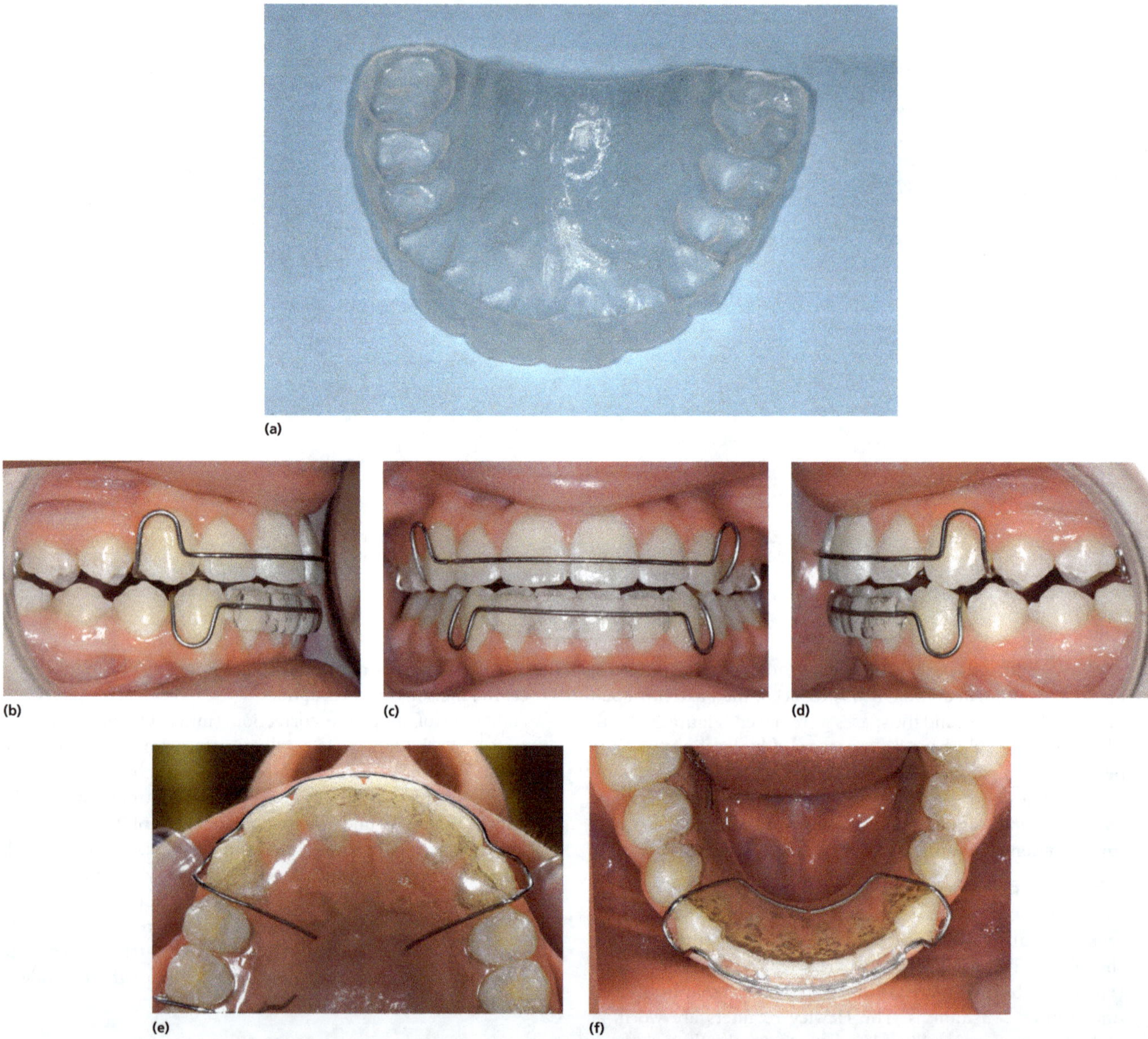

Figure 2.43 A deep bite retention protocol: (a) vacuum-formed retainers are initially worn during the day, (b–f) Hawley retainers, with maxillary anterior biteplate to disclude the posterior teeth, are worn at night for life.

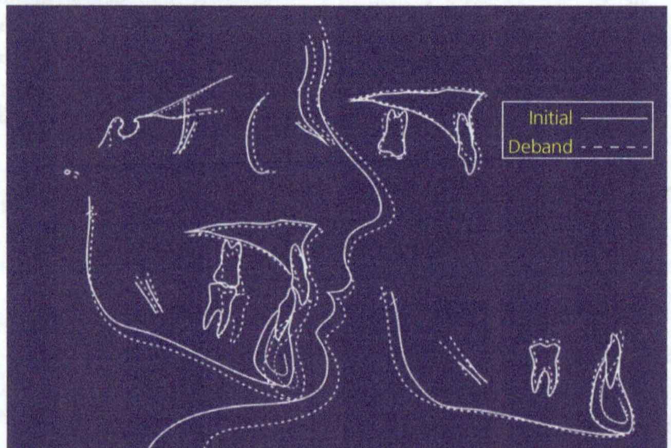

(a)

Figure 2.44 Long-term deep bite correction stability: (a) cephalometric superimposition of deep bite correction, (b) initial deep bite, (c) OB correction at deband, and (d) 10–20% OB increase 10 years later.

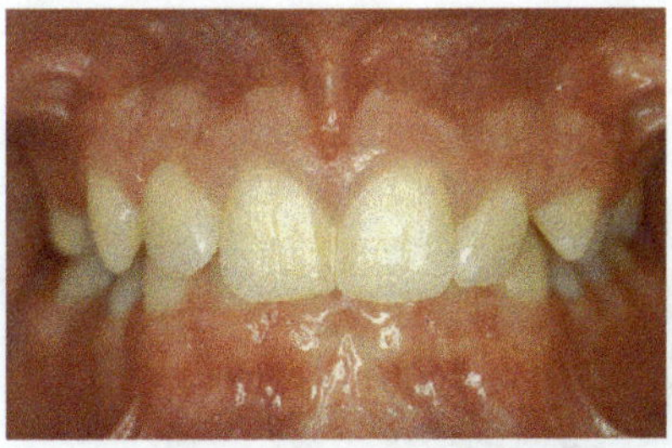

(b)

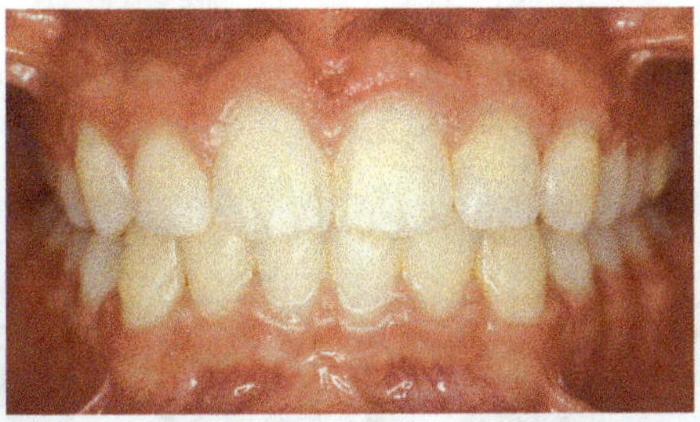

(c)

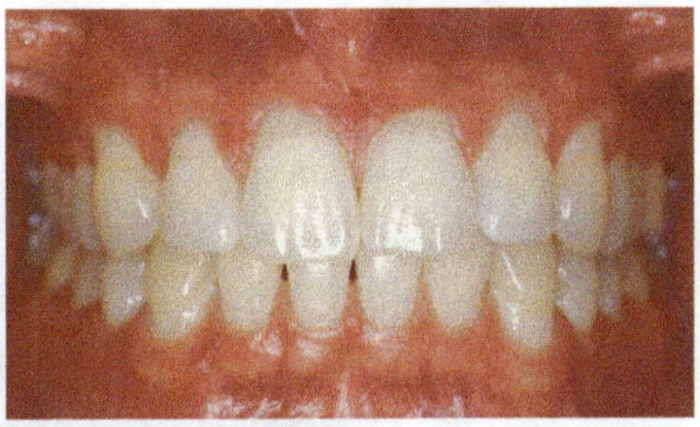

(d)

Figure 2.44 (Continued)

Q: In summary, what are your "take-home messages" regarding etiology, identifying, treating, and retaining dental deep bite patients?

A: Take-home messages:

- Dental deep bites result from excessive maxillary and mandibular anterior tooth eruption.
- The hallmark of a *dental* deep bite is excessive OB in a patient who is otherwise normal in the vertical dimension.
- To evaluate the specific teeth involved in causing the dental deep bite, have the patient open and examine the relationship: between the mandibular incisors and mandibular canines, between the maxillary incisors and maxillary canines, from the mandibular canines to the mandibular second molars, and from the maxillary canines to the maxillary second molars.
- Dental deep bites are corrected, ideally, by intruding maxillary and mandibular anterior teeth.
- Deep bites are also corrected by proclining anterior teeth—which is desirable if incisors are initially upright but undesirable if incisors are initially proclined.
- Dental deep bites are also corrected by eruption of premolars/molars (elimination of the COS), but this action tends to increase the LAFH and rotate the mandible down and back.
- Overall, OB correction stability is good in dental deep bite patients with good retainer wear, but some relapse should be anticipated. For that reason, overcorrection is reasonable (perhaps finishing with as little as 10% OB). Avoid incisor protrusion during treatment, when possible. Your patient should be retained, for life.

Case Andrew

Andrew is a 10-year-old boy (Figure 2.45) who presents to you with the chief complaint, "I need braces." His PMH, PDH, and TMJ evaluation are WRN. He has thin labial attached tissue over the root of the mandibular left central incisor (Figure 2.45h) and CR=CO.

Q: List diagnostic findings/problems. What is your diagnosis? (Note: The Appendix includes a Diagnostic Findings/Problems List Template that you may copy and use as a worksheet to help organize your thoughts.)

A: See Table 2.2

Q: Is Andrew's deep bite a *skeletal* deep bite, a *dental* deep bite, or a combination of both? What is the etiology of his deep bite?

A: Andrew's deep bite is a dental deep bite. Andrew's vertical relationships appear normal. He presents with normal vertical soft tissue proportions (Figure 2.45a, soft tissue Glabella–Subnasale approximately equal to Subnasale–soft tissue Menton). Although his MPA is steeper than average FMA (31°)/SNMP (38°), his LAFH/TAFH is ideal (ANS-Menton/Nasion-Menton ~55%). His deep bite is a result of maxillary incisor overeruption (Figure 2.45l–n and q) coupled with mandibular incisor overeruption (Figure 2.45s–u, COS of ~3 mm). *He has a dental deep bite.*

Q: Why is it important to look at molar AP relationships, not only from the buccal, but also from the *lingual* of the models?

A: If the maxillary first molars were actually Class I but *rotated mesially*, then they could appear to be Class II when viewed from the buccal. But when viewed from the lingual, the maxillary first molars lingual cusps would still be properly seated in the mandibular first molar central fossa. As shown in Figure 2.46a and b, Andrew's maxillary first molar lingual cusps are *not* properly seated in the mandibular first molar central fossa. This view confirms the fact that Andrew has a true Class II molar relationship.

Q: Do Andrew's dental arch asymmetries reflect the difference between his right and left AP molar relationships?

A: Yes. Andrew does not appear to have a skeletal asymmetry (Figure 2.45a and b). Therefore, his mild dental arch asymmetries (Figure 2.45o and p: maxillary left first molar ahead/mandibular right first molar ahead) reflect exactly the mild AP molar relationship differences: Class II (1–2) II (1–2) II (3–4) II (3–4). That is, these slight dental asymmetries explain why Andrew is more Class II on his left side.

Q: As seen on the panoramic image (Figure 2.45f), what does mild overlap of the permanent maxillary right canine crown over the root of the permanent maxillary right lateral incisor suggest?

A: Three factors measurable on panoramic radiographs can be used to assess the potential for impaction of a developing permanent canine: (i) the vertical distance of the developing permanent canine cusp tip to the occlusal plane, (ii) the angle formed between the long axis of the developing permanent canine and the maxillary midline, and (iii) the amount of overlap of the crown of the developing permanent canine with the root of the adjacent permanent lateral incisor [36]. That is, *the overlap suggests the possibility that the permanent canine could eventually become impacted. The greater the overlap, the greater the risk.*

Q: Should you extract Andrew's *primary* maxillary right canine (or primary maxillary right canine plus primary right first molar) to increase the probability that the permanent maxillary right canine will erupt?

A: No, not yet, not in this particular case. Why not? Looking at Andrew's panoramic radiograph (Figure 2.45f), the right permanent canine appears to overlap 30 to 50% of the root of the right permanent lateral incisor, but has minimal deviation in its long axis compared to the maxillary midline. The left permanent canine shows minimal overlap with the root of the left permanent lateral incisor, and has approximately 10° of angulation toward the maxillary midline. Given these findings, coupled with the anterior position of the permanent canine crowns viewed in the cephalometric radiograph (Figure 2.45d) and the prominence of the crowns in the labial alveolar plate (palpable during the clinical exam), you judge that Andrew's

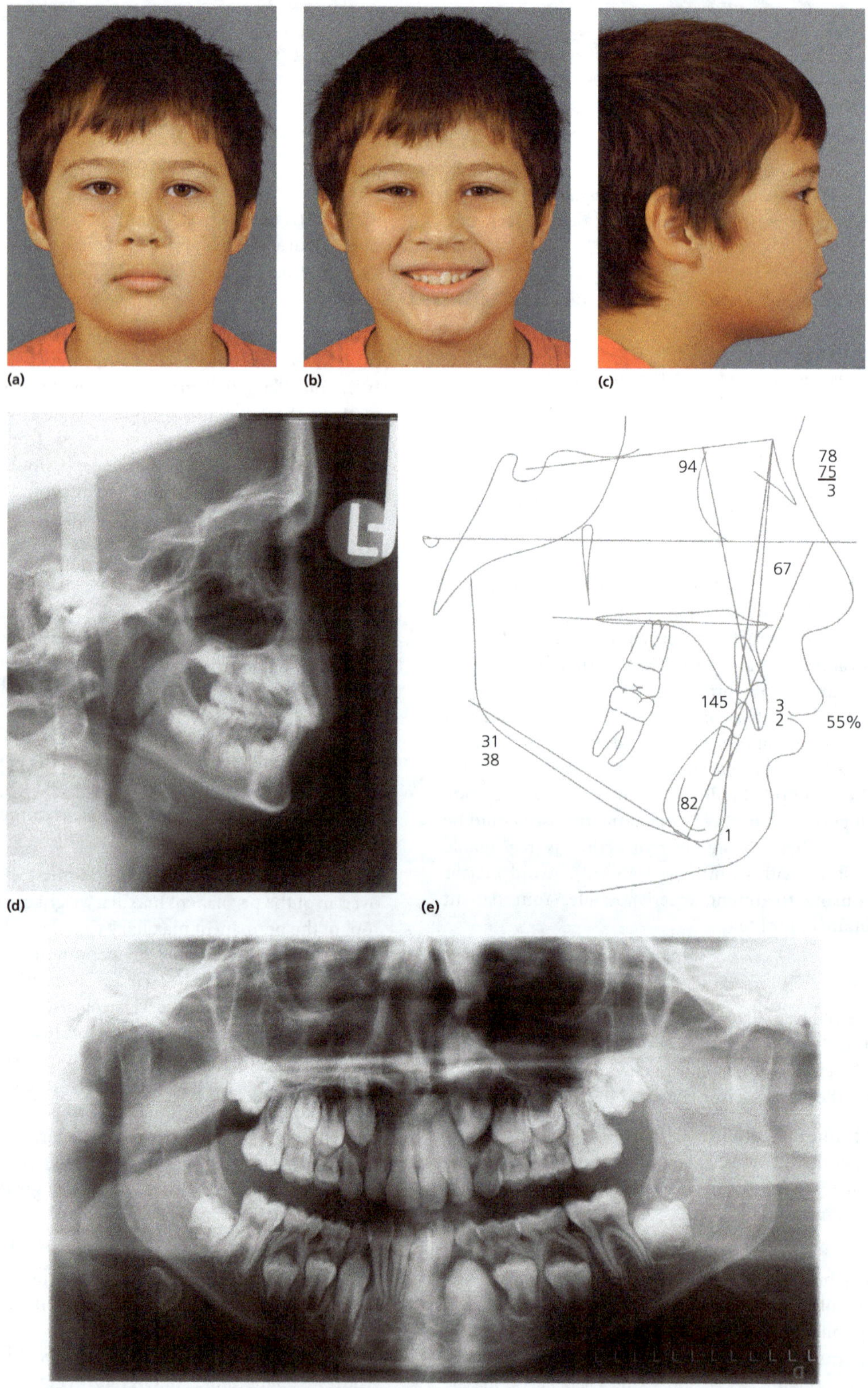

Figure 2.45 Initial records of Andrew: (a–c) initial facial photographs, (d) lateral cephalograph, (e) cephalometric tracing, (f) pantomograph, (g–k) intraoral photographs, (l–p) model photographs, and (q–u) separated model views.

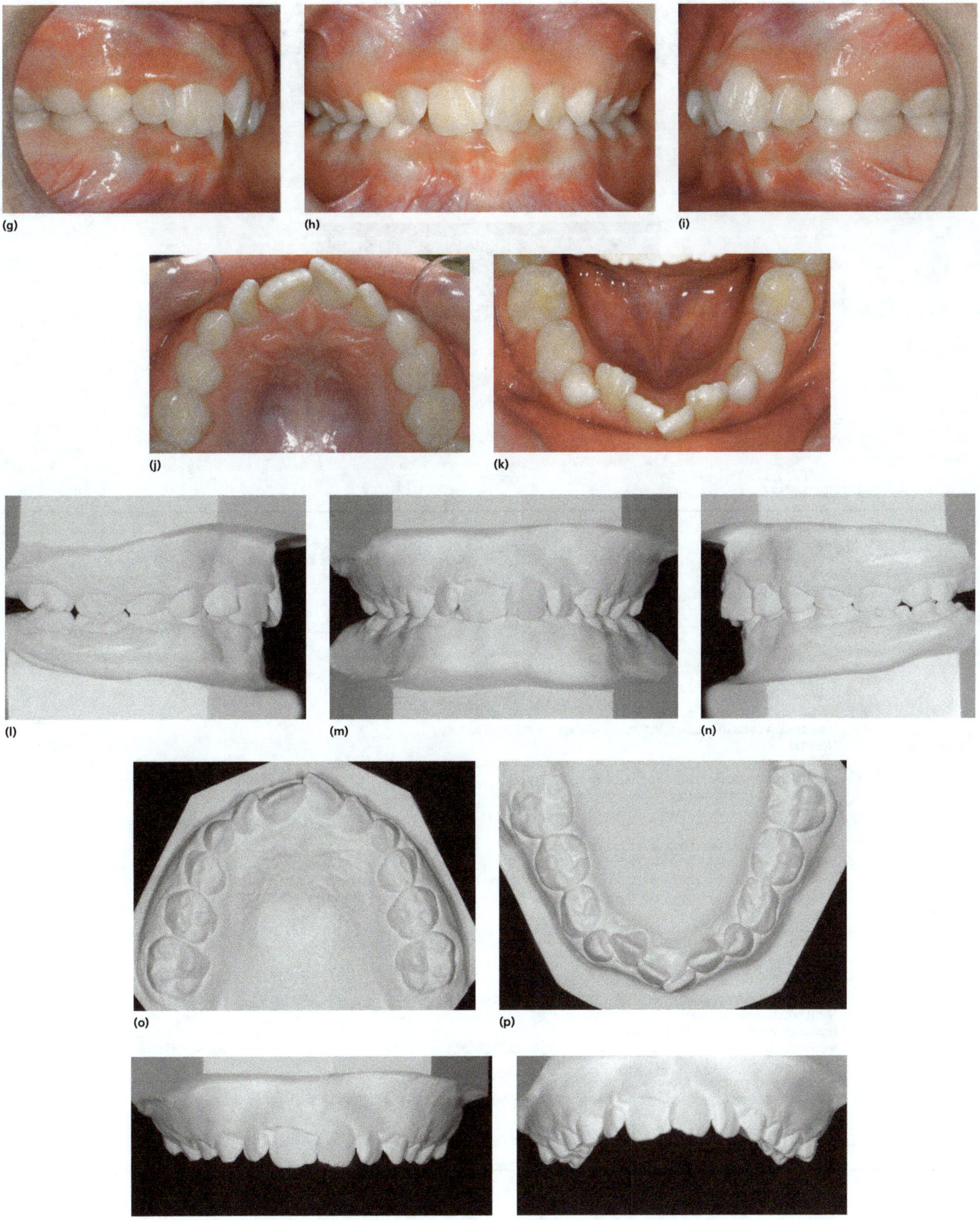

Figure 2.45 (Continued)

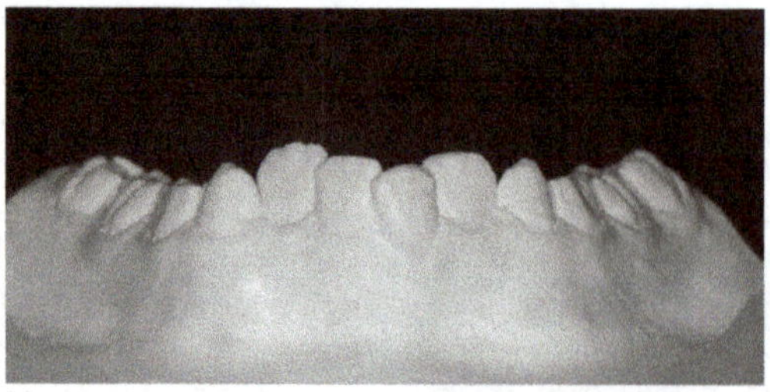

(s)

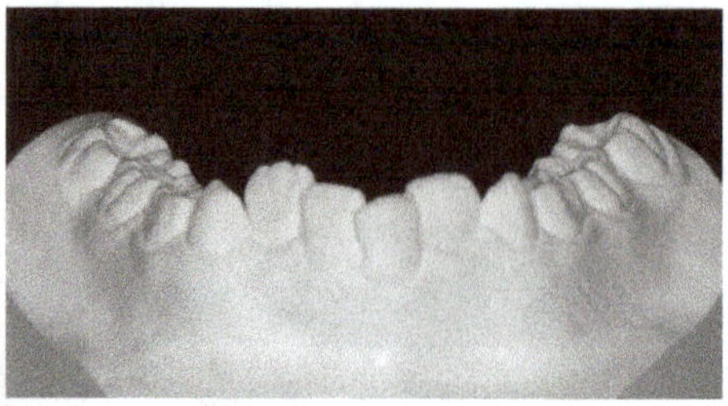

(t)

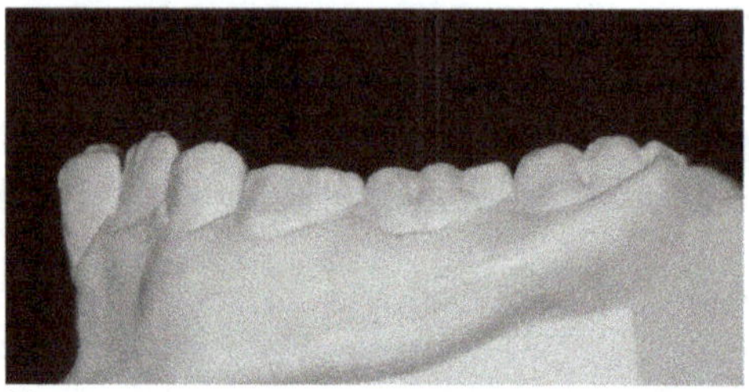

(u)

Figure 2.45 (Continued)

Table 2.2 Diagnostic findings and problem list for Andrew.

Full face and profile	**Frontal view** Face is symmetric Vertical facial proportions appear WRN (Figure 2.45a, soft tissue Glabella—Subnasale approximately equal to Subnasale–soft tissue Menton) Absence of interlabial gap Prominent buccal corridors UDML: WRN Excessive gingival display in posed smile (central incisor gingival margins inferior to vermillion border of maxillary lip) **Profile view** Obtuse naso-labial angle (NLA) with upturned nose Convex profile Retrusive chin Mildly deep labiomental sulcus Differential fullness of maxillary and mandibular lips (mandibular lip fuller)
Ceph analysis	**Skeletal** Maxillary anteroposterior position is retrusive (A-point lies behind Nasion-perpendicular line) Mild mandibular retrusion (ANB = 3°, but maxilla is retrusive) LAFH/TAFH: ideal (ANS-Menton/Nasion-Menton ~55%) Steep mandibular plane (FMA = 31°; SNMP = 38°) **Dental** Upright maxillary incisors (Mx central incisor to SN = 94°) Mandibular incisors: WRN (FMIA = 67°)
Radiographs	Early mixed dentition transitioning into late mixed dentition as the mandibular canines erupt in the next few months Small overlap of maxillary right permanent canine crown over root of maxillary permanent lateral incisor
Intraoral photos and models	Angle Class II division 2 Iowa Classification: II (1–2) II (1–2) II (3–4) II (3–4) OJ: ~3 mm OB: ~100% COS: ~3 mm, mandibular anterior teeth over-erupted Maxillary incisors are stepped down relative to the posterior maxillary occlusion Slight buccal crown torque maxillary first molars Lingual crown torque mandibular first molars Moderate mandibular and maxillary anterior crowding (since the permanent canines are unerupted and the leeway space is still present, it is difficult to estimate the precise tooth size arch length deficiency) Midlines are not coincident (LDML to right of UDML by 1–2 mm) Dental arches demonstrate a slight maxillary asymmetry (maxillary left first molar ahead) and mandibular asymmetry (mandibular right first molar ahead)
Other	None
Diagnosis	Angle Class II division 2 malocclusion Dental deep bite

maxillary permanent canines are not erupting to the palatal. Additionally, the primary canines appear to be resorbing normally. Further, there appears to be adequate room for at least initial eruption of the permanent canines (Figure 2.45j). So, there is no need to extract primary teeth at this time.

Q: If you suspect maxillary right permanent canine impaction (palatal or labial), is there anything you could do to increase the chance for spontaneous eruption?

A: Yes, *extract the primary maxillary right canine and create space for the permanent canine* using [37–47] the following:

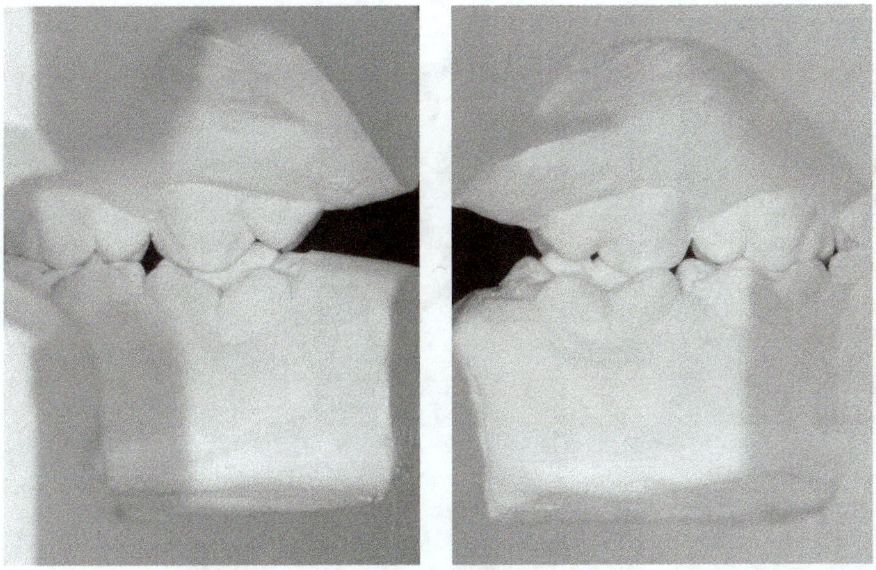

(a) (b)

Figure 2.46 (a, b) Andrew's models as viewed from the lingual.

- Fixed orthodontic appliances. Trapping an open-coil spring between the posterior teeth and the lateral incisor can be effective. However, the spring force should be kept light, and the lateral incisor bracket should be tipped so as to *move the lateral incisor root mesial* (away from the erupting permanent canine crown).
- RME followed by TPA.
- Distal movement of the posterior teeth using headgear.
- Extraction of the primary maxillary first molar in addition to the primary canine.
- Localized permanent tooth extractions.
- Extraction of the primary canines plus placement of a TPA. A recent study suggests that this is as effective as extraction of the primary canines plus RME plus TPA [48].

Q: Define your treatment goals for Andrew.

A: Improve his profile (increasing chin projection), reduce his incisal/gingival display, decrease his buccal corridors, achieve Class I canine and molar relationships, and achieve ideal OB and OJ.

Q: Which facial dimensions have apical base discrepancies?

A: AP only (mandibular AP hypoplasia)

Q: What are Andrew's major, or *primary*, problems in each dimension (plus other problems)?

A: See Table 2.3

Q: How can you address Andrew's AP apical base discrepancy?

A: *Orthopedics* (restrict maxillary growth while permitting the mandible to continue growing forward and/or accelerate mandibular growth). The advantage of orthopedic treatment is that Andrew's molar relationship could be corrected and his profile esthetics potentially improved. Orthopedic options:

- Headgears (Figure 2.47): High-pull headgear effects in growing individuals (Figure 2.47c and e) include distalization of the maxillary molars through the maxillary alveolar process bone (creating space for Andrew's crowded maxillary canines and incisors), while at the same time potentially restricting maxillary forward growth. In the vertical dimension, a high-pull headgear may reduce descent of the maxillary corpus and may reduce eruption of the maxillary first molars [49, 50].

Table 2.3 Primary problems list for Andrew *(apical base/skeletal discrepancies italicized)*.

AP	II (1–2) II (1–2) II (3–4) II (3–4) *Mandibular skeletal retrusion*
Vertical	100% OB due to 2–3 mm deep curve of Spee (overerupted mandibular anterior teeth) and overerupted maxillary incisors
Transverse	Absence of posterior cross bites, but presence of mandibular first molar lingual crown torque
Other	—

These effects of high-pull headgear, along with favorable mandibular growth, will facilitate correction of Andrew's Class II molar relationship and potentially improve his chin projection. In a study of high-pull headgears in monkeys, cephalometric and histologic analysis actually revealed posterior and superior maxillary corpus displacement [51]. Due to Andrew's excessive maxillary gingival and incisal display, a cervical headgear (Figure 2.47b) should not be used. Why? Cervical-pull headgear effects in growing individuals (Figure 2.47d and f) include anterior palatal plane downward rotation, which could increase his gingival and incisal display [50, 52]. Cervical-pull headgears also restrict forward maxillary growth and retract maxillary first molars. Surprisingly, less than 1 mm of molar extrusion occurs.

- Functional appliances: With relatively upright mandibular incisors (FMIA of 67°) Andrew would be a good candidate for a functional appliance, such as a twin block (Figure 2.48a) or bionator (Figure 2.48b). Class II functional appliances posture the mandible forward, distracting the condylar head out of the glenoid fossa (Figure 2.48c). As the mandible is held forward, the stretched musculature and other soft tissues attempt to retract the mandible, producing the following effects to varying degrees depending on the appliance used: retraction of maxillary posterior teeth, uprighting of maxillary incisors, mesial movement of mandibular posterior teeth, proclination of mandibular incisors, acceleration of condylar growth, and anterior displacement of the glenoid fossae in growing individuals [53, 54].

Correction of a Class II malocclusion using a fixed functional appliance, a Herbst appliance, is illustrated in Figure 2.49. The adolescent patient had an impacted maxillary left central

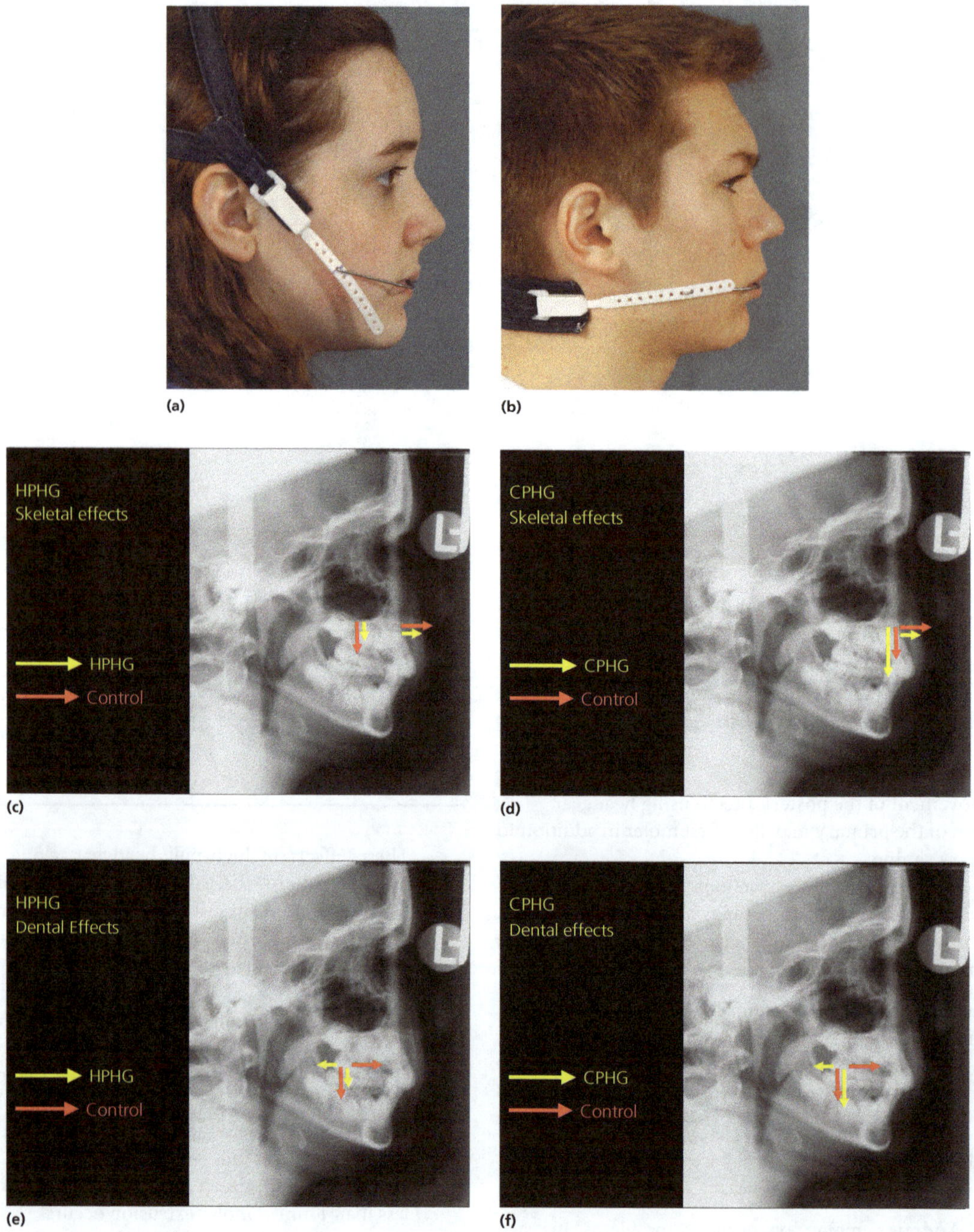

Figure 2.47 (a, c, and e) Skeletal and dental effects of high-pull headgears (HPHG) and (b, d, and f) cervical-pull headgears (CPHG) compared to controls.

incisor, which was first erupted (Figure 2.49g and h), at which time the Herbst appliance was delivered (Figures 2.49i–m). The Herbst appliance held the mandible forward in a Class III canine relationship for 9 months. The Herbst appliance was removed, fixed orthodontic appliances were placed, and the arches leveled/aligned and finished. Significant growth occurred during treatment (Figure 2.49n), and an excellent result was achieved (Figure 2.49o–t).

Care must be taken to minimize posterior tooth eruption with functional appliances. As the mandible is postured forward in deep bite patients, a temporary posterior open bite may occur, posterior teeth may then erupt, and the mandible may undergo backward rotation. To help minimize posterior tooth eruption during functional appliance treatment, maxillary fixed appliances may be placed to advance the maxillary incisors and open spaces between the maxillary lateral incisors and maxillary canines, creating OJ, and permitting the mandible to be postured forward while maintaining posterior occlusal contact. Or, the posterior teeth in one jaw can be "capped" with the appliance acrylic to prevent eruption. Functional appliances *do* accelerate mandibular growth in growing individuals. However, they do *not* enhance mandibular horizontal growth beyond that found in control subjects [55]. As they have been shown to promote condylar growth in a posterior direction, the increase in mandibular length gained by functional appliance treatment may not improve chin projection [56–58].

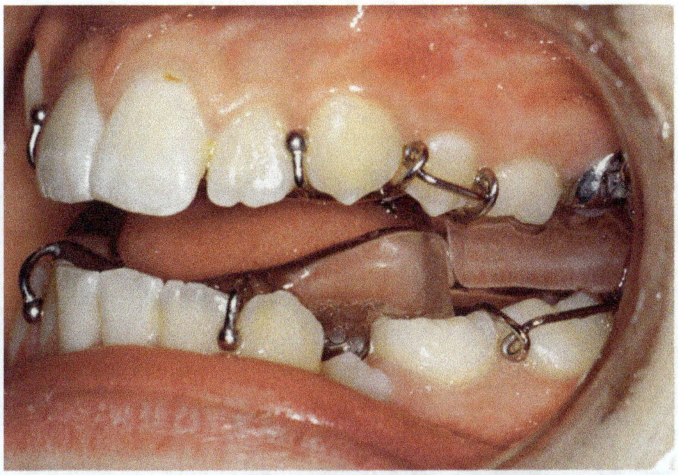

(a)

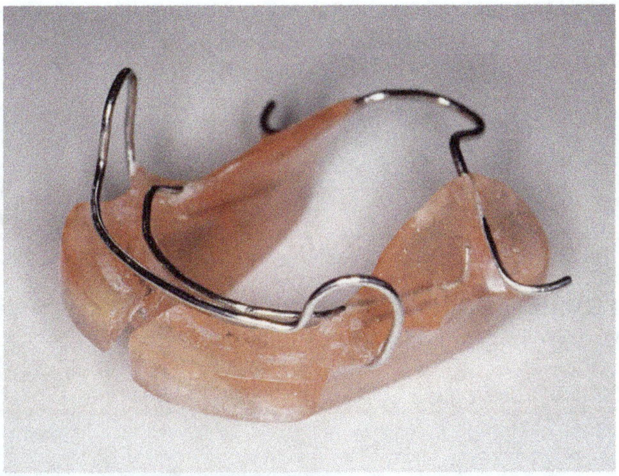

(b)

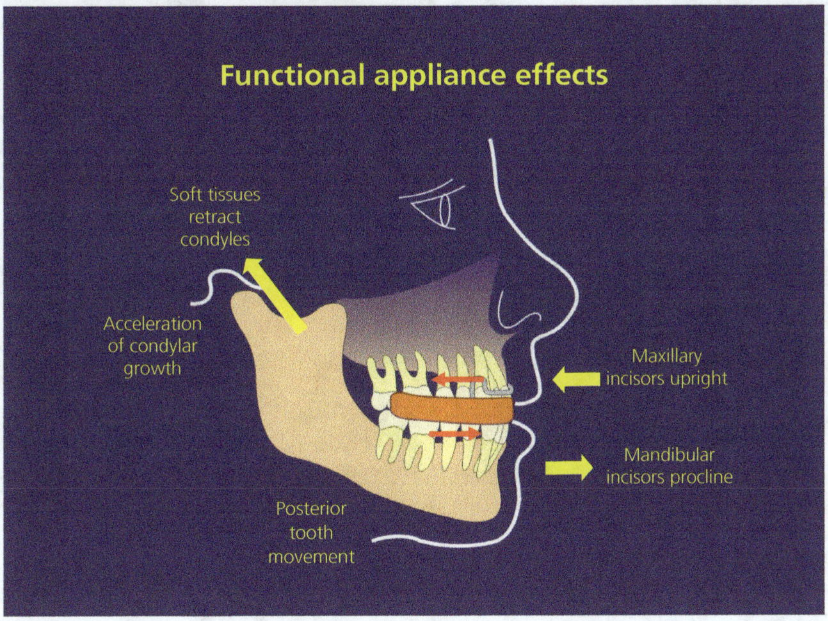

(c)

Figure 2.48 Effects of Class II functional appliances, such as a (a) twin block or (b) bionator, as the mandible is held forward (c).

Masking or camouflage (achieving a Class I canine relationship without addressing the underlying apical base discrepancy) could correct Andrew's molar and canine relationships to Class I but would not improve his profile esthetics (chin projection). Masking would be considered if Andrew was uncooperative with headgear or functional appliance treatment.

Masking options:

- Extraction of maxillary first premolars (see Figure 2.50, a temporary anchorage device is being used for anchorage), which would permit retraction/alignment of the maxillary anterior teeth (ending with Class I canines and Class II molars). The drawback of this approach is that Andrew's maxillary incisors are already upright—any retraction of maxillary incisors could result in further incisor uprighting and bite deepening. See Figure 2.51—in the top left illustration, maxillary first premolars have been extracted and the maxillary canines have been retracted. Activating the closing loops results in a retraction force at the brackets of the maxillary incisors (Figure 2.51, top center left). This force is equivalent to the same retraction force plus a counter clockwise (CCW) moment at the incisors' center of resistance (CR) (Figure 2.51, top center right). The retraction force at CR translates the incisors distally, but the CCW at CR uprights the incisors (Figure 2.51, top right). This uprighting can be prevented (Figure 2.51, bottom) by filling the bracket slot with a large rectangular archwire (to reduce "play" between the archwire and bracket), placing lingual root torque in the archwire, decreasing the retraction force magnitude (so that the CCW moment at CR is reduced), and giving the archwire adequate time to drive the roots through the bone.
- Use of a temporary anchorage device (TAD) to retract the entire maxillary arch to Class I without extractions. In Figure 2.52, a TAD was placed in the maxillary buccal left and used as anchorage to drive the maxillary left molars

distally to Class III with an open coil spring (Figure 2.52b and c). The TAD was then removed and the space closed, reciprocally, to retract the canine/premolars to Class I and protract the molars forward to Class I (Figure 2.52d).

- Use of Class II elastics (Figure 2.53a), Class II springs (Figure 2.53b), or other interarch Class II correctors (e.g., Jasper Jumpers, Eureka Springs, etc.) to make the correction.

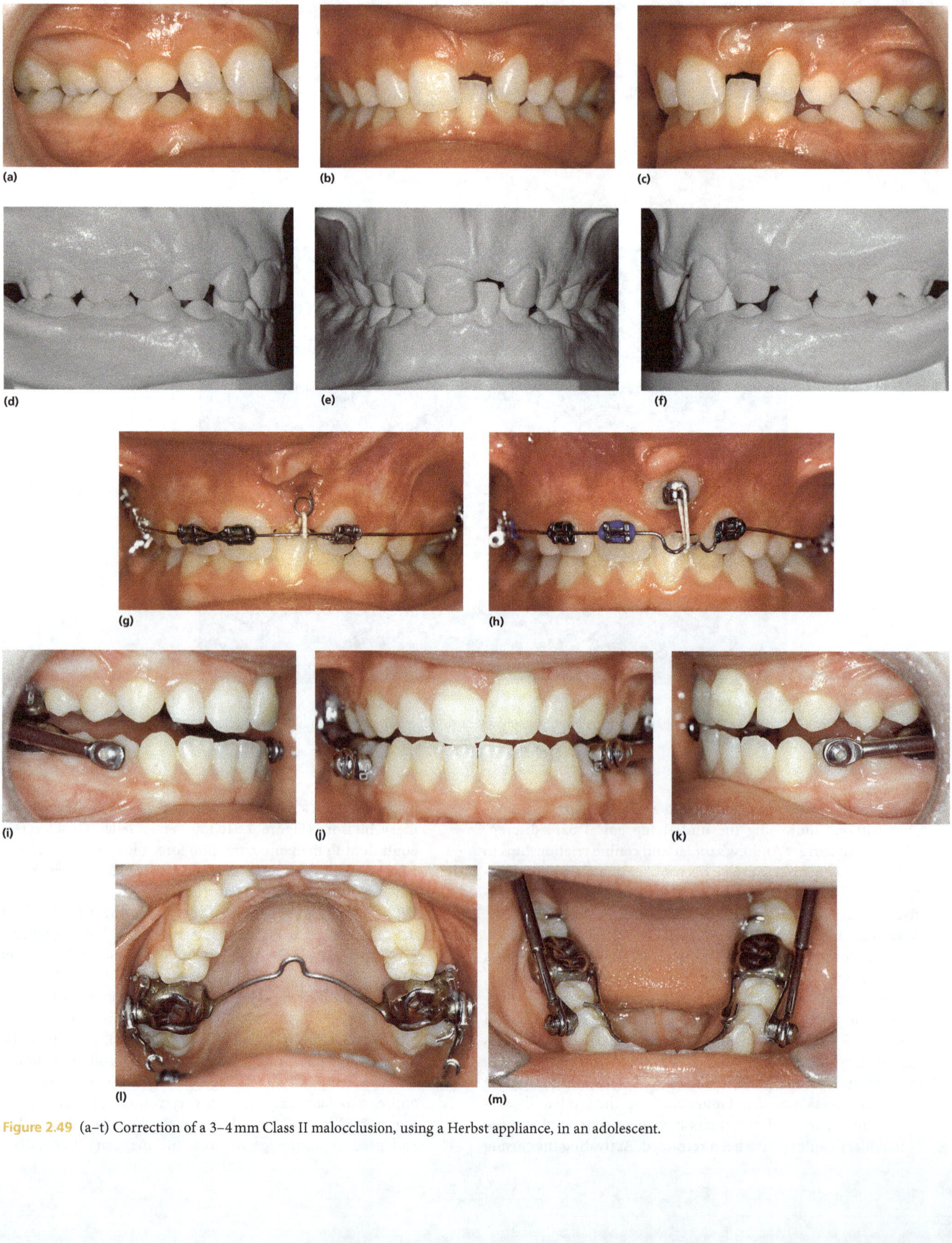

(a) (b) (c) (d) (e) (f) (g) (h) (i) (j) (k) (l) (m)

Figure 2.49 (a–t) Correction of a 3–4 mm Class II malocclusion, using a Herbst appliance, in an adolescent.

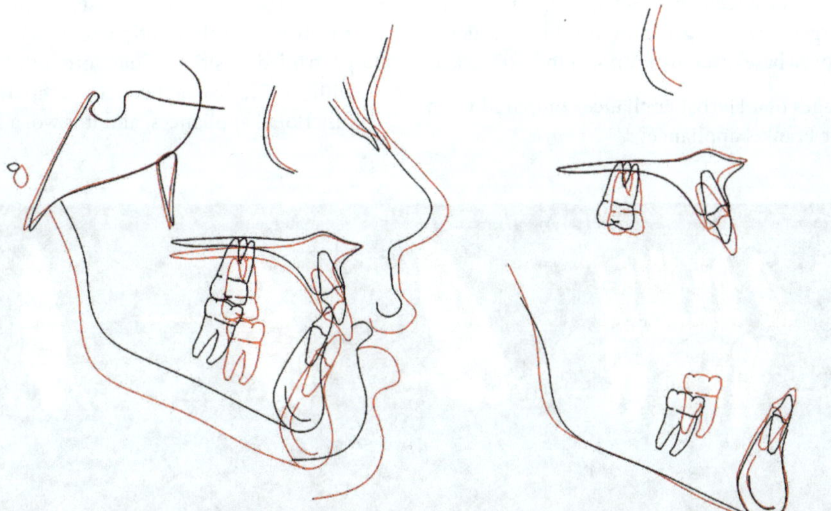

(n)

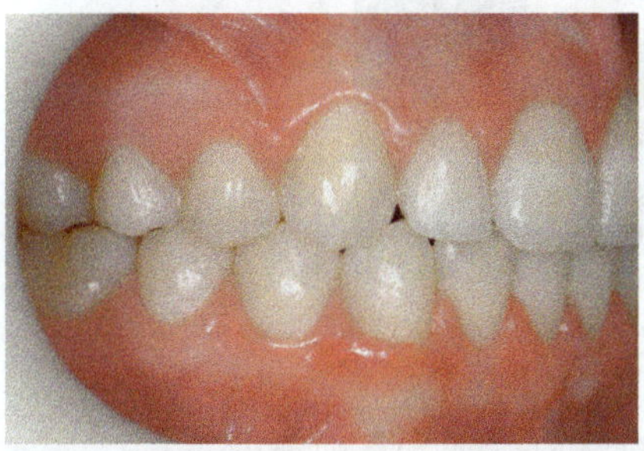

(o)

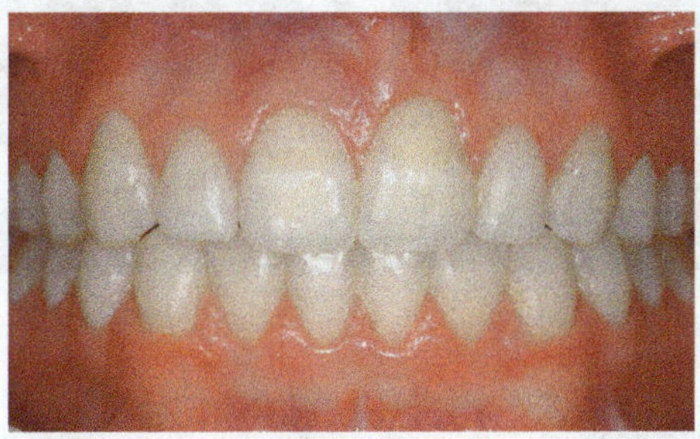

(p)

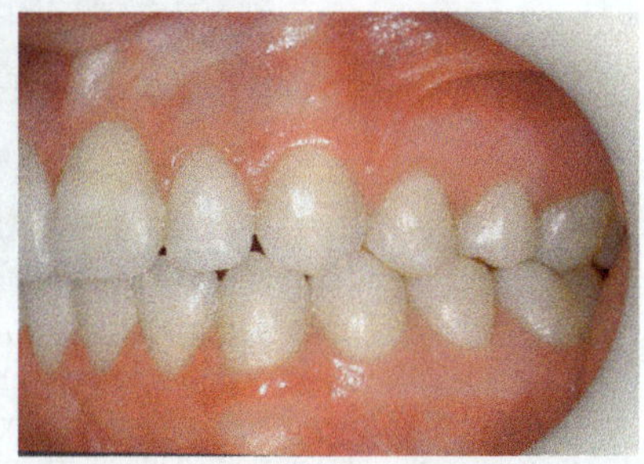

(q)

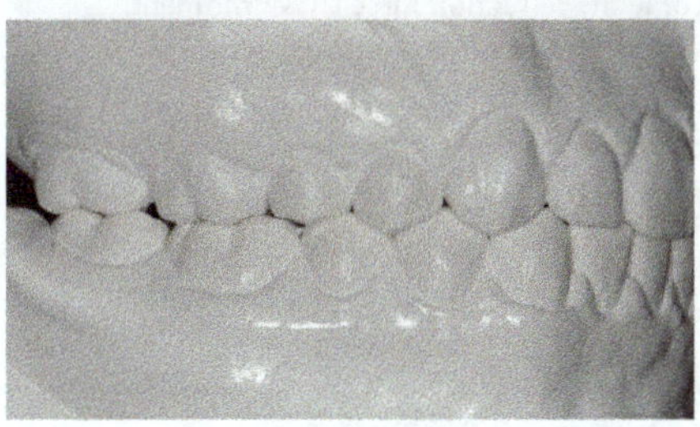

(r)

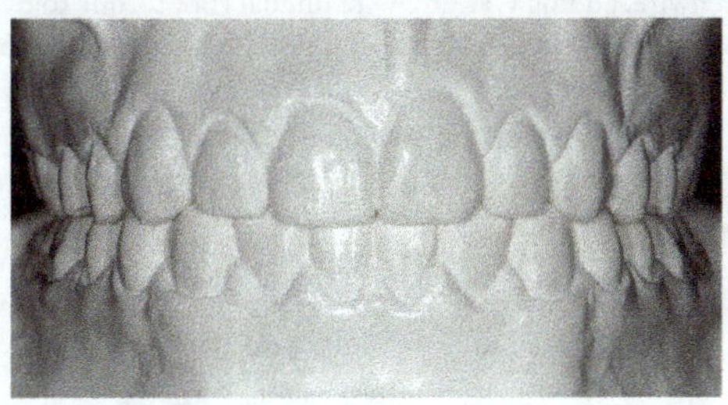

(s)

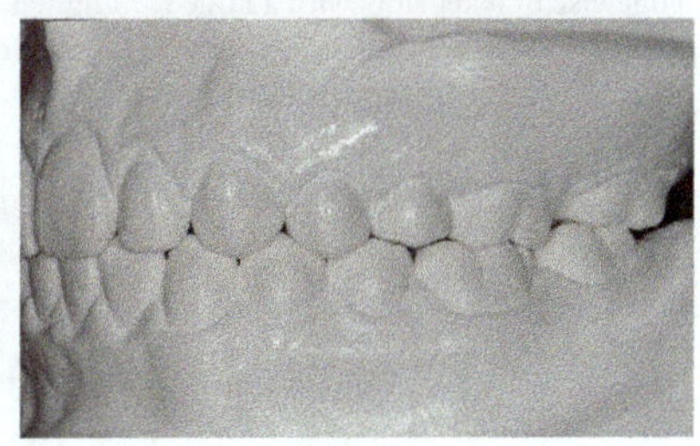

(t)

Figure 2.49 (Continued)

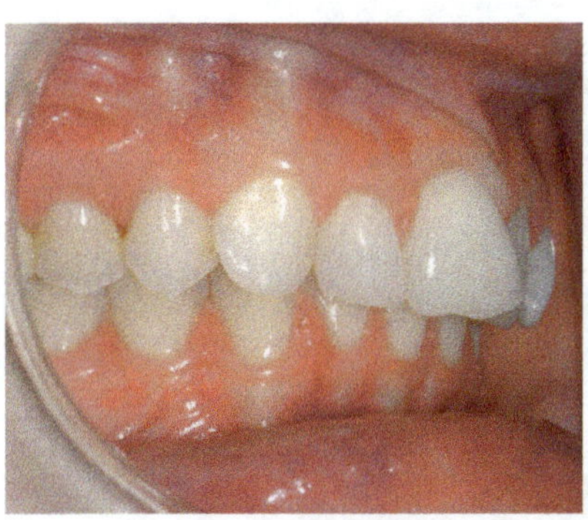

(a)

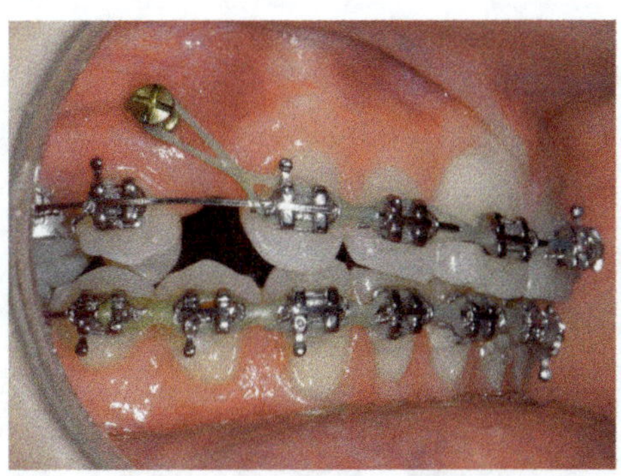

(b)

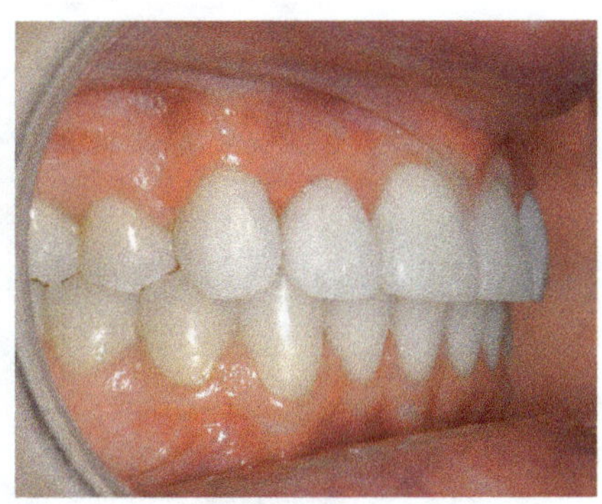

(c)

Figure 2.50 Masking, or camouflage, of a Class II (mandibular deficient) patient by extraction of maxillary first premolars: (a) initial Class II relationship, (b) extraction of maxillary first premolars and retraction of maxillary anterior teeth using TADs as anchorage, and (c) final Class I relationship.

Surgery (mandibular advancement—Figure 2.54a initial, Figure 2.54b post-surgery) would generally not be considered with Andrew's mild apical base discrepancy nor at this young age.

Q: What are the advantages of a Herbst appliance compared to an activator, Bionator, or Frankel appliance?

A: The Herbst appliance consists of a bilateral telescope mechanism attached to orthodontic bands, which keep the mandible in a protruded position. Therefore, minimal cooperation is needed with a Herbst appliance compared to other (removable) functional appliances, and it is worn 24 h per day.

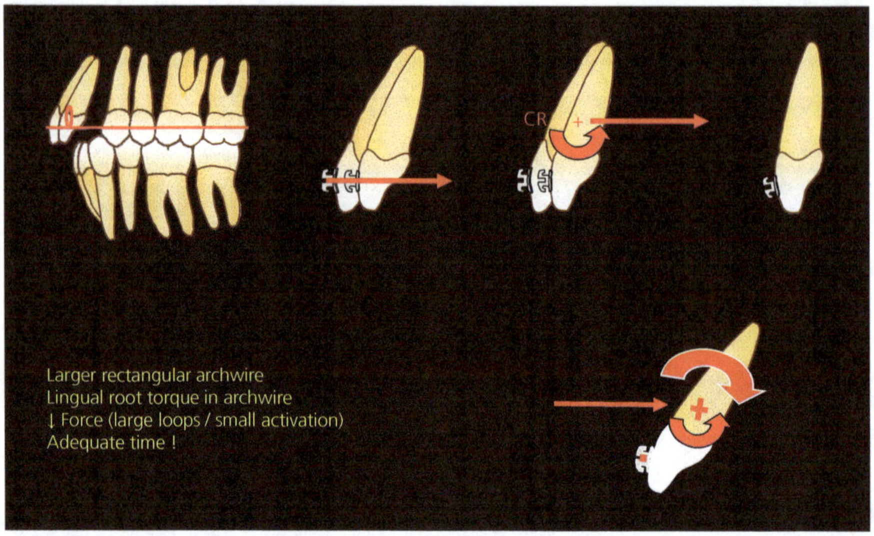

Figure 2.51 Tendency for maxillary incisors to upright during retraction: (top left) maxillary incisors to be retracted using a closing loop archwire, (top center left) opening the closing loop results in a retraction force being applied against the maxillary incisor brackets, (top center right) at the center of resistance (CR) this retraction force is equivalent to the same retraction force translating the incisors distally plus a CCW moment tending to upright the incisors, (top right) uprighted maxillary incisors, (bottom) this tendency for maxillary incisors to upright can be reduced by filling the incisor edgewise bracket slots with a large rectangular archwire, adding CW archwire lingual root torque to overcome the retraction force CCW moment, decreasing the retraction force magnitude so its CCW moment is reduced, and providing adequate time for the incisor roots to move through the maxillary alveolar process bone.

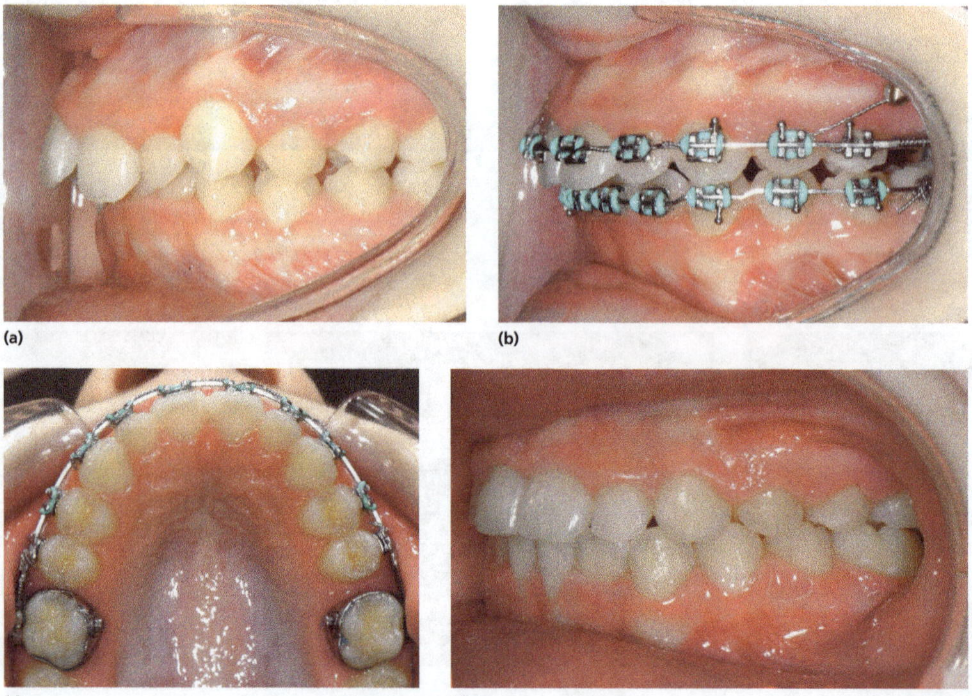

Figure 2.52 Masking, or camouflage, of a Class II (mandibular deficient) patient by retracting the entire maxillary arch: (a) initial Class II relationship, (b and c) distalization of maxillary molars to Class III with an open-coil spring—the more anterior teeth are held in place with a steel ligature to a left buccal TAD, and (d) following TAD removal and reciprocal space closure, a Class I relationship was achieved.

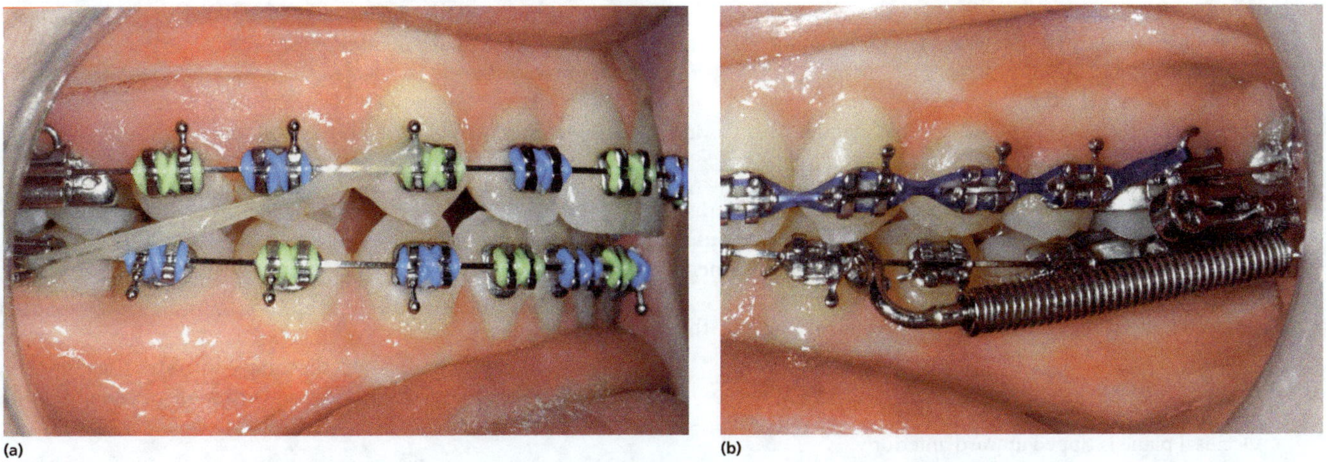

Figure 2.53 Masking, or camouflage, of a Class II (mandibular deficient) patient by use of interarch Class II mechanics: (a) elastic and (b) spring.

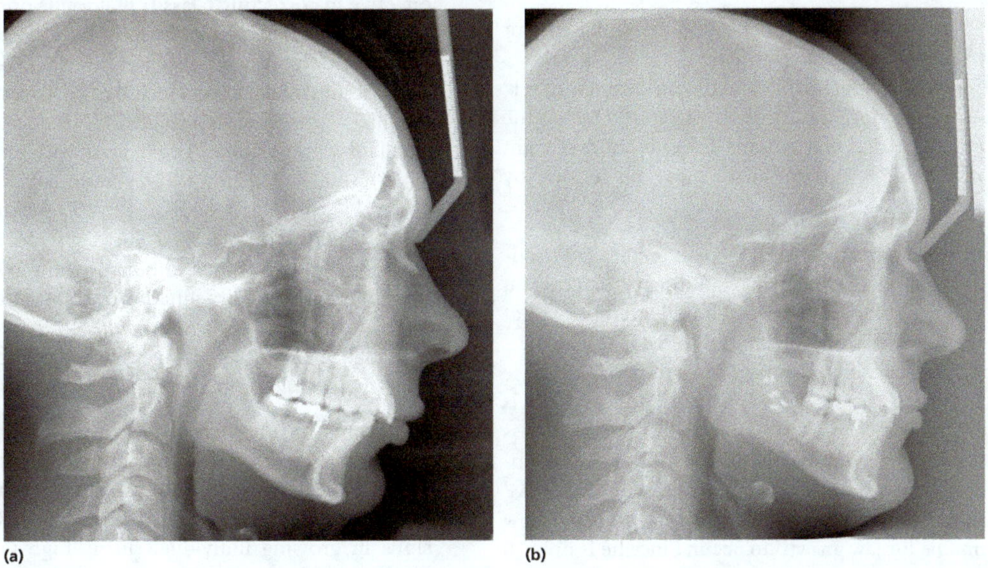

Figure 2.54 Surgical correction of a Class II (mandibular deficient) patient with a BSSO mandibular advancement osteotomy: (a) initial relationship and (b) final relationship.

Q: Is the Herbst appliance indicated in the deciduous or mixed dentition? What is the usual active treatment time when using a Herbst appliance?

A: There is controversy in the literature regarding this question. It has been suggested that the Herbst appliance is not recommended in the deciduous or mixed dentition stages of development. Why? Because a stable intercuspation is difficult to achieve during these dentition stages and the desired orthopedic effects of Herbst therapy are maximized when stable intercuspation can be achieved during the post-treatment period. Instead, *the Herbst appliance is indicated in the permanent dentition at, or just after, the pubertal peak of growth* [53, 59]. Treatment at this time will have the greatest effect on mandibular growth with the least amount of mandibular incisor proclination. *A total of 6–9 months of wear is normally indicated with a Herbst appliance.* By contrast, successful correction of Class II molar relationships by Herbst therapy in the mixed dentition has been shown to remain stable throughout the transitional dental period. However, the skeletal response in these subjects was primarily maxillary restraint and mandibular vertical development, with little effect on sagittal mandibular projection [60].

Q: You provide a Herbst appliance to an 11-year-old Class II patient. You have designed the appliance to keep the patient in a slightly Class III (1 mm) molar relationship, and you leave the appliance in for nine months. What skeletal and dental changes do you expect to see?

A: Skeletal and dental changes with Herbst treatment include the following:

- Inhibition of maxillary growth
- Distal movement of maxillary teeth

- Maxillary molars are intruded in majority of patients
- Occlusal plane is tipped down in the anterior in the majority of patients
- Acceleration of mandibular growth
- Mesial movement of mandibular teeth (mandibular incisors procline) [53]

Q: For a typical 11-year-old Class II patient treated with a Herbst appliance, it is estimated that 90% of post-treatment occlusal changes occur during the first 6 months after Herbst treatment is discontinued. What are these post treatment changes?

A: Post-treatment changes after Herbst treatment include the following:
- Mesial movement of maxillary teeth
- Maxillary molars erupt
- Occlusal plane is tipped upward anteriorly
- Distal movement of mandibular teeth (mandibular incisors upright)
- Less mandibular length increase compared to control subjects [53]

Q: What is the effect of Herbst treatment on mandibular incisor proclination? What is seen post treatment?

A: During treatment, lower incisors procline an average of 11° and the incisal edges move anteriorly by 3.2 mm. During the first post-treatment period of 6 months, lower incisors upright an average of 8° and the incisal edges move posteriorly by 2.5 mm [61].

Q: If you are considering treating Andrew orthopedically (headgear or functional appliance), are there guiding principles you should follow in deciding *whether* you should attempt to treat him orthopedically and *when* you should initiate treatment?

A: Yes. First, you must consider the *magnitude* of his apical base discrepancy. In Andrew's case, the AP apical base discrepancy is relatively mild (ANB angle of 3° with a retrusive maxilla, Class II molar relationship of 2–4 mm). Because of this, if he is cooperative, you have a reasonable chance of making a full AP correction using orthopedics. Second, you must consider how much *time* remains for jaw growth to occur. Since he is only 10 years old, you have significant time to utilize orthopedics. Next, you must decide *when* to begin Class II treatment. There is generally no advantage to beginning Class II treatment in the early mixed dentition [62–65], but Andrew is about ready to enter the late mixed dentition stage of development. Now is the time to begin. An important point—timing Class II orthopedic treatment to coincide with the late mixed dentition dental stage is to be taken as a broad guideline and not a fixed rule. Dental stage is poorly correlated with skeletal growth—so you must use your own judgment in deciding when to initiate orthopedic treatment. Average onset of the statural growth spurt is a little more than 9 years for girls and a little less than 12 years for boys; peak of the statural growth spurt is about 1½–2 years later; facial skeletal growth peaks later; but, there is considerable variation in these times amongst patients [66]. *Even if Andrew was in the early mixed dentition, but his parents told you he was beginning to enter his growth spurt, then you should consider initiating orthopedic treatment immediately.* In summary, considering his mild AP apical base discrepancy and his future growth potential, Andrew is a good candidate for orthopedic treatment. As he is entering the late mixed dentition stage of treatment, begin orthopedic treatment now.

Q: Regarding growth during adolescent orthopedic treatment, when is growth hormone released?

A: Growth hormone is released, in a pulsatile fashion, typically with a large bolus as a child goes to sleep in the early evening, sometimes with pulses in the later sleep cycle [67, 68].

Q: When does tooth eruption occur?

A: Nearly, all tooth eruption occurs between 8 PM and midnight, and often some intrusion during the early morning [69, 70].

Q: Based on the above two questions, when might we speculate would be the optimal time to apply orthopedic treatment each day?

A: Between early evening and morning—to restrict jaw growth, accelerate jaw growth, restrict tooth eruption, or enhance tooth eruption.

Q: Are headgears and functional appliances equally effective in correcting Class II malocclusions in children (before comprehensive treatment)? Are headgears and functional appliances, followed by fixed orthodontic appliances, equally effective in correcting Class II malocclusions in children?

A: *Before comprehensive treatment—yes, headgears and functional appliances are equally effective* [63–65, 71–78]. Unequivocal short-term skeletal effects include a small restriction in forward maxillary growth with headgear (SNA decreases 0.5–3°) and a small forward positioning of B-point with functional appliances (1–2°), resulting in an ANB improvement in Class II patients of about 1° with either appliance. A significant portion of the Class II correction is distal maxillary molar movement with headgears and mesial mandibular molar movement (along with mandibular incisor proclination) with functional appliances.

Following comprehensive treatment—unknown. Higher levels of evidence are missing to answer the question of whether their effects *following* comprehensive treatment are equal.

Q: What are the long-term (post-retention) skeletal effects of treatment for Class II malocclusions in growing individuals using cervical traction headgear? What are the long-term (post-retention) skeletal effects of treatment for Class II malocclusions in growing individuals using high-pull or vertical-pull headgear? What are the long-term (post-retention) skeletal effects of treatment for Class II malocclusions in growing individuals using functional appliances?

A: *Cervical traction*—the available evidence, based largely on retrospective nonrandomized studies, suggests that reduction of the SNA angle by treatment is largely stable, the SNB angle is largely unaffected by treatment or continued growth, and any increase in mandibular plane angle caused by treatment is recovered during continued facial growth. The question of whether cervical traction causes a clinically significant change in vertical facial proportions remains equivocal [78].

High-pull or vertical-pull—The immediate skeletal effects of high-pull and vertical-pull headgear are thought to be different from that of cervical traction headgear. However, at present, a similar analysis of high-pull or vertical-pull headgear is not possible because no long-term evaluations involving the exclusive use of these treatment modalities with or without edgewise treatment are available [78].

Functional appliances—the available evidence, based largely on retrospective nonrandomized studies, suggests that, over the long-term, functional appliances do not modify the inherited facial growth pattern significantly. A lasting enhancement of horizontal mandibular growth is not supported for Bionator, Headgear-Activator, or Herbst appliances, and remains equivocal for the Fränkel FR-2 appliance [78].

Q: Is profile improvement better in growing Class II patients treated with headgear or Herbst appliances?

A: *Both treatments result in significantly improved profiles that are similarly attractive* [79]. For example, Figure 2.55 top illustrates the profile silhouettes of a Class II patient with an average amount of esthetic improvement when treated with headgear (before left, after right). Figure 2.55 bottom illustrates the profile silhouettes of a Class II patient with an average amount of esthetic improvement when treated with a Herbst appliance (before left, after right). Both final profiles were judged similarly attractive.

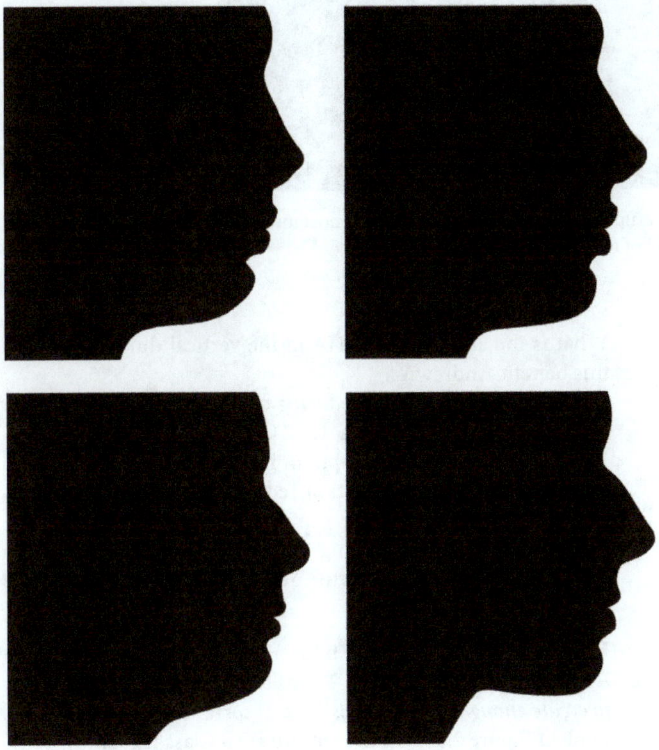

Figure 2.55 Before (left) and after (right) silhouettes of patients having average profile improvements when using headgear (top) and Herbst (bottom) appliances.

Q: What are the effects Class II springs (e.g., Forsus™ appliance)?

A: Maxillary molar distal movement, mandibular molar mesial movement, maxillary incisor retrusion, mandibular incisor proclination, and mandibular incisor intrusion [80, 81]. Restriction of the maxilla [1] has also been reported (an orthopedic effect), but Forsus springs are not generally used for long enough periods of time for this effect to be significant.

Q: What are the effects of Class II elastics?

A: Mainly dentoalveolar: maxillary incisor eruption and lingual tipping, mandibular incisor labial tipping, mandibular molar eruption, and mesial movement [82]. For example, look at the illustration in Figure 2.56. This high MPA patient wore heavy Class II elastics for many months. The mandibular molar erupted and moved mesially; the maxillary incisors erupted and moved lingually; and the mandible rotated down and back increasing the patient's facial height and worsening his profile. Class II elastics have their place. Most orthodontists use them in many Class II patients. But be careful of using heavy Class II elastics in steep MPA patients for extended periods of time. *Principle of Class II treatment: avoid treatments that tend to rotate the mandible down and back. Why? Rotating the mandible down and back worsens the Class II relationship).*

Q: What is the difference between masking Andrew's Class II apical base discrepancy using *intra-arch* mechanics (e.g., extraction of maxillary first premolars, using a headgear to distalize his maxillary teeth, or using a palatal TAD to retract the entire maxillary arch) and masking using *inter-arch* mechanics (e.g., Class II springs, Jasper jumpers, etc.)?

A: With *intra-arch* mechanics, no tooth movement will occur in the mandibular arch. Mandibular incisors are unmoved, so maxillary incisors are retracted to the same position against the mandibular incisors no matter what maxillary intra-arch treatment is chosen (non-extraction or extraction). Likewise, maxillary canines are moved from a Class II to a Class I relationship, the same amount, no matter what maxillary intra-arch treatment was chosen.

With *inter-arch* mechanics, tooth movement occurs in both arches. Maxillary incisors are retracted, but to a lesser extent than with intra-arch mechanics, since the mandibular teeth are advanced. Maxillary canines are retracted, but to a lesser extent than with intra-arch mechanics, since mandibular canines are advanced.

Q: Let's move from discussing Andrew's Class II treatment options to discussing other problems. How would you address Andrew's moderate mandibular anterior crowding?

A: Serial extraction would not be advised. Why? Because he is Class II, premolar extractions plus reciprocal mandibular space could result in an even worse canine Class II relationship. However, premolar extractions could be considered *after* Andrew was converted to a Class I molar/canine relationship with orthopedics and *after* all permanent teeth had erupted (so the amount of crowding could be accurately assessed). A prudent approach would be to first place Andrew in an LLHA and later re-evaluate mandibular crowding once the second molars erupted.

Q: How does a LLHA work?

A: *Without an LLHA*, when the mandibular primary molars exfoliate, leeway space is created—the incisors tip lingually and the molars drift mesially [83, 84]. The mesial drift of the molars can benefit an "end-on" molar relationship (moving the molars into a Class I relationship), but the mesial drift uses space that could aid anterior tooth alignment. *With an LLHA*, almost all of the leeway space is used by transeptal fibers to move the premolars and canines distally and improve alignment of the anterior teeth, spontaneously (see Figure 2.57a and b). Depending on the mesio-distal width of the second premolars, approximately 5 mm of space can be obtained in the mandibular arch using this approach [85]. Of course, an end-on molar relationship will not be corrected through mesial drift with this approach and will need to be corrected some other way (headgear, functional appliance, Class II elastics, Class II springs, etc.).

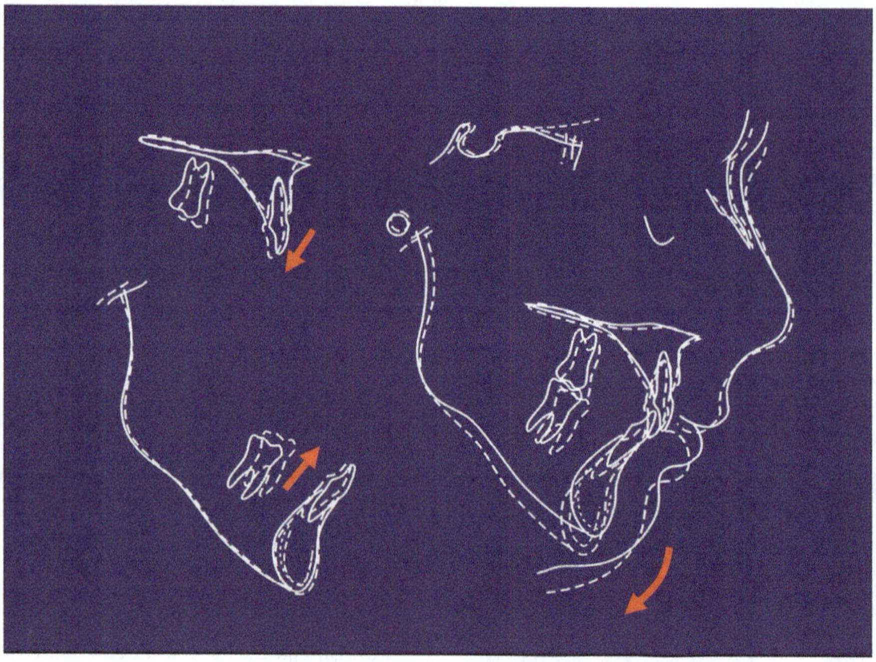

Figure 2.56 Maxillary incisor eruption and lingual tipping, mandibular molar eruption, mandibular molar mesial movement, and CW (down and back) rotation of mandible following heavy Class II elastic use for an extended period of time.

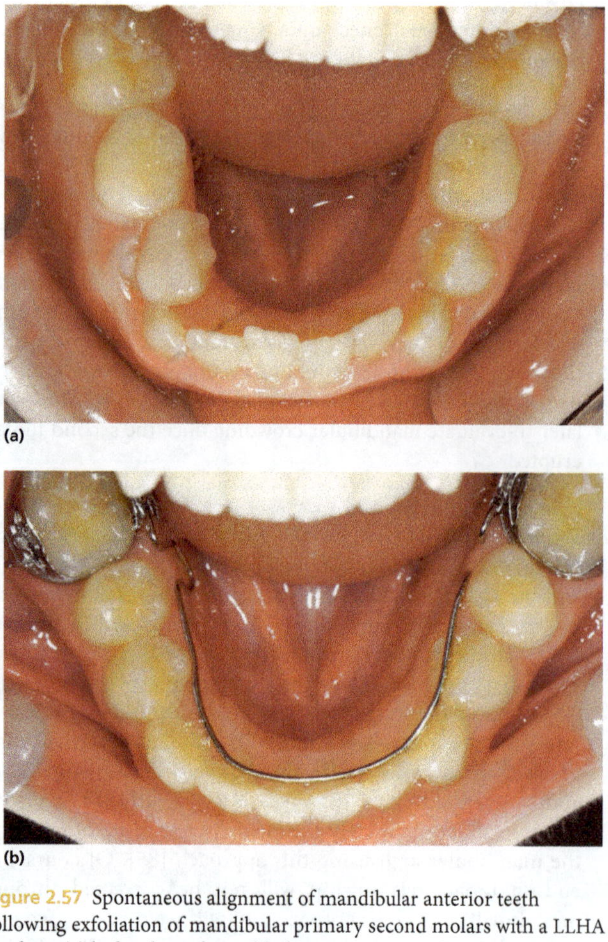

Figure 2.57 Spontaneous alignment of mandibular anterior teeth following exfoliation of mandibular primary second molars with a LLHA in place: (a) before loss of mandibular primary second molars and (b) after loss of mandibular primary second molars.

Q: What is the effect of an LLHA in the vertical dimension? Will this benefit Andrew?

A: The LLHA is effective in *reducing eruption of mandibular first molars* to 0.3 mm during a 12–24 month period versus 1.2–2.1 mm of first molar eruption in controls [86]. This is a significant amount of eruption reduction. Reduction of mandibular first molar eruption can potentially help the mandible to rotate forward (improving a Class II relationship), during mandibular condylar growth. Yes, this vertical effect could benefit Andrew.

Q: *Why* correct Andrew's deep bite?

A: Andrew's 100% OB (Figure 2.45h) must be eliminated in order *to create enough OJ so that his Class II correction can be achieved.* Look at Figure 2.58. On the left, we see a Class II (3 mm), 100% deep bite, malocclusion like Andrew has. To correct this Class II relationship, we must first "open the bite." Once the bite is opened (center), OJ is created, maxillary teeth can be retracted and/or mandibular teeth can be advanced. The result (right): a Class I occlusion with ideal OJ and ideal OB.

Q: *How* will you correct Andrew's deep bite?

A: Intruding/proclining Andrew's overerupted maxillary incisors with fixed orthodontic appliances (Figure 2.59, top left) will open his bite. A reciprocal, extrusive, force will be applied against the maxillary posterior teeth, and the maxillary arch will become level (top right). Leveling Andrew's 3 mm COS with fixed orthodontic appliances (Figure 2.59, bottom left to bottom right) results primarily through premolar extrusion (growing mandibular alveolar process bone) [14], uprighting/erupting mandibular molars, and intruding/proclining mandibular anterior teeth. Any posterior tooth eruption will rotate his mandible down and back (yellow arrow)—tend to counter forward mandibular growth and worsen his Class II relationship.

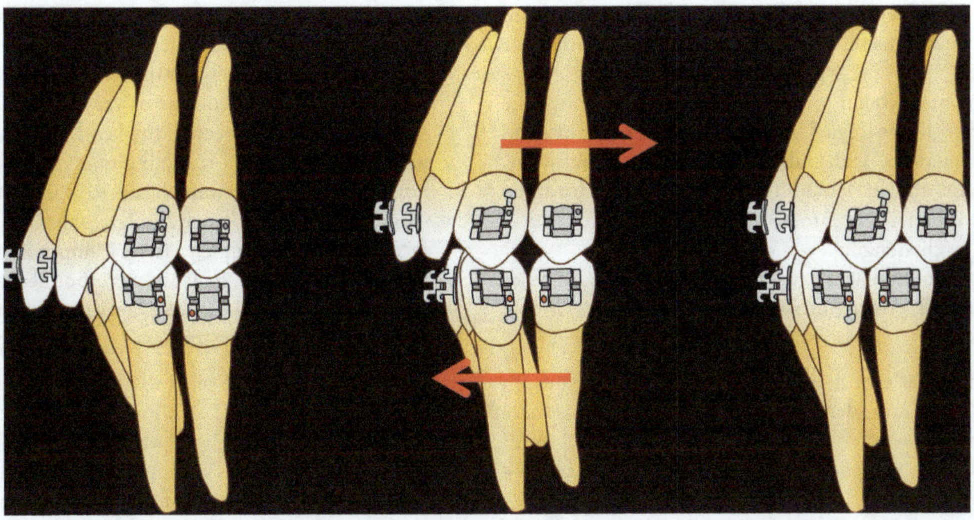

Figure 2.58 Why we need to correct Andrew's deep bite: with a deep bite (left), Andrew lacks the OJ to correct his Class II relationship; by opening his bite (center), OJ is created to allow his maxillary teeth to move distally and/or his mandibular teeth to move mesially—resulting in (right) a Class I occlusion with ideal overbite.

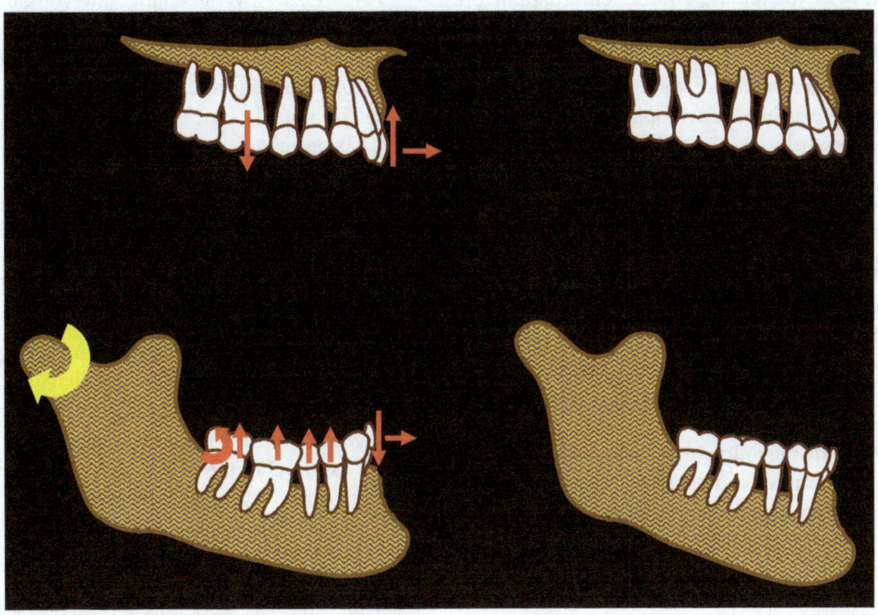

Figure 2.59 Tooth movements to correct Andrew's deep bite include leveling his maxillary arch (top, left to right) by intruding/proclining his maxillary incisors and erupting posterior teeth; leveling his mandibular curve of Spee (bottom, left to right) by intruding/proclining his mandibular incisors, and erupting his mandibular premolars and uprighting/erupting his mandibular molars. Any posterior tooth eruption will rotate his mandible CW, worsening his Class II relationship.

Q: Would you recommend RME to reduce Andrew's buccal corridors (Figure 2.45b)?

A: No, a pressing need to reduce Andrew's buccal corridors is not evident. Lay persons prefer a broader smile (smaller buccal corridors) as contrasted to a narrower smile (larger buccal corridors). Therefore, you need to identify prominent buccal corridors during your clinical exam and include this finding in the patient's problem list [87]. However, maxillary expansion is rarely warranted for the *sole* purpose of reducing large buccal corridors. On the other hand, RME may be indicated if large buccal corridors are the result from a constricted maxilla. In Andrew's case, a posterior cross bite is absent, and his maxillary arch is not constricted (Figure 2.45o). An argument could be made for RME to create posterior OJ to allow uprighting his mandibular first molars (they have significant lingual crown torque, Figure 2.45s and t).

Q: What options can your recommend for addressing Andrew's mandibular first molars lingual crown torque?

A: Options include the following:

- Expansion with an LLHA or a removable appliance (e.g., Schwartz appliance) could upright the mandibular molars. However, if the mandibular molars are uprighted by expanding them laterally, then the maxillary arch will also need to be expanded (using an RME appliance, expanded TPA, or expanded maxillary archwire) to maintain adequate posterior OJ.

- Maintain the mandibular arch width, but try to remove the mandibular posterior lingual torque using an LLHA, or fixed edgewise appliances with full-size rectangular archwires, to torque the molar roots lingually. However, torquing mandibular molar roots through thick mandibular cortical bone could be challenging.
- Maintain the mandibular arch width and leave the mandibular posterior lingual crown torque as it is. This option is a compromise.

Q: With every new patient, it is a good habit to ask yourself whether you should consider the possibility of surgery. Is there a possible need for surgery with Andrew, now or in the future? Should you discuss the possibility of surgery with Andrew's parents?

A: No. There is no need to discuss surgery or the possibility of surgery with Andrew's parents. He is too young, and the magnitude of his apical base discrepancies is too small to warrant surgery.

Q: Are there any unknowns you should address/eliminate before doing something irreversible (e.g., extracting permanent teeth) or before you define Andrew's final treatment plan?

A: Yes. *Growth and treatment compliance are significant unknowns in Andrew's case*—especially if orthopedic treatment is attempted. Will Andrew help us in correcting his AP? If he is compliant, will he have adequate mandibular growth (magnitude *and* direction) to correct his AP? Other unknowns include maintenance of good hygiene and the presence of an undetected AP shift.

Q: Before establishing a final treatment plan, you should always ask yourself what are the advantages/disadvantages of treating the patient nonextraction, with extraction of anterior teeth, or with extraction of different combinations of posterior teeth. What do you recommend in Andrew's case?

A: Treatment options include the following:

- Nonextraction: *if* Andrew can achieve orthopedic AP correction to Class I, and *if* space can be created for alignment of the maxillary anterior teeth by distal movement of the maxillary posterior teeth, and *if* mandibular leeway space results in minimal mandibular anterior crowding—then a nonextraction approach to treatment would be reasonable.
- Extraction of anterior teeth: although his maxillary laterals do look small (Figure 2.45j and o), it is too early to consider extracting a mandibular incisor to alleviate crowding because the permanent canines are unerupted (an anterior Bolton discrepancy cannot be calculated).
- Extraction of different combinations of posterior teeth: although extraction of maxillary first premolars or a combination of maxillary first premolars and mandibular second premolars may be a viable alternative at some future date, it is just too early to consider these alternatives.

Andrew and his parents should be informed that depending on his growth and compliance, any of the aforementioned options may be considered at some future date.

Q: What treatment do you recommend?

A: *A decision was made to reduce the unknowns we were facing before making a final treatment decision.* Andrew was placed on an HPHG to correct his AP relationship and reduce his profile convexity (with mandibular growth). Headgear was worn every day with approximately 300 g of force per side from 8 PM until the next morning. Andrew was very compliant. Once his molar AP position was corrected, the headgear was worn only to bed with a minimum of force to maintain the corrected molar relationship. An LLHA was placed to utilize mandibular leeway space and reduce mandibular anterior crowding as his secondary teeth erupted. After 7 months of headgear/LLHA wear, the maxillary incisors were bonded and aligned. "Tip-back" or "V" bends were placed in the maxillary archwire mesial to the maxillary molars.

Q: What is the effect of placing a "tip-back" or "V" bend in the archwire just mesial to the maxillary molar brackets, like Andrew had?

A: An intrusive force is applied to the maxillary incisors (Figure 2.60), an extrusive force is applied to the maxillary first molars, and a tip-back moment is applied to the maxillary first molars.

Q: After 1 year, 5 months of headgear and LLHA wear, progress models and a cephalometric radiograph were made of Andrew (Figure 2.61). What changes do you note?

A: Andrew's progress records indicate the following:

- Andrew's face and jaws grew minimally downward and forward (Figure 2.61c).
- The maxilla (A-point) grew forward less than the mandible (B-point).
- The mandible translated minimally downward in conjunction with the maxillary corpus descending and the mandibular molars erupting.
- The mandibular body grew minimally (note little ramus change on the mandibular superimposition).
- The maxillary molars showed no eruption, while the mandibular molars showed mild eruption—an indication of good vertical control of maxillary first molars with the use of HPHG.
- Maxillary molars were distalized mildly.
- Mandibular molars were carried forward with mandibular growth.

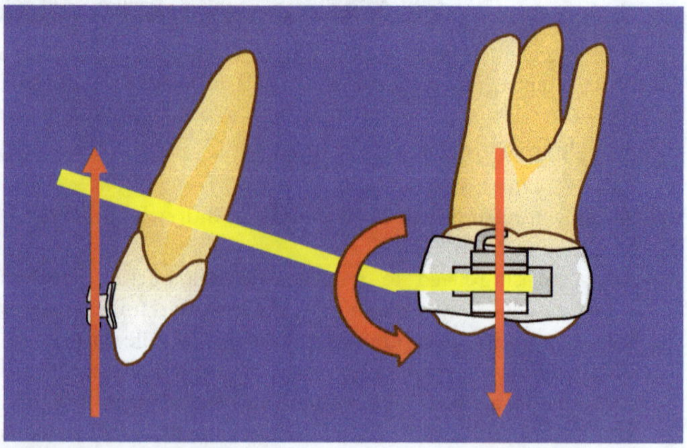

Figure 2.60 A "tip back" or "V" bend placed in the archwire, just mesial to the maxillary molar bracket, results in an intrusive force against the incisors, an extrusive force against the molars, and a CCW moment (as shown in this view) against the molars.

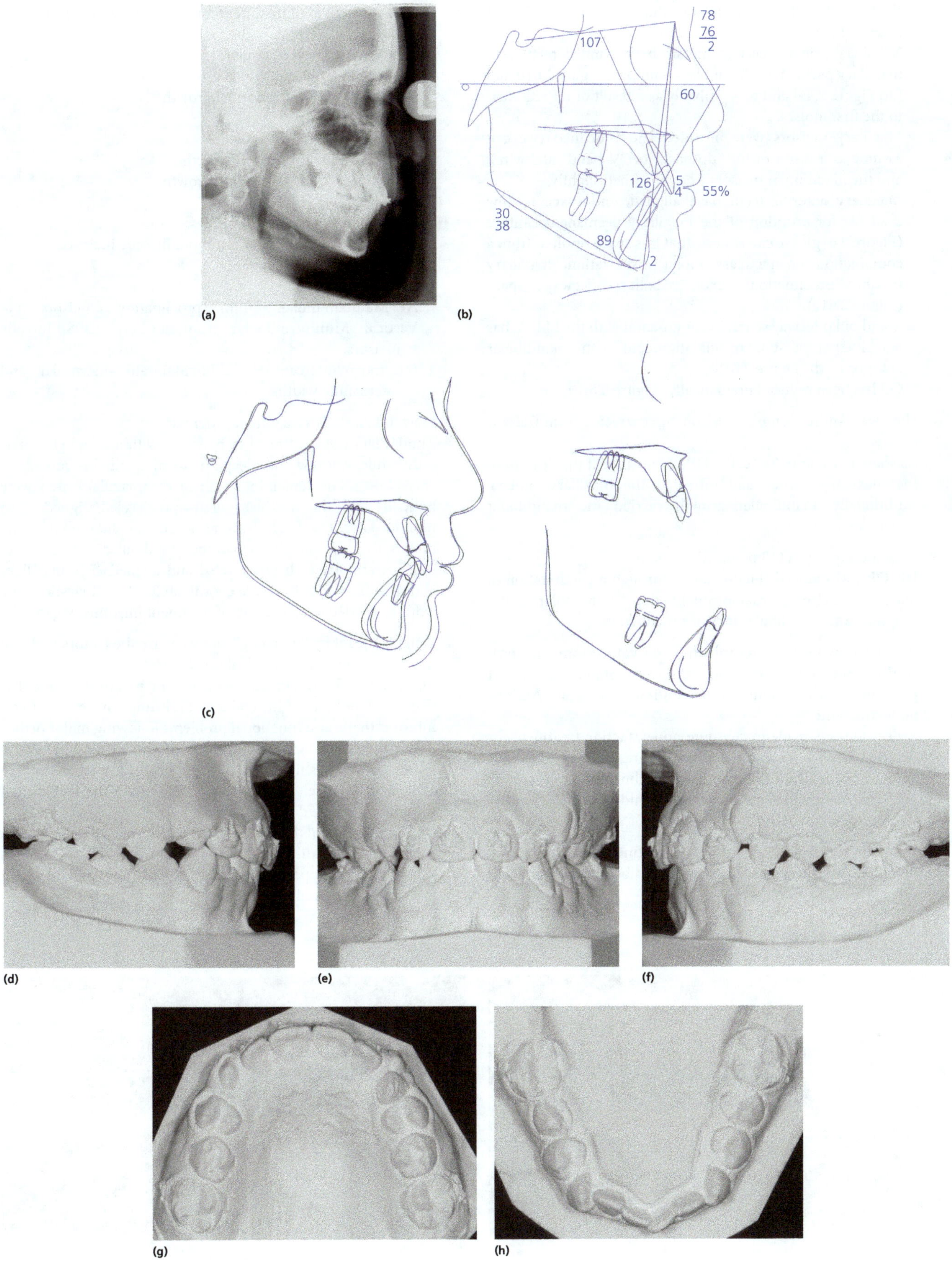

Figure 2.61 (a–h) Progress records of Andrew.

- Right and left molar relationships are now Class I (Figure 2.61d–f).
- Maxillary primary second molars have erupted relative to maxillary permanent first molars (compare Figure 2.61d and f to Figure 2.45l and n)—probably as a result of HPHG wear to the first molars.
- Maxillary incisors were intruded and proclined (we can assume as a result of the "tip-back" or "V-bend" archwire), and the mandibular incisors were proclined slightly.
- Maxillary anterior teeth have aligned, and space is now available for eruption of the maxillary permanent canines (Figure 2.61g). We can assume that this space resulted from a combination of maxillary molar distalization, maxillary incisor proclination, and maxillary leeway space (Figure 2.61c).
- Mandibular leeway space, in conjunction with the LLHA, has permitted some spontaneous alignment of the mandibular anterior teeth (Figure 2.61h).
- OB has been reduced dramatically (Figure 2.61e).

Q: How was Andrew's molar relationship corrected from Class II to Class I?

A: As shown in Figure 2.61c, the HPHG restrained the descent of the maxillary corpus and retracted the maxillary molars. Additionally, mandibular growth carried the mandibular molars forward.

Q: How was Andrew's OB reduced?

A: His OB was reduced (Figure 2.61c) through a combination of maxillary incisor intrusion/proclination, mandibular molar eruption, and mandibular incisor proclination.

Q: Based on his progress records, how do you recommend proceeding? Should you extract anterior teeth? Should you extract posterior teeth? Should you continue to treat Andrew nonextraction?

A: A decision was made to continue nonextraction treatment for Andrew. Why? His mandibular incisors are still at a good angulation, although he exhibits mild mandibular anterior crowding. The mandibular anterior teeth could be slenderized by interproximal reduction (IPR) as needed.

Q: What are the specific objectives of treatment for the maxilla, mandible, maxillary dentition, and mandibular dentition in all three planes of space?

A: Specific objectives of treatment for Andrew are as follows:

Maxilla
- AP: Restrict forward growth.
- Vertical: Restrict downward growth.
- Transverse: Allow for normal growth.

Mandible
- AP: Allow for normal growth.
- Vertical: Allow for normal growth.
- Transverse: Allow for normal growth.

Maxillary dentition
- AP: Distalize molars and canines.
- Vertical: Minimize molar eruption. Intrude incisors.
- Intermolar width: Maintain.

Mandibular dentition
- AP: Maintain molar. Minimize proclination of incisors.
- Vertical: Minimize molar eruption. Level COS. Intrude incisors.
- Intermolar/intercanine width: Maintain intermolar and intercanine widths.

Q: How did Andrew's treatment progress?

A: The HPHG was continued to be worn, with a very light force, only while Andrew was sleeping (to maintain his molar AP correction). The remaining teeth in the maxillary arch were bonded, and the maxillary arch was leveled/aligned. Two months later, the LLHA was removed, the mandibular first molars banded, and the remaining mandibular teeth bonded. The mandibular arch was leveled and aligned. The maxillary and mandibular arches were coordinated, Class II elastics were worn as needed, and a period of treatment finishing began.

Q: What is meant by "finishing" and what are the factors that you must examine to achieve ideal finishing?

A: Finishing is the final stage in treatment before the patient is debanded and placed in retainers. Finishing corrects relatively minor esthetic and functional problems following major orthodontic correction in the anteroposterior, vertical, and transverse dimensions. Finishing is a very important aspect of care to achieve excellence. The following are some of the factors that should be evaluated:

- Incisal display at rest with the lips slightly parted and position of maxillary midline relative to the face (Figure 2.62a). In this patient, there appears to be about 3–4 mm of incisal display at rest and the maxillary midline is "on" with the face.

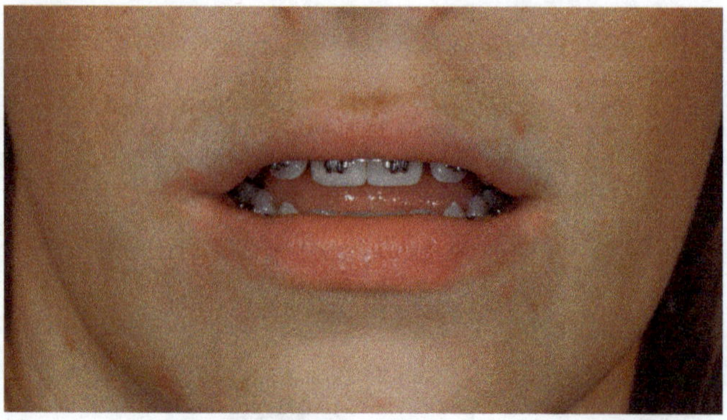
(a)

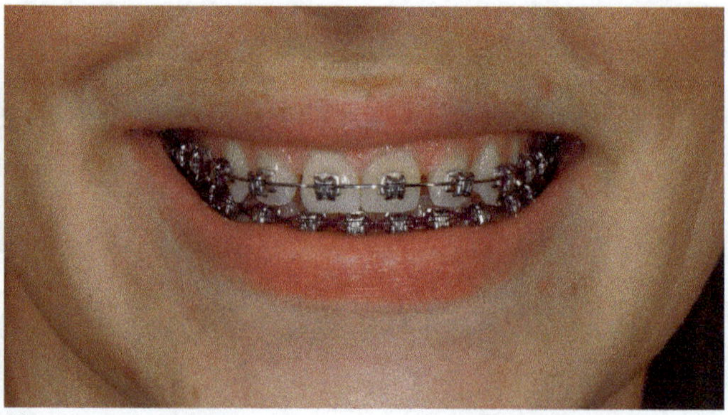
(b)

Figure 2.62 Evaluation of some frontal features important to finishing: (a) at rest with lips slightly parted and (b) in a posed smile.

- In a posed smile (Figure 2.62b), the position of the maxillary lip vermillion relative to the maxillary central incisor gingival margins. In this figure, the gingival margin of the maxillary right central incisor is well positioned, but the gingival margin of the maxillary left central incisor appears to be below the maxillary lip vermillion. Note that the asymmetric elevation of the upper lip contributes to this disparity. Smile symmetry is always an important factor to consider when evaluating incisal display.
- Congruence of the maxillary anterior smile arc with the mandibular lip (Figure 2.62b) plus the presence (or absence) of significant buccal corridors. In this figure, the maxillary anterior smile arc is approximately congruent with the mandibular lip and significant buccal corridors are absent.
- Class I canines with proper interdigitation of posterior teeth (Figure 2.63a and c).
- Minimal OB (Figure 2.63b) in deep bite cases or more OB in initially open bite patients; coordination of maxillary and mandibular canines; maxillary central incisor even gingival levels, slightly more incisal lateral incisor gingival levels plus slightly higher canine gingival levels ("high–low–high"); absence of gingival embrasures (black triangles); and absence of incisal embrasures. In this figure, minimal OB is present, the patient's right canines are coordinated, the patient's left canines do not appear to be coordinated, relative gingival levels appear fine, but large incisal embrasures are seen.
- Arch alignment without spacing, rotations, or slipped contacts (Figure 2.64).
- With the patient open (Figure 2.65), maxillary and mandibular incisal edge shape; the relative position of incisors to canines in each arch; the presence of a COS (or compensating

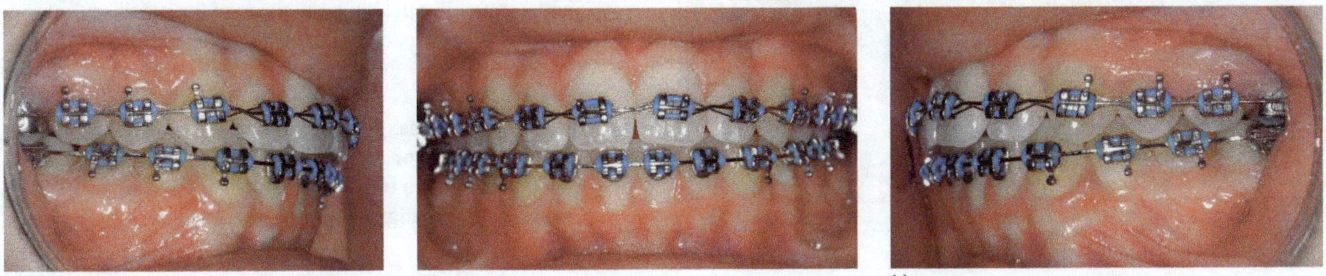

(a) (b) (c)

Figure 2.63 Evaluation of dental features viewed from (a) the right, (b) front, and (c) left.

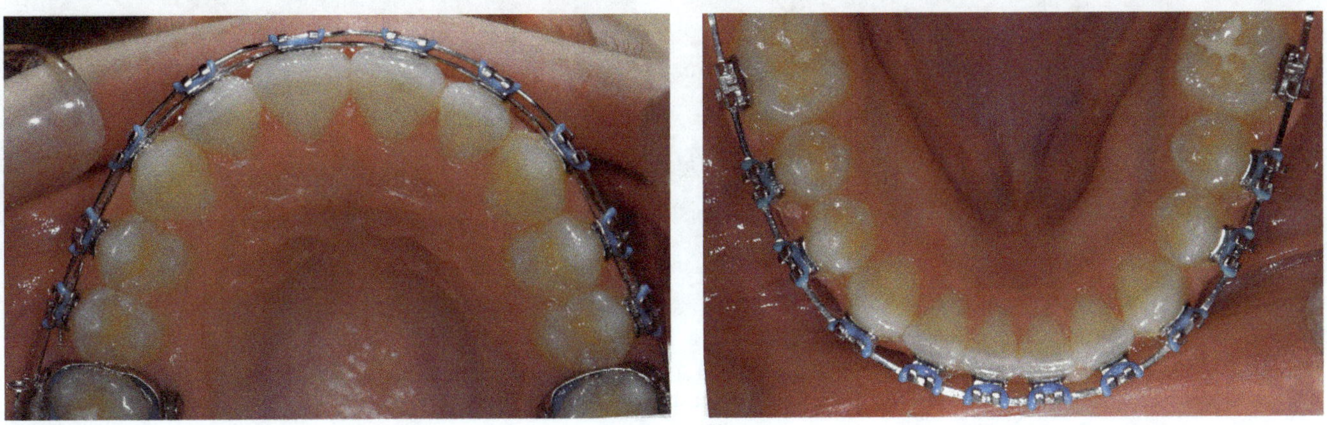

(a) (b)

Figure 2.64 (a, b) Evaluation of dental features viewed from occlusal.

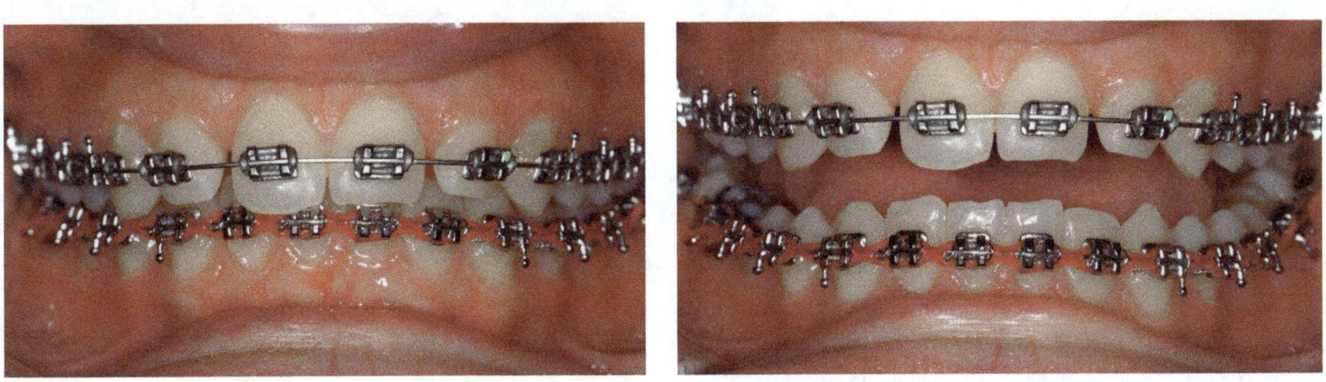

(a) (b)

Figure 2.65 Evaluation of dental features (a) when closed and (b) open.

curve in the maxillary posterior arch); presence of vertical steps due to bonding errors; and posterior crown torque. In this figure, *having the patient open provides excellent contrast* between the incisors and the oral cavity. As seen, the incisal edges are terribly irregular, a significant COS is still present, the mandibular incisors are stepped up relative to the canines, significant mandibular lingual posterior crown torque exists, and the maxillary lateral incisal edges are stepped up relative to the maxillary canines.

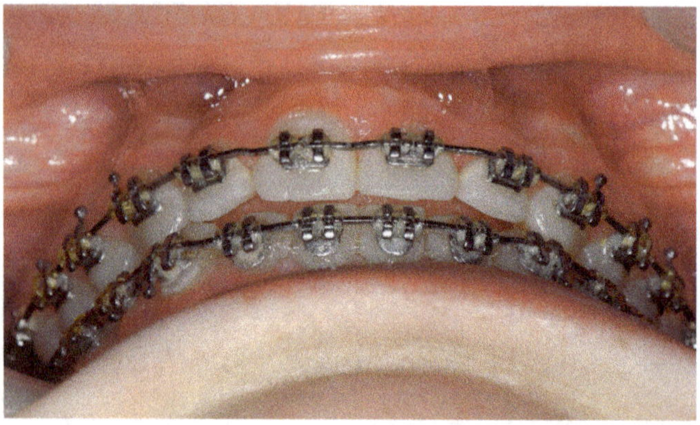

Figure 2.66 Determining the magnitude of OJ.

- Presence or absence of OJ (Figure 2.66). In this figure, 1–2 mm of OJ is present.
- Presence of absence of a CR—CO shift (Figure 2.67a and b). In these figures, a previously undetected CR—CO shift of 3–4 mm was found.
- Proper buccal-lingual crown torque of posterior, and anterior, teeth. In Figure 2.68, the maxillary left central incisor demonstrates excessive lingual crown torque compared to the maxillary right central incisor.

Q: Now let's more closely examine esthetics of the maxillary anterior teeth (Figure 2.69). What additional finishing goals can you suggest, in terms of the maxillary anterior teeth? (G.L. Denehy, University of Iowa College of Dentistry, personal communication, January 15, 2012.)

A: Finishing goals for maxillary anterior teeth include the following:

- Shade: generally speaking, the shade of the maxillary anterior teeth should approach the whiteness of eye sclera.
- Coincidence of maxillary and mandibular midlines (Figure 2.70).
- Equal widths of maxillary central incisors (Figure 2.70).
- Ideal central incisor width/length ratio of 4/5 (Figure 2.71a).
- Golden proportion of maxillary anterior teeth (Figure 2.71b).
- Proper long axis alignment (Figure 2.72a).

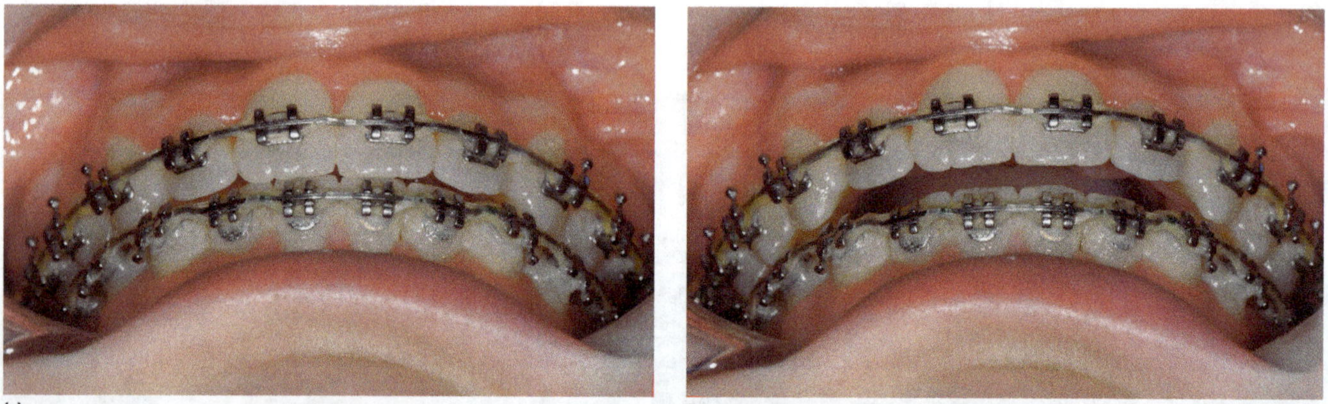

(a) (b)

Figure 2.67 The importance of examining the patient for a CR—CO shift at every appointment cannot be overstated. (a) Here a CR—CO shift went undetected for many months. (b) The discovery of this shift completely changed the treatment plan.

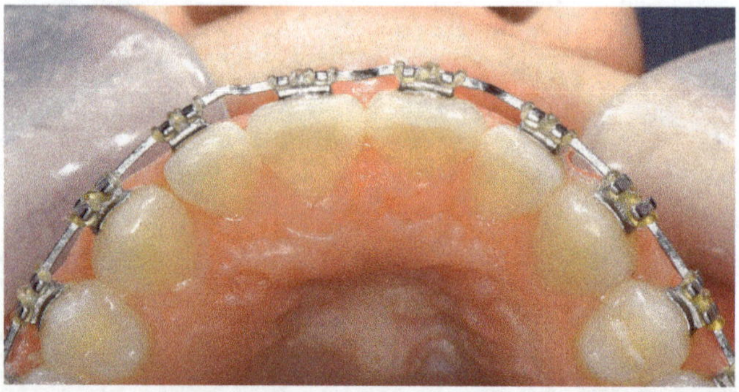

Figure 2.68 Inadequate lingual root torque of the maxillary left central incisor. Not only should buccal-lingual crown torque of posterior teeth be checked, but buccal-lingual crown torque of anterior teeth must also be checked.

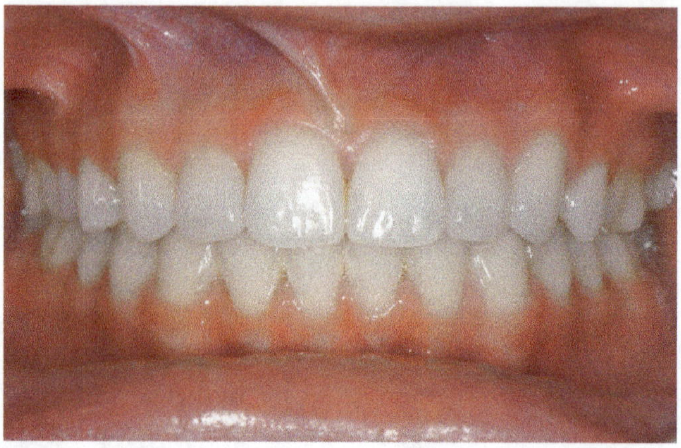

Figure 2.69 Evaluating esthetic features of the maxillary anterior teeth. Ideal shade is probably the most important of all features.

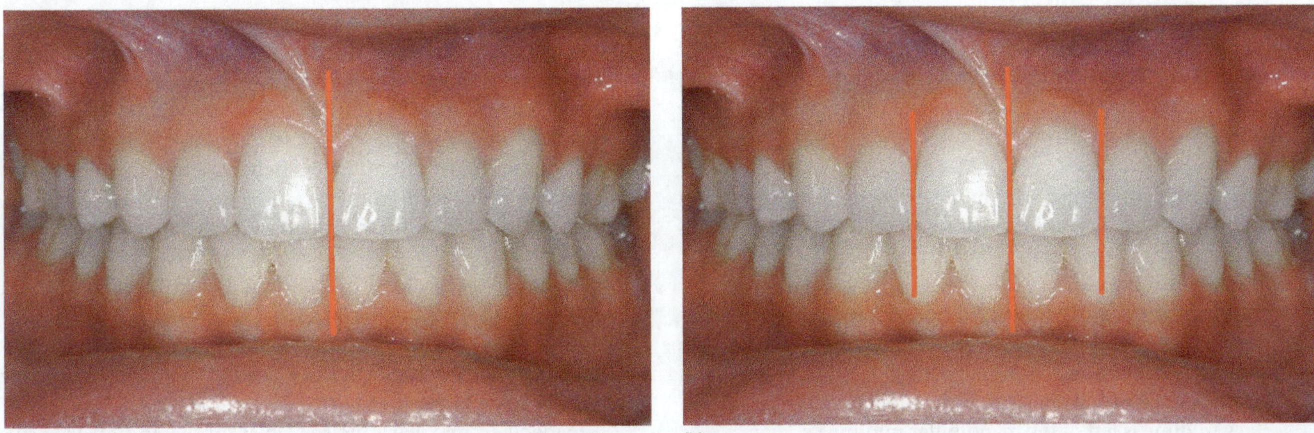

(a) (b)

Figure 2.70 (a) Maxillary and mandibular midlines should be coincident and (b) the maxillary central incisor widths should be equal.

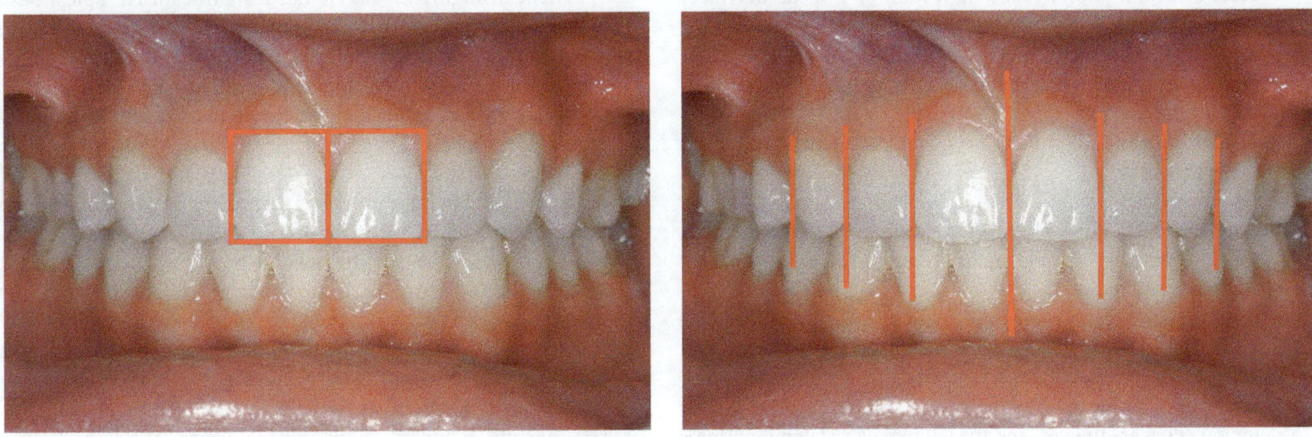

(a) (b)

Figure 2.71 (a) Width/length ratio of the maxillary incisors should be 4/5, and (b) tooth widths from central incisor to canine should be follow the golden proportion.

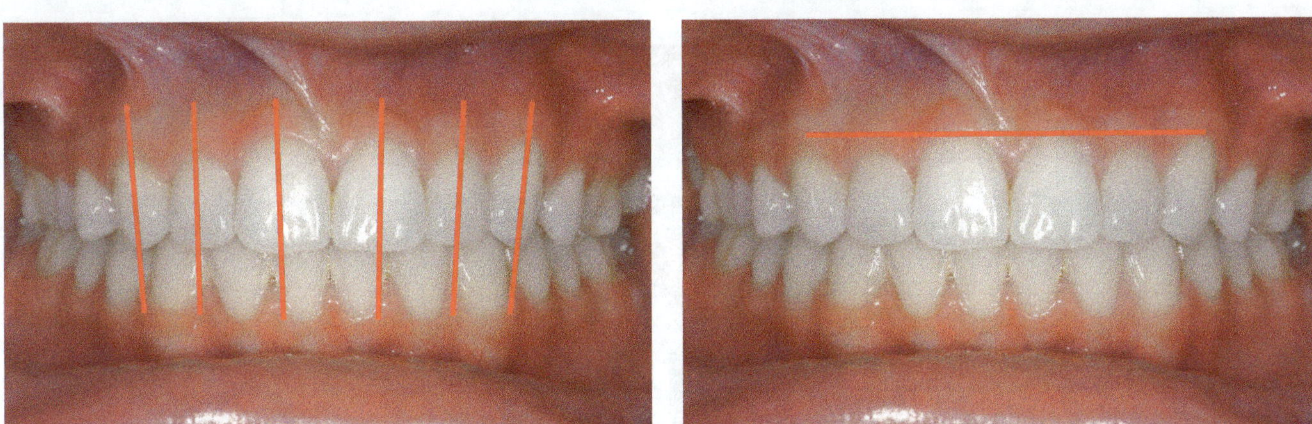

(a) (b)

Figure 2.72 (a) Proper mesio-distal long axis alignment should exist. (b) Gingival margins of the maxillary central incisors should be even, the maxillary lateral incisor gingival margins should be slightly more incisal, and the canine gingival margins should be at the same level as the central incisors.

- Even maxillary central incisor gingival margins (Figure 2.72b). Note that the maxillary lateral incisor gingival margins are slightly more incisal than the maxillary central incisor gingival margins. Note that the maxillary canine gingival margins are slightly more apical than the lateral gingival margins. Moving from the central incisor to lateral incisor to canine gingival margin heights, the effect should be "high–low–high." In this example, the maxillary right canine gingival margin should (ideally) be more apical.

- Even maxillary incisor incisal edges. Lateral incisor edges should be at the same level or slightly stepped up. Maxillary central incisor edges, maxillary lateral incisor edges, and canine cusp tips should, ideally, lay along a gentle arc (the smile arc) congruent with the lower lip.

Q: With these esthetic goals in mind, what do you observe in Andrew's six maxillary anterior teeth at this point in his finishing stage of treatment (Figure 2.73)?

A: Observations include the following:
- Shade: it is too early to determine the need for tooth lightening—wait until Andrew is debanded and the brackets are not in the way.
- Coincidence of maxillary and mandibular midlines: maxillary midline is left of the mandibular midline.
- Equal maxillary central incisor widths: maxillary central incisors widths are approximately equal.
- Ideal central incisor width/length ratio of 4/5: the maxillary right central incisor is too short, and the maxillary left central incisor has a nearly ideal ratio.
- Golden proportion of maxillary anterior teeth: lateral incisors are too narrow.
- Proper long axis alignment: no major problems with mesiodistal tip are noted.
- Even maxillary central incisor gingival margins: maxillary central incisor gingival margins are uneven, lateral incisor gingival margins are too incisal, and right canine gingival margin is too incisal.
- Even incisal edge relationships: these relationships should be evaluated with the patient opened slightly, so a nice contrast exists between the white maxillary teeth and the dark oropharynx. In Figure 2.73b, it appears that the central incisor incisal edges are uneven, and the left maxillary lateral incisor is stepped down. We are unable to judge the presence or absence of a smile arc in this image (relative to the lower lip).

Q: Looking at Andrew's maxillary occlusal image (Figure 2.73d), notice the ~2 mm spaces distal to the maxillary lateral incisors. This is a classic problem of *space distribution* during finishing. That is, if you have spaces like these, you will have to decide where to put these spaces (i.e., where best to hide them or restore them). What are reasons why you end up with spaces like these at deband?

A: Reasons why you finish treatment with spacing in the maxillary anterior teeth:
- Excess OJ still exists. This OJ should be reduced/eliminated as the spaces are further closed.
- An anterior Bolton tooth size discrepancy exists (maxillary anterior tooth size deficiency and/or mandibular anterior tooth size excess).
- Inadequate maxillary incisor labial torque and/or excessive mandibular incisor labial torque. As an example, look at the initial cephalometric tracing from a Class II adolescent patient in Figure 2.74a. He has a significant AP apical base discrepancy (normally positioned maxilla/retrusive mandible) and bimaxillary dental protrusion. Because his proclined mandibular incisors were initially well aligned (Figure 2.74b), a decision was made to treat him nonextraction (orthopedically) with a HPHG and fixed orthodontic appliances.

In his deband lateral cephalometric tracing (Figure 2.75a), note the improved apical base relationship (ANB angle reduced from 6° to 4°). Note also that the maxillary incisors were uprighted and the mandibular incisors were proclined. *Because the mandibular incisors are very proclined, the mandibular incisal edges are more forward than if they were upright—so the maxillary incisors contact the mandibular incisal edges, during retraction, long before all maxillary spaces can be closed.* This relationship, coupled with a maxillary anterior Bolton deficiency (small maxillary lateral incisors, Figure 2.75e), resulted in maxillary anterior spacing (Figure 2.75b and d).

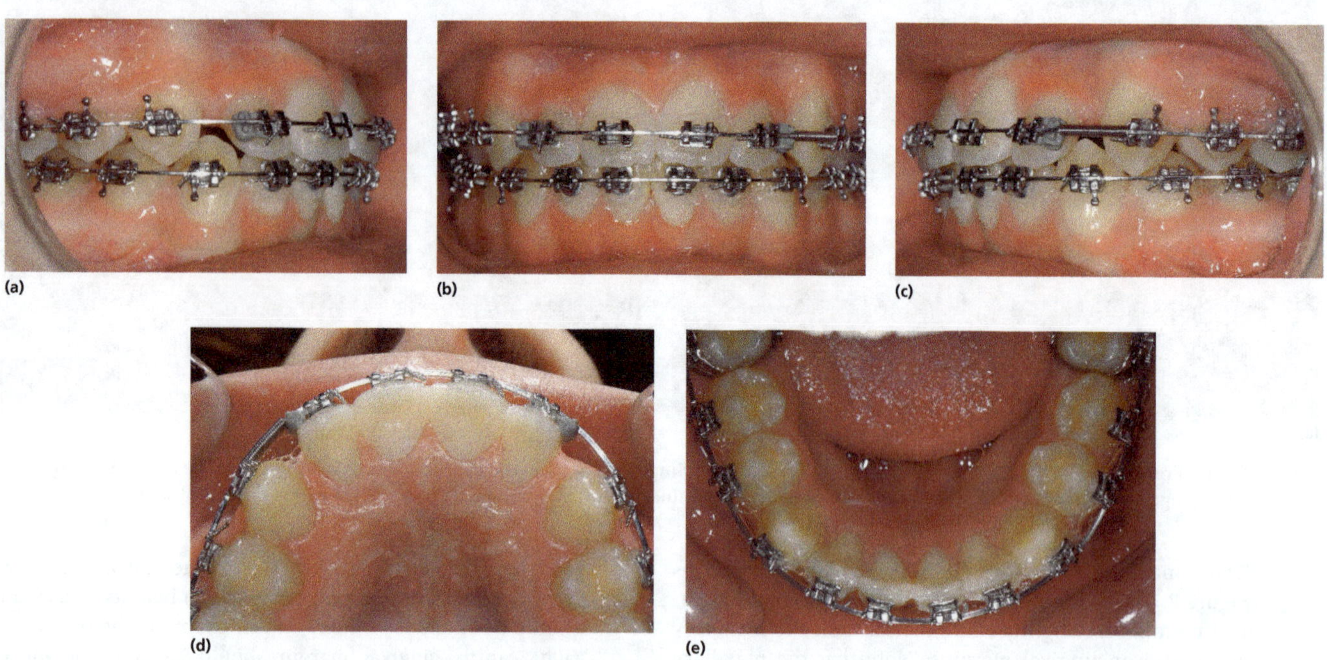

Figure 2.73 (a–e) Progress intraoral photographs of Andrew.

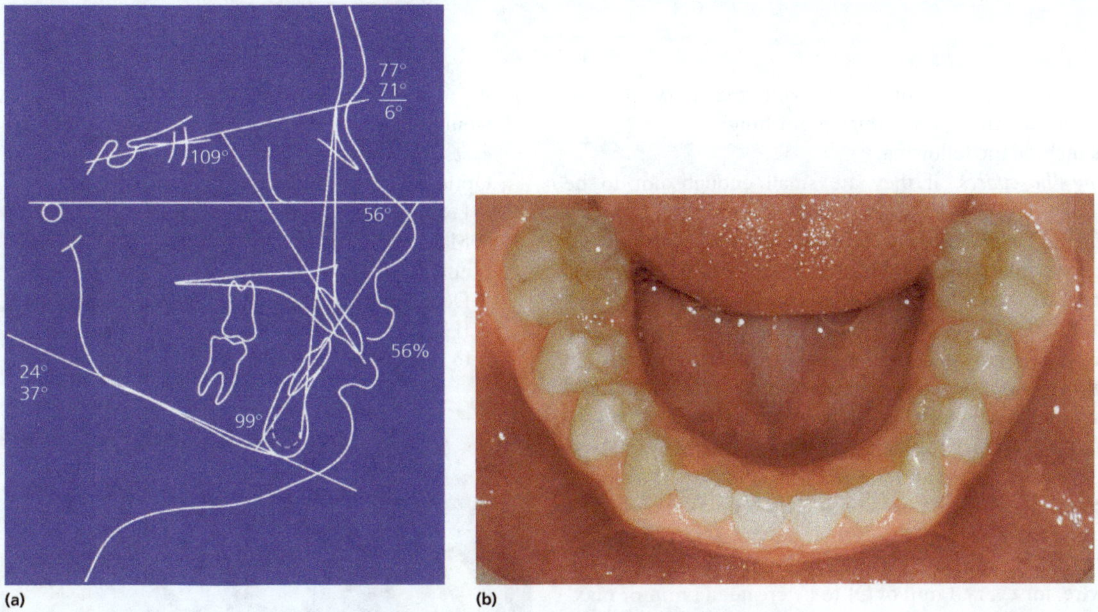

Figure 2.74 (a, b) Initial records of a Class II adolescent patient treated nonextraction with orthopedics and fixed orthodontic appliances.

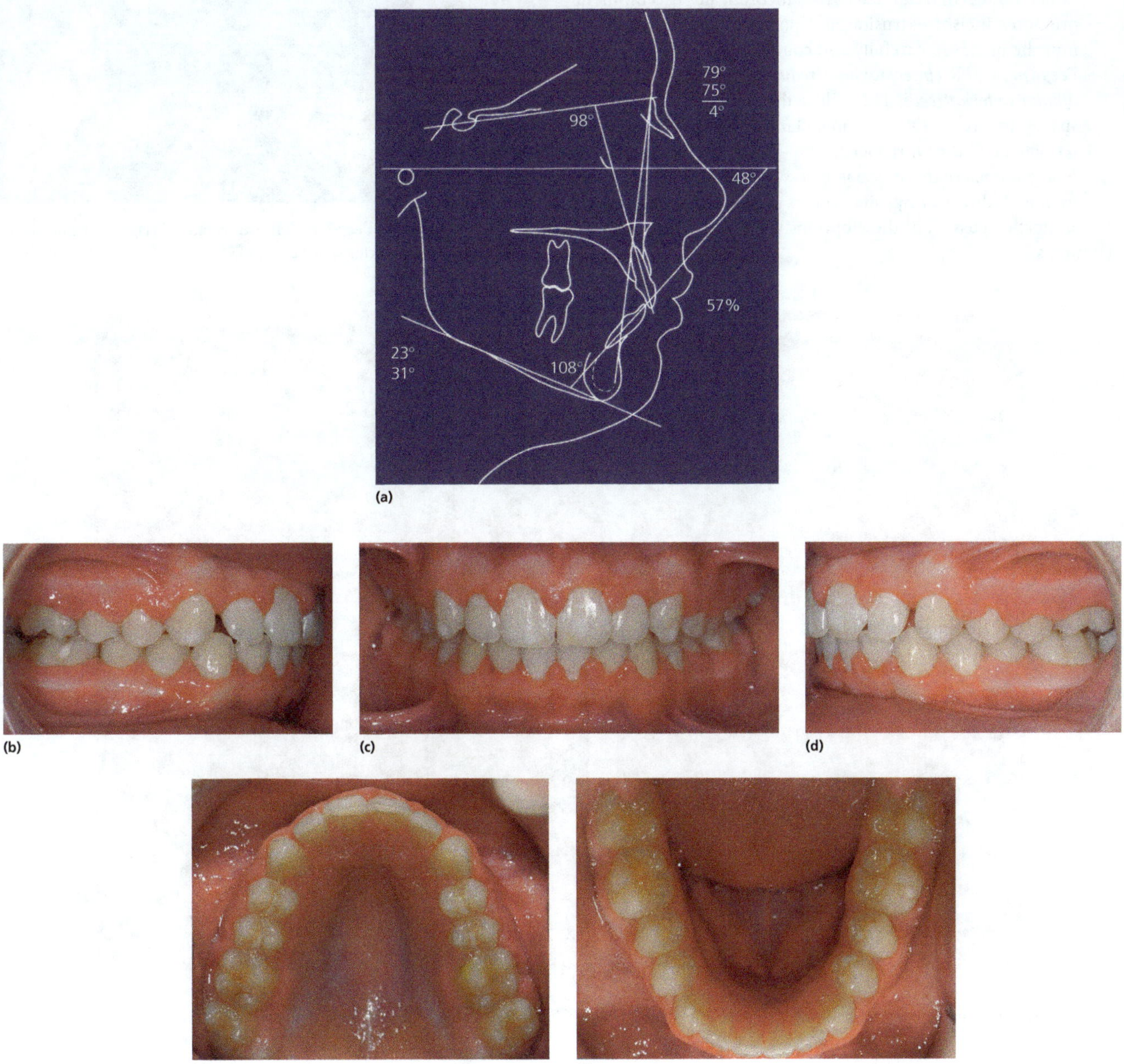

Figure 2.75 Deband records of the same patient. (a) Note the upright maxillary incisors, the very proclined mandibular incisors, and (b–e) the spacing distal to the maxillary lateral incisors.

Q: What are your options for *dealing* with maxillary anterior spacing, such as Andrew has, during finishing?

A: Options include the following:

- *Leaving the spaces,* if they are small enough not to be noticeable. This is not the case with Andrew.
- *Positioning the maxillary canines slightly ahead (slightly Class II)* to close small spaces (Figure 2.76, note the Class II canines, the small maxillary lateral incisors, and absence of OJ).
- If a deep bite is present (Figure 2.77, left), *opening the bite* (Figure 2.77, right) to create OJ to permit space closure.
- *Placing anterior labial crown torque (lingual root torque) in a cinched maxillary rectangular archwire* (Figure 2.78a) to rotate the maxillary incisal edges labially (creating OJ) and the roots lingually around the archwire (Figure 2.78b and c). The resulting OJ can be used for incisor retraction and space closure (Figure 2.78d). The problem with creating OJ this way is that because we are rotating the incisors around the archwire, for every 1 mm of OJ to be created (1 mm of maxillary incisor edge mesial movement), the maxillary incisor root tips must move distally 10+ mm (requiring many additional months of treatment). Also, theoretically, this moment promotes incisor extrusion and posterior intrusion, which must be observed carefully and countered, if it occurs [88].
- *Performing IPR (interproximal reduction) between the mandibular anterior teeth.* Then, close these mandibular anterior spaces to create OJ. The maxillary incisors can then be retracted and the OJ reduced.
- *Filling the maxillary anterior spaces by restoring the adjacent teeth* with direct composite veneers or porcelain veneers.

You must discuss all of these options with the Andrew and his parents.

Q: As an aside, let's consider the opposite problem. What options would you have in finishing a case with Class I canines, *excess OJ,* and no spaces?

A: Options include the following:

- Leaving the patient with excess OJ
- Making the patient slightly Class III at the canines to reduce anterior OJ
- Deepening the bite (e.g., by erupting mandibular incisors)
- IPR of the maxillary anterior teeth, then closing these spaces to reduce OJ

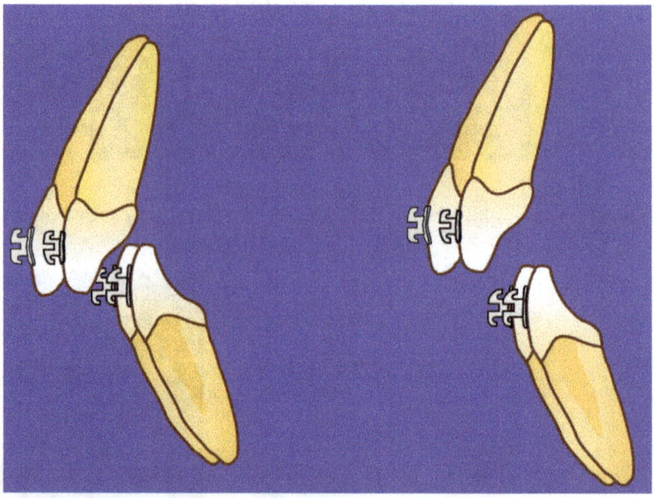

Figure 2.77 Opening a deep bite (left) can create OJ (right) for maxillary incisor retraction (anterior space closure).

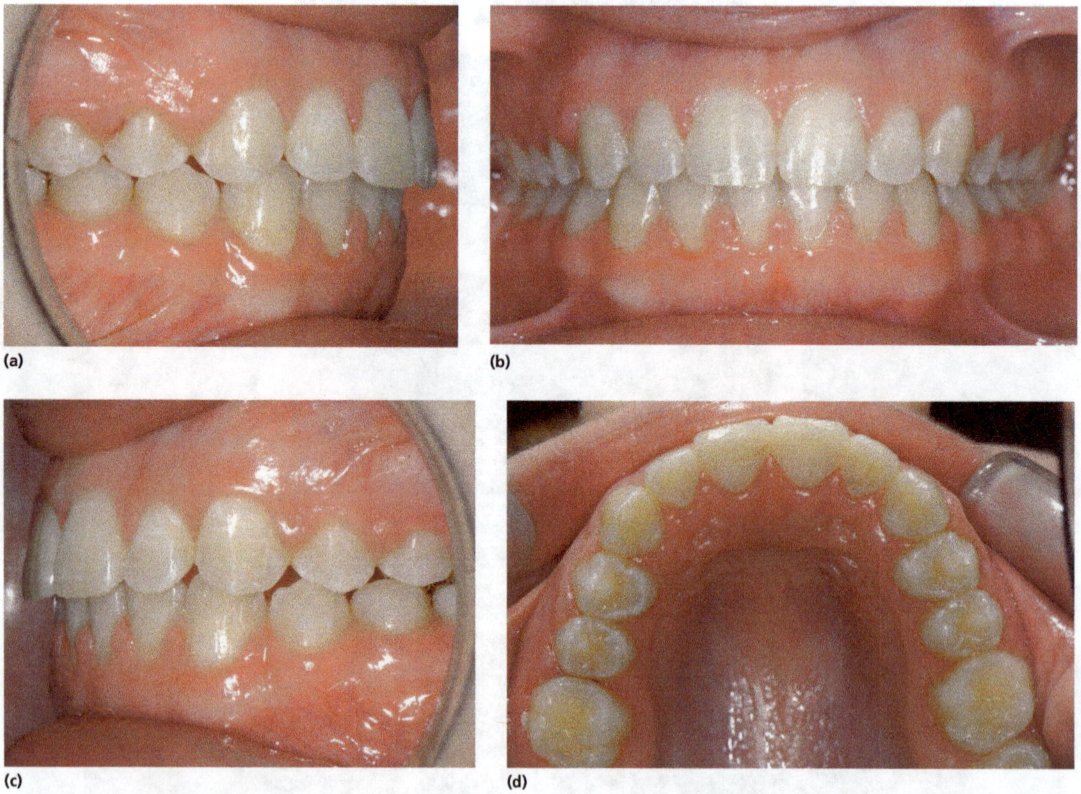

(a) (b) (c) (d)

Figure 2.76 (a–d) Example of a patient with small maxillary lateral incisors who chose to be left slightly Class II in order to avoid anterior spacing.

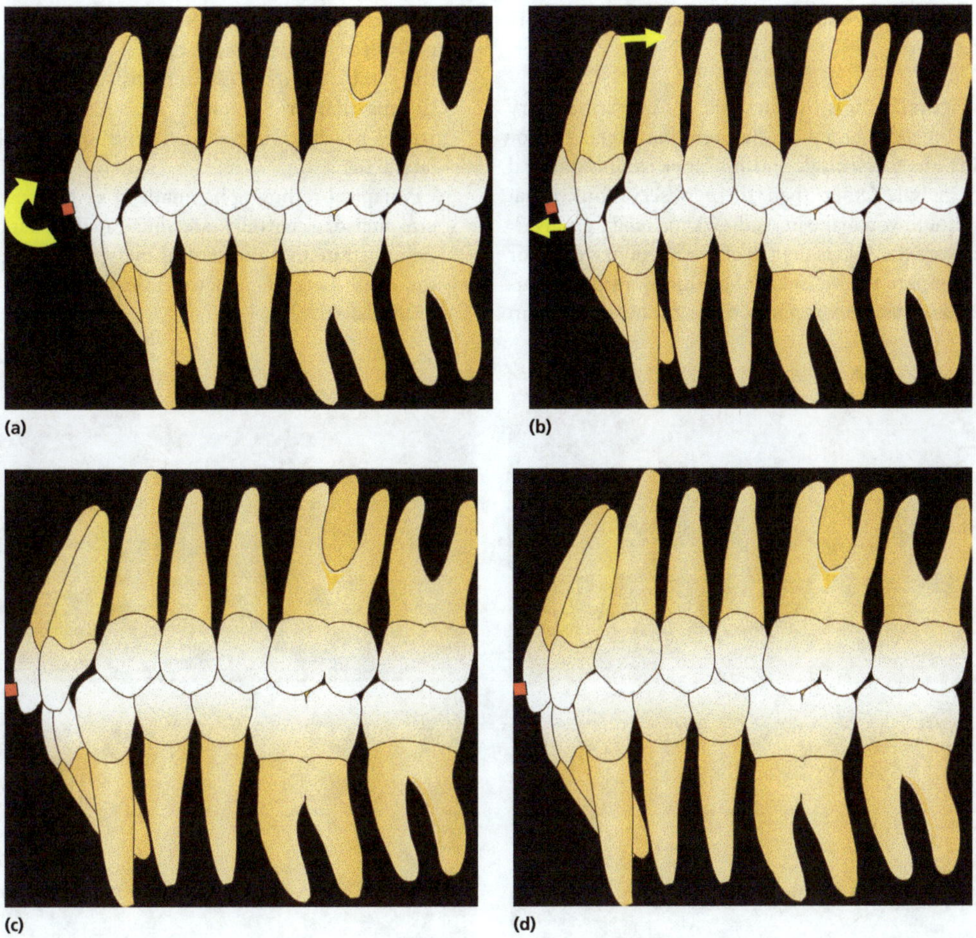

Figure 2.78 Creating OJ for space closure: (a and b) placing anterior labial crown torque (lingual root torque) in the maxillary archwire can create OJ (c), which can be used for space closure (d).

- Opening spaces between the mandibular anterior teeth to advance them and reduce OJ (and building up the spaces with direct composite veneers or porcelain veneers)

Q: Back to Andrew, if you decide to close his maxillary spaces by restoring the teeth (with direct composite veneers or porcelain veneers), are there any guidelines you should follow for distributing the space among the maxillary anterior teeth at finishing?

A: Yes. The guidelines include the following:

- First, *confirm that you have a Class I canine relationship and no OJ in CR.*
- Try to minimize the number of teeth and teeth surfaces to be restored. The more space that exists, the more that space must be distributed, and the more teeth surfaces that must be restored.
- If there is minimal space remaining—leave the space distal to the maxillary laterals.
- If there is much more space remaining—consider "centering" the maxillary laterals in the space (lateral incisor restorations on the mesial and distal surfaces).
- Try to place restorations more posteriorly, so they are less visible.
- Greater tooth length *and* flat tooth contours make it easier to close space with restorations. Short teeth with curved proximal contours tend to result in "over contouring" of interproximal surfaces.

Q: You discuss options for dealing with his spaces (Figure 2.73d) with Andrew and his parents. They wish to have his spaces closed, restoratively. How would you apply the above restorative guidelines to Andrew?

A: Restorative guidelines as they pertain to Andrew:

- A Class I canine relationship is evident in CR (Figure 2.73a and c).
- The minimum number of surfaces that would need to be presently closed include the distal of both laterals and perhaps the mesial of the canines, but the ~2 mm of space right and left (Figure 2.73d) is simply too wide to close restoring just the distal of the lateral incisors and mesial of the maxillary canines. Other teeth will also need to be restored to distribute this space.
- There is too much space to simply leave the space distal to the maxillary lateral incisors.
- Moving the maxillary lateral incisors distally, "centering" the maxillary lateral incisors in the space, is the best option (restoration will then be distributed to the distal of the central incisors, mesial of the lateral incisors, distal of the lateral incisors, and mesial of the canines).
- Lateral incisor centering is, overall, the most posterior positioning possible.
- An attempt will be made to add most of the restorative material to interproximal surfaces which have greater tooth length *and* flatter tooth contours.

Andrew and his parents chose to have the lateral incisors centered and restored.

Q: Also noted in Figure 2.73b is the fact that Andrew's maxillary central incisor gingival margins are uneven, his lateral incisor gingival margins are too incisal, and his right canine gingival margin is too incisal. Other than these observations, what measurements should you make in Andrew's maxillary gingiva?

A: You should measure the sulcus depths of the maxillary anterior teeth and also compare the incisor CEJ positions, radiographically. Figure 2.79a illustrates a periodontal probe with 3 mm demarcations, Figure 2.79b demonstrates a 1 mm sulcus depth of Andrew's maxillary left central incisor (left lateral incisor was the same), Figure 2.79c demonstrates a 2 mm sulcus depth of the maxillary right central incisor, and Figure 2.79d demonstrates nearly a 3 mm sulcus depth of tooth the maxillary right lateral incisor.

Periapical radiographs, made after moving his maxillary lateral incisors centrally, are illustrated in Figure 2.80a–c. They demonstrate that the central incisor CEJs are at approximately the same heights, and the maxillary lateral incisor CEJs are more incisal.

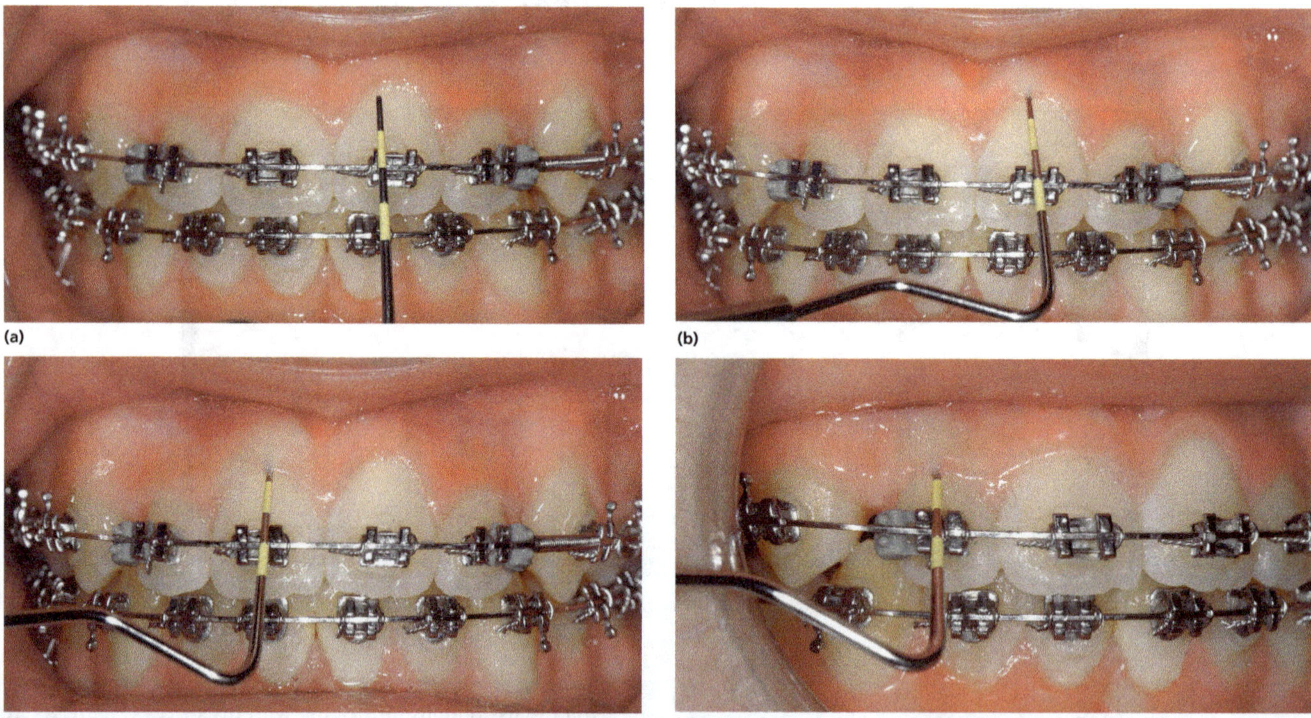

(a) (b) (c) (d)

Figure 2.79 (a–d) Clinical examination of Andrew's gingival sulcus depths.

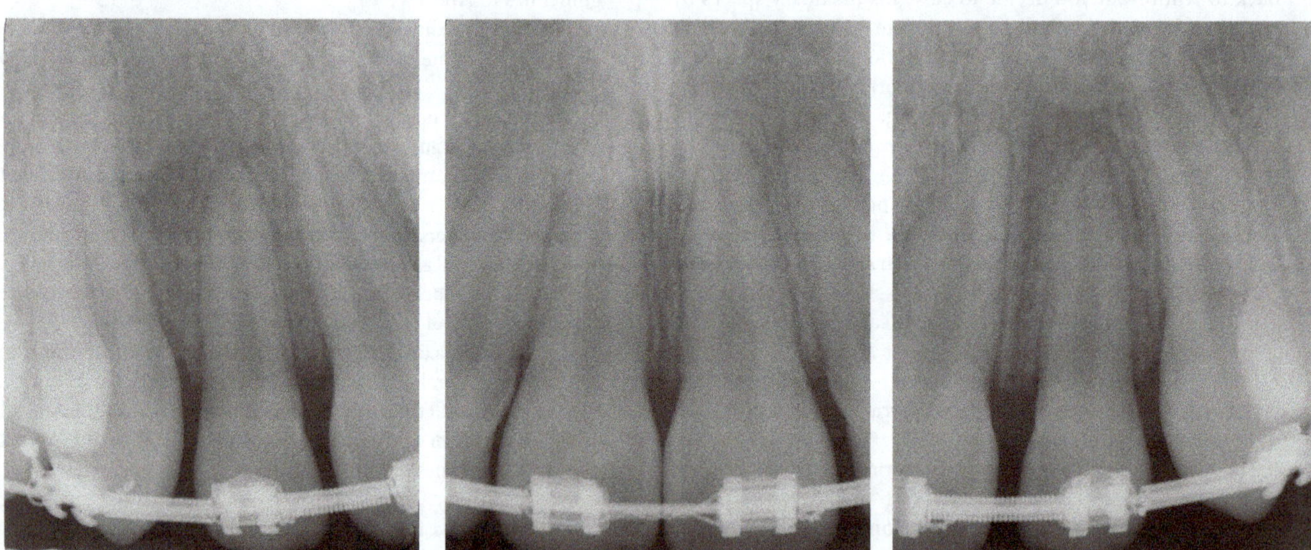

(a) (b) (c)

Figure 2.80 (a–c) Periapical radiographs of Andrew's maxillary incisors to compare CEJ levels.

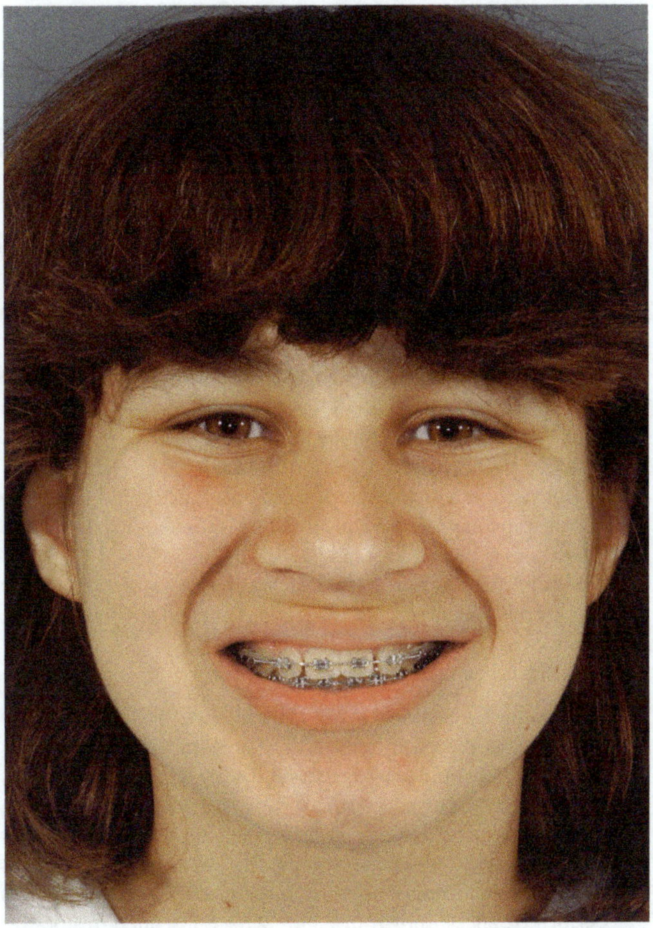

Figure 2.81 Because Andrew has a low smile line, you could choose to leave his central incisor gingival margins uneven.

Q: How can you deal with Andrew's discrepancy in gingival heights?

A: One option is to do nothing, especially if Andrew has a low smile line (Figure 2.81).

However, if Andrew and his parents wish to have even central incisor gingival margins, then this can be achieved with laser gingivoplasty since the sulci of the maxillary right lateral and right central incisors are deep. He and his parents chose to have this done. Since the CEJs are at normal levels (no vertical orthodontic movement required), then the procedure can be postponed until after deband.

Q: Intraoral views during distal movement of the maxillary lateral incisors (to center the lateral incisors in the spaces) are shown in Figure 2.82. Take a look. *I made a mistake during this space distribution treatment.* Can you tell what it was?

A: Look closely at the amount of maxillary incisor OJ that is still present (Figure 2.82a and c). It is significant. The lateral incisor spaces could (*should*) have been reduced, simply by eliminating this OJ.

Q: In addition to confirming that Andrew had Class I canines in CR, how should I have checked him to look at OJ?

A: Have him tilt his head back in CR. Figure 2.83 illustrates his OJ in CR, clearly. This view should have been examined (but was not) when the anterior esthetics were being analyzed. A quick *assessment of OJ magnitude must be made—in CR—at every patient appointment.* If the large OJ had been noticed, then the next step would have been to eliminate the OJ by reducing the spaces distal to the lateral incisors.

Q: How should you proceed now?

A: Close the maxillary anterior spaces until you eliminate the OJ. Then distribute the remaining spaces.

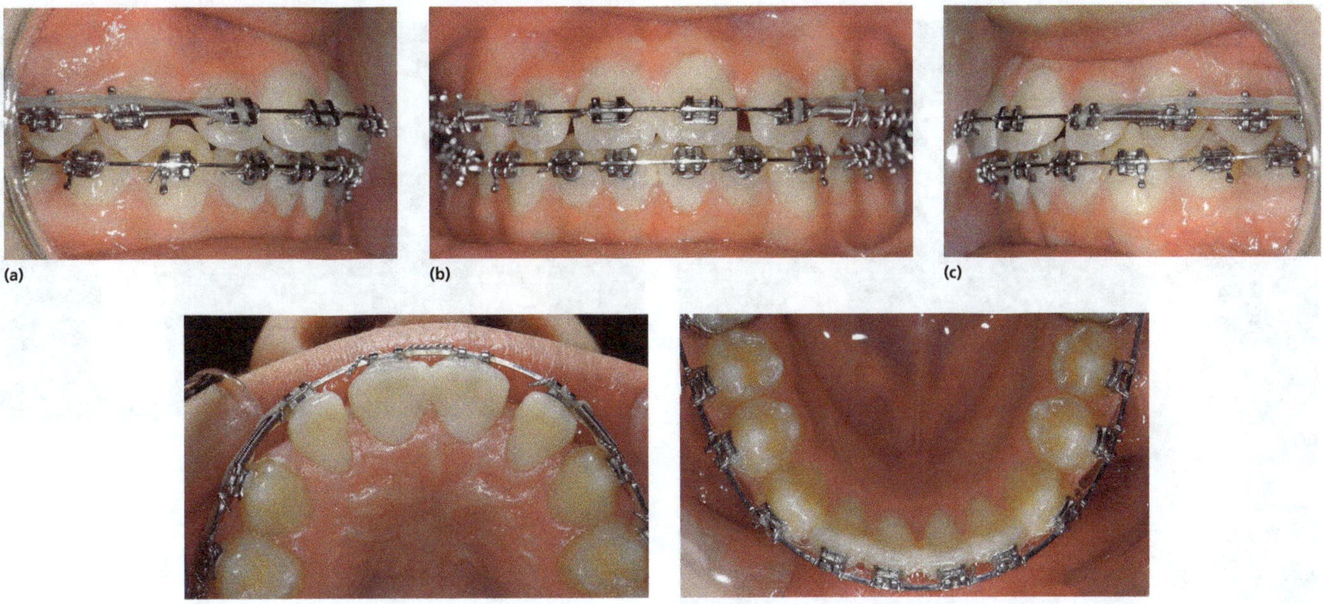

(a) (b) (c) (d) (e)

Figure 2.82 (a–e) Progress intraoral photographs of Andrew while his maxillary lateral incisors are being centered in the anterior spaces.

Q: Can you eliminate Andrew's maxillary anterior spaces entirely? In other words, how does an orthodontist determine *how much OJ is needed to close anterior spaces entirely?*

A: If (Figure 2.84a) you have 2 mm of space distal to both maxillary lateral incisors, then you need 2 mm of OJ to retract the incisors and eliminate the OJ (Figure 2.84b).

If you have *fewer* than 2 mm of OJ, then you will not be able to close 2 mm of bilateral space. If you have *more* than 2 mm of OJ, then you will close the space with excess OJ remaining. Finally, if you have 2 mm of *unilateral* space, then you only need 1 mm of OJ to close the space (2 mm of unilateral space is equivalent to shifting the space until you have 1 mm of space, bilaterally).

Q: In Figure 2.85, Andrew's OJ has been completely eliminated and the maxillary incisal spaces greatly reduced. What must you do now—in terms of communication with the restorative dentist?

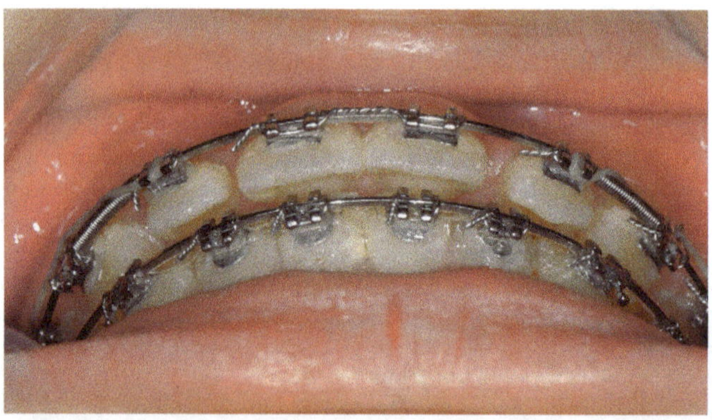

Figure 2.83 Andrew had significant OJ in CR which should have been eliminated before dealing with any residual spaces.

A: Have him or her examine Andrew and give final approval for the anterior tooth positions and space distribution before you deband Andrew. This was done and approval for deband was obtained.

Q: Deband records are shown in Figure 2.86. What do you see?

A: Observations include the following:

- A Class I canine relationship has been achieved (Figure 2.86a and c).
- Maxillary canines appear well coordinated with mandibular canines (Figure 2.86b).
- Maxillary canines are tucked in nicely at the distal—not "rolled out" at the distal (Figure 2.86b and d).
- Molars are now Class I (Figure 2.86g, i, l, and m).
- An ideal OB (~10%) is evident.
- UDML and LDML are coincident.
- Roots are fairly parallel (Figure 2.86f). Mandibular incisor roots appear shortened, but this appearance could be due to their proclination. Periapical radiographs should be made to assess true incisor root length.
- Maxillary posterior buccal crown torque and mandibular posterior lingual crown torque is still present (Figure 2.86n and o).
- COS has been eliminated (Figure 2.86p).

Q: What retention protocol should you follow?

A: Andrew was placed in temporary (vacuum-formed) retainers the day of deband. He wore these full-time, except when eating, until his restorative treatment was complete. Whenever a restorative procedure was done, a new temporary retainer was fabricated if the old retainer did not fit. Laser surgery, to address Andrew's inadequate/uneven incisor crown lengths, was performed and is shown in Figure 2.87. Subsequent restorative treatment with direct composite veneers (before and after) is shown in Figure 2.88.

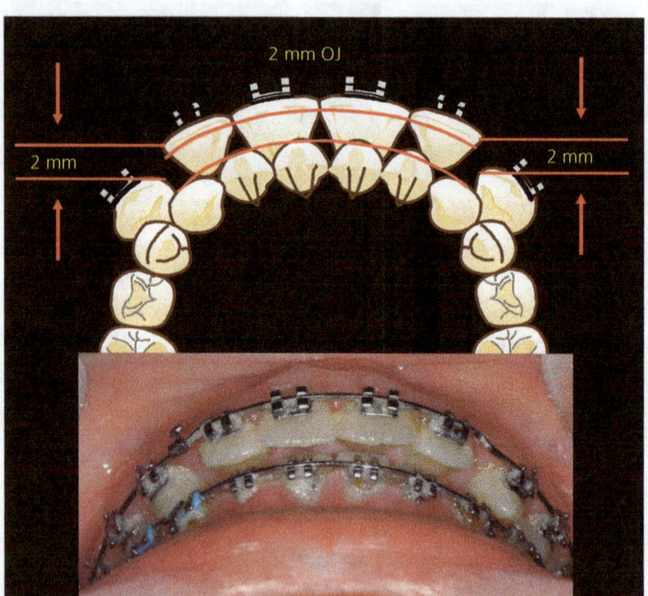

(a)

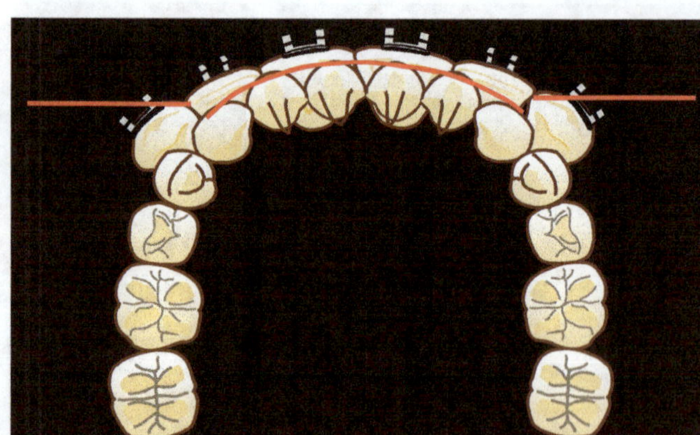

(b)

Figure 2.84 (a, b) If you have 2 mm of bilateral maxillary spaces to close, then you need 2 mm of OJ to close the spaces entirely.

After all restorative treatment was completed, Andrew was placed in removable maxillary and mandibular Hawley retainers. His maxillary retainer was fabricated with an anterior biteplate to disclude his posterior teeth slightly and improve the chance of maintaining his deep bite correction. He was advised to wear the Hawley retainers every night for life.

Q: Final records are shown in Figure 2.89. (Figure 2.89f is a cephalometric superimposition from progress to deband, and Figure 2.89g is a cephalometric superimposition from initial to deband). What do you observe?

A: Changes noted include the following:

- The change in Andrew's facial appearance is dramatic. He now has a wonderful smile, and the gift dentistry has given him is reflected in his enhanced self-confidence.
- His smile arc, formed by the edges of his maxillary anterior teeth, is congruent with his lower lip.
- Large buccal corridors are still present.
- Andrew still has a convex profile and retrusive chin, but his facial convexity has been reduced slightly (compare Figure 2.45c to Figure 2.89c).

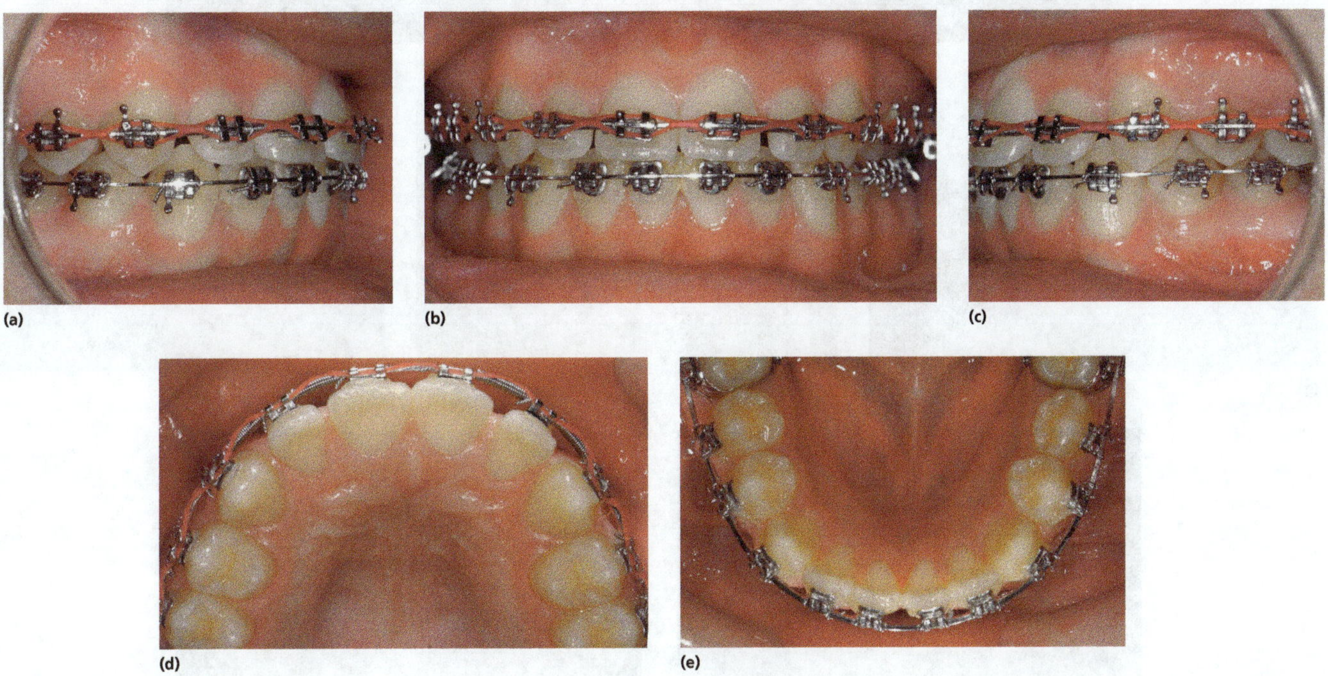

Figure 2.85 (a–e) Progress intraoral photographs of Andrew after his OJ has been eliminated and his maxillary anterior spaces reduced.

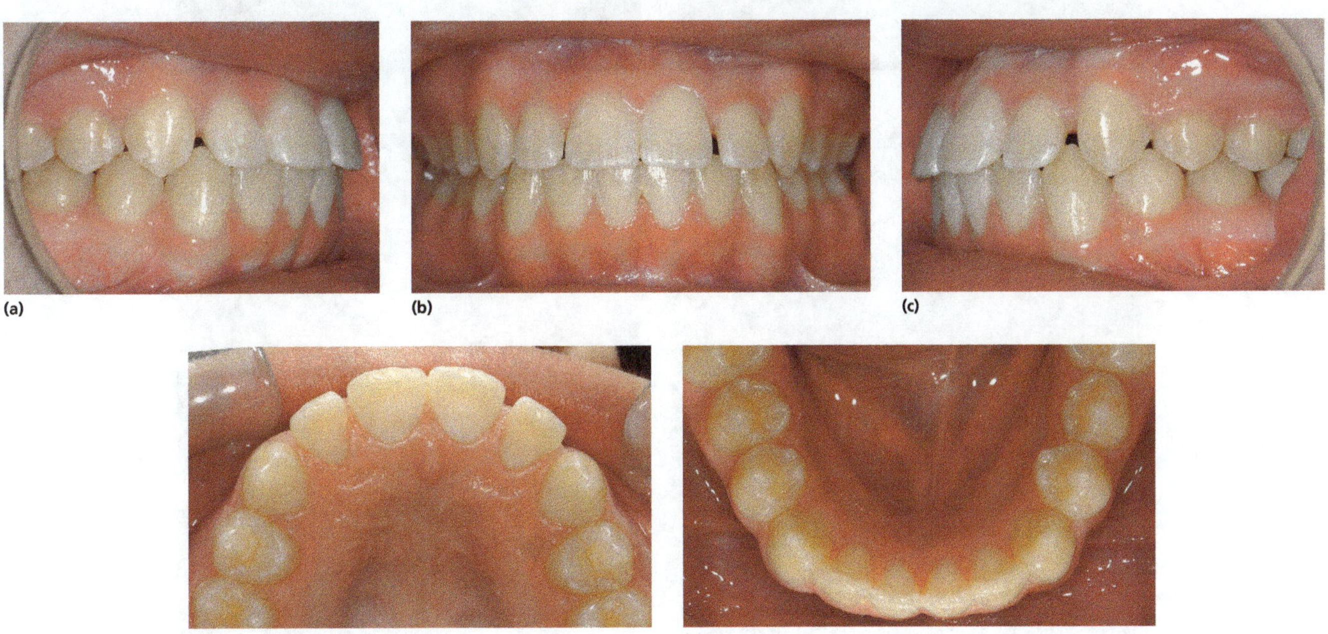

Figure 2.86 (a–p) Deband records of Andrew.

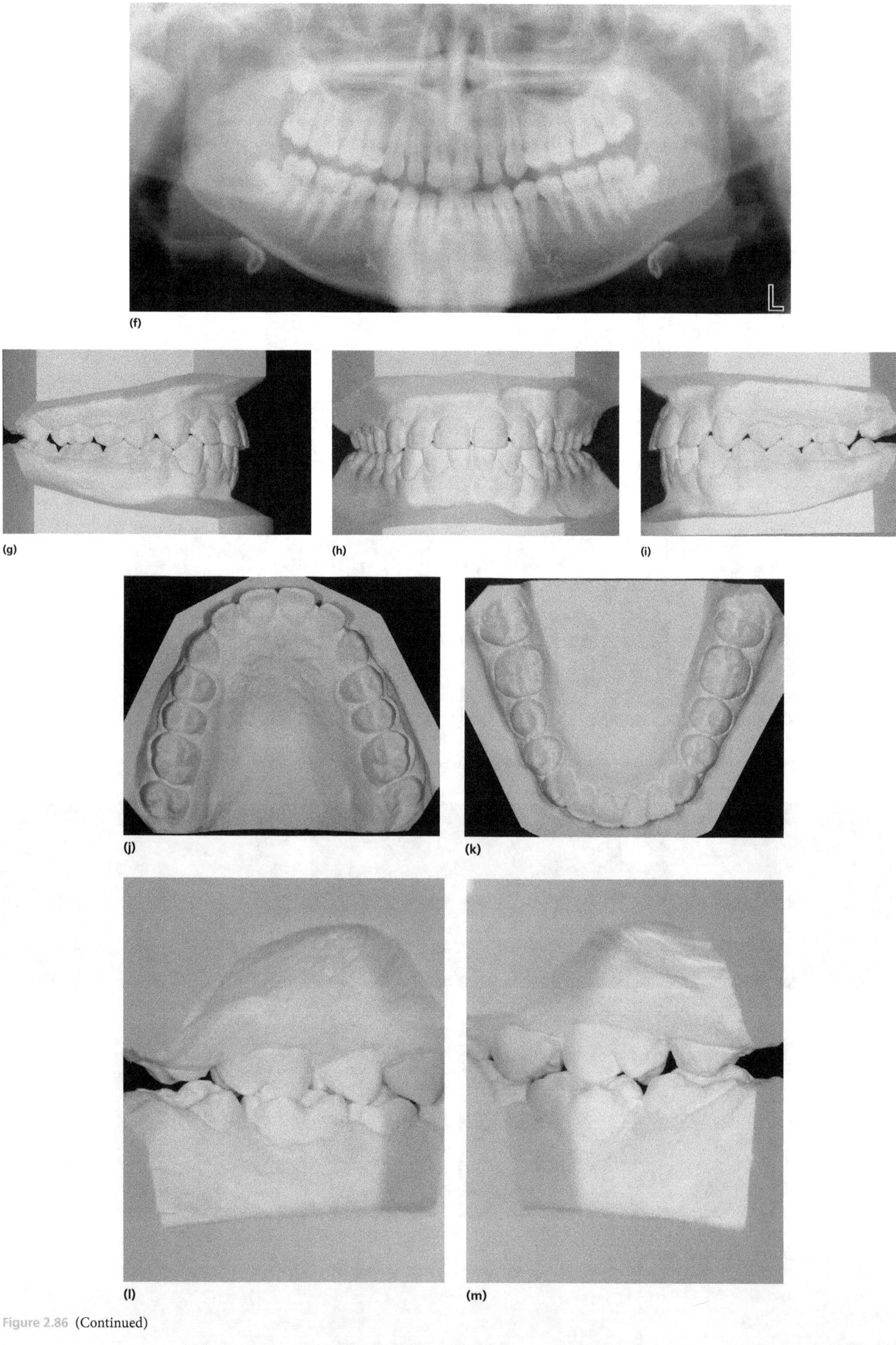

Figure 2.86 (Continued)

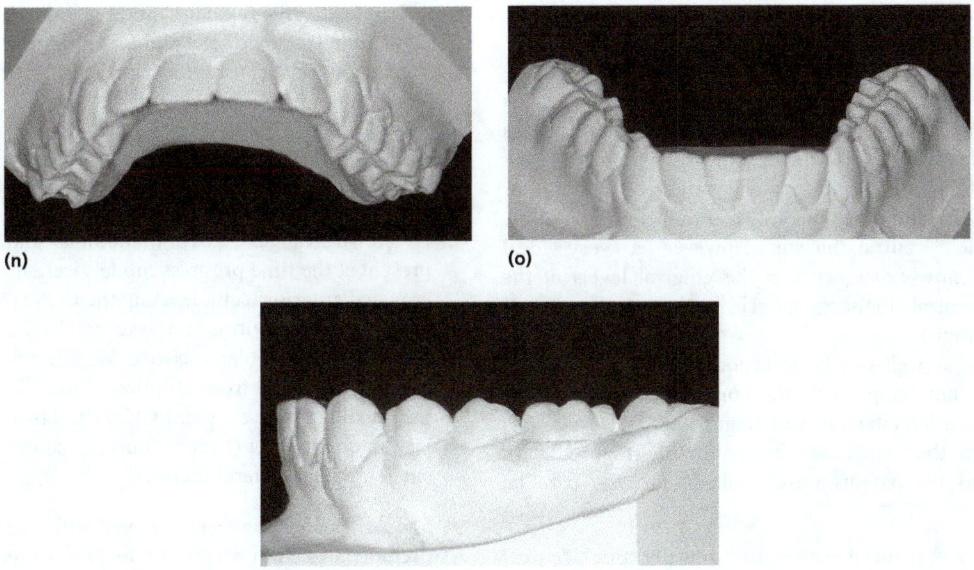

(n) (o) (p)

Figure 2.86 (Continued)

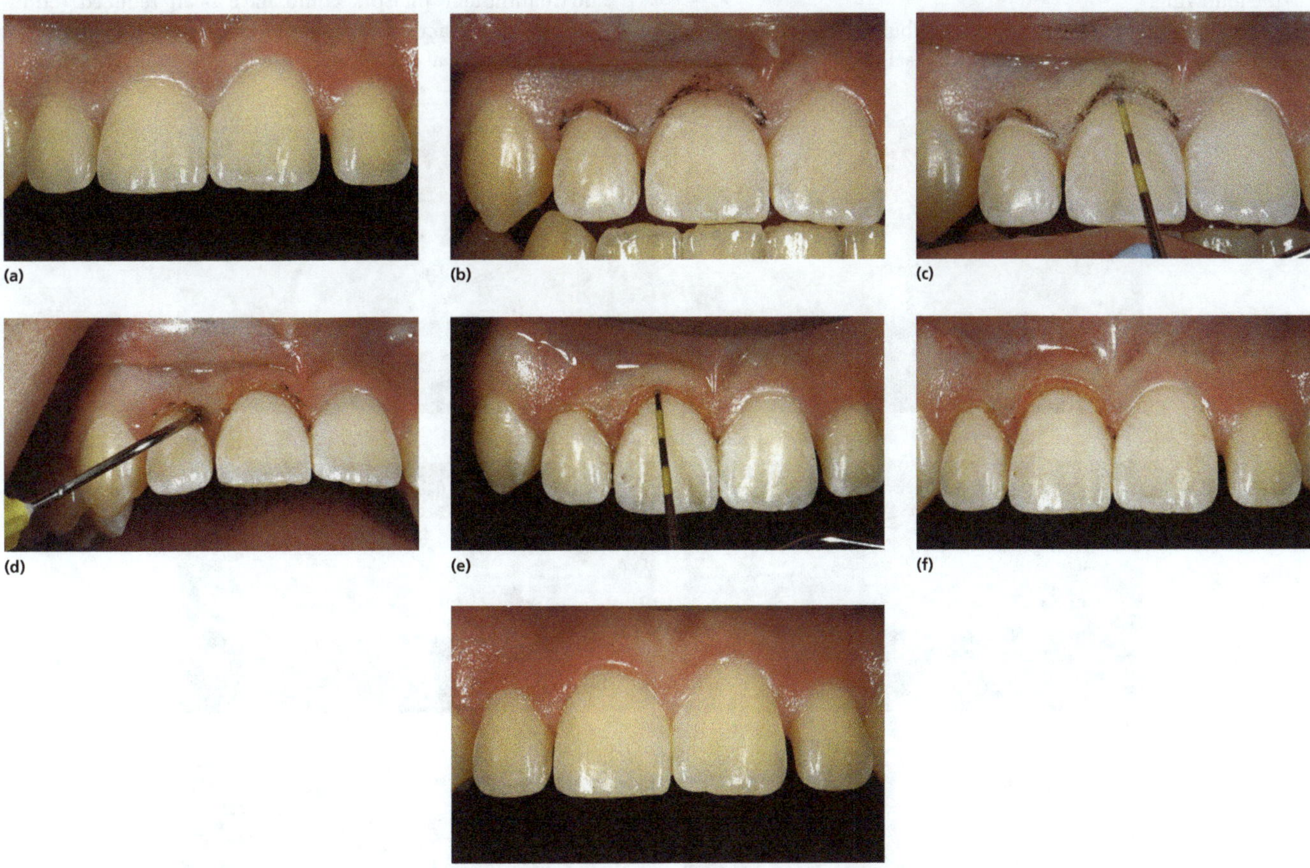

(a) (b) (c) (d) (e) (f) (g)

Figure 2.87 (a–g) Because Andrew's right central incisor and right lateral incisor gingival sulci were deep, laser gingivoplasty was used to improve his gingival margin positions.

- His maxilla and mandible are both retrusive (Figure 2.89e), and he is dentally bimaxillary protrusive.
- Progress to deband lateral cephalometric superimposition (Figure 2.89f) demonstrates significant mandibular growth.

The mandibular plane descended and flattened slightly with this growth (Figures 2.45e and 2.89e, f: FMA decreased from 30° to 29°, while SNMP decreased from 38° to 35°). Andrew's face grew downward and forward. His labiomental sulcus opened up slightly. The maxillary corpus descended. A-point and B-point moved downward and forward with the mandible displaced forward almost twice the amount of maxillary forward displacement. Maxillary and mandibular molars erupted. Maxillary incisors proclined. Mandibular incisors erupted and proclined (FMIA increased from 60° to 50°).

- The gingival margin of the maxillary right central incisor (Figure 2.89i) is improved but still slightly below that of the maxillary left central incisor. However, a very ideal relationship now exists between the gingival levels of the maxillary central incisors, lateral incisors, and canines (high–low–high).
- Andrew has a well-seated occlusion, but the restorative dentist was not happy with the composite veneer (black triangle) of the left lateral incisor (Figure 2.88f). Despite this self-criticism, the triangle was not noticeable (Figure 2.89j). Andrew and his parents were thrilled with the care he received.

Q: Andrew's OB was reduced even more from the time progress records were made until he was debanded (Figure 2.89f). How was his OB reduced *during this time*?

A: Andrew's OB was reduced from progress records to deband by the following:

- Proclination of maxillary and mandibular incisors
- Slight intrusion of the maxillary incisal tips
- Eruption of maxillary and mandibular molars during mandibular downward and forward growth (Note that mandibular incisors erupted during this time period, which would not help to open the bite.)

Q: *Why* were the mandibular and maxillary incisors proclined from the time of the progress cephalometric radiograph until deband (Figure 2.89f)?

A: As shown in Figure 2.61h, mandibular anterior crowding was present at the time progress models were made. Aligning these crowded anterior teeth, leveling the COS (Figures 2.61d, f, and 2.86p) with archwires, and wearing Class II elastics proclined Andrew's mandibular incisors. Maxillary incisor proclination may have resulted from eruption of maxillary molars (rotating the maxillary occlusal plane CCW) and from creation of maxillary anterior spaces (to accommodate composite veneers for the small maxillary lateral incisors).

Q: Should Andrew have been treated with extraction of four first premolars (or four second premolars) instead of being treated nonextraction?

A: An excellent outcome may have resulted with premolar extractions. Bimaxillary protrusion of Andrew's maxillary and mandibular incisors could have been reduced (eliminated) with extraction of premolars and retraction of anterior teeth. However, at the initial workup it was simply too early

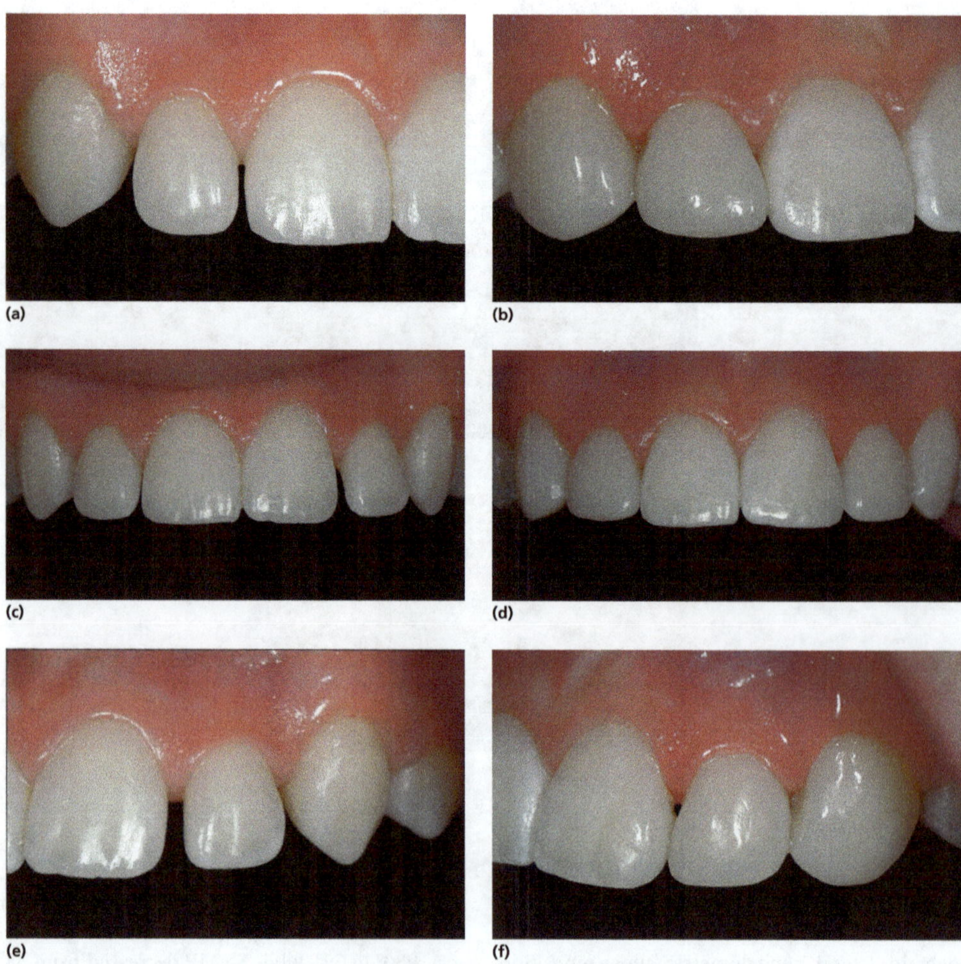

Figure 2.88 (a–f) Placement of direct composite veneers permitted closure of remaining anterior spaces.

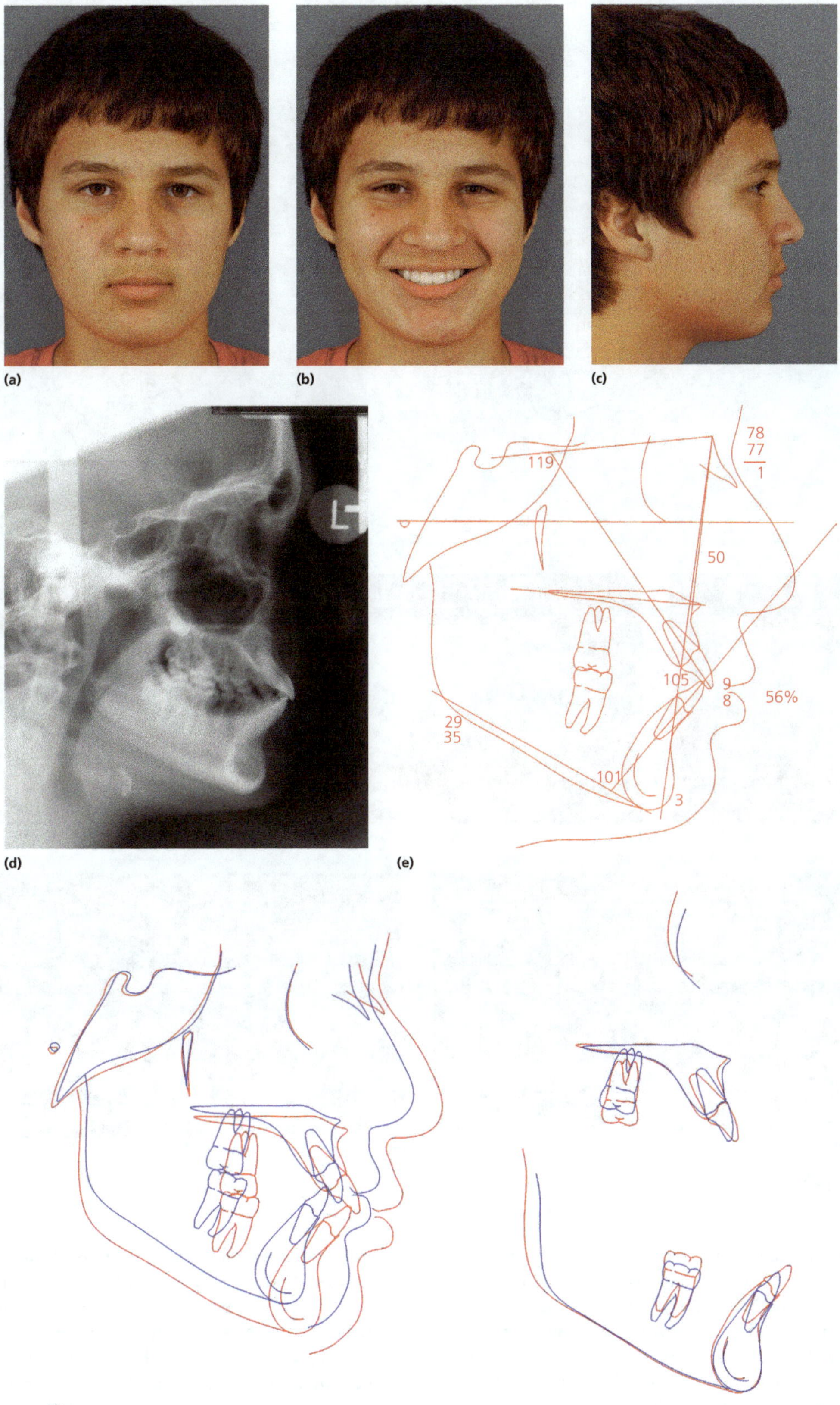

Figure 2.89 (a–l) Andrew's final records.

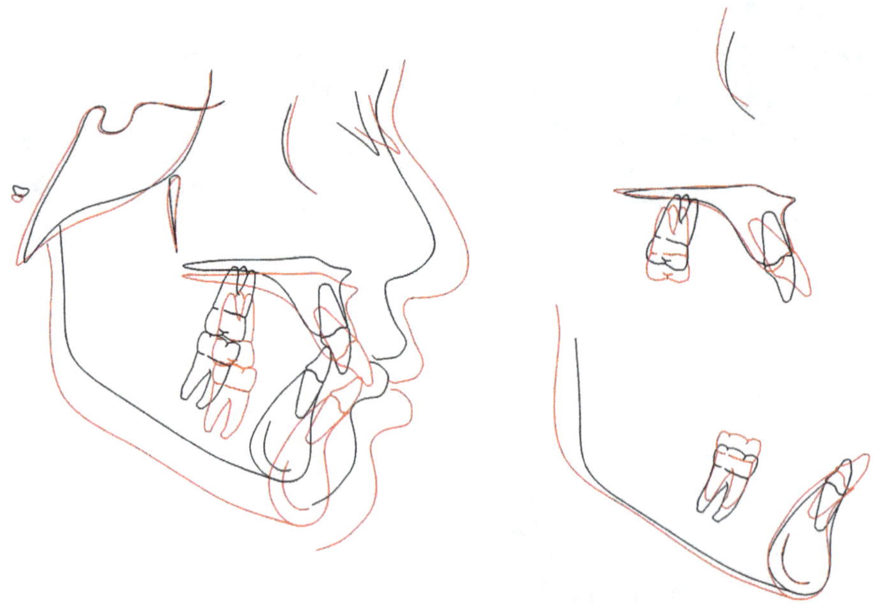

(g)

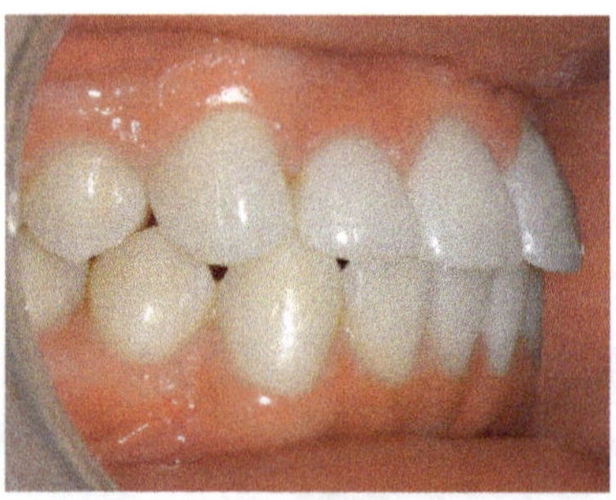

(h)

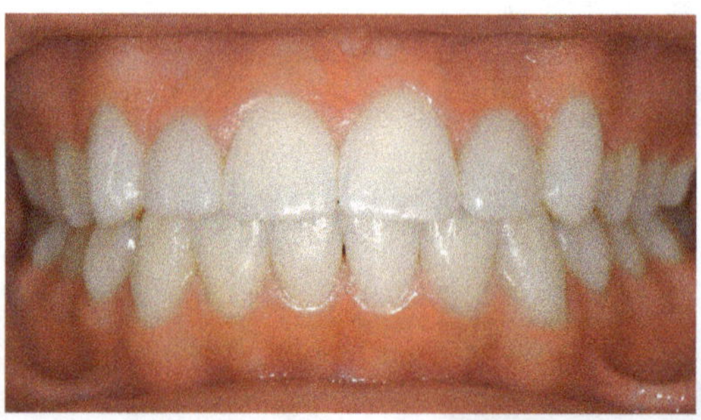

(i)

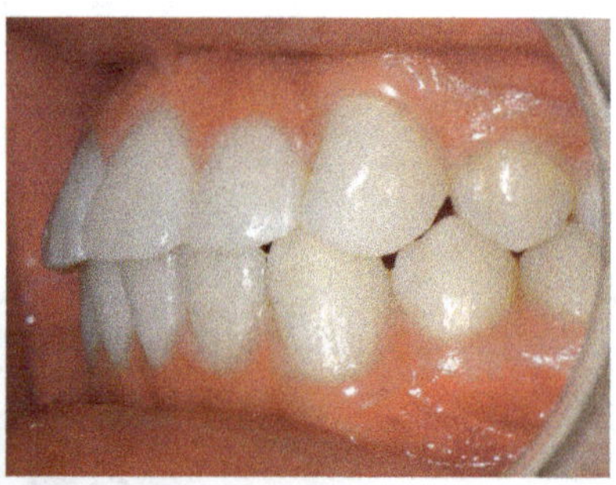

(j)

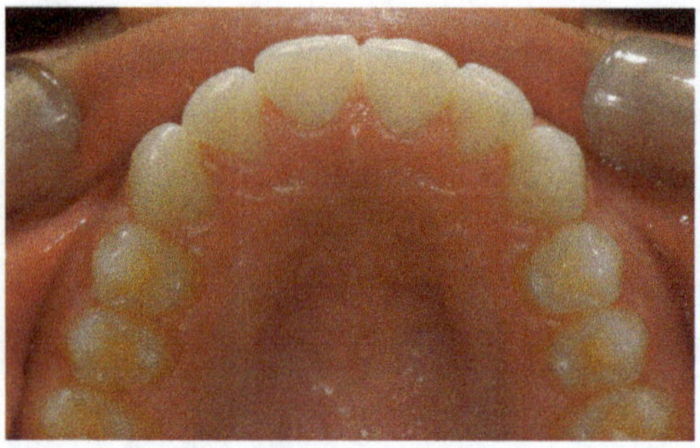

(k)

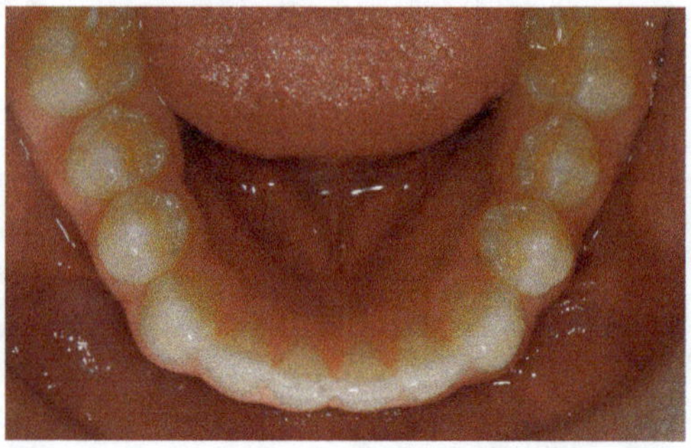

(l)

Figure 2.89 (Continued)

to make a decision regarding extraction of first premolars. It would have been ill-advised to extract mandibular first premolars at the time because Andrew was Class II. That is, without a guarantee of good growth and compliance, you may never have been able to correct his Class II relationship if mandibular canines were retracted through extraction spaces the same amount as maxillary canines. Andrew did not really begin growing until the time between progress records and deband. At the time of progress records (Figure 2.61b and h), the mandibular incisors still had a good angulation (FMIA was 60°) and the mandibular anterior crowding was mild. So the decision to continue treating him nonextraction was reasonable. Andrew still has a slightly upturned nose with good maxillary lip support. Extraction of first premolars plus incisor retraction could have reduced that support. Nonextraction treatment resulted in a pleasing profile, good maxillary lip support, beautiful smile, and healthy tissue. Extraction of four premolars could have produced as good, or even better, result. But, you cannot treat the same patient twice.

Q: Would postretention crowding be less if Andrew had been treated with premolar extractions instead of being treated nonextraction?

A: No. *Long-term (lifetime) orthodontic retention is the only guarantee that an excellent orthodontic result will be maintained.* Whether patients are treated with premolar extractions, treated with a lower incisor extraction, or treated nonextraction, the same post-treatment (postretention) changes tend to occur over time compared to untreated normal subjects, including arch length decrease and mandibular intercanine width reduction (whether or not the arch was expanded during treatment). Mandibular anterior crowding continues well into the 20–40 years age bracket and likely beyond [89].

Q: Should Andrew have been expanded with an RME appliance?

A: Yes. Andrew still has large buccal corridors and posterior transverse dental compensations. Buccal corridors and transverse compensations could have been reduced if he had been expanded with an RME appliance and his mandibular molars uprighted. In addition, widening the arches could have possibly reduced his incisor proclination. How can we say this? Well, every millimeter of maxillary premolar width increase produces a 0.7 mm increase in available maxillary arch perimeter, and it can be assumed that increasing mandibular posterior arch width (by uprighting mandibular posterior teeth) would likewise increase mandibular arch perimeter [90]. Generating perimeter could reduce incisor proclination.

Q: What "take-home" messages can you draw from Andrew's treatment?

A: Take-home messages include the following:

- Andrew presented with a dental deep bite. His vertical skeletal facial proportions were normal, but his maxillary and mandibular incisors were overerupted (COS of ~3 mm). Together, this incisor overeruption resulted in his 100% OB. His deep bite was corrected through a combination of maxillary incisor intrusion and proclination, mandibular incisor proclination, molar eruption, and mandibular downward and forward growth.
- Treatment decisions should be made with great care using the best scientific evidence available, your clinical experience, and patient desires. Whenever possible, reduce unknowns before committing to a nonreversible treatment step. In Andrew's case, each decision made, at each time point, was reasonable. He had a very nice result, but as doctors, you must always strive to learn from your care and to improve the treatment you are providing.
- Should Andrew's orthopedic treatment have been delayed? As noted earlier, compared to the lateral cephalometric superimposition from initial to progress (Figure 2.61c), the lateral cephalometric superimposition from progress to final (Figure 2.89f) demonstrated significant mandibular growth. Clearly, it may have been efficacious to delay the start of orthopedic treatment to capture this growth. So, should orthopedic treatment have been delayed? The answer is no. One of the challenges facing orthodontists is our inability to precisely predict the onset, magnitude, and direction of future growth for an individual. We know as a general rule that delaying the start of Class II treatment until the late mixed dentition stage is prudent. But even this rule is not cast in stone. If a patient is in the early mixed dentition, and the parents say that the patient has started his or her growth spurt, then it would be foolish not to initiate orthopedic treatment at that time. In Andrew's particular case, he was just entering the late mixed dentition stage and orthopedic treatment initiation was justified. We just missed out on timing his growth, exactly.
- HPHG was a good orthopedic appliance choice (he was very compliant in wearing it). Andrew's mandibular incisors would have proclined even more if a functional appliance had been worn.
- For less compliant patients, a fixed orthopedic appliance (e.g., Herbst appliance) may be better. If you place a patient on headgear, be sure to set a fixed length of time (3–4 months?) to judge their compliance with it. If compliance is not forthcoming, switch to another treatment approach.
- Considering his large buccal corridors (Figure 2.89b) and transverse dental compensations present at the end of treatment (Figure 2.86n and o), initial maxillary expansion with an RME appliance may have been justified and beneficial.
- Orthodontists should belong to teams (orthodontists, restorative dentists, periodontists, oral surgeons, pediatric dentists) who act together to provide the highest level of care to their patients. Communication between each team member is of paramount importance. The excellent care provided to Andrew was a direct result of teamwork.
- It was prudent to correct Andrew's OB to 10%. Why? No matter how you retain him, you should expect 10–20% increase in his OB with time. *Principle: overcorrect deep bites to a shallow OB, overcorrect open bites to a deep bite.*

Case Emma

Emma is an 11-year-old girl who presents to you with her parents' chief complaint, "Emma needs orthodontic treatment." Her PMH, PDH, and TMJ evaluation are WRN. She is without periodontal problems (her hygiene is not ideal) and CR=CO (Figure 2.90).

Q: List diagnostic findings/problems. What is your diagnosis?

A: See Table 2.4

Q: Although Emma has an initial ANB angle of only 2°, she appears mildly retrusive in her profile view (Figure 2.90b). Why?

A: Two reasons are as follows:

1. As seen on her cephalometric radiograph, her maxilla is slightly retrusive, which reduces her ANB angle. If her maxilla were in an ideal position, then her ANB angle would be larger.
2. Due to the presence of her blocked out mandibular permanent canines, Emma's B-point was hard to locate. The position of B-point chosen on her cephalometric radiograph (Figure 2.90e) is probably ahead of where B-point should be located. Consequently, ANB is probably larger than measured.

Based on her clinically retrusive appearance, and the above observations, we can conclude that Emma's mandible is mildly retrusive.

Q: What is the etiology of Emma's deep bite? Should it be classified as a *skeletal* deep bite or a *dental* deep bite?

A: Skeletally, Emma is normal in the vertical dimension. She presents with normal vertical soft tissue proportions (Figure 2.90a, soft tissue Glabella–Subnasale approximately equal to Subnasale–soft tissue Menton), and normal vertical skeletal proportions (Figure 2.90e, LAFH/TAFH ~56%, FMA 19°, SNMP 28°). The etiology of her deep bite is dental, overeruption mandibular incisors (resulting COS ~2–3 mm deep).

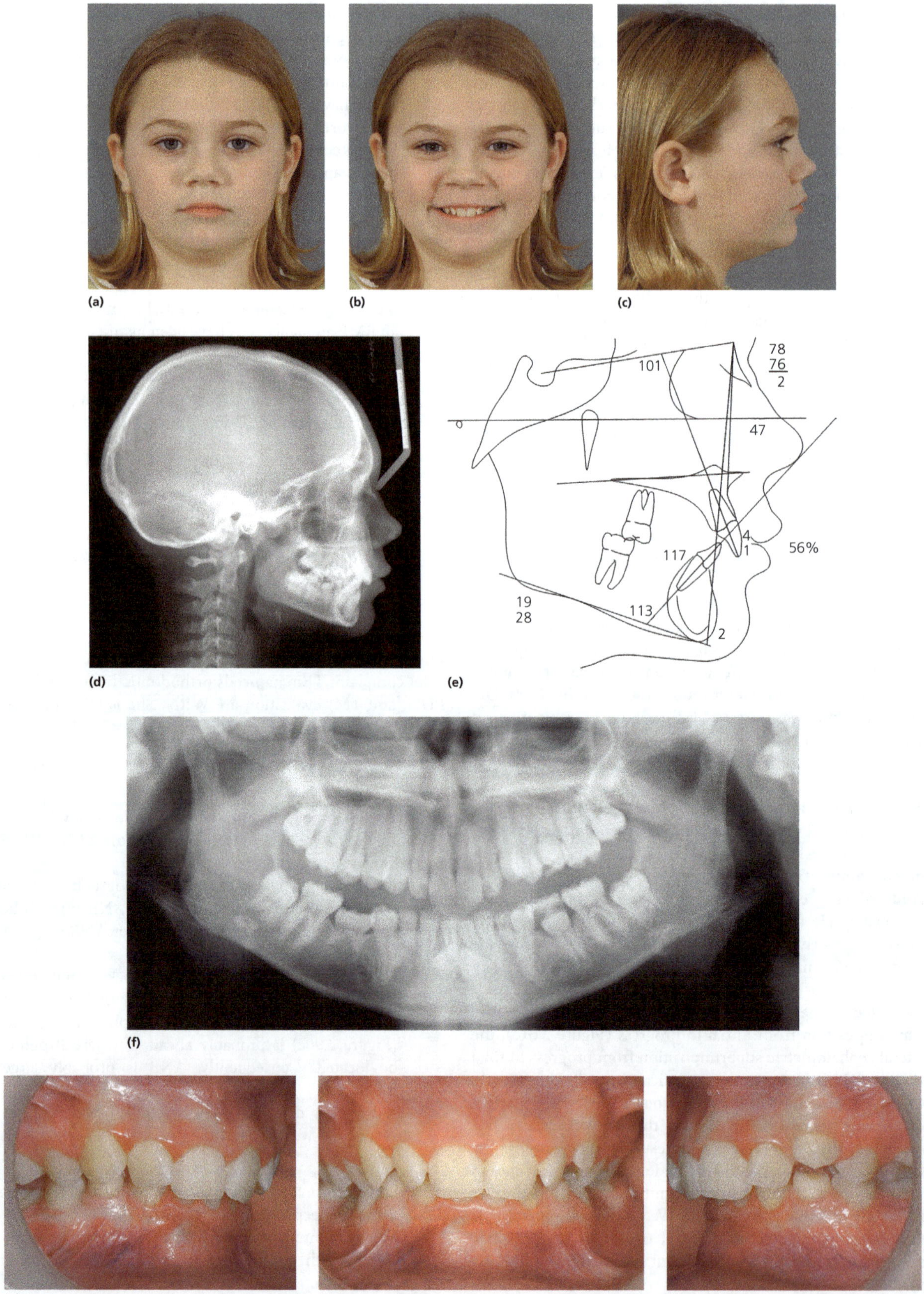

Figure 2.90 Initial records of Emma: (a–c) facial photographs, (d) lateral cephalograph, (e) cephalometric tracing, (f) pantomograph, (g–k) intraoral photographs, (l–p) model photographs, and (q–t) separated model views.

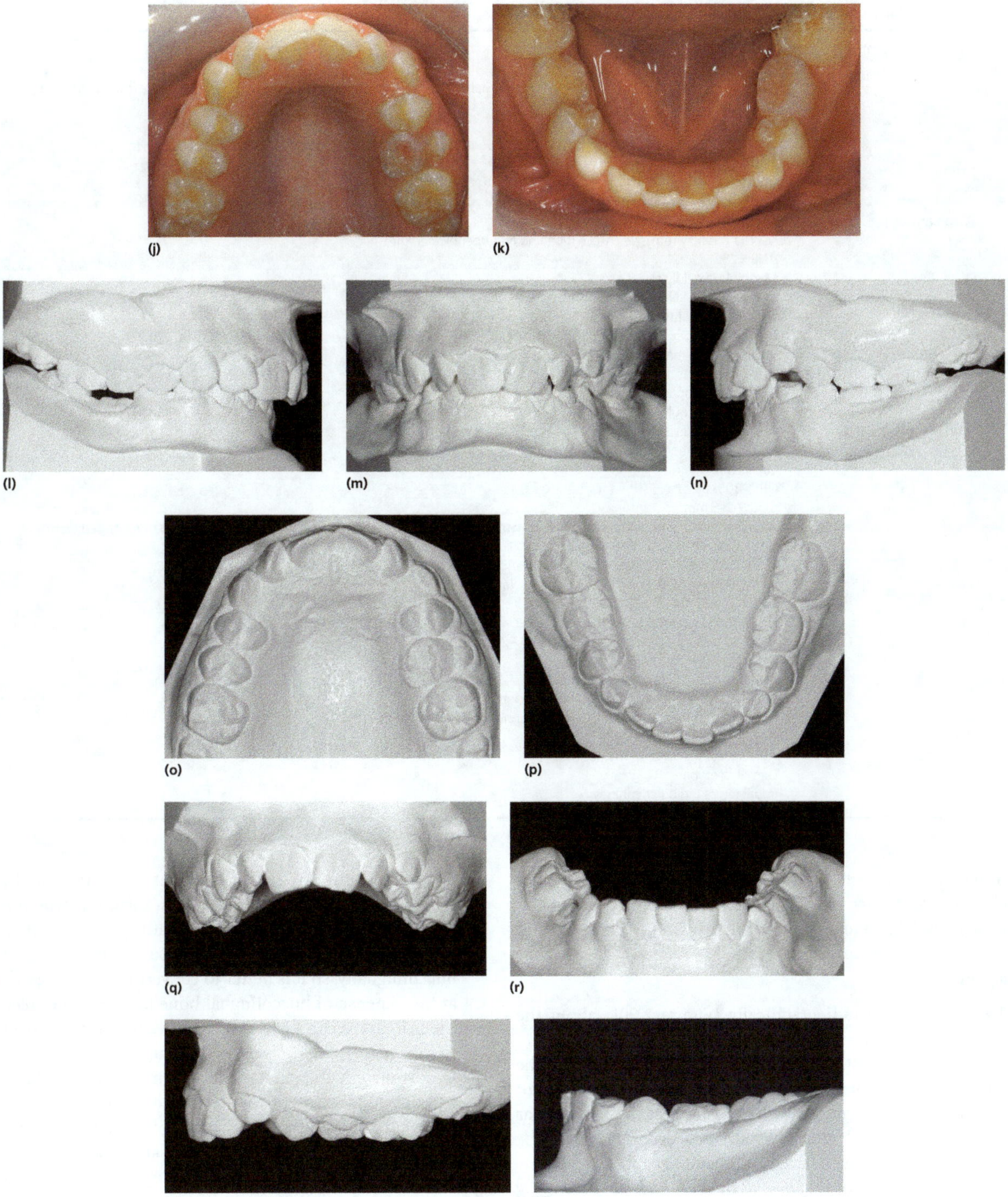

Figure 2.90 (Continued)

This pattern of vertical drift of tooth and alveolar bone has resulted in excess OB. Emma has a *dental* deep bite.

Q: What do you note, from her model (Figure 2.90l), about the mandibular right primary second molar?

A: It is *stepped down*, occlusally, from the mandibular first molar and first premolar.

Q: What can you conclude about the mandibular right primary second molar from its appearance on the model?

A: Most of us are quick to incorrectly conclude that the mandibular right primary second molar must be ankylosed because it is stepped down—but be careful of drawing this conclusion. Primary second molars typically have *shorter clinical crowns* than permanent teeth. This height difference can lead to an occlusal step between the mandibular permanent first molars and primary second molars. However, looking at her left primary second molar (Figure 2.90n), you note that its clinical occlusal level appears similar to the mandibular left permanent

Table 2.4 Diagnostic findings and problem list for Emma.

Full face and profile	**Frontal view** Face is symmetric Normal vertical facial proportions (soft tissue Glabella–Subnasale approximately equal to Subnasale–soft tissue Menton) Absence of interlabial gap UDML: WRN Central incisor gingival margins correctly positioned at vermillion border of maxillary lip in a posed smile **Profile view** Upturned nose Mildly convex profile and retrusive chin
Ceph analysis	**Skeletal** Maxilla is mildly retrusive (A-point behind N-perpendicular line) ANB = 2° Mandible is mildly retrusive LAFH/TAFH: WRN (ANS-Menton/Nasion-Menton ~56%) MPA slightly flat (FMA = 19°; SNMP = 28°) **Dental** Very proclined mandibular incisors (FMIA = 47°)
Radiographs	Late mixed dentition Blocked out/impacted mandibular canines Missing mandibular right second premolar
Intraoral photos and models	Angle Class II division 2 Iowa Classification: II (5–6) II (5–6) II (5–6) II (5–6) OJ: ~3 mm OB: ~80% COS: ~2–3 mm Maxillary incisors are approximately level with the posterior maxillary occlusion (neither stepped up nor stepped down) Lingual crown torque mandibular first molars Slight buccal crown torque maxillary first molars Lingual crown torque maxillary first premolars UTSALD ~5 mm LTSALD mild crowding, but mandibular leeway space still present LDML to the right of UDML (and face) by ~2 mm Dental arches reasonably symmetric Retained mandibular primary canines Retained mandibular right primary second molar Maxillary and mandibular left primary second molars nearly exfoliated
Other	—
Diagnosis	Angle Class II division 2 malocclusion Dental deep bite Impacted mandibular canines

first molar—there is no occlusal step on the left (Figure 2.90r and t). *Based on her models (clinical impression), you cannot conclude that her mandibular right primary second molar is ankylosed, but you are correct in suspecting that it might be ankylosed.*

Q: What do you note radiographically (Figure 2.90f) about the mandibular right primary second molar?

A: The mesial and distal alveolar process bone levels of the mandibular right primary second molar are lower than that of the adjacent permanent teeth—indicating that the mandibular right primary second molar has stopped erupting, while the adjacent permanent teeth have continued to erupt. *The best way to confirm ankylosis of erupting teeth is to look for developing discrepancies in alveolar crest levels with adjacent teeth.* The mandibular right primary second molar is *ankylosed.*

Q: How would you deal with this ankylosed mandibular right primary second molar?

A: Extract it. If you leave the ankylosed right primary second molar in the arch, then a major *vertical* bone discrepancy will result as the adjacent permanent teeth continue to erupt with growth. This vertical bone defect could be very difficult to correct (graft) when Emma is older. It is true that if you extract the ankylosed primary second molar now, you will develop a buccal-lingual narrowing of the edentulous site. But, if you extract it, then the alveolar ridge crest should actually move *occlusally* as the adjacent permanent teeth erupt, and pull the bone up with periosteal pull [91]. In turn, this would improve the potential for successful bone grafting later. In other words, it is harder to achieve successful bone grafting vertically than buccolingually, so it is better to get vertical bone growth now—at the expense of buccolingual bone loss. For example, look at the primary second molar in Figure 2.91a. Do you see the step in alveolar bone height mesial and distal to this tooth? Unfortunately, the primary second molar was retained during orthodontic treatment until the second radiograph was made one year later (Figure 2.91b); note the very large mesial and distal bone step as the first premolar and first molar continue to erupt. It was determined that the primary second molar was ankylosed at this time, and it was extracted. Two years later (Figure 2.91c), see how the alveolar crest at the primary second molar has returned to a satisfactory level (use the ghosts of the retained primary molar root tips as a reference).

Q: Extracting the mandibular right primary second molar at 11 years of age makes sense to prevent worsening of her vertical bony discrepancy. But would you extract this primary second molar if Emma was 17 years old and had finished growing?

A: Not necessarily. If Emma had finished growing (no further anticipated worsening of the bony defect) and the primary second molar had a good crown (no caries, no large restorations), good roots (minimal or no root resorption), and good bone (minimal

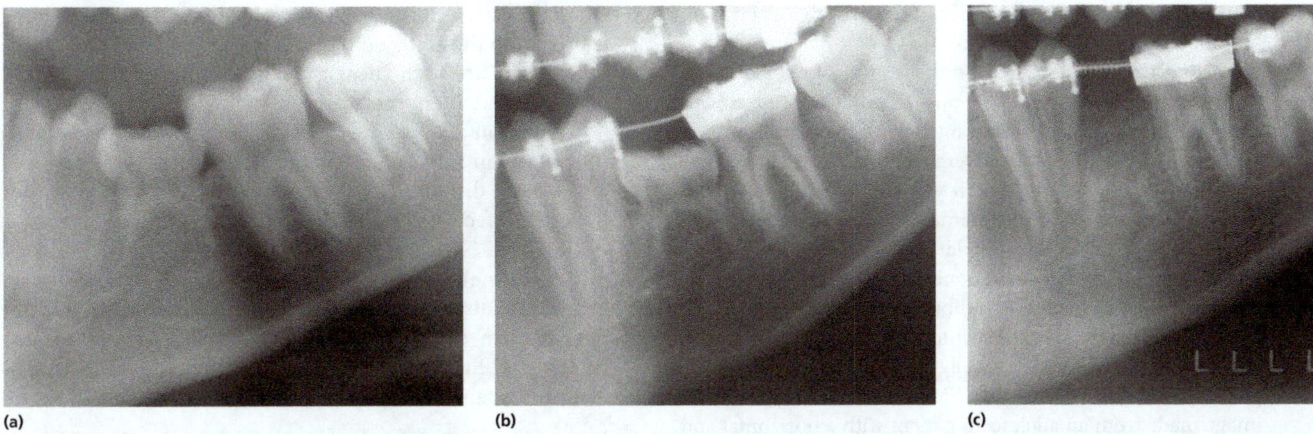

Figure 2.91 (a) If a mandibular primary second molar is ankylosed, then (b) a vertical bone defect will develop during adolescence as the second premolar and permanent first molar continue to erupt. (c) However, if the ankylosed primary second molar is extracted, then the alveolar ridge crest should move occlusally to a satisfactory level for later bone grafting.

vertical bony discrepancy), a viable alternative would be to retain it [92]. Of course, that is assuming that the vertical bone height discrepancy is small enough that Emma is able to maintain hygiene of the primary tooth easily. If this were the case, you would probably need to tip the permanent first molar distally in order to build up the primary second molar (see Figure 2.90f), so the opposing permanent tooth does not super-erupt.

Q: If you extract her mandibular right primary second molar, what are your options for dealing with the resulting space?

A: If you determine that Emma requires bilateral extractions in the mandibular arch, you could extract the ankylosed primary second molar on the right, extract a premolar on the left, and close the spaces. If you determine that Emma does not require extractions in the mandibular arch, then you could

- Protract the right mandibular molars to close the extraction space, using a TAD or protrusive Class II springs as anterior anchorage.
- Replace the missing second premolar with a FPD or implant/crown.

Q: You note that the mandibular permanent canines are unerupted/impacted (Figure 2.90f and h). Which are the most frequently impacted teeth, and how does the incidence of mandibular canine impaction compare?

A: Third molars, maxillary canines, maxillary and mandibular premolars, and maxillary central incisors are the most frequently impacted teeth [93]. The prevalence of impacted maxillary canines is 0.9–2.2%, but prevalence of impacted mandibular canines is much lower (0.07–1.3%) [94–98].

Q: What are your treatment options for Emma's unerupted/impacted mandibular canines?

A: You could retain the canines in their current position (observation), extract them, transplant them, or retain them but attempt to move them into the arch in their correct position.

Q: How do you decide which of these treatment options to pursue?

A: Options include the following:

- Retaining the permanent mandibular canines in their current position is not a good idea because they could eventually resorb the mandibular incisor roots. You should inform Emma's parents that resorption may have already occurred

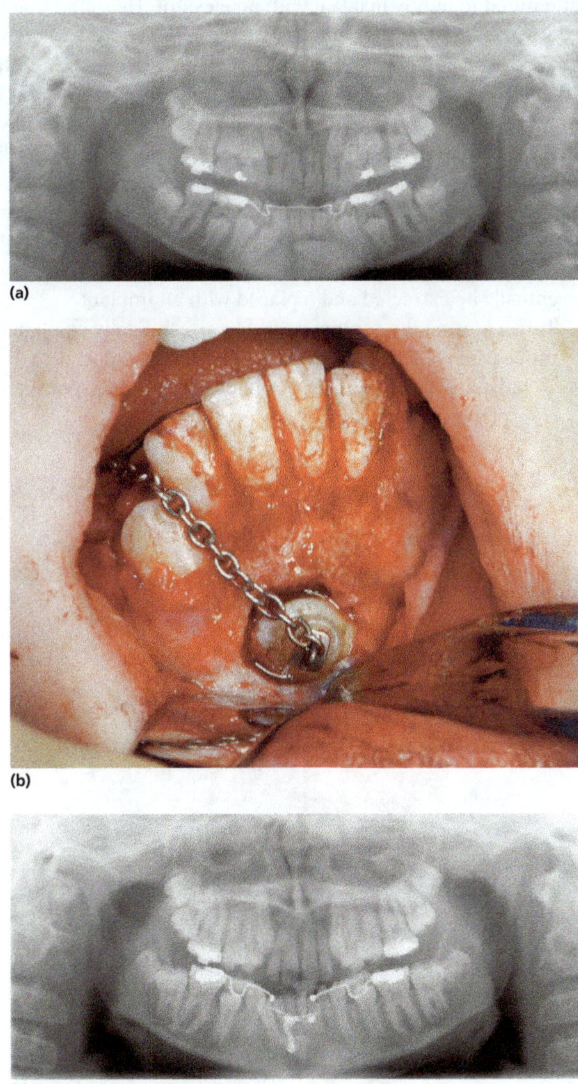

Figure 2.92 Adolescent with a deeply impacted mandibular left canine: (a) initial panoramic image, (b) surgical exposure of the mandibular canine, and (c) eruption of the mandibular canine was unsuccessfully attempted for 1 year and the canine was subsequently extracted.

(you will need a CT scan in order to confirm that resorption has not already occurred).

- Extracting the canines could be the option of choice, if the canines were more unfavorably positioned, if anterior crowding of the mandibular arch warranted permanent tooth extractions anyway, or if the canines were ankylosed (which you may only be able to determine when you attempt to luxate them during surgery or when you attempt to move them orthodontically). If the retained mandibular primary canines had good crowns, good roots, and good bone, then one option would be to extract the permanent mandibular canines and retain the primary canines in their place (informing the patient and parents that implants may eventually be required to replace the primary canines). For example, Figure 2.92a is the panoramic image made from an adolescent patient with a horizontal and deep impacted mandibular left permanent canine. Because the canine root appeared to be in a good position, a decision was made to expose it and attempt to upright it.

When the surgeon exposed the canine crown (Figure 2.92b), he attempted to lightly luxate it with an elevator. He stated that the canine was mobile, not ankylosed. We thought we had a good chance of bringing it into the arch. However, after applying labial traction to the crown for one year without any success erupting it, a follow-up panoramic radiograph was made which showed that the canine had not moved (Figure 2.92c). The left mandibular permanent canine was subsequently extracted, and the left mandibular primary canine (which had a good crown, root, and bone) was retained as a substitute. However, years later, we noted mobility of the primary canine due to root resorption. It will eventually be extracted and replaced with an implant.

- Transplanting the canines would be a technically challenging procedure. Furthermore, their root apices appear to have already closed (Figure 2.90f) making long-term success of a transplantation questionable.
- Retaining the permanent mandibular canines and moving them into the arch could be a viable alternative. The canine cusp tips are high (near the cervical line of the adjacent teeth), and their roots are positioned to the distal. This orientation allows for a more simple tipping movement to bring them into an acceptable arch position—as opposed to a more difficult translational (bodily) movement if they were perfectly upright in the center of the symphysis. Moreover, neither canine has transmigrated (crossed the midline).

You need to discuss these options with the parents and patient—inform them of the benefits and risks of each option. The parents and Emma elected to expose the permanent mandibular canines and attempt to move them into the arch.

Q: Let's talk for a few minutes about impacted teeth. What is a common error for initial movement of blocked out/impacted teeth such as these mandibular permanent canines?

A: A major error: *pulling the impacted tooth crown across the root of an adjacent tooth,* which can result in resorption of the adjacent toot root [99].

Q: In treatment of the palatally impacted canine shown in Figure 2.93a, what is the mistake being made?

A: The elastic force is pulling the impacted maxillary left canine crown not only distally but also labially, *into the root* of the lateral incisor, possibly causing resorption of the root. Furthermore, the lateral incisor is bonded so that its root has even less chance of moving out of the way of the canine crown without being resorbed. A wiser approach is to initially move the impacted canine crown *away* from the incisor roots (example Figure 2.93b; also note that the lateral incisors are *not* bonded, are free to move). Later, the canines can be moved laterally and positioned into the arch (Figure 2.93c).

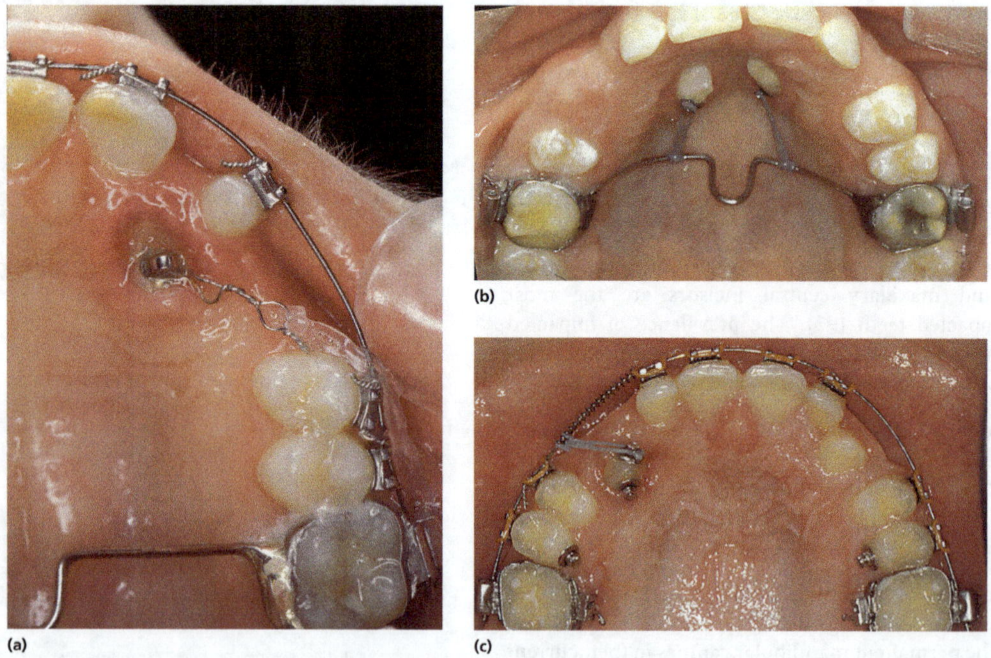

Figure 2.93 The wrong and right ways to initially move a palatally impacted maxillary canine crown: (a) the wrong way, dragging the canine crown across the lateral incisor root and potentially resorbing the root, (b) the right way, moving the canine crown initially *away* from the incisor roots until they are clear of the roots, (c) and then moving the canine crowns buccally into position.

Q: What is the first principle to follow during early movements of impacted teeth?

A: Always attempt to move the impacted tooth crown *away* from any adjacent tooth roots. Once the impacted tooth crown is clear of neighboring roots, it can be moved toward its future position in the arch without causing potential damage to adjacent tooth roots.

Q: For example, a 12-year-old female is referred to you for treatment of her left impacted maxillary canine, which you determine, using digital radiography, to be positioned labially (Figure 2.94a). It appears that resorption of the left central incisor root has already occurred. Are there any tests that you would like to make for the central incisor? What recommendations do you have for treatment? If you attempt to bring the canine into the arch, then what biomechanical principles should be followed?

A: It would be reasonable to perform a vitality test of the central incisor. This was done, and the central incisor was found to be vital. A CBCT image of the anterior maxilla could confirm possible resorption of the central incisor. However, even if resorption is found, it would be reasonable to attempt to retain the incisor. Since the crown of the impacted canine is much higher than the mucogingival junction, a closed exposure (Figure 2.94b and c), as opposed to an open exposure, should be attempted as this improves the potential for keratinized tissue to form properly during the forced eruption of the tooth. If keratinized tissue is inadequate after the tooth is brought into the arch, then a subsequent periodontal procedure may be necessary to create attached, keratinized gingiva. An apically positioned flap should *not* be used in a case of impaction this high, since significant stretching of the attached, keratinized tissues will occur, with potential upward relapse once the canine is brought into position. Biomechanically, the crown of the canine should be initially moved *labially*, away from the incisor roots (in this case using segmental mechanics, Figure 2.94c), and not dragged across the incisor roots. Later, when the impacted canine crown is clear of the incisor roots, it can be moved distally and coronally (Figure 2.94d) into its final position (Figure 2.94e). Note the extensive root resorption of the (still vital) maxillary left central incisor (Figure 2.94f).

Q: In Emma's case, in what direction should you initially attempt to move the crowns of her mandibular canines?

A: Labially, not distally across the roots of the mandibular incisors.

Q: Do you have any creative suggestions on how to initially move the exposed mandibular permanent canines labially?

A: To pull the exposed mandibular canines labially, you will need to have a wire, or bar, labial to the canine crowns. A lower arch lip bumper, or variant of a lip bumper, is well suited for this task. The exposed canines can be, initially, pulled toward the lip bumper (and later, pulled to the distal along the lip bumper).

Q: What are your treatment *goals* for Emma?

A: To improve her profile (increased chin projection), attempt to retain/properly position her permanent mandibular canines, achieve a Class I canine and molar relationship, and achieve

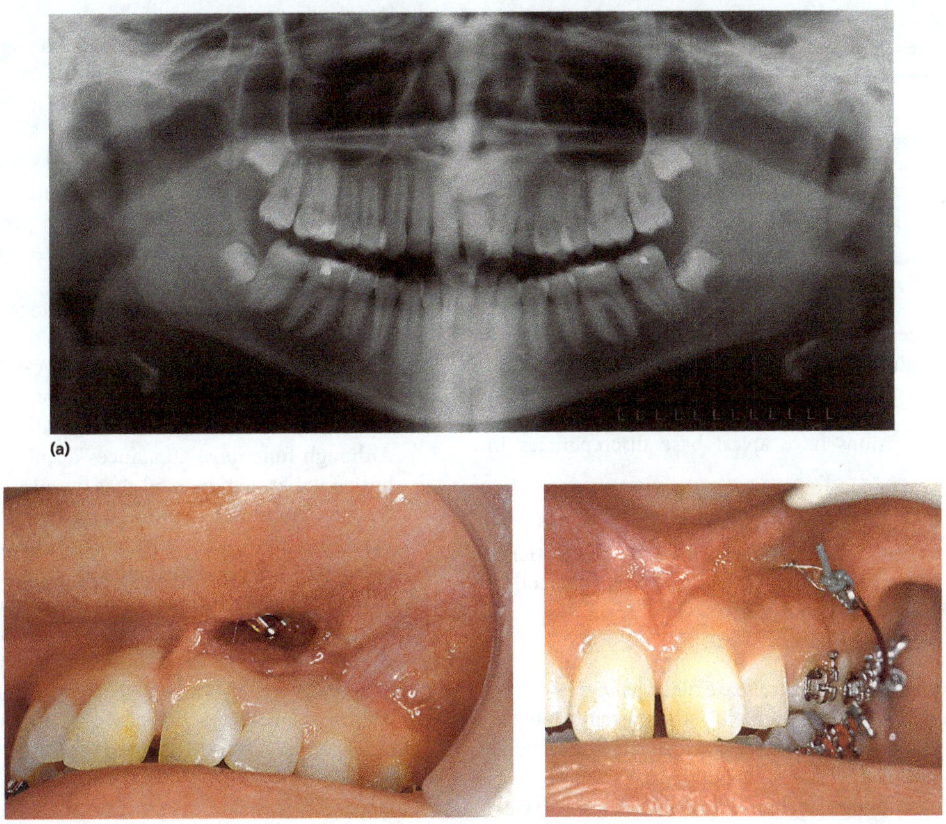

Figure 2.94 Forced eruption of a buccally impacted canine: (a) panoramic image reveals a high impaction of the maxillary left permanent canine which is resorbing the central incisor root; (b and c) a bracket is attached to the canine crown and a segmental wire used to initially move the canine crown *buccally*—away from the incisor roots; and (d–f) later, the left primary canine is extracted and the permanent canine erupted and moved distally into its correct position.

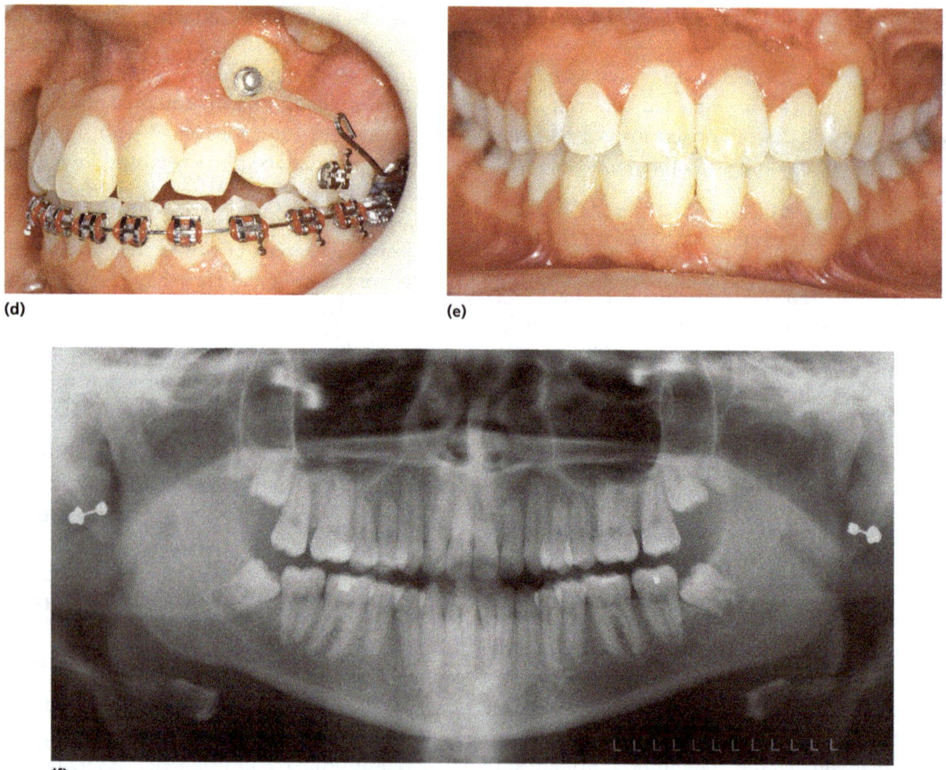

(d) (e) (f)

Figure 2.94 (Continued)

Table 2.5 Primary problems list for Emma *(apical base/skeletal discrepancies italicized).*

AP	II (5–6) II (5–6) II (5–6) II (5–6) *Mild maxillary and mandibular skeletal retrusion*
Vertical	80% OB due to 2–3 mm deep curve of Spee
Transverse	Absence of posterior cross bites, but presence of significant mandibular lingual crown torque
Other	Impacted mandibular canines and ankylosed mandibular right primary second molar

ideal OB (correct her deep bite) and ideal OJ. Finally, to prepare the mandibular right ankylosed primary first molar extraction space for eventual implant replacement or space closure.

Q: Which facial dimensions have apical base discrepancies in Emma?
A: AP only.

Q: The orthodontist must always stay focused on the patient's major, or *primary*, problems in each dimension (plus other problems). What are these in Emma?
A: See Table 2.5

Q: How can you address her AP apical base discrepancy?
A: *Orthopedics* (restrict maxillary growth while permitting the mandible to continue growing and/or accelerate mandibular growth). Orthopedic options are as follows:

- Headgears: A headgear (highpull, straightpull, or cervical pull) would tend to distalize the maxillary molars through the maxillary alveolar process bone (creating space for the anterior maxillary crowding) while at the same time restricting maxillary forward growth and allowing the mandible to continue growing downward and forward. A high-pull headgear may reduce descent of the maxillary corpus and maxillary first molars during growth, improving the mandibular AP skeletal relationship compared to if the maxilla/maxillary molars descended more [49, 50, 52, 55, 100]. A cervical-pull headgear would reduce the forward growth of the maxillary corpus while increasing the descent of the maxillary first molars (on average by <1 mm) and producing a slight CW rotation of the palatal plane [2–4]. A straight-pull headgear would produce an effect somewhere between that of a high-pull headgear and a cervical-pull headgear.
- Functional appliances: Emma has a flat (low) MPA but very proclined mandibular incisors (FMIA = 47°), so she would not be an ideal candidate for a Herbst or other functional appliance (the mandibular incisors would procline even further). Although functional appliances do not enhance mandibular horizontal growth beyond that found in control subjects [5], the acceleration of mandibular growth found when using a functional appliance may offer an advantage in treatment planning. (After 9–12 months of wear, you may have a good assessment of the expected chin projection in the profile.)

Masking or camouflage (achieving a Class I canine relationship without addressing the underlying skeletal apical base discrepancy) could be used to correct her molar and canine relationships dentally, especially if Emma turned out to be noncooperative or if her growth was poor. Options include the following:

- Intra-arch mechanics: extraction of maxillary first premolars to permit retraction of the maxillary anterior teeth (resulting in Class I canines, but leaving molars Class II). If you attempt this approach, you must be very wary of uprighting Emma's incisors more (and deepening her bite) during incisor retraction.

- Intra-arch mechanics: using maxillary TADs to distalize the entire maxillary arch.
- Inter-arch mechanics: Class II elastics or other inter-arch Class II correctors (e.g., Jasper Jumpers, Eureka Springs, Forsus) could correct her dental AP relationship, but mandibular incisor proclination will worsen as the mandibular teeth move forward unless the Class II elastics or inter-arch Class II correctors are connected to TADs (not teeth) in the mandible.

Surgery (mandibular advancement) would generally not be considered with this mild of an apical base discrepancy nor at this age.

Q: What two factors must be considered in the decision to treat a patient using orthopedics?

A: The *magnitude of the apical base discrepancy* and the *estimated time for growth to occur*. If the magnitude of the apical base discrepancy is small, and if the patient is young (and cooperative), then a full AP correction with orthopedics is probable. If the magnitude of the apical base discrepancy is large and the patient is older (or noncooperative), then a full AP correction with orthopedics is improbable.

Q: Based on these factors, is Emma a good candidate for attempting orthopedics?

A: Yes. The magnitude of her AP discrepancy is moderate (5–6 mm Class II at the molars), but she is only 11 years old, and significant facial growth is anticipated. There is no guarantee that Emma will have enough growth to obtain a full orthopedic AP correction, nor is there a guarantee that she will cooperate. But, you could discuss this option with her. If she is willing to try orthopedics, then it would be worth attempting. If you achieve *any* orthopedic correction, but not a full AP correction, then that amount of correction will only help you if you need to mask the remaining AP discrepancy.

Q: If orthopedics is instituted, when should you begin Emma's Class II correction?

A: Immediately. There is generally no advantage to beginning Class II treatment in the early mixed dentition stage of treatment [62–65, 74, 101, 102], but Emma is in the late mixed dentition. Even if Emma was in the early mixed dentition, if her parents told you that she was showing signs of a growth spurt, then you should initiate Class II treatment. Waiting to begin treatment until late mixed dentition is a good general principle to follow, but use your own judgment—dental stage is poorly correlated with skeletal growth.

Q: Emma has a mildly retrusive maxilla. Since headgears restrict forward maxillary growth, should you be concerned about using headgear therapy to correct her AP relationship? Will using headgear therapy adversely impact her facial esthetics?

A: No. In groups of Class II growing patients with protrusive, normally positioned, or retrusive maxillae, headgear treatment used in conjunction with fixed orthodontic appliances was found to be effective in improving facial profile esthetics in *all* groups. No significant correlations were found between initial anteroposterior position of the maxilla (FH-NA) and initial, final, or change in profile esthetic score. There was an average improvement with headgear treatment in profile esthetics for all groups [103].

Q: How should you treat Emma's deep bite?

A: Emma exhibits normal vertical soft tissue and skeletal proportions (Figure 2.90a and e). So, any treatment to decrease her OB by intentionally increasing her vertical dimension would be inappropriate. On the other hand, her 80% OB must be reduced in order to create incisal OJ for correction of her Class II relationship. Leveling the COS will open her bite. Leveling the COS with archwires results in premolar extrusion [1], mandibular incisor intrusion/proclination, and molar uprighting/eruption, which tends to rotate the mandible down and back. Her mandibular incisors are already so proclined that further proclination would not be welcomed. We must take this fact into consideration when we define our final treatment plan. Of course, the future direction and amount of maxillary and mandibular growth will affect Emma's OB.

Q: How would you address Emma's transverse problem (excessive lingual crown torque of mandibular first molars, slight buccal crown torque of maxillary first molars)?

A: Options include:

- The lower molars could be uprighted, to the buccal, with an LLHA or a removable Schwartz appliance. However, if the mandibular molars are uprighted, then the maxillary arch will need to be expanded (RME) in order to maintain posterior OJ. Or, you could expand the maxilla with an RME appliance and (simultaneously) upright the mandibular molars using cross-bite elastics worn from lingual buttons on the mandibular molars to the buccal of the RME appliance.
- An attempt to upright the molars could be made using maxillary and mandibular coordinated rectangular archwires and edgewise appliances, alone. However, this approach would involve torquing the mandibular molar roots lingually, through lingual cortical bone—which could be heroic. If this was attempted and the mandibular molar crowns began expanding buccally, then cross-bite elastics would need to be worn (maxillary molar lingual to mandibular molar buccal) to prevent the development of a posterior crossbite.
- Last, you could choose to leave the mandibular posterior lingual crown torque. This is a compromise.

Q: It is always important to at least consider the possibility of surgery. Is there a possible need for surgery and should you discuss this with Emma's parents?

A: No. There is no need to discuss surgery or the possibility of surgery with Emma's parents. Her skeletal discrepancy is simply too mild to warrant surgery.

Q: It is also important to consider unknowns you face in treating each patient. Specifically, are there any unknowns that you should reduce before doing something irreversible (e.g., extracting permanent teeth) or before you define a final treatment plan?

A: Yes. Unknowns include the following:

- Growth and compliance. If you attempt orthopedics, will Emma help us in correcting her AP? If she will be compliant, will she have adequate mandibular growth magnitude and direction to (partially) correct her AP?
- Impacted canines. Can the impacted mandibular canines be brought into the arch? Are they ankylosed, or will they ankylose when you are trying to move them?
- Hygiene. Will she improve her hygiene or will she need to be debanded early because of gingival overgrowth, white spot lesions, and caries?
- CR/CO shift. Is there an undetected shift?

Q: Should Emma be treated without extraction of permanent teeth?

A: In theory, every patient can be treated nonextraction, even those whose teeth are severely crowded, if you expand the arches enough. However, the cost for treating nonextraction may be too high (excessive labial/buccal tooth tipping, adverse effects on the periodontium, unsightly esthetic results). In Emma's case, if the AP can be corrected by distal movement of the maxillary molars; and if the mandibular canines can be brought into the arch without excessive dental arch expansion, then Emma could be treated nonextraction. A critical factor will be maintaining anchorage during retraction of the mandibular canines. Loss of anchorage (mesial movement of her mandibular posterior teeth), would limit the use of leeway space for uprighting mandibular incisors. TADs could be used in the mandible as anchorage to support retracting the impacted canines. The mandibular right primary second molar would eventually require prosthetic replacement.

Q: Should Emma be treated with extraction of anterior permanent teeth or some combination of posterior permanent teeth?

A: Extraction options include the following:

- Extract the impacted mandibular canines and retain the primary mandibular canines (if the primary canine crowns, roots, and supporting bone are WRN, as seen on periapical radiographs). Orthopedics to improve Emma's apical base relationships and Class II molar relationship, as considered for nonextraction treatment, would still apply. Mandibular leeway space could be used to upright mandibular incisors, but this would require retracting the mandibular primary canines (always dangerous, due to the potential for root resorption). Emma and her parents must be informed that the primary canines could eventually be lost and require implant replacement.
- Extraction the maxillary first premolars. If the mandibular canines are brought into the arch, this could allow finish to Class I canines (plus ideal OJ). Maxillary and mandibular molar anchorage would be critical with this approach (mandibular TADs? maxillary TADs or headgear?).
- Extract the maxillary first premolars, mandibular right primary second molar and mandibular left second premolar. Her full-step, bilateral Class II relationship (5–6 mm Class II) would require considerable mesial protraction of the mandibular first molars to achieve Class I molars. The amount of mandibular molar protraction needed would depend on Emma's compliance with headgear to hold/distalize maxillary first molars and upon mandibular forward growth. If headgear compliance were poor, then maximum mandibular molar protraction would be required to obtain Class I molars/canines, which would further limit our ability to retract mandibular canines and upright mandibular incisors.

Q: After everything we have discussed so far is considered, what treatment do you recommend?

A: After prosthodontic and periodontic consults were obtained, we decide to first reduce our major unknowns—growth/compliance, movement of the impacted canines, and hygiene. Emma began treatment nonextraction and was placed on an HPHG to improve her AP relationship and, with mandibular growth, reduce her profile convexity. A lower lingual holding arch was placed first molar to first molar, a lip bumper was fitted and tied back to the mandibular first molars bands, and her mandibular primary canines/primary molars were extracted. Her mandibular permanent canines were surgically exposed using an open procedure without an apically positioned flap (Figure 2.95a).

Q: What are the specific objectives of treatment for the maxilla, mandible, maxillary dentition, and mandibular dentition in all three planes of space?

A: Specific objectives of treatment for Emma are as follows:

Maxilla

AP: Restrict forward growth.
Vertical: Restrict downward growth.
Transverse: Allow for normal growth.

Mandible

AP: Allow for normal growth.
Vertical: Allow for normal growth.
Transverse: Allow for normal growth.

Maxillary dentition

AP: Distalize molars and canines. Maintain incisor inclination.
Vertical: Minimize molar eruption. Relative incisor intrusion.
Intermolar width: Maintain.

Mandibular dentition

AP: Maintain molars while retracting canines. Minimize incisor proclination.
Vertical: Minimize molar eruption. Level COS. Intrude incisors.
Intermolar/intercanine width: Maintain intermolar and intercanine widths.

Q: How did Emma's treatment progress?

A: The canine crowns were first pulled *labially* toward the lip bumper (Figure 2.95b), away from the mandibular incisor roots. Then, the canine crowns were moved distally. Distal movement of the canines continued using power chain (Figure 2.95c–e) and later using an open-coil spring between the canines (Figure 2.95f). Note spreading of the lower incisor crowns. Also note reciprocal proclination of the incisor crowns by the LLHA as the canines are retracted distally (compare Figure 2.95d and f).

Fixed appliances were placed, arches leveled and aligned (leveling the COS) with increasingly larger and stiffer archwires, and the spaces closed between the mandibular incisors (Figure 2.96). It took almost 3 years to retract the permanent mandibular canines.

Q: Remember, always *check primary problems in each dimension (plus other major problems) in CR, in each patient, at every appointment*. What do you see in Figure 2.96?

A: Emma is still Class II (~2 mm) at the left canines and Class II (~3–4 mm) at the right canines. Compliance and response to the use of headgear has been less than anticipated. Her transverse looks fine, she still has a deep OB, and she has mandibular right spacing. Also, poor hygiene is evident despite repeated instructions on proper oral hygiene.

Q: Observe the very hyperemic tissue seen mesial to the mandibular canines (Figure 2.96a–c) and the "bunching up" of the tissue distal to the canines. Is this a concern?

A: Not necessarily. It is not unusual to see hyperemic gingival tissue immediately in the wake of a translated tooth. This capillary rich tissue should remodel as the tissue matures. Bunching up of tissue can be a problem in terms of stability. Monitor this for now. A periodontic evaluation may be required at a later date.

Q: Let's re-group. What "in-treatment" recommendations do you now suggest?

A: Recommendations include the following:

- In terms of her AP, options considered and discussed with Emma included continued headgear wear, placement of TADs to retract the maxillary teeth en masse, premolar extractions, Class II elastics, or Class II springs. Emma chose interarch springs and elastics.

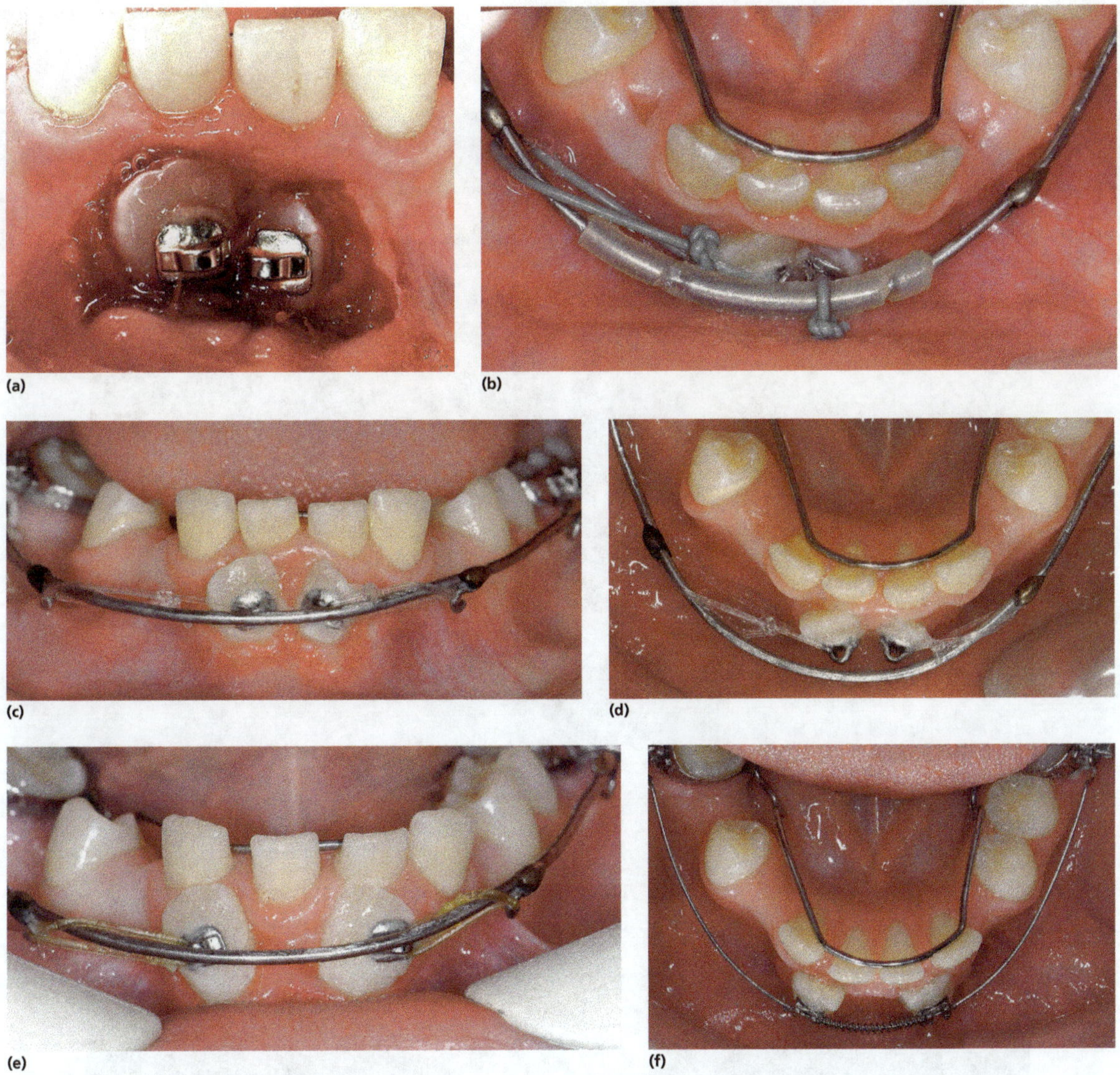

Figure 2.95 (a) Open surgical exposure and (b–f) initial orthodontic movement of Emma's impacted mandibular canines. To avoid incisor root resorption, the canine crowns were first moved toward the lip bumper (away from the incisor roots) before being moved distally. Also note reciprocal proclination of the incisor crowns by the LLHA (which is moving mesially) as the canines are retracted distally.

- In terms of her vertical, she was currently in light wires. Her archwires were gradually increased to maxillary and mandibular stainless steel archwire sizes of 0.019 × 0.025 inches. Maxillary and mandibular incisor steps were placed to open her bite (but maintain adequate maxillary incisor display).
- Mandibular spaces were closed to achieve canine symmetry and a 7 mm space for the (eventual) mandibular right second premolar implant.

An interarch Class II spring (Forsus®) was placed on Emma's left side and Class II elastics were worn on her right. Lingual crown torque was placed in the mandibular incisors. Following AP correction, artistics were placed, the prosthodontist was consulted to approve the premolar implant space, and Emma was debanded.

Q: What retention protocol would you suggest for Emma?

A: Emma was asked to wear Hawley retainers every night for a lifetime. Specifically, her retainers were designed with an anterior biteplate to disclude her posterior teeth and improve the chance of maintaining his deep bite correction. She could have been placed in a fixed mandibular canine to canine retainer, but she would still need to wear a maxillary retainer every night to guarantee long-term stability

Q: Total treatment time was 5 years. Deband records are shown in Figure 2.97. First, what do you note regarding the periodontium of her mandibular canines? Do you have any recommendations?

A: Although the mandibular canine gingival tissue (Figure 2.97g and i) shows a reduction in hyperemia and tissue bunching, the tissue looks very thin and lacks keratinization. Also, root exposure appears present on the mandibular left permanent canine. A periodontist was consulted and a subepithelial connective tissue graft was performed at this site.

Q: Do you have any recommendations regarding the right mandibular edentulous ridge?

A: As anticipated, the right mandibular edentulous ridge narrowed (compare Figure 2.90k to Figure 2.97k, q), but the alveolar bone

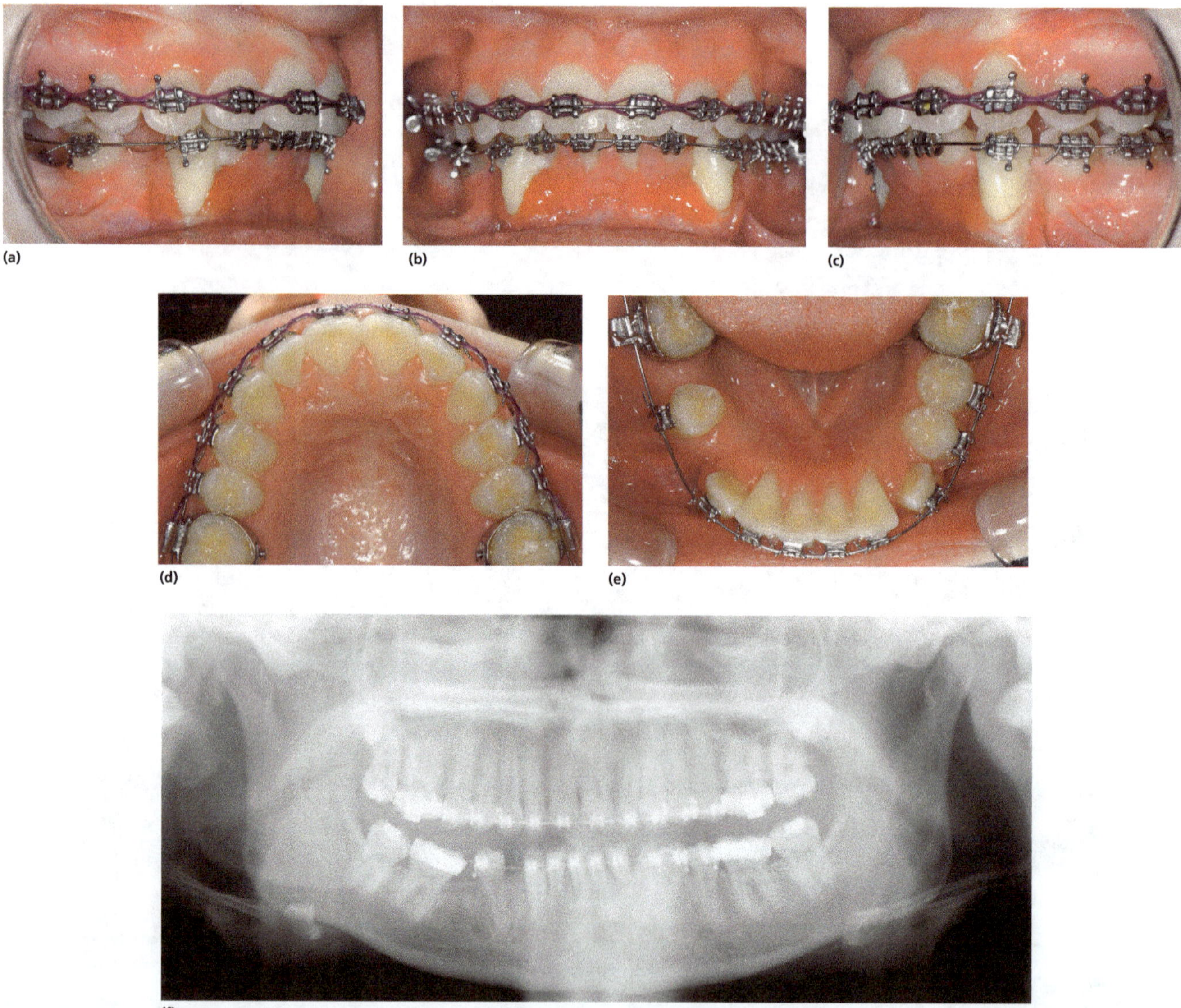

Figure 2.96 (a–f) Progress records of Emma.

vertical defect was eliminated (compare Figure 2.90f to Figure 2.97l). Extracting the ankylosed primary second molar reduced the need for bone grafting in a *vertical* direction. A cortical bone allograft was completed to prepare the ridge for an implant. Some months later, an implant was placed.

Q: Postprosthodontic treatment photographs are shown in Figure 2.98 (retainer wear was not ideal). Between her deband and postprosthodontic treatment records, what else do you observe?

A: Observations include the following:

- Emma has a beautiful smile with a noticeable reduction in buccal corridor size (compare Figure 2.90b to Figures 2.97b and 2.98b).
- Her maxillary central incisor gingival levels are ideally positioned (congruent with the maxillary lip vermillion border in a posed smile).
- Her profile esthetics are quite pleasing. She maintains an upturned nose. Chin projection has improved, but her labiomental sulcus is a little deep.
- Significant mandibular growth occurred during treatment (Figure 2.97f, B-point grew down and forward). Of course, this would be expected during ages 11–16 years. The mandibular plane descended in a parallel fashion. The maxilla descended. Maxillary molars erupted vertically, while mandibular molars moved mesially. Maxillary incisors erupted and moved mesially. Mandibular incisors intruded slightly and moved mesially.
- There has been a slight uprighting of her mandibular incisors (Figure 2.97f, FMIA increased from 47° to 53°). Her mandibular incisors translated, mesially.
- A Class I canine relationship was achieved (Figure 2.97g and i).
- Canines appear coordinated (Figures 2.97h, n, and 2.98f).
- Maxillary canines show distal-out rotations (Figure 2.97h and j)—this could have been corrected with IPR on the distal of the canines and rotation mechanics (placement of a rotation barrel on the distal?) to better align these teeth.
- Gingival tissue coverage of the mandibular permanent canine roots is improved (Figure 2.98e and g) following the gingival grafting.
- An ideal OB (~10%) and ideal maxillary incisal display is seen at deband (Figure 2.97h) but has deepened to 20% by the completion of prosthodontic treatment (Figure 2.98f).

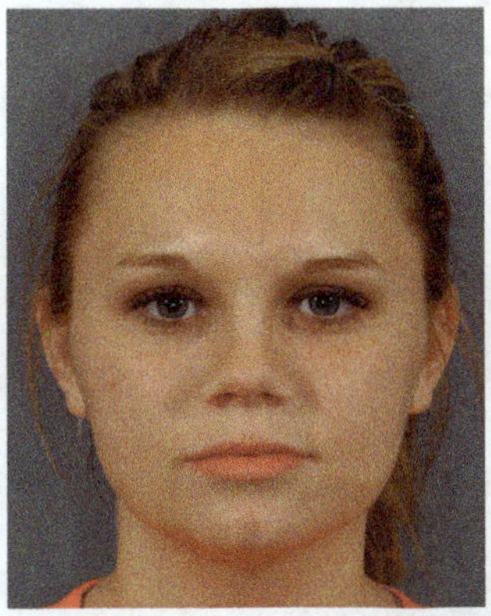
(a)

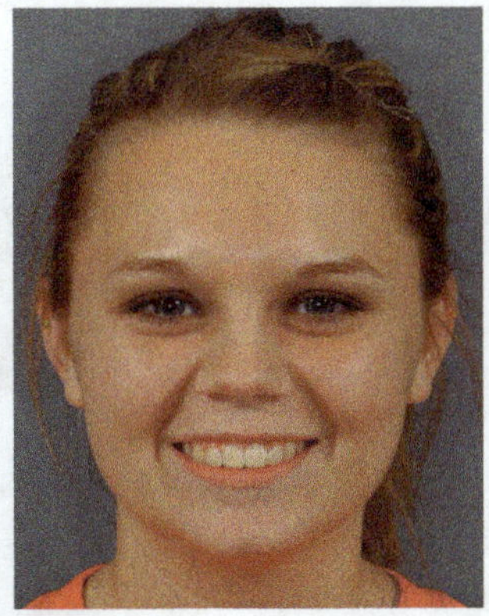
(b)

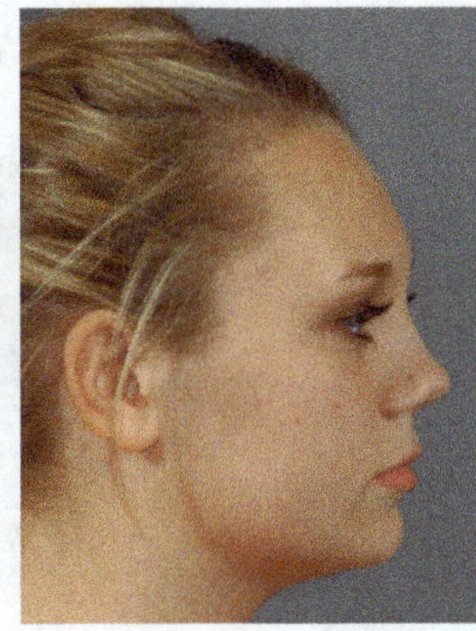
(c)

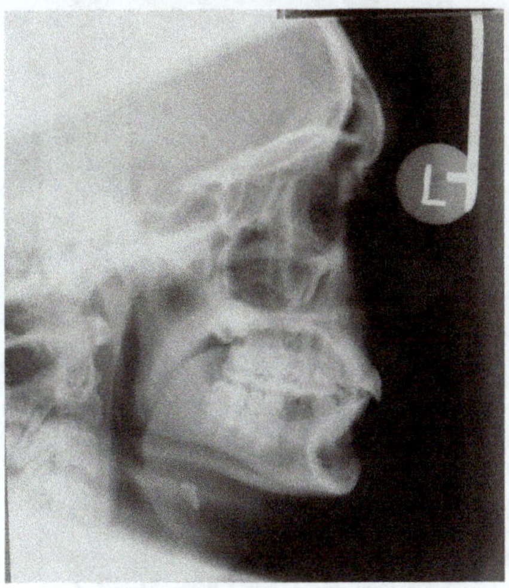
(d)

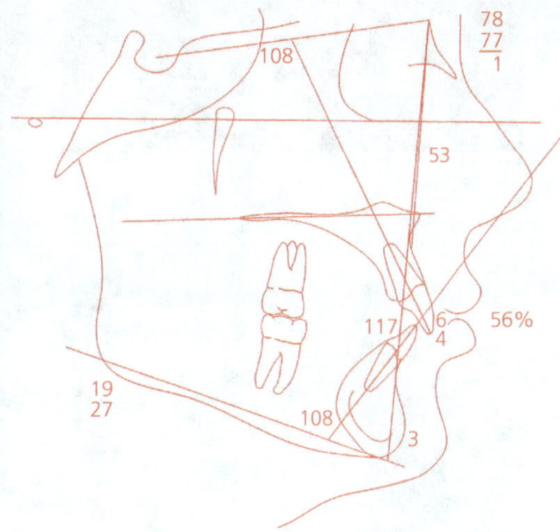

(e)

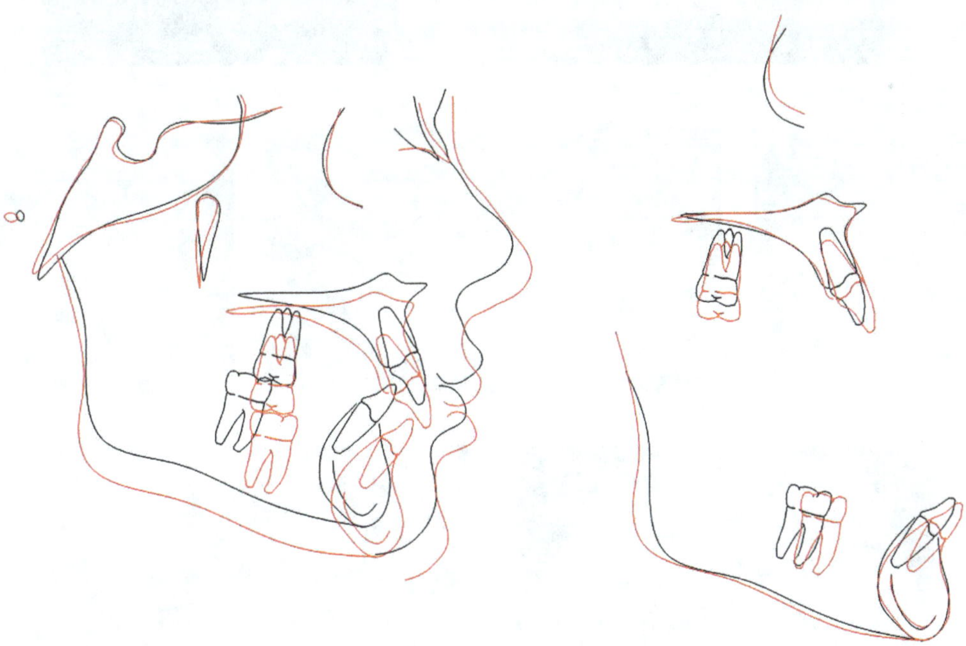
(f)

Figure 2.97 (a–u) Deband records of Emma.

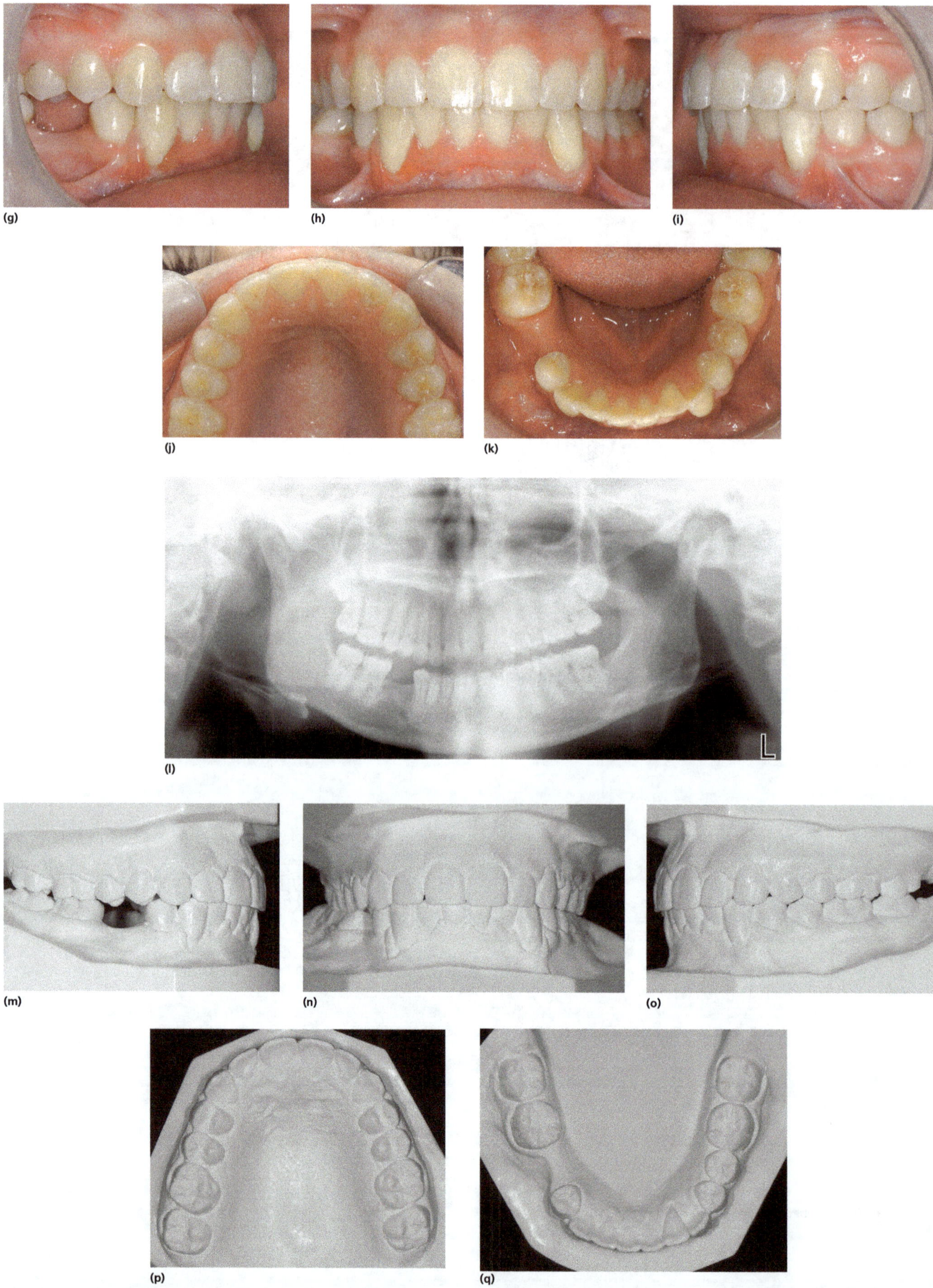

Figure 2.97 (Continued)

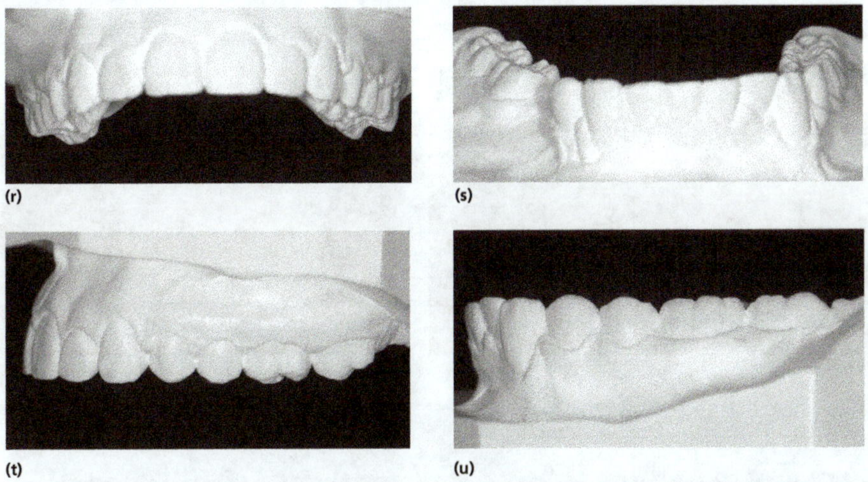

Figure 2.97 (Continued)

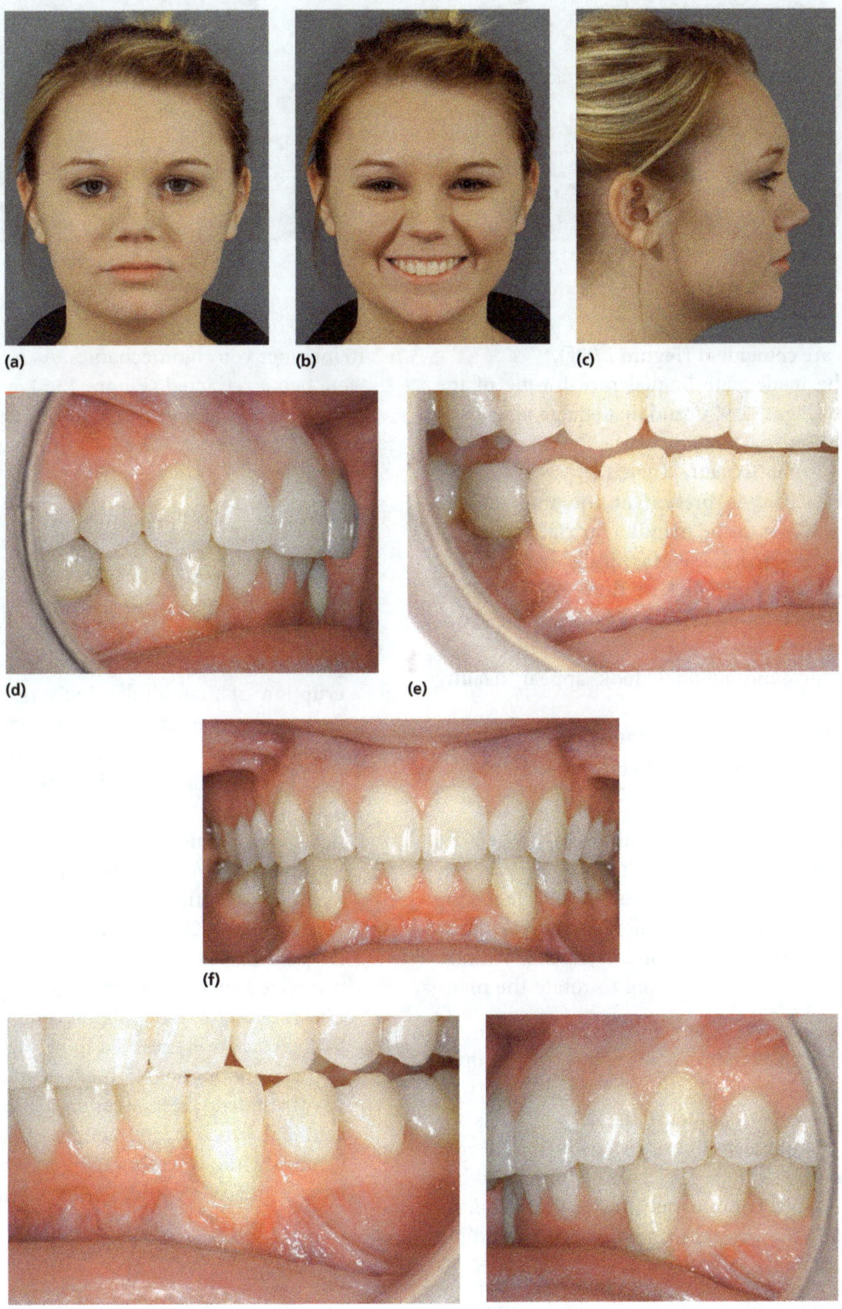

Figure 2.98 (a–k) Final records of Emma.

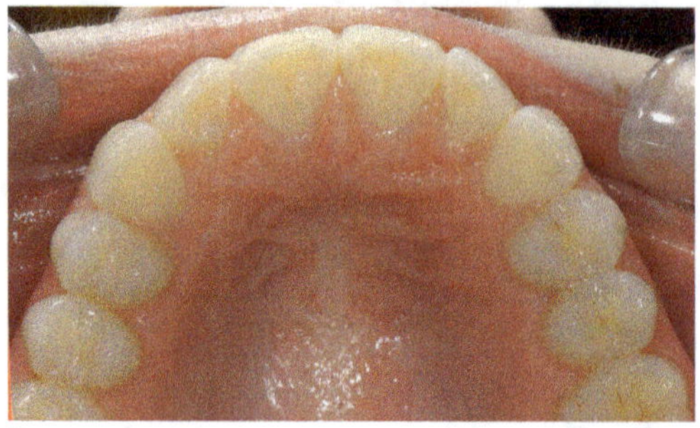

(i)

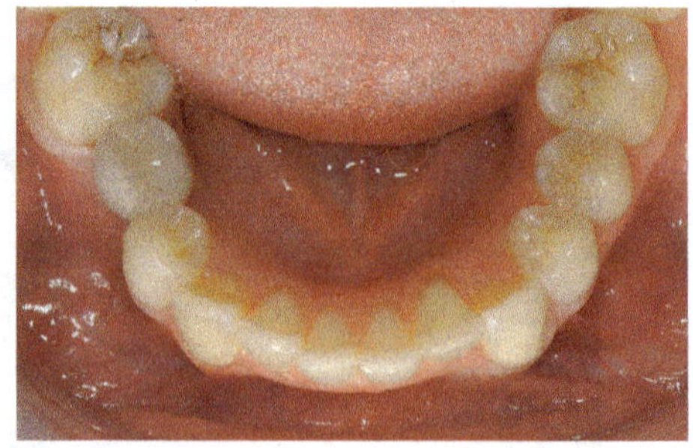

(j)

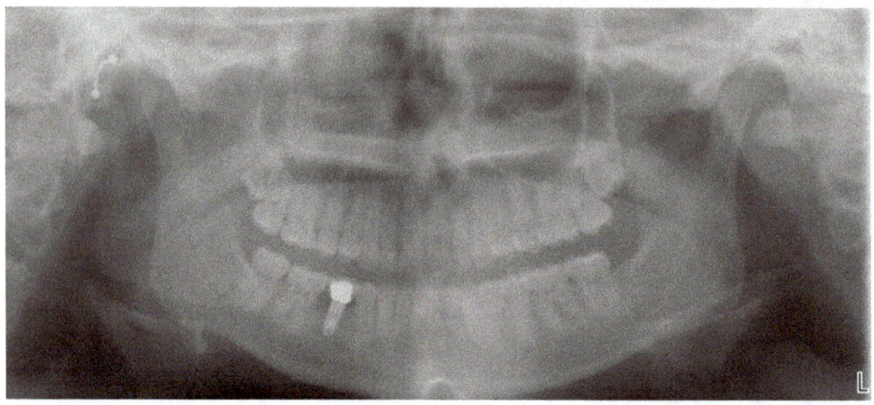

(k)

Figure 2.98 (Continued)

- UDML and LDML are coincident (Figure 2.98f).
- There appears to be inadequate lingual root torque of the mandibular canines (Figure 2.97k) and inadequate labial root torque of the mandibular lateral incisors. The mandibular right central incisor is not perfectly aligned.
- Adequate root parallelism is present at the implant site (Figure 2.97l), but the root of the mandibular right first premolar is not properly aligned. Radiographically, the mandibular incisors appear foreshortened as they are proclined (periapical radiographs should be made to examine their root lengths).
- The implant and surrounding bone look appear healthy (Figure 2.98e and k).
- Maxillary posterior buccal crown torque and mandibular posterior lingual crown torque is still evident (Figure 2.97r and s).
- The COS has been eliminated (Figure 2.97u).

Q: Based on her cephalometric superimposition (Figure 2.97f), how was Emma's AP relationship corrected?

A: Her Class II molar relationship was corrected to Class I by mandibular forward growth and mandibular molar mesial movement. Downward maxillary descent and maxillary molar eruption opposed this correction—tending to rotate the mandible down and back.

Q: Based on the cephalometric superimposition, how was Emma's deep bite corrected?

A: The effect of incisor movements on her initial deep bite was not particularly helpful. Mandibular incisors were intruded only slightly and uprighted slightly. Maxillary incisors proclined but erupted. What really opened her bite was growth. Emma's maxilla grew down, her maxillary molars erupted, and her mandible grew downward and forward.

Q: Why did Emma's mandibular incisors translate mesially (Figure 2.97f)?

A: Remember your biomechanics. As Emma's mandibular canines were being retracted (Figure 2.95), a reciprocal force from the LLAH tended to move her molars and incisors forward. Also, use of the interarch Class II springs and Class II elastics would do the same.

Q: What other "take-home" messages can you draw from Emma's treatment?

A: Take-home messages include the following:

- Emma presented with a dental deep bite. She had normal vertical soft tissue proportions and normal vertical skeletal proportions. The etiology of her deep bite was dental, over-eruption of mandibular incisors (resulting COS ~2–3 mm deep). She was treated non-extraction with leveling and aligning of her arches, using fixed appliances, to open her bite. Her mandibular incisors were intruded, slightly. But her deep bite was corrected by growth—her maxilla grew down, her maxillary molars erupted, and her mandible grew downward and forward. Incisor movements had minimal effect, overall, in opening her bite.
- Her initial 80% OB was reduced to 10% at deband, but it quickly relapsed to ~20% by the time prosthodontic treatment was completed (poor retainer wear). *Try to overcorrect your deep bites to a shallow OB at the end of treatment—expect relapse.*
- Compliance was expected to play a major part in the outcome of this orthodontic treatment plan. The ideal treatment would have included HPHG wear until Emma achieved Class I molar/canine correction, retraction of her impacted mandibular canines without anchorage loss, and use of the mandibular leeway space to permit uprighting mandibular incisors. Instead, final AP correction was achieved using a Class II protrusive spring and Class II elastics, which protracted her mandibular molars and left less space for mandibular incisor uprighting. In retrospect, we would consider placing TADs, for anchorage, in Emma's mandible during canine retraction.

- Of the four alternatives to dealing with an impacted mandibular canine (observation, extraction, transplantation, and orthodontic movement), the optimal choice depends on the canine position (vertical, horizontal, axis inclination), presence of an open or closed canine apex, determination of whether the patient requires extractions in the mandibular arch, and patient choice. If extraction of the impacted mandibular canines is warranted in a nonextraction mandibular arch, and if the primary mandibular canines are intact (good crown, root, and bone), retention of the primary mandibular canines may be a worthwhile option.
- Orthodontic movement of some impacted mandibular canines can take years and be heroic. Here, total treatment time was 5 years. Initial movement of the canine crown should be away from the incisor roots to avoid (further) root resorption, which can occur if the canine crown is dragged across the incisor roots.
- Exposing and moving impacted teeth (without adequate attached tissue) can be problematic and result in the teeth roots lacking keratinized tissue coverage.
- Ideal buccal uprighting of Emma's mandibular molars would have necessitated maxillary expansion with an RME appliance to maintain posterior OJ. This would have been a reasonable option.
- Regarding her ankylosed primary molar—extraction was the correct decision (as adjoining teeth erupted, their periosteal pull returned the alveolar crest bone height to a normal level).
- Although often considered a lesser problem, poor oral hygiene should always be considered a primary problem by orthodontists. White spot lesions, decay, and premature debanding can result from poor hygiene.
- Retainer wear noncompliance could eventually result in anterior tooth crowding and deepening of Emma's bite. Perhaps, a fixed mandibular canine to canine retainer should be advised for Emma.

References

1 Burstone CJ. Lip posture and its significance in treatment planning. *Am J Orthod.* 1967;**53**:262–84.

2 Formby WA, Nanda RS, Currier GF. Longitudinal changes in the adult face profile. *Am J Orthod Dentofacial Orthop.* 1994;**105**:464–76.

3 Lapatki B, Klatt A, Schulte-Monting J, Jonas I. Dentofacial parameters explaining variability in retroclination of the maxillary central incisors. *J Orofac Orthop.* 2007;**68**:109–23.

4 Lapatki BG, Mager AS, Schulte-Moenting J, Jonas IE. The importance of the level of the lip line and resting lip pressure in Class II division 2 malocclusion. *J Dent Res.* 2002;**81**:323–8.

5 Johnston DJ, Millett DT, Ayoub AF, Bock M. Are facial expressions reproducible? *Cleft Palate Craniofac J.* 2003;**40**:291–6.

6 Fudalej P. Long-term changes of the upper lip position relative to the incisal edge. *Am J Orthod Dentofacial Orthop.* 2008;**133**:204–9.

7 Marshall SD, Caspersen M, Hardinger RR, Franciscus RG, Aquilino SA, Southard TE. Development of the curve of Spee. *Am J Orthod Dentofacial Orthop.* 2008;**134**:344–52.

8 Farella M, Michelotti A, van Eljden TM, Martina R. The curve of Spee and craniofacial morphology: a multiple regression analysis. *Eur J Oral Sci.* 2002;**110**:277–81.

9 Demisch A, Ingerwall B, Thuer U. Mandibular displacement in Angle Class II division 2 malocclusion. *Am J Orthod Dentofacial Orthop.* 1992;**102**:509–18.

10 Ingervall B. Studies of mandibular positions in children. *Odontol Revy Suppl.* 1968;**15**:1–53.

11 Ingervall B. Relation between retruded contact, intercuspal, and rest positions of mandible in children with angle class II, division 2 malocclusion. *Odontol Revy.* 1968;**19**:293–310.

12 Ingervall B. Recording of retruded positions of mandible in children. *Odontol Revy.* 1968;**19**:65–82.

13 Ng J, Major PW, Heo G, Flores-Mir C. True incisor intrusion attained during orthodontic treatment: a systematic review and meta-analysis. *Am J Orthod Dentofacial Orthop.* 2005;**128**:212–9.

14 Bernstein R, Preston C, Lampasso J. Leveling the curve of Spee with a continuous archwire technique: a long term cephalometric study. *Am J Orthod Dentofacial Orthop.* 2007;**131**:363–71.

15 De Praeter J, Dermaut L, Martens G, Kulipers-Jagtman AM. Long-term stability of the leveling of the curve of Spee. *Am J Orthod Dentofacial Orthop.* 2002;**121**:266–72.

16 Al-Baraiki H. Sadowsky C, Schneider B. The effectiveness and long-term stability of overbite correction with incisor mechanics. *Am J Orthod Dentofacial Orthop.* 2005;**127**:47–55.

17 Shannon KR, Nanda RS. Changes in the curve of Spee with treatment and at 2 years post treatment. *Am J Orthod Dentofacial Orthop.* 2004;**125**:589–96.

18 Baccetti T, Franchi L, Guintini V, Masucci C, Vangelisti A, Defraia E. Early vs late orthodontic treatment of deepbite: a prospective clinical trial in growing subjects. *Am J Orthod Dentofacial Orthop.* 2012;**142**:75–82.

19 Dake ML, Sinclair PM. A comparison of the Ricketts and tweed-type arch leveling techniques. *Am J Orthod Dentofacial Orthop.* 1989;**95**:72–8.

20 Weiland FJ, Bantleon HP, Droschl H. Evaluation of continuous arch and segmented arch leveling techniques in adult patients—a clinical study. *Am J Orthod Dentofacial Orthop.* 1996;**110**:647–52.

21 AlQabandi A, Sadowsky C, Sellke T. A comparison of continuous archwires and utility archwires for leveling the curve of Spee. *World J Orthod.* 2002;**3**:159–65.

22 Binda SK, Kuipers-Jagtman AM, Maertens JK, Van 't Hof MA. A long-term cephalometric evaluation of treated Class II division 2 malocclusions. *Eur J Orthod.* 1994;**16**:301–8.

23 Devreese H, De Pauw G, Van Maele G, Kuipers-Jagtman AM, Dermaut L. Stability of upper incisor inclination in Class II division 2 patients. *Eur J Orthod.* 2007;**29**:314–20.

24 Schütz-Fransson U, Bjerklin K, Lindsten R. Long-term follow-up of orthodontically treated deep bite patients. *Eur J Orthod.* 2006;**28**:503–12.

25 Kim TW, Little RM. Postretention assessment of deep overbite correction in Class II division 2 malocclusion. *Angle Orthod.* 1999;**69**:175–86.

26 Kale Varlik S, Onur Alpakan O, Turkoz C. Deepbite correction with incisor intrusion in adults: a long-term cephalometric study. *Am J Orthod Dentofacial Orthop.* 2013;**144**:414–9.

27 Huang GJ, Bates SB, Ehlert AA, Whiting DP, Chen SS, Bollen AM. Stability of deep-bite correction: a systematic review. *J World Fed Orthod.* 2012:**1**:e89–e96.

28 Riedel RA. A review of the retention problem. *Angle Orthod.* 1960;**30**:179–99.

29 Ludwig M. A cephalometric analysis of the relationship between facial pattern, interincisal angulation and anterior overbite changes. *Angle Orthod.* 1967;**37**:194–204.

30 Simons ME, Joondeph DR. Change in overbite: a ten-year postretention study. *Am J Orthod.* 1973;**64**:349–67.

31 Canut JA. Arias S. A long-term evaluation of treated Class II, division 2, malocclusions: a retrospective study model analysis. *Eur J Orthod.* 1999;**21**:377–86.

32 Lapatki BG, Baustert D, Schulte-Monting J, Frucht S, Jonas IE. Lip-to-incisor relationship and postorthodontic long-term stability of overbite treatment. *Angle Orthod.* 2006;**76**:942–9.

33 Pollard D, Akyalcin S, Wittshire WA, Rody W. Relapse of orthodontically corrected deepbites in accordance with growth pattern. *Am J Orthod Dentofacial Orthop.* 2012;**141**:477–83.

34 Nanda R. Correction of deep overbite in adults. *Dent Clin North Am.* 1997;**41**:67–87.

35 McLaughlin RP, Bennett JC, Trevisi H. *Systemized orthodontic treatment mechanics.* 1st ed. Edinburgh, Scotland: Mosby, 2001.

36 Sajnani AK, King NM. Early prediction of maxillary canine impaction from panoramic radiographs. *Am J Orthod Dentofacial Orthop.* 2012;**142**:45–51.

37 Power SM, Short MB. An investigation into the response of palatally displaced canines to the removal of deciduous canines and an assessment of factors contributing to favourable eruption. *Br J Orthod.* 1993;**20**:215–23.

38 Kettle MA. Treatment of the unerupted maxillary canine. *Dent Pract.* 1958;**8**:245–55.

39 Jacobs SG. Palatally impacted canines: aetiology of impaction and scope for impaction. Report of cases outside the guidelines of interception. *Aust Dent J.* 1994;**39**:206–11.

40 Olive RJ. Orthodontic treatment of palatally impacted maxillary canines. *Aust Orthod J.* 2002;**18**:64–70.

41 Leonardi M, Armi P, Franchi L, Baccetti T. Two interceptive approaches to palatally displaced canines: a prospective longitudinal study. *Angle Orthod.* 2004;**74**:581–6.

42 Baccetti T, Leonardi M, Armi P. A randomized clinical study of two interceptive approaches to palatally displaced canines. *Eur J Orthod.* 2008;**30**:381–5.

43 Baccetti T, Mucedero M, Leonardi M, Cozza P. Interceptive treatment of palatal impaction of maxillary canines with rapid maxillary expansion: a randomized clinical trial. *Am J Orthod Dentofacial Orthop.* 2009;**136**:657–61.

44 Alessandri Bonetti G, Incerti Parenti S, Zanarini M, Marini I. Double vs single primary teeth extraction approach as prevention of permanent maxillary canines ectopic eruption. *Pediatr Dent.* 2010;**35**:407–12.

45 Armi P, Cozza P, Baccetti T. Effect of RME and headgear treatment on the eruption of palatally displaced canines: a randomized clinical study. *Angle Orthod.* 2011;**81**:370–4.

46 Sigler LM, Baccetti T, McNamara JA Jr. Effect of rapid maxillary expansion and transpalatal arch treatment associated with deciduous canine extraction on the

eruption of palatally displaced canines: a 2-center prospective study. *Am J Orthod Dentofacial Orthop*. 2011;**139**:e235–44.

47 Alessandri Bonetti G, Zanarini M, Incerti Parenti S, Mairini I, Gatto MR. Preventive treatment of ectopically erupting maxillary permanent canines by extraction of deciduous canines and first molars: a randomized clinical trial. *Am J Orthod Dentofacial Orthop*. 2011;**139**:316–23.

48 Baccetti T, Sigler LM, McNamara JA Jr. An RCT on treatment of palatally displaced canines with RME and/or transpalatal arch. *Eur J Orthod*. 2011;**33**:601–7.

49 Firouz M, Zernik J, Nanda R. Dental and orthopedic effects of high-pull headgear in treatment of Class II, division 1 malocclusion. *Am J Orthod Dentofacial Orthop*. 1992;**102**:197–205.

50 Baumrind S, Korn EL, Isaacson RJ, West EE, Molthen R. Quantitative analysis of the orthodontic and orthopedic effects of maxillary traction. *Am J Orthod*. 1983;**84**:384–98.

51 Elder JR, Tuenge RH. Cephalometric and histologic changes produced by extraoral high-pull traction to the maxilla in Macaca mulatta. *Am J Orthod*. 1974;**66**:599–617.

52 Kirjavainen M, Kirjavainen T, Hurmerinta K, Haavikko K. Orthopedic cervical headgear with an expanded inner bow in Class II correction. *Angle Orthod*. 2000;**70**:317–25.

53 Pancherz H. The effects, limitations, and long-term dentofacial adaptations to treatment with the Herbst appliance. *Semin Orthod*. 1997;**3**:232–43.

54 Le Cornu M, Cevidanes LH, Zhu H, Wu CD, Larson B, Nguyen T. Three-dimensional treatment outcomes in Class II patients treated with the Herbst appliance: a pilot study. *Am J Orthod Dentofacial Orthop*. 2013;**144**:818–30.

55 Huang G, English J, Ferguson D, Kulbersh R, Osterle L, Nah HD, et al. Ask us—functional appliances and long-term effects on mandibular growth. *Am J Orthod Dentofacial Orthop*. 2005;**128**:271–2.

56 Pancherz H, Ruf S, Kohlhas P. Effective condylar growth and chin position changes in Herbst treatment: a cephalometric roentgenographic long-term study. *Am J Orthod Dentofacial Orthop*. 1998;**114**:437–46.

57 Araujo AM, Buschang PH, Melo AC. Adaptive condylar growth and mandibular remodeling changes with bionator therapy—an implant study. *Eur J Orthod*. 2004;**26**:515–22.

58 Ruf S, Baltromejus S, Pancherz H. Effective condylar growth and chin position changes in activator treatment: a cephalometric roentgenographic study. *Angle Orthod*. 2001;**71**:4–11.

59 Konik M, Pancherz H, Hansen K. The mechanism of Class II correction in late Herbst treatment. *Am J Orthod Dentofacial Orthop*. 1997;**112**:87–91.

60 Croft RS, Buschang PH, English JD, Meyer R. A cephalometric and tomographic evaluation of Herbst treatment in the mixed dentition. *Am J Orthod*. 1999;**116**:435–43.

61 Hansen K, Koutsonas TG, Pancherz H. Long-term effects of Herbst treatment on the mandibular incisor segment: a cephalometric and biometric investigation. *Am J Orthod Dentofacial Orthop*. 1997;**112**:92–103.

62 Proffit WR, Tulloch JF. Preadolescent Class II problems: treat now or wait? *Am J Orthod Dentofacial Orthop*. 2002;**121**:560–2.

63 Tulloch JF, Proffit WR, Phillips C. Outcomes in a 2-phase randomized clinical trial of early Class II treatment. *Am J Orthod Dentofacial Orthop*. 2004;**125**:657–67.

64 Ghafari J, Shofer FS, Jacobsson-Hunt U, Markowitz DL, Laster LL. Headgear versus functional regulator in the early treatment of Class II division 1 malocclusion: a randomized clinical trial. *Am J Orthod Dentofacial Orthop*. 1998;**113**:51–61.

65 Keeling SD, Wheeler TT, King GJ, Garvan CW, Cohen DA, Cabassa S, et al. Anteroposterior skeletal and dental changes after early Class II treatment with bionators and headgear. *Am J Orthod Dentofacial Orthop*. 1998;**113**:40–50.

66 Mellion ZJ, Behrents RG, Johnston LE Jr. The pattern of facial skeletal growth and its relationship to various common indexes of maturation. *Am J Orthod Dentofacial Orthop*. 2013;**143**:845–54.

67 Born J, Muth S, Fehm HL. The significance of sleep onset and slow wave sleep for nocturnal release of growth hormone (GH) and cortisol. *Psychoneuroendocrinology*. 1988;**13**:233–43.

68 Postel-Vinay MC, Djiane J. Growth hormone and prolactin: biochemistry and physiology. In: Bertrand J, Rappaport B, Sizonenko PC, eds. *Pediatric endocrinology, physiology, pathophysiology, and clinical aspects*. 4th ed. Baltimore, MD: Williams & Wilkins, 1993. p. 210–20.

69 Lee CF, Proffit WR. The daily rhythm of human premolar eruption. *Am J Orthod Dentofacial Orthop*. 1995;**107**:38–47.

70 Risinger R, Proffit W. Continuous overnight observation of human premolar eruption. *Arch Oral Biol*. 1996;**41**:779–89.

71 Jakobsson SO. Cephalometric evaluation of treatment effect on Class II, division 1 malocclusions. *Am J Orthod*. 1967;**53**:446–57.

72 Tulloch JF, Phillips C, Koch G, Proffit WR. The effect of early intervention on skeletal pattern in Class II malocclusion: a randomized clinical trial. *Am J Orthod Dentofacial Orthop*. 1997;**111**:391–400.

73 Wheeler TT, McGorray SP, Dolce C, Taylor MG, King GJ. Effectiveness of early treatment of Class II malocclusion. *Am J Orthod Dentofacial Orthop*. 2002;**121**:9–17.

74 Dolce C, McGorray SP, Brazeau L, King GJ, Wheeler TT. Timing of Class II treatment: skeletal changes comparing 1-phase and 2-phase treatment. *Am J Orthod Dentofacial Orthop*. 2007;**132**:481–9.

75 Almeida-Pedrin RR, Almeida MR, Almeida RR, Pinzan A, Ferreira FP. Treatment effects of headgear biteplane and bionator appliances. *Am J Orthod Dentofacial Orthop*. 2007;**132**:191–8.

76 Thurman MM, King GJ, Ramsay DS, Wheeler TT, Phillips C. The effect of an anterior biteplate on dental and skeletal Class II correction using headgears: a cephalometric study. *Orthod Craniofac Res*. 2011;**14**:213–21.

77 Baccetti T, Franchi L, Stahl F. Comparison of 2 comprehensive Class II treatment protocols including the bonded Herbst and headgear appliances: a double-blind study of consecutively treated patients at puberty. *Am J Orthod Dentofacial Orthop*. 2009;**698**:e1–10; discussion 698–9.

78 Southard TE, Marshall SD, Allareddy V, Moreno Uribe LM, Holton NE. An evidence-based comparison of headgear and functional appliance therapy for the correction of Class II malocclusions. *Semin Orthod*. 2013;**19**:174–95.

79 Sloss EA, Southard KA, Qian F, Stock SE, Mann KR, Meyer DL, et al. Comparison of soft-tissue profiles after treatment with headgear or Herbst appliance. *Am J Orthod Dentofacial Orthop*. 2008;**133**:509–14.

80 Franchi L, Alvetro L, Giuntini V, Masucci C, Defraia E, Baccetti T. Effectiveness of comprehensive fixed appliance treatment used with the Forsus Fatigue Resistant Device in Class II patients. *Angle Orthod*. 2011;**81**:678–83.

81 Heinig N, Goz G. Clinical application and effects of the Forsus spring. A study of a new Herbst hybrid. *J Orofac Orthop*. 2001;**62**:436–50.

82 Janson G, Sathler R, Fernandes TM, Branco NC, Freitas MR. Correction of Class II malocclusion with Class II elastics: a systematic review. *Am J Orthod Dentofacial Orthop*. 2013;**143**:383–92.

83 Rebellato J, Lindauer SJ, Rubenstein LK, Isaacson RJ, Davidovitch M, Vroom K. Lower arch perimeter preservation using the lingual arch. *Am J Orthod Dentofacial Orthop*. 1997;**112**:449–56.

84 Viglianisi A. Effects of lingual arch used as space maintainer on mandibular arch dimension: a systematic review. *Am J Orthod Dentofacial Orthop*. 2010;**138**:382e1–4; discussion 382–3.

85 Moyers RE, van der Linden FPGM, Riolo ML, McNamara JA. *Standards of human occlusal development*. Ann Arbor, MI: Center for Human Growth and Development, University of Michigan; 1976. 371 p.

86 Villalobos FJ, Sinha PK, Nanda RS. Longitudinal assessment of vertical and sagittal control in the mandibular arch by the mandibular fixed lingual arch. *Am J Orthod Dentofacial Orthop*. 2000;**118**:366–70.

87 Moore T, Southard KA, Casko JS, Qian F, Southard TE. Buccal corridors and smile esthetics. *Am J Orthod Dentofacial Orthop*. 2005;**127**:208–13.

88 Isaacson RJ, Lindauer SJ, Rubenstein, LK. Moments with the edgewise appliance: incisor torque control. *Am J Orthod Dentofacial Orthop*. 1993;**103**:428–38.

89 Little RM. Stability and relapse of mandibular anterior alignment: University of Washington studies. *Semin Orthod*. 1999;**5**:191–204.

90 Adkins MD, Nanda RS, Currier GF. Arch perimeter changes on rapid palatal expansion. *Am J Orthod Dentofacial Orthop*. 1990;**97**:194–9.

91 Ostler MS, Kokich VG. Alveolar ridge changes in patients congenitally missing mandibular second premolars. *J Prosthet Dent*. 1994;**71**:144–9.

92 Sletten DW, Smith BM, Southard KA, Casko JS, Southard TE. Retained deciduous mandibular molars in adults: a radiographic study of long-term changes. *Am J Orthod Dentofacial Orthop*. 2003;**124**:625–30.

93 Rajic S, Muretic Z, Percac S. Impacted canine in a prehistoric skull. *Angle Orthod*. 1996;**66**:477–80.

94 Grover PS, Lorton L. The incidence of unerupted permanent teeth and related clinical cases. *Oral Surg Oral Med Oral Pathol*. 1985;**9**:420–5.

95 Chu FC, Li TK, Lui VK, Newsome PR, Chow RL, Cheung LK. Prevalence of impacted teeth and associated pathologies—a radiographic study of the Hong Kong Chinese population. *Hong Kong Med J*. 2003;**9**:158–63.

96 Rohrer A. Displaced and impacted canines. *Int J Orthod Oral Surg Radiogr*. 1929;**15**:1003–20.

97 Aydin U, Yilmaz HH, Yildirim D. Incidence of canine impaction and transmigration in a patient population. *Dentomaxillofac Radiol*. 2004;**33**:164–9.

98 Yavuz MS, Aras MH, Buyukkurt MC, Tozoglu S. Impacted mandibular canines. *J Contemp Dent Pract*. 2007;**8**:78–85.

99 Woloshyn H, Årtun J, Kennedy DB, Joondeph DR. Pulpal and periodontal reactions to orthodontic alignment of palatally impacted canines. *Angle Orthod*. 1994;**64**:257–64.

100 Melsen B. Effects of cervical anchorage during and after treatment: an implant study. *Am J Orthod*. 1978;**73**:526–40.

101 O'Brien K. Is early treatment for Class II malocclusions effective? Results from a randomized controlled trial. *Am J Orthod Dentofacial Orthop*. 2006;**129**:S64–5.

102 O'Brien K, Wright J, Conboy F, Appelbe P, Davies L, Connolly I, et al. Early treatment for Class II division 1 malocclusion with the Twin-block appliance: a multi-center, randomized, controlled trial. *Am J Orthod Dentofacial Orthop*. 2009;**135**:573–9.

103 Mann KR, Marshall SD, Qian F, Southard KA, Southard TE. Effect of maxillary anteroposterior position on profile esthetics in headgear-treated patients. *Am J Orthod Dentofacial Orthop*. 2011;**139**:228–34.

CHAPTER 3

Skeletal Deep Bites

Introduction

Haley (Figure 3.1) is 13 years 4 months old and presents to you with the CC, "I want to fix my front teeth. These ones (pointing to her maxillary lateral incisors) go behind the front ones." PMH includes headaches. Her periodontal tissues are healthy, and centric relation = centric occlusion (CR=CO).

Q: What features would lead you to classify her as a dental deep bite? A skeletal deep bite?

A: *Dental* deep bite features: OB 70% (Figure 3.1h) partially due to stepped down maxillary incisors (overerupted relative to posterior teeth, Figures 3.1h and 3.1l) and stepped up mandibular incisors (overerupted relative to posterior teeth, curve of Spee (COS) approximately 3 mm, Figure 3.1m). *Skeletal* deep bite features include overclosed appearance (everted mandibular lip, deep labiomental sulcus); short soft tissue LAFH (Subnasale–soft tissue Menton < soft tissue Glabella–Subnasale); minimally adequate posed smile incisal display (Figure 3.1b) despite the fact that Haley has stepped down maxillary incisors plus a short upper lip length (~14 mm in length, contrasted with a normal adolescent female length of 17–23 mm) [1]; and vertical skeletal deficiency (short skeletal LAFH/TAFH = 49%, Figure 3.1e), flat MPA (FMA = 20°, SNMP = 25°; and SN, FH, and MP nearly parallel.)

Q: What is "lip trapping," and how does it contribute to Haley's overclosed appearance?

A: Haley exhibits a redundancy of her lower facial soft tissue, especially eversion of her lower lip. This is primarily due to "lip trapping." Look at the lateral cephalometric radiograph (Figures 3.1d and e). Notice how, with her retrusive mandible, the lower lip curls under the maxillary incisors. This is "lip trapping," and it forces her lower lip down, everting the lip and creating a deep labiomental sulcus (overclosed appearance).

Q: Does Haley exhibit adequate incisal display when relaxed (~2 mm, Figure 3.2a) and in a posed smile (Figure 3.2b)? Why or why not?

A: No. Although Haley presents with approximately 2 mm of incisal display at rest, an ideal amount of incisal display at rest for an adolescent female would be 3–4 mm, and in a young woman, 3 mm [2–4]. In addition, her maxillary incisors are stepped down relative to her maxillary posterior teeth (Figure 3.1l), a feature leading us to expect her to exhibit excess incisal display. We conclude that *her incisal display at rest is inadequate*. Ideally, when Haley smiles, the maxillary lip vermillion border should be congruent with her maxillary central incisor gingival margins [5]. Instead, her maxillary lip vermillion is incisal to her maxillary incisor gingival margins. *She exhibits inadequate incisal display in a posed smile.* Factors that typically contribute to inadequate incisal display at rest and in a posed smile include inadequate vertical maxillary skeletal growth, a long maxillary lip, stepped up maxillary incisors, and hypoactivity of (smiling) facial muscles. Of these factors, Haley demonstrates inadequate vertical maxillary skeletal growth and is probably demonstrating hypoactivity of her smiling musculature (lack of effort in smiling, not uncommon for someone who is self-conscious of her smile).

Q: How likely are skeletal deep bite patients to complain of an overclosed facial appearance?

A: Not likely (clinical opinion). In contrast to skeletal open bite patients (who often express concerns about their excessive incisal/gingival display and inability to achieve lip competence), our clinical impression is that skeletal deep bite patients rarely express concern about their short LAFH. Instead, they will often express concern regarding dental features: excess depth of their bite, mandibular incisor palatal impingement, and so on.

Q: Haley asks if her headaches are related to her deep bite. You ask her to describe the headaches more fully (history, frequency, severity, duration, precipitating factors). She states that she has had headaches for years, they occur on only one side of her head, and can be severe. She often sees flashing lights before she gets a headache, feels sick to her stomach, and she usually has to lie down when she gets them. She gets them about once every couple of months. What is your tentative diagnosis?

A: Migraine headaches. Migraines are typically unilateral, pulsating, and associated with nausea, vomiting, photophobia, or phonophobia. The pain can be aggravated by physical activity. Up to one-third of patients with migraine headaches perceive an aura: a transient visual, sensory, language, or motor disturbance, which signals that the headache will soon occur [6].

Q: What is the cause of migraine headaches?

A: The exact mechanisms of migraines are not known. They are considered to be a neurovascular disorder [7]. The primary theory is related to increased excitability of the cerebral cortex and abnormal control of pain neurons in the trigeminal nucleus of the brainstem [8].

Orthodontics in the Vertical Dimension: A Case-Based Review, First Edition. Thomas E. Southard, Steven D. Marshall and Laura L. Bonner.

Q: What is the recommended management of migraines?

A: Initial recommended management is with simple analgesics (e.g., ibuprofen and acetaminophen) for the headache, an antiemetic for the nausea, and avoidance of triggers. Other agents may be used by those for whom simple analgesics are not effective.

Q: List other neurovascular disorders.

A: cluster headache, cranial arteritis, and carotidynia [9].

Q: Are Haley's migraines related to her deep bite?

A: Although chronic TMD patients have been found to have psychosocial and behavioral characteristics similar to patients with lower back pain and headaches, *the literature and scientific studies do not support the role, in general, of malocclusion as a primary etiologic factor in TMD and headaches* [10–14]. Haley's migraines are of neurovascular origin and unrelated to her deep bite.

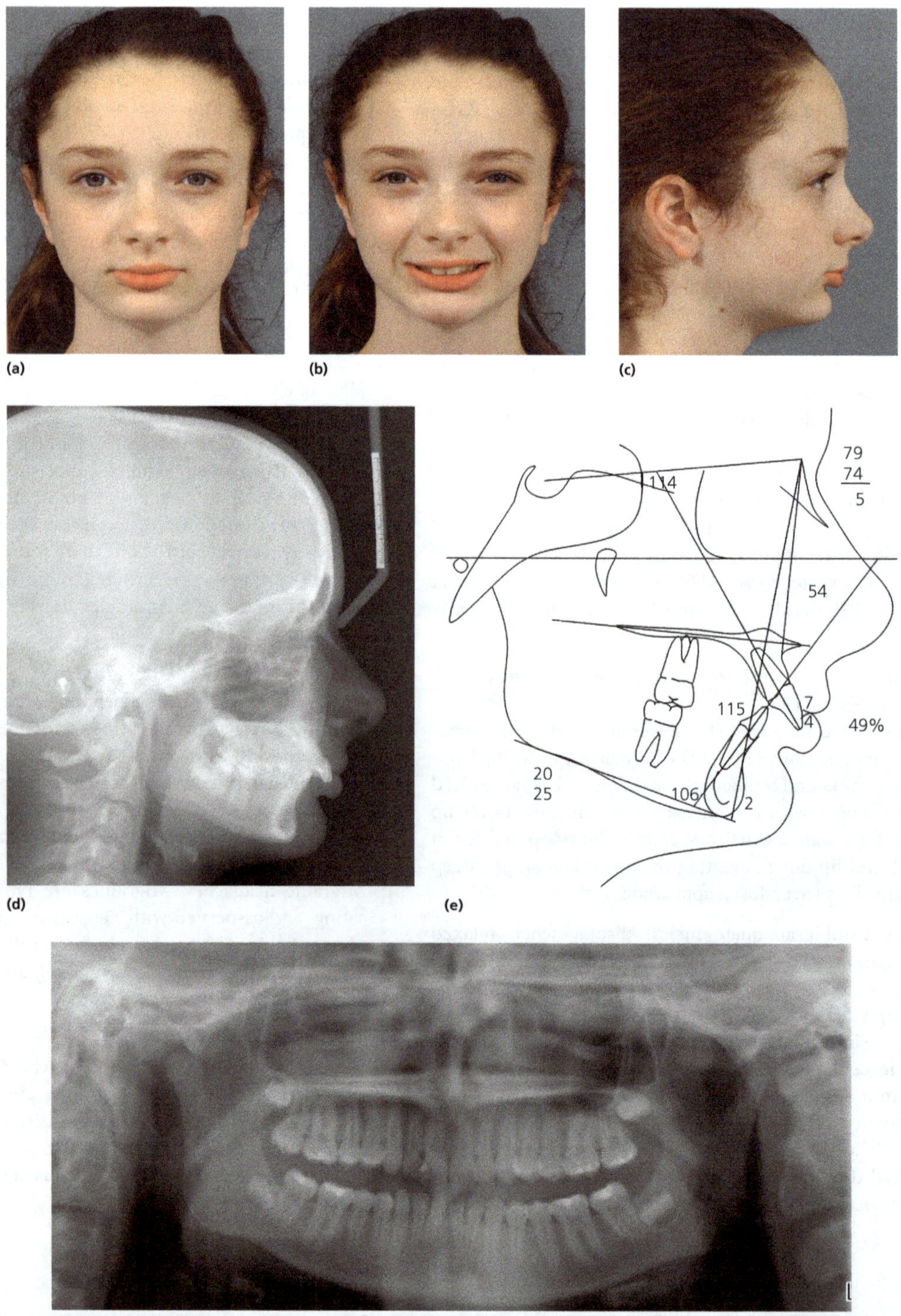

Figure 3.1 Initial records of Haley: (a–c) initial facial photographs, (d) lateral cephalograph, (e) cephalometric tracing, (f) pantomograph,

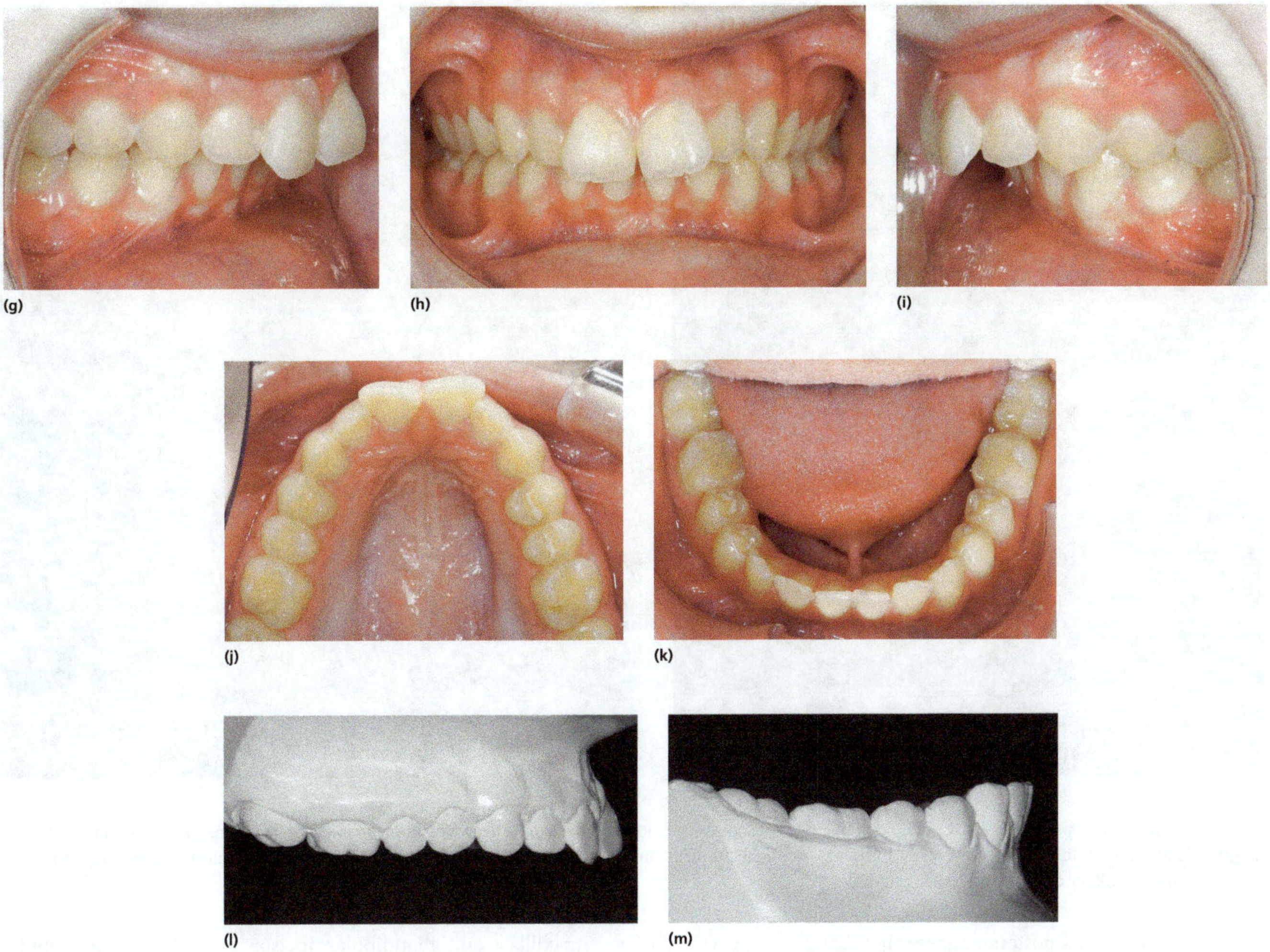

Figure 3.1 (Continued) (g–k) intraoral photographs, and (l–m) right buccal view of maxillary and mandibular models.

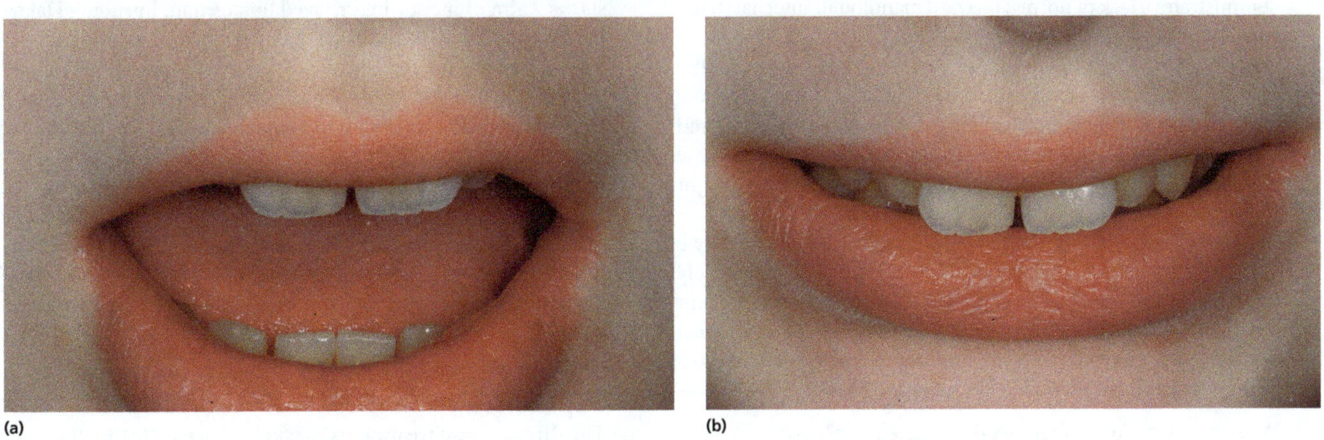

Figure 3.2 Close-up of Haley's maxillary incisal display with (a) lip relaxed and (b) in a posed smile.

Q: Does Haley have a skeletal deep bite, a dental deep bite, or a combination of both?

A: Haley has a *combination* of skeletal and dental deep bite. Skeletally, she has a short lower anterior face height with a resulting overclosed appearance. Dentally, she has excessive OB (70%) partially resulting from stepped down maxillary incisors and stepped up mandibular incisors.

Q: Contrast the etiology of a skeletal open bite (long face) to the etiology of a skeletal deep bite (short face) like Haley's.

A: Vertical growth of the lower anterior face depends on a number of variables: magnitude and direction of condylar growth, vertical descent of the maxillary corpus, maxillary/mandibular bony surface apposition/resorption, and maxillary/mandibular molar eruption [15–21]. In a *skeletal anterior open bite growth pattern*:

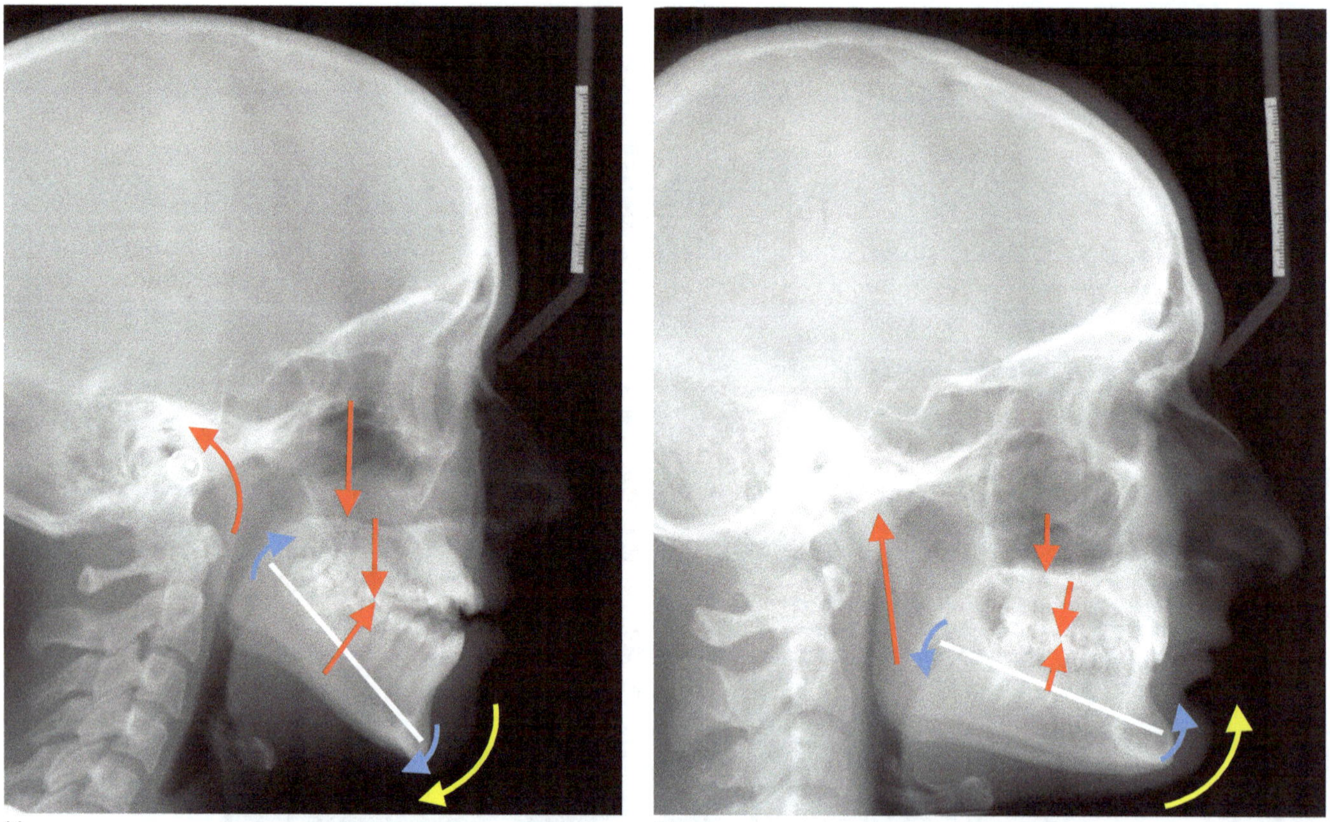

(a) (b)

Figure 3.3 The growth pattern of (a) skeletal open bite patients contrasts with (b) the skeletal growth pattern of skeletal deep bite patients in terms of magnitude and direction of condylar growth, maxillary, and mandibular bony surface apposition/resorption (mandibular internal/true rotation), vertical descent of the maxillary corpus, and molar eruption.

the condyle grows posterior-superiorly (Figure 3.3a, curved red arrow); a reference line (white line), drawn from the anterior contour of the chin to the contour of the mandibular canal [19], demonstrates a lack of normal forward mandibular internal (true) rotation or even a backward internal (true) rotation (curved blue arrows); there is a lack of posterior face height development; the maxilla descends more than normal (palatal plane may rotate down posteriorly); and molars often erupt more than normal (red arrows). As the mandible rotates backward (yellow arrow), the mandibular plane angle steepens, the anterior face height increases, and an anterior open bite results.

In a *skeletal deep bite growth pattern* (Figure 3.3b), the condyle grows more vertically, the mandible rotates forward excessively (internally) the maxilla descends less, and molars often erupt less than normal. As the mandible rotates upward and forward (yellow line), a deep bite results from increased vertical overlap of the incisors.

Q: What is the etiology of Haley's dental deep bite?

A: Her maxillary and mandibular anterior teeth have overerupted, probably due to the fact that she has a retrusive mandible and the incisors continued to erupt without contacting the opposing dentition.

Q: What treatment would you consider for Haley's *dental* deep-bite component?

A: You would treat her dental deep bite (overeruption of maxillary and mandibular incisors, deep COS) in the same way you would treat dental deep bites in patients with normal vertical facial dimensions: maxillary and mandibular incisor intrusion [22], maxillary and mandibular incisor proclination, mandibular premolar eruption [23], and mandibular molar eruption as molars tip back/upright during COS leveling. But remember, Haley only shows 2 mm of incisor in a relaxed lip position. Intruding Haley's maxillary incisors as you level and align her maxillary arch will likely eliminate any maxillary incisal display—giving her an aged appearance. We will need to level Haley's maxillary arch. But, if we must intrude incisors more to open her bite, then intrude her mandibular incisors, if you have a choice. Why? Maintaining any maxillary incisor display will help her esthetic outcome. An additional point—the only one of the above treatment effects that could possibly benefit her vertical dimension would be mandibular posterior tooth eruption (rotating her mandible down and back/ increasing her LAFH). But the cost of mandibular rotation down and back is—a worsening of her Class II relationship.

Q: What *general* treatments would you consider for Haley's *skeletal* deep bite component?

A: The three general treatments for skeletal deep bites are the same as for any apical base discrepancy—whether in the vertical, transverse, or anteroposterior dimension: orthopedics, camouflage/masking, or surgery.

Q: Describe principles for treating skeletal deep bites with orthopedics.

A: Orthopedic skeletal deep bite treatment consists of (Figure 3.4) enhancing downward maxillary corpus growth, increasing maxillary molar eruption, and increasing mandibular molar eruption—all of which tend to lengthen the lower anterior face height, increase the mandibular plane angle, open the deep bite,

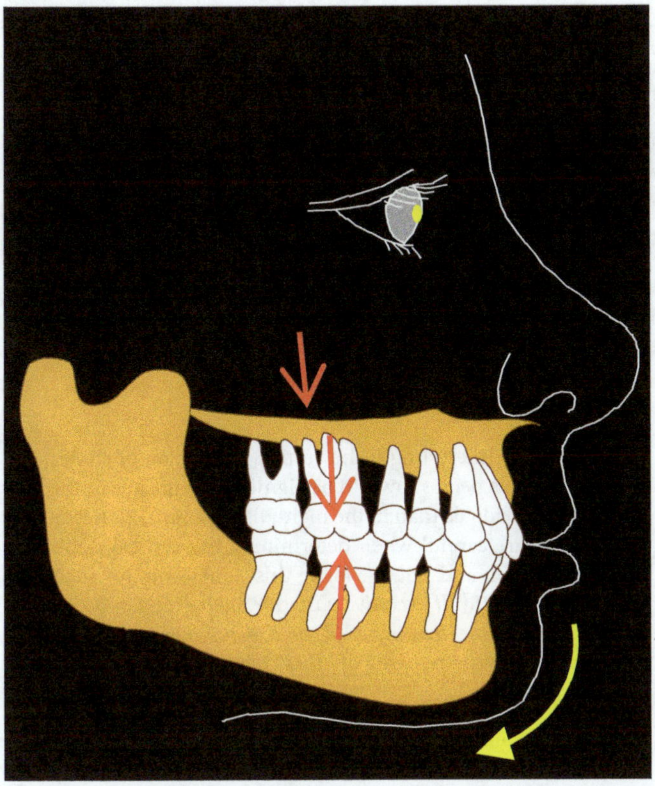

Figure 3.4 Orthopedic correction of a skeletal deep bite is aimed at enhancing maxillary corpus downward growth and molar eruption—resulting in downward/backward mandibular rotation, increased LAFH, and bite opening.

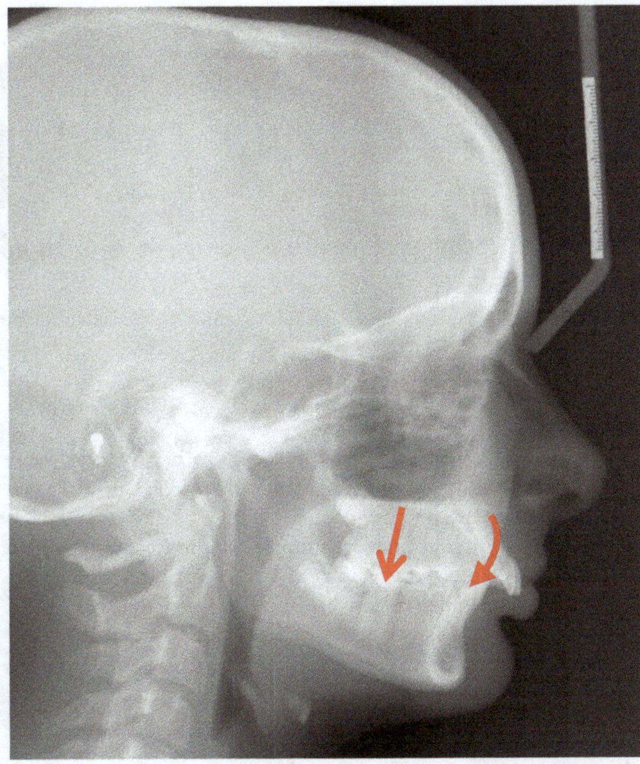

Figure 3.5 Cervical-pull headgears tend to rotate the anterior palatal plane downward and backward, increasing LAFH and gingival display, plus erupting maxillary first molars slightly (less than 1 mm, on average).

eliminate lip redundancy, and eliminate an overclosed appearance. The mandible will tend to rotate down and back (yellow line)—worsening a Class II molar relationships but improving a Class III molar relationship. Of course, unfavorable vertical condyle growth, or excessive forward mandibular internal (true) rotation, can oppose these efforts.

Q: Exhaustively list and discuss orthopedic appliances/techniques to potentially increase downward maxillary growth, increase maxillary molar eruption, and/or increase mandibular molar eruption during adolescence—to increase lower anterior face height and correct skeletal deep bites.

A: Appliances/techniques include the following:

- Cervical-pull headgears during Class II correction. CPHG's rotate the anterior palatal plane downward and backward (Figure 3.5) [24, 25], potentially increasing lower anterior facial height and gingival display. In addition to restricting forward maxillary growth and retracting maxillary first molars, cervical pull headgears also erupt maxillary first molars, although by less than 1 mm, on average. Using Björk-type implants in cervical headgear patients, Melsen [26] identified this downward and backward maxillary rotation, and a similar indirect effect on the mandible. However, the skeletal headgear effect appeared to be temporary. Studies have reported that the effects of cervical pull (Kloehn) headgears range from a slight increase in vertical when measured at Menton [27], and a slight increase in the SN–MP angle [28], to no increase in the MPA [29–31]. *The question of whether cervical traction causes a clinically significant change in vertical facial proportions remains equivocal* [32].
- Headgears with biteplates. Studies have reported headgear/biteplate treatment effects to range from a slight increase in mandibular plane angle (1.3°) [31] to nonsignificant changes in the mandibular plane angle and LAFH [33]. We consider these findings equivocal.
- Straight-pull headgear. One study reported a slight increase in SN–MP angle (1°) [28]. We consider this finding equivocal.
- Activators/bionators during Class II correction. The reported effects range from a slight vertical increase when measured at Menton [27], to nonsignificant changes in the mandibular plane angle and LAFH [31, 33]. We consider these vertical effects equivocal.
- The Frankel regulator (FR-II). One study reported a slight decrease in the SN–MP angle (decrease of 0.6°) [28]. We consider this result equivocal.
- Leveling the COS. Mandibular premolars are erupted [23] (alveolar process bone is grown) as the COS is leveled. Likewise, mandibular molars are tipped distally and erupted. Eruption of posterior teeth can potentially increase the vertical facial dimension.
- Anterior bite plates (Figure 3.6a–c). Bite plates disclude posterior teeth, which assist leveling the COS/erupting posterior teeth by eliminating occlusal forces.
- Anterior bite plates used in conjunction with posterior vertical elastics can accelerate posterior tooth eruption (alveolar bone growth), potentially increasing the vertical facial dimension.

In summary, the above treatments may help to increase the LAFH in adolescent skeletal deep bite patients. However, even with aggressive treatment, increasing the LAFH in short face patients can be challenging.

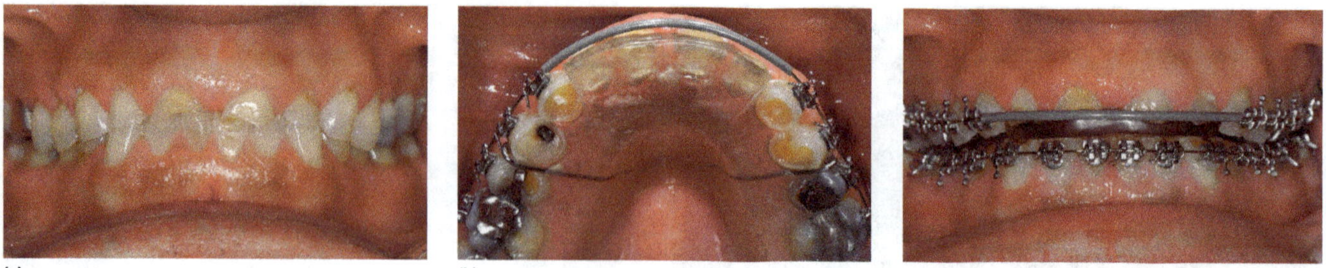

(a) (b) (c)

Figure 3.6 (a–c) By separating posterior teeth slightly, anterior biteplates remove posterior occlusal forces and assist in the eruption of posterior teeth during curve of Spee leveling.

Q: How can the patient's mandibular growth, in a favorable direction and magnitude, improve LAFH/TAFH in a skeletal deep bite patient?

A: Look at the initial and deband cephalometric tracings of a skeletal deep bite patient, Vaughn, shown in Figure 3.7a and b. Treatment included a cervical-pull headgear. Because of his significant condylar posterior–superior growth, normal mandibular internal (true) rotation (Figure 3.7c), and significant molar eruption, Vaughn achieved both AP correction and an improvement in his LAFH/TAFH—from 53 to 55%. This was despite mandibular incisor eruption. Likewise, Margaret, a skeletal deep bite patient treated with an LSU activator and bionator (Figure 3.7d), underwent significant condylar posterior–superior growth, normal mandibular internal (true) rotation, and mandibular molar eruption—increasing her LAFH/TAFH, dramatically. In both patients, mandibular growth resulted in LAFH increasing more than midface height. *Favorable mandibular growth can play a major role in improving LAFH in skeletal deep bite adolescent patients. Likewise, unfavorable mandibular growth can play a major role in worsening LAFH in skeletal deep bite patients.*

Q: Is there a potential problem with erupting posterior teeth to increase LAFH?

A: Yes, there can be a problem. Whereas the eruption of posterior teeth may be the treatment of choice in growing patients, if one wishes to increase lower face height, steepen the mandibular plane, correct lip redundancy, and/or increase facial convexity, the *stability* of erupting posterior teeth has been questioned [34].

Q: What is probably the limiting factor in erupting posterior teeth during orthopedic correction of skeletal deep bites?

A: Stretching of the masseter muscles, medial pterygoid muscles, temporalis muscles, and other facial soft tissues is probably the limiting factor. We do not fully understand how vertical growth of the facial bones and musculature is controlled, but we can speculate that there is probably a limit as to how far these tissues can be stretched with forced posterior tooth eruption. At the physiologic resting length, the muscle is capable of exerting maximal force and maximal velocity under isometric and isotonic conditions. This ability is explained by the sliding filament theory of muscle contraction which postulates that the maximal availability of cross-bridge reactive sites is present at a muscle's physiologic resting length [35]. When the mandible is in its physiologic rest position, the interocclusal distance, or separation, between the occlusal surfaces of the teeth is termed the "freeway" space, which has been reported to range from 2 to 7 mm [36]. Interestingly, the vertical dimension of clinical rest position has been shown to be significantly greater in the low-angle individuals than in the high-angle group [37]. Restorative dentists are careful when determining the vertical dimension of occlusion, and not to violate this dimension, for successful prostheses [38]. *If excessive posterior tooth eruption occurs during orthodontic treatment (beyond what the musculature can tolerate), then relapse of this tooth eruption should be anticipated.*

Q: You are considering treating an adolescent skeletal deep bite patient orthopedically. What two factors could persuade you to attempt orthopedic treatment or should dissuade you from attempting orthopedic treatment?

A: The two factors are *magnitude* of the skeletal discrepancy and *time* of remaining potential growth. If the patient has a mild (borderline) skeletal deep bite and many years of anticipated growth, then you could attempt orthopedic treatment. If the patient has a very severe skeletal deep bite with little future anticipated growth, then it would be heroic to attempt orthopedic correction. In this latter situation, if the short facial height is a concern of the patient's, then surgery to increase the facial height should be considered.

Q: Is Haley a good candidate for orthopedic treatment?

A: No. On the one hand, the magnitude of Haley's vertical problem is moderate. She has a short LAFH, but it is not severe. She has an overclosed appearance but this is due, in part, to her lip trapping. On the other hand, she is 13 years and 4 months old. You inquire and discover that she reached menarche when she turned age 12. Remember, for girls the peak rate of stature increase is reached *prior* to menarche [39]. With the onset of menses, the rate of change in height drops to prepubertal levels and decreases sharply to an adult rate of change during the subsequent 2 years. So, we do not expect much more growth for Haley. Furthermore, Haley's anteroposterior apical base discrepancy (retrusive maxilla and mandible) is *severe*—so, orthopedics would be contraindicated to achieve correction in that dimension. At best, with the understanding that you are only trying to improve (not correct) her vertical and AP with orthopedics, you could attempt orthopedic treatment for a set period of time (6–9 months?) and then re-evaluate for either masking or surgery.

Q: What is masking (camouflage) of a skeletal deep bite?

A: Masking a skeletal deep bite is reduction/correction of the overbite without addressing the vertical apical base discrepancy

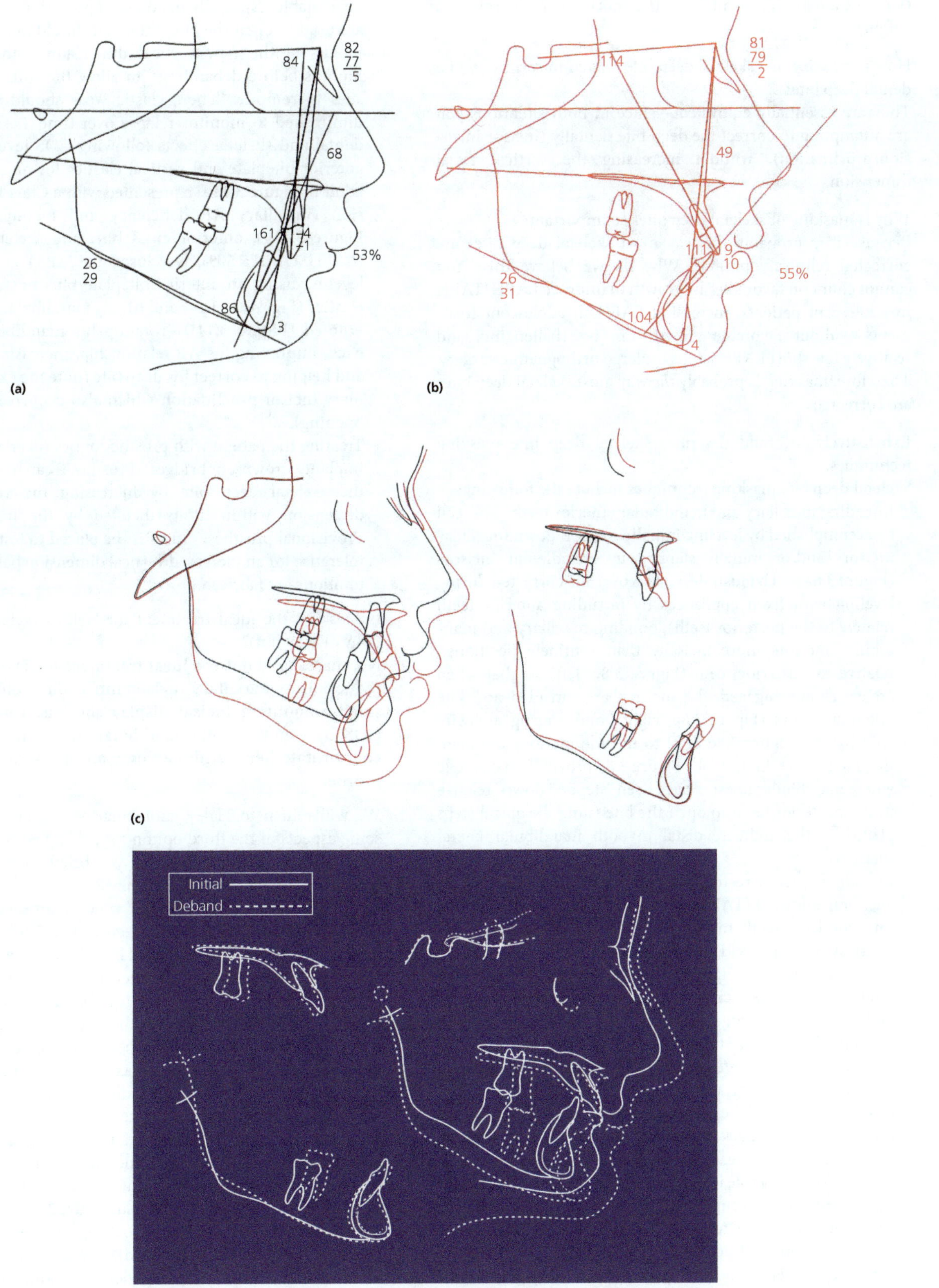

Figure 3.7 Favorable mandibular growth can improve LAFH/TAFH in skeletal deep bite patients: (a–c) Vaughn, a skeletal deep bite patient treated with a cervical-pull headgear and (d) Margaret, a skeletal deep bite patient treated with an LSU activator and bionator. Both had favorable mandibular growth with LAFH increasing more than midface height. Of course, unfavorable adolescent growth can worsen LAFH.

(without attempting to increase the short lower anterior face height).

Q: How is *masking* of a skeletal deep bite related to *correction* of a dental deep bite?

A: They are essentially equivalent—since in both situations you are attempting to correct the deep bite dentally (incisor intrusion/proclination), without increasing the vertical facial dimension.

Q: Why is masking of skeletal deep bites so important?

A: Because it is probably the way most skeletal deep bites are corrected (clinical opinion). Why do we believe this? You cannot count on favorable jaw growth to improve LAFH/TAFH in adolescent patients, increasing LAFH in adolescent treatments without favorable growth can be challenging, and relatively few short LAFH adults undergo orthognathic surgery. Therefore, masking is probably *the* way most skeletal deep bites are corrected.

Q: Exhaustively list (and describe) skeletal deep bite masking techniques.

A: Skeletal deep bite masking techniques include the following:

- Intruding maxillary and mandibular anterior teeth. This can be accomplished by leveling initially stepped down maxillary incisors and/or initially stepped up mandibular incisors (Figure 3.8a and b illustrate a 100% overbite corrected during leveling with fixed appliances by intruding anterior teeth relative to the posterior teeth); bonding maxillary and mandibular incisors more incisally than routinely positioned relative to posterior teeth (Figure 3.8c, left) so that when archwires are engaged, the incisors are intruded and bite opening occurs (Figure 3.8c, right); and placing archwire apical steps (Figure 3.8d, left) to intrude incisors and open the bite (Figure 3.8d, right). Figure 3.8e provides an example where mandibular incisors have been "stepped down" relative to the posterior teeth to open the bite (note the apical steps placed in the archwire distal to both mandibular lateral incisors).
- Intruding anterior teeth using clear aligners with temporary anchorage devices (TADs) for intrusion anchorage and buttons bonded directly to the clear aligners (Figure 3.9, photos courtesy of Dr. Laurel Leslie-Martin).
- Proclining incisors (Figure 3.10a) during alignment, which tends to rotate the incisors about their apicies (red crosses) and opens the bite (Figure 3.10b).
- Leveling the COS by eruption of mandibular premolars [23] or by distally tipping/erupting mandibular molars that are mesially tipped. Since alveolar process bone is grown during tooth eruption, and the LAFH can increase as the mandible is rotated down and back, it could be argued that this is orthopedic treatment (increasing the LAFH). Notes: the muscles of mastication play a role in determining how much mandibular posterior teeth can erupt during COS leveling; and, whereas eruption of posterior teeth may be helpful in some growing patients, eruption of posterior teeth may not be appropriate for every patient—and the stability of erupting posterior teeth has been questioned [34]. This is especially true for adult patients.
- Leveling the COS using anterior bite plates (or anterior biteplates together with posterior vertical elastics) to disclude posterior teeth. Again, eruption of posterior teeth may be unstable, especially in adults. If posterior vertical elastics are used to open the bite, then you should hold the erupted molars at the new vertical dimension with elastics for months before debanding—to allow the soft and hard tissues to remodel. Then, elastic wear should be gradually diminished to monitor relapse over time. Let's look at the dental and skeletal effects following COS leveling with an anterior biteplate and vertical elastics for one patient. The adult in Figure 3.11a–c presented with a Class III malocclusion (maxillary *AP* deficiency and mandibular excess, Figure 3.11g), anterior cross bite, and skeletal deep bite (LAFH/TAFH = 50%, overclosed, flat MPA). Following COS leveling using an anterior biteplate plus posterior vertical elastics (Figure 3.11d–f and h), his mandibular molars were erupted (Figure 3.11i)—rotating his mandible down and back, improving his AP relationship, increasing his LAFH, and helping to correct his deep bite (note the excessive maxillary incisor proclination which also occurred during bite opening).
- Treating the patient with prosthodontics (overlay prosthesis, implants, crowns, or bridges). Prostheses can be used to mask the skeletal deep bite by increasing the vertical facial dimension within limits dictated by the freeway space. Provisional prostheses can first be placed to test the patient's tolerance for an increased vertical dimension before final restorations are fabricated.

Q: Is masking the ideal treatment for Haley's skeletal deep bite (why or why not)?

A: No, masking is not the ideal treatment for Haley. Overbite reduction by maxillary incisor intrusion could reduce the small amount of incisal display she has. Correcting her COS by erupting her mandibular premolars and molars could rotate her mandible down and back, worsening her profile.

Q: We will return to Haley, momentarily. For now, let's review some aspects of the third option for dealing with skeletal deep bites, orthognathic surgery. Can you briefly describe the surgical correction of skeletal deep bites?

A: Unlike orthopedics—the goal of which is to increase vertical facial growth—or masking—the goal of which is to open the bite without addressing the short LAFH—the goal of surgery is to increase the vertical facial dimension by grafting bone to the maxilla. The Le Fort I osteotomy is the surgical procedure commonly used to do this. Look at the Class III skeletal deep bite patient in Figure 3.12a who has been prepared for surgery and who will undergo a Le Fort I maxillary downgraft osteotomy. During surgery, a horizontal maxillary bony cut is made above the palate and at a safe distance from the teeth root apices (Figure 3.12b). The nasal septum and lateral nasal walls are separated from the palate, and the maxilla is downfractured (Figure 3.12c). The exact amount of bone grafting material is interposed (and the maxilla fixated, Figure 3.12d) to provide an ideal vertical facial dimension, postsurgically. As the maxilla is downgrafted (moved downward), the mandible will rotate down and back around the condyles. Depending on the anteroposterior position of the mandible following this rotation, a mandibular advancement or setback osteotomy may be required to correctly relate the dental arches anteroposteriorly (note in this patient the maxilla was also advanced, as was the chin, Figure 3.12e).

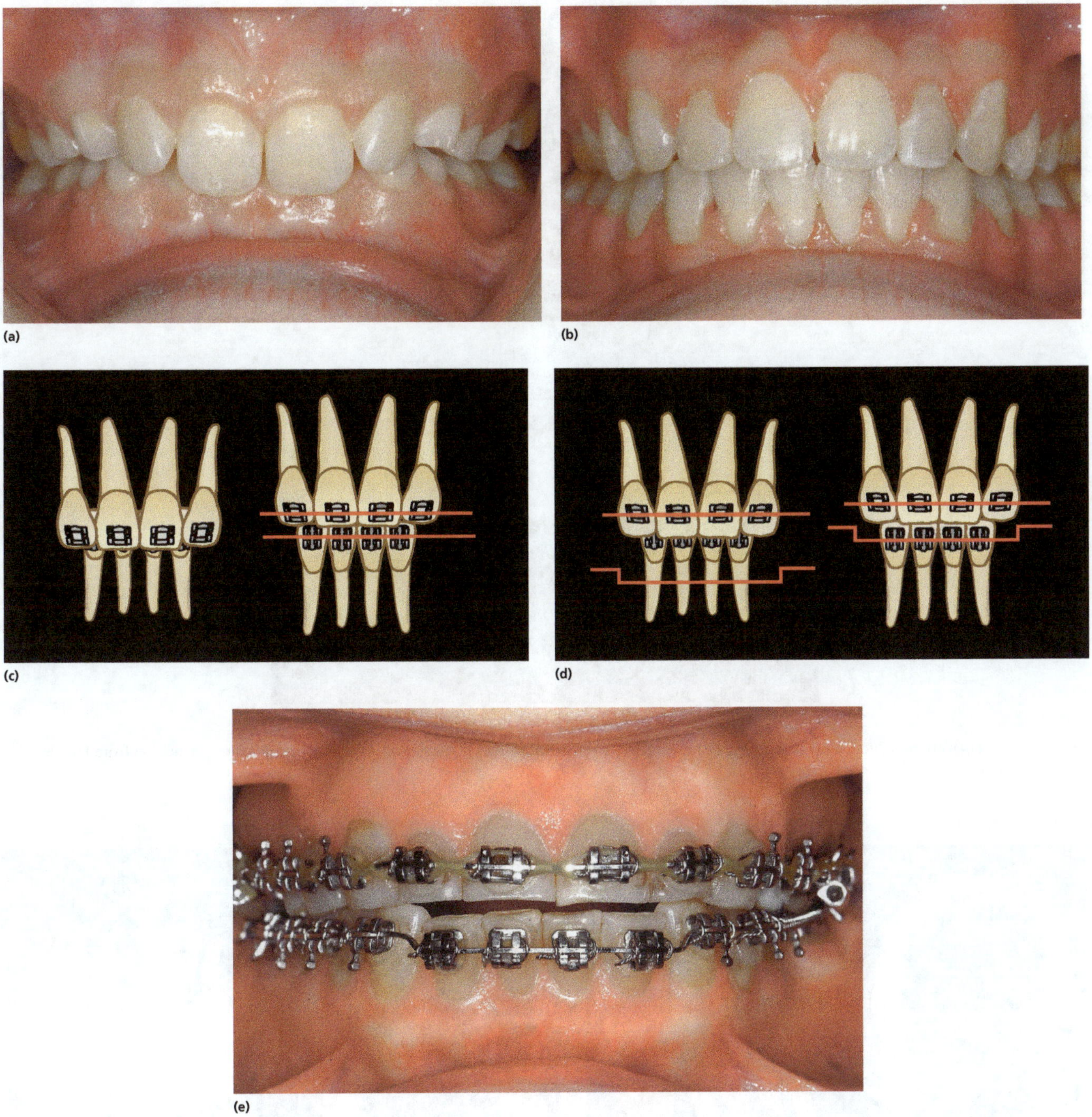

Figure 3.8 Masking a skeletal deep bite consists of reducing the overbite without addressing the short LAFH—and is therefore equivalent to dental deep bite correction. Overbite may be reduced by (a and b) intruding anterior teeth relative to posterior teeth using fixed orthodontic appliances and increasingly stiffer archwires; (c, left to right) using fixed appliances, enhancing this bite opening by bonding anterior teeth more incisally; or (d, left to right) enhancing this bite opening by placing "steps" in the archwire. (e) Example of mandibular incisors stepped down by placing archwire "steps" distal to the mandibular lateral incisors (to open the bite in preparation for maxillary incisor restorative treatment).

Q: Briefly describe another surgical procedure to treat mild adult skeletal deep bite patients who are also mandibular deficient.

A: If a patient has acceptable maxillary incisal display (following maxillary arch leveling), then a *tripod mandibular advancement* could be used to treat a mild LAFH deficiency in a patient who also presents with mandibular anteroposterior deficiency. In a tripod advancement, you do not level the COS prior to surgery (the mandibular arch is leveled *after* surgery) [40].

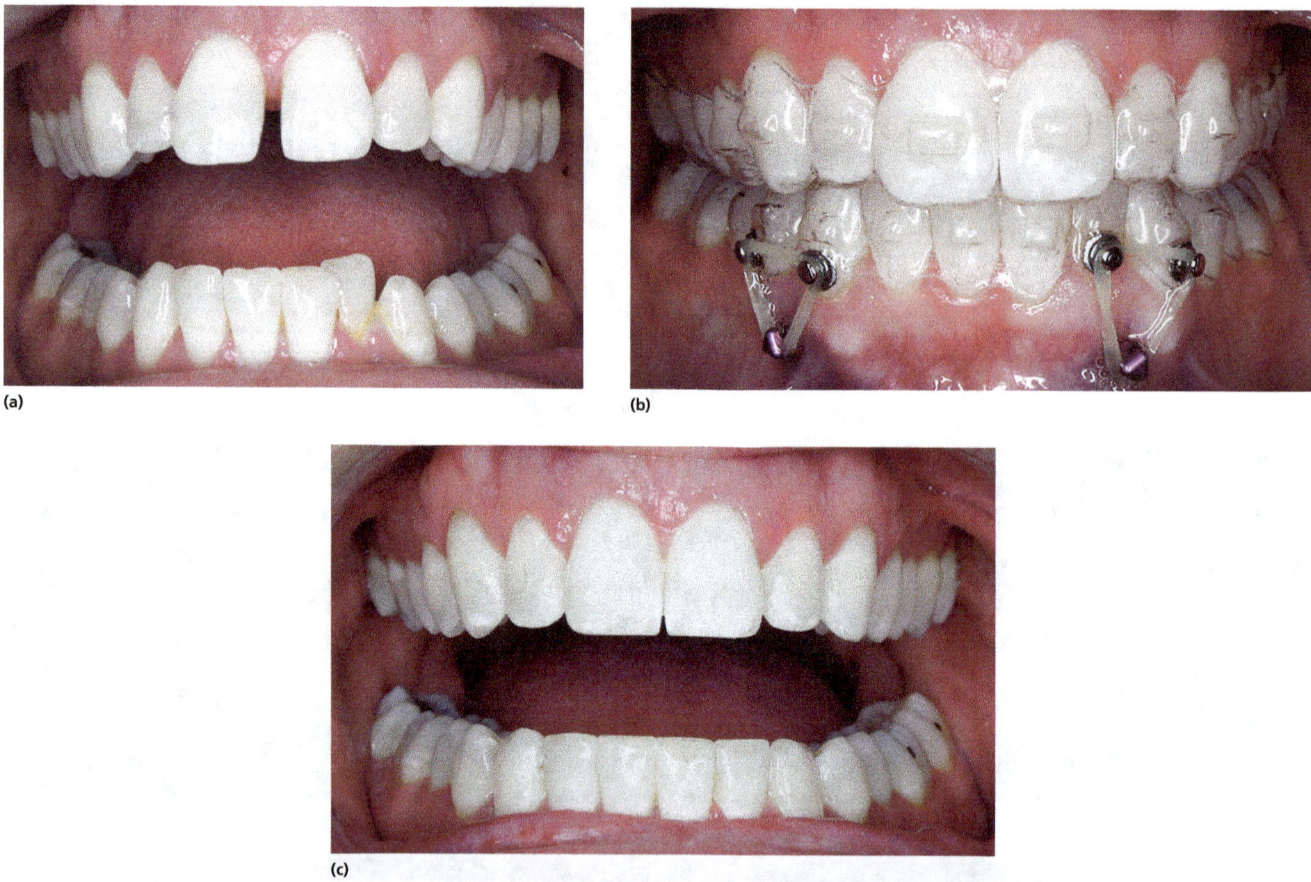

Figure 3.9 (a–c) Overbite reduction by intruding mandibular anterior teeth with clear aligners and TADs (Reproduced with permission from Dr. Laurel Leslie-Martin.).

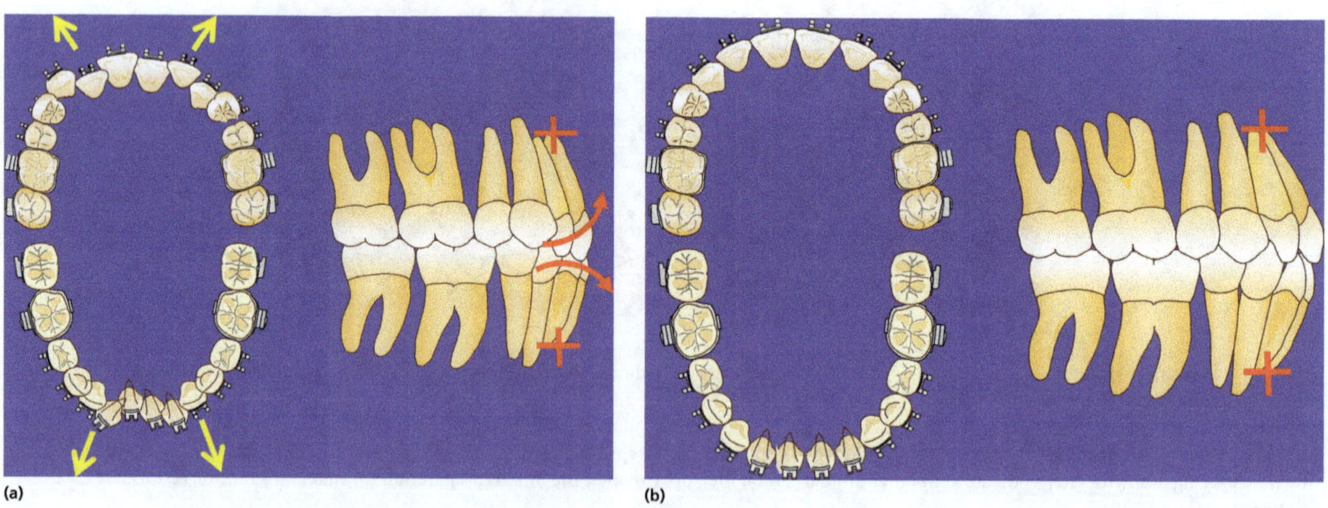

Figure 3.10 (a, b) Overbite reduction by proclination of anterior teeth during alignment.

As the mandible is lengthened during surgery (Figure 3.13, top left), the stepped up mandibular incisors "ride down" the lingual surfaces of the maxillary incisors (Figure 3.13, bottom), increasing LAFH. The advanced mandibular arch contacts the maxillary arch at three points only, the right and left second molars and incisors—hence the name, "tripod advancement" (Figure 3.13, top right).

Q: How much additional facial height does the tripod advancement give you?

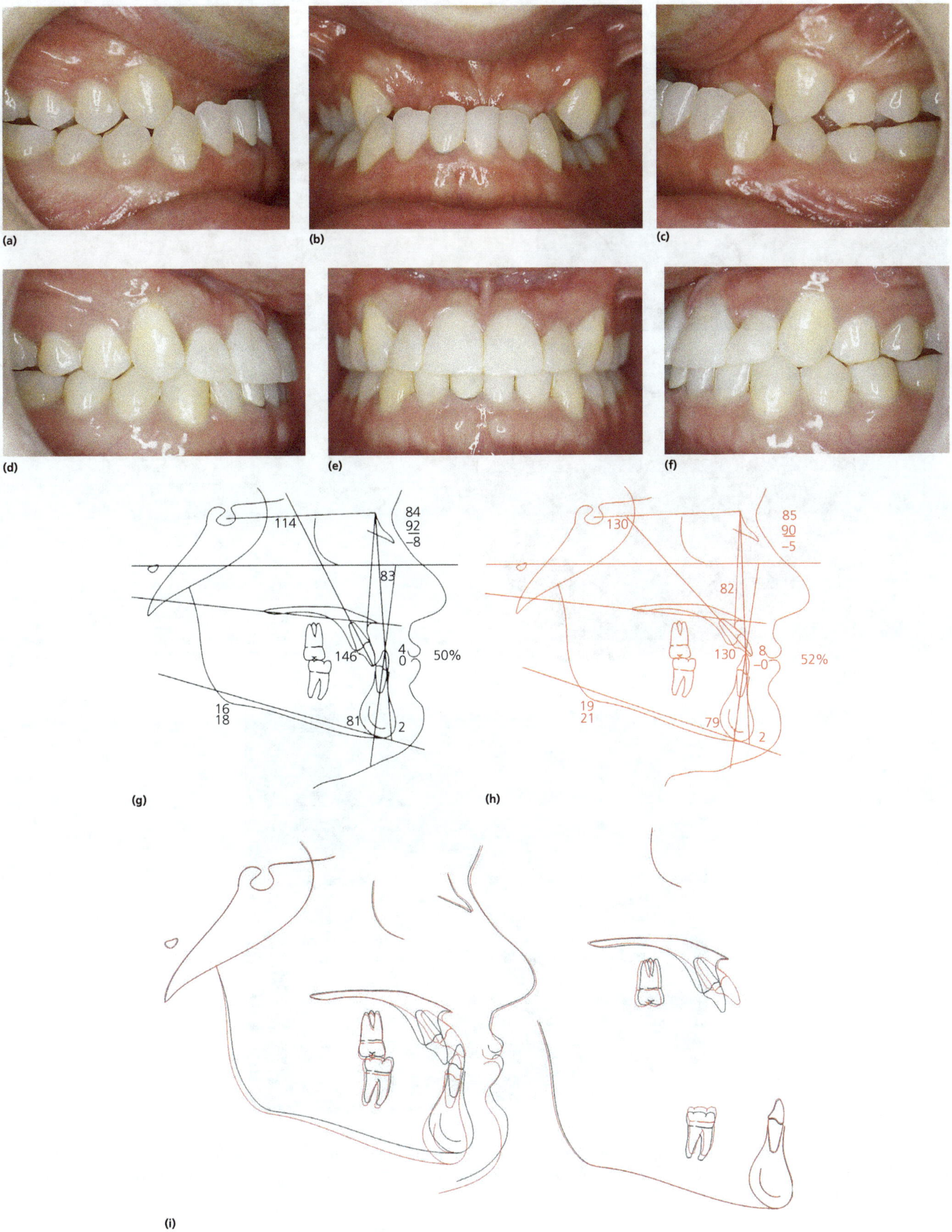

Figure 3.11 (a–i) Following curve of Spee leveling using an anterior biteplate plus posterior vertical elastics, this adult Class III patient's mandibular molars erupted, rotating the mandible down and back, improving his AP relationship, increasing his LAFH, and helping to correct his deep bite (under bite). Excessive maxillary incisor proclination also helped open his bite.

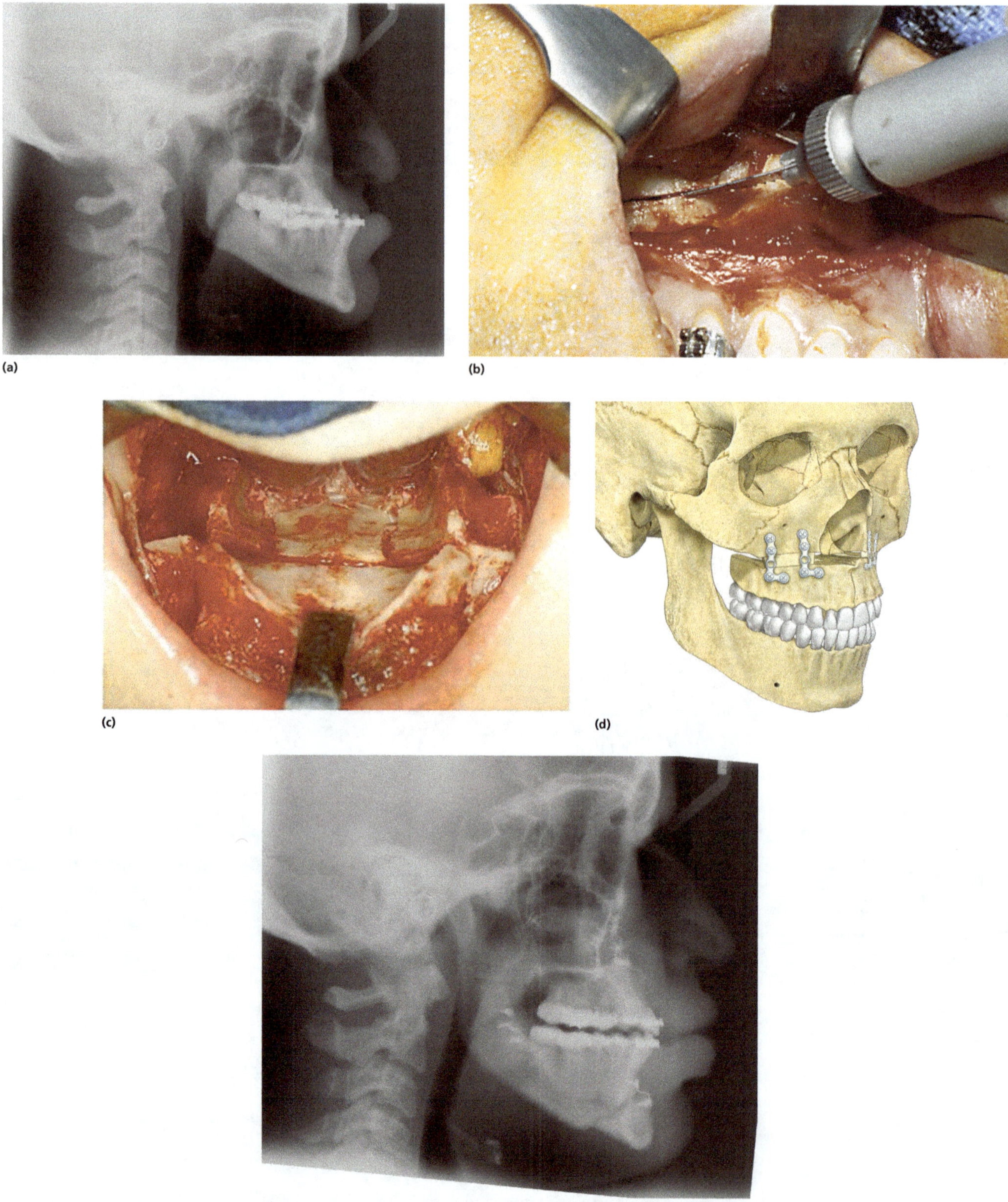

(a) (b) (c) (d) (e)

Figure 3.12 (a–e) The Le Fort I maxillary downgraft osteotomy is the surgical procedure traditionally used to treat vertically deficient LAFH (skeletal deep bite) patients. The patient illustrated here also underwent maxillary advancement, mandibular setback, and genioplasty advancment osteotomies.

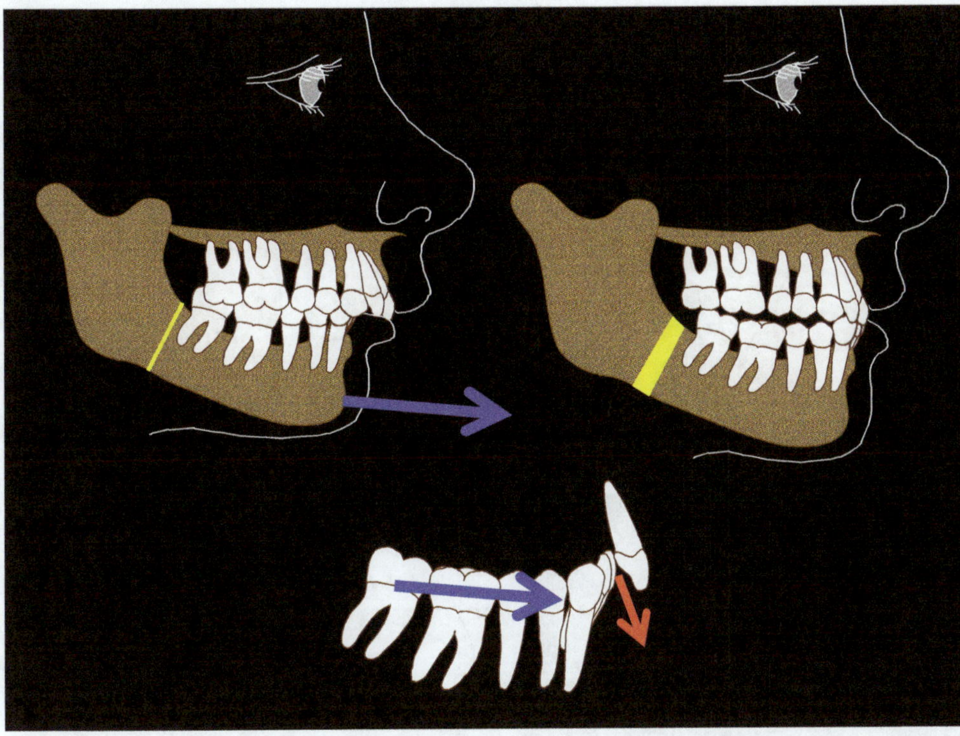

Figure 3.13 A tripod mandibular advancement (top left to top right) increases LAFH slightly as the mandible is advanced. It does this because the curve of Spee is *not* leveled before surgery. Therefore, the mandibular incisors are left stepped up (bottom), and they "ride down" the lingual surfaces of the maxillary incisors as the mandible is advanced—increasing the LAFH.

A: It gives you additional LAFH equal to the amount the mandibular incisors would have been intruded during leveling (a few millimeters).

Q: What is the goal of presurgical orthodontics?

A: Presurgical orthodontic treatment positions the teeth so that ideal facial balance and ideal occlusion can be achieved when the jaws are repositioned during surgery.

Q: What dental movements are typically performed during presurgical orthodontics?

A: The most frequent presurgical orthodontic movements aim to *reduce or eliminate dental compensations,* which resulted from growth abnormalities. For example, Michael (Figure 3.14) presents with concerns that his top teeth stick out and his chin sits back. Michael's maxilla and mandible are retrusive, he has a steep mandibular plane, his maxillary incisors are at a good angulation, and his mandibular incisors are very proclined (FMIA = 42°). His mandibular incisors erupted in a proclined angulation as compensation for the AP apical base discrepancy that developed between his maxilla and mandible. That is, during development, incisors erupt in the soft tissue trough between the lips/cheeks and tongue. If the mandible is deficient, then the tongue may tend to posture forward, maintaining a patent airway, while the maxillary lip may tend to pull back to maintain contact with the mandibular lip. This soft tissue positioning forces the mandibular incisors to procline and maxillary incisors to upright as they erupt. Presurgically, mandibular-deficient patients, such as Michael, usually need to have their mandibular incisors uprighted, and their maxillary incisors proclined, in order to create enough overjet to allow the mandibular advancement and fully seated Class I canines. Mandibular premolars may need to be extracted to create enough space to permit retraction/uprighting of mandibular incisors.

Q: If you are considering mandibular advancement surgery, you should take a photo with the patient postured forward until his/her canines are in a Class I relationship. When you juxtapose their initial profile image and their image postured forward, you are better able to judge whether this amount of surgical advancement will be adequate. For example, when Michael was shown his initial profile (Figure 3.15a) compared to his profile when postured forward into a Class I canine relationship (Figure 3.15b), he said he preferred his profile when postured forward but wanted an even stronger chin projection. Based on Michael's profile improvement when postured forward to Class I canines (Figure 3.15b), together with his lower incisor proclination (Figure 3.14e), and his mild mandibular anterior crowding, would you recommend presurgical *nonextraction* treatment for Michael or presurgical mandibular first premolar *extraction* treatment?

A: Although Michael's profile is indeed improved when postured forward into a Class I canine relationship, he still looks retrusive (Figure 3.15b). Michael could benefit from advancing his mandible even more than shown. If you extract mandibular first premolars, then you will have extraction space to upright his mandibular incisors (eliminating the incisor proclination and crowding) as you retract his mandibular canines distally. Extracting Michael's mandibular first premolars, and retracting

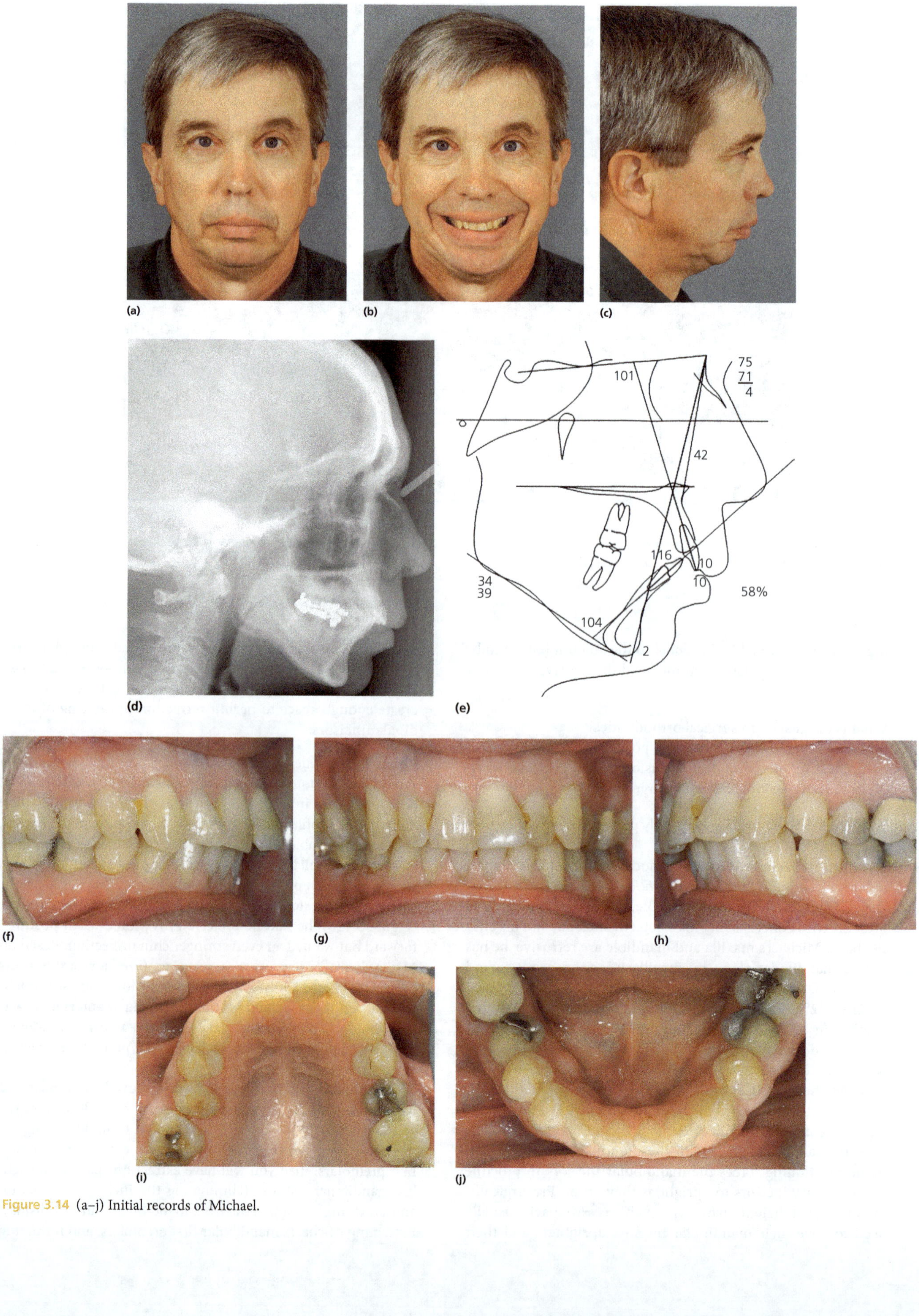

Figure 3.14 (a–j) Initial records of Michael.

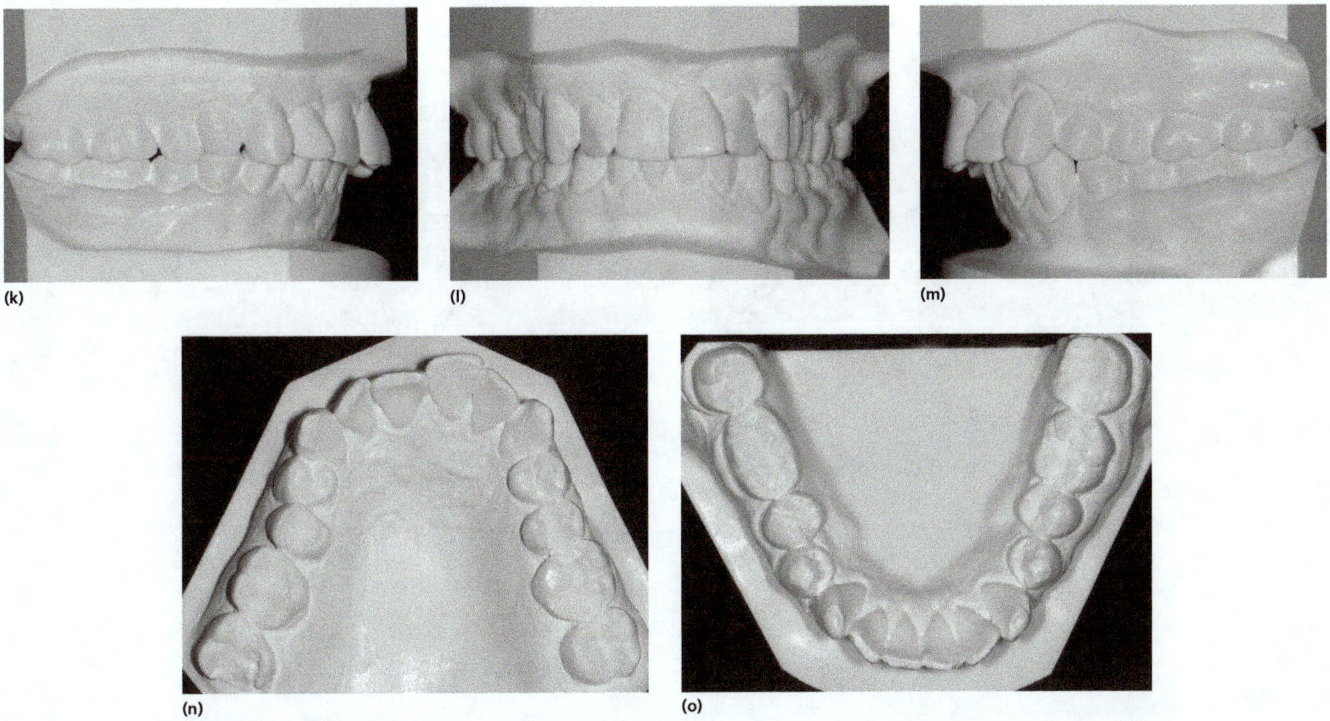

Figure 3.14 (Continued)

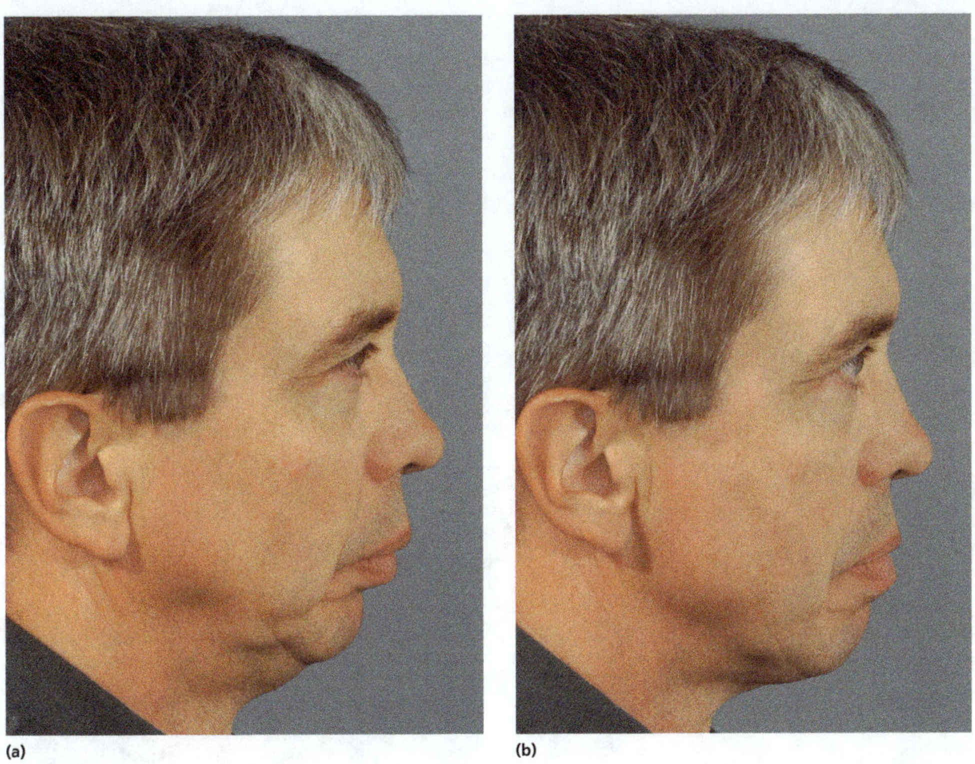

Figure 3.15 Profile photos of Michael: (a) initial and (b) postured forward into a Class I canine relationship.

his canines through the extraction space, will make Michael even more Class II at the canines and force the surgeon to give Michael an even greater mandibular advancement/stronger chin projection when the mandibular canines are brought forward, surgically, into a Class I relationship.

Q: Fixed orthodontic appliances were placed in Michael, maxillary and mandibular dental arches were leveled and aligned, mandibular first premolars were extracted, mandibular canines were retracted distally through the extraction spaces, and the mandibular incisors were retracted/uprighted (Figure 3.16).

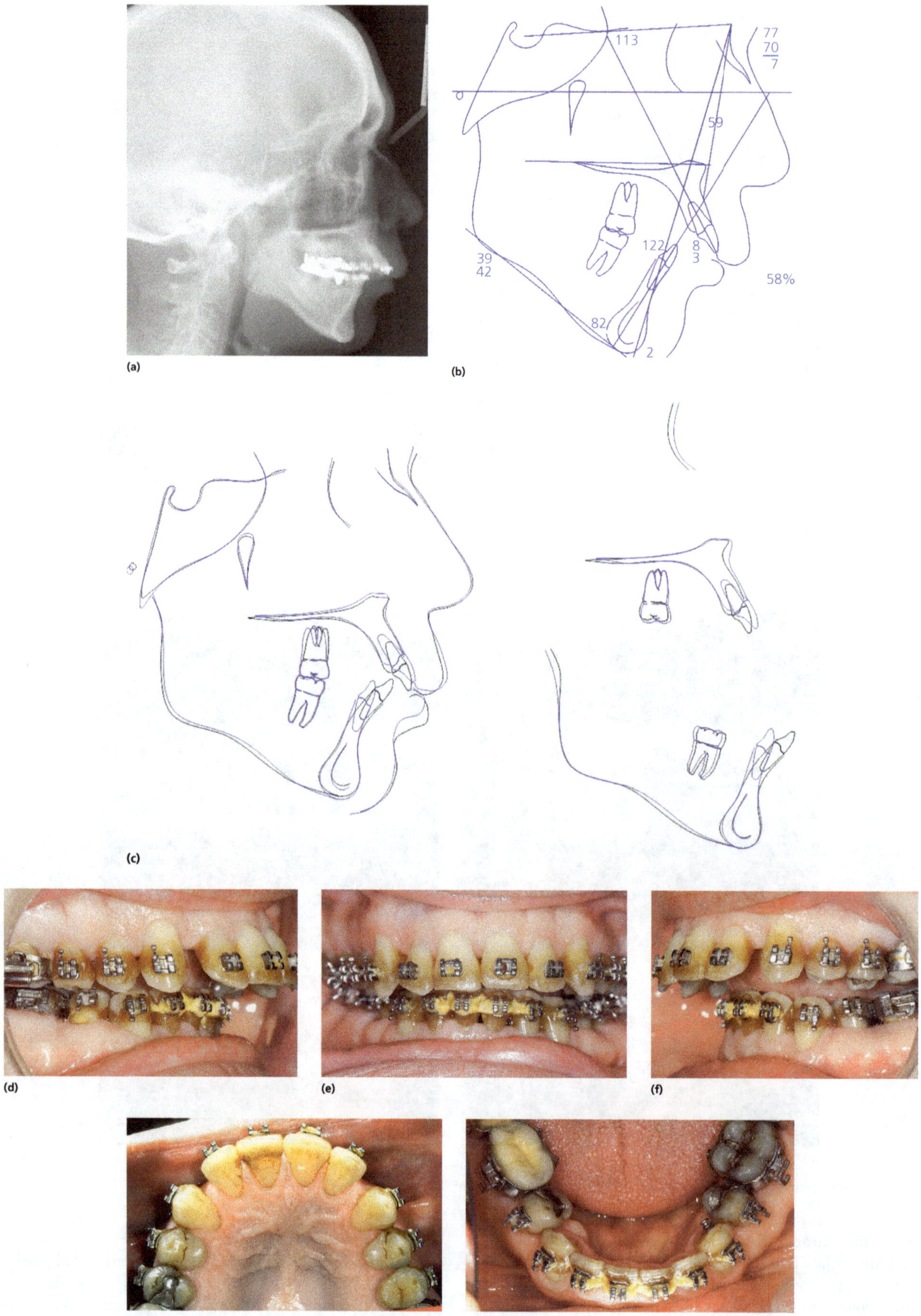

Figure 3.16 (a–h) Michael's presurgical records.

Note in Figure 3.16g that spaces have been opened mesial to the maxillary lateral incisors (Iowa spaces, which are closed postsurgically). The purpose for these spaces it to provide adequate overjet so that the surgeon can advance the mandible to a Class I canine relationship without any concern for incisor interference (especially in cases of anterior tooth size discrepancies). How can you tell if your presurgical orthodontic treatment has succeeded in preparing Michael for surgery?

A: Your initial treatment planning was based on the facial changes and occlusal changes you intended to make with orthodontics/surgery. At this juncture, you want to check how the maxillary and mandibular arches you have prepared fit together. Make a set of models, and see how they articulate. You could hand-articulate them or, better yet, attach them to an articulator (Figure 3.17). As a result of presurgical orthodontic treatment, *presurgical models of the patient should articulate perfectly, in all three planes of space.*

Q: But *how* do you articulate presurgical models, and what do you look for?

A: Articulate presurgical models so that *the canines are seated in a Class I relationship with the best transverse fit you can achieve* (Michael's presurgical models, Figure 3.18). In a nonextraction case, the molars should also articulate in a Class I relationship. If mandibular first premolars were extracted (and no teeth were extracted in the maxillary arch), then the mandibular molars will articulate in a Class III relationship, and the maxillary second molars will be unopposed. The models should coordinate beautifully with perfect dental interdigitation in all three dimensions. We see that Michael's right side articulates fairly well (Figure 3.18a), but his left side has a posterior open bite in the premolar area (Figure 3.18c). This could be corrected by rebonding the mandibular left second premolar (and releveling the arch) or "stepping up" the mandibular left second premolar with a step-up bend in the archwire. Michael's posterior transverse dimension appears to have minimal overjet. Should we have expanded Michael with a SARME? In terms of cost/benefit, probably not. Although a SARME would have helped improve posterior overjet, it would have been a second surgical procedure. Should we expand Michaels' maxillary transverse dimension with a multiple-piece maxillary osteotomy? Again, in terms of cost/benefit, a maxillary multiple-piece osteotomy would help improve posterior overjet, but the amount of improvement needed does not warrant an additional (separate jaw) surgical procedure. Instead, based on the magnitude of the additional posterior OJ needed, we felt that the transverse overjet could be addressed postsurgically, by increasing the dental compensations slightly with cross-bite elastics.

Looking from the occlusal (Figure 3.19), we see that Michael has reasonably good arch alignment and symmetry. Iowa spaces (which will be closed postsurgically) are seen mesial to the maxillary canines. After the coordination of Michael's models was shown to the surgeon, it was agreed that Michael was ready for surgery. Michael underwent a BSSO mandibular advancement and genioplasty advancement.

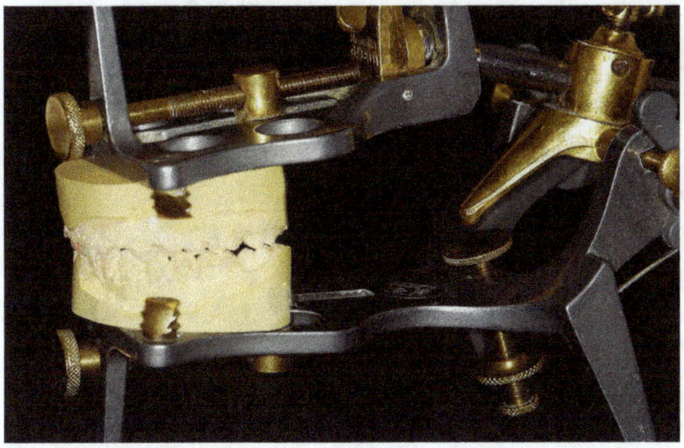

Figure 3.17 Presurgical models mounted on a Galetti articulator.

Q: What is the goal of postsurgical orthodontic treatment?

A: The goal of postsurgical orthodontics is to finish treatment, providing a perfect occlusion. In Michael's case, this consisted of stepping up the mandibular left second premolar, using cross-bite elastics to increase posterior transverse compensations/increase posterior overjet, and closing the Iowa spaces until anterior overjet was eliminated (composite veneers closed small residual spaces). Postsurgically, the orthodontist and surgeon continue to work as a team. If surgical complications arose during surgery, preventing a perfect surgical result, then the team works together to optimize the outcome for the patient.

Q: Initial, presurgical, and deband profile photos (along with deband intraoral photos) of Michael are shown in Figure 3.20. What do you observe?

A: Comparing Michael's initial to deband views, it is apparent that a significant profile improvement has resulted. He has a reasonably well-finished occlusion, but the left premolar open bite is still present.

Q: What if, postsurgically, you noticed Michael relapsing 1–2 mm to Class II. What are the possible immediate, intermediate, and long-term causes of postsurgical relapse?

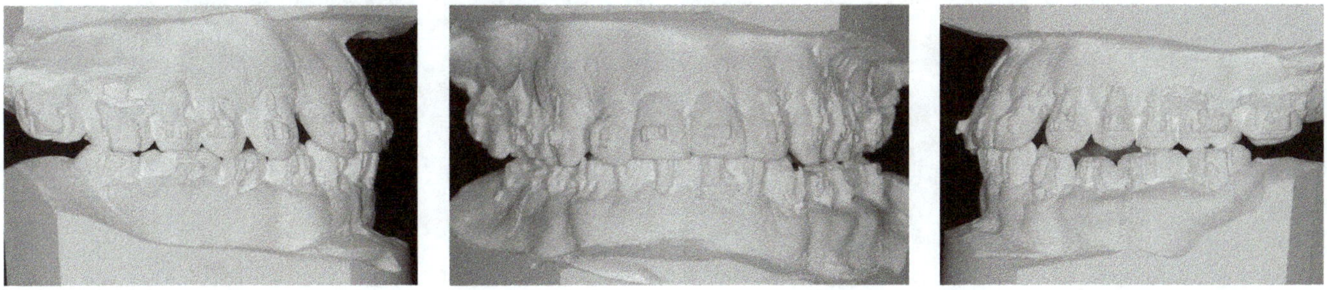

(a) (b) (c)

Figure 3.18 (a–c) Michael's presurgical articulated models.

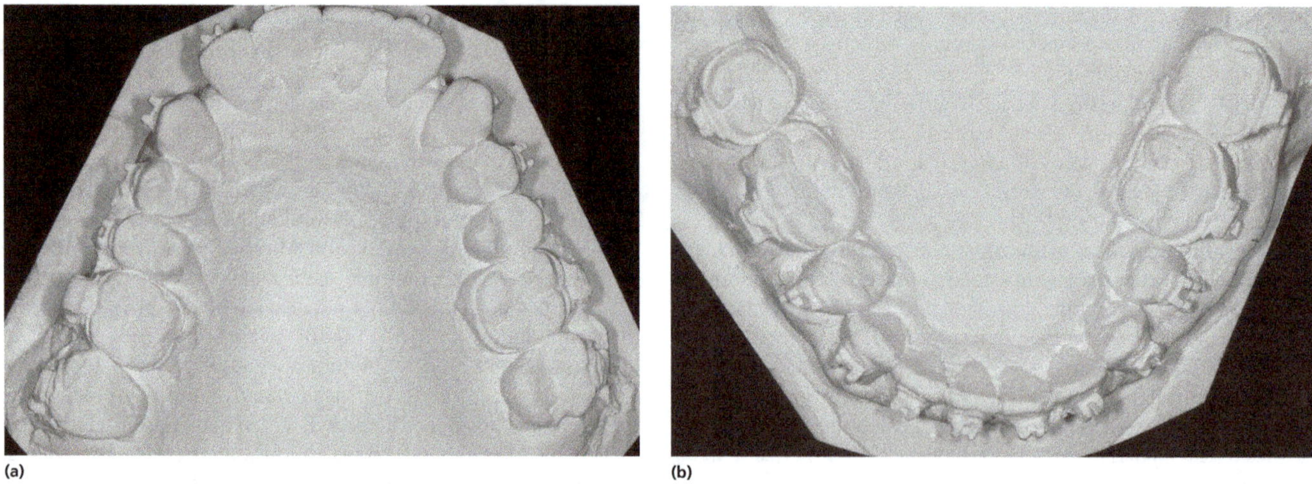

Figure 3.19 (a–b) Michael's presurgical maxillary and mandibular models.

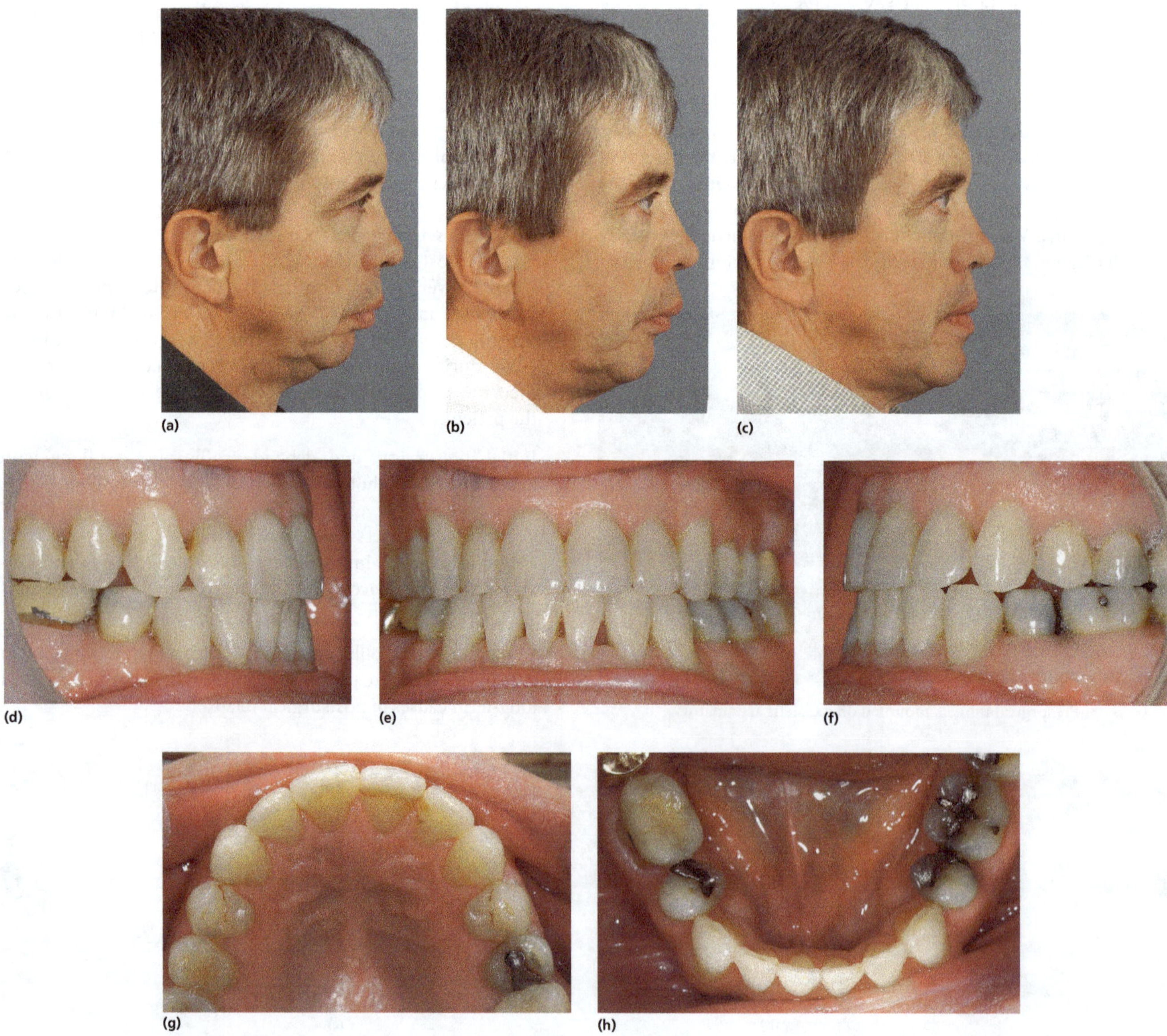

Figure 3.20 (a) Initial, (b) presurgery, and (c) deband profile photos of Michael. (d–h) Deband intraoral photos.

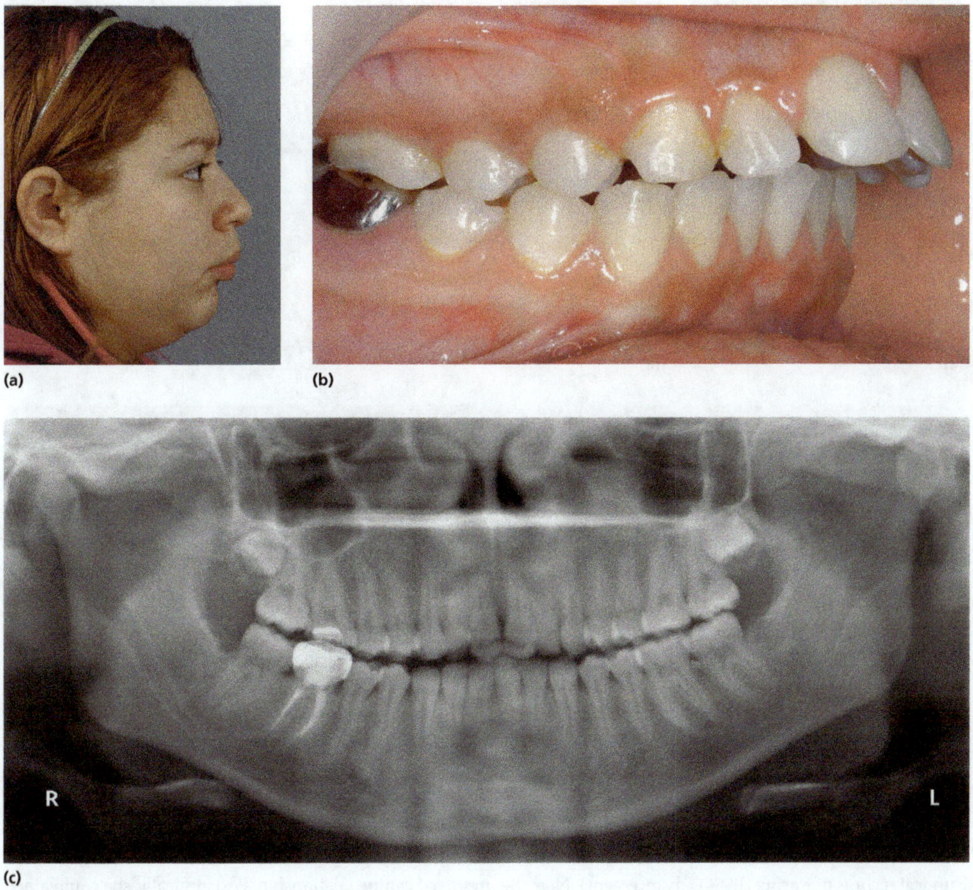

Figure 3.21 (a–c) Initial records of Karina.

A: Possible causes of postsurgical relapse include:
- *Immediate:* failure to seat the condyles properly in the glenoid fossa during surgery, swelling/edema, muscle spasm or muscle posturing, and/or fixation hardware failure.
- *Intermediate:* bony remodeling as the stretched musculature (pterygomasseteric sling and soft tissue stretch) pulls the bone back through the fixation screws.
- *Long term:* continued jaw growth, condylar degeneration (in a conversation with a colleague from the University of Iowa College of Dentistry, Department of Oral & Maxillofacial Surgery (Stein KM 2013), oral communication, September 16).

Q: Karina is an adult who presented with a Class II dental relationship secondary to mandibular skeletal AP hypoplasia (Figure 3.21). Her PMH and TMJ status were noncontributory. She underwent a BSSO mandibular advancement (Figure 3.22) but, postsurgically, complained of bilateral intermittent TMJ pain. What does the literature say about the relationship between orthognathic surgery and TMD?

A: Onizawa et al. [41] reported no significant difference in the incidence of TMJ sounds, deviation of mouth opening, or tenderness of TMJ and masticatory muscles between orthognathic surgery patients and healthy volunteers; patients did not report TMJ symptoms significantly more often than the control subjects. In a prospective follow-up study examining the influence of contemporary orthognathic treatment on signs and symptoms of TMJ dysfunction, Panula et al. [42] reported that TMJ functional status can be significantly improved, pain levels reduced, and the risk for new TMD extremely low with orthognathic surgery. Dervis and Tuncer [43] found that, at initial examination, orthognathic surgery patients did not report TMD signs and symptoms significantly more often than healthy subjects and, at final examination, improvements in TMD symptoms of orthognathic surgery patients were found when compared with healthy subjects. In summary, *it appears that orthognathic surgery patients do not present with increased TMJ problems either before, or after, surgery compared to healthy subjects.*

Q: Karina missed further appointments. She returned to the clinic 1 year later asking to have her braces removed. Records were made (Figure 3.23). What do you observe?

A: Karina has significant relapse (3–4 mm anteroposteriorly plus the development of an open bite).

Q: *Why* did Karina have relapse?

A: Comparing the shape of her condyles 1 year post surgery (Figure 3.23c) to the initial shape of her condyles (Figure 3.21c) and to the shape of her condyles immediately post surgery (Figure 3.22c), it is apparent that Karina has had significant bilateral condylar resorption. This resorption has resulted in Karina's AP relapse and open bite development—as her mandible rotated down and back around her condyles.

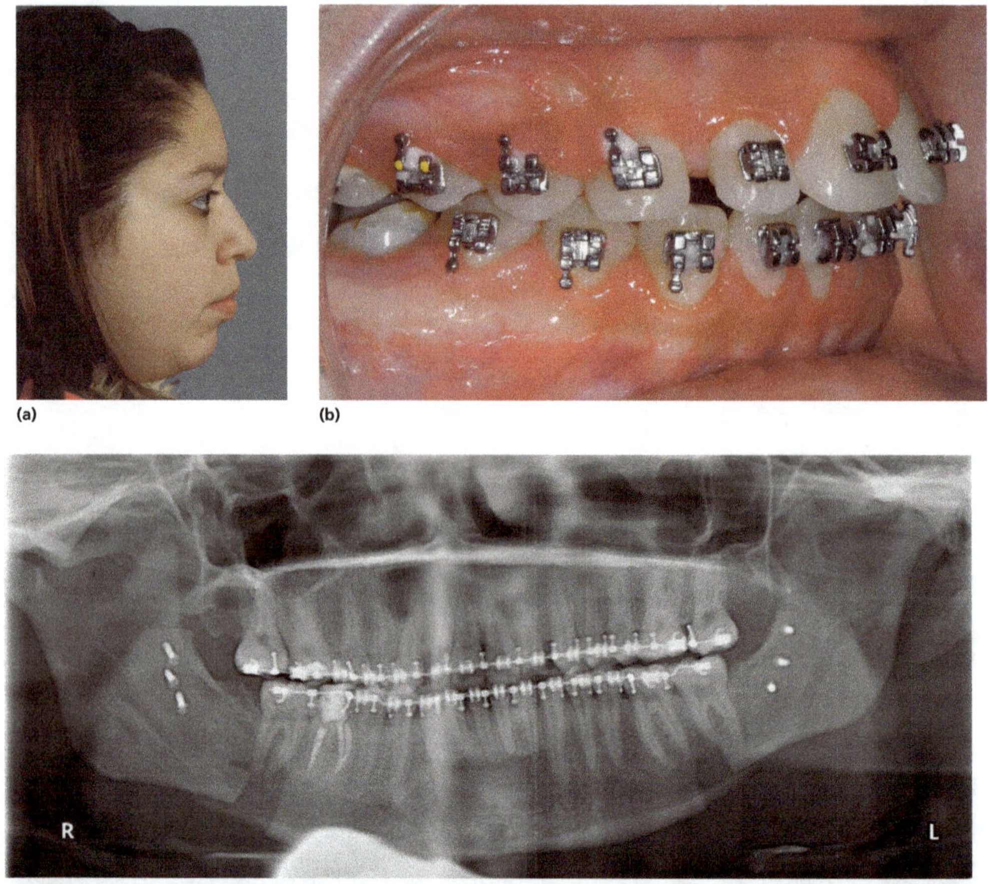

(a) (b) (c)

Figure 3.22 (a–c) Postsurgical records of Karina (BSSO advancement). Note the improved canine relationship. Postsurgically, she complained of bilateral TMJ pain.

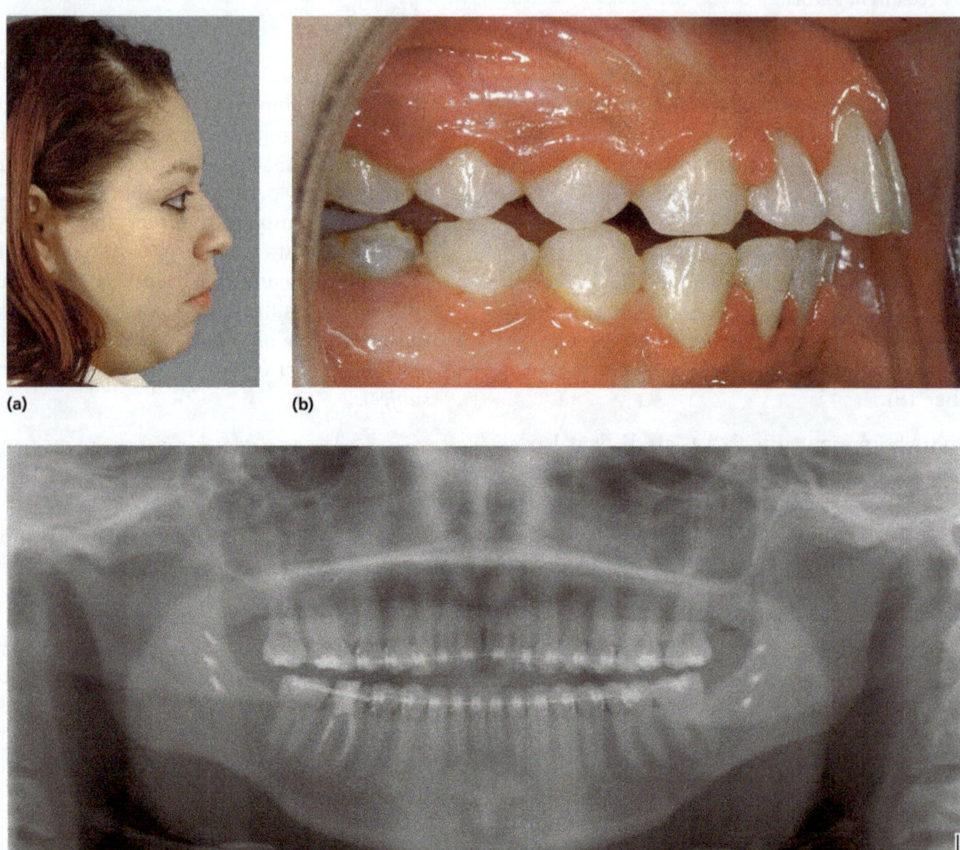

(a) (b) (c)

Figure 3.23 (a–c) Records of Karina 1 year post surgery. She had missed all appointments since her postsurgical visit (Figure 3.22) and requested that her braces come off.

Q: What does the literature say about the development of condylar resorption following orthognathic surgery?

A: Condylar resorption is an idiopathic condition in which one or both of the mandibular condyles are (partially) resorbed. It is nine times more likely to be present in females than males (hormonal mediation may be involved) [44]. Strain on the temporomandibular joint from orthognathic surgery (or orthodontics) may be related to the condition, and reactive arthritis, rheumatoid arthritis, or psoriatic arthritis are other possible causes [45]. Bouwman et al. [46] found that the avoidance of intermaxillary fixation seemed to reduce the incidence of condylar resorption in patients with a mandibular deficiency and high mandibular plane angle. In another study, 31% of high-angle mandibular deficiency surgery patients, all female, were found to develop ramus resorption of more than 2 mm (there was no correlation between resorption and age, the amount of retrognathism, or the presence of preoperative temporomandibular joint dysfunction) [47]. The authors concluded that female patients with high-angle retrognathism should be informed of the possibility of postoperative condylar resorption and should be followed with radiographic controls for at least 2 years after surgery. Simmons et al. [48] reported that about 10% of mandibular advancement patients show a modest long-term shortening of mandibular length, whether or not simultaneous maxillary surgery was carried out. Proffit et al. [49] reported that two-jaw open bite patients showed a mean increase in Condylion-Pogonion dimensions in the long term, suggesting that in long-face, high mandibular plane angle patients with significant anterior open bite, two-jaw surgery with mandibular advancement is not a risk factor for condylar remodeling and resorption beyond 1 year post surgery. Finally, Grammer et al. [50] postulated that avascular condylar necrosis could be the etiology in major resorption cases. In summary, *orthognathic surgery patients should be informed of the risk of condylar resorption and should be followed for at least 1–2 years postsurgically.*

Q: How should you proceed with Karina and the resorption you detected?

A: Inform Karina of the relapse and condylar resorption. You should not consider additional surgical retreatment until documentation (serial panoramic images or CBCT images) clearly shows that the resorptive process has stopped. Furthermore, if you decide to re-treat Karina, then you would be prudent to consider only maxillary surgery or genioplasty surgery (avoiding disruption of the ramus and condylar blood supply/rotation of the condylar heads). Treatment of condylar resorption may include: monitoring the patient for progressive joint changes, prescribing anti-inflammatory medications, orthodontic treatment to address the patient's occlusion, and possible TMJ reconstruction (very severe cases). Discussions regarding treatment should be held between the orthodontist, oral surgeon, family physician, and rheumatologist.

Q: Now, finally, back to Haley. What other facial views should you examine if you are considering surgical treatment?

A: Other useful views include the following:

- Haley with her mandible postured forward. If you are considering a mandibular advancement osteotomy, have Haley posture forward to judge the effect this movement would have on her profile (Figure 3.24a shows Haley in CR, and Figure 3.24b shows Haley postured forward until her canines are Class I). As was the case with Michael, having the mandibular-deficient patient posture forward can help you decide not only the effect of a BSSO advancement on the profile, but it can also help you to decide whether you should extract mandibular premolars. If her profile looks good when postured forward to a Class I canine relationship, then you can consider treating Haley without extractions (assuming extractions are not required to alleviate crowding or for other reasons). Postured forward into a Class I canine relationship, Haley's profile looks improved and acceptable. Even though

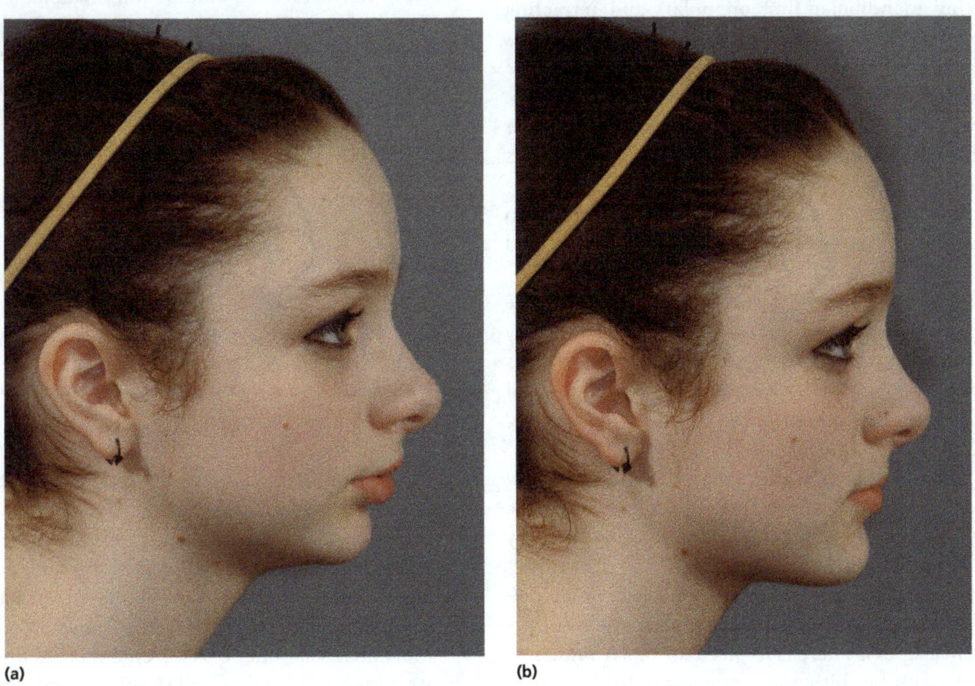

Figure 3.24 Judging the impact of a mandibular advancement osteotomy on Haley's profile: (a) initial photo of Haley in CR and (b) postured forward until canines are Class I.

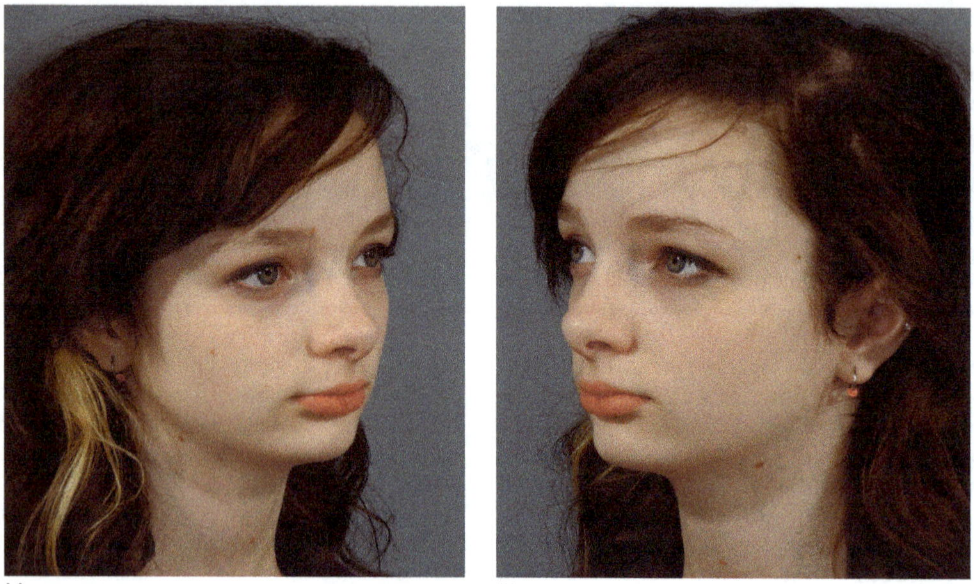

(a) (b)

Figure 3.25 (a) Right and (b) left three-quarter facial views of Haley (45° views).

her mandibular incisors are proclined (Figure 3.1e, FMIA = 54°), they are relatively well aligned (Figure 3.1k). If Haley undergoes surgery, then she should be treated without extracting mandibular premolars. On the other hand, if Haley had looked better when she was postured forward to a Class III (3–4 mm) canine relationship, then extracting mandibular premolars would be prudent so that you could reciprocally close the extraction spaces and retract the mandibular canines—thereby forcing the surgeon to lengthen the mandible even more in order to surgically bring the mandibular canines to Class I. If Haley looked even better when she was postured forward to a Class III (7–8 mm) canine relationship, then extracting mandibular first premolars and retracting canines through the *entire* extraction space using TADs as anchorage may be justified. Of course, the preceding logic assumes the surgical advancement is within the acceptable BSSO advancement limits of 10 mm for steep mandibular plane patients or 15 mm for flat mandibular plane patients like Haley. One final note: notice the improvement, not only in Haley's chin projection when postured forward, but also the improvement in her vertical dimension when postured forward (as the mandibular incisors slide down along the lingual surfaces of the maxillary anterior teeth). Finally, in some patients the incorporation of an advancement genioplasty can also be considered to improve their chin projection. This is not the case for Haley. In summary, *based on* Figure 3.24 *Haley could benefit from a nonextraction BSSO advancement osteotomy (but without a genioplasty).*

- 45°views (Figure 3.25) to examine Haley's malar (zygomatic/cheek) projection and determine a need for malar implants. Even though Haley's maxilla is deficient anteroposteriorly (Figure 3.1e, A-point sits behind, not on, a line drawn perpendicular to Frankfort through Nasion), her 45° views look acceptable (her cheeks project beyond a line drawn vertically from her corneal apex). There is no need for malar implants.
- A frontal view with her biting a tongue blade from right to left in the posterior to check for an occlusal cant. An occlusal cant is demonstrated by the tongue blade not being parallel to her interpupillary line. This view was not made for Haley.

Q: What is one more important view, specifically useful when considering a maxillary downgraft osteotomy?

A: A frontal photo should be made with the teeth separated to the point where Haley's lips are just touching (just achieving lip competence). This view illustrates any discrepancy between the facial soft tissue vertical and the facial skeletal vertical. This view was not made for Haley. As a substitute, a second lateral cephalometric radiograph could be made with the teeth separated to the point where the lips are just touching. Such a view can reveal the amount the maxilla should be surgically downgrafted. For example, look at the initial lateral cephalometric radiographs of the skeletal deep bite patient shown in Figure 3.26. On the left (a), the patient is biting together. On the right (b), the patient has opened, just enough, to where her lips are just touching. The posterior interocclusal gap created provides a guide as to how much the maxilla will needed to be downgrafted (or the posterior teeth erupted) to support the ideal facial soft tissue vertical. Of course, to avoid development of an interlabial gap (lip incompetence), *the maxilla should not be downgrafted beyond the point where the relaxed lips just touch.*

Q: In preparation for a maxillary downgraft osteotomy, should incisal display be judged based on relaxed lip position from initial records, smile position from initial records, relaxed lip position after the maxillary arch is leveled, or smile position after the maxillary arch has been leveled?

A: In preparation for a maxillary downgraft osteotomy, you must judge how far down you want the anterior maxilla to move. Incisal display influences this decision. Incisal display should be judged based on relaxed lip position after leveling the arches. Surgical movements should be based on hard and soft tissue structural relationships, not neuromuscular activity. So surgical movements should be based on a relaxed lip position, which is structure, and *not* on a smile (which is neuromuscular function). Additionally, maxillary anterior teeth can initially be stepped

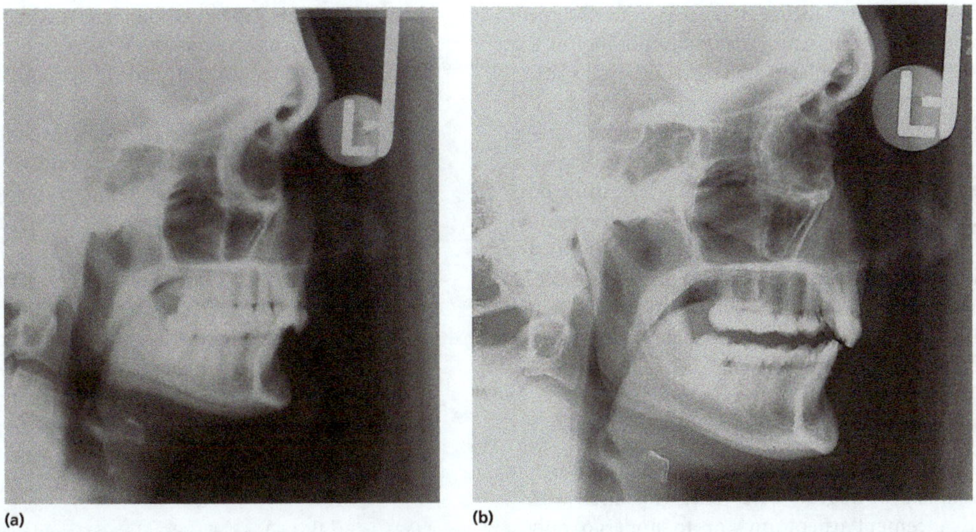

Figure 3.26 Initial lateral cephalometric radiographs of a skeletal deep bite patient: (a) in maximum intercuspation, (b) with her teeth separated to where her relaxed lips are just touching. The interocclusal gap created provides a guide as to how much the maxilla will needed to come down (or the maxillary/mandibular teeth erupted) to support the facial soft tissue drape adequately.

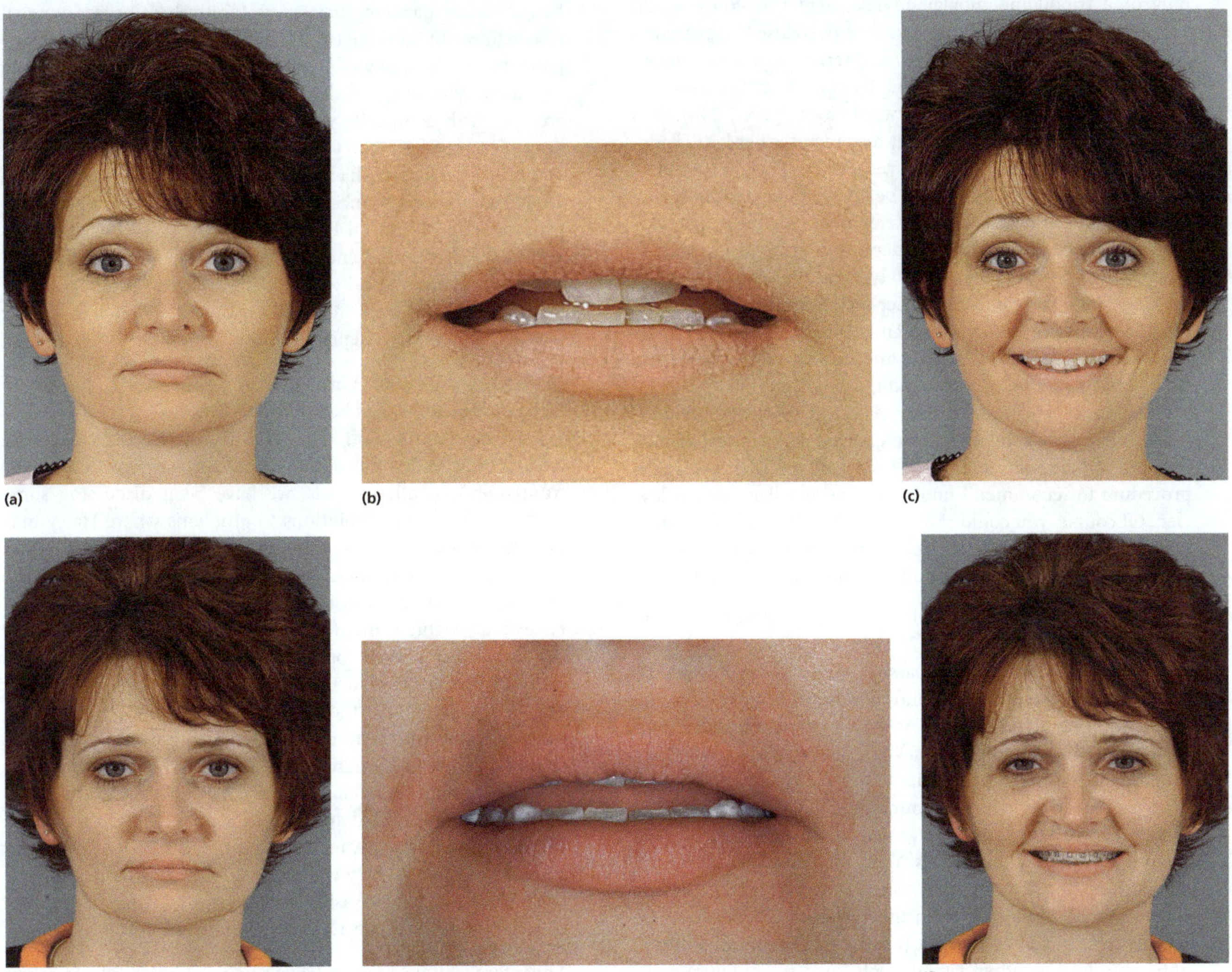

Figure 3.27 Judging maxillary incisal display: (a) initial frontal photo, (b) initial relaxed lip position, (c) initial posed smile, (d) postleveling of arches frontal photo, (e) postleveling relaxed lip position, (f) postleveling posed smile. Note that her incisal display was reduced following maxillary arch leveling because her maxillary central incisors were initially stepped down.

up or stepped down relative to the maxillary posterior teeth, which can give a false impression of the amount of incisor that will be displayed after maxillary arch leveling. So, surgical movements should be based on incisal display in a relaxed lip position *after* the arches are leveled. As an example, look at Kim's (Figure 3.27a) initial maxillary central incisor display in relaxed lip position (Figure 3.27b) and initial posed smile position (Figure 3.27c). Her incisal display looks pretty normal, doesn't it? Now look at her maxillary incisor display following maxillary arch leveling in relaxed lip position (Figure 3.27e) and smiling position (Figure 3.27f). She demonstrates inadequate incisal display (virtually no incisal display) in a relaxed lip position, and only marginally adequate incisal display in a posed smile. *Judge adequacy of incisal display in a relaxed lip position after the maxillary arch is leveled.*

Q: What factors would influence you to encourage Haley to undergo a maxillary downgraft osteotomy (together with a mandibular advancement osteotomy) or to undergo only a tripod mandibular advancement osteotomy?

A: Her LAFH is short (Subnasale–soft tissue Menton < soft tissue Glabella–Subnasale; skeletally, LAFH/TAFH = 49%), and she has an overclosed appearance. Either a maxillary downgraft osteotomy or a tripod mandibular advancement osteotomy would increase her LAFH and decrease her overclosed appearance. *Deciding which surgery is a question of vertical deficiency magnitude and patient desires.* If you think that her vertical relationship looks good when she postures forward now (Figure 3.24b), then a tripod mandibular advancement may increase her LAFH adequately. If you feel that even more vertical facial height is needed, then a maxillary downgraft may be appropriate (assuming you can maintain lip competence). Remember, her maxillary incisors are stepped down relative to her posterior occlusion with an incisal display of only approximately 2 mm (lips relaxed). When her maxillary arch is leveled, her maxillary incisors will be intruded, possibly by that entire 2 mm (see Figure 3.1h), leaving her with no incisal display at rest and inadequate incisal display in a posed smile. A tripod mandibular advancement will not increase maxillary incisal display. A maxillary downgraft (plus mandibular advancement) will increase maxillary incisal display. So, you should not make the final call on which surgical procedure to recommend until after the maxillary arch is leveled. Of course, you could chose not to level her maxillary arch completely in order to give her some incisal display if she is willing to only undergo a tripod mandibular advancement.

Q: If you treat Haley surgically, what factor determines *when* you can perform surgery?

A: Completion of growth. At 13 years, 4 months of age, it would be reasonable to begin leveling and aligning her arches now, in anticipation of surgery. Why? As a rule of thumb, individuals with (vertical or anteroposterior) *deficiencies* of jaw growth are expected to finish growing earlier than individuals with normal, or excessive, jaw growth. Of course, age alone is no guarantee that Haley will have completed growth by the time you are done leveling and aligning her arches. You should also talk to her and her parents to ask if she is finished growing. If there is any question of whether she has finished growing, then it would be wise to wait to begin treatment (or at least to perform surgery) until you take another lateral cephalometric radiograph in 9–12 months, superimpose the radiographs, and confirm that growth is complete. If the superimposed lateral cephalograms demonstrate that growth is complete, then you can proceed with surgery. If the superimposed lateral cephalograms demonstrate an unexpected amount of growth during that time, then you could chose to postpone surgery (leaving the braces on) or deband her and place her in retention (as long as the presurgical arches fit perfectly). She can then undergo surgery when she has completed growth. As we mentioned earlier, Haley reached menarche when she turned age 12. For girls, the peak rate of statural increase is reached prior to menarche [39]. With the onset of menses, the rate of change in height drops to prepubertal levels and decreases sharply to an adult rate of change during the subsequent 2 years. So, we do not expect much more growth for Haley. One final note: if Haley's dentofacial deformity was so severe (which it is not, in our opinion) that psychosocial pressures justified surgery before growth was completed—then you would need to inform Haley and her parents that she could grow out of the surgical correction and require a second surgery later.

Q: Here is a clinical pearl: when a patient lacks adequate incisal display following treatment, for instance, if you leveled Haley's maxillary arch (intruding her maxillary incisors) and she later complained of inadequate maxillary incisal display, what could you do to improve her display?

A: Lengthen her maxillary incisors, restoratively. Whereas our goal is to achieve an ideal OB (minimal or 10%) in initially deep bite patients, in situations of inadequate incisal display following treatment, you can consider lengthening the maxillary incisor crowns (with composite veneers or porcelain veneers). As an example, consider Justin (deband photos shown in Figure 3.28a and c). At deband, he had minimal OB but expressed concern about his inadequate incisal display when smiling. Composite veneers were placed on his maxillary incisors (Figures 3.28b and 3.28d), which deepened his overbite but improved his smiling esthetics, dramatically. Of course, another option would be to put the patient back in maxillary braces and step down the maxillary incisors to deepen the bite and increase incisal display.

Q: In deciding on a final treatment plan for Haley, what important factor must be revisited before proceeding?

A: Haley's chief complaint: "I want to fix my front teeth. These ones (points to her maxillary lateral incisors) go behind the front ones." In other words, we have been discussing some sophisticated surgical solutions to problems where Haley may not see problems (e.g., overclosed appearance, short LAFH, and minimally adequate incisal display). Haley may only desire maxillary anterior tooth alignment. In fact, if this is all that Haley truly wanted, and if simple alignment would not prevent her from seeking more comprehensive treatment later, then the orthodontist is justified in proceeding with tooth alignment only. However, the orthodontist must (tactfully) discuss all problems, and treatment options, with the patient and parents so that they can make an informed decision. Following multiple discussions with Haley and her parents, covering all treatment options, Haley decided to proceed with orthodontics and a tripod mandibular advancement surgery. Orthodontics was started now, but surgery will be postponed until after she is at least age 15. A final decision regarding a maxillary downgraft osteotomy will be made after the maxillary arch is leveled.

Q: The interocclusal rest space (freeway space) is the difference between the vertical dimension of rest and the vertical dimension in occlusion. Prosthodontists, and other restorative dentists, are

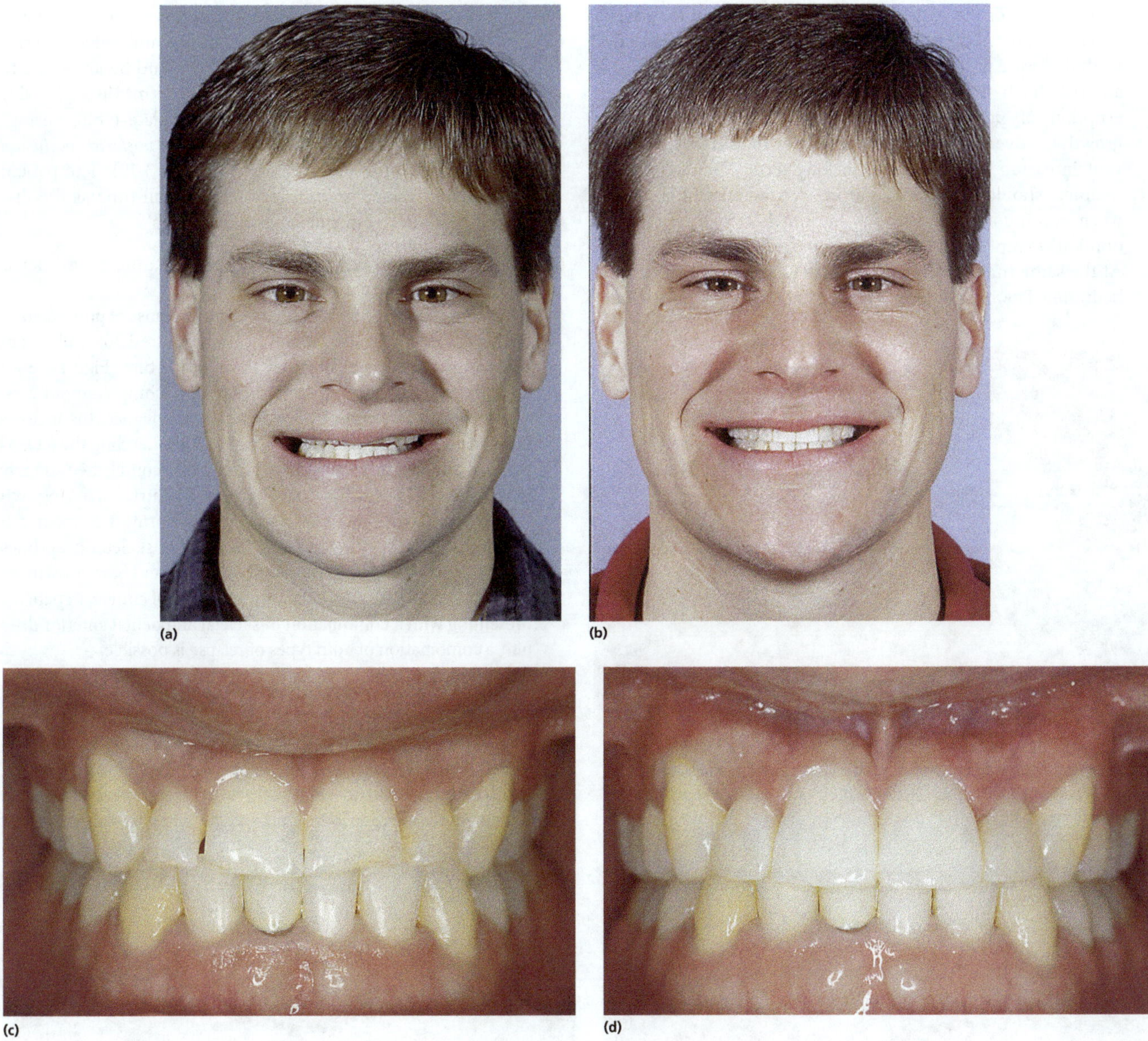

Figure 3.28 Restorative treatment to increase incisal display: (a and c) initial photos of Justin who was finished with minimal OB but was concerned with his lack of incisal display, (b and d) improvement in his incisal display by lengthening his maxillary incisors (but deepening his bite), restoratively.

careful not to violate this space. And yet, with orthodontic treatment (e.g., erupting posterior teeth during leveling) and with surgical treatment (e.g., maxillary downgraft osteotomies), we routinely violate this space. How is this possible?

A: We can speculate that, with orthodontic treatment, the vertical changes are occurring slowly enough that some form of adaptation occurs. But surgery is instantaneous, like an immediate full-mouth rehabilitation that increases the vertical dimension. So, the answer to this question is not fully known.

Q: Assuming that all your treatment goals have been achieved, when can you safely deband a skeletal deep bite patient and begin retention?

A: For adolescent patients, discontinuing treatment before growth is complete is always a stability gamble. Unfavorable growth could deepen the bite and ruin an excellent finish. If possible, do not deband until growth is complete. But, if growth has slowed dramatically and you decide to deband, then monitor the patient carefully for signs of deep bite relapse. In a surgically treated skeletal deep bite patient, or any surgery patient for that matter, keep the patient in fixed orthodontic appliances at least 4–6 months after surgery. These months are needed for postsurgery bony remodeling to occur. With any adolescent or adult patient, treated with surgery or without surgery, *once you have finished treatment to an ideal result, it is a good idea to maintain that patient in fixed orthodontic appliances for 2–4 months (clinical opinion) to allow bony and soft tissues time to remodel before debanding. This 2–4 month period is called "active retention."*

Q: What is an effective retention protocol for enhancing skeletal deep bite correction stability?

A: Retention protocol for skeletal deep bites is the same as for dental deep bites—the key is patient compliance. Retention is a major part of orthodontic care, and nightly retainer wear must be part of the patient lifestyle to guarantee a long-term, excellent result. Our goal is to prevent uprighting of anterior teeth that were proclined during treatment, prevent eruption of anterior teeth that were intruded during treatment, permit eruption of posterior teeth during remaining mandibular growth or adverse bony remodeling following surgery, and prevent intrusion of posterior teeth long term. Vacuum-formed retainers should be fabricated at the deband appointment and worn continuously during the day for 2–3 months (clinical opinion) except when eating or when drinking something hot. At the same time, Hawley retainers are fabricated and worn at bedtime. The mandibular Hawley retainer design includes HIGH acrylic on the lingual of the anterior teeth, plus a band of acrylic along the labial bow of the mandibular anterior teeth. Or, a fixed lingual retainer, from mandibular canine to mandibular canine, can be substituted. The maxillary Hawley retainer should include an anterior bite plate ("bite-raising" design) [51, 52] which *slightly discludes the posterior occlusion* when the patient wears it at night (Figure 3.29). The patient should NOT wear the maxillary retainer full time as the discluded posterior teeth will supererupt.

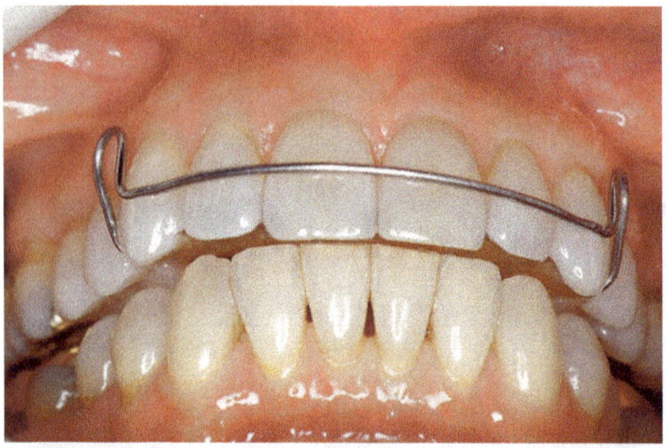

Figure 3.29 Retention of a skeletal deep bite patient should include a maxillary Hawley retainer incorporating an anterior bite plate ("bite-raising" design) which slightly discludes the posterior occlusion when the patient wears it at night.

Q: How can relapse of skeletal deep bite patients differ from relapse of dental deep bite patients?

A: Relapse of dental deep bites usually occurs because of poor retainer wear. As an example, the patient shown in Figure 3.30a underwent orthodontic treatment in order to open his bite (Figure 3.30b) and make space for restorative material (composite veneers, Figure 3.30c). Because of poor retainer compliance, his incisors erupted and his bite deepened (Figure 3.30d). Leveling the COS is generally stable [53], probably because it is accomplished so early in treatment and held. But, incisors that were intruded during arch leveling can erupt, and incisors proclined during treatment can upright, thus deepening the bite. Relapse of skeletal deep bites occurs with continued unfavorable adolescent jaw growth or unfavorable postsurgical bone remodeling. Of course, in patients presenting with a combination of skeletal and dental anterior deep bite, a combination of both types of relapse is possible.

Q: *How* does continued growth contribute to deep-overbite relapse in skeletal deep bite patients?

A: The unfavorable growth pattern, which initially caused the skeletal deep bite, can continue to cause the retention deep bite. Posttreatment relapse results from a greater posterior facial height increase than combined sutural and alveolar growth of

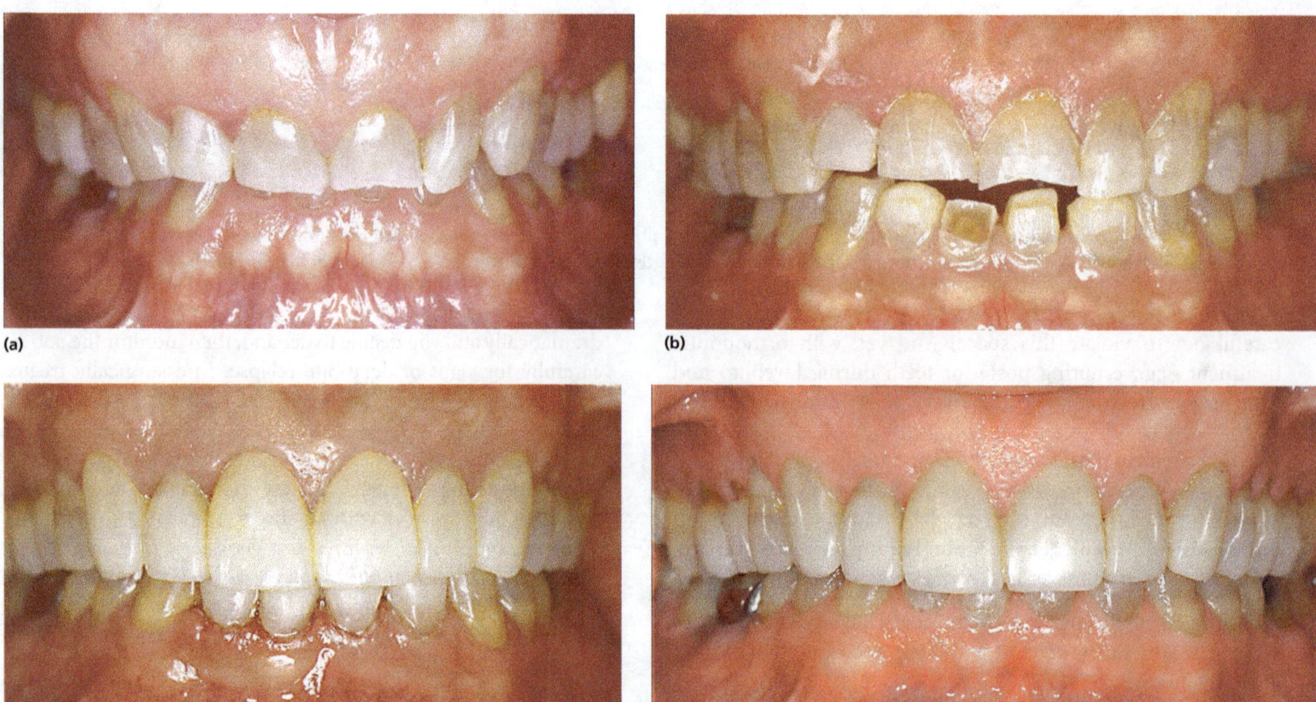

(a) (b) (c) (d)

Figure 3.30 A patient whose dental deep bite was opened to make room for restorative material: (a) initial deep bite, due to overerupted maxillary and mandibular incisors, (b) bite opened, and (c) restorative material placed. (d) Poor retainer wear resulted in deepening of his bite.

the maxilla plus alveolar growth of the mandible [18]. As the mandible rotates upward and forward, increased vertical incisor overlap occurs (the bite deepens).

Q: In terms of orthopedic or masking treatment stability, what should you tell parents of adolescent skeletal deep bite patients before beginning treatment?

A: Despite your best efforts, and the best efforts of the patient, continued unfavorable growth could eventually result in the need for orthognathic surgery to achieve an ideal occlusal and esthetic result.

Q: Is nonsurgical skeletal deep bite correction stable?

A: Although the literature lacks an investigation specifically addressing nonsurgical skeletal deep bite stability, one could assume that (if growth is complete) the stability of successful skeletal deep bite treatment would approach the stability of successful dental deep bite treatment—that is, be reasonably stable [51, 54–57]. If growth is not complete, then growth is one more unknown which could adversely impact stability. If you deband a skeletal deep bite adolescent before growth is complete, then you should carefully monitor that patient while he or she is still growing.

Q: Is surgical correction of skeletal deep bites by Le Fort I downgrafts stable? Is surgical correction by mandibular tripod advancements stable?

A: Stability of maxillary downgrafts is good, if *rigid* fixation is used. It was previously reported that maxillary downgrafting was the least stable of various surgical movements [58], especially when performed with wire fixation (relapse rates ranged from 0 to 100%) [59–63]. Stability was said to be improved if the vertical ramus musculature was not altered with inferior repositioning of the maxilla, but stability worsened if the lower facial height was increased greater than the freeway space (maxillomandibular fixation and suspension wires) [64]. Recently [65], maxillary downgrafts with *rigid* fixation were reported as having good stability (80% of cases showing relapse of 2 mm or fewer superior movement). The mean amount of postoperative relapse represented 28% of the surgical downgraft. In this later study, no correlation was found between the amount of the maxillary downgraft and the subsequent postsurgical vertical stability of the maxilla. No difference was found in the vertical stability of the maxilla comparing one-jaw and two-jaw procedures. No study has addressed stability of tripod mandibular advancement surgery, specifically. However, we speculate that mandibular tripod advancement surgery mirrors mandibular advancement surgery stability—which is very good [66].

Q: In summary, what are your "take-home messages" regarding etiology, identifying, treating, and retaining skeletal deep bite patients?

A: Take-home messages include the following:

- Skeletal deep bites result from a pattern of growth, including a more vertically growing condyle, excessive forward mandibular internal (true) growth rotation, less maxillary corpus descent, and/or less molar eruption. As a result, the mandible rotates upward and forward increasing incisor vertical overlap (increasing OB). Skeletal deep bites can present combined with dental deep bites (which result from overeruption of incisors).
- Contrasted with dental deep bites (identified by stepped down maxillary incisors, stepped up mandibular incisors, and a deep COS), the identifying features of skeletal deep bites include a short soft tissue LAFH, an overclosed appearance, a short skeletal LAFH/TAFH, a flat MPA, nearly parallel MPA-FH-SN planes, and inadequate incisal display (not due to stepped up maxillary incisors).
- Orthopedic adolescent treatment of skeletal deep bites consists of attempting to enhance downward maxillary growth plus increasing molar eruption.
- Masking treatment of skeletal deep bites is equivalent to correcting dental deep bites and consists of intruding/proclining anterior teeth while not addressing the short LAFH. Leveling the COS can, potentially, increase the LAFH.
- Surgical treatment of skeletal deep bites consists of grafting additional maxillary bone to move the maxilla inferiorly, and allowing the mandible to rotate down and back to increase the LAFH.
- Retaining skeletal deep bites is similar to retaining dental deep bites. Skeletal deep bite correction stability is reasonable, but some relapse should be anticipated. The difference is that with skeletal deep bites, you should anticipate *both* dental relapse (uprighting of anterior teeth that were proclined during treatment, eruption of anterior teeth that were intruded during treatment, intrusion of posterior teeth that were erupted during treatment) *and* skeletal relapse (continued unfavorable growth in adolescents or vertical skeletal closure in maxillary downgraft patients). Stability of skeletal deep bite correction by eruption of molars in adults (especially with low to average mandibular plane angles) is questionable. *Deep bite overcorrection (perhaps finishing with 10% OB or less) is a good idea. Once you have finished treatment to an ideal result, you should maintain a finished patient in fixed orthodontic appliances for 2–4 months before debanding (active retention).* Compliance with night-time retainer wear (maxillary anterior biteplate to slightly disclude posterior teeth) is of paramount importance. Your patient should be retained, for life.

Case Adam

Adam is a 10-year-old male (Figure 3.31) who presents to you for "correction of my bite." His PMH, PDH, and TMJ evaluation are WRN. His periodontal evaluation is WRN and CR=CO.

Q: List all diagnostic findings/problems. What is your diagnosis?

A: See Table 3.1

Q: Which dimensions have apical base discrepancies?

A: AP and vertical

Q: In order to determine the etiology of Adam's deep bite, how should you proceed?

A: Evaluate his features, which define either a skeletal or dental deep bite. *Skeletal deep bite features*: evaluate his vertical lower facial third—clinically and cephalometrically. Is his soft tissue LAFH shorter than his soft tissue midface height? If yes, by how much? Is his skeletal LAFH/TAFH <55%? If yes, by how much? Is his MPA flat and his MP relatively parallel to his FH and SN lines? *Dental deep bite features*: have Adam open slightly to evaluate the vertical position of his mandibular incisors relative to the mandibular canines (mandibular incisors should be stepped down slightly relative to his canines), mandibular canines relative to his mandibular posterior teeth (all cusp tips should lie on the same plane), maxillary incisors relative his maxillary canines (maxillary incisors should be stepped up slightly relative to his canines), maxillary canines relative to his maxillary posterior teeth (all cusp tips should lie on the same plane), and the presence of a COS (the deeper the COS, the deeper the dental deep bite).

Q: We lack a frontal (intraoral) photograph of Adam, with his teeth separated, to help judge his dental vertical relationship. But, we can separate his models to take a look. What do you see (Figure 3.32)?

A: Adam's mandibular permanent incisors are stepped up relative to his primary canines, the mandibular posterior cusp tips do not lie on the same plane, and a deep COS exists. Adam's maxillary lateral incisors are stepped down slightly relative to his

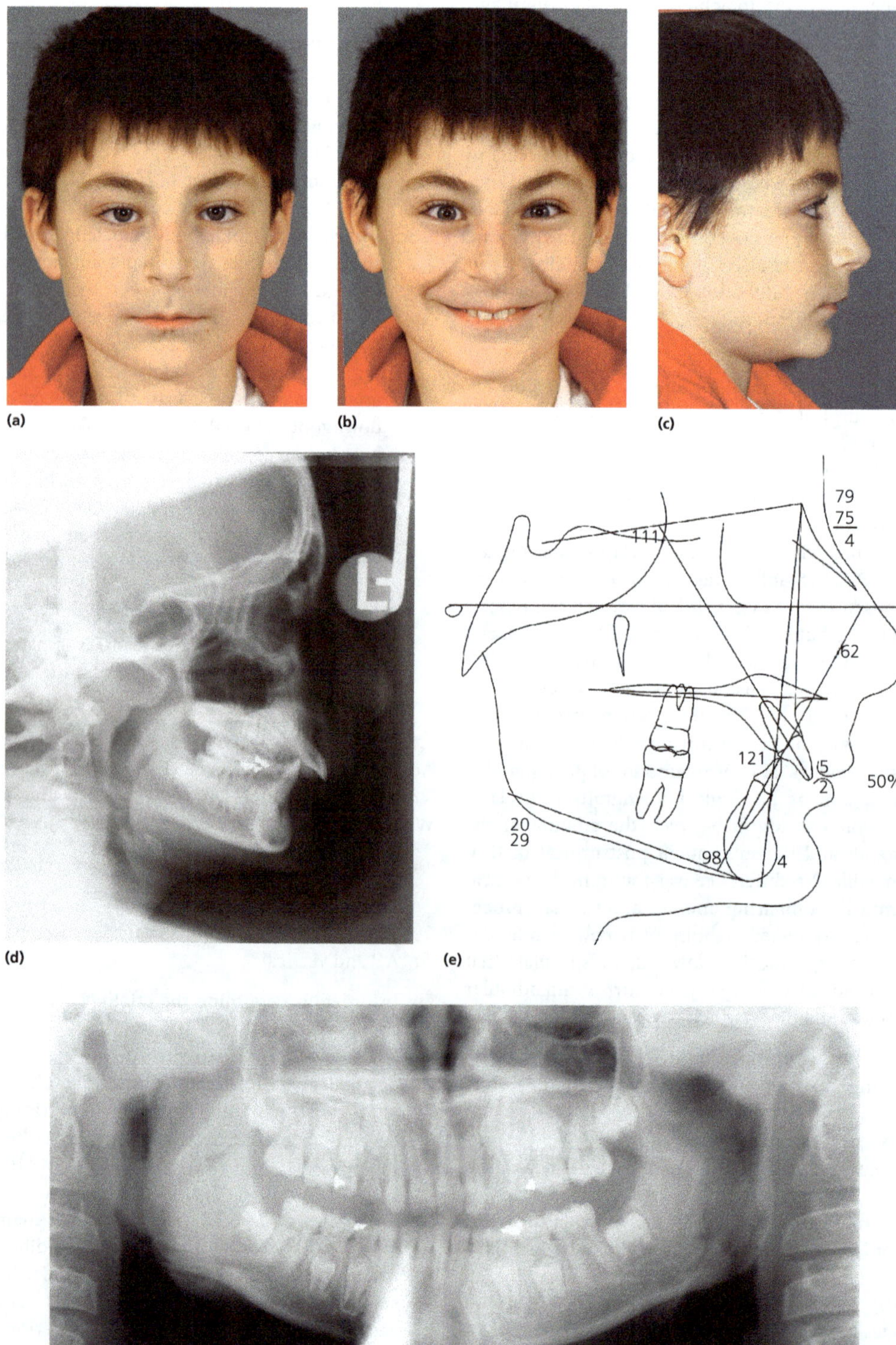

Figure 3.31 Initial records for Adam: (a–c) initial facial photographs, (d) lateral cephalograph, (e) cephalometric tracing, (f) pantomograph,

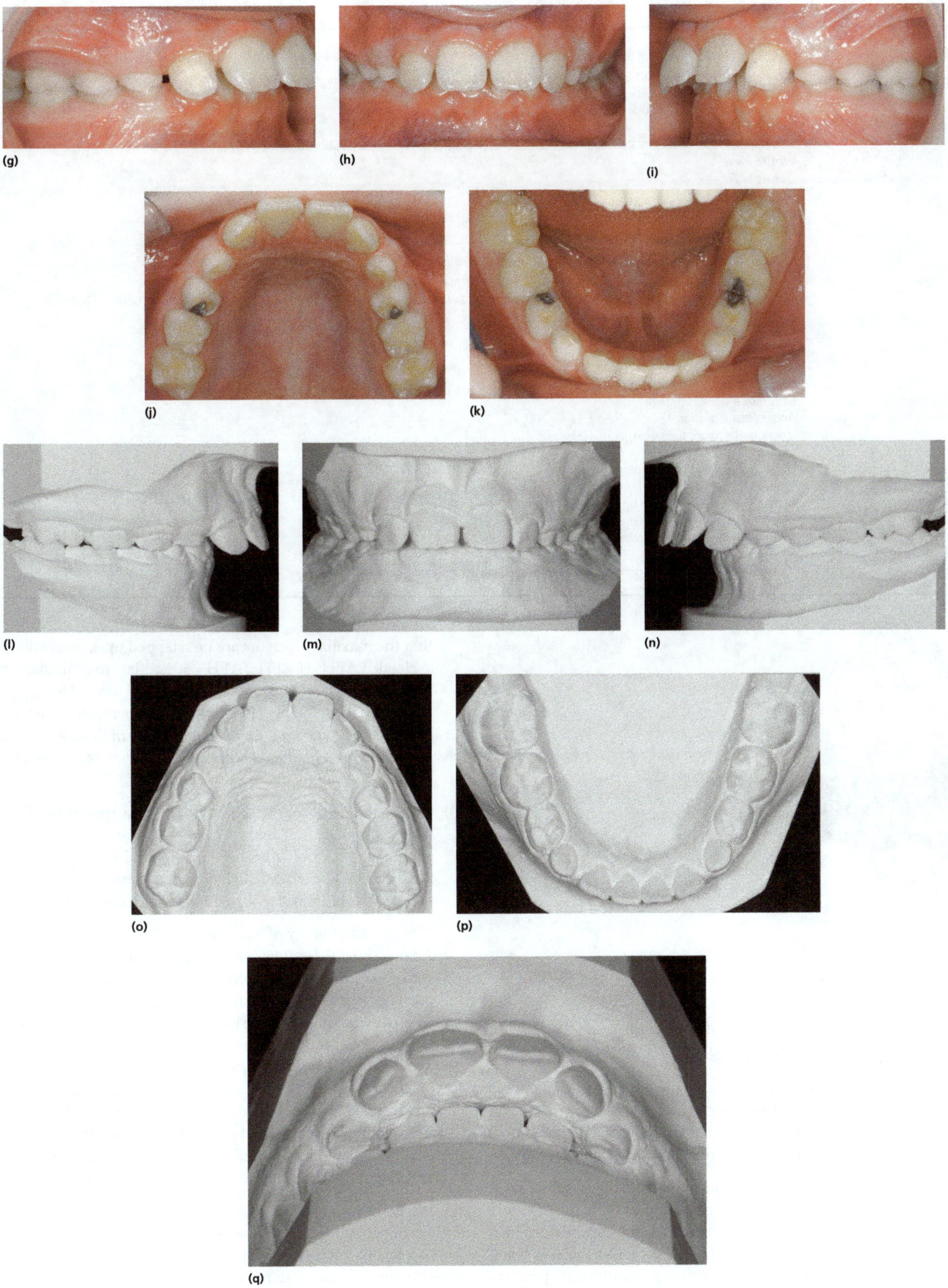

Figure 3.31 (Continued) (g–k) intraoral photographs, (l–p) models, and (q) articulated models tipped up.

Table 3.1 Diagnostic findings and problem list for Adam.

Full face and profile	**Frontal view**
	Face is symmetric
	Short LAFH (Subnasale—soft tissue Menton slightly shorter than soft tissue Glabella—Subnasale)
	Absence of an interlabial gap
	Thin maxillary and mandibular lip vermillion
	UDML: WRN
	Inadequate incisal display in a posed smile (central incisor gingival margins are positioned above vermillion border of maxillary lip)
	Profile view
	Obtuse NLA
	Convex profile
	Retrusive chin
	Deep labiomental sulcus
Ceph analysis	**Skeletal**
	Normal maxillary AP position (NA to FH approximately 90°)
	Mild mandibular skeletal AP hypoplasia (ANB = 4° with a normal maxillary AP position)
	Vertical skeletal deficiency (LAFH/TAFH = 50%; flat mandibular plane angles with FMA = 20° and SNMP = 29°; relatively parallel SN, FH, and MP lines)
	Mandibular lip trapping
	Prominent soft tissue Pogonion
	Dental
	Proclined maxillary incisors (maxillary incisor to SN = 111°)
	Mildly proclined mandibular incisors (FMIA = 62°)
Radiographs	Early mixed-dentition stage
Intraoral photos and models	Angle Class II division 1
	Iowa Classification: II (5) II (5) II (5) II (5)
	OJ: 10 mm
	OB: 100% (palatal impingement)
	3 mm COS
	Mandibular incisors stepped up relative to mandibular primary canines
	Mild maxillary and mandibular anterior spacing
	Midlines are approximately coincident
Other	—
Diagnosis	Angle Class II division 1 malocclusion. Skeletal and dental deep bite

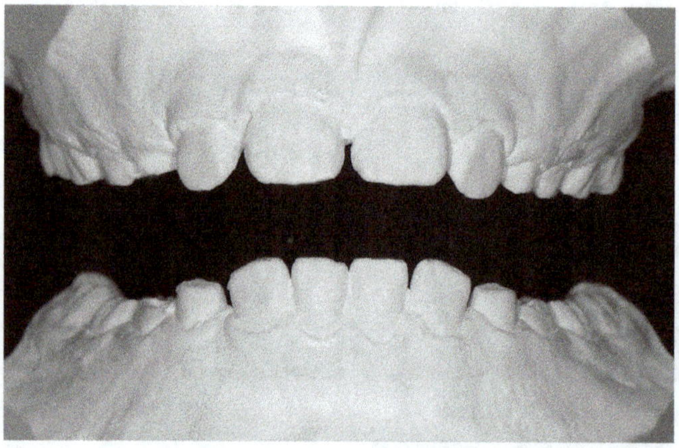

Figure 3.32 Adam's separated models viewed from the front.

maxillary central incisors, but all his maxillary posterior teeth lie approximately on the same plane.

Q: Adam lacks posterior cross bites. But, what do you think of his mandibular and maxillary posterior crown torque (Figure 3.32)?

A: Adam exhibits significant mandibular posterior lingual crown torque. His maxillary posterior crown torque appears reasonable.

Q: Is Adam's 100% OB (with palatal impingement) a *dental* deep bite, a *skeletal* deep bite, or a combination of both?

A: Adam's deep bite is a combination dental and skeletal deep bite. His *dental deep bite features* include mandibular incisors being stepped up (overerupted) relative to mandibular primary canines and mandibular posterior teeth (deep COS). His *skeletal deep bite features* include a short soft tissue LAFH, inadequate maxillary incisal display in a posed smile despite the fact that the maxillary incisors are not stepped up, a markedly short skeletal LAFH (LAFH/TAFH = 50%, flat mandibular plane angles). *Adam is classified as a skeletal deep bite especially because his skeletal LAFH is markedly deficient. He is classified as a dental deep bite because his mandibular incisors have erupted above his mandibular canines and posterior teeth. Adam is a combination dental and skeletal deep bite.*

Q: Can you think of another photograph/measurement that should have been made on Adam?

A: A photograph should have been made with his teeth slightly separated and his lips relaxed/slightly parted to evaluate incisal display at rest. Also, his maxillary lip length should have been measured.

Q: What is the etiology of Adam's deep bite?

A: Adam's *skeletal deep bite* (Figure 3.33) probably resulted from his condyles growing more vertically than normal (as opposed to posterior-superiorly), his mandible rotating forward (internally, true rotation) more excessively than normal (blue arrows), his maxilla descending less than normal, and his molars erupting less than normal. As his mandible rotated upward and forward (yellow arrow), his skeletal deep bite resulted. Adam's *dental deep bite* resulted from excess mandibular incisor eruption. Why did his mandibular incisors erupt excessively? Because he is significantly Class II, his mandibular incisors were unopposed and kept erupting until they occluded with his palate (Figure 3.31q).

Q: What are your treatment goals for Adam?

A: To improve his profile and smile. Ideally, this could include increasing his lower anterior facial height, improving his chin projection, and reducing his labiomental sulcus depth. Additionally, we would like to position his canines (and maxillary molars if he is treated nonextraction) into a Class I relationship and obtain minimal overbite and overjet.

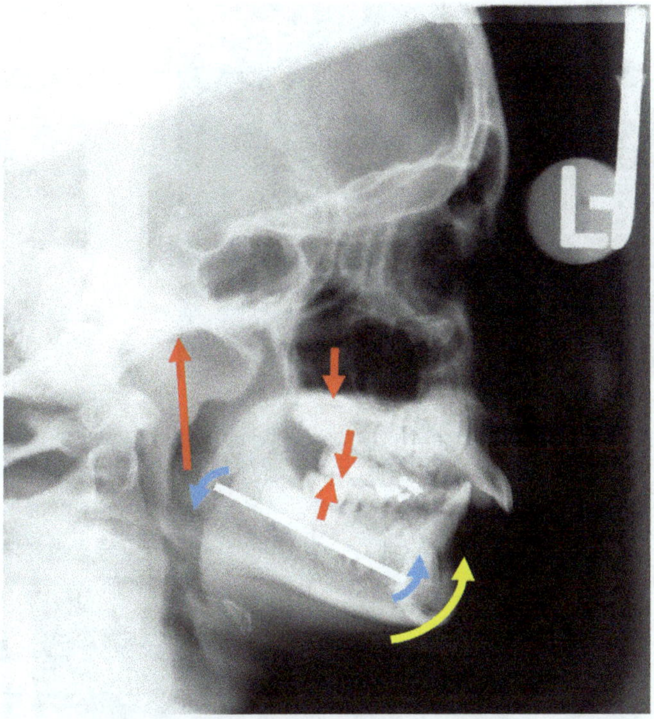

Figure 3.33 Adam probably illustrates the classic growth features found in a skeletal deep bite patient: condyles growing more vertically than normal, mandible rotating forward (internally, true rotation) more excessively than normal (blue arrows), maxilla descending less than normal, and molars erupting less than normal. His skeletal deep bite resulted as his mandible rotated upward and forward (yellow arrow) producing excessive incisal vertical overlap. Excessive eruption of his mandibular incisors contributed to this deep bite as a dental deep bite component.

Table 3.2 Primary problems list for Adam *(apical base/skeletal discrepancies italicized).*

AP	II (5) II (5) II (5) II (5) *mandibular skeletal retrusion*
Vertical	*Skeletal* and dental deep bite
Transverse	—
Other	—

Q: ***First Principle** of orthodontic treatment: define the patient's **primary** problems in each dimension (plus other major problems) and stay focused on these problems throughout treatment. At every appointment, check primary problems in CR.* Considering problems of the face and dentition in each dimension, plus other pertinent problems, what are your primary problems for Adam?

A: His primary problems include the following: See Table 3.2

Q: What are the three general ways that you can treat his AP apical base discrepancy? List specific treatments for each of these three.

A: *Orthopedics* (restrict maxillary growth, while permitting the mandible to continue growing, or accelerate mandibular growth). Options include the following:

- Headgears: The advantage of using either a high-pull, straight-pull, or cervical-pull headgear is that it would distalize the maxillary molars through the maxillary alveolar process bone, restrict maxillary forward growth, and allow the mandible to continue growing forward. In addition, a high-pull headgear may reduce descent of the maxillary corpus and maxillary first molars, potentially further improving AP correction by relative mandibular CCW rotation [24, 67]. A cervical-pull headgear rotates the palatal plane CW and slightly extrudes (<1 mm) the maxillary molars [24, 25]. Since Adam does not demonstrate excessive incisal display, the palatal rotation is of little consequence (or actually helpful in terms of improving his incisal display). A straight-pull headgear would be expected to produce an effect somewhere between that of a high pull and a cervical pull.
- Functional appliances: Since Adam has a low MPA, proclined maxillary incisors, and only slightly proclined mandibular incisors (FMIA = 62°), he would be a good candidate for a Herbst appliance or other functional appliance. Although functional appliances do not enhance mandibular horizontal growth (long term) beyond that found in control subjects [68], the advantage of using a functional appliance would be acceleration of mandibular growth. That is, after 9–12 months of functional appliance wear, you could have a good idea of Adam's final mandibular length and AP correction.

Masking or camouflage (achieving a Class I canine relationship without addressing the underlying AP apical base discrepancy). Masking could be considered later, especially if Adam turned out to be noncooperative or if his mandibular forward growth was poor. At that time, options will include the following:

- Intra-arch mechanics with extraction of maxillary first premolars to permit retraction of the maxillary anterior teeth (leaving molars Class II).
- Intra-arch mechanics using TADs to distalize the entire maxillary arch. As an example, consider using a maxillary noncompliance Class II appliance (i.e., a pendulum appliance) supported by TADs attached to the palatal acrylic button. Noncompliance appliances *without* TAD support (Figure 3.34) are also capable of distalizing molars (red arrows) but at the expense of reciprocal moderate anchorage loss (yellow arrows) which must later be recaptured with headgears or Class II elastics [69–71].
- Interarch mechanics using Class II elastics or Class II springs.

Surgery (mandibular advancement) would generally not be considered with this mild of an apical base discrepancy nor at this age.

Q: Let's take a minute to compare and contrast the *short-term skeletal and dental* effects of headgears and functional appliances in correcting Class II malocclusions in adolescents. How do they work, and how do they differ?

A: Short-term *skeletal* effects include a small restriction in forward maxillary growth with headgears (SNA decreases 0.5°–3°) and a small forward positioning of B-point with functional appliances (1–2°), resulting in an ANB improvement of about 1° in Class II patients with either appliance. A significant portion of the Class II correction with either headgears or functional appliances is *dental*: distal maxillary molar movement with headgears and mesial mandibular molar movement (along with mandibular incisor proclination) with functional appliances [27–31, 33, 72, 73].

Q: What are the *long-term skeletal* effects of treatment for Class II malocclusions in adolescents using cervical-pull headgear, high-pull headgear, or functional appliances?

A: The available evidence, based largely on retrospective nonrandomized studies, suggests that reduction of the SNA angle by cervical pull headgear treatment is largely stable, the SNB angle is largely unaffected by treatment or continued growth, and any

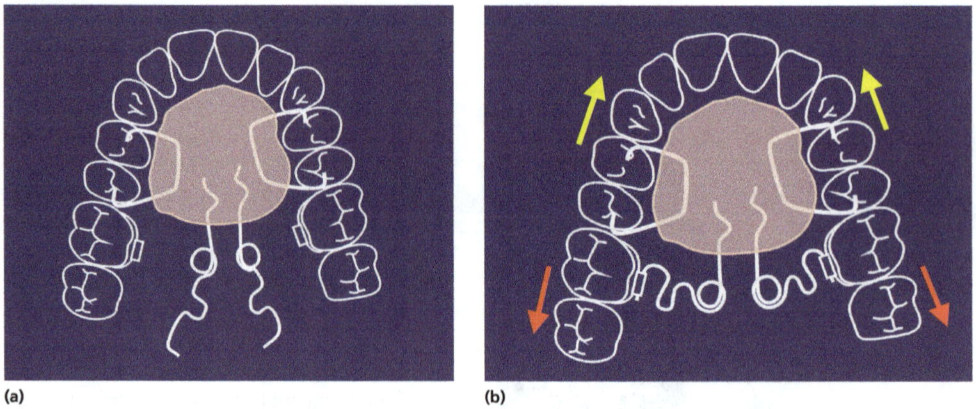

Figure 3.34 Noncompliance Class II molar distalizers, such as the Pendulum appliance (a), are capable of driving the maxillary molars distally when activated (b, red arrows). However, this effect comes at the expense of reciprocal mesial anchorage loss of the anterior teeth (b, yellow arrows). To prevent such anchorage loss, TADs must be placed in the palate and secured to the palatal acrylic of the appliance.

increase in mandibular plane angle caused by treatment is recovered during continued facial growth [26, 74, 75]. The question of whether cervical traction causes a clinically significant change in vertical facial proportions remains equivocal. A similar analysis of the long-term skeletal effects of high-pull headgear is not possible because no long-term evaluations involving its exclusive use are available. The available evidence, based largely on retrospective nonrandomized studies, suggests that over the long-term functional appliances do not modify the inherited facial growth pattern significantly [32]. A lasting enhancement of horizontal mandibular growth is not supported for Bionator, Headgear-Activator, or Herbst appliances, and remains equivocal for the Fränkel FR-2 appliance.

Q: Are headgears and functional appliances, followed by fixed orthodontic appliances, equally effective in correcting Class II malocclusions in adolescents?

A: Headgears and functional appliances (used in conjunction with fixed orthodontic appliances) can effectively correct Class II malocclusions. But higher levels of evidence are missing to answer the question of whether their effects are equal.

Q: *When* should Adam's Class II correction begin?

A: Generally, Class II correction should be delayed until the patient is in the late mixed dentition of development, as opposed to the early mixed dentition [28, 29, 31, 73, 76–78]. But, this rule of thumb is based on dental stage, which is poorly correlated with skeletal growth. *Even if the patient is in the early mixed dentition stage of development, if the patient is beginning to show signs of his/her adolescent growth spurt, you should consider initiating Class II treatment.*

Q: Adam's parents state that he has not begun his adolescent growth spurt. Should you begin Class II or wait?

A: You should wait to begin his Class II correction until either (i) he reaches his late mixed dentition stage of development, or (ii) his parents state that he has begun his adolescent growth spurt (they can begin making monthly height measurements now).

Q: What are the three *general* ways that you can treat Adam's vertical apical base discrepancy? List specific treatments for each of these three ways.

A: *Orthopedics* (Figure 3.35, enhancing downward maxillary corpus growth, increasing maxillary molar eruption, and increasing mandibular molar eruption—all of which would tend rotate the mandible down and back, lengthen his LAFH, increase his mandibular plane angle, and open his deep bite). Options include the following:

- Cervical-pull headgear: In addition to restricting forward maxillary growth and retracting maxillary first molars, a cervical-pull headgear could rotate Adam's anterior palatal plane downward and backward (Figure 3.36, curved arrow) [24, 25], increasing his LAFH and gingival display. CPHGs also erupt maxillary first molars (Figure 3.36, straight arrow), although by less than 1 mm, on average. Using Björk-type implants in cervical headgear patients, Melsen [26] identified this downward and backward maxillary rotation, and a similar indirect effect on the mandible. However, the skeletal headgear effect appeared to be temporary. Studies have

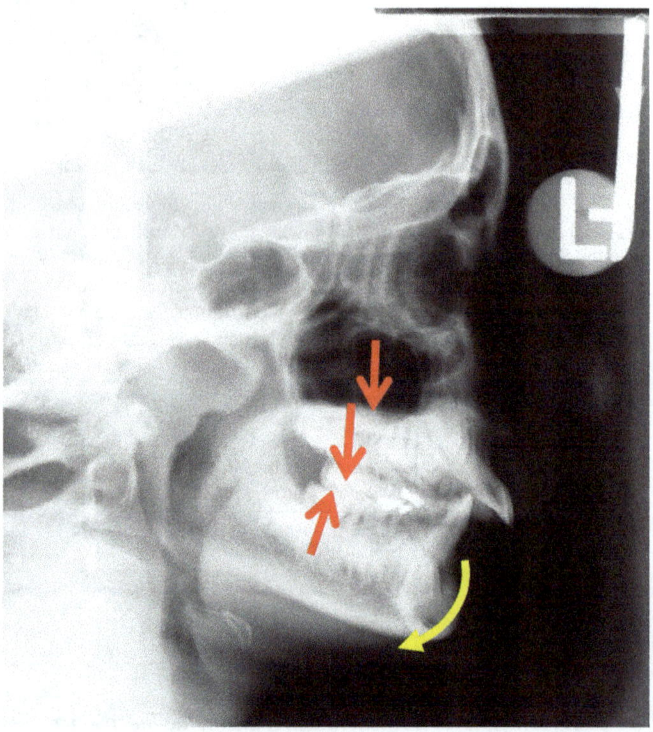

Figure 3.35 Orthopedic changes to improve Adam's short skeletal LAFH would include enhancing maxillary corpus downward growth and increasing molar eruption. As a result, his mandible would tend to rotate down (and back), thereby increasing his LAFH.

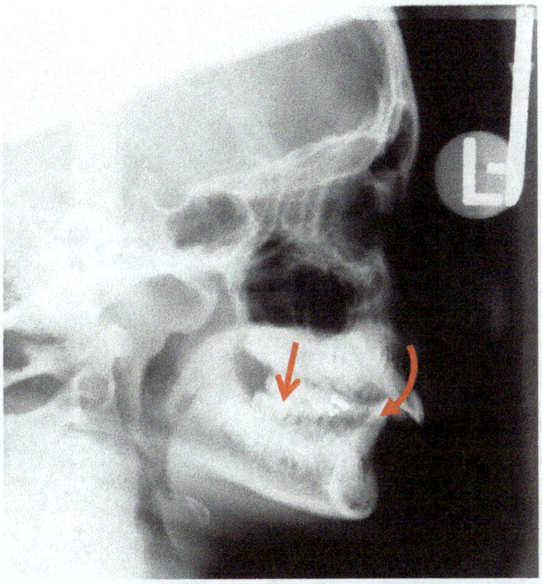

Figure 3.36 Potential vertical effects of cervical-pull headgears include rotating the anterior palatal plane downward and backward, increasing lower anterior facial height and gingival display, plus erupting maxillary first molars slightly (less than 1 mm, on average).

reported that the effects of cervical-pull (Kloehn) headgears range from a slight increase in vertical when measured at Menton [27], and a slight increase in the SN-MP angle [28], to no increase in the MPA [29–31]. *The question of whether cervical traction causes a clinically significant change in vertical facial proportions remains equivocal* [32].

- Straight-pull headgear: For a Class II patient like Adam, a straight-pull headgear could be employed. One study reported a slight increase in SN-MP angle (1°) using straight-pull headgears [28], but we consider this finding equivocal.
- Head gear with a bite plate: Studies have reported headgear/biteplate treatment effects to range from a slight increase in mandibular plane angle (1.3°) [31] to nonsignificant changes in the mandibular plane angle and LAFH [33]. We consider these results equivocal.
- Functional appliances: We also consider equivocal the vertical changes reported with functional appliance use in Class II patients. Activators/bionators are found to have effects ranging from a slight vertical increase when measured at Menton [27], to nonsignificant changes in the mandibular plane angle and LAFH [31, 33]. One study reported a slight decrease in the SN-MP angle (decrease of 0.6°) when using a Frankel regulator [28].
- Leveling the COS: Leveling the COS with archwires occurs primarily through premolar extrusion [11] (alveolar process bone growth). In addition, incisors are intruded/proclined, mesially tipped mandibular molars are uprighted/tipped distally/erupted—potentially increasing the vertical facial dimension.
- Anterior bite plates: Anterior bite plates (or anterior bite turbos) can be used to disclude posterior teeth and assist leveling the COS/eruption of posterior teeth by eliminating occlusal loading. Vertical elastics can be used with, or without (Figure 3.37), anterior biteplates to accelerate posterior tooth eruption (grow alveolar bone) potentially increasing the vertical facial dimension. However, such tooth extrusion may not be stable, long term. If posterior vertical elastics are used to open the bite, you are advised to hold the erupted molars at the new vertical dimension with elastics for some time before debanding—to allow the soft and hard tissues to remodel. Once results are achieved, elastic wear should be gradually diminished to monitor relapse over time.

Masking or camouflage (reducing/correcting Adam's overbite without addressing his vertical skeletal discrepancy. *This is essentially equivalent to correction of a dental deep bite.*) Options include the following:

- Intruding maxillary and mandibular anterior teeth by leveling stepped down maxillary anterior teeth or leveling stepped up mandibular anterior teeth with fixed orthodontic appliances, bonding maxillary and mandibular incisors more incisally than usual, and placing bends (steps) in the archwires to intrude anterior teeth.
- Proclining incisors rotates them forward around their apicies—opening the bite.
- Leveling the COS by eruption of mandibular premolars [23] or by distally tipping/erupting mandibular molars that are mesially tipped, opens the bite. Since alveolar process bone is grown during tooth eruption, and the LAFH can increase as the mandible is rotated down and back, it could be argued that this is orthopedic treatment.
- Discluding posterior teeth with an anterior bite plate, or an anterior biteplate used in conjunction with posterior vertical elastics, can assist leveling the COS/erupting posterior teeth by eliminating occlusal forces. This can help open the bite. Although such treatment can be effective in correcting deep bites, eruption of posterior teeth to increase the vertical facial dimension is really orthopedics and may be unstable, especially in adults.
- Treating Adam prosthodontically to increase his vertical dimension would not be reasonable.

Surgery (increasing Adam's vertical facial dimension by grafting bone to the maxilla). Considering the mild-to-moderate magnitude of Adam's vertical discrepancy, surgery would not be considered, especially at his age. Depending on how unfavorably he grows, surgery could be an option later in life.

Q: Why is it challenging to achieve correction in *both* the anteroposterior and vertical dimensions for Class II skeletal deep bite patients, like Adam?

A: It is hard because of the interrelationship between anteroposterior treatment and vertical treatment. On the one hand, if you do everything you can in an attempt to lengthen Adam's LAFH, then his mandible will rotate CW (down and back), worsening his Class II relationship. On the other hand, if you do everything you can in an attempt to maximize his Class II correction, say by preventing eruption of his posterior teeth so his growing mandible tends to rotate CCW (up and forward), then his LAFH may worsen. Let's illustrate this concept in Figure 3.38. At the top left, we have an adolescent Class II skeletal deep bite patient where the orthodontist is attempting to lengthen the LAFH by increasing maxillary corpus descent and increasing molar eruption. Although an increase in LAFH is achieved (top right), as the mandible rotates downward and backward around the condyle, the Class II relationship worsens. In the bottom left, the orthodontist is hoping to maximize Class II correction as the mandible grows by trying to prevent maxillary corpus descent and prevent molar eruption. Class II correction is maximized (bottom right), but the patient's LAFH remains short.

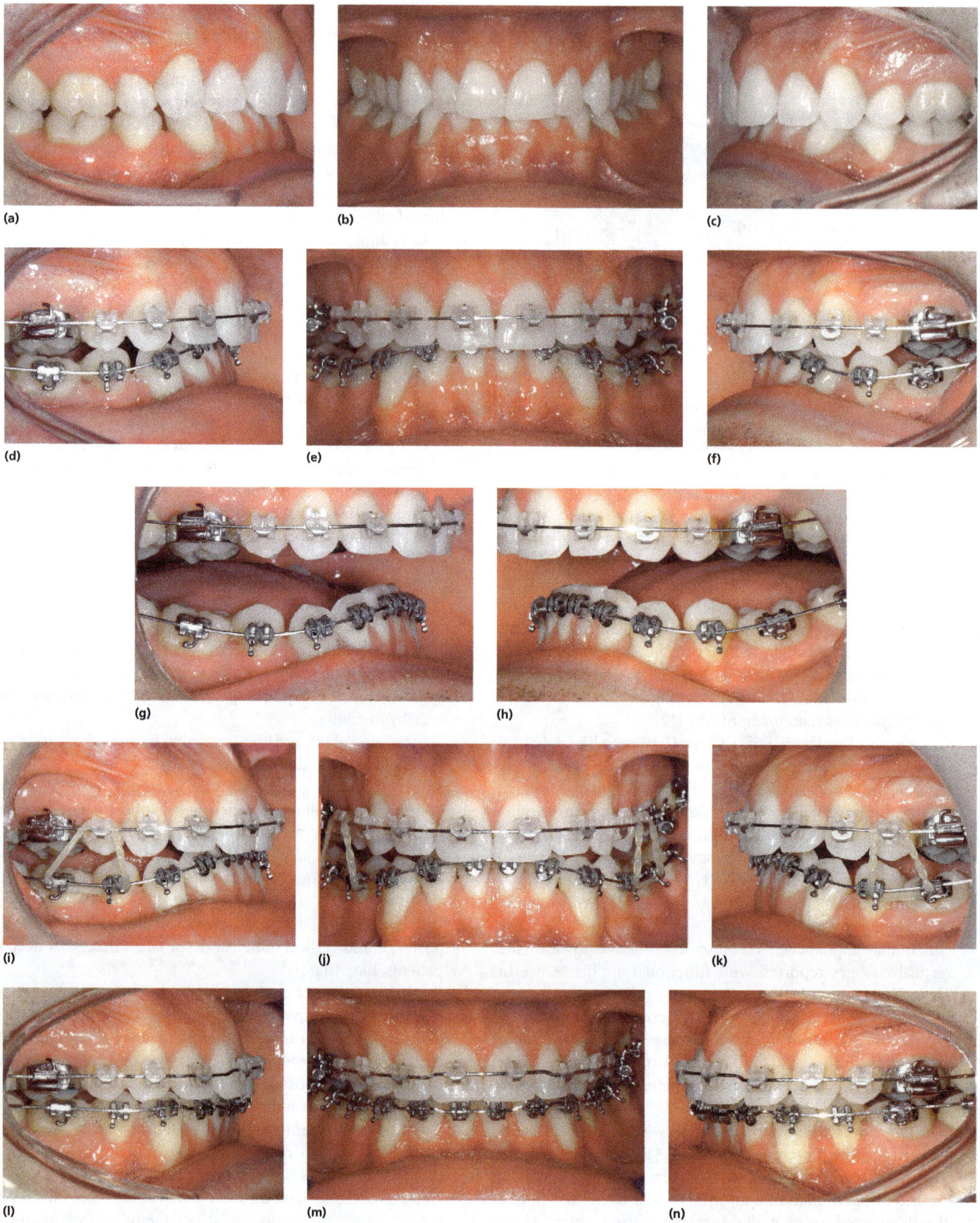

Figure 3.37 (a–n) Use of vertical elastics to assist leveling the curve of Spee. Eruption of posterior teeth potentially increases the vertical facial dimension.

Q: So, which dimension should take priority when treatment planning for Adam?

A: The answer to this question depends on the individual patient—on their chief complaint and magnitude of vertical and Class II discrepancies. In Adam's case, his chief complaint (correction of my bite) involved both the AP relationship and OB, but no concern was expressed regarding his short LAFH. Furthermore, Adam's short soft tissue LAFH was relatively mild, not moderate or severe. Therefore, in treatment planning for Adam, we decided to focus on correcting his deep bite, his AP relationship, but not his short soft tissue LAFH.

In our experience, the majority of Class II mild-to-moderate skeletal deep bite patients (and their parents) focus on having

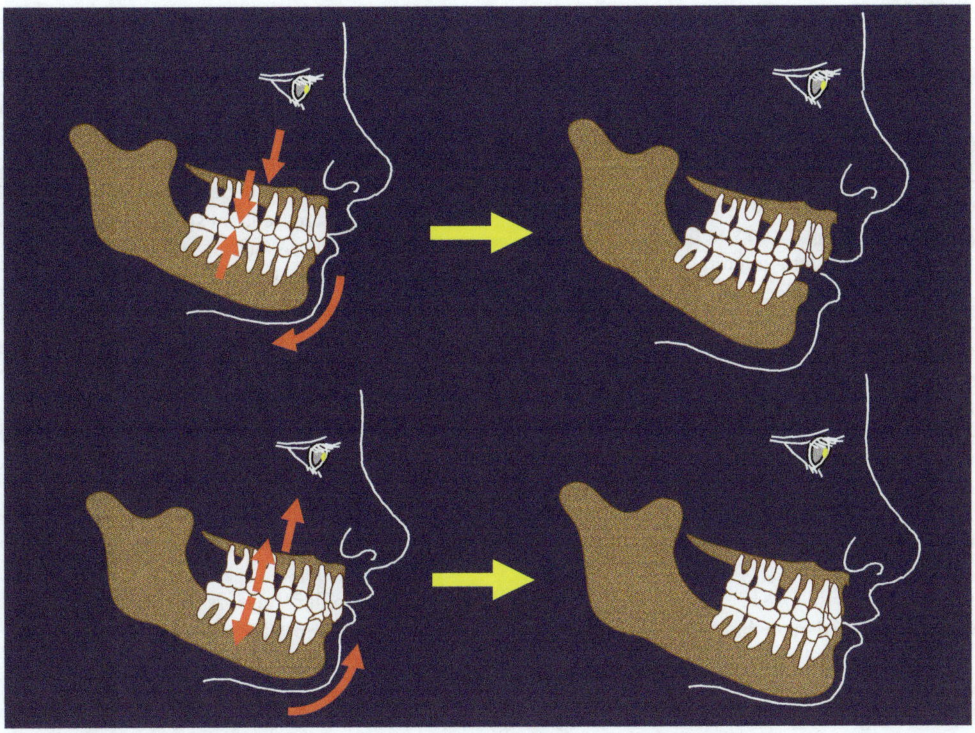

Figure 3.38 The dilemma of trying to achieve correction in *both* the anteroposterior and vertical dimensions for Class II skeletal deep bite adolescent patients, like Adam. If you attempt to lengthen Adam's LAFH (top, left-to-right), then his mandible will rotate CW (down and back), worsening his Class II. If you attempt to maximize his Class II correction, say by preventing eruption of his posterior teeth (bottom, left-to-right), then his growing mandible will tend to rotate CCW, worsening his LAFH.

their anteroposterior relationship (OJ, deficient chin projection) corrected and their deep bite corrected. Most patients and parents do not focus on their short soft tissue LAFH.

However, some patients are concerned with their vertical skeletal deficiency. For patients who present with a short soft tissue LAFH, but who fail to identify this feature as being a concern, you should discuss this finding with them—sensitively. Phrase this finding in such a way that it *does not become* a concern. For example, "Mr. Doe, as your orthodontist it is important that I discuss all clinical findings I have made with you. However, I have to be careful not to convert a finding that was not a concern to you into a finding that is a concern. A range of attractiveness exists in any one facial feature. Does that make sense to you? You have a handsome face. The lower part of your face did not grow quite as much for you as the middle part of your face. To many of my patients, this would not be a concern, but to some it might. Do you have any thoughts about it?" Or, one trick to find out if this has ever been a concern to Mr. Doe is to ask him, "Mr. Doe, have you ever looked in the mirror and thought that you wanted to change this feature?" If Mr. Doe says no, then that is a pretty good indication that his short soft tissue LAFH is not a concern to him. For patients who are concerned with a short LAFH, you should discuss options to address it, or discuss leaving it as a compromise.

Q: In an adolescent, like Adam, how can the effect of future growth impact your treatment outcome?

A: If, during his remaining growth, Adam's condyles grow more vertically than normal, if his mandible rotates forward (internally, true rotations) more excessively than normal, if his maxilla descends less than normal, and if his molars erupt less than normal, then his skeletal deep bite could worsen. On the other hand, if during his remaining growth, Adam's condyles grow more posteriorly-superiorly than before, if his mandible rotates forward (internally, true rotation) less than before, if his maxilla descends more than before, or if his molars erupt more than before, then his skeletal deep bite (short LAFH) could improve. Of course, if his mandible grows forward more than before, then his Class II relationship will tend to improve. If his mandible grows forward less, then his Class II relationship could worsen.

Q: Does Adam have a possible need for surgery, and should you mention this to his parents?

A: Yes. Although Adam is too young to consider a surgical solution now, depending on his (unfavorable) future growth and treatment compliance, he may be a candidate for surgery at a future date to achieve an ideal outcome. This fact should be mentioned to Adam's parents.

Q: What unknowns do you face in treating Adam? Especially, are there any *unknowns you should eliminate* before doing something irreversible (e.g., extracting teeth) or before you establish a final treatment plan?

A: Yes. It would be prudent to ascertain Adam's compliance, amount of growth, direction of growth, and presence of an undetected CR–CO shift before instituting any irreversible treatment or establishing a final treatment plan.

Q: Should Adam be treated without extraction of permanent teeth, with extraction of anterior permanent teeth, or with extraction of posterior permanent teeth?

A: With the mild spacing between anterior teeth and relatively favorable inclination of his mandibular incisors (FMA = 62°), a nonextraction treatment option would be reasonable. However, depending on growth and compliance, later extraction of teeth (possibly maxillary first premolars molars to position his canines into a Class I relationship and to reduce his overjet) may be necessary.

Q: Considering everything we have discussed up to this point, should you begin Adam's treatment now or wait? If you begin now, then what do you recommend doing? If you wait, then what do you recommend doing when you begin?

A: We recommend waiting. As Adam entered his late mixed dentition stage of treatment, he was placed on a high-pull headgear along with an anterior biteplate. He was asked to wear the bite plate all the time (encouraging molar eruption) and his headgear every night from about eight o'clock until the next morning—until his molars were corrected to Class I.

Q: What are the specific objectives of treatment for the maxilla, mandible, maxillary dentition, and mandibular dentition in all three planes of space?

A: Specific objectives of treatment for Adam are as follows:

Maxilla

AP: Restrict forward growth.

Vertical: Restrict downward growth.

Transverse: Allow for normal growth.

Mandible

AP: Allow for normal growth.

Vertical: Allow for normal growth.

Transverse: Allow for normal growth.

Maxillary dentition

AP: Distalize molars and canines. Retract (upright) incisors

Vertical: Minimize molar eruption. Incisor eruption with retraction.

Intermolar width: Maintain.

Mandibular dentition

AP: Maintain molars and canines. Minimize proclination of incisors.

Vertical: Encourage molar eruption and incisor intrusion.

Intermolar/Intercanine width: Maintain intermolar and intercanine widths.

Q: How did Adam's treatment proceed?

A: His cooperation was outstanding. The new Class I molar position was held with a light headgear force when sleeping until all permanent teeth (including his second molars) erupted. At this time, fixed appliances were placed, his arches were leveled and aligned, finishing was completed, and he was debanded. Note: the later decision to place Adam on an anterior biteplate (to encourage molar eruption) contradicts our original plan to focus on Adam's AP relationship and deep bite (but not focus on his short LAFH). By encouraging molar eruption, we are attempting to increase his LAFH by rotating his mandible CW (potentially worsening his Class II relationship). This is somewhat of a growth gamble—you will be hoping for even more mandibular growth than you would have needed to achieve Class I if you had not encouraged mandibular molar eruption.

Q: Adam's deband records are presented in Figure 3.39. What changes do you note? Judge his treatment outcome.

A: Adam achieved a nice orthodontic result. Observations include the following:

- Adam's nose grew downward and forward, his maxillary corpus (A-point) grew nearly straight down, and his mandible (B-point) grew down and slightly forward.
- His profile appears slightly less convex (Figure 3.39c).
- Considering the amount of mandibular ramus/condylar growth Adam had (mandible superimposition), B-point would have come forward more (and his profile would have been even less convex), if Adam's maxilla had not descended as much and his mandibular molars had not erupted as much (tending to rotate his mandible down and back).
- LAFH increased, but so did his midface height (Figure 3.39f), leaving his cephalometric LAFH/TAFH at 50%.
- ANB angle was reduced from 4°to 3° (as anticipated for HPHG wear).
- His Class II dental relationship was corrected through differential mandibular forward growth and not by maxillary molar distalization (Figure 3.39f); OJ was corrected through differential mandibular forward growth plus uprighting of maxillary incisors.
- Inadequate incisal display in a posed smile is still noted (Figure 3.39b).
- Mandibular molars erupted significantly more than the maxillary molars.
- Mandibular incisors erupted much less than mandibular molars erupted.
- OB decreased from 100 to 40%.
- Lip trapping was corrected as the OB and overjet were reduced.
- Midlines are not congruent by approximately 1 mm.
- A number of roots are not parallel (Figure 3.39g).
- Maxillary canines appear to have inadequate mesiodistal tip, especially the maxillary left canine (Figure 3.39h and j).
- Excessive buccal OJ is noted on the left second molars (Figure 3.39o).

Q: How was Adam's deep bite corrected?

A: As shown in his initial-to-deband superimpositions, Adam's mandibular incisors were neither erupted nor intruded. His maxillary incisors were slightly erupted (tending to deepen his bite) as they were retracted. Our point is, Adam's OB was *not* reduced from either incisor intrusion or protrusion. Instead, his mandible descended much more than the maxilla descended (the mandibular incisors descended much more than the maxillary incisors)—opening his bite. Another way of saying this is that *Adam's downward and forward mandibular growth, coupled with his mandibular molar eruption—opened his bite.*

Q: Would a Herbst appliance have been as equally effective in treating Adam as the HPHG was?

A: Yes [32].

Q: To review: what are the skeletal and dental effects of Herbst appliances in growing Class II patients? What are the posttreatment changes during the first 6 months after Herbst treatment is discontinued?

A: Skeletal and dental effects of a Herbst appliance during treatment include the following:

- Inhibition of maxillary growth
- Distal movement of maxillary teeth
- Maxillary molars are intruded in majority of patients
- Occlusal plane is tipped down in the anterior in the majority of patients
- Acceleration of mandibular growth
- Mesial movement of mandibular teeth (mandibular incisors procline) [1]

Post treatment changes include the following:

- Mesial movement of maxillary teeth
- Maxillary molars erupt
- Occlusal plane is tipped upward anteriorly
- Distal movement of mandibular teeth (mandibular incisors upright)
- Less mandibular length increase compared to control subjects [79]

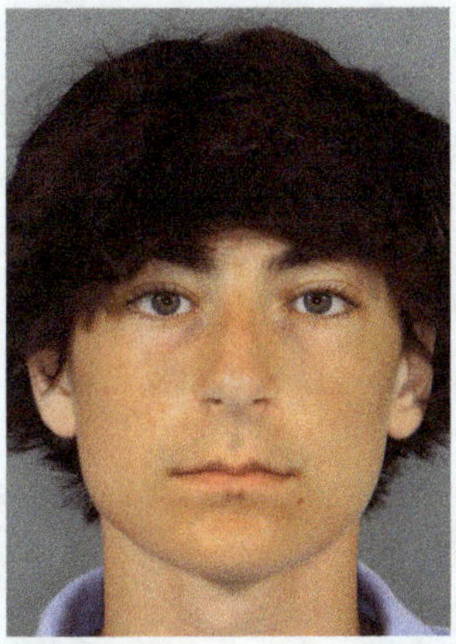

(a)

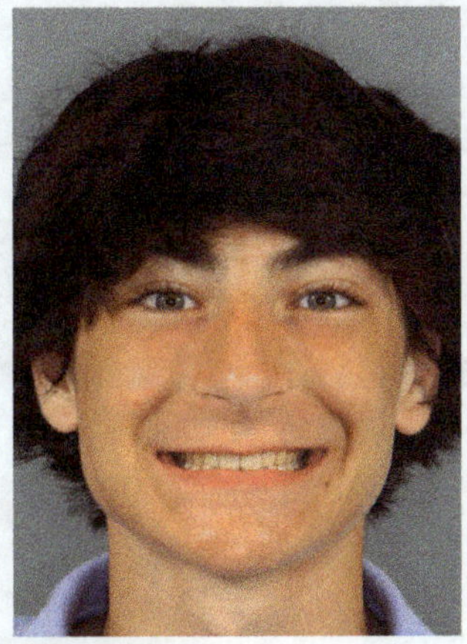

(b)

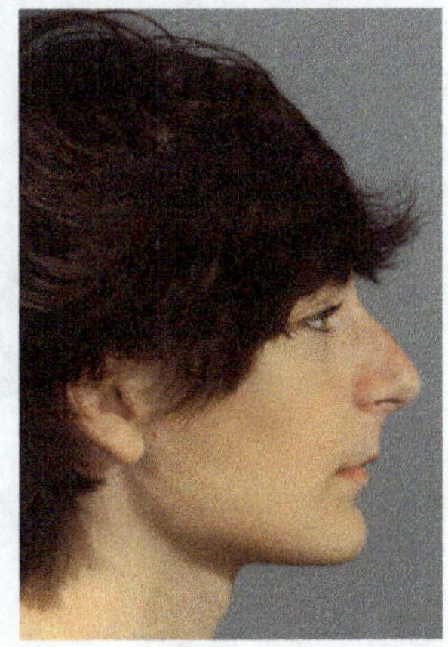

(c)

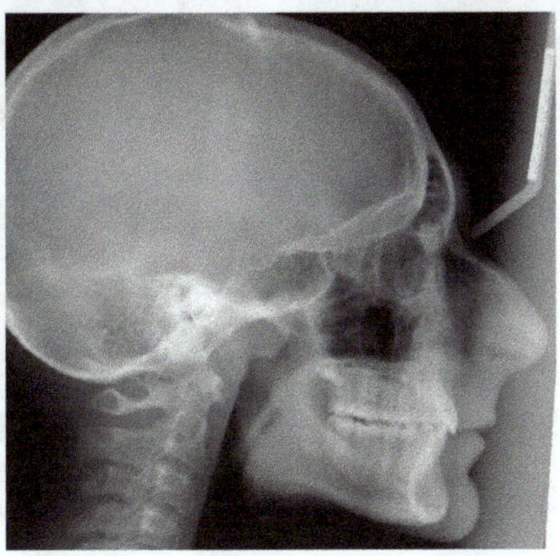

(d)

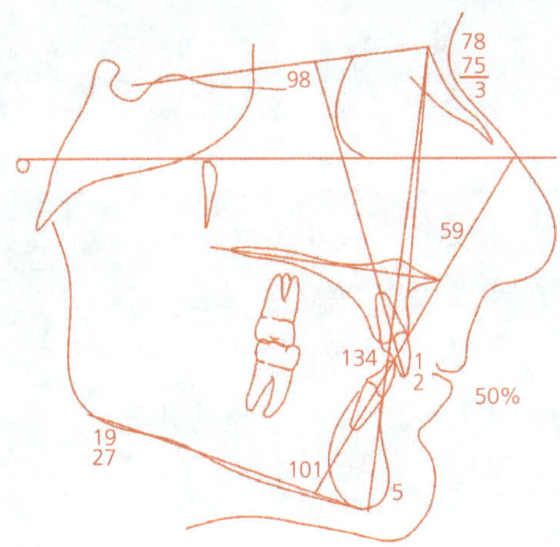

(e)

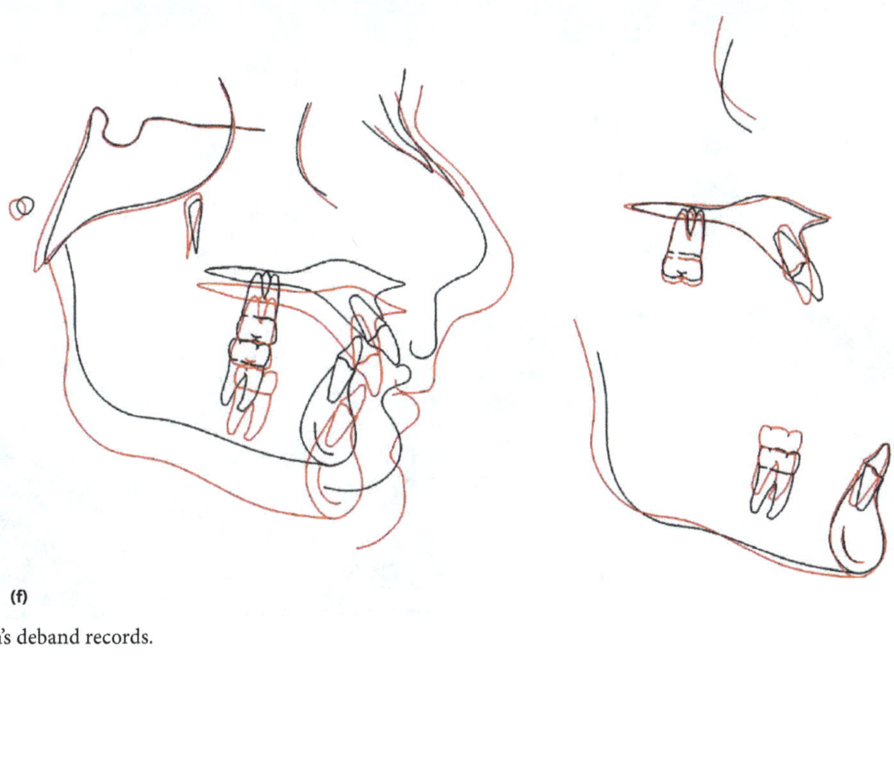

(f)

Figure 3.39 (a–q) Adam's deband records.

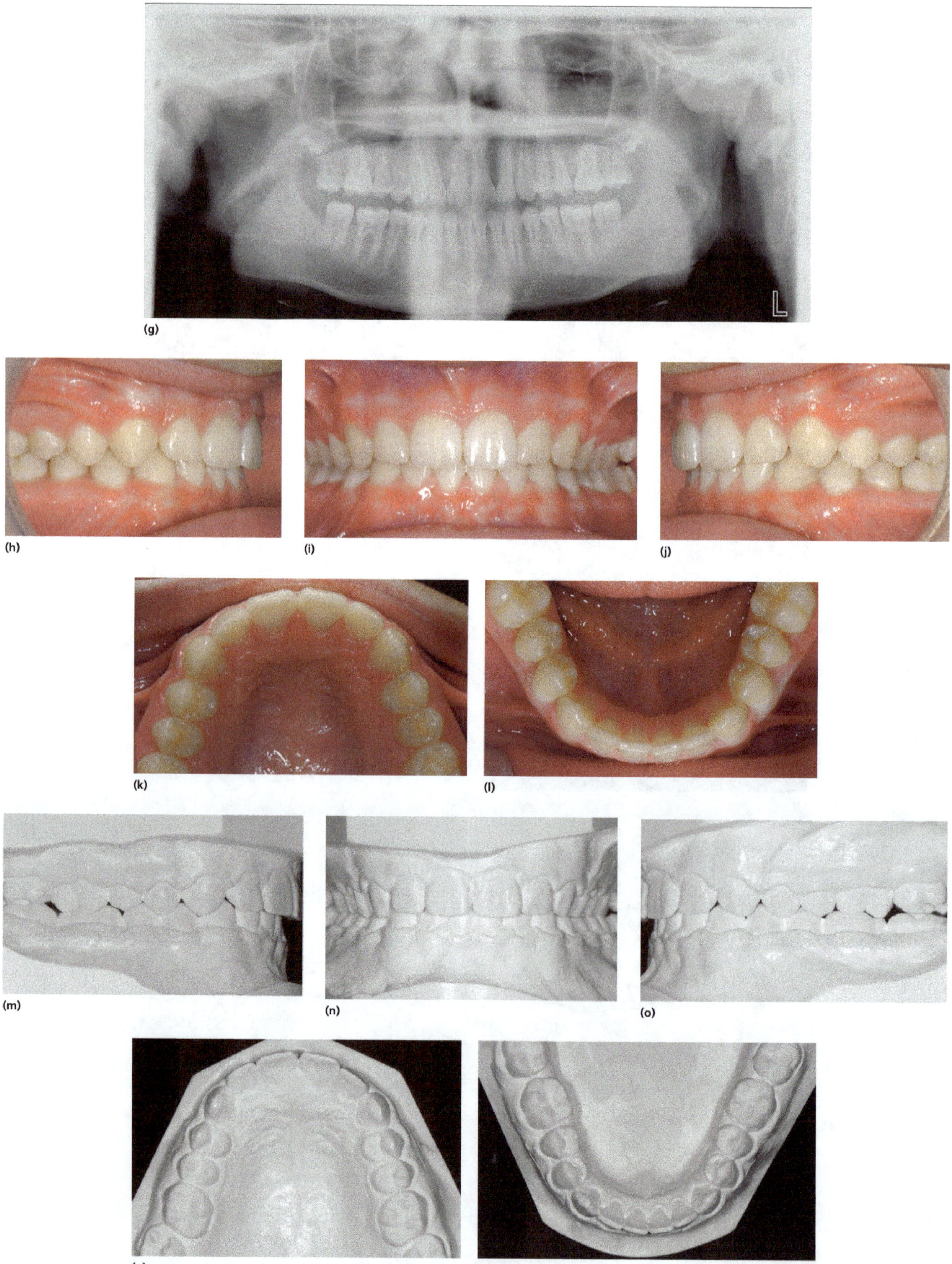

(g) (h) (i) (j) (k) (l) (m) (n) (o) (p) (q)

Figure 3.39 (Continued)

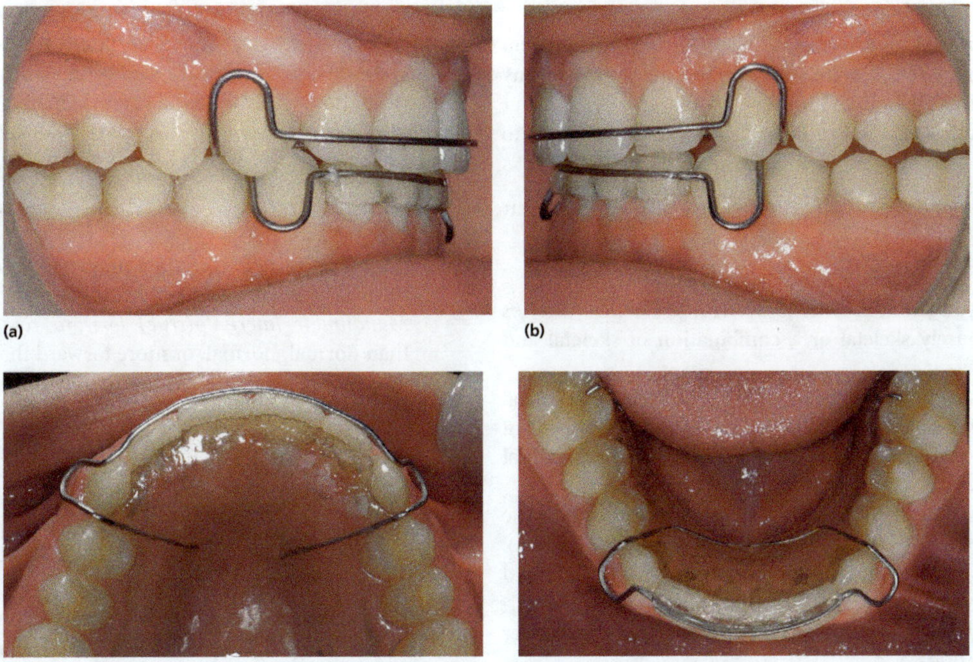

Figure 3.40 (a–d) Adam was placed in maxillary and mandibular Hawley retainers to be worn at night. His maxillary retainer includes an anterior biteplate that discludes his posterior teeth slightly when worn—improving his chances of maintaining OB correction.

Q: Is profile improvement better in growing Class II patients treated with headgear or Herbst appliances?

A: Both treatments result in significantly improved profiles that are similarly attractive [80].

Q: What retention protocol would you suggest for Adam?

A: Adam was asked to wear Hawley retainers every night for a lifetime. Specifically, his maxillary retainers were designed with an anterior biteplate (bite-raising appliance) to disclude his posterior teeth (Figure 3.40) when he wears them at night. This design could improve the chance of maintaining his deep bite correction [51, 52]. His mandibular Hawley retainer has acrylic added labially to insure incisor alignment. This labial acrylic could also have been added to his maxillary Hawley retainer. A fixed mandibular canine-to-canine retainer would also be acceptable in place of a mandibular Hawley retainer, but nighttime wear of the bite-raising Hawley retainer would still be required.

Q: What "take-home" messages can you draw from Adam's treatment?

A: Take-home messages include the following:

- Adam presented with a combination of dental and skeletal deep bite (100% OB with mandibular incisor palatal impingement). His dental deep bite resulted from overeruption of mandibular incisors. His skeletal deep bite (inadequate skeletal LAFH) probably resulted from his condyles growing more vertically, his mandible rotating forward (internally, true rotation) more excessively, his maxilla descending less, and his molars erupting less than normal. As his mandible rotated upward and forward, a deep overbite resulted.
- Orthopedic treatment consisted of high-pull headgear and anterior biteplate wear. The anterior biteplate discluded his posterior teeth. Mandibular molars erupted more than maxillary molars, probably as a result of the high-pull headgear reducing maxillary molar eruption and the anterior biteplate permitting mandibular molar eruption.
- Adam's Class II relationship was corrected from forward mandibular growth and restriction of maxillary growth (ANB reduced from 4° to 3°).
- Adam wore the headgear until a Class I molar relationship was obtained. When using headgears, Herbst appliances, Class II elastics, or other Class II correctors, it is prudent to overcorrect the molar relationship slightly—then hold this correction and monitor the patient for stability.
- If Adam's forward mandibular growth had been less, then an ideal canine and molar relationship may not have been achieved. In this case, either masking (e.g., extraction of maxillary first premolars or Class II elastic wear) or surgery (BSSO advancement) may have been required.
- Adam's OB was corrected by mandibular downward and forward growth—coupled with significant mandibular molar eruption. However, Adam's vertical facial proportions remained approximately the same. He still has less than ideal incisal display when smiling.
- Ideally, his OB should have been corrected even more—to 10%, in anticipation of some relapse during retention.
- The favorable posterior–superior direction of mandibular condylar growth during treatment (Figure 3.39f) aided OB correction. Unfavorable (vertical condylar) growth would have hindered Adam's vertical and anteroposterior treatment.
- The decision to postpone Class II orthopedic treatment until Adam's late mixed dentition stage of development was prudent because we confirmed that Adam had not begun his growth spurt until the late mixed dentition.
- Should Adam have been treated *without* an anterior biteplate? Perhaps. Doing so may have resulted in his lower molars not erupting as much—and B-point coming forward more.

Case Valerie

Valerie is a 14-year-old female (Figure 3.41) who presents to you with the chief complaint, "I want to get braces to straighten my teeth" Her PMH, PDH, and TMJ evaluation are WRN. Her periodontal evaluation is WRN and CR=CO. Valerie is reluctant to smile.

Q: List your diagnostic findings/problems. What is your diagnosis?
A: See Table 3.3

Q: What should you check in order to determine whether Valerie's deep bite is purely skeletal or a combination of skeletal and dental?
A: Not only should you evaluate her soft tissue LAFH and skeletal (cephalometric) LAFH to evaluate the skeletal component of her deep bite, you should also look for the presence of a dental component by evaluating

- Vertical position of the mandibular incisors relative to the mandibular canines (incisors stepped up or stepped down). Ideally, her mandibular incisors would be slightly stepped down relative to the canines. In a dental deep bite, the incisors are overerupted (stepped up by themselves or together with the canines).
- Vertical position of the mandibular canines relative to the mandibular posterior teeth. Ideally, all cusp tips lay on a flat plane. In a dental deep bite, a deep COS may be present.
- Vertical position of the maxillary incisors relative to maxillary canines (incisors stepped up or stepped down). Ideally, the maxillary incisors would be slightly stepped up relative to the canines. In a dental deep bite, the incisors may be overerupted (stepped down by themselves or together with the canines).
- Vertical position of the maxillary canines relative to maxillary posterior teeth. Ideally, all cusp tips lay on a flat plane.

Q: Looking at Valerie's models (Figure 3.42), what do you note?
A: Observations include the following:

- Mandibular incisors are stepped up relative to the mandibular canines.
- A deep (approximately 3 mm) COS is present.
- Maxillary incisors are stepped down relative to the maxillary posterior teeth.
- A relatively flat maxillary occlusal plane is present from maxillary canines to maxillary molars.

Q: When you have Valerie open slightly with lips relaxed (not smiling), what do you note (Figure 3.43)?
A: Minimal incisal display. Whereas a young woman should ideally display between 2 and 4 mm of incisor at rest with lips relaxed, Valerie shows only 1–1.5 mm.

Q: What do the stepped down maxillary incisors mean in terms of anticipated incisal display following maxillary arch leveling?
A: Since the maxillary incisors are stepped down relative to the maxillary posterior teeth, you can anticipate that the maxillary incisors will be intruded following leveling of the maxillary arch and that the amount of her incisal display will diminish.

Q: Is Valerie's deep bite a pure dental deep bite, a pure skeletal deep bite, or a combination of both? What features define either, or both, in Valerie?
A: Valerie presents with a combination of both dental and skeletal deep bites. Her *dental* deep bite features include stepped up mandibular incisors, a deep COS, and stepped down maxillary incisors. Valerie's *skeletal* deep bite features include a mildly overclosed clinical appearance together with a short soft tissue LAFH, short skeletal LAFH (LAFH/TAFH 50%), flat mandibular plane angles, and relatively parallel SN, FH, and MP.

Q: For each of the following four bulleted options, what is the growth pattern (select one) which produced Valerie's skeletal deep bite?

- *Condylar growth direction*: more superior–posterior than normal, normal, or more vertical than normal
- *Mandibular internal (true) forward rotation*: less forward than normal, normal, or more forward than normal
- *Maxillary corpus descent*: less descent than normal, normal, or more descent than normal
- *Molar eruption*: less than normal, normal, or more than normal

A: In a skeletal deep bite patient like Valerie (Figure 3.44), condyles grow more vertically than normal, mandibles rotate forward (internally, true rotation) more than normal, maxillae descend less, and molars often erupt less than normal. As Valerie's mandible rotated upward and forward (yellow arrow), a deep bite resulted from increased vertical incisor overlap.

Q: Valerie is Class II by 3 mm at the right first molar (Figure 3.41m) and Class II by 5 mm on the left (Figure 3.41o). How should you interpret this difference?
A: A difference between right and left molar relationships indicates either a skeletal asymmetry, a dental asymmetry, a lateral CR–CO shift, or a combination. Since Valerie is skeletally symmetric (Figure 3.45) and does not exhibit a lateral CR–CO shift, then a mandibular and/or maxillary dental arch asymmetry *must* be present.

Q: Does the dental arch asymmetry you initially noted (Table 3.3) make sense in view of Valerie's right and left molar Class II magnitude?
A: Yes. You initially noted her maxillary left first molar slightly ahead and her mandibular right first molar slightly ahead compared to their contralateral sides. These dental arch asymmetries result in a worse Class II molar relationship on her left side than on her right side.

Q: Look at Marissa (Figure 3.46) who lacks a CR–CO shift. How does Valerie's dental asymmetry contrast with Marissa's asymmetry?
A: Like Valerie, Marissa differs in her right and left dental AP relationships. Valerie was more Class II on the left than on the right, due to *dental* arch asymmetries. Marissa is Class III on the right, but Class I on her left (Figure 3.46c and e), due to a *skeletal* asymmetry. Her mandibular right condyle grew more than her left condyle (Figure 3.46h), which advanced her mandibular right dentition into a Class III relationship (Figure 3.47), deviated her chin to the left (Figure 3.46a), deviated her mandibular dental midline 3–4 mm left of her maxillary dental midline, and put her into a left posterior cross bite. Her maxillary dental arch is actually symmetric (Figure 3.46f), and there is only a slight mandibular dental arch asymmetry (right posterior ahead, Figure 3.46g), which worsens her right Class III relationship.

Q: So, Valerie had a pure dental arch asymmetry, and Marissa had a skeletal (and slight dental) asymmetry. Both conditions led to

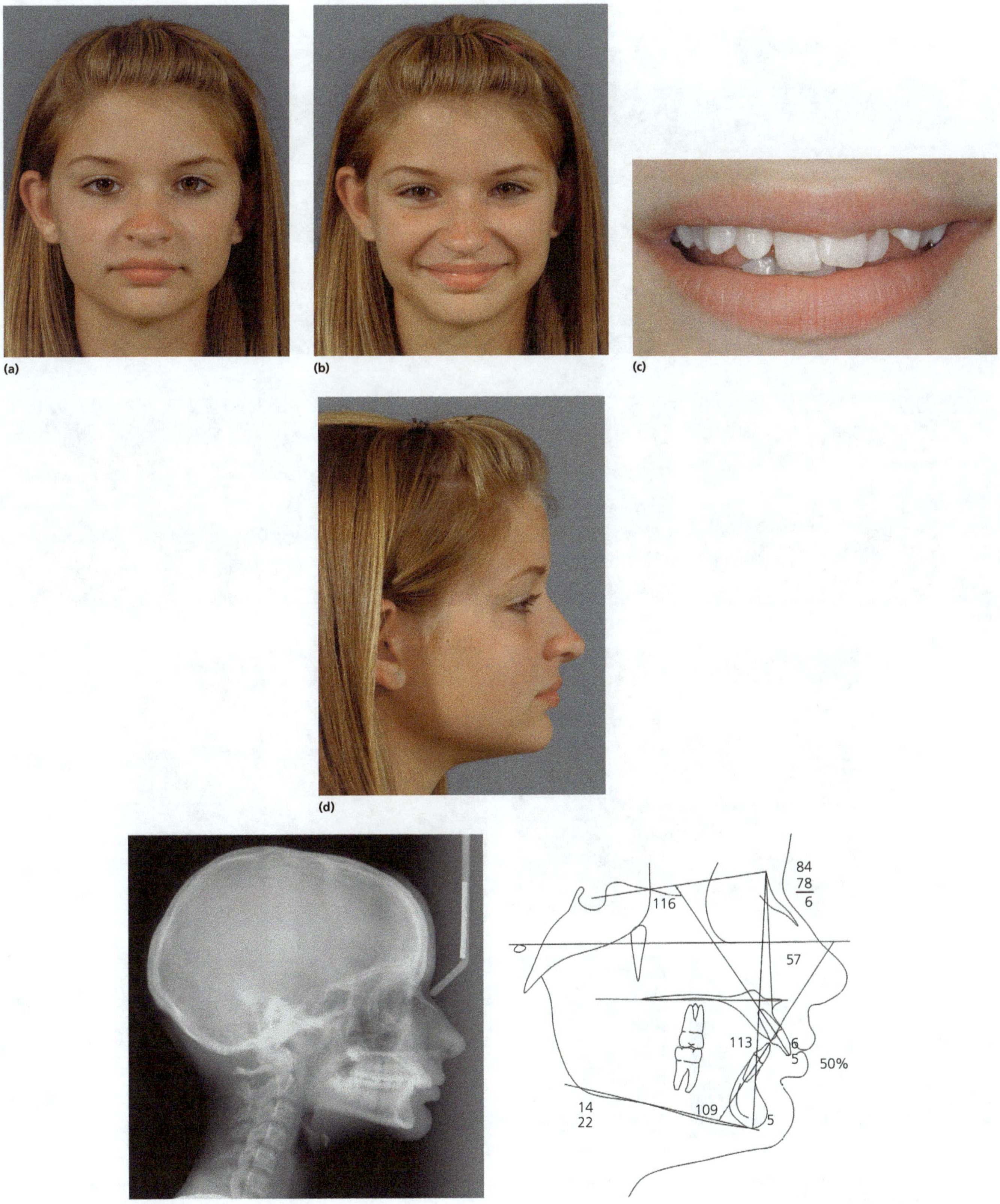

Figure 3.41 Initial records for Valerie: (a and b) facial photographs, (c) close-up posed smile, (d) profile, (e) lateral cephalograph, (f) cephalometric tracing,

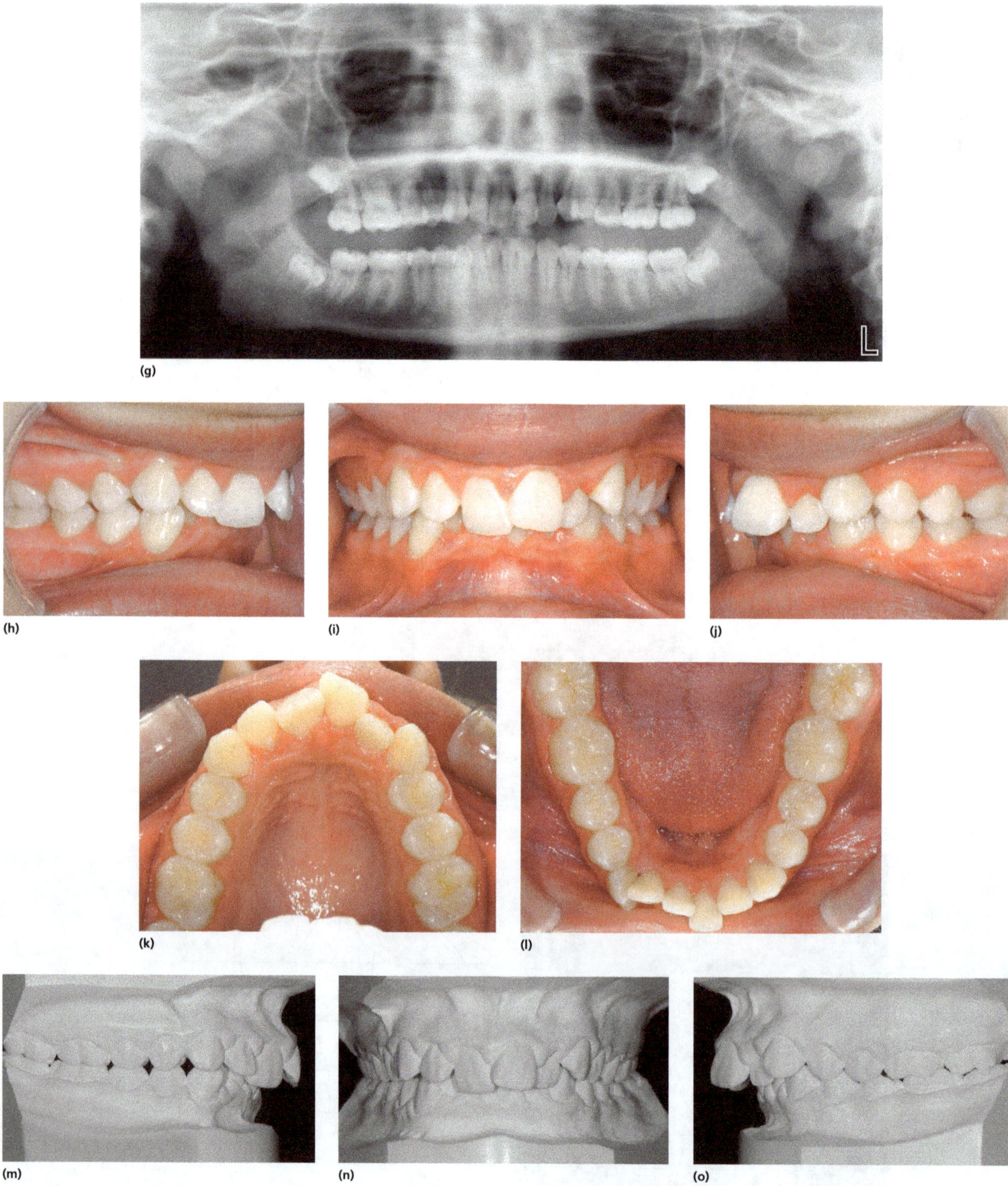

Figure 3.41 (Continued) (g) pantomograph, (h–l) intraoral photographs, (m–q) model photographs, (r and s) occlusal view with lines to determine arch symmetry, and (t) overjet assessment.

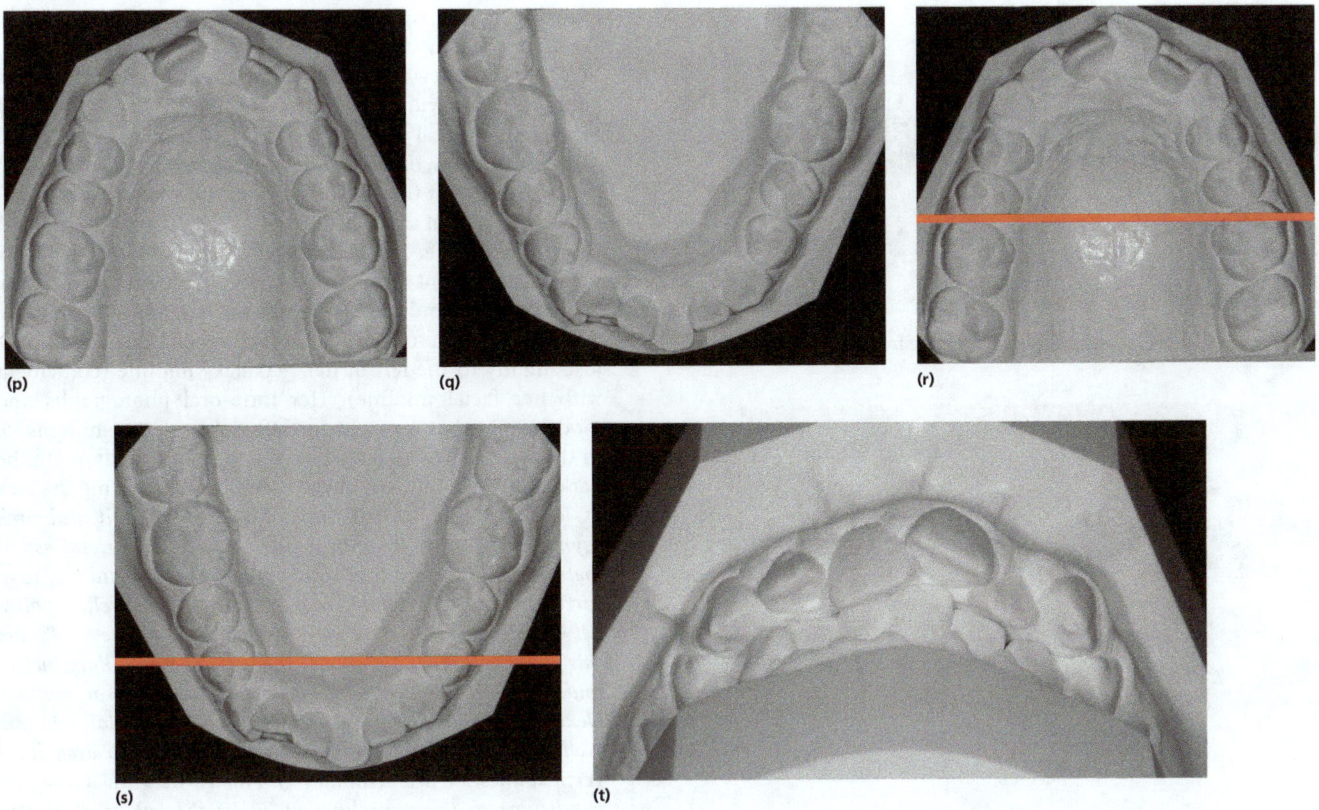

Figure 3.41 (Continued)

Table 3.3 Diagnostic findings and problem list for Valerie.

Full face and profile	**Frontal view**
	Face is symmetric
	Mildly overclosed appearance (everted lower lip, deep labiomental sulcus)
	Mildly short LAFH (Subnasale to soft tissue Menton < soft tissue Glabella to Subnasale)
	Inadequate incisal display during posed smile (maxillary incisors are not fully exposed nor is the maxillary lip vermillion congruent with the maxillary central incisor gingival margins)—despite the fact that maxillary incisors are stepped down
	UDML approximately centered with philtrum
	Profile view
	Chin projection appears adequate
	Obtuse NLA
	Deep labiomental sulcus
	Everted lower lip
Ceph analysis	**Skeletal**
	Slightly prognathic maxilla (NA to FH is slightly > 90°)
	Mandibular skeletal AP hypoplasia (ANB = 6° with slightly protrusive maxilla)
	Vertical skeletal deficiency (LAFH/TAFH = 50%, low mandibular plane angles with FMA = 14° and SNMP = 22°, relatively parallel SN, FH, and MP lines)
	Mandibular lip trapping
	Prominent bony and soft tissue Pogonion
	Dental
	Proclined maxillary incisors (upper incisor to SN = 116°)
	Proclined mandibular incisors (FMIA = 57°)
Radiographs	Permanent dentition stage
	Developing third molars
Intraoral photos and models	Angle Class II division 1
	Iowa Classification: II (3) II (3–4) II (5) II (5)
	OJ: 0–4 mm
	OB: 100% (palatal impingement)
	2–3 mm COS
	UTSALD ~ 4–5 mm
	LTSALD ~ 3–4 mm
	Mandibular midline to right of maxillary midline by ~ 1–2 mm
	Maxillary dental arch asymmetric with left posterior slightly ahead
	Mandibular dental arch slightly asymmetric with right posterior slightly ahead
Other	—
Diagnosis	Angle Class II division 1 malocclusion
	Skeletal and dental deep bite

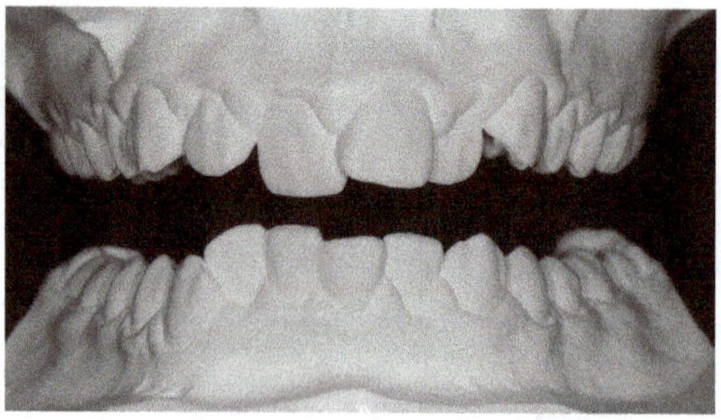

Figure 3.42 Valerie's separated models from the front.

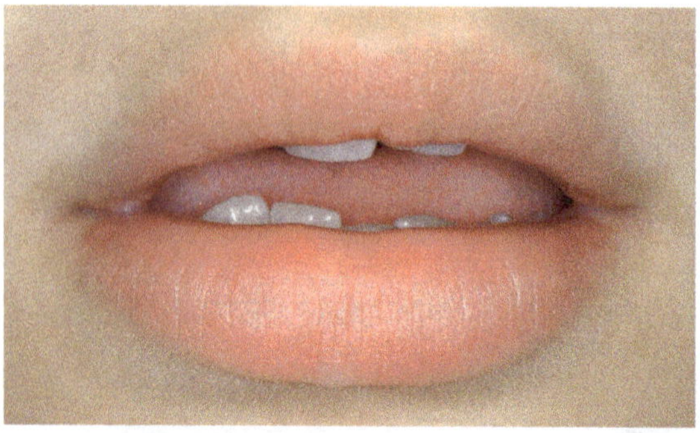

Figure 3.43 Valerie with her relaxed lips and teeth/lips parted slightly.

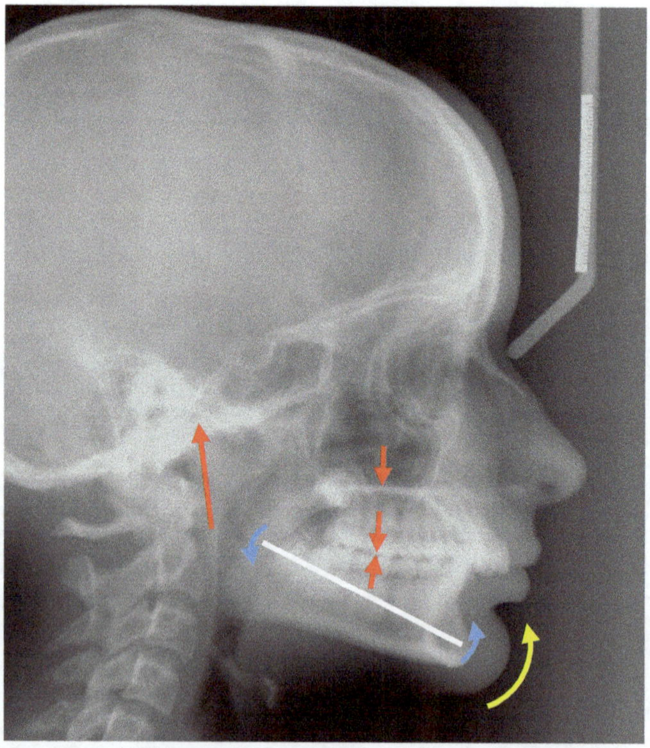

Figure 3.44 Classic patterns of growth which result in skeletal deep bites, like Valerie's: condyles growing more vertically than normal, mandible rotating forward (internally, true rotation) more excessively than normal (blue arrows), maxilla descending less than normal, and molars erupting less than normal. As a result, Valerie's mandible rotates upward and forward (yellow arrow), resulting in a skeletal deep bite (excessive incisor vertical overlap). Her excess maxillary and mandibular incisor eruption added a dental deep bite component.

a difference in right versus left molar AP relationships. Asymmetries play a very important role in orthodontic practice. Let's take a few minutes to talk more about them. What if a patient presents with right and left first molar relationships that *match* in the buccal view (e.g., Class I molars bilaterally, Class II (2 mm) bilaterally, or Class III (1 mm) bilaterally). Does the fact that right and left first molar relationships match always indicate the *absence* of an asymmetry?

A: Not in every case. For instance, examine Taylor, a skeletally symmetric patient who lacks a CR–CO shift (Figure 3.48). Her maxillary midline is slightly to the right of her facial midline (1–2 mm to the right), and her mandibular midline is just slightly to the left of her maxillary midline (coincident with her facial midline). Her intra-oral photographs and models show that her right and left molar relationships *match* in the buccal view (Class II by 1–2 mm, bilaterally; note the dark "Class II windows" at the premolars illustrating the lack of ideal occlusal articulation). Now, *to detect dental arch asymmetries, we first confirm the absence of a skeletal asymmetry. Next, we transfer the patient's facial midline to a corresponding point on the incisors of her models (yellow points between central incisors, Figure* 3.48*j and k). Notice for Taylor, this facial midline is 1–2 mm to the left of her maxillary incisor midline and coincident with her mandibular incisor midline. Next, we imagine a line drawn from those facial midlines (yellow points) running along the midline of each arch (blue vertical lines, Figure* 3.48*j and k). Finally, we draw a line perpendicular to these midlines at either the left or right first molar/second premolar contact (red horizontal lines, Figure* 3.48*j and k)*. Based on these red horizontal lines, we see that Taylor does have a maxillary and mandibular dental asymmetry. In fact, Taylor's right and left first molars' AP

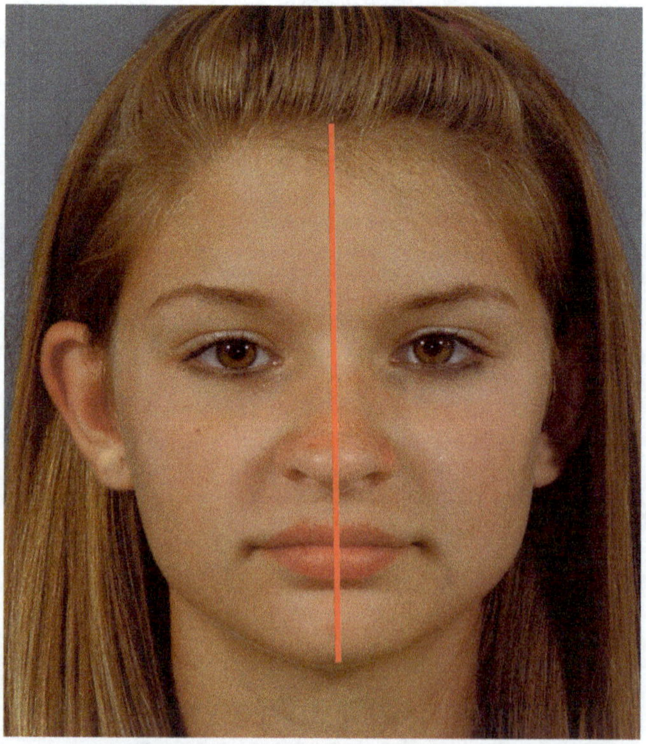

Figure 3.45 Valerie's brow, nose, philtrum, lips, and chin are all symmetric. She is skeletally symmetric.

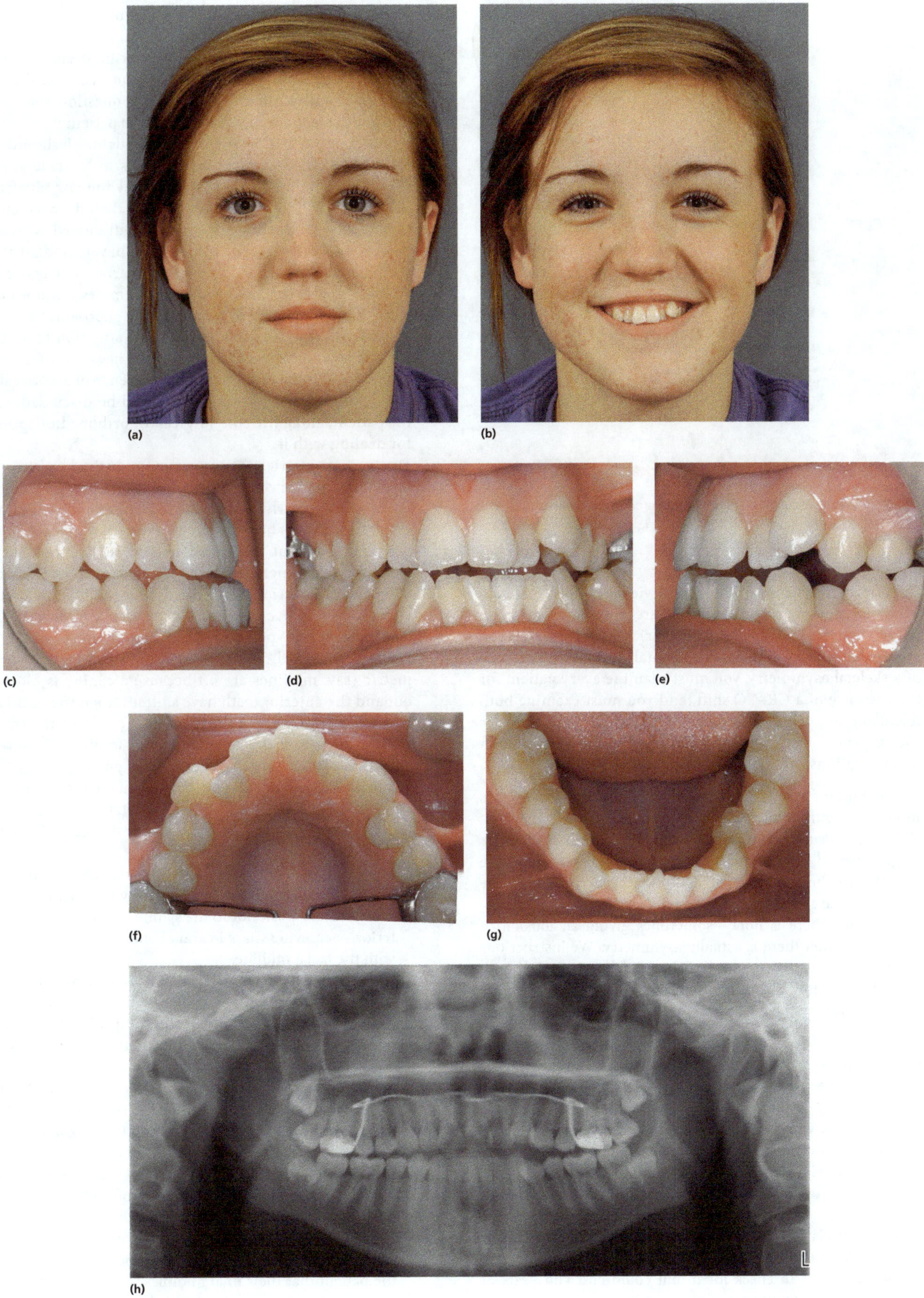

Figure 3.46 (a–h) Initial records of Marissa.

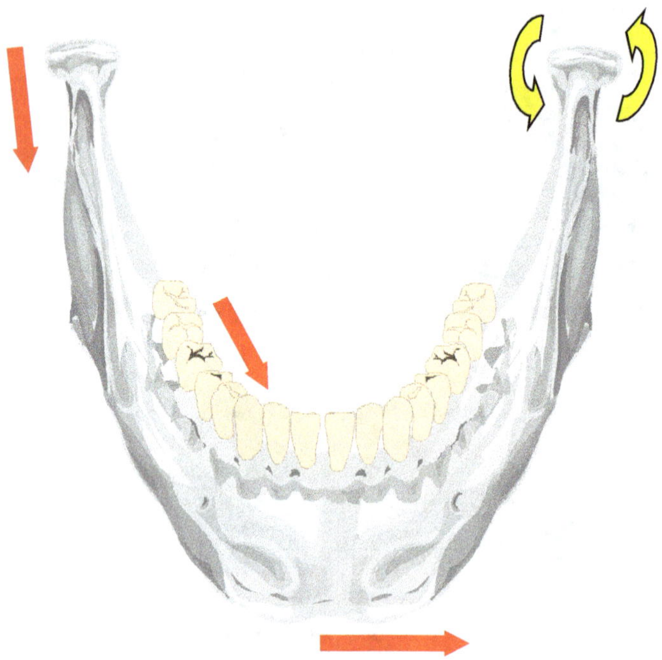

Figure 3.47 Marissa's excessive right mandibular condylar growth produced a Class III dental relationship on her right, deviation of her chin to the left, and a left posterior cross bite.

classification matches in the buccal view only because *both* maxillary and mandibular arches are equally asymmetric (right posterior ahead of left posterior). Our point is that you must examine each patient in the frontal view for the presence of a skeletal asymmetry, you must examine every patient for the presence of a CR–CO shift, and you must examine both maxillary and mandibular models from the occlusal view for the existence of a dental asymmetry even if the right and left molar relationships match in the buccal view.

Q: One important note: we did not include the "heels" of Taylor's models in Figure 3.48j and k. Why not?

A: The *heels of dental models should never be used as references for judging dental arch asymmetries*. Why? Your lab may have trimmed the heels at an angle instead of perpendicular to the midline of the arch —sometimes giving an illusion of an asymmetry when there is none—sometimes giving an illusion of symmetry when there is actually asymmetry. We instruct our residents to cover up the heel of the model with their thumb when looking for left to right dental asymmetries, so they are not led astray by the heel of the model having been trimmed incorrectly.

Q: Ok, let's assume that you have followed the aforementioned steps and detected a skeletal and/or dental asymmetry. What are your next steps in treating asymmetries?

A: Steps to follow when treating asymmetries:

- First, always *confirm the absence of a CR–CO shift*. An undetected CR–CO shift can give the false impression of an asymmetry where one does not exist. If you detect a shift, then eliminate the CR–CO shift before establishing your final treatment plan. *You should make it a habit to routinely check for a CR–CO shift in every patient at every appointment*. It only takes 10 s to check for it, but could cost you years of additional treatment time, if you miss it.
- Skeletal asymmetries: Identify the magnitude of the asymmetry, which is key to managing asymmetries. No person is perfectly symmetric. So, if you look hard enough, you will find a facial asymmetry in everyone. Is a mild skeletal asymmetry worth treating? This is a question that only you and the patient can answer. Ask the patient if he or she has ever looked in a mirror and thought, "I should do something about the way my chin sits to the side," or "I should do something about the way my top jaw tilts from left-to-right." If they have thought this, then the correction of the skeletal asymmetry should be discussed with the patient and the surgeon. If they have never thought this, then maybe the asymmetry does not warrant correction. If a person has a very mild skeletal asymmetry but does not bring it up as a concern, then you may choose not to even discuss it. Why? As soon as you draw attention to a mild skeletal asymmetry, some patients will negatively focus on it, forever. On the other hand, the presence of a noticeable (moderate) skeletal asymmetry should be discussed with the patient, along with the surgical (or orthopedic) options for dealing with it.
- Dental asymmetries: There are many orthodontists who immediately worry about dental midlines being off to the facial midline early in treatment. You shouldn't. Do not focus on midlines being off to the face, or off to each other early in treatment. Instead, focus your attention on the symmetry/asymmetry of the posterior portion of the arch. Why? The posterior occlusion is the foundation of the arch. *Your objective is to achieve symmetry of the posterior dentition*. If the posterior dentition in both arches is symmetric, but the anterior dentition is initially asymmetric (say, midlines are off because a canine is blocked out and the anterior teeth have shifted), then the midlines should end up being coincident at the end of treatment (unless, of course, an anterior Bolton tooth size discrepancy exists). On the other hand, if the posterior dentition is initially asymmetric, you must either try to improve/correct it, or leave it and settle for dental midlines ending up off to the facial midline when the case is done. Guidelines include the following:
  1. If the mandibular posterior arch is *symmetric* to the face, but the maxillary posterior arch is *asymmetric*, then treat the maxillary posterior to the symmetric mandibular posterior—achieving Class I canines and midlines coincident with the facial midline.
  2. If the mandibular posterior arch is *asymmetric*, then you have two options: either treat the maxillary arch to the asymmetric mandibular arch (finishing with dental midlines coincident but off to the facial midline), or improve/correct the mandibular asymmetry and treat the maxillary arch to it. For a *mild mandibular posterior asymmetry*, try to incorporate biomechanics, which could improve it. If this is not possible, consider treating the maxillary dentition to the mild mandibular asymmetry. Why? If you leave the mild mandibular asymmetry and treat the maxillary arch to it, then the midlines will end off to the facial midline—but lay persons will be unlikely to notice this (even if the midlines are off to the face by > 4 mm) [81, 82]. If you chose to leave the mild asymmetry, be sure to explain to the patient that their final midlines will be off to the face. For a *moderate to severe mandibular posterior asymmetry*,

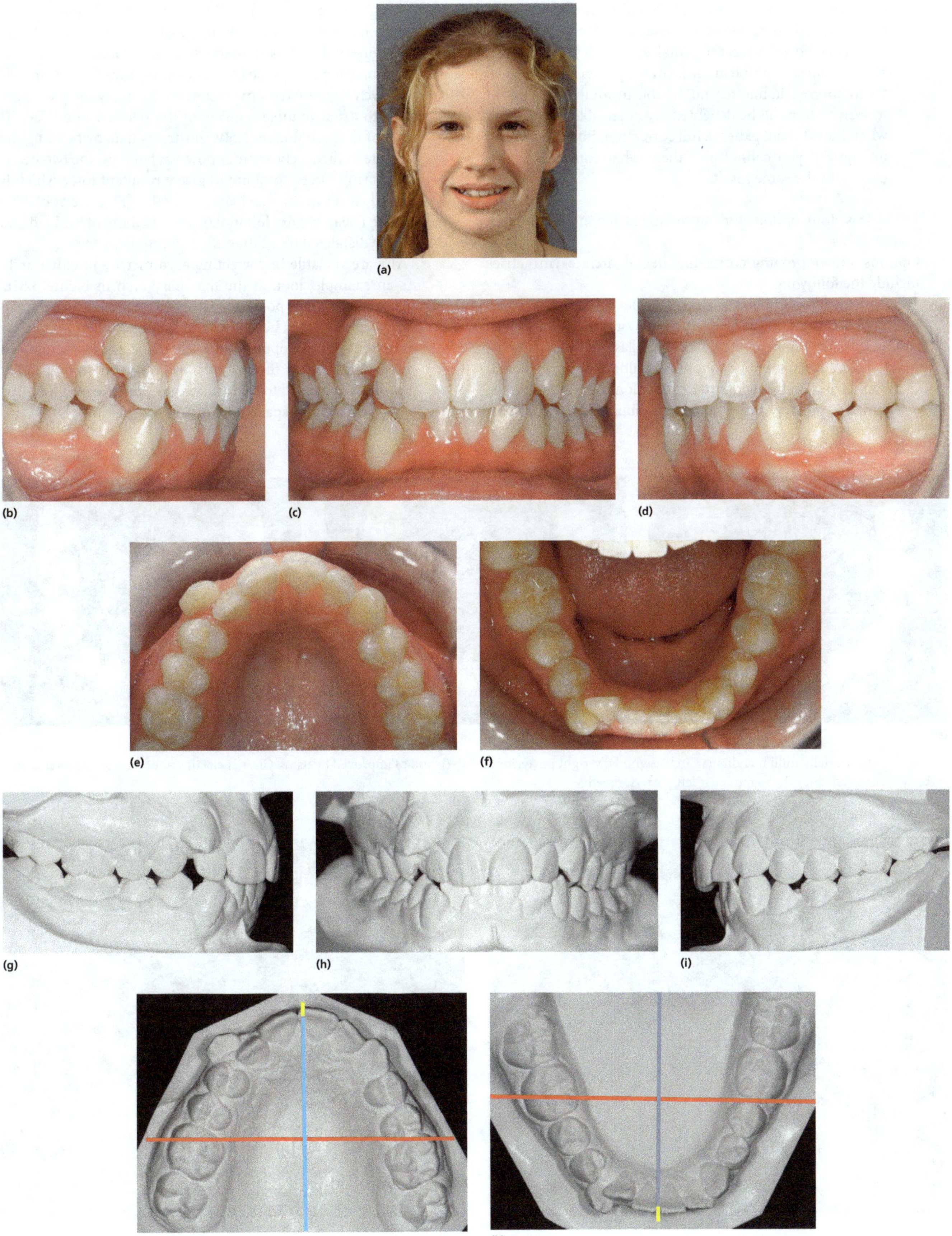

Figure 3.48 (a–k) Taylor's initial records. Taylor is skeletally symmetric, lacks a CR–CO shift, and has an identical dental arch asymmetry in the maxilla and mandible (right posterior slightly ahead of left), resulting in matching right and left first molar relationships (Class II by 1–2 mm) when viewed from the buccal.

try to correct or improve it, and treat the maxillary arch to the improved/corrected mandibular asymmetry.

3 When trying to correct a dental asymmetry (or frankly, any orthodontic problem), inform the patient that you will try to improve it, but may not be able to completely correct it. Why? They will be delighted if you are able to correct it when they did not expect a full correction. But, they will be unhappy if you cannot give them what you promised—even with the same result.

Q: List at least four options for improving/correcting dental arch asymmetries.

A: Options for improving/correcting dental arch asymmetries include the following:

1 Inter-arch biomechanics such as unilateral Class II elastics, Class III elastics, other Class II force systems (Forsus appliances, Jasper Jumpers, etc.), or other Class III force systems (DynaFlex springs, etc.) can improve mild to moderate dental asymmetries in the appropriate situations. As an example, Figure 3.49 illustrates a very mild mandibular arch asymmetry (patient's right posterior slightly ahead of left) improved by advancing the left mandibular posterior dentition slightly using one of the Class II interarch force systems.

2 Asymmetric facebow headgears can improve Class II maxillary arch asymmetries by preferentially applying a stronger force to distalize molars more on the selected side (Class II side) of the arch. Figure 3.50a illustrates that, by bending the left side of the facebow outer bow out laterally, the two headgear spring forces combine to give a resultant force which is shifted closer to the maxillary left molar (Figure 3.50b). The result? The maxillary left molar receives more of the load and will be distalized more than the right molar.

3 TADs are versatile in correcting asymmetries in either arch. As an example, look at the maxillary arch in Figure 3.51a. The patient's right posterior is slightly ahead of her left. To complicate matters, her left lateral incisor and left first molar were considered hopeless and scheduled for extraction. To complicate matters further, her maxillary left second molar (not shown) needed to be advanced to close the resulting first molar extraction space. Following extraction of the two

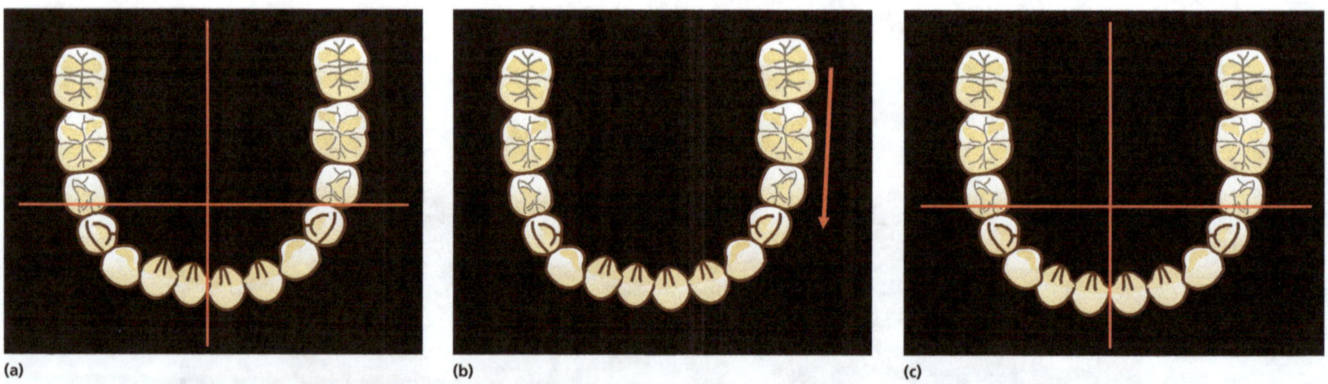

Figure 3.49 (a) Initially mild mandibular arch asymmetry, right posterior ahead, (b and c) improved by using Class II elastics or other Class II interarch force systems to advance the mandibular left posterior teeth.

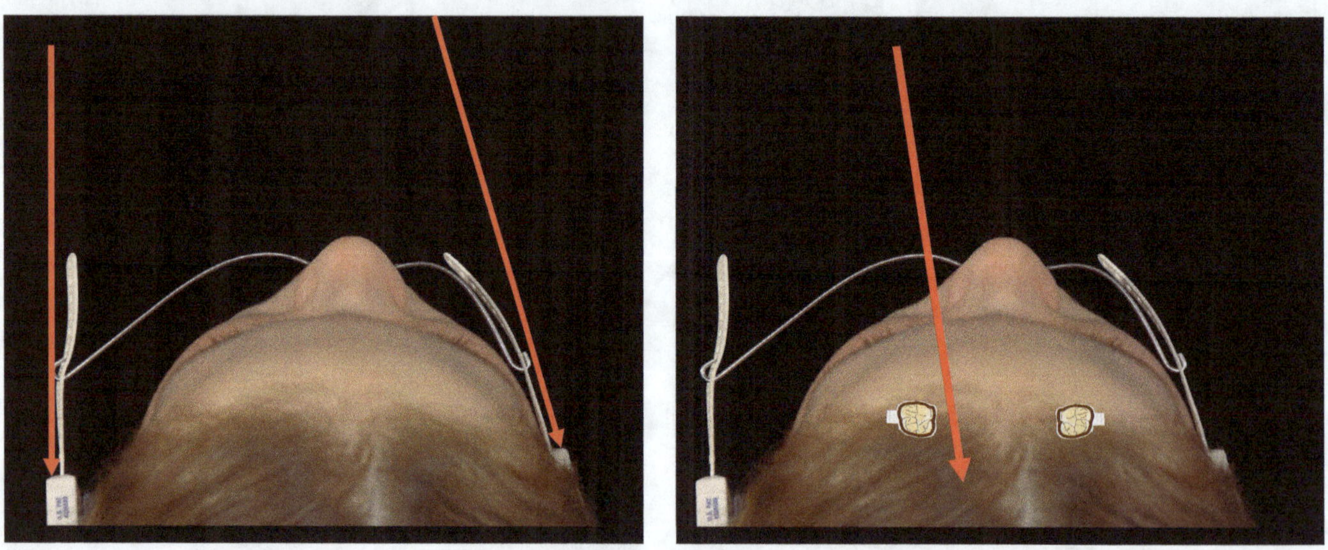

Figure 3.50 (a) An asymmetric left facebow headgear is created by bending the left arm of the facebow laterally. (b) The resultant force vector is brought closer to the left molar—loading and distalizing it more.

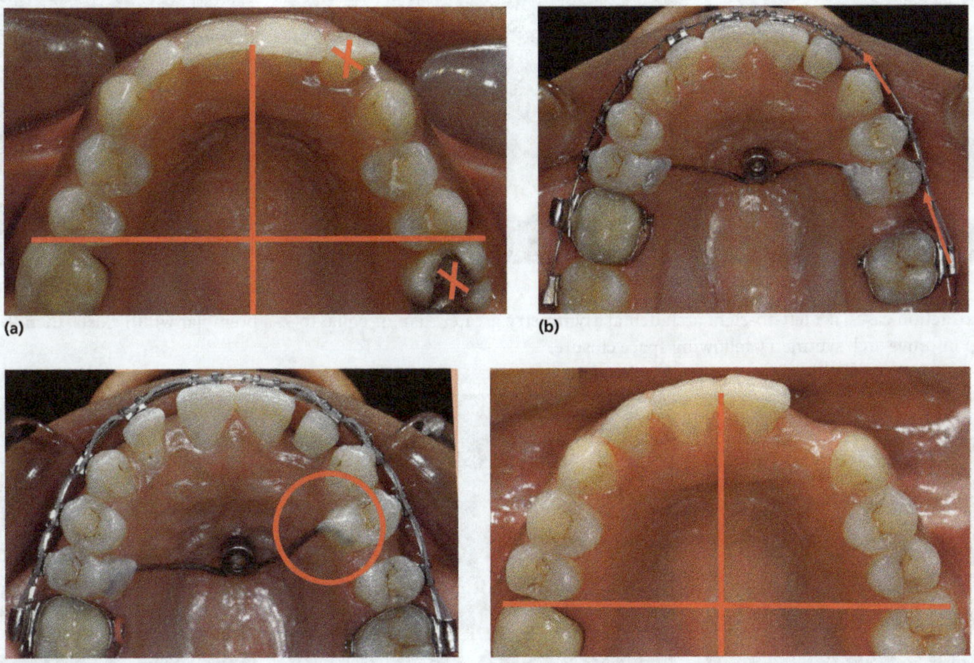

(a) (b) (c) (d)

Figure 3.51 TADs can useful in correcting dental asymmetries: (a) in this case, a slight maxillary (right posterior ahead) asymmetry exists and the maxillary left lateral incisor plus left first molar were deemed hopeless and extracted; (b–d) a palatal TAD was used to move the left canine and premolars forward into symmetry with the right—and to move the maxillary left second molar forward to replace the extracted left first molar.

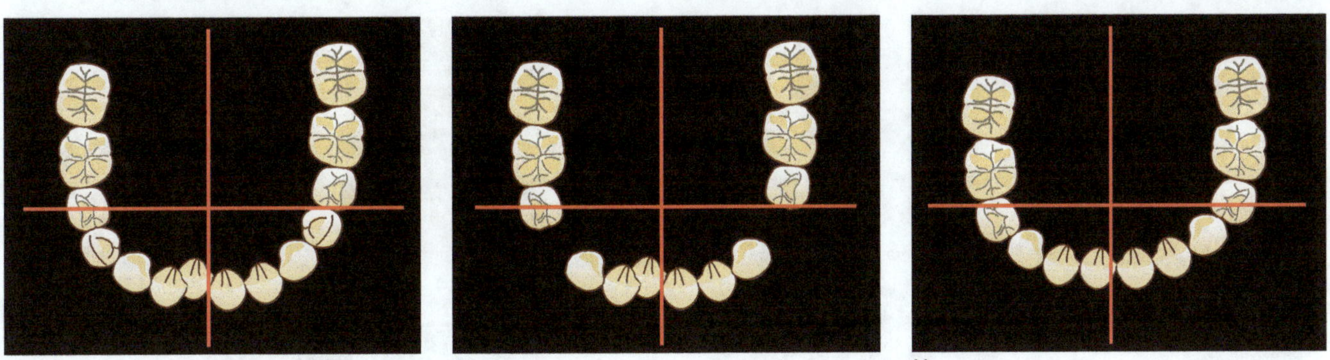

(a) (b) (c)

Figure 3.52 (a) In extraction cases, if a left-to-right dental arch asymmetry less than or equal to ½ a premolar width exists, then (b and c) it is generally best to extract symmetrically and improve the arch asymmetry using biomechanics.

teeth, and using a palatal TAD as anchorage connected to the second premolars (Figure 3.51b), the left canine and left first premolar were advanced into a symmetrical position with the right canine and right first premolar. Protraction of the left second molar was then begun. Later, the TAD was reattached to the maxillary left first premolar (Figure 3.51c), and the maxillary left second premolar and second molar were advanced. The asymmetry was corrected nicely (slightly overcorrected, Figure 3.51d). Without the use of this TAD, space closure on the patient's left could have resulted in a severe asymmetry.

4 In extraction cases, thoughtful extraction choices can improve arch asymmetries. *If the left-to-right arch asymmetry is less than or equal to ½ a premolar width (Figure 3.52a), it is generally best to extract symmetrically* and improve the asymmetry using biomechanics (e.g., Class II elastics and TADs). Of course, you should inform the patient that the asymmetry may be improved but not fully corrected (Figure 3.52b and c).

5 *In extraction cases, with a left-to-right arch asymmetry greater than or equal to ½ a premolar width (Figure 3.53a), consider extracting asymmetrically.* For example, extraction of a first premolar on the more mesially positioned side, and extraction of a second premolar on the more distally positioned side (Figure 3.53a) can result in more advancement of the molars on the more distally positioned side—and help correct the asymmetry with reciprocal space closure (Figure 3.53c).

6 If the left-to-right arch asymmetry is a full premolar width, then a single premolar extraction may be ideal. However, for asymmetries less than a full premolar width (Figure 3.54a), extraction of a single premolar on the more mesially positioned side can create an equal, but reversed, asymmetry on

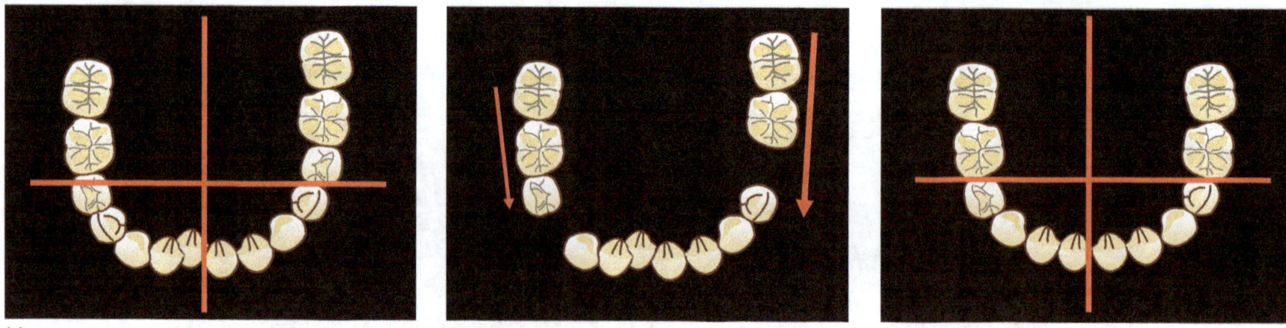

(a) (b) (c)

Figure 3.53 (a) In extraction cases, if a left-to-right arch dental asymmetry greater than or equal to ½ a premolar width exists, then (b and c) asymmetric extractions may help improve arch symmetry following space closure.

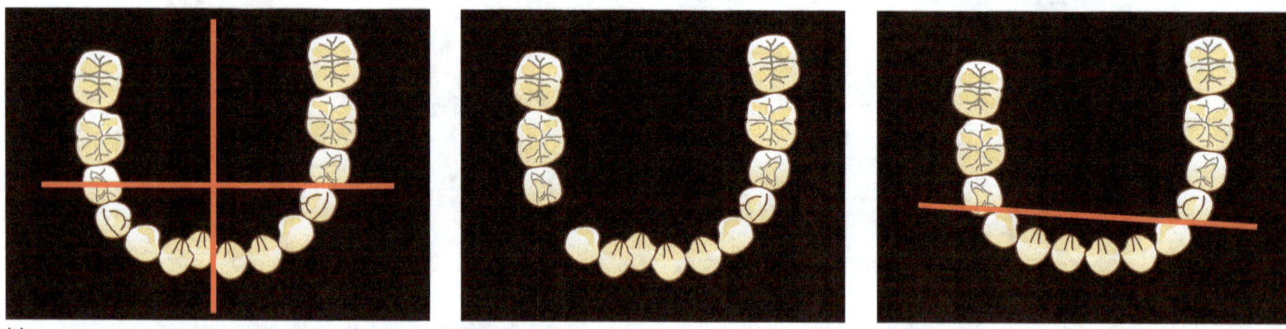

(a) (b) (c)

Figure 3.54 Single premolar extractions should be reserved for severe arch asymmetries (e.g., a left-to-right full premolar width asymmetry): (a and b) a single premolar extraction in a case less than a full premolar width asymmetry can create (c) a reversed arch asymmetry following space closure.

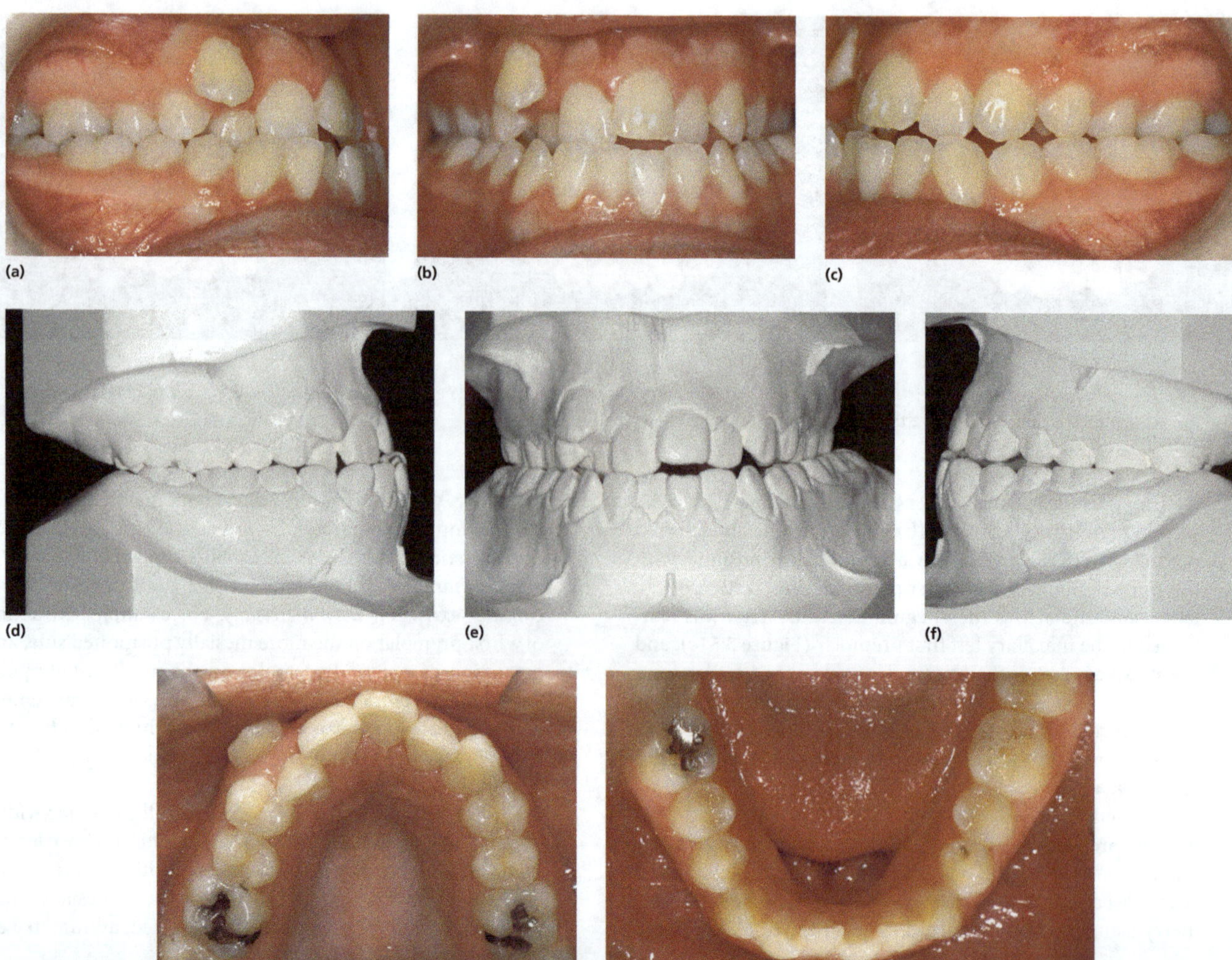

(a) (b) (c) (d) (e) (f) (g) (h)

Figure 3.55 (a–h) Initial records of a four-premolar extraction patient with a symmetric mandibular arch and an asymmetric maxillary arch (patient's right posterior ahead).

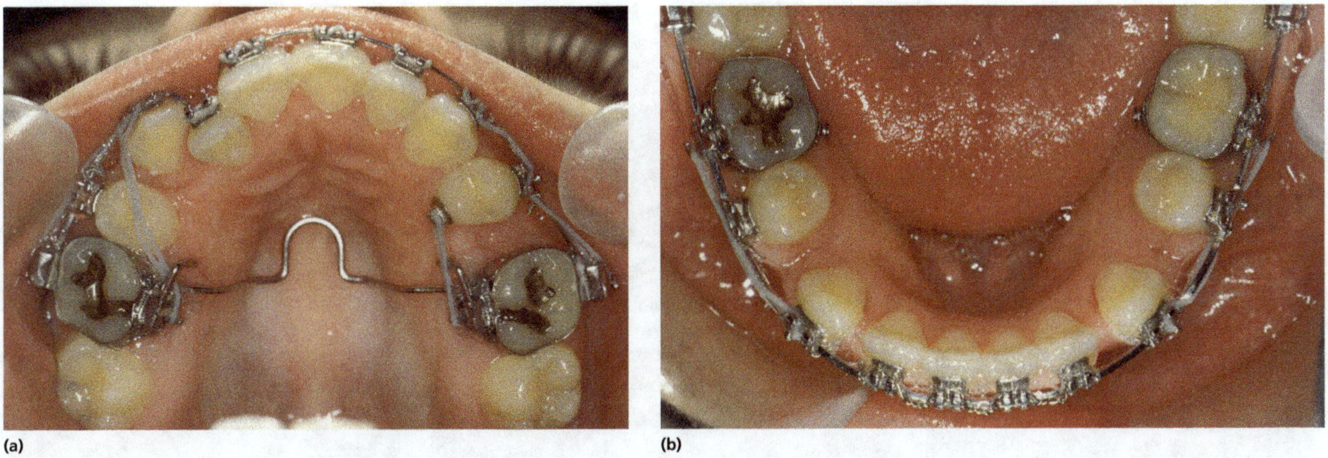

Figure 3.56 (a–b) Progress records of the patient in Figure 3.55. The maxillary right first premolar, maxillary left second premolar, and mandibular first premolars were extracted. Reciprocal space closure is proceeding.

the contralateral side following space closure (Figure 3.54c). This approach should generally be avoided.

Q: As an example of extractions in an arch asymmetry patient, consider the CR occlusion of a 16-year-old girl shown in Figure 3.55. A skeletal asymmetry was absent and she was Class III (1 mm) at her right first molars and Class III (4 mm) at her left first molars. Her mandibular arch was symmetric, but her maxillary arch was asymmetric with her maxillary right first molar ahead of the left by 3 mm. It was decided that she required RME to correct her cross bite plus extraction of premolars in all four quadrants. Can you suggest a four premolar extraction pattern to address her asymmetry *and* Class III relationship?

A: Realize, we have already decided that this patient requires premolar extractions in all four quadrants, and that decision was made using information from her facial photographs and cephalometric radiographs—information you do not have here. That said, since her mandibular arch is symmetric, then symmetric extractions in the lower arch would be prudent. Mandibular first premolars were extracted to permit retraction of her mandibular anterior teeth to correct her Class III relationship and alleviate crowding. A maxillary right first premolar was extracted to provide space for the blocked out maxillary right canine and to match extraction of the mandibular right first premolar (keeping the right posterior occlusion nearly the same). Now, to address her maxillary asymmetry, the maxillary left *second* premolar was extracted to provide more mesial movement of the maxillary left first molar (less retraction of the maxillary left canine) compared to the right, to improve her left Class III relationship during reciprocal space closure (Figure 3.56), and to improve her maxillary arch asymmetry.

Space closure resulted in a Class I relationship, symmetric arches, and coincident midlines (Figure 3.57).

Q: Now, back to our patient, Valerie. How do the above asymmetry considerations relate to Valerie's treatment?

A: Since Valerie's mandibular asymmetry is *mild*, you should incorporate biomechanics to improve it. Treat the maxillary dentition to the mandibular arch to achieve Class I canines and coincident midlines.

Q: You noted that Valerie's chin projection appears adequate. What *soft tissue* reference do you use to judge chin (soft tissue Pogonion) projection? What *skeletal* reference do you use to judge chin (bony Pogonion) projection?

A: *Zero meridian line is used to judge soft tissue Pogonion projection.* The zero meridian line is a line drawn perpendicular to the Frankfort horizontal line, passing through soft tissue Nasion, and used to measure the position of the chin. The chin should lie on this line or just short of it [83, 84]. Note, in Figure 3.58, that Valerie's chin (soft tissue Pogonion) lies just anterior to zero meridian. So, her chin projection is adequate. An effective *bony* (cephalometric) Pogonion is defined as one that lies at or anterior to a line drawn from Nasion—B-point. An ineffective bony Pogonion is defined as one that lies posterior to a line from Nasion—B-point. As shown in Figure 3.41f, Valerie possesses an effective bony pogonion.

Q: Considering problems of the face and teeth in each dimension, and other pertinent problems, what are the primary problems you should focus on when treating Valerie?

A: See Table 3.4

Q: What are your treatment goals for Valerie?

A: To address her chief complaint by aligning her teeth, reducing her OJ and OB to minimal, and obtaining Class I canines. Ideally, you would like to increase her LAFH slightly, reduce her labiomental sulcus depth, and increase her amount of maxillary incisal display.

Q: Which dimensions have apical base discrepancies in this patient?

A: AP and vertical.

Q: You speak to Valerie's parents about her growth. They tell you Valerie is still growing, but she achieved menarche about a year ago. That said, what are the three *general* ways you can treat her *AP* apical base discrepancy? For each of these three, list specific treatments.

A: *Orthopedics* (restrict maxillary AP growth while permitting the mandible to continue growing, or accelerate mandibular growth). The problem with attempting orthopedics is Valerie's maturity. For girls, the peak rate of statural increase is reached prior to menarche; and with the onset of menses, the rate of change in height drops to prepubertal levels, decreasing sharply to an adult rate of change during the subsequent 2 years [39]. Since Valerie reached menarche a year ago, and considering the magnitude of her AP problem (molar correction of 3–4 mm

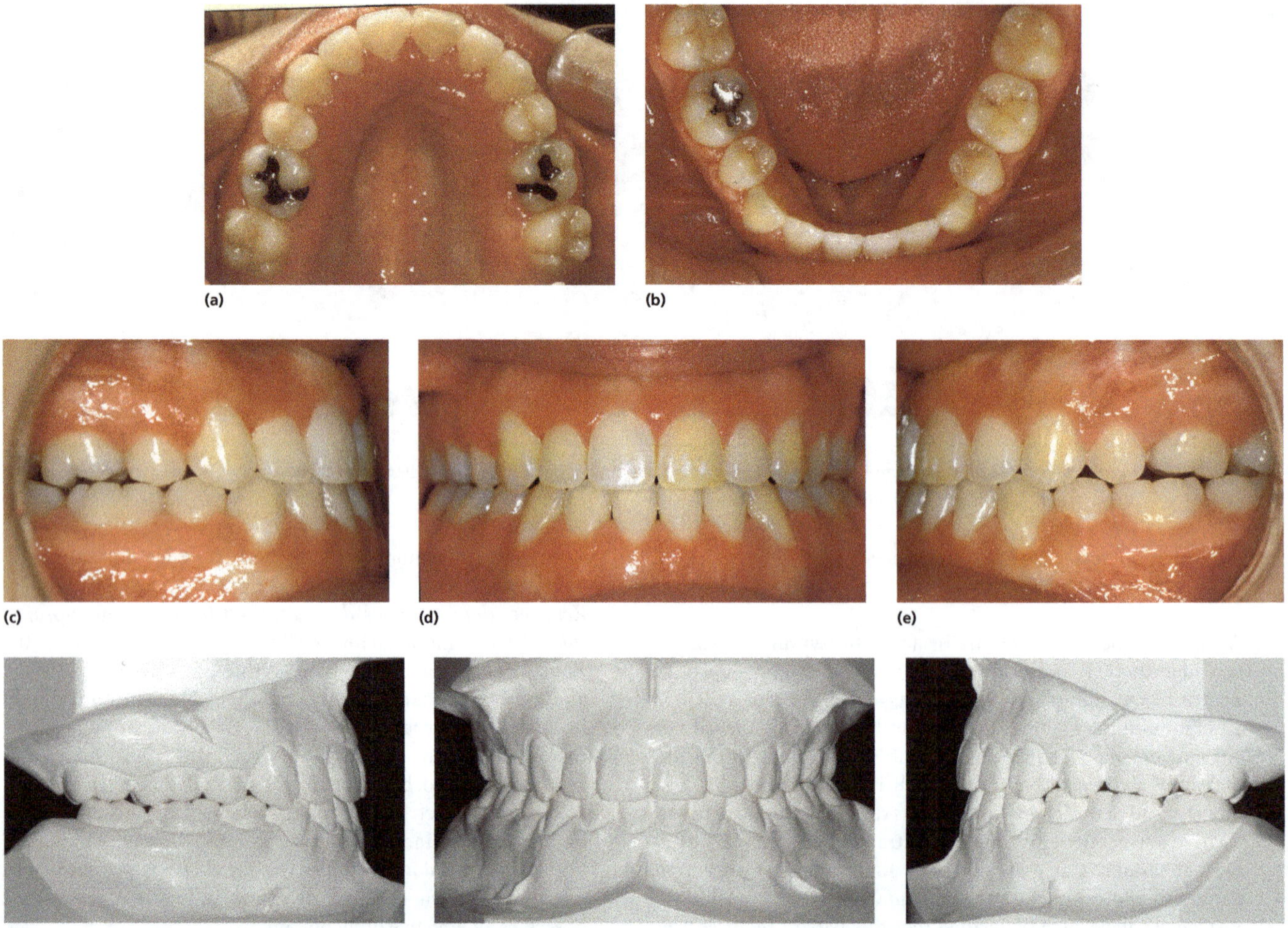

Figure 3.57 (a–h) Final records of the patient from Figure 3.55.

needed on the right and 5 mm needed on the left, ANB angle of 6°), Valerie *probably* does not have enough growth remaining to achieve a full AP correction. But, she *possibly* could. This fact should be explained to Valerie and her parents. If Valerie is interested in attempting orthopedics for 6–9 months, then you could do so and evaluate her improvement at the end of that time. Orthopedic options include the following:

- Headgears: A high-pull headgear restricts forward maxillary growth, and may reduce maxillary descent and maxillary first molar eruption [24, 67]. Given any remaining mandibular growth, these effects would improve Valerie's Class II relationship (but not help her vertical). Due to Valerie's inadequate incisal display, a cervical headgear could also be used. Why? Cervical-pull headgears restrict forward maxillary growth, but also tip the anterior palatal plane downward, which could increase her gingival and incisal display [24, 25]. Both cervical-pull and high-pull headgears distalize maxillary first molars—improving her Class II relationship with or without mandibular growth.
- Functional appliances: With proclined mandibular incisors (FMIA of 57°), Valerie is not an ideal candidate for a functional appliance (as her mandibular incisors will procline more). On the other hand, she has proclined maxillary incisors, a deep bite, and a short LAFH, which, generally, are ideal for Class II correction with a functional appliance. If you are willing to sacrifice some additional mandibular incisor proclination, then you could attempt Class II correction with a bionator, Herbst, Frankel, activator, or other functional appliance. With any of these appliances, you are aiming for dental movement (uprighting of maxillary incisors, distalization of maxillary posterior teeth, mesial movement of mandibular posterior teeth) and *acceleration* of any remaining mandibular growth—not enhanced mandibular growth [68].

Masking or camouflage (achieving a Class I canine relationship without addressing the underlying apical base discrepancy). Masking options include the following:

- Extraction of maxillary first premolars to permit retraction/alignment of the maxillary anterior teeth. This alternative would result in Class I canines/Class II molars. It could improve her profile by reducing OJ, eliminating lip trapping, and by opening her labiomental sulcus. Since Valerie is already a full-cusp Class II on the left, and cannot afford mesial movement of her maxillary molars, some form of maxillary anchorage support (TADs or headgear) will be necessary to hold the molar positions during reciprocal space closure. The drawback of this treatment approach is that as the maxillary incisors are retracted and uprighted, the maxillary incisors will tend to rotate around their apices—deepening her bite. Also, the mandibular incisors (anterior crowding, deep COS) will be proclined to a greater degree.
- Extraction of maxillary first premolars to permit retraction of the maxillary anterior teeth plus extraction of one mandibular

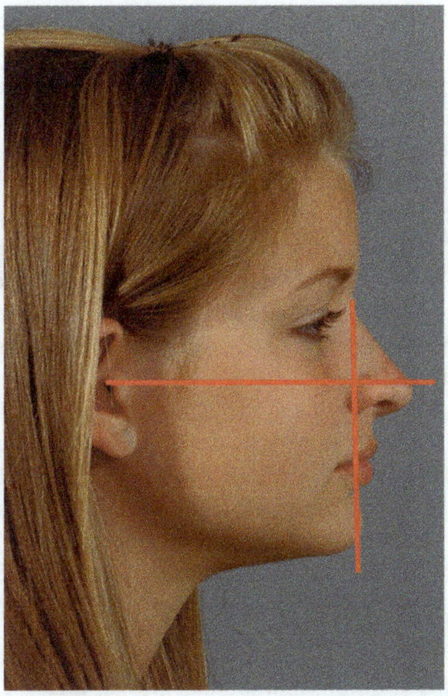

Figure 3.58 Zero meridian line is drawn perpendicular to FH at soft tissue Nasion. The chin should lie on or just short of zero meridian line to be considered effective.

Table 3.4 **Primary problems list for Valerie** *(apical base/skeletal discrepancies italicized).*

AP	II (3) II (3–4) II (5) II (5) *mandibular skeletal retrusion*
Vertical	*skeletal* and dental deep bite
Transverse	—
Other	—

incisor to alleviate the mandibular anterior crowding (without incisor proclination). A diagnostic wax setup would be recommended if this approach was undertaken—in order to insure that the resulting final anterior OJ would not be excessive. If the diagnostic wax setup showed too much final overjet, then interproximal reduction (IPR, slenderizing) of the mandibular incisors could be a reasonable alternative to an incisor extraction.

- Extraction of maxillary first premolars to permit retraction of the maxillary anterior teeth plus extraction of mandibular second premolars to permit advancement of her mandibular molars into a Class I relationship. This option is not recommended. Why? Her maxillary left first molars are a "full step" Class II. To correct the left side to Class I molar you would need to use the *entire* left second premolar extraction space to protract the mandibular left molars to Class I. There is no advantage in doing this. No studies exist which demonstrate occlusal/functional superiority of having Class I versus Class II molars. Further, there is always the concern that the mandibular canines could actually be retracted into part of that second premolar extraction space (leaving the canines and molars in a Class II relationship following space closure).
- High-pull or cervical-pull headgears—not used for orthopedics, but simply to distalize the maxillary molars into a Class I relationship. This approach offers the advantage of no teeth being extracted, but the drawback is the magnitude of the (heroic) distalization needed. Concern still exists regarding excess incisor proclination of the mandibular arch if it is treated nonextraction.
- TADs to distalize the entire maxillary arch. Since the maxillary canines will end up in a Class I relationship, this approach would produce the same result as extracting the maxillary first premolars (but without loss of permanent teeth) or retraction with headgears. That is, both approaches are intra-arch mechanics.
- Class II elastics, or other inter-arch Class II correctors, could improve Valerie's Class II relationship. The drawback of inter-arch mechanics is further mandibular incisor proclination.

Surgery (mandibular advancement) should be considered as an option, especially if Valerie has profile concerns (she does not). However, if this approach is taken, then her growth should be monitored while the arches are leveled and aligned. If she grows favorably, there is the possibility that the need for surgery could be eliminated.

The surgical option requires that a decision be made about how much advancement is desirable (by having Valerie posture her mandible forward into a Class I canine relationship, or beyond, as you examine her profile). Based on the amount of advancement you want, you could chose to

- Treat her mandibular arch nonextraction (4–5 mm advancement at the canines, but leaving mandibular incisor proclination).
- Extract mandibular first premolars, close the spaces reciprocally, and retract the anterior teeth (forcing the surgeon to advance the mandible further, 9–11 mm).
- Extract mandibular first premolars and place TADs in the mandible as anchorage (or use mandibular J-hook headgear) to retract the canines the entire first premolar extraction space. The result would be a maximum surgical advancement (11–12 mm of advancement)
- Extract the mandibular second premolars and close reciprocally (resulting in more advancement that nonextraction, but less than advancement following first premolar extraction, 7–8 mm).

Even looking at Valerie's initial profile (Figure 3.41d and f), which appears reasonable—if we advance her mandible, a nonextraction approach would be chosen. A setback genioplasty may also be considered.

Q: What are the three general ways to treat Valerie's *vertical* apical base discrepancy? List specific treatments for each.

A: *Orthopedics* (Figure 3.59, enhancing downward maxillary corpus growth, increasing maxillary molar eruption, and increasing mandibular molar eruption could lengthen her short LAFH, increase her mandibular plane angle, open her deep bite, help eliminate lip redundancy, and eliminate her overclosed appearance). The ideal vertical treatment goal would be to increase her LAFH, but not to the point where Valerie develops an ILG. If these vertical movements are successful, then her mandible will rotate down and back—tending to worsen Valerie's Class II molar relationship. The problems with attempting orthopedics are Valerie's maturity and the potentially poor stability of such correction, especially molar eruption. Considerations include the following:

- Since Valerie is Class II, a cervical-pull headgear could be used to rotate the anterior palatal plane downward and backward [24–26], potentially increasing her lower anterior facial height and incisor display. However, this effect appears to be temporary [26], and the question of whether cervical traction causes a clinically significant change in vertical facial proportions remains equivocal [32].

- The vertical effects of straight-pull headgear [28], headgear with a biteplate [31, 33], activators, bionators [27], and Frankel appliances [28] remain equivocal.
- Leveling the COS with archwires occurs primarily through premolar extrusion [23] (alveolar process vertical bone growth, orthopedics), plus incisor intrusion (masking), plus incisor proclination (masking), and uprighting/distal tipping of mesially tipped mandibular molars (alveolar process vertical bone growth, orthopedics).
- Anterior bite plates (or anterior bite turbos) disclude posterior teeth and can assist leveling the COS/eruption of posterior teeth by removing occlusal forces. Posterior vertical elastics can be used with, or without, anterior biteplates to aid this leveling. The stability of posterior tooth eruption in someone as old as Valerie is questionable, but increasing LAFH by erupting posterior teeth could be attempted. If you are successful in using posterior vertical elastics to erupt posterior teeth and open her bite, do not discontinue the elastics as soon as you achieve your result. Instead, maintain her on them for some time afterward and slowly reduce elastic wear as you monitor relapse.

Masking or camouflage (reducing/correcting Valerie's deep bite without addressing her vertical skeletal discrepancy). Such treatment is analogous to correcting a *dental* deep bite. Options include the following:

- Intruding Valerie's stepped down maxillary incisors and intruding her stepped up mandibular incisors with fixed orthodontic appliances and archwires. This process may be aided by bonding maxillary and mandibular incisors more incisally than normal or by placing archwire steps specifically to intrude anterior teeth.
- Proclining incisors to rotate them forward around their apicies. This approach is *not recommended* for Valerie because her incisors are already proclined.
- Erupting mandibular premolars [23] or distally tipping/erupting mandibular molars that are mesially tipped will open her bite during COS leveling–with or without anterior bite plates to disclude posterior teeth or posterior vertical elastics (eruption of posterior teeth to increase the vertical dimension may be unstable, especially in adults, and can be considered orthopedics).
- Increasing Valerie's vertical dimension and opening her deep bite through prosthodontic treatment would not be reasonable.

Surgery (maxillary downgraft to lengthen her LAFH)—it is very important to consider the magnitude of her vertical problem. Surgery would generally not be considered with Valerie's mild-to-moderate vertical apical base discrepancy unless this was a specific concern of hers (and only if the LAFH can be lengthened without creating an interlabial gap).

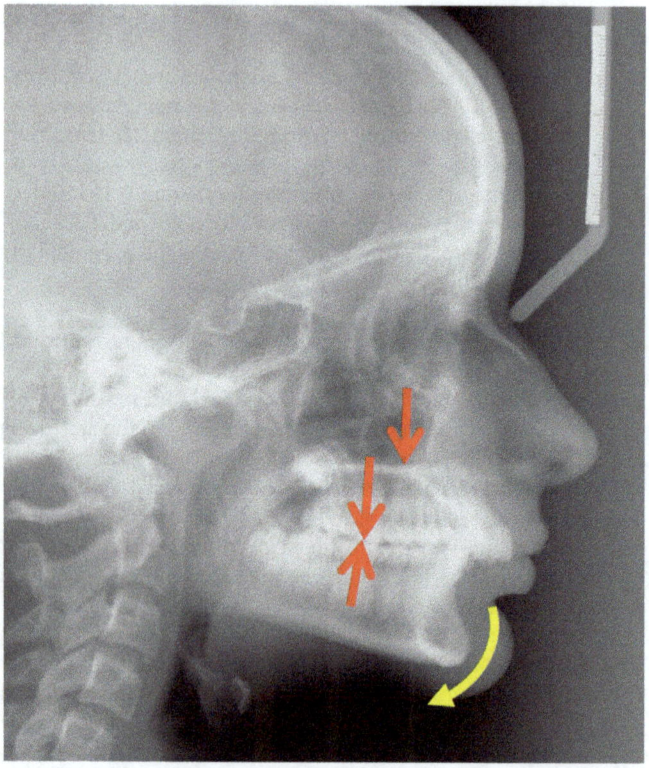

Figure 3.59 Orthopedically increasing maxillary corpus downward growth and increasing molar eruption would improve Valerie's short skeletal LAFH, but her mandible would tend to rotate down (and back) worsening her Class II relationship.

Q: How can remaining mandibular growth affect Valerie's treatment outcome?

A: If during any remaining growth, Valerie's condyles grow more vertically than normal, if her mandible rotates forward (internally, true rotation) more excessively than normal, if her maxilla descends less than normal, and if her molars erupt less than normal, then her skeletal deep bite could worsen—making treatment to open her bite more difficult. But, if during any remaining growth, Valerie's condyles grow more posteriorly superiorly than before, if her mandible rotates forward (internally, true rotation) less than before, if her maxilla descends more than before, and if her molars erupt more than before, then her skeletal deep bite (and treatment to open her bite) could improve. Of course, forward mandibular growth could aid in the correction of her Class II relationship. Lack of forward mandibular growth could make Class II correction more difficult.

Q: Treatment changes in Valerie's vertical dimension are intimately related to changes in the anteroposterior dimension. Can you visualize and discuss this relationship? How do changes directed at improving Valerie's short LAFH affect her Class II correction?

A: Schudy [15] brought attention to the interrelationship between anteroposterior and vertical facial changes, in terms of growth. If the vertical components of growth are held constant (no maxillary corpus descent, no maxillary molar eruption, no mandibular molar eruption), then mandibular growth should result in B-point moving forward and the mandibular plane rotating CCW. On the other hand, for the same amount of mandibular growth, if the maxillary molars erupt, if the mandibular molars erupt, and if the maxillary corpus descends, then the mandibular plane could rotate CW, and B-point could rotate down and back. This same relationship between AP and vertical applies in the absence of growth. If the maxilla is brought down or molars are erupted, the mandible will rotate downward and backward making the patient more Class II. If the maxilla is moved upward or molars are intruded, the mandible will rotate upward and forward making the patient more Class III. So, for Valerie, attempts to lengthen her short LAFH by molar eruption or maxillary corpus descent will tend to rotate her mandible down and back—worsening her Class II relationship.

Q: Can you explain how vertical molar movement and the resulting mandibular rotation are related to the *vertical and horizontal distances between the condyle and B-point*?

A: During initial jaw opening, B-point rotates down and back *perpendicular to a line drawn between the condyle and B-point*, as viewed in the sagittal plane on a lateral cephalometric radiograph (blue arrow, Figure 3.60a). For this reason, the relationship between vertical molar movement and mandibular rotation is dependent on the vertical and horizontal distances between the condyle and B-point. In short-faced individuals (Figure 3.60b), where the horizontal distance (H) between B-point and condyle is greater than the vertical distance (V) between B-point and condyle (H>V), molar eruption has greater effect on *vertical* (B-point moving down, bite opening) than on AP (B-point moving back, Class II worsening). However, in long-faced individuals (Figure 3.60c), the horizontal distance is smaller than the vertical distance (H<V), and molar eruption has less effect on vertical (B-point moving down, bite opening) and greater effect on *AP* (B-point moving back, Class II worsening). For Valerie, 3 mm of vertical molar extrusive movement will produce −1°change in SNB.

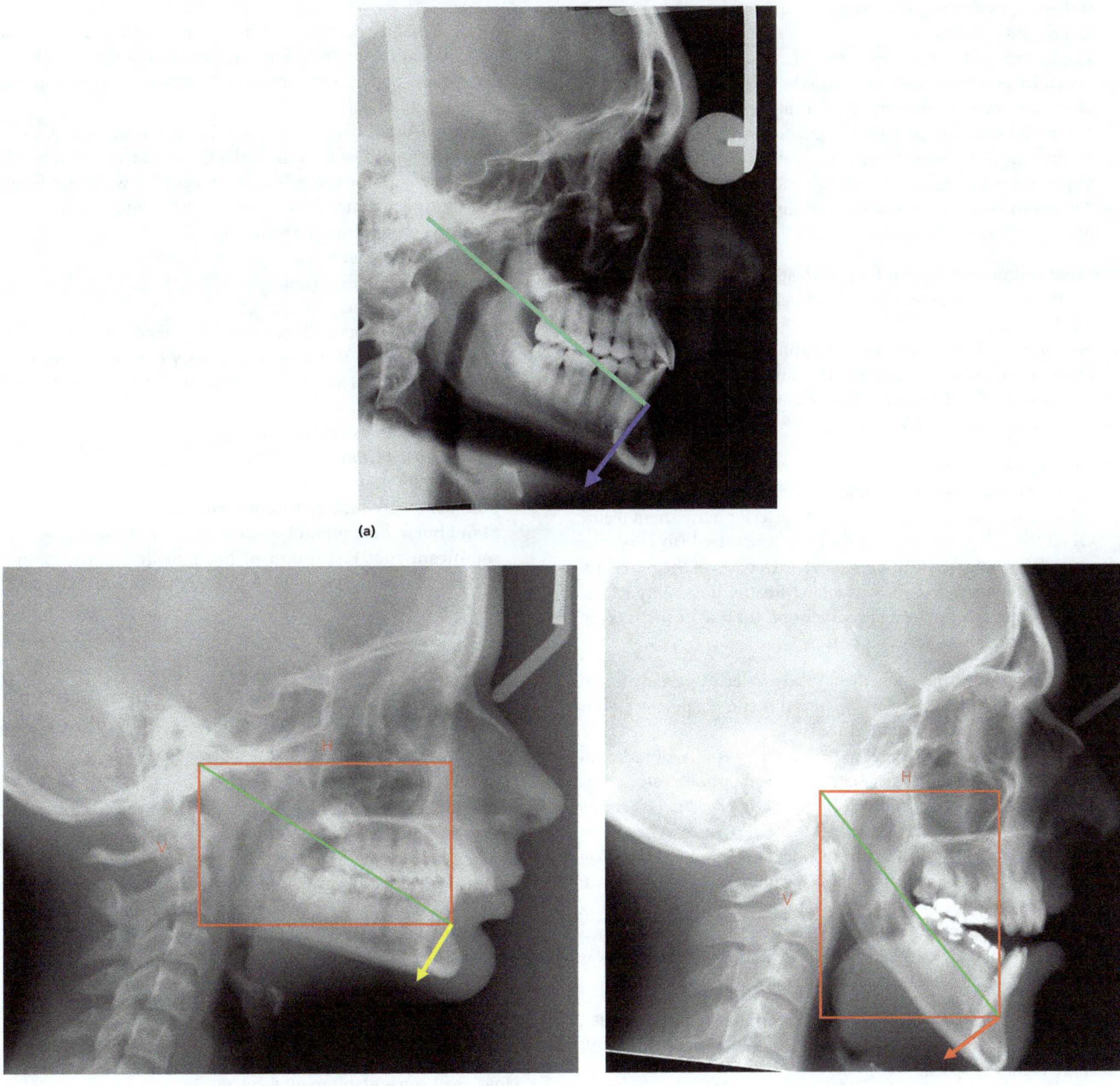

Figure 3.60 (a) During initial opening, B-point moves in a direction (blue arrow) perpendicular to a line drawn from the condyle to B-point. For this reason, the vertical and horizontal distances from the condyle to B-point determine the direction B-point moves if molars are erupted; (b) in short face patients, molar eruption results in greater downward movement of B-point (bite opening) and less backward movement of B-point (Class II worsening). In long-face patients (c), molar eruption results in less bite opening and greater Class II worsening.

Q: Since the vertical and anteroposterior dimensions are so interrelated, which dimension should be emphasized in treating a Class II skeletal deep bite patient, such as Valerie?

A: The answer depends on the patient's chief complaint and the magnitude of the vertical and AP problems. For many borderline vertical deficiency (short LAFH, skeletal deep bite) patients, we have found there may be little concern expressed for the facial vertical deficiency. The chief complaint is usually AP (overjet) or the OB. For those patients who do express concern of moderate to severe facial vertical deficiency, it should be addressed. In Valerie's case, a discussion was held with her and her parents—and a decision was made to focus on her AP correction.

Q: Is there a possible need for surgery and should you mention this to Valerie's parents?

A: Yes. It should be mentioned to Valerie and her parents that depending on her desires, she could be a candidate for mandibular advancement surgery (including setback genioplasty?). You could have her posture her jaw forward until the canines are in a Class I position and show Valerie and her parents the improvement in facial balance this movement would provide. Also, with future growth still remaining, her desire for orthognathic surgery could increase.

Q: What unknowns do you face in treating Valerie? Specifically, are there any unknowns you should eliminate before irreversible treatments?

A: Yes, it would be ideal to determine Valerie's compliance, amount/direction of growth remaining, and confirm the absence of a CR-CO shift - before any irreversible treatments (e.g., tooth extractions).

Q: Should Valerie be treated without extraction of permanent teeth, with extraction of anterior permanent teeth, or with extraction of other combinations of posterior permanent teeth?

A: Of all the extraction options we have considered (to mask the underlying apical base discrepancy), extraction of the maxillary first premolars is the most viable (with the possibility of the additional extraction of a lower incisor if the diagnostic wax-up looked promising—in terms of final OJ).

Q: Let's bring everything together. When Valerie's parents asked you what treatment you would recommend if she were your daughter, how would you respond?

A: A nonextraction, orthopedic treatment was attempted, and Valerie and her parents declined a surgical option. Valerie was placed on a CPHG and in fixed orthodontic appliances. Her arches were leveled/aligned with increasingly stiffer archwires. When it was confirmed that mandibular growth would not provide a complete orthopedic correction, her maxillary first premolars were extracted. Maxillary canines and incisors were retracted, and finishing completed. Extraction of a mandibular incisor was not deemed necessary, but some slenderizing of the mandibular incisors was performed. Class II elastics were worn as needed during finishing.

Q: What are the specific objectives of treatment for the maxilla, mandible, maxillary dentition, and mandibular dentition in all three planes of space?

A: Specific objectives of treatment for Valerie are as follows:

Maxilla

AP: Restrict any remaining forward growth.
Vertical: Allow for remaining downward growth.
Transverse: Allow for remaining growth.

Mandible

AP: Allow for remaining growth.
Vertical: Allow for remaining growth.
Transverse: Allow for remaining growth.

Maxillary dentition

AP: Protract molars. Retract canines and incisors.
Vertical: Maintain molars and incisors.
Intermolar width: Maintain.

Mandibular dentition

AP: Maintain molars. Minimize proclination of incisors.
Vertical: Level COS. Intrude incisors.
Intermolar/Intercanine width: Maintain intermolar and intercanine widths.

Q: Valerie's deband records are presented in Figure 3.61. What changes do you note, and what was the effect of treatment?

A: Valerie was cooperative throughout treatment. Observations include the following:

- Anteroposterior correction (Class I canine relationship, Class II molar relationship, minimal OJ) was achieved through maxillary anterior tooth retraction coupled with significant and unexpected mandibular jaw growth (Figure 3.61f).
- ANB angle was reduced from 6° to 3°.
- Lip trapping was corrected.
- Chin projection increased.
- Labiomental sulcus was opened.
- B-point came forward because her mandibular condylar growth exceeded downward maxillary corpus growth plus molar eruption (which would rotate B-point down and back).
- LAFH/TAFH was unchanged.
- OB decreased from 100 to 10%.
- Midlines are now coincident.
- Mild dental asymmetries were corrected.
- Mandibular first premolar roots are not parallel, she had significant root resorption of her maxillary incisors, and her third molars must be followed for future extraction (Figure 3.61g).

Q: Were your treatment goals achieved?

A: No, not all of them. Her profile and smile were improved, although she still exhibits minimal incisal display when smiling. Her LAFH was not increased. Class I canines, minimal OB, and minimal OJ were achieved.

Q: How was Valerie's deep bite corrected?

A: Figure 3.61f illustrates slight maxillary corpus descent and slight mandibular molar eruption—both movements that would tend to open her bite. However, the *major* factors included maxillary incisor intrusion coupled with mandibular downward and forward growth (carrying B-point downward and forward and decreasing OB).

Q: We expected her mandibular incisors to procline with nonextraction, but they did not (Figure 3.61f). Why?

A: Probably because the mandibular anterior teeth were "slenderized" (IPR) to create room for their alignment.

Q: How was Valerie's labiomental sulcus opened?

A: Reduction in OJ (elimination of lip trapping) combined with mandibular downward and forward growth.

Q: Would a purely orthopedic (nonextraction) treatment with a headgear or Herbst appliance have worked?

A: Only if her treatment had started at a younger age when she had more growth remaining. Nonextraction treatment with a headgear or Herbst appliance would have restrained maxillary forward growth, distalized maxillary molars, allowed (or accelerated) mandibular forward growth, and (in the case of the Herbst appliance) moved mandibular teeth mesially/proclined mandibular incisors. A successful, nonextraction, result could very possibly have been achieved, if we had started treatment at a younger age (especially prior to menarche). However, it was wise to attempt orthopedics while we were leveling/aligning her arches since we were not sure how much growth she had remaining. And, it was wise to consider masking once we saw that a full correction would not be made with orthopedics. Again, the principle is: reduce

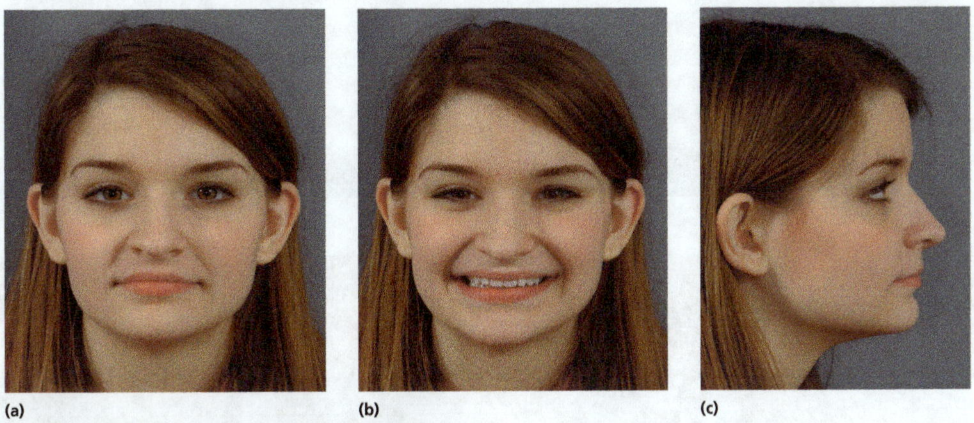

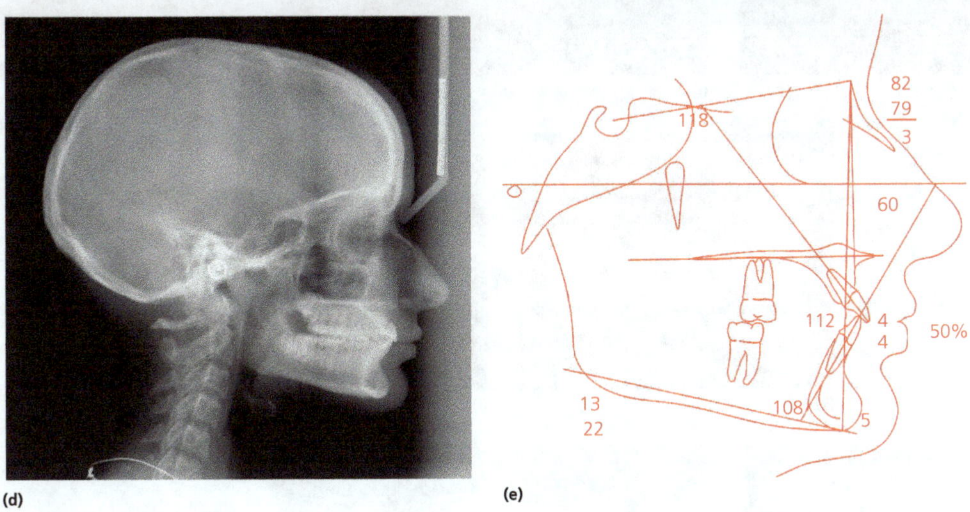

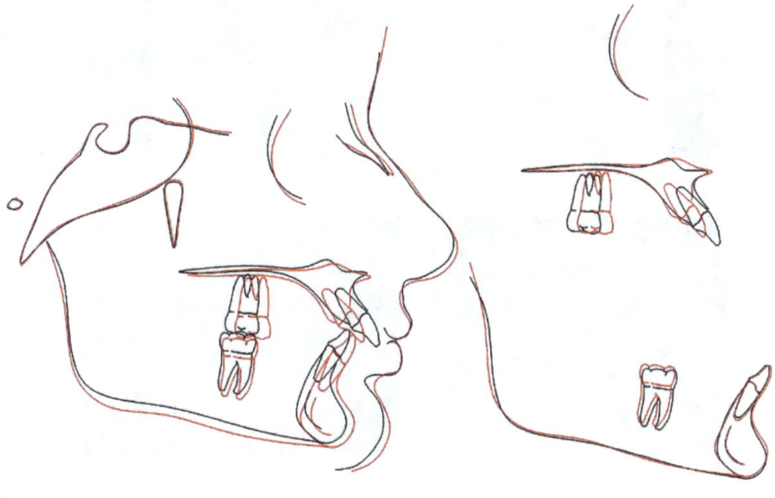

Figure 3.61 (a–q) Deband records of Valerie.

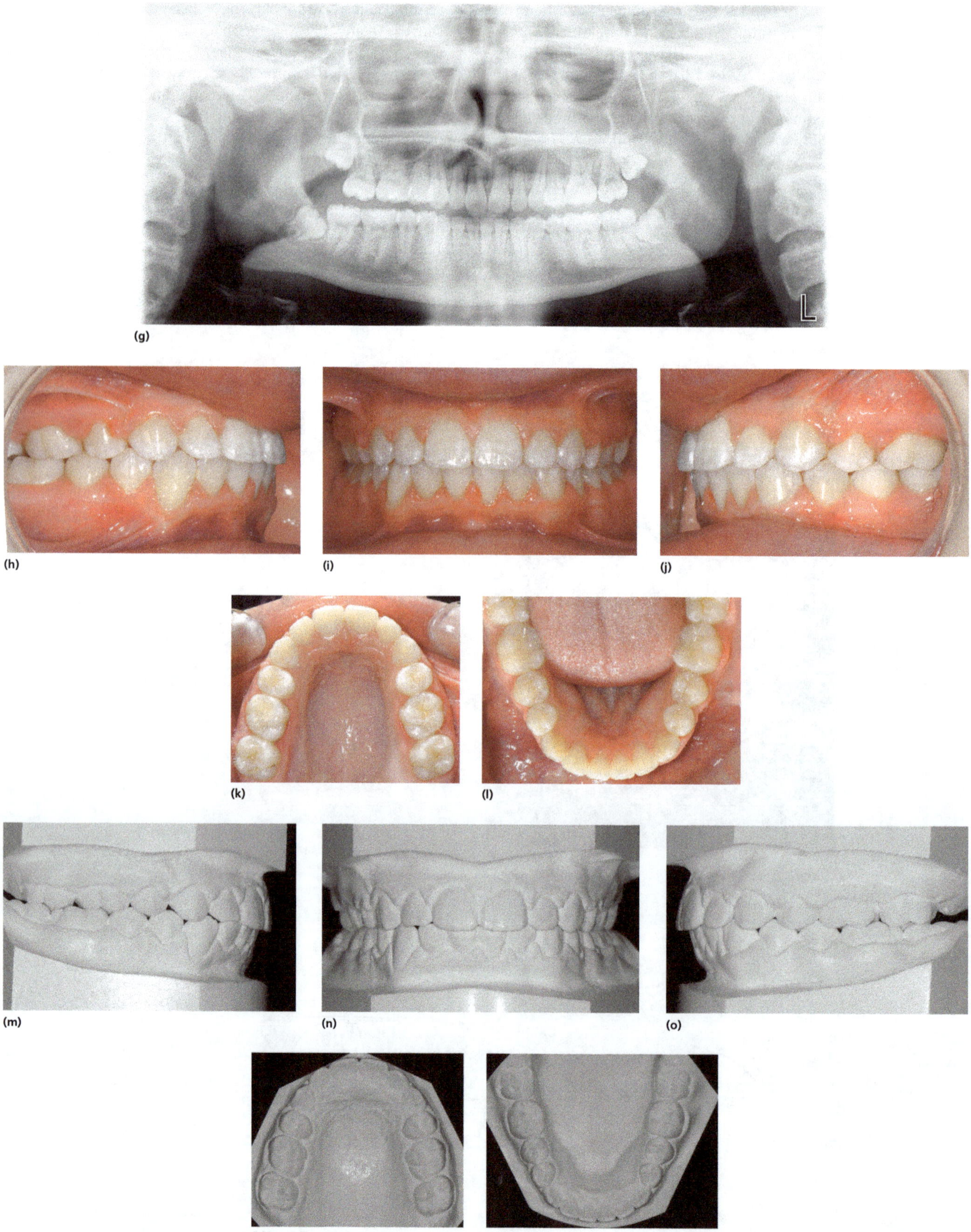

Figure 3.61 (Continued)

your unknowns before defining your final treatment plan or doing anything irreversible.

Q: Maxillary incisor root resorption was significant (Figure 3.61g). How do you deal with it?

A: It is very important that Valerie and her parents were informed about the possibility of root resorption *before* treatment began. In fact, you should discuss the risks and benefits of orthodontic treatment with every patient before beginning treatment. At this juncture, Valerie and her parents should be informed that root resorption did occur, that it will not worsen in retention, and that it will not affect the longevity of her teeth (as long as she practices good hygiene).

Q: Could Valerie's external apical root resorption have been predicted?

A: The state of the art does not permit us to predict root resorption for an individual at the initiation of treatment. *Examining tooth roots, radiographically, 6–9 months after the initiation of orthodontic treatment appears to be a useful predictor of severe resorption at the end of treatment* [85]. Why? A risk of severe resorption is seen in teeth with minor resorption after 6–9 months. No severe resorption is found after treatment in teeth without resorption after 6–9 months. So, on the one hand, radiographs could have been made of Valerie's teeth after 6–9 months of treatment to look for resorption. However, her maxillary first premolars were already extracted at that time, and the extraction spaces still needed to be closed. Of course, a decision could have been made to discontinue treatment (leaving extraction spaces) if severe resorption was found at that time.

Q: Are there any risk factors that could help us predict future external apical root resorption?

A: Yes, although it seems that for every risk factor one study reports to be related to root resorption, another study will report that factor not to be related. Examples of factors that have been reported to be related to orthodontically induced root resorption include *total apical displacement of the tooth root, treatment duration, and the presence of teeth with blunt or pipette-shaped roots* [85, 86]. Genetic factors account for at least 50% of the variation in root resorption. Future estimation of susceptibility to root resorption will likely require the analysis of a suite of genes, root morphology, skeletodental values, and the treatment method to be used—or essentially the amount of tooth movement planned for treatment [87].

Q: What retention protocol would you suggest?

A: Valerie was asked to wear Hawley retainers every night for a lifetime. Her maxillary retainer was designed with an anterior biteplate to disclude her posterior teeth to improve the chance of maintaining her deep bite correction. A fixed mandibular canine–canine retainer would also be acceptable in place of a mandibular Hawley retainer.

Q: What "take-home" messages can you glean from this case?

A: Take-home messages include the following:

- Valerie presented with 100% OB, a combination of skeletal and dental deep bite. Her dental deep bite resulted from over-eruption of mandibular and maxillary incisors. Her skeletal deep bite (mildly overclosed clinical appearance, mildly short soft tissue LAFH, short skeletal LAFH, flat mandibular plane angles, and relatively parallel SN, FH, and MP) probably resulted from a combination of her condyles growing more vertically; her mandible rotating (internally, true rotation) forward more excessively; her maxilla descending less; and her molars erupting less than normal. As her mandible rotated upward and forward, a skeletal deep bite resulted, which exacerbated her dental deep bite. Valerie was treated with fixed orthodontic appliances, a CPHG, and extraction of maxillary first premolars to provide space to retract her maxillary canines into a Class I relationship and to retract her maxillary incisors to a minimal OJ. Some slenderizing of her mandibular anterior teeth was performed.
- OB was corrected by a combination of slight maxillary corpus descent and slight mandibular molar eruption. However, the *major* factors included maxillary incisor intrusion coupled with mandibular downward and forward growth (carrying B-point downward and forward and decreasing OB).
- Correcting her OB with maxillary incisor intrusion did not help increase her amount of incisal display when smiling (compare Figures 3.41c and 3.61b).
- Correcting her OB from 100 to 10% was prudent in terms of anticipated, long-term, OB relapse (10–20%).
- Considering the fact that Valerie reached menarche 1 year before treatment began, the amount of mandibular growth (Figure 3.61f) she had during treatment was surprising. There is no way to predict this individual jaw growth (magnitude and direction). For over 40 years, various radiographic methods have been promoted purporting the ability to predict individual jaw growth (including the CVM method)—but none has survived. The pearl here is this: *if there is any chance that the patient is still growing, then you must take that potential growth into consideration during treatment planning and retention planning.*
- In deciding whether to treat a patient with orthopedics, the orthodontist must take the *magnitude* of the skeletal problem into account and the amount of *time* of potential growth remaining into account. With Valerie, we anticipated that she did not have much growth remaining, but we were not sure. Starting treatment with fixed appliances and orthopedics—then re-evaluating months later—was smart.
- At that time, a decision to switch to a masking approach for AP correction was appropriate and provided an excellent result. Masking, orthopedics, and surgery all have their place in your armamentarium.
- The *ideal* vertical facial proportions include an LAFH equal to midface height (Subnasale to soft-tissue Menton = soft-tissue Glabella to Subnasale). And yet, there is a *range* of vertical proportions, which are deemed attractive. Valerie's vertical facial proportions (Figure 3.61a, b, and f) did not change—she still has a short LAFH. And yet, she is a very attractive young woman with a pretty smile.
- In many adolescent Class II patients with mild-to-moderate skeletal deep bites, it is wise to focus on correcting the AP relationship. Of course, in severe skeletal deep bites the vertical dimension should be addressed directly.
- In cases of mild mandibular arch asymmetries such as Valerie's, you can treat the maxillary dentition to the mandibular asymmetry (achieving Class I canines and leaving dental midlines off slightly to the face), or you can attempt to improve the mandibular asymmetry biomechanically and treat the maxillary dentition to the corrected mandibular arch. This latter approach was taken with Valerie. Class II elastic wear corrected her mild mandibular asymmetry.
- It is unusual to have only one correct treatment approach in orthodontics. Often, a beautiful and functional outcome can be achieved through any number of treatment options.

Case Shawn

Shawn (Figure 3.62) is a 15-year and 4-month-old male who presents to you with a CC, "Please correct my bite and straighten my teeth." PMH, PDH, and TMJs are WRN. His periodontal evaluation is WRN.

Q: List diagnostic findings/problems. What is your diagnosis?
A: See Table 3.5

Q: What *major* clinical finding is missing from the above?
A: Shawn was not examined for a CR–CO shift. Not detecting a CR–CO shift can invalidate your diagnosis and treatment plan.

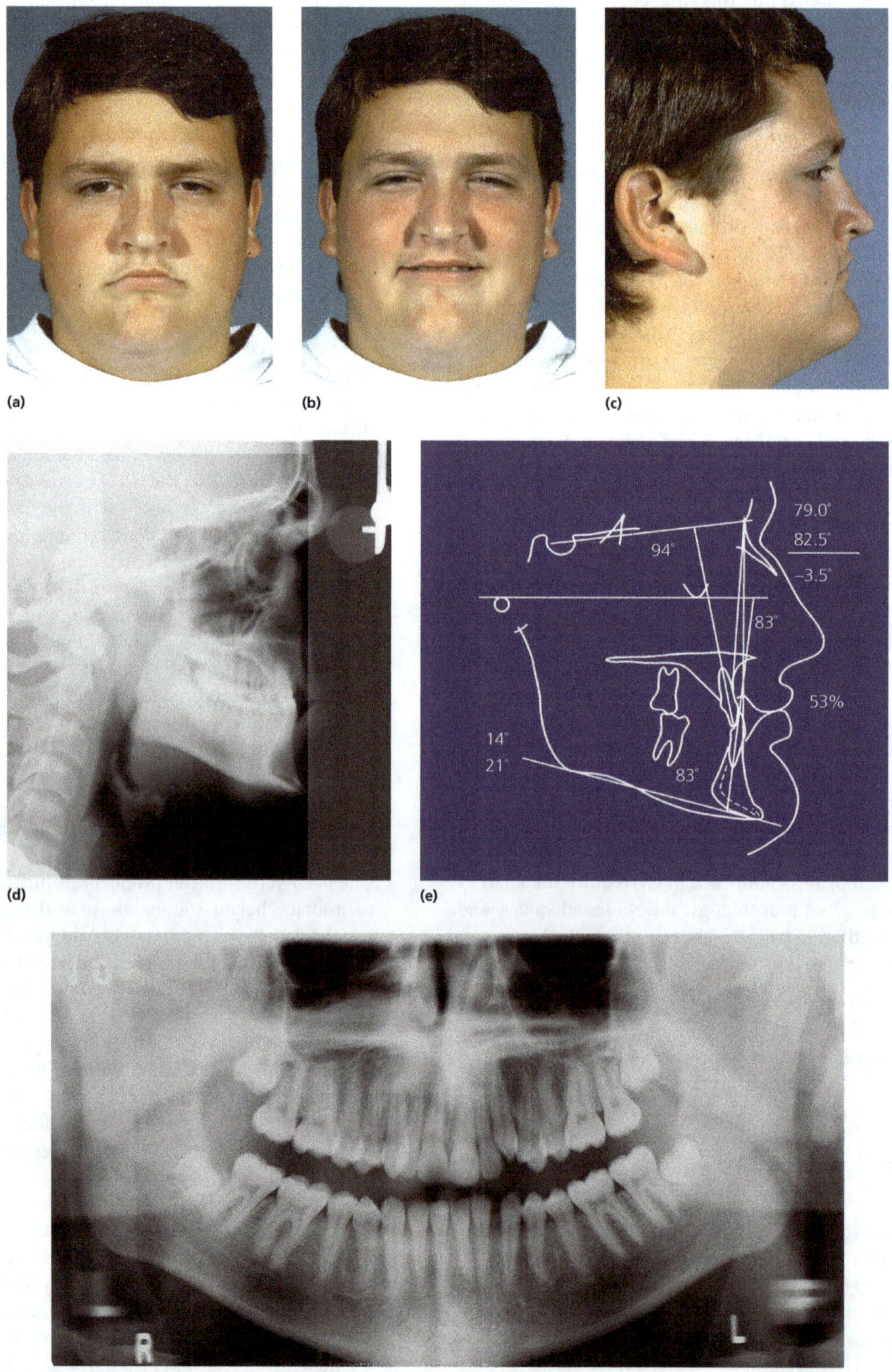

Figure 3.62 Initial records of Shawn: (a–c) facial photographs, (d) lateral cephalograph, (e) cephalometric tracing, (f) pantomograph,

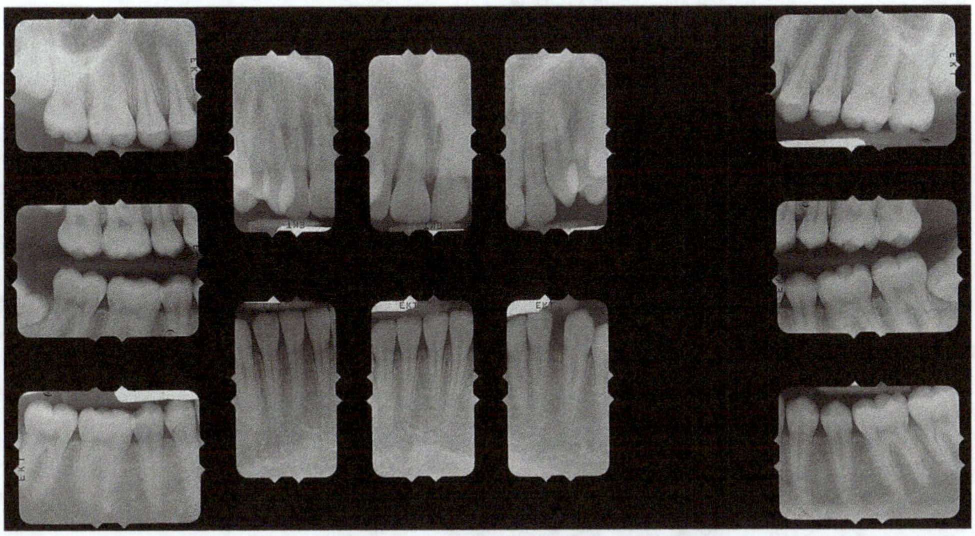

(g)

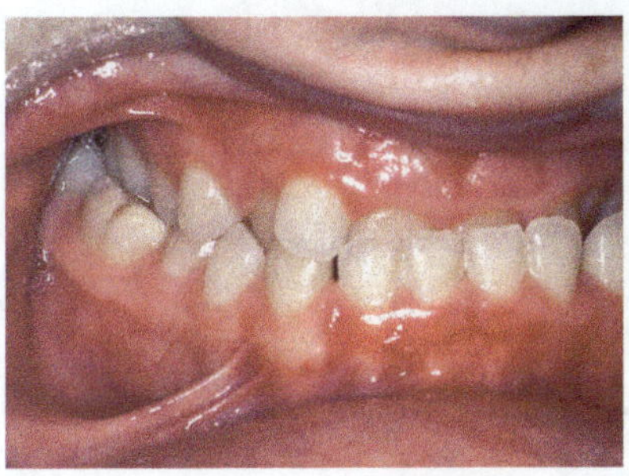

(h)

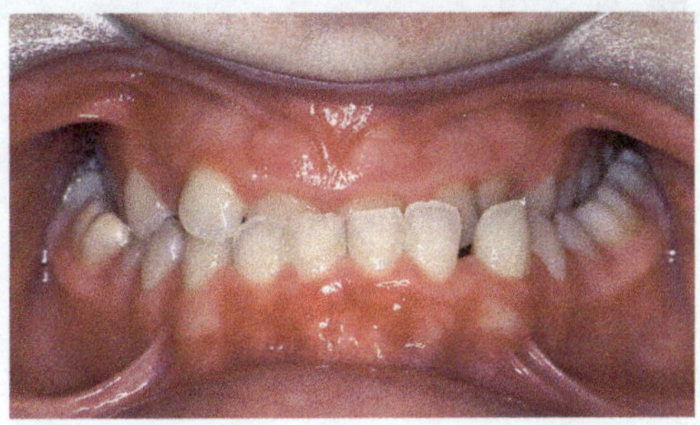

(i)

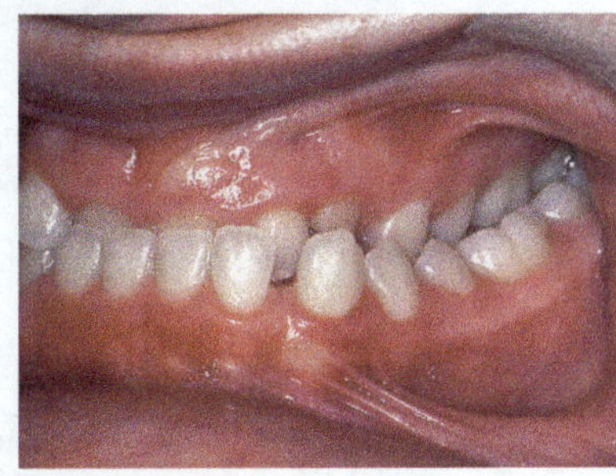

(j)

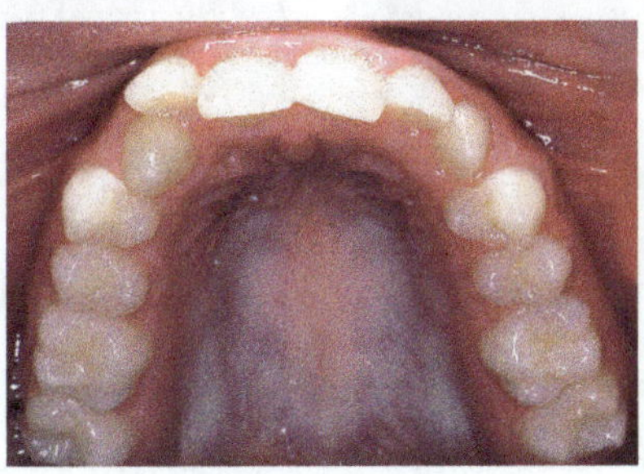

(k)

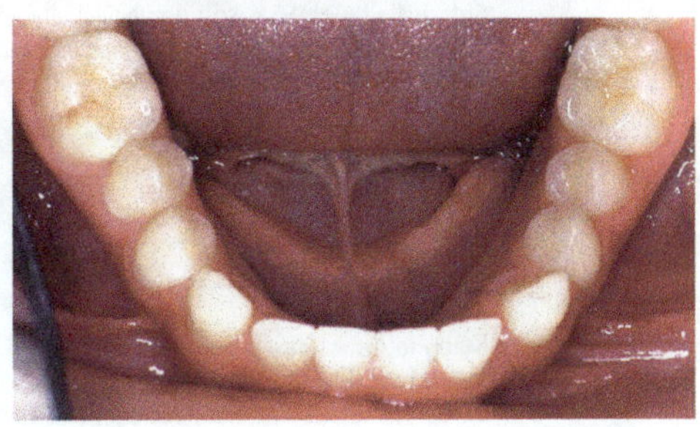

(l)

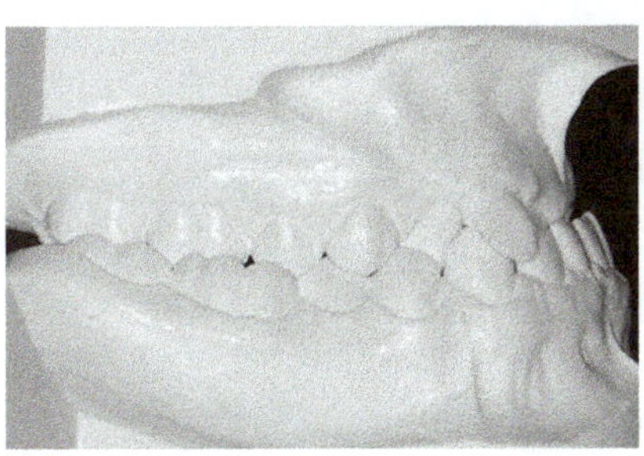

(m)

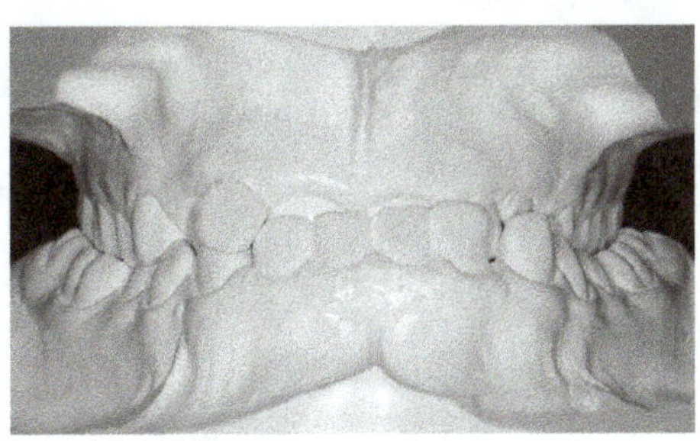

(n)

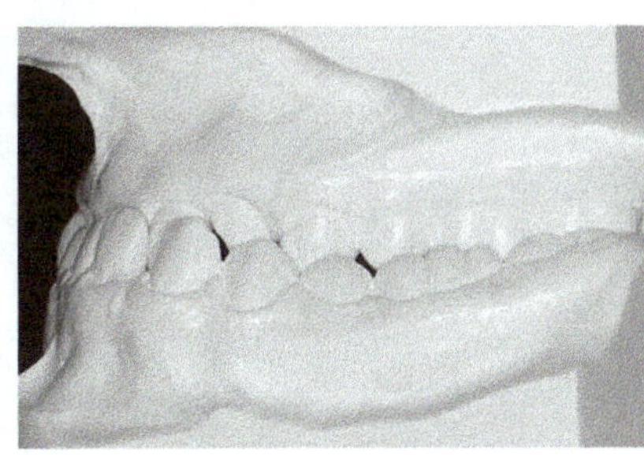

(o)

Figure 3.62 (Continued) (g) complete mouth series of dental radiographs, (h–l) intraoral photographs, and (m–r) model photographs.

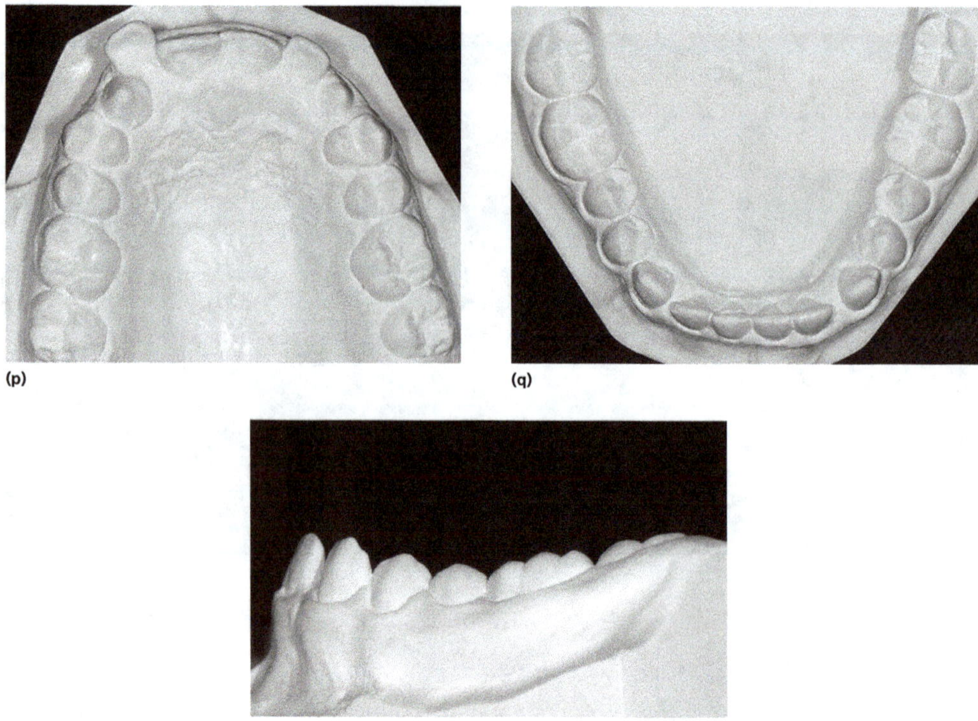

(p) (q) (r)

Figure 3.62 (Continued)

Table 3.5 Diagnostic findings and problem list for Shawn.

Full face and profile	**Frontal view** Face is symmetric Overclosed appearance Soft tissue LAFH WRN (soft tissue Glabella—Subnasale approximately = Subnasale to soft tissue Menton) Incisal display on posed smile appears adequate (difficult to judge in Figure 3.62b) UDML right of facial midline ~ 2 mm Everted lower lip **Profile view** Concave profile Deep labiomental sulcus Prominent chin Obtuse lip-chin-throat angle
Ceph analysis	**Skeletal** Mildly retrusive maxilla Mildly protrusive mandible Borderline vertical skeletal deficiency (LAFH/TAFH = 53%; SN-MP = 21°; FMA = 14°; SN, FH, and MP nearly parallel) Effective and prominent bony Pogonion Robust soft tissue chin thickness **Dental** Upright maxillary incisors (maxillary incisor to SN = 94°) Upright mandibular incisors (FMIA = 83°)
Radiographs	Permanent dentition stage Wisdom teeth developing Caries on maxillary left first molar
Intraoral photos and models	Angle Class III Iowa Classification: III (3) I III (2) III (3) OJ: −1 mm 100% underbite COS ~ 3 mm Complete lingual cross bite except maxillary right first premolar and right lateral incisor Maxillary first molar intermolar width 44.8 mm (between palatal cusps) Mandibular first molar intermolar width 51.3 mm (between central fossae) UTSALD − 4.3 mm (crowding) LTSALD + 3.3 mm (spacing) Anterior Bolton tooth size discrepancy: 1.4 mm mandibular anterior excess Maxillary midline right of mandibular midline by 2–3 mm Maxillary and mandibular dental arches appear symmetric Maxillary left first molar rotated forward slightly
Other	—
Diagnosis	Angle Class III malocclusion Skeletal and dental deep bite Maxillary skeletal transverse deficiency

Later, a significant CR–CO shift was identified in Shawn, and in CR (Figure 3.63), his left central incisors were found to make contact. From CR to CO (compare Figure 3.63 to 3.62i), Shawn shifts forward 2 mm and left 2 mm. We wish to underscore the importance of making a *CR–CO evaluation for every patient at every appointment.*

Q: How will the identification of this shift affect Shawn's findings/problem list?

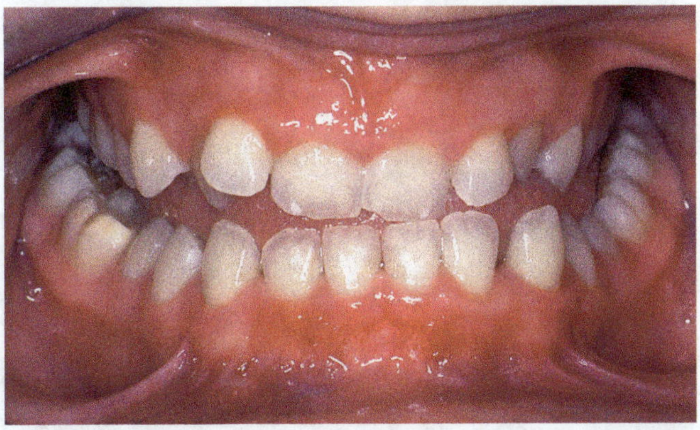

Figure 3.63 When Shawn was re-examined, he displayed a sizable CR–CO shift. In CR, his left central incisors contacted. Note that his mandibular incisors appear overerupted but that his maxillary incisors do not.

A: The identification of this shift not only reduces Shawn's Class III relationship but also reduces his transverse problem as a narrower (anterior) part of his mandibular arch is positioned posteriorly in CR. However, in CR (Figure 3.63), Shawn is still in complete lingual posterior cross bite.

Q: Two patients, hypothetically, present to you for treatment. The first is Class II in CO, and second is Class III in CO. If both have a forward shift from CR to CO, then how will this shift affect your treatment for each?

A: In the first patient, the Class II relationship will worsen in CR, making your treatment more difficult. In the second patient, the Class III relationship will improve in CR, making your treatment potentially easier.

Q: What other occlusal factors must be examined in Shawn (and every patient) using models?

A: Additional occlusal factors needing examination include the following:

- Posterior transverse compensations. Note (Figure 3.64) that Shawn exhibits significant maxillary posterior buccal crown torque and mandibular posterior lingual crown torque.
- AP molar relationships viewed from the lingual. Note that Shawn looks more Class III on his left (Figure 3.65a) than on his right (Figure 3.65b).

Q: Shawn's Iowa Classification is III (3) I III (2) III (3). That is, both first molars appear Class III by 3 mm when viewed from

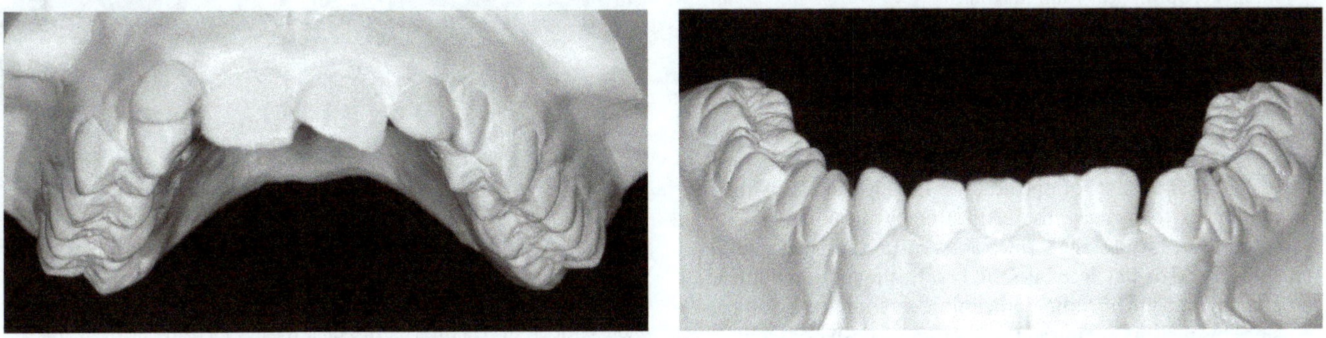

(a) (b)

Figure 3.64 (a, b) Separated models view of Shawn.

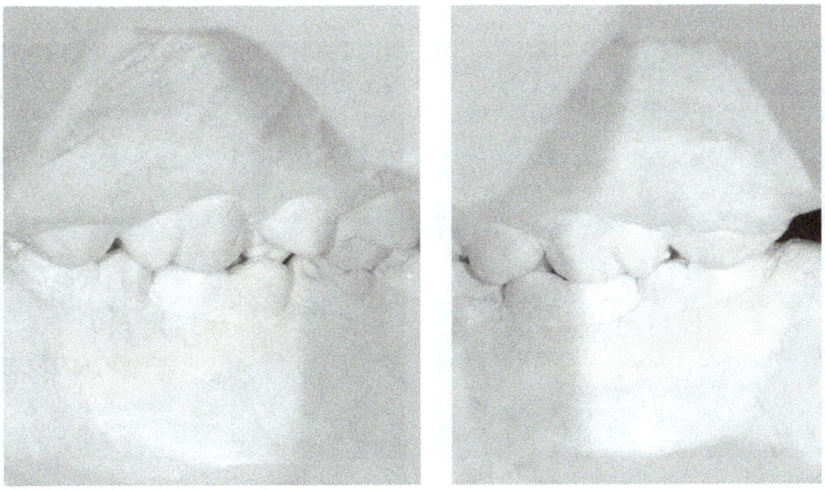

(a) (b)

Figure 3.65 Shawn's models viewed from the lingual: (a) left side and (b) right side the buccal. Why then does Shawn appear more Class III on the left when his models are viewed from the lingual?

A: Because Shawn's maxillary left first molar is rotated forward slightly, it appears less Class III when viewed from the buccal than it really is (when viewed from the lingual).

Q: Is Shawn's deep bite (under bite) a *skeletal* deep bite, a *dental* deep bite, or a combination of both?

A: A combination of both. Shawn presents with borderline *skeletal* deep bite features: soft tissue overclosed appearance (everted lower lip, deep labiomental sulcus) and borderline short skeletal LAFH (LAFT/TAFH = 53%; FMA = 14°; SN-MP = 21°; and SN, FH, and MP nearly parallel). His *dental* deep bite features include excessively erupted mandibular incisors and a deep (3 mm) COS.

Q: What is the etiology of Shawn's deep bite?

A: His dental deep bite resulted from his Class III relationship and anterior cross bite. Because the mandibular incisors were habitually positioned ahead of the maxillary incisors, the mandibular incisors had nothing to prevent their eruption. As a result, the mandibular incisors overerupted, creating a dental deep bite (under bite) and an exaggerated COS. Shawn's borderline skeletal deep bite probably occurred when his mandible rotated upward and forward (yellow arrow, Figure 3.66) as a result of his condyles growing more vertically than normal, mandible rotating forward (internally, true rotation) more excessively than normal, maxilla descending less than normal, and/or molars erupting less than normal.

Q: In basic terms, how are dental and skeletal deep bites treated? In general terms, how would you treat Shawn's deep bite?

A: Ideally, dental deep bites (normal LAFH) are corrected by intruding/proclining overerupted anterior teeth (not altering the LAFH). Skeletal deep bites (short LAFH) are corrected by erupting posterior teeth (orthopedically/surgically/possibly with prosthodontics to increase the LAFH) or by intruding/proclining anterior teeth (masking). Since Shawn is a combination of both skeletal and dental deep bites, his best treatment would include a combination of intruding/proclining anterior teeth (especially since his incisors are upright) and erupting posterior teeth.

Q: If stable eruption of Shawn's posterior teeth could be achieved, would this hurt or help his Class III relationship?

A: If stable eruption of Shawn's posterior teeth could be achieved, then the mandible would rotate down and back (Figure 3.67), helping to reduce his Class III relationship, increase his LAFH, reduce his overclosed appearance, and open his bite.

Q: What are your primary problems in each dimension (plus other) that you must stay focused on when treating Shawn?

A: See Table 3.6

Q: What are your treatment goals?

A: Ideally, reduce Shawn's overclosed appearance (or at least not worsen it) by increasing his LAFH, reducing his lower lip prom-

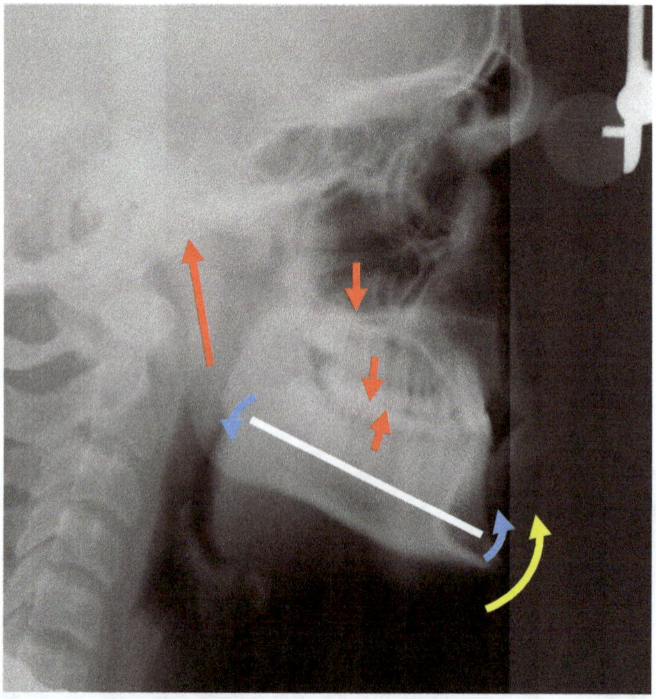

Figure 3.66 Borderline skeletal deep bites, like Shawn's, result from the same underlying growth patterns as more severe skeletal deep bites: condyles growing more vertically than normal, the mandible rotating forward (internally, true rotation) more than normal (blue arrows), the maxilla descending less than normal, and/or molars erupting less than normal. As a result, the mandible rotates upward and forward (yellow arrow), deepening the bite.

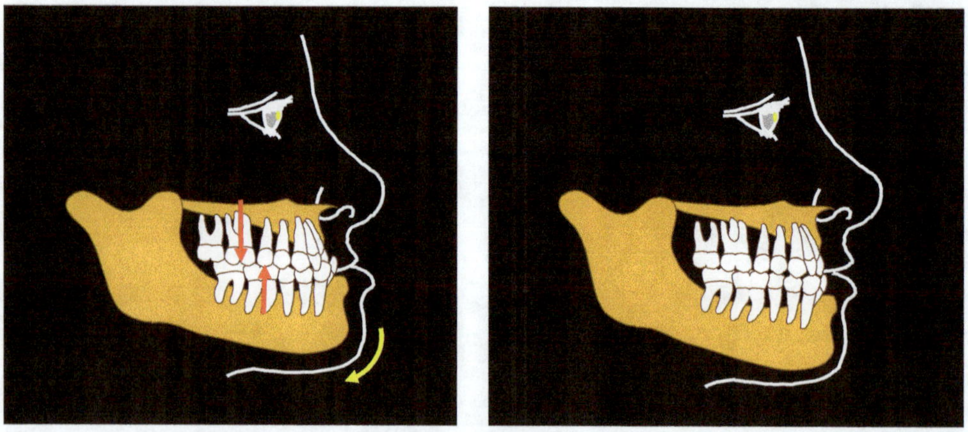

(a) (b)

Figure 3.67 (a, b) If you could (stably) erupt Shawn's posterior teeth, Shawn's mandible would rotate down and back—improving his Class III relationship, LAFH, and underbite.

inence, and reducing his labiomental sulcus depth. Additionally, we would like to position his canines (and maxillary molars if he is treated without extractions) into a Class I relationship, obtain minimal OB and minimal OJ, and correct his cross bites.

Q: Which dimensions have apical base discrepancies in Shawn?
A: All three—AP, vertical, and transverse.

Q: Of the three, general, ways to treat Shawn's Class III skeletal discrepancy (orthopedics, masking, surgery), let's talk about orthopedics first. What is the objective of orthopedics, and what are two problems in attempting an orthopedics solution on Shawn?
A: Orthopedic objectives for Shawn include restricting mandibular forward growth while permitting the maxilla to continue growing forward and/or enhancing maxillary forward growth. Problems in attempting an orthopedic solution with Shawn are his age and his anterior cross bite. First, at 15 years of age we do not know how much more Shawn will grow. He may be finished growing, or he could have significant Class III growth for years to come. You ask Shawn's parents, and they tell you that he has already passed his growth spurt and is no longer growing very much. That is good news, but you must not be complacent about monitoring his future growth. Second, because of his anterior cross bite, his front teeth could get in the way of your AP orthopedic treatment.

Table 3.6 **Primary problems list for Shawn** *(apical base/skeletal discrepancies italicized).*

AP	III (3) I III (2) III (3) *Mild maxillary skeletal retrusion* *Mild mandibular skeletal protrusion*
Vertical	*Borderline skeletal* deep bite and dental deep bite
Transverse	Bilateral cross bites secondary to *maxillary skeletal transverse deficiency*
Other	—

Q: Considering the existence of his significant CR–CO shift, and his incisor edge-to-edge relationship in CR, what will be the first thing you must consider doing with Shawn?
A: *Correct his anterior cross bite.* Before deciding whether to institute AP orthopedic treatment, or before deciding what specific orthopedic treatment to institute, the first thing you should do is to correct his anterior cross bite, eliminate his CR–CO shift, and re-evaluate his AP relationship.

Q: Once his anterior cross bite (CR–CO shift) is corrected, if you decide to attempt orthopedics, then what specific orthopedic treatments would you consider using?
A: As Shawn presents with a mildly deficient maxilla and (possibly) mildly protrusive mandible, possible orthopedic options would include RPHG, high-pull chin cup, or Class III elastics worn between TADs.

Q: Why did we say "possibly" mildly protrusive mandible?
A: Because the finding of a mildly protrusive mandible was determined using his initial lateral cephalometric radiograph, made in CO. Once the CR–CO shift is eliminated, his mandible may be considered normal.

Q: Allison (Figure 3.68) presented with a deficient maxilla, posterior lingual cross bite, anterior cross bite, and Class III dental relationship. She was initially treated with an RME appliance and RPHG. Note that the anterior cross bite has been corrected (Figure 3.68e). What are the effects of RPHGs?
A: The effects of RPHG [88, 89] wear (6 months, 380 gms of force per side) following RME are, on average, as follows

- 1.8 mm forward maxillary growth
- Increased fullness of maxillary lip
- Downward and backward mandibular rotation
- Mandibular MPA increase of 1.5°

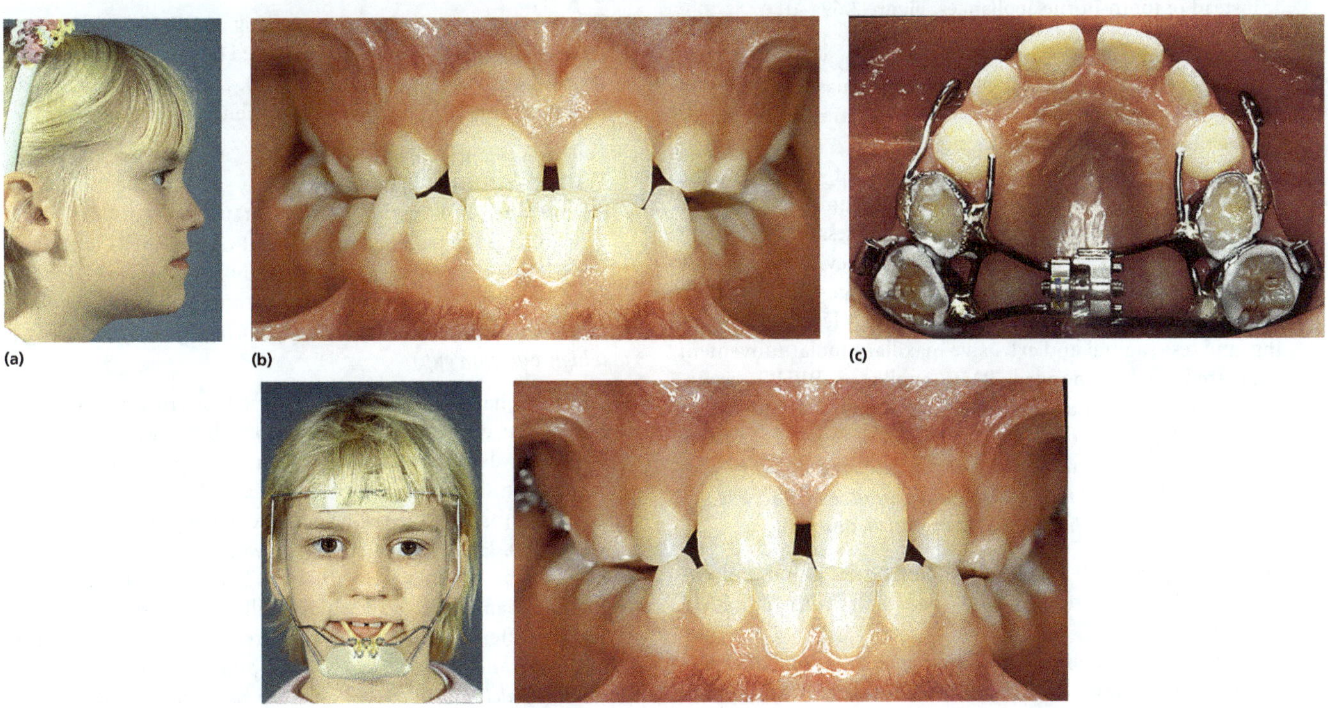

(a) (b) (c) (d) (e)

Figure 3.68 (a–e) Allison is a 7-year-old Class III patient (deficient maxilla, normal mandible), initially treated with RME and RPHG (elastics running between the RPHG and attachments on the RME) which corrected her anterior cross bite.

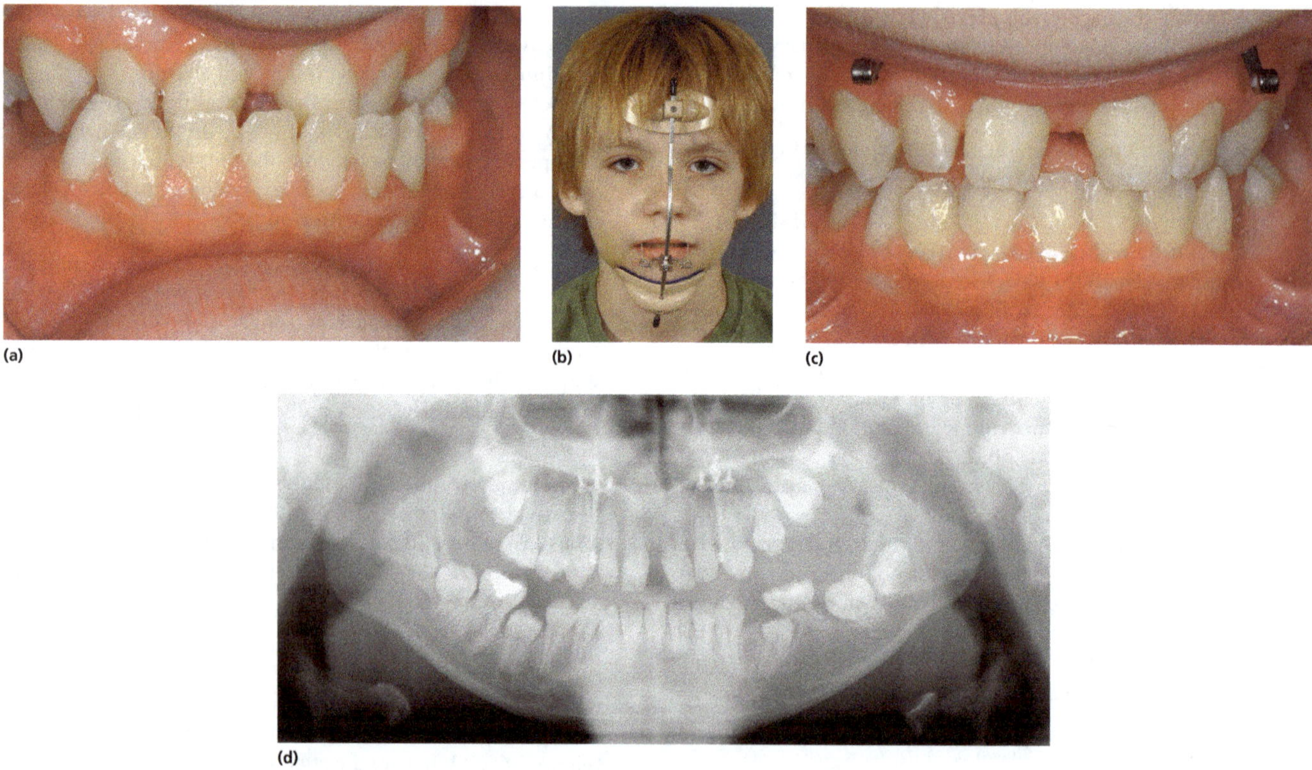

Figure 3.69 (a–c) Marc is a 12-year-old Class III patient (deficient maxilla, normal mandible), initially treated with RPHG (elastics running between the RPHG and maxillary anterior miniplates) which corrected his anterior cross bite.

- LAFH increase of 2.9 mm
- Lingual movement of mandibular incisors
- Labial movement of maxillary incisors (maxillary tooth movement is eliminated if miniplates are used for anchorage instead of tooth-borne appliances, Figure 3.69a–d)

Q: How does maxillary facemask protraction with miniplate anchorage compare to conventional facemask protraction (tooth-borne) where both groups first undergoing rapid maxillary expansion with a bonded appliance?

A: In the miniplate anchorage RPHG group of one study, the maxilla moved forward more and without significant anterior rotation, the mandible rotated posteriorly less, facial height increased less, and no dental movement was evident [90]. In a similar study [91], the miniplate anchorage RPHG group showed more forward maxillary movement, less FMA opening, and less sagittal and extrusive maxillary molar movement compared to the bonded RME appliance RPHG group. Following a meta-analysis [92], the authors concluded that approximately *3 mm of horizontal A-point movement is reliably attainable with skeletal (miniplate) anchorage maxillary protraction—which is 1 mm greater than what can be expected with tooth-borne anchored maxillary protraction* [93].

Q: When using an RPHG, does A-point advance more if the circumaxillary sutures are loosened first with an RME appliance?

A: Although some studies report no difference in A-point advancement with or without RME [93–95], at least one study reported that A-point advances more if the RPHG (300–500 gms/side, 12 h/day until the cross bite is corrected) is applied ***during*** RME, less after RME, and even less without RME [96].

Q: Is there a difference in treatment effects between early and late maxillary RPHG protraction treatment in growing patients?

A: Yes. The skeletal effects of RPHGs are less in patients greater than 10 years of age [97–99].

Q: What does this mean in terms of using an RPHG on Shawn?

A: At over 15 years of age, if RPHG is used to correct Shawn's Class III relationship (maxillary retrusion), then the correction will be made, primarily, by dental movements (not skeletal).

Q: Is RPHG therapy stable?

A: Yes and no. Although the maxillary advancement may not relapse after it is used, RPHG therapy does not normalize growth, and the patient can grow out of the RPHG correction [99–101]. *The key to using an RPHG on growing Class III maxillary deficient patients is overcorrecting and maintaining correction until the patient is done growing (often by switching to a high-pull chin cup).*

Q: Once you have corrected Shawn's anterior cross bite, you may decide to use a high-pull chin cup to orthopedically correct his Class III dental relationship. For example, the Class III adolescent shown in Figure 3.70a and b presented with an anterior cross bite, maxillary AP deficiency, and mandibular AP excess. His anterior cross bite was first corrected using a mandibular bite plate (to disclude his teeth) plus maxillary fixed appliances to advance his maxillary incisors (Figure 3.70c and d). After his cross bite was corrected, we re-evaluated his occlusion and *placed him on a high-pull chin cup* (Figure 3.70e and f), *which he wore until growth was complete* (Figure 3.70g and h). His AP was corrected and he desired no additional treatment. What are the effects of high-pull chin cup wear in an adolescent?

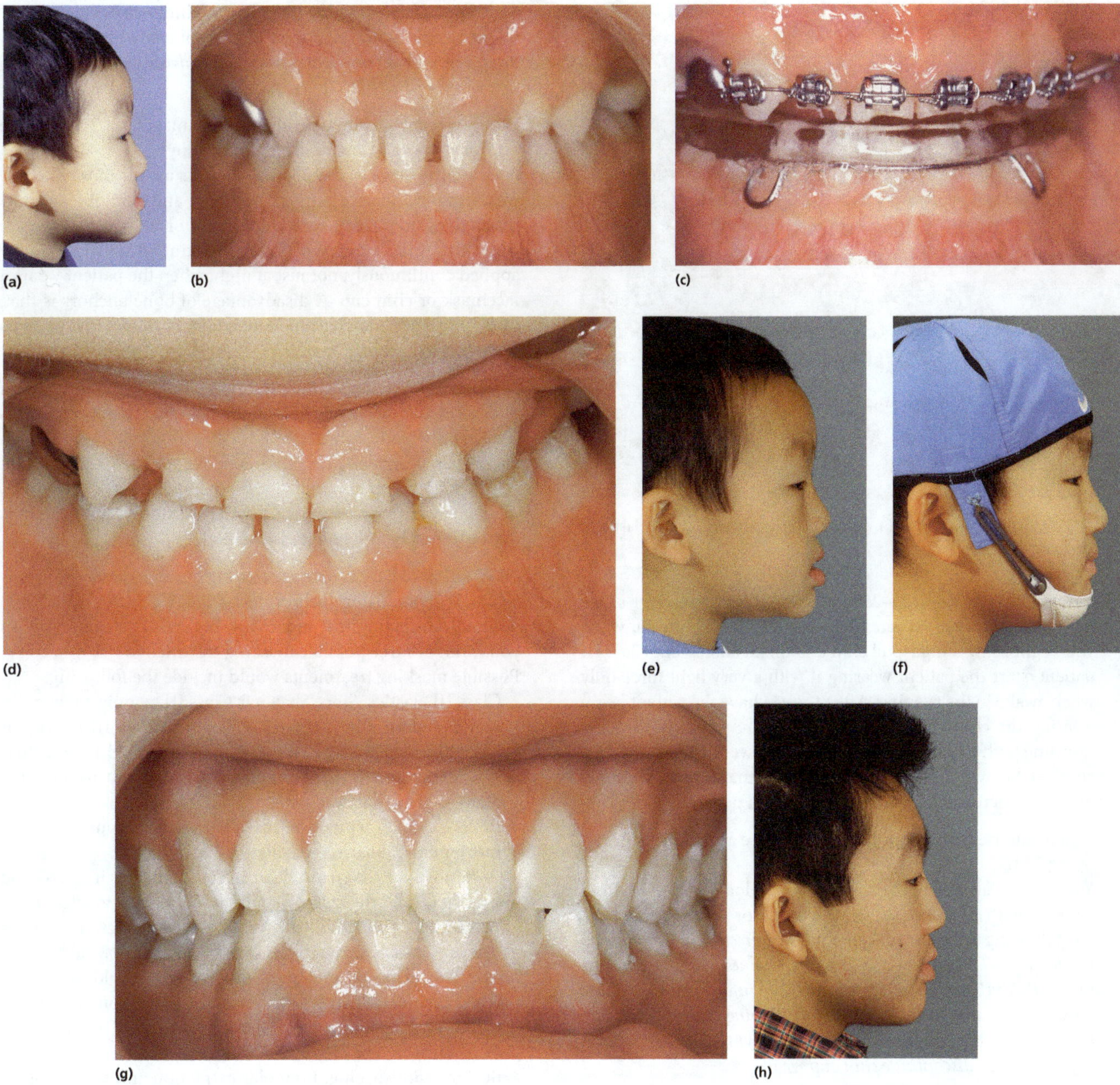

Figure 3.70 (a–h) After his anterior cross bite was corrected using a mandibular biteplate and fixed orthodontic appliances, this Class III adolescent (maxillary AP deficiency, mandibular AP excess) patient was placed on a high-pull chin cup until growth was complete. No additional treatment was requested or instituted. Note the dramatic improvement with this treatment.

A: *High-pull* chin cup effects (14 h/day of chin cup wear for 2 years plus chin cup wear during sleep for three additional years) include the following [102]:
- ANB improvement (compared to controls)
- Chin position improvement
- Inhibition of mandibular ramal height and mandibular body length growth (maxilla can continue to grow forward)
- Backward rotation of mandible
- Closure of gonial angle
- Mandibular plane angle (FMA) flattened in chin cup patients while control group subjects opened
- LAFH not increased [103]

However, wearing a chin cup (like wearing a RPHG) does not normalize growth. The listed changes will not be maintained if chin cup wear is discontinued before facial growth is complete [104]

Q: What is the effect of light-force (125–250 gm) chin cup wear on growing Class III patients? How much force should you apply with a high-pull chin cup?

A: In a recent study, although a slight decrease in SNB angle was noted, fewer than 50% of patients treated with a light-force chin cup had favorable clinical outcomes [105]. There were significant dentoalveolar changes, particularly uprighting of the mandibular incisors. *The ideal force for chin cup therapy is still unknown,*

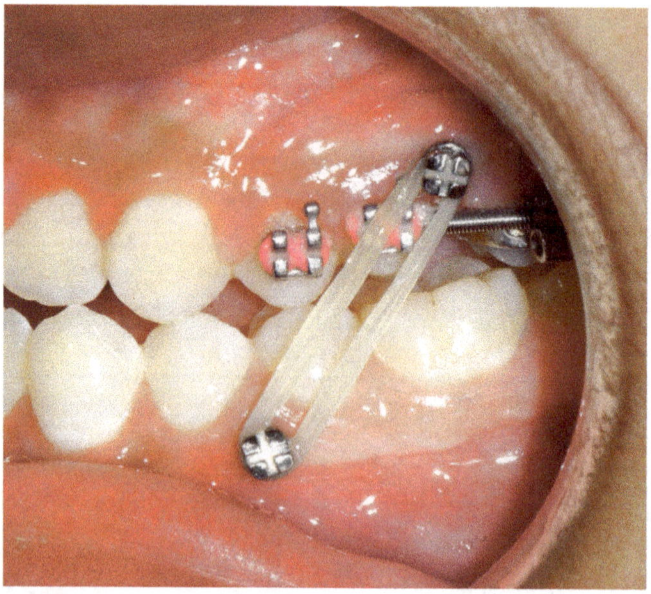

Figure 3.71 Orthopedic Class III treatment consisting of Class III elastics worn between TADs.

but a force exceeding 125–250 gm, measured at the center of the chin cup, appears to be necessary. In our clinical opinion, when you begin using a high-pull chin cup on an adolescent Class III patient, start the patient wearing it with a very light force only when awake in the evening. After 1 week, have the patient begin wearing the chin cup starting at about 7–8 pm until the next morning with a light force for a period of weeks. Once they are comfortable with that regimen, maintain that time of wear but gradually increase the force level to 250 gm per side.

Q: When you use a high-pull chin cup, is there a concern of developing TMD?

A: You should always be concerned about loading the TMJs—whether with chin cups, Class III elastics, or soft tissue stretching following BSSO advancements. *In our clinical opinion, do not load the TMJs using chin cups in patients who initially present with TMJ pain or restricted function; inform patients of the possibility of transient symptoms developing during chin cup treatment; in patients who develop TMD symptoms during chin cup treatment, discontinue chin cup wear.*

Q: A relatively new orthopedic treatment for Class III adolescents consists of wearing Class III elastics between TADs in both jaws (Figure 3.71). An advantage of this technique is that *unilateral* mandibular hyperplasias can be treated using it. How does growth of untreated Class III subjects compare to growth of Class III patients treated with bone-anchored maxillary protraction (Class III elastics worn between maxillary and mandibular TADs)?

A: Compared with growth in untreated Class III subjects, bone-anchored protocol patients have an average maxillary advancement of 4 mm and B-point improvement of 2 mm [106].

Q: Which treatment results in greater maxillary advancement in prepubertal patients: RME followed by RPHG or Class III elastic worn between infrazygomatic and anterior mandibular miniplates?

A: *Class III elastics worn between miniplates,* initially applied with a force of 150 grams and gradually increased to 250 grams after 3 months, coupled with a bite plate to eliminate occlusal interference in the incisor region until anterior cross-bite correction, *produced over 2 mm greater maxillary advancement than RME followed by RPHG* [107].

Q: What are the advantages and disadvantages of TAD (bone anchor) Class III elastic correction therapy?

A: A clear advantage is compliance. Patients are far more likely to wear intraoral elastics between maxillary and mandibular miniplates than they are to wear a facemask or high-pull chin cup. Also, the force from the Class III intraoral elastics can be applied continuously, not just at night when the patient wears a facemask or chin cup. A disadvantage of bone anchors is that, over time, they may become embedded in adolescent bone as bony surface apposition occurs.

Q: No matter what Class III adolescent orthopedic treatment you attempt, what fact must you remember after the correction is successfully made, long term?

A: Fact: Class III orthopedic treatment does *not* normalize growth. A Class III correction will not be maintained if RPHG wear, high-pull chin cup wear, or Class III elastics wear to TADs is discontinued before growth is complete.

Q: Next, let's move from orthopedics to consider *masking* Shawn's Class III relationship (achieving a Class I canine relationship without addressing his underlying skeletal discrepancy). Can you think of three possible masking treatments?

A: Possible masking treatments would include the following:

- Class III elastics. Since Shawn is Class III by only a few millimeters (3 mm minus the CR–CO shift), Class III elastics or Class III springs (e.g., Dynaflex springs) could be effective, *after* the cross bites are corrected and *only* if you are sure that Shawn's growth is complete.
- RPHG, which could be used to achieve purely dental movement of Shawn's maxillary arch.
- Posterior (ramal) mandibular TADs could be inserted and used to retract the entire mandibular dentition to Class I.
- Extraction of mandibular premolars and retraction of mandibular canines through the extraction spaces would *not* be justified. Why? So much extraction space would be created with premolar extractions that the mandibular canines would end up being retracted into a Class II relationship. Furthermore, Shawn's mandibular incisors are already very upright *with* spacing. Premolar extraction and space closure would result in mandibular incisors uprighting even more.

Q: The horizontal effects of Class III elastics are (Figure 3.72a) protraction of maxillary teeth and retraction mandibular teeth—improving the patient's Class III relationship. The horizontal effects of Class II elastics are (Figure 3.72b) retraction of maxillary teeth and protraction of mandibular teeth—improving the patient's Class II relationship. The vertical effects of Class III and Class II elastics tend to rotate the occlusal plane (which aids in improving the respective AP relationships, but may relapse since it is based on erupting teeth) and to rotate the mandibular plane. Contrast the effects of Class III elastics on the occlusal and mandibular planes with the effects of Class II elastics on the occlusal and mandibular planes. How do they differ?

A: Both Class III elastics (blue line, Figure 3.72c left) and Class II elastics (blue line, Figure 3.72d left) tend to erupt molars, and thereby rotate the mandibular plane down and back (yellow arrows Figure 3.72c and d). Class III elastics erupt maxillary

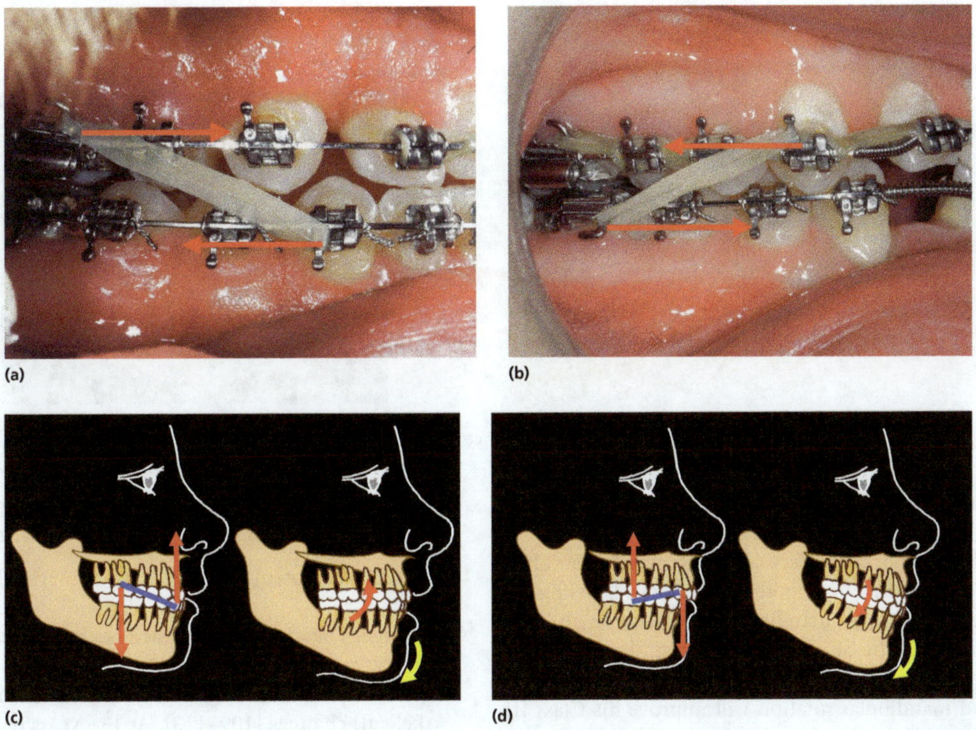

Figure 3.72 Class III elastics (a, c) tend to protract maxillary teeth, retract mandibular teeth, erupt maxillary molars, erupt mandibular anterior teeth, rotate the mandibular plane CW, and rotate the occlusal plane CCW. Class II elastics (b, d) tend to retract maxillary teeth, protract mandibular teeth, erupt mandibular molars, erupt maxillary anterior teeth, rotate the mandibular plane CW, and rotate the occlusal plane CW.

molars, while Class II elastics erupt mandibular molars. Because they also erupt mandibular anterior teeth, Class III elastics tend to rotate the occlusal plane CCW (curved red arrow Figure 3.72c, right). Because they also erupt maxillary anterior teeth, Class II elastics tend to rotate the occlusal plane CW (curved red arrow Figure 3.72d, right).

Q: Finally, let's consider surgery to correct Shawn's Class III relationship. What surgery might you consider?

A: Depending on Shawn's desires, position of the jaws once the CR–CO shift is corrected, and the amount of growth Shawn has remaining, a maxillary advancement osteotomy could be an option. But, quite frankly, Shawn is a handsome young man, and surgery to correct his AP relationship would be unreasonable.

Q: What are the general ways that you can treat Shawn's borderline skeletal deep bite? List specific treatment options for each. Recall that our ideal goal is to increase Shawn's LAFH *slightly* to decrease his overclosed appearance (but not enough to create an ILG).

A: *Orthopedics* (enhance downward growth of the maxillary corpus, enhance maxillary alveolar growth by erupting maxillary posterior teeth, or enhance mandibular alveolar growth by erupting mandibular posterior teeth). Once again, the problem in attempting an orthopedic solution is Shawn's age and the fact that he is no longer growing very much. Options include the following:

- RPHG. Since Shawn has a mildly deficient maxilla, an RPHG could increase LAFH, increase the MPA, and result in downward and backward mandibular rotation [88, 89, 108]. But the skeletal effects of RPHGs are less in patients older than 10 years of age [97–99], so this treatment may be ineffective.
- Leveling the mandibular COS with archwires occurs primarily through premolar eruption (growing mandibular alveolar process bone) [23]. Mandibular molars (tipped mesially with the COS, see Figure 3.62r) will tip distally during arch leveling. As they tip distally, they will erupt—potentially increasing his vertical facial dimension. However, molar eruption could be unstable in someone approaching adulthood. Leveling the COS also proclines and intrudes mandibular anterior teeth, which is a dental (masking) approach to opening the deep bite.
- An anterior biteplate (to disclude the posterior teeth) coupled with vertical elastics to erupt the maxillary and mandibular posterior teeth (grow posterior alveolar process bone). This could be performed in conjunction with COS leveling to lengthen the LAFH, although such short-term tooth eruption may not be stable in the long term, especially in someone approaching adulthood.

Masking or camouflage (opening Shawn's overbite, dentally, but not trying to change his borderline skeletal vertical deficiency). You could mask Shawn's skeletal deep bite in the same way you would ideally correct a dental deep bite: maxillary and mandibular incisor intrusion/proclination [22]. Intruding maxillary or mandibular anterior teeth will open Shawn's bite. However, you must be careful not to overintrude his maxillary incisors because he could end up with inadequate incisal display. In cases like Shawn's, when you intrude incisors to open the bite, try to intrude mandibular incisors, if you have a choice—in order to maintain maxillary incisor display. Proclining Shawn's incisors would help open his bite, and could be desirable since his incisors are upright. Aligning the crowded maxillary anterior teeth will procline them. However, proclining Shawn's mandibular anterior teeth is not likely, since he has anterior spacing. Closing spaces between Shawn's mandibular anterior teeth will upright them, tending to deepen the bite. Leveling the mandibular COS

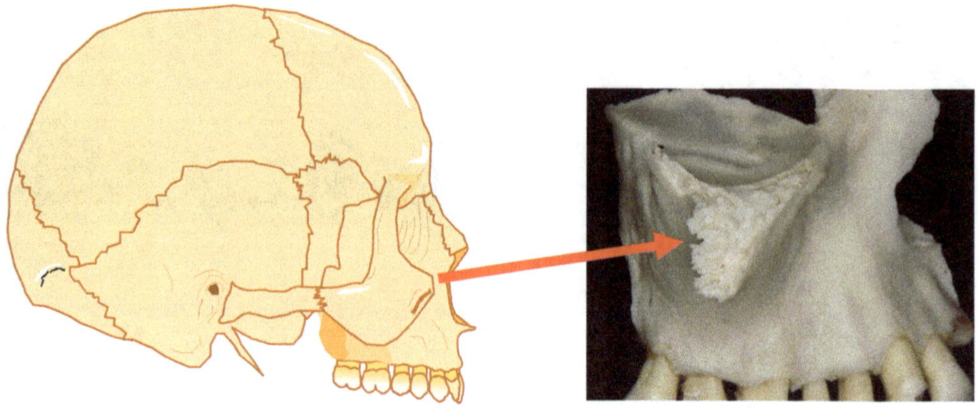

Figure 3.73 The zygomatic buttress—considered the primary skeletal resistance site to RME.

intrudes/proclines the mandibular anterior teeth but occurs primarily through eruption of mandibular premolars, which could be considered an orthopedic effect (growing mandibular alveolar process bone, tending to lengthen the LAFH). Leveling the COS also uprights/erupts mandibular molars, which may lengthen the LAFH. The beauty of increasing Shawn's LAFH through COS leveling (posterior tooth eruption) is that downward/backward mandibular rotation will improve his Class III relationship. Considering the fact that Shawn has a borderline skeletal deep bite, *masking seems to be a viable alternative.*

Surgery (maxillary downgraft to lengthen Shawn's LAFH). Although surgery is an option, it is important to reflect on the magnitude of Shawn's vertical deficiency. Surgery would generally not be considered with his mildly short LAFH unless this was a specific concern of Shawn's (and only if his LAFH could be lengthened without producing an interlabial gap).

Q: How would you address Shawn's transverse apical base discrepancy?

A: *Orthopedics* (widening the maxilla by separating the hemimaxillae at the midpalatal suture). Successful RME could result in both maxillary skeletal and dental expansion. If the maxillary dental arch is widened, then enough posterior OJ could be created to permit uprighting maxillary and mandibular posterior teeth (removing transverse dental compensations) and coordinating the arches.

Masking or camouflage (creating posterior OJ by increasing transverse compensations and not by addressing the underlying transverse skeletal discrepancy—maxillary transverse deficiency). The magnitude of Shawn's transverse discrepancy is so large (Figure 3.63, 6.5 mm discrepancy between maxillary and mandibular intermolar widths), and he already has such significant transverse dental compensations (Figure 3.64), that increasing/worsening posterior compensations is not advised.

Surgery options include the following:

- SARME would achieve adequate maxillary expansion. However, a SARME should be considered only if RME failed to achieve a midpalatal split.
- MPMO would be reasonable if a maxillary downgraft osteotomy was already part of the treatment plan. But remember, unlike a SARME (which grows bone and soft tissue), the magnitude of maxillary transverse expansion is limited with an MPMO, because you are stretching the palatal soft tissue, at surgery, instantaneously. Up to 8 mm of transverse correction may be possible in some patients with high palatal vaults and upright maxillary molars, but stretching the palatal soft tissue too much can compromise the blood supply.

Q: What is the potential problem in attempting RME expansion in Shawn?

A: His age. *The most marked RME skeletal effect occurs before/during the pubertal growth spurt*, and expansion after the pubertal growth spurt results in mainly dentoalveolar (not orthopedic/skeletal) changes [109–113]. At 15+ years of age, Shawn's facial maturation may be too advanced, and offer too much skeletal resistance, to permit separation of his midpalatal suture. However, you can attempt RME at the rate of 0.25 mm per day, or 0.25 mm every other day when starting, and monitor if the midpalatal suture separates.

Q: Is the midpalatal suture, itself, considered the major site of skeletal resistance to RME?

A: No. If the midpalatal suture was the major site of skeletal resistance to RME, then once the suture was opened, the skeletal resistance would drop dramatically. However, Isaacson and Ingram [114] reported no significant change in the RME opening force during the time the suture opened. It is currently believed that the zygomatic buttress (Figure 3.73) is the major skeletal resistance site to RME [115].

Q: If you attempt RME on Shawn, how will you know if his midpalatal suture separates?

A: The most obvious sign that the midpalatal suture has separated during RME is the formation of a maxillary midline diastema. If a midline diastema does not form, then look for other signs that the suture is not splitting which include the following:

- Absence of a clear bony midpalatal split when viewed on an occlusal radiograph
- Impingement of the RME appliance's metal arms on the palatal soft tissue (indicating lateral dental movement in the absence of lateral maxillary bone movement)
- Sensation of continued pressure from the screw more than 5 or 10 min beyond expansion screw activation
- Pain

Q: If Shawn activates the RME screw for 1 or 2 weeks, but the midpalatal suture does not separate, what can you do?

A: The answer depends on whether you have already achieved significant dental expansion of the maxillary molars with the RME appliance. If only minimal expansion has occurred (and you require over 6.5 mm of transverse expansion in Shawn), then you could consider either surgical intervention (SARME or multiple-piece maxillary osteotomy) or leaving Shawn in posterior cross bite. If significant dental expansion had already occurred, and if the posterior buccal periodontium appeared robust (lots of buccal bone, lots of thick keratinized attached tissue), then you could consider continuing dental expansion with the RME appliance (albeit slowly, at the rate of 0.25 mm or 0.5 mm *per week*). However, Shawn (Figure 3.62p) does not appear to have wide thicknesses of bone buccal to his maxillary posterior teeth. *Considering the magnitude of the transverse correction Shawn needs and the magnitude of the transverse compensations he already has, we would not recommend expanding him dentally if the RME appliance failed to achieve a midpalatal split.*

Q: Could Shawn be left in cross bite without attempting RME?

A: Yes. However, all treatment options should be presented to him and his parents. Leaving Shawn in cross bite is a compromise. Generally, we will consider leaving an adult in posterior cross bite only if the canines can be coordinated properly (clinical opinion).

Q: Is surgical treatment an option for Shawn?

A: Although Shawn could be treated with surgery in all three planes of spaces (maxillary downgraft to lengthen his LAFH, maxillary advancement or possible mandibular setback to correct his AP, and SARME or MPMO to widen his maxilla), considering the magnitude of his discrepancies, it would be reasonable to first attempt nonsurgical treatment. However, surgical options must be discussed with Shawn and his parents.

Q: What unknowns do you face? Specifically, what unknowns should you try to eliminate before defining a final treatment plan or doing something irreversible (e.g., extractions or surgery) for Shawn?

A: Unknowns include the following:

- An undetected CR–CO shift. You should reassess Shawn's AP and transverse relationships *after* you are confident his shift is eliminated.
- Growth. How long and how much will Shawn continue to grow Class III?
- Cross-bite correction. Can Shawn's posterior cross bite be corrected with an RME appliance? Can a midpalatal split be achieved?
- Patient cooperation and hygiene.

Q: Would a nonextraction treatment plan be justified, or should anterior or posterior teeth be extracted?

A: Considering his mandibular anterior spacing, uprightness of his incisors, and need for maxillary expansion, a nonextraction treatment plan would make sense. Extraction of permanent teeth would not be reasonable.

Q: Taking all of our previous discussion into consideration, and reflecting on all of your options, what treatment do you recommend? How do you think Shawn was treated?

A: First, maxillary expansion with an RME appliance (Figure 3.74) was attempted, and a midpalatal suture split was (thankfully) achieved. RME continued until overcorrection was reached (maxillary first molar lingual cusps on end with mandibular first molar buccal cusps). Three months later, the RME appliance was removed. Fixed appliances were bonded on the maxillary arch, and the maxillary anterior teeth were proclined to correct the anterior cross bite. (A biteplate was worn on the posterior teeth to open the anterior bite during cross-bite correction.) After the anterior cross bite was corrected, Shawn's AP was reassessed. Growth was again discussed with his parents, and they stated that he was no longer growing. In CR, Shawn was now found to be Class III by only 1–2 mm, bilaterally, at the first molars. A decision was made to finish his treatment nonextraction, without orthopedics, without tooth extractions, and without surgery.

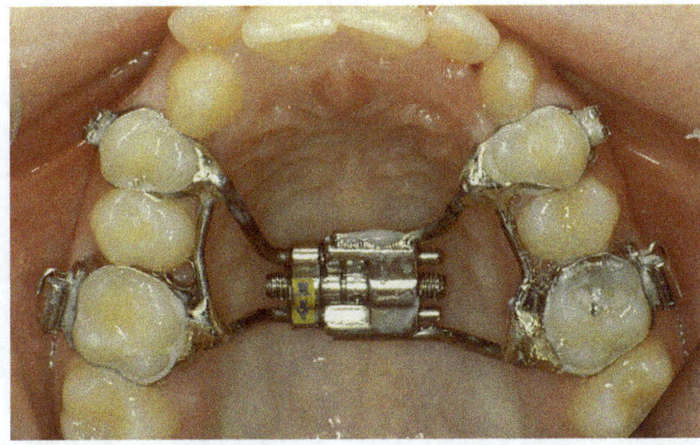

Figure 3.74 Maxillary expander cemented in Shawn.

Q: What are the specific objectives of treatment for the maxilla, mandible, maxillary dentition, and mandibular dentition in all three planes of space?

A: Specific objectives of treatment for Shawn are as follows:

Maxilla

AP: Allow for any remaining forward growth.
Vertical: Allow for any remaining downward growth.
Transverse: Increase width to establish normal transverse relationship.

Mandible

AP: Monitor growth and possibly restrict remaining growth.
Vertical: Allow for any remaining growth.
Transverse: Allow for any remaining growth.

Maxillary dentition

AP: Class I molars. Procline incisors.
Vertical: Slightly erupt molars and maintain incisors.
Intermolar width: Increase width to establish normal transverse relationship.

Mandibular dentition

AP: Class I molars. Upright incisors.
Vertical: Level COS. Intrude incisors.
Intermolar/Intercanine width: Maintain molars. Maintain intercanine widths.

Q: How did Shawn's treatment progress?

A: The mandibular arch was bonded and all spaces closed. Class III elastics were worn. Arches were coordinated and finished.

Q: Deband photographs, radiographs, and cephalometric tracings are shown in Figure 3.75. (Initial facial photographs in Figure 3.75a, c, and e are included for comparison.) What changes are evident?

A: Changes from Shawn's initial to deband records include the following:

- Shawn's initially overclosed appearance has been improved and chin projection softened. Why? Eruption of the maxillary molars (Figure 3.75i) from Class III elastic wear has resulted in a down-and-back rotation of the mandible,

opening of the mandibular plane angle by 2–3°and slightly increasing LAFH/TAFH from 53% to 55%.
- A more confident smile.
- His maxillary incisors have been proclined (Figure 3.75i) and the anterior cross bite has been corrected.
- The transverse cross bite has been corrected (except for the right second molars), but the transverse OJ appears minimal. (Shawn is "tight" in the transverse.)
- His final overbite is improved, about 40%, but is deeper than ideal 10% (Figure 3.75l and q).
- AP correction (Class I canines) has been achieved.
- Maxillary posterior buccal crown torque and mandibular posterior lingual crown torque is still evident (Figure 3.75u and v).
- COS has been greatly reduced (Figure 3.75w).
- The root of the maxillary left second premolar appears to be dilacerated and third molar eruption will need to be monitored (Figure 3.75j)

Q: How was Shawn's deep bite corrected?
A: Primarily, by maxillary first molar eruption (Figure 3.75i), which rotated his mandible down and slightly back, opening his bite. Also, proclination of his maxillary incisors (to correct his cross bite) helped to open his bite. Although only a small amount of mandibular molar eruption is evident cephalometrically, eruption of the mandibular molars and premolars probably occurred to level the COS (Figure 3.75w), which also contributed to opening the bite.

Q: Were your treatment goals achieved?
A: For the most part, yes. His facial balance, profile, and smile were improved. Class I canines and cross-bite correction was obtained. Overbite was decreased, but not to the 10% ideal. Posterior teeth have *minimal* OJ.

Q: What retention protocol would you suggest?
A: Shawn was asked to wear Hawley retainers every night for a lifetime. His maxillary retainer was designed with an anterior biteplate to disclude his posterior teeth and improve the chances of maintaining his deep bite correction.

Q: Can you think of something that was overlooked in terms of his retention protocol?
A: Yes. *Shawn should have been placed on a high-pull chin cup as part of his retention protocol.* Shawn had a small amount of mandibular growth during treatment (Figure 3.75i), and we do not know if he is still growing (despite the fact that his parents claimed he had finished growing). Until we are absolutely sure that he has finished growing, we are gambling with his outcome if he is not wearing a chin cup at night.

Q: What "take-home" messages should be emphasized here?
A: Take-home messages include the following:
- Shawn presented with a Class III deep bite (under bite), and nearly complete lingual cross bite, malocclusion. His anteroposterior relationship resulted from a mildly deficient maxilla and a mildly protrusive mandible. His deep bite was a combination borderline skeletal deep bite (overclosed appearance; flat SN–MP angle; flat FMA; LAFT/TAFH = 53%; and SN, FH, and MP nearly parallel) plus dental deep bite (excessively erupted mandibular incisors, deep COS). His borderline skeletal deep bite occurred as a result of his condyles growing more vertically than normal, his mandible rotating forward (internally, true rotation) more excessively than normal, his maxilla descending less than normal, and/or his molars erupting less than normal. His dental deep bite resulted from his anterior cross bite with his mandibular incisors free to overerupt. His posterior cross bite resulted from a maxillary transverse skeletal discrepancy and from his Class III relationship (wider part of mandibular dental arch postured forward). Shawn was treated with RME to correct his posterior cross bite, fixed orthodontic appliances to

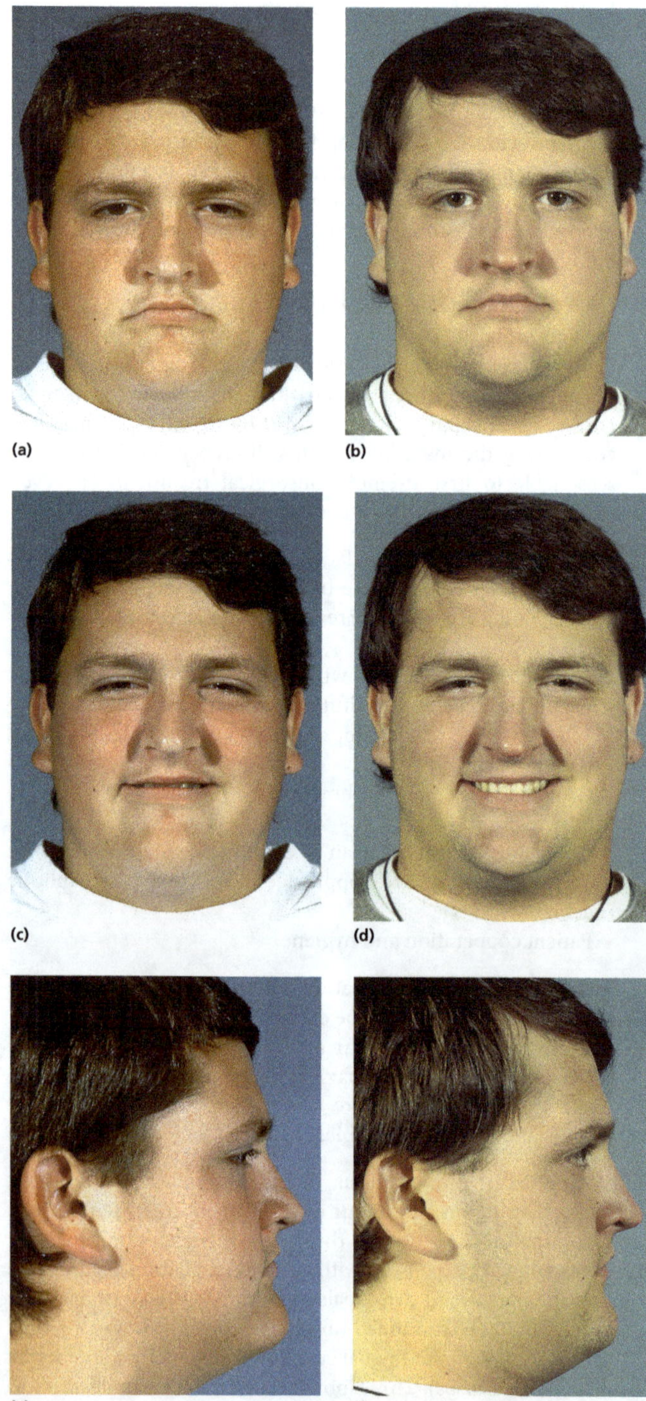
(a) (b) (c) (d) (e) (f)

Figure 3.75 Deband records of Shawn: (a, c, e) initial facial photographs and (b, d, f) final facial photographs. (g–w) final records.

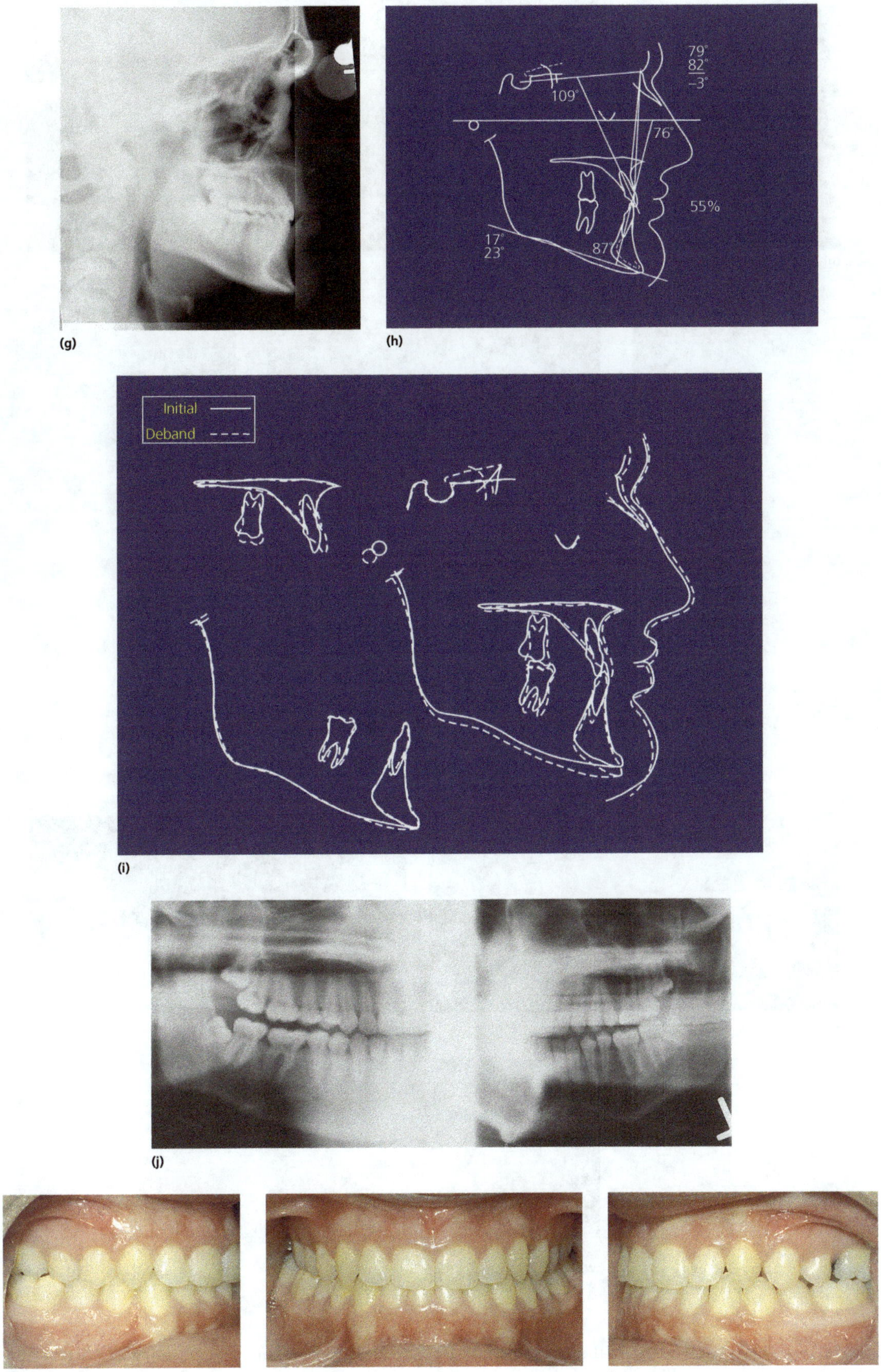

Figure 3.75 (Continued)

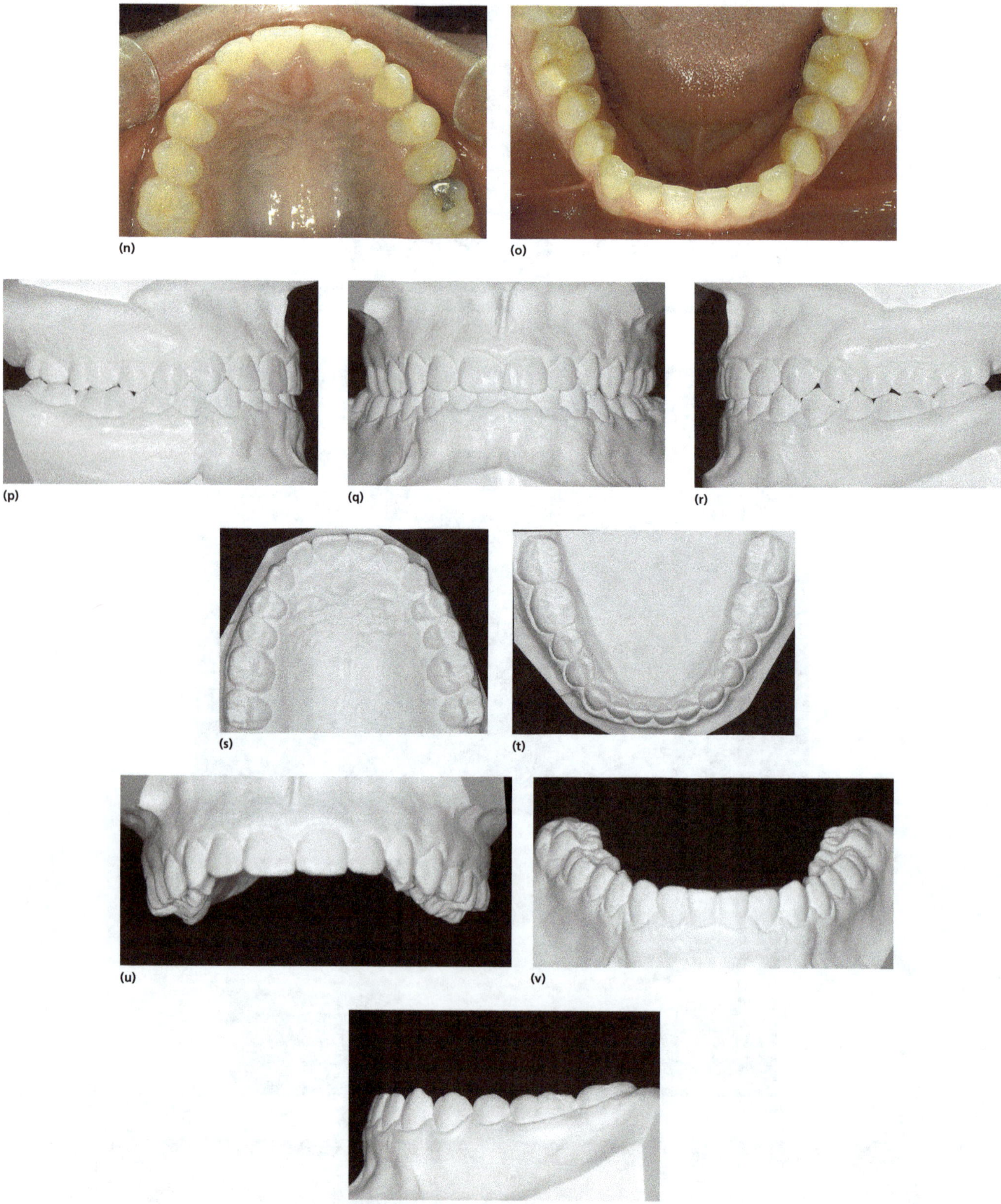

Figure 3.75 (Continued)

correct his anterior cross bite, and Class III elastics (masking) to correct his Class III relationship.

- Always, always, *always* ask yourself if there are any unknowns that should be eliminated before defining your final treatment plan or performing any irreversible treatment. Patients and parents will appreciate and understand your need to reduce/eliminate unknowns before defining a final treatment plan. Shawn's major unknowns included a CR–CO shift, response to RME, and future growth. His actual AP position could only be determined after his anterior cross bite was eliminated. Thankfully, he was minimally Class III after his shift was eliminated. (If a lateral cephalometric radiograph had been taken after cross-bite elimination, it would have shown a reasonably normal mandible.) His response to RME could only be determined by attempting RME. Thankfully, he responded well to RME, he had a mid-palatal split, and his posterior cross bite was corrected. If he had not responded well to RME, then you could have considered SARME or MPMO to make the posterior transverse correction, leaving him in posterior cross bite, or trying to correct the cross bite dentally (not recommended). Finally, Shawn had only minimal additional mandibular growth during treatment. If, during treatment, we had found his Class III relationship worsening, then we could have considered placing him on a high-pull chin cup. It was wise not to do anything irreversible until you were sure his growth was under control or complete. In summary, reducing Shawn's unknowns by correcting his cross bite first, then reassessing his AP jaw relationships before defining his final treatment plan, was brilliant.

- Since some mandibular growth was detected when his deband cephalometric tracing was superimposed on his initial deband tracing, Shawn should have been placed on a high-pull chin cup during retention to protect your result—until you were absolutely sure he was done growing.
- RME was overcorrected to the point where the lingual cusps of the maxillary molars occluded with the buccal cusps of the mandibular molars. This is generally adequate, but in Shawn's case this was inadequate. Why? This amount of RME expansion is adequate only if the mandibular molars are upright. Shawn's mandibular molars had significant lingual crown torque. The *mandibular molars should have been uprighted (all lingual crown torque removed) during RME, requiring you to expand the maxilla even more.* If this had been done, then the final transverse relationship would not have ended with minimal overjet.
- Following RME, the expander should have been left in place (or converted to a TPA by removing arms to the premolars) for as long as possible. *Hold your RME correction with a TPA as long as possible.*
- Contrasted with deep bite correction in Class II patients, deep bite correction in Class III patients can benefit AP correction. Why? Treatment that results in skeletal and dental deep bite correction (e.g., molar eruption during COS leveling) tends to rotate the mandible down and back—worsening a Class II relationship but improving a Class III relationship (tending to change a Class III into a Class I relationship).
- Treatment that tends to rotate the mandible down and back can improve frontal facial esthetics for patients with an overclosed appearance (short LAFH, everted lower lip, deep labiomental sulcus). It was wonderful to see that increasing Shawn's LAFT/TAFH ratio from 53 to 55% dramatically improved his facial esthetics (contrast Figure 3.75a and b).
- OB correction from 100 to 40% was good. Ideally, it should have been reduced to approximately 10% by completely leveling the COS (Figure 3.75w). You would not want to reduce Shawn's OB by intruding his maxillary incisors (decreasing his incisal display even more).
- *First principle: Overcorrect and hold in active retention.* When you treat a deep bite, overcorrect to a shallow bite. When you treat an open bite, overcorrect to a deep bite. The same principle applies to AP and transverse correction. And after you have made the correction, do not deband the patient immediately. Instead, monitor the patient in the corrected state for some months before removing the braces (active retention).

Case Megan

Megan (Figure 3.76) is a 16-year-old girl and presents to you with the CC: "I do not like my smile." PMH, PDH, and TMJs are WRN. Her periodontal evaluation is WRN and CR=CO.

Q: List your diagnostic findings/problems. What is your diagnosis?

A: See Table 3.7

Q: What other features must be examined using her models?

A: Features to examine include the following:

- Posterior transverse compensations (Figure 3.77a and b). Note that Megan exhibits significant maxillary *lingual* posterior crown torque and mandibular lingual posterior crown torque. This is an interesting finding. Normally, you find maxillary posterior *labial* crown torque in constricted maxillae.
- COS magnitude (Figure 3.77c). Note that it is 1–2 mm deep.
- Right and left molar AP position viewed from the lingual. Note (Figure 3.77d and e) that Megan's molars are significantly Class II when viewed from the lingual. Thus, she is truly Class II and not just appearing to be Class II in the buccal views as a result of forward maxillary first molar rotation around the maxillary first molar palatal roots.
- Incisors stepped up or stepped down relative to the posterior dentition. Her maxillary incisors are stepped *down* relative to her maxillary posterior teeth (Figure 3.76j and l). Mandibular incisors are stepped up (COS) relative to her mandibular posterior teeth.

Q: Are there additional frontal photos or radiographs you wish to make?

A: Yes. Additional photos/radiographs to take include the following:

- Since Megan is overclosed, have her separate her teeth until her lips are just touching. This image shows where her soft tissue vertical should be, ideally. Note that when this was done (Figure 3.78a), Megan actually opened a little too much, and her lips are actually slightly separated. However, from this image you can note the absence of any incisal display with lips relaxed.
- Have her bite on a tongue blade in the posterior to help judge the presence of an occlusal cant (Figure 3.78b, Megan has a right-to-left occlusal cant).
- Photographs taken at 45°angles (3/4 facial views, Figure 3.78c–d) help judge malar (cheek) prominence, which appears adequate on Megan. In other words, her malar soft tissue projects further forward than a vertical line drawn down from her corneal apex.
- Considering the right-to-left asymmetry that was seen on the frontal photograph, a PA film (Figure 3.78e and f) or CBCT scan would be useful. A right-to-left mandibular border asymmetry is seen on the PA film. In fact, if you look closely,

you'll note that her left nasal cavity looks slightly larger than the right. On her panoramic image, the left condyle and left maxillary sinus looked larger than the right. (Could Megan be mildly hemifacial hypoplastic?)

- Figure 3.78g–j illustrate making profile photographs and lateral cephalometric radiographs on a patient with a short LAFH—when he is closed and when he is opened to where his lips are just touching. These radiographs can be useful in determining the amount of downward maxillary movement required during surgery (or mandibular molar/premolar eruption required during leveling) to obtain an ideal LAFH. Notice, in this particular patient, how a significant portion of the vertical problem lies in the *mandibular* dentition being vertically underdeveloped.

Q: Christy (Figure 3.79) presents to you for treatment. What do you observe in her frontal views?

A: Her overall vertical facial proportions are normal and her lips are competent. Her chin is deviated to her right. Her left mandibular border is lower than her right mandibular border.

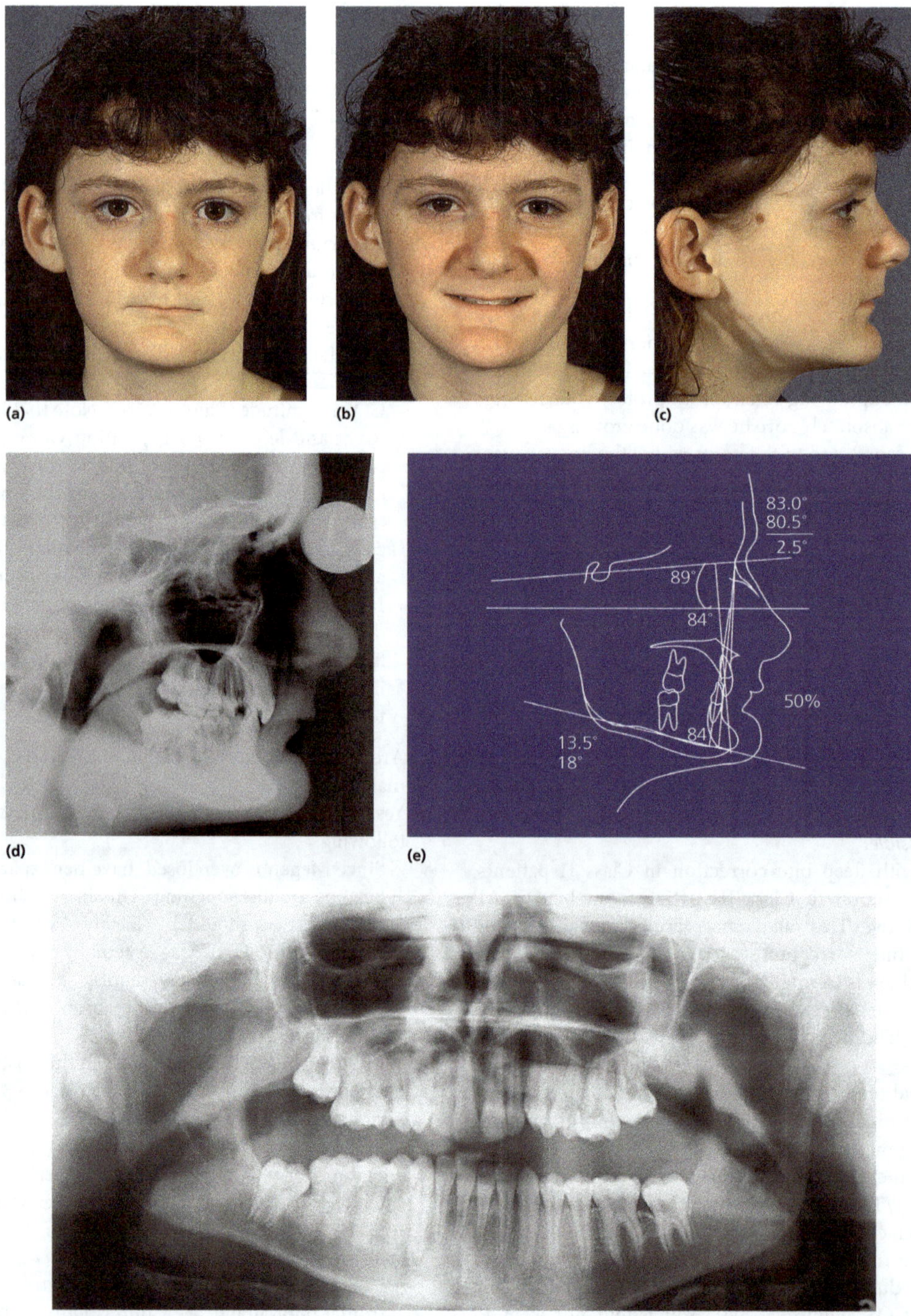

Figure 3.76 Initial records for Megan: (a–c) initial facial photographs, (d) lateral cephalograph, (e) cephalometric tracing, (f) pantomograph,

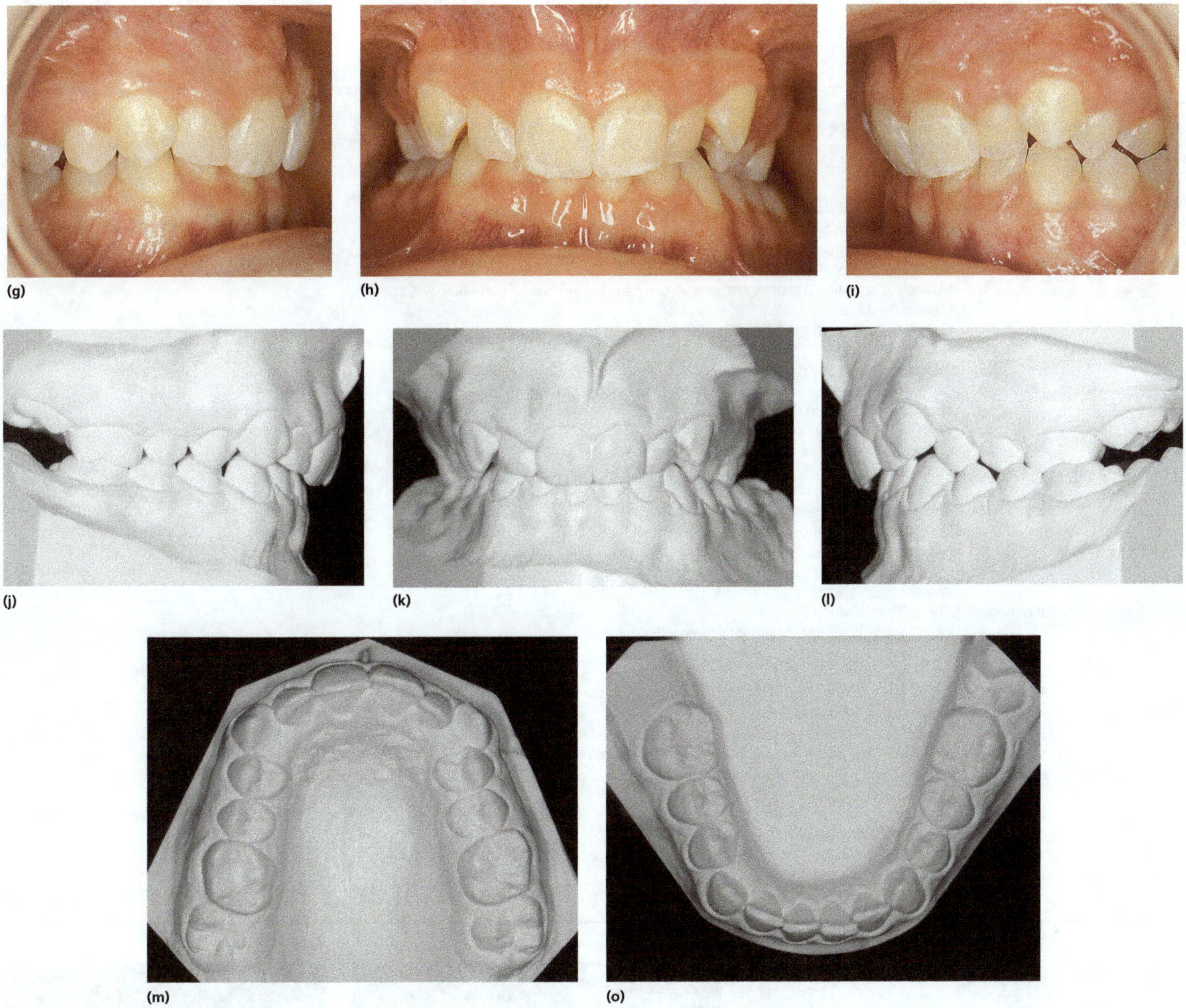

Figure 3.76 (Continued) (g–i) intraoral photographs, and (l–n) models.

Her maxillary midline is coincident with her facial midline, but her mandibular midline is 2–3 mm to the right of her maxillary midline. Compared to her interpupillary line, she has a distinct right-to-left occlusal cant with her maxillary left dentition erupted down more than her right maxillary dentition.

Q: Megan and Christy have right-to-left occlusal cants. What are possible causes of occlusal cants?

A: Possible causes of occlusal cants include the following:

- Asymmetric condylar and ramus growth. Based on a study of adolescent monkeys following condylar resection, Sarnat [116] concluded that vertical growth of the ramus initiates growth of the maxilla and mandible in height which, in turn is necessary for the free vertical eruption of teeth. For example, look at Christy's panoramic and lateral cephalometric images (Figure 3.80). Greater vertical growth of her left condyle (Figure 3.80a, red arrow) than her right condyle (yellow arrow) resulted in greater eruption of her mandibular left molars (red arrow) than her mandibular right molars (yellow arrow). Also, note in Figure 3.80b the resulting difference in right and left mandibular lower border heights (red arrow). The point is that Christy's asymmetric condylar and ramus growth produced her occlusal cant.
- Iatrogenic causes. During attempted eruption of Thomas's maxillary right canine (Figure 3.81), the doctor failed to notice that the maxillary right canine had ankylosed. He continued trying to erupt the maxillary right canine for years using fixed appliances plus vertical elastics between the maxillary right canine and mandibular right canine. As a result, the maxillary right teeth intruded, and the mandibular right teeth erupted. A significant right-to-left occlusal cant resulted (Figure 3.81c; compare Thomas's interpupillary line to his maxillary and mandibular occlusal planes). Also note (Figure 3.81e) the extreme posterior-to-anterior occlusal plane tip that resulted as the right mandibular teeth erupted.

Q: Describe the general orthodontic/surgical movements required to correct a right-to-left occlusal cant.

A: First, you must determine whether the occlusal cant resulted from inadequate tooth eruption on one side of the maxillary arch,

Table 3.7 Diagnostic findings and problem list for Megan.

Full face and profile	**Frontal view**
	Left to right cant of the lower border of mandible and lips
	Overclosed appearance (deep labiomental sulcus)
	Short LAFH (Subnasale–soft tissue Menton < soft-tissue Glabella–Subnasale)
	Thin vermillion
	Minimal incisal display in a posed smile (the gingival margins of the maxillary central incisors should be congruent with the maxillary vermillion border—here the gingival margins cannot be seen)
	UDML: WRN (coincident with facial midline)
	Profile view
	Retrusive soft tissue B-point
	Obtuse NLA
	Deep labiomental sulcus
	Very prominent chin
	Acute lip–chin–throat angle
Ceph analysis	**Skeletal**
	Maxillary AP position is slightly retrusive (A-point sits behind Nasion perpendicular) but WRN
	Mandibular AP position is WRN
	Vertical deficiency (short LAFH/TAFH = 50%)
	Flat MPA (FMA = 13.5°, SNMP = 18°)
	SN, FH and MP nearly parallel
	Obtuse NLA due to poor maxillary lip support (upright maxillary incisors)
	Robust soft tissue chin thickness
	Very prominent bony Pogonion
	Left occlusal plane lower than right occlusal plane
	Left mandibular border lower than right mandibular border
	Dental
	Upright maxillary incisors (upper incisor to SN = 89°)
	Upright mandibular incisors (FMIA = 84°)
Radiographs	Permanent Dentition
	Mandibular second molars not fully erupted
	Wisdom teeth are missing
Intraoral photos and models	Angle Class II division 2
	Iowa Classification: II (4–5) II (4–5) II (5–6) II (5–6)
	OJ: 1 mm
	OB: 70%
	Deep COS
	Left posterior lingual cross bite
	Maxillary arch constricted: maxillary first molar intermolar width = 29 mm (between palatal cusp tips)
	Mandibular first intermolar width: 36 mm (between central fossa)
	Mild maxillary and mandibular anterior crowding
	Maxillary and mandibular midlines approximately coincident
	Maxillary and mandibular dental arches appear symmetric
	Unerupted second molars
Other	—
Diagnosis	Angle Class II division 2 malocclusion
	Skeletal and dental deep bite

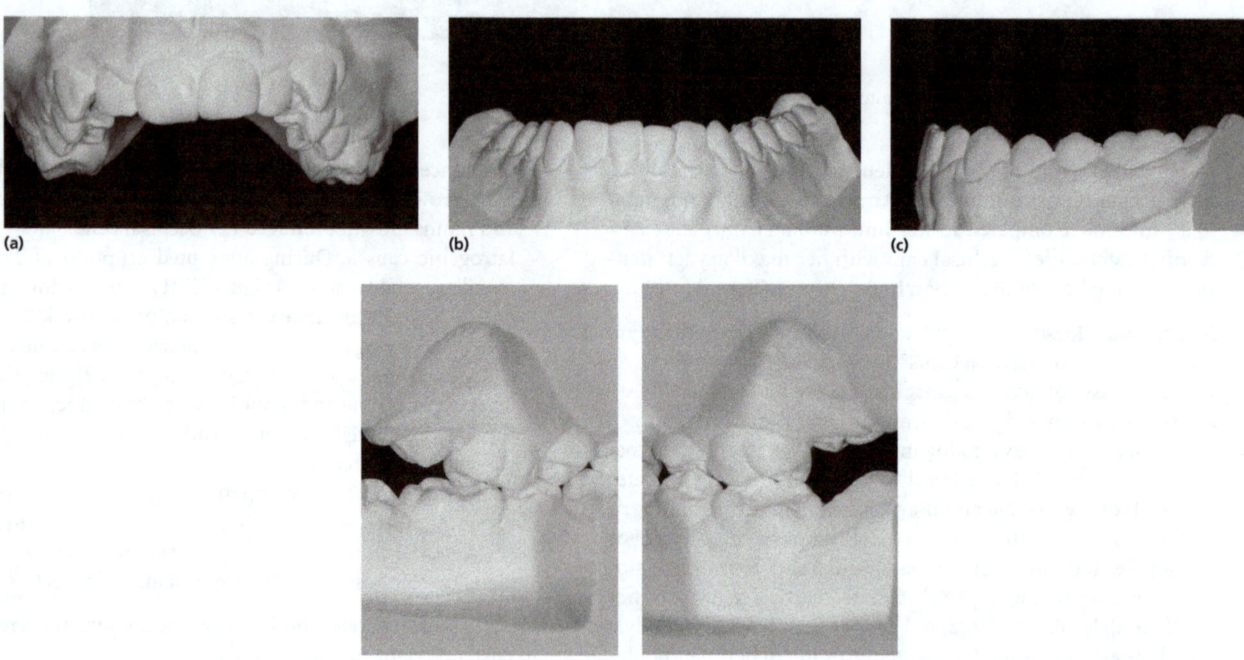

Figure 3.77 (a–e) Additional model views for Megan: (d) left molar relationship viewed from the lingual and (e) right molar relationship viewed from the lingual.

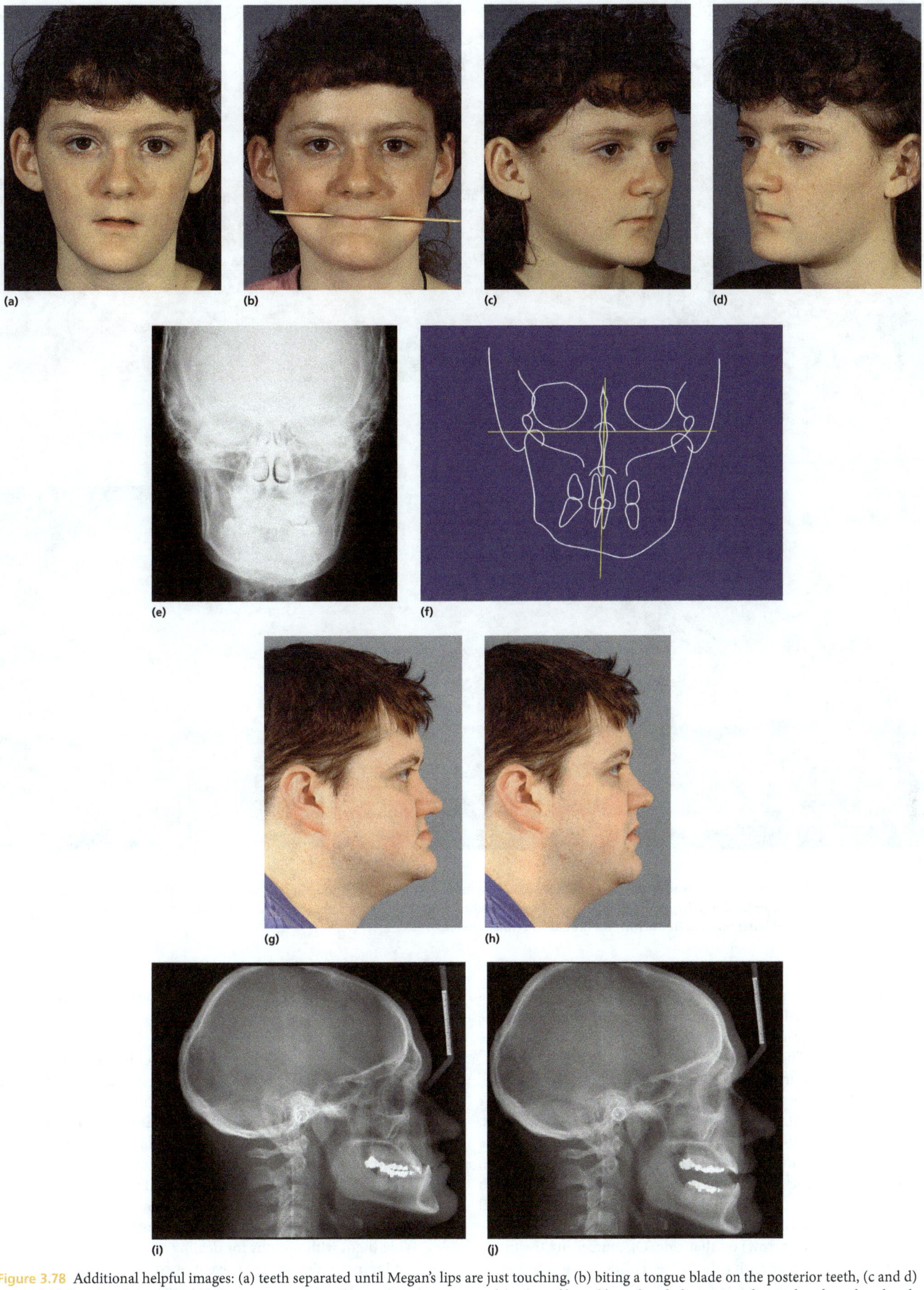

Figure 3.78 Additional helpful images: (a) teeth separated until Megan's lips are just touching, (b) biting a tongue blade on the posterior teeth, (c and d) right and left ¾ facial views, (e and f) posteroanterior radiograph and tracing, and (g–j) profile and lateral cephalometric radiographs when closed and with teeth separated until the lips are just touching.

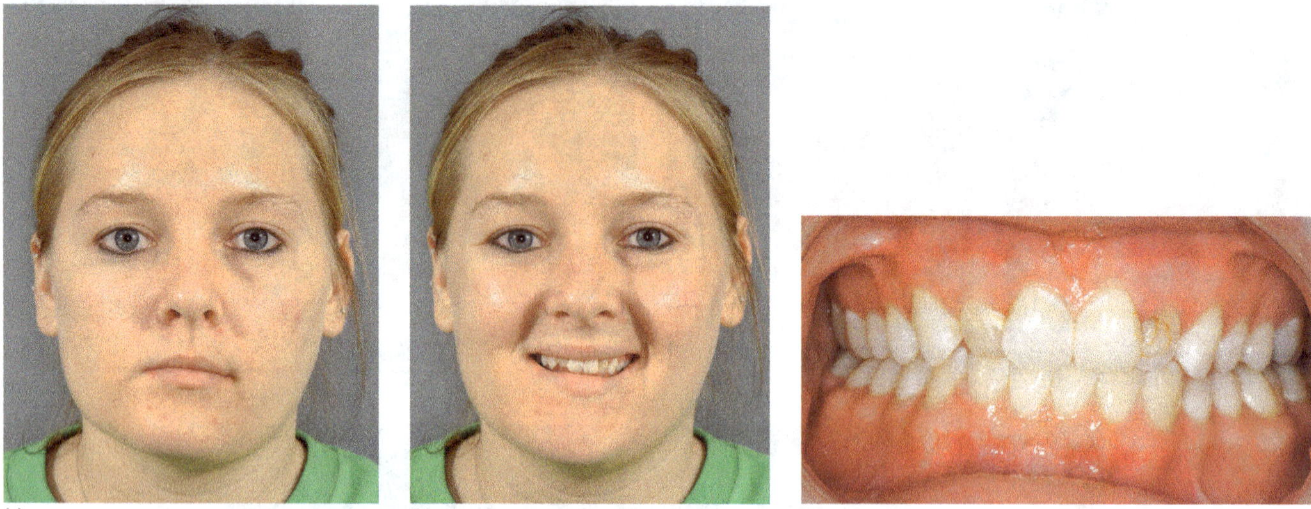

(a) (b) (c)

Figure 3.79 (a–c) Christy presents with a significant maxillary occlusal cant.

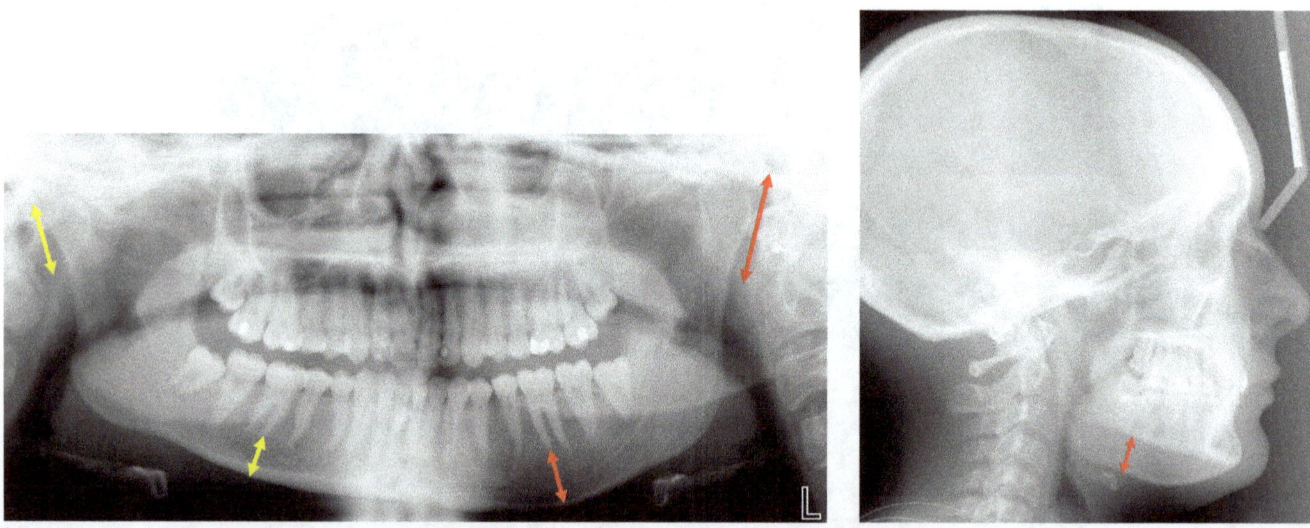

(a) (b)

Figure 3.80 Christy's radiographs demonstrate the skeletal nature of her asymmetry: (a) her pantomograph shows a longer left condyle and greater distance from the left inferior border of her mandible to left root apices (red arrows) than on the right (yellow arrows); (b) notice the discrepancy in right-to-left inferior mandibular borders (red arrow) on the lateral cephalograph.

excessive tooth eruption on the other side, or a combination of both. Looking at the patient from the front, confirm the presence of an occlusal cant by comparing the interpupillary line to the occlusal plane. Then, examine the patient's right and left LAFHs, right versus left incisal display with relaxed lips following arch leveling, and look for an ILG. As illustrated in Figure 3.82, if one side of the maxillary arch has inadequate vertical development, then orthodontic/surgical treatment is aimed at lowering the occlusal plane (increasing the facial height, yellow arrow) on that side. On the other hand, if one side of the maxillary arch has excessive vertical development, then orthodontic/surgical treatment is aimed at raising the occlusal plane (decreasing the facial height, red arrow) on that side. Of course, any treatment aimed at lowering or raising the occlusal plane requires treatment in *both* jaws to achieve proper occlusal interdigitation.

Q: What are your specific options for treating right-to-left occlusal cants?

A: Options include the following:

- *Leave the cant; do not treat it.* Remember, 7% of the population has an occlusal cant [117], and a maxillary right-canine-to-left-canine cant of at least 3 mm is required for lay persons to rate it as noticeable [82]. If the patient does not express concerns about a cant, be careful when deciding whether to bring it to their attention or not. If they present with a cant being a concern, ask them if they have ever looked in a mirror and thought they should have it corrected. If they have thought they should have the cant corrected, then provide them with options for dealing with it, so they can make an informed decision to leave it or treat it. Otherwise, advise them that only severe cants are noticed by lay persons.

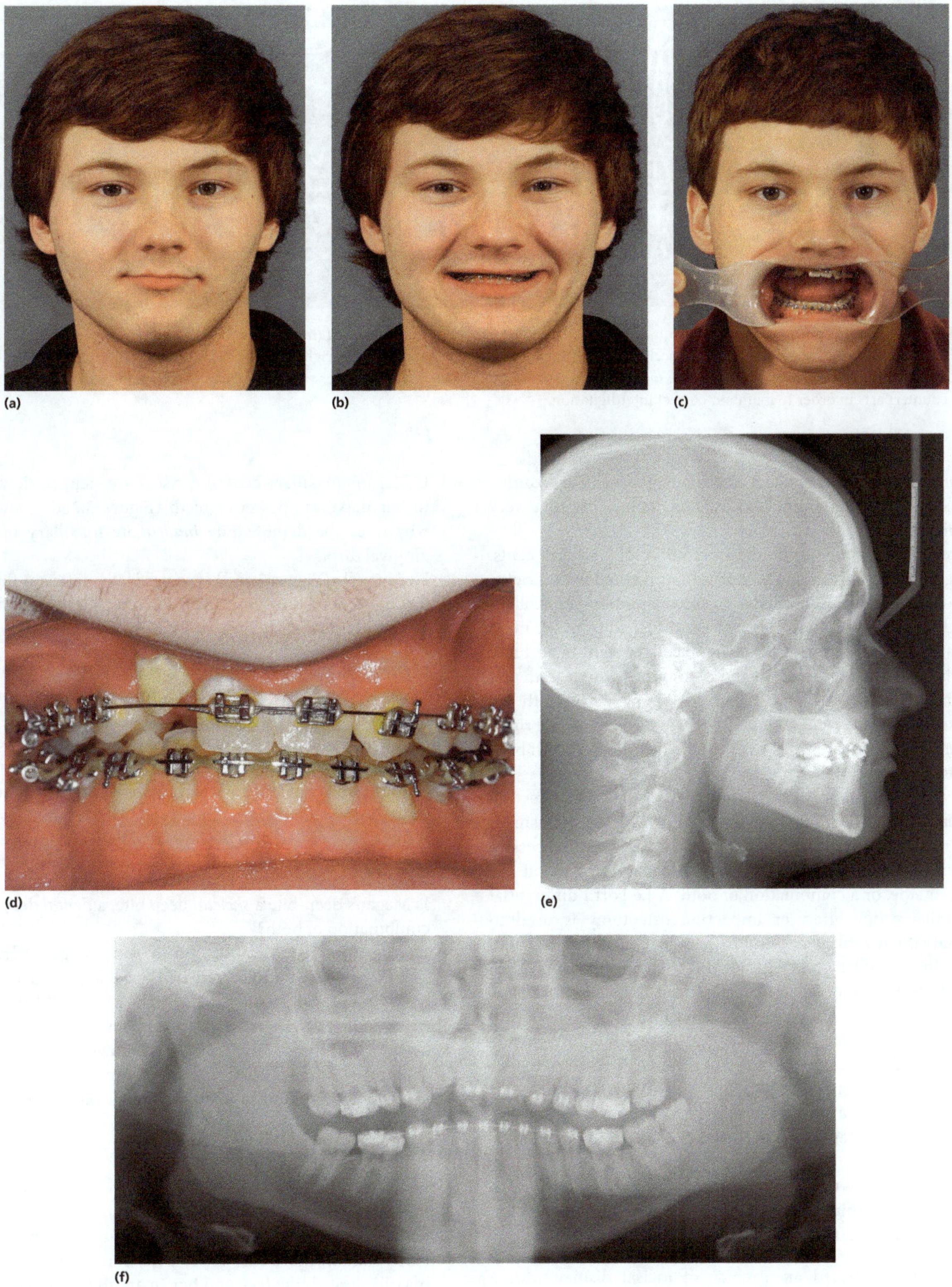

Figure 3.81 (a–f) Iatrogenic right-to-left occlusal cant resulting from prolonged attempted eruption of an ankylosed maxillary right canine. Attempting to erupt the ankylosed canine with fixed appliances and vertical elastics resulted in intrusion of the maxillary right incisors and maxillary right premolars and eruption of the mandibular right incisors, canines, and premolars.

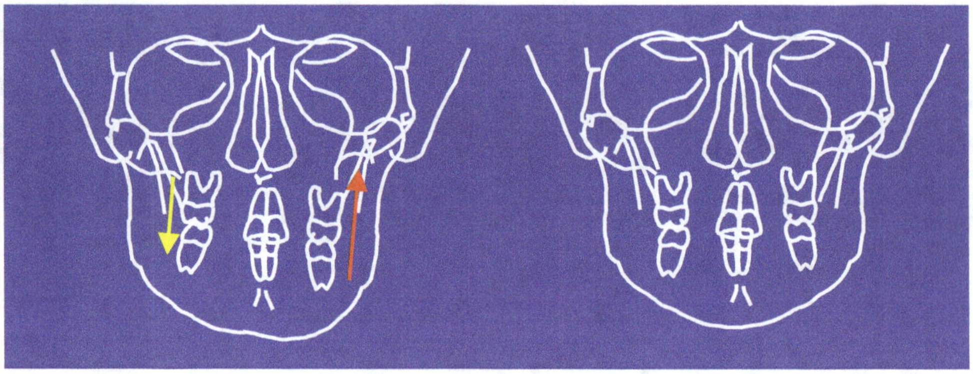

Figure 3.82 Correction of an occlusal cant. Inadequately erupted maxillary right teeth are erupted (left, yellow line) or excessively erupted maxillary left teeth are intruded (left, red line), resulting in an occlusal plane parallel to the interpupillary line (right), ideal LAFH, ideal maxillary incisal display in relaxed lip position, and absence of an ILG. These movements are accomplished orthodontically or surgically. Mandibular teeth must follow their maxillary counterparts in order to maintain correct interdigitation.

- *Enameloplasty* of maxillary incisor edges/maxillary canine cusp tips can sometimes be used to slightly improve very mild cants.
- *Use of TADs* to aid in the correction of occlusal cants. Figure 3.83a illustrates a patient who presented with a right-to-left 3 mm occlusal cant due to excess eruption of maxillary right teeth. Elastomeric chains were stretched from the maxillary right posterior teeth to the maxillary right buccal and palatal TADs (Figure 3.83b and c) to intrude these teeth and correct her cant (Figure 3.83d–f). As maxillary teeth are intruded on the right, an open bite will develop on the right. Vertical elastics are worn to erupt the mandibular teeth back into occlusion.
- *Orthognathic surgery* (the traditional occlusal cant correction treatment). Following completion of growth, an assessment is made to determine whether the cant is due to excessive facial growth on the one side, inadequate growth on the other side, or a combination of both. A Le Fort I differential maxillary downgraft or impaction osteotomy is used to rotate the maxillary occlusal plane into a position parallel to the interpupillary line with ideal LAFH, absence of an ILG, and ideal incisal display at rest. A mandibular osteotomy is then performed to permit proper occlusal interdigitation of both arches. Kim (Figure 3.84) illustrates this approach. She presented with a maxillary occlusal cant as a result of inadequate vertical growth on the left side of her face. She was treated with a Le Fort I differential maxillary downgraft osteotomy (bone graft added to the left, Figure 3.84h), a mandibular BSSO osteotomy to properly articulate the mandibular dentition with the new maxillary occlusal plane, and a differential genioplasty (Figure 3.84j) to lengthen her chin height on the left side.

Q: Megan demonstrated an absence of incisal display with a relaxed maxillary lip (Figure 3.78a) and inadequate incisal display in a posed smile (Figure 3.76b). By contrast, the patient in Figure 3.85 displays excessive incisal display in relaxed lip position and excess incisal and gingival display when smiling. List the reasons why a patient could present with excess incisal display. What are the reasons why a patient could present with inadequate incisal display?

A: See Table 3.8

Q: If Megan's maxillary central incisors are stepped down relative to her maxillary posterior teeth (Figure 3.76d, j, and l), then why does she demonstrate *inadequate* maxillary incisor and gingival display?

A: Her maxilla (Figure 3.76d) is so vertically deficient that despite having stepped down maxillary incisors, she still exhibits inadequate incisal display.

Q: Megan's maxilla was said to be slightly retrusive, but WRN. What influence do Megan's upright maxillary incisors play in defining her maxillary AP position?

A: In patients with upright incisors, A-point is positioned forward of where it will be after treatment. Why? During treatment, as the upright maxillary incisor roots are torqued lingually to a more normal angulation, the alveolar process bone will follow, A-point will follow, and Megan's maxilla will appear even more deficient, anteroposteriorly.

Q: Is Megan's deep-bite a *skeletal* deep bite, a *dental* deep bite, or a combination of both?

A: Her deep bite is a combination of both. Megan's *skeletal deep bite features include* an overclosed facial appearance, short soft tissue LAFH, short skeletal LAFH (LAFH/TAFH = 50%, flat MPA, and relatively parallel SN, FH, and MP). Megan's *dental deep bite features include* stepped down maxillary incisors (Figure 3.76j and l) plus stepped up mandibular incisors (Figure 3.77c). She is a combination skeletal and dental deep bite patient.

Q: What is the etiology of her deep bite?

A: Her skeletal deep bite (Figure 3.86) resulted from her condyles growing more vertically than normal (as opposed to posterior-superiorly), her mandible rotating forward (internally, true rotation) more excessively than normal (blue arrows), her maxilla descending less, and her (mandibular) molars erupting less than normal. As Megan's mandible rotated upward and forward (yellow arrow), a deep overbite resulted. Megan's dental deep bite resulted from excess maxillary and mandibular incisor eruption (as Class II, Megan's incisors did not make contact with opposing incisors to stop eruption).

Q: All of Megan's growth characteristics fit a classic skeletal deep bite growth pattern—except for one. What is it?

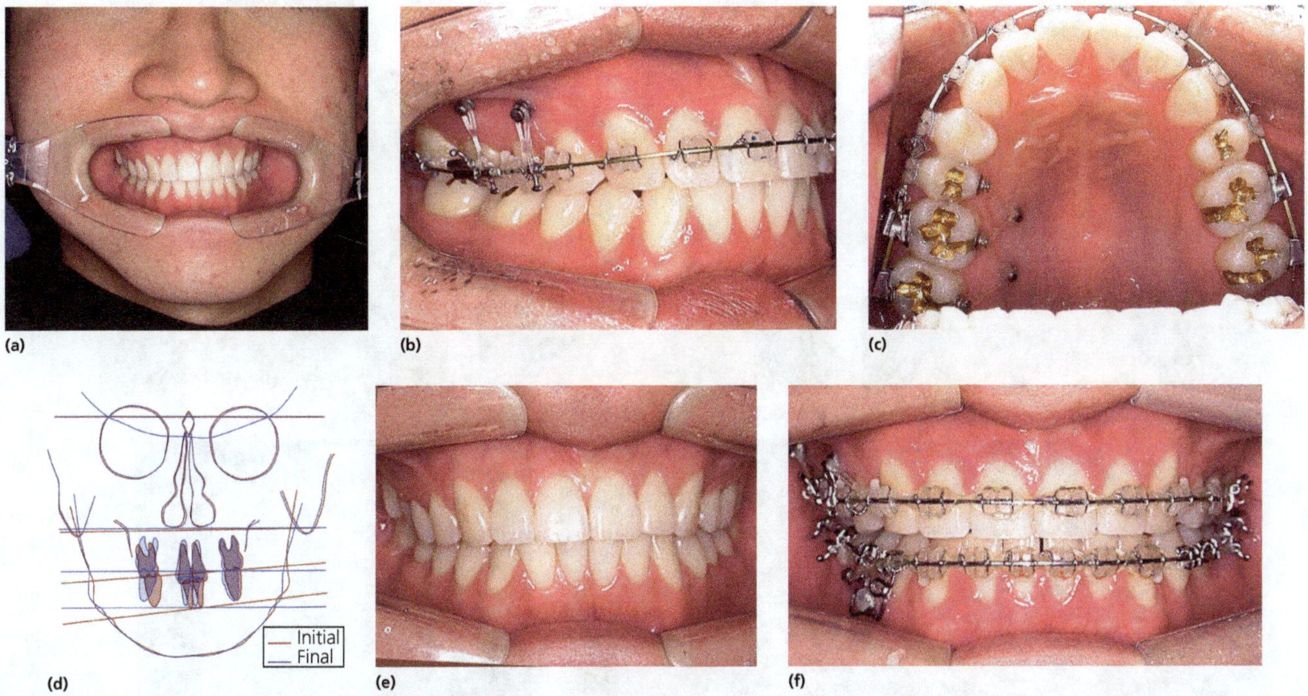

Figure 3.83 TADs used to intrude excessively erupted maxillary right teeth and correct an occlusal cant: (a) patient presents with a right-to-left occlusal cant, (b and c) elastomeric chains stretched between the maxillary right posterior teeth and TADs inserted into the buccal and palatal alveolar processes, (d) posteroanterior initial-to-final cephalometric superimposition showing leveling of the occlusal plane by intrusion of the maxillary right teeth plus eruption of the mandibular right teeth (using vertical elastics), (e) initial frontal photo showing canted occlusal relationship, and (f) final corrected occlusal relationship (Dr. Young Chel Park, DDS, PhD. Reproduced with permission from Dr. Young Chel Park).

A: Surprisingly, Megan's maxillary first molars apicies have erupted well below her palatal plane (Figure 3.86), but we would have expected them to have erupted *less* than normal in a skeletal deep bite growth pattern. This is an example of a preponderance of features leading to a diagnosis—without all features needing to be present.

Q: Remember, there are only two general approaches to correcting deep bites—describe them. How do you decide which approach to use for a particular patient?

A: *Erupting posterior teeth:* opens the bite by *increasing LAFH* (Figure 3.87a). This can be done orthodontically—say, by erupting posterior teeth during COS leveling in an adolescent. Or, it can be done surgically—by downgrafting the maxilla. Figure 3.87b illustrates the initial osteotomy cuts for a Le Fort I downgraft. Figure 3.87c illustrates allogenic bone being prepared for interpositional insertion in the downfractured maxilla (Figure 3.87d) to increase LAFH. *Intruding/proclining anterior teeth* (Figure 3.87e): which will *not increase LAFH*. In deciding which approach to use, you must consider the etiology of the deep bite and patient desires. Erupting posterior teeth would be appropriate in an overclosed skeletal deep bite when the patient was concerned about their short LAFH. Intruding/proclining anterior teeth would be appropriate in a dental deep bite to correctovererupted incisors.

Q: Which of these two general approaches would be the best in correcting Megan's deep bite?

A: Since Megan presents with both a skeletal and a dental deep bite, her ideal treatment would include both approaches.

Q: Concerning growth and development, what questions do you want to ask Megan and her parents?

A: Is Megan still growing? When did she reach menarche? You learn that she has not grown for at least a year and reached menarche at age 13 years.

Q: In what dimensions does Megan present with *apical base* discrepancies?

A: Vertical and transverse. However, her maxilla (A-point) may be judged retrusive once the maxillary dental arch is level and the maxillary incisor roots are torqued lingually (bringing A-point lingual).

Q: What are your primary problems in each dimension (plus other) that you must stay focused on when treating Megan?

A: See Table 3.9

Q: What are your treatment goals?

A: To address her chief complaint and maximally improve her smile: reduce Megan's overclosed appearance, increase her LAFH, provide her with ideal (2–4 mm of) incisor show at rest, and increase her incisal display when smiling. Also, to position her canines (and maxillary molars if she is treated nonextraction) into a Class I relationship and to obtain minimal OB and OJ.

Q: What are the general ways to correct Megan's 4–6 mm Class II molar and canine relationship? Describe specific treatments you would use for each.

A: Even though Megan does not present with an anteroposterior apical base discrepancy, let's approach her significant

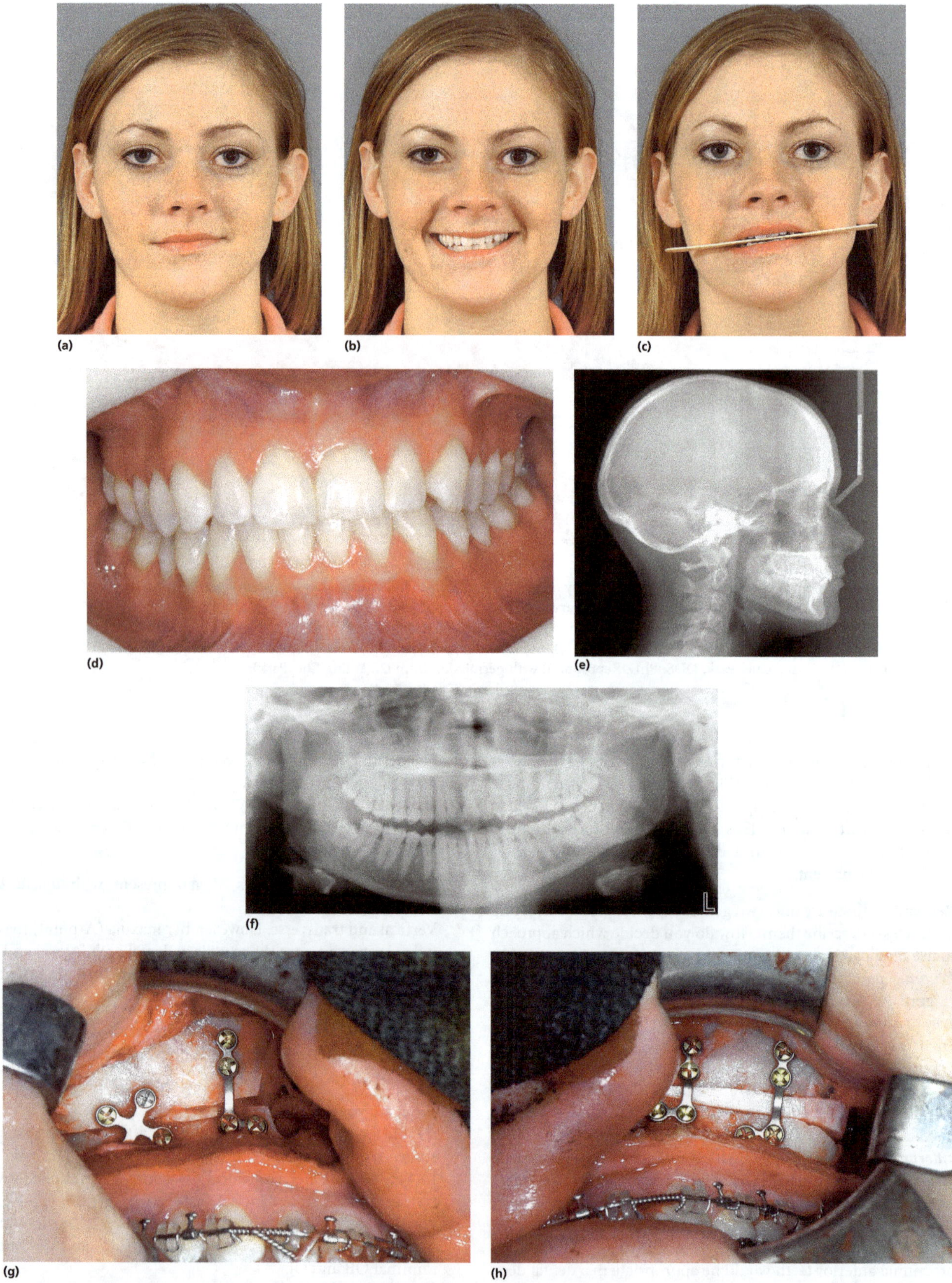

Figure 3.84 Orthognathic surgery used to correct an occlusal cant: (a–f) patient presents with a right-to-left occlusal cant of approximately 3 mm. Her right maxillary dentition appears to have erupted normally. Her left dentition appears undererupted. Note (e) the difference in height between her left and right mandibular skeletal border, (f) the shorter left condylar length, the shorter left ramal height, and the shorter distance between the left posterior teeth apicies and the mandibular border then, the right; (g–j) surgical correction consisted of a Le Fort I differential maxillary downgraft osteotomy with her left side inferiorly repositioned, (i) a mandibular BSSO to articulate the mandibular occlusion into the newly positioned maxillary occlusion, and (j) a differential downgraft genioplasty to enhance her chin symmetry. (i) Note improved coincidence of Kim's mandibular lower borders postsurgically; (l–m) initial and final posteroanterior radiographs illustrating surgical correction of her occlusal cant; and (n–p) final facial photographs demonstrating cant improvement (a very slight right-to-left occlusal cant is still evident).

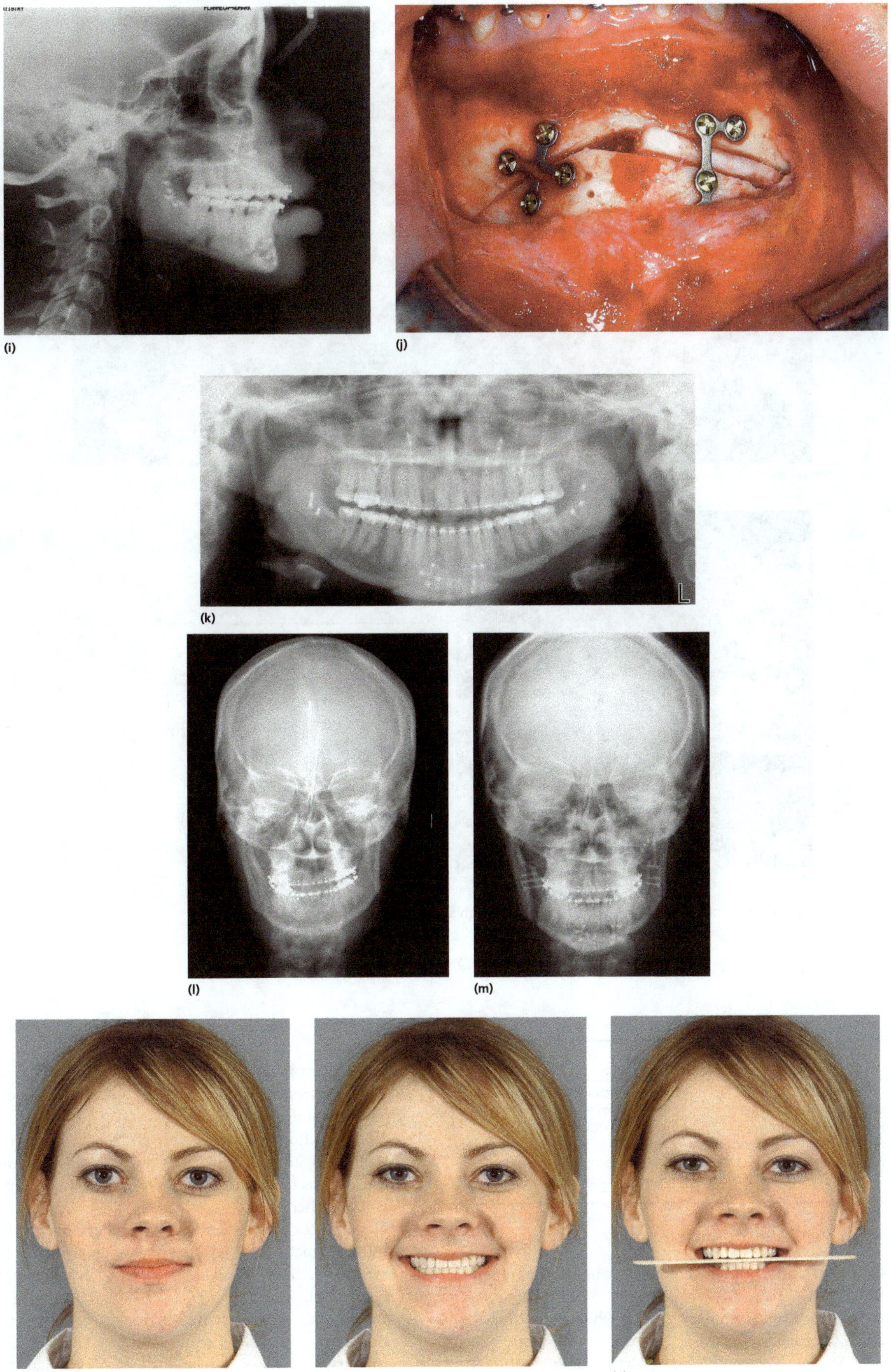

Figure 3.84 (Continued)

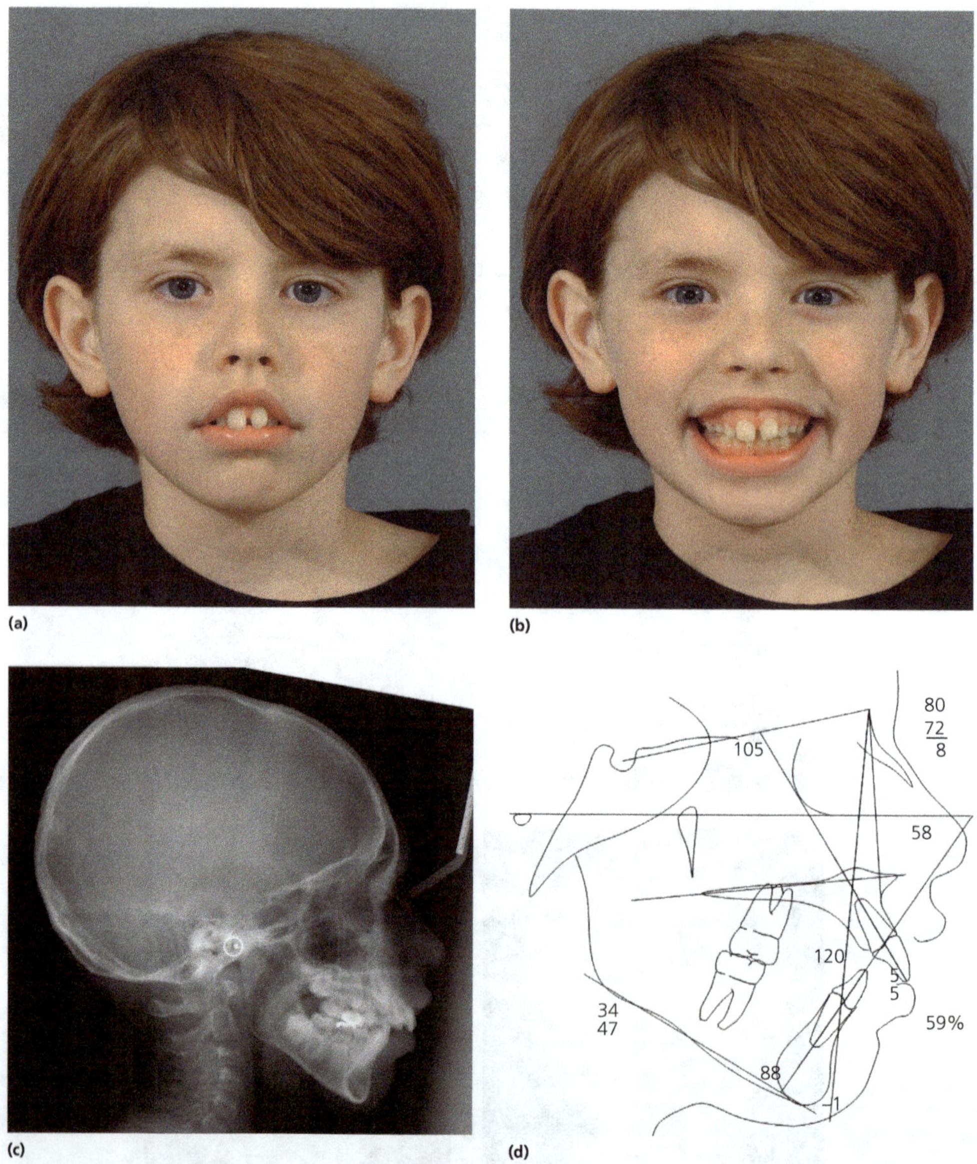

Figure 3.85 (a–d) Adolescent patient exhibiting excessive incisal and gingival display.

Table 3.8 Possible reasons for excessive or inadequate incisal/gingival display.

Excess incisal/gingival display	Inadequate incisal display
• Excess maxillary vertical growth • Short maxillary lip (philtrum) length • Stepped down maxillary incisors • Hyperactivity of facial (smiling) muscles • Excessively long maxillary incisor crowns • Delayed passive eruption (excess gingiva)	• Inadequate maxillary vertical growth • Long maxillary lip length • Stepped up maxillary incisors • Hypoactivity of facial (smiling) muscles • Short maxillary incisor crowns

Class II molar and canine discrepancy using the same logic as if she did.

Orthopedics (restrict maxillary growth while permitting the mandible to continue growing, or accelerate mandibular growth): Megan has completed growth, so attempting to correct her Class II relationship with orthopedics is not reasonable.

Masking or camouflage (achieve a Class I canine relationship without addressing the underlying apical base discrepancy). Options include the following:

- Nonextraction treatment with HPHG, CPHG, or straight-pull headgear could retract her maxillary molars and canines into a Class I relationship. However, the compliance required would be heroic.
- Nonextraction treatment using maxillary palatal, buccal, or infrazygomatic crest TADs as anchorage to retract her entire maxillary dental arch could be effective in achieving a Class I relationship.
- Extraction of maxillary first premolars could permit retraction of her maxillary canines into a Class I relationship (molars in a Class II relationship). Megan has such poor

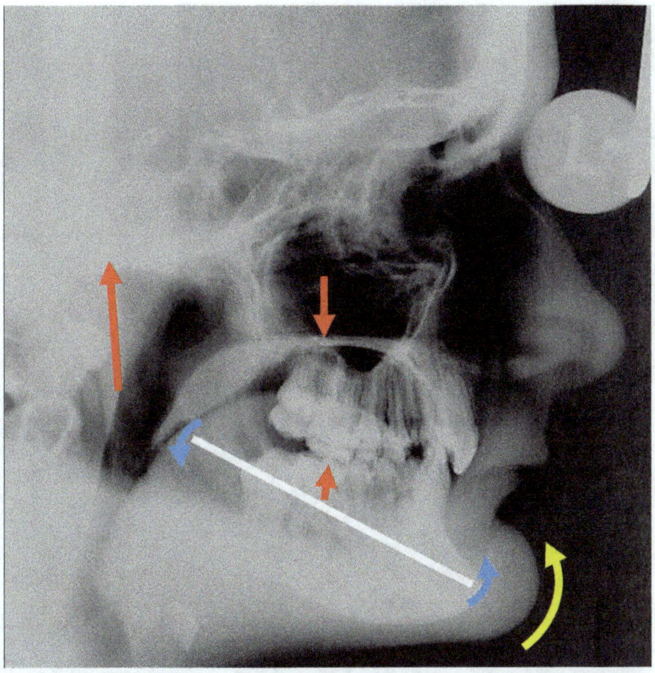

Figure 3.86 Megan represents a classic skeletal deep bite growth pattern: condyles growing more vertically than normal, mandible rotating forward (internally, true rotation) more than normal (blue arrows), maxilla descending less, and (mandibular) molars erupting less than normal. Consequently, her mandible rotated upward and forward (yellow arrow), resulting in excessive incisal overlap (a skeletal deep bite).

maxillary lip support (due, in part, to her upright incisors) that you must take care not to retract her incisors much more. However, as shown in Figure 3.76d, she has such a small amount of OJ (~1 mm) that her maxillary incisors cannot be retracted very much anyway without putting her in anterior cross bite. The principle maxillary incisor movement during space closure would be lingual torqueing of maxillary incisor roots.

- Nonextraction interarch treatment such as with Class II elastics, Jasper Jumpers, MARA appliances, Forsus, Herbst appliances, or similar interarch mechanics could achieve a Class I relationship through a combination of maxillary distal and mandibular mesial dental movement. The good news is that Megan's mandibular incisors are very upright and can afford to be proclined. However, you must carefully monitor the periodontium covering her mandibular incisors during such treatment to avoid recession.

Surgery (mandibular advancement) could be an option to correct her AP molar relationship, especially since B-point looks retrusive on her profile view (Figure 3.76c). If her maxilla was concurrently downgrafted (increasing her LAFH, but rotating the mandible down and back), then there would be an even greater need to perform a mandibular advancement. However, if a mandibular advancement were performed, then some form of genioplasty setback would be necessary to prevent her chin from becoming too prominent.

Q: If you decide to treat Megan's Class II relationship by masking, then compare and contrast the resulting maxillary and mandibular AP tooth movements when using intra-arch versus interarch mechanics.

A: Whether you treat Megan by retracting maxillary teeth with headgear, by retracting maxillary teeth using TADs, or by retracting maxillary anterior teeth following extraction of maxillary premolars, the AP correction made is entirely *intra-arch* (Figure 3.88a, no mandibular tooth movement). So with each technique, the maxillary canines will be retracted the same amount (to the point where they are Class I with the mandibular canines), and the maxillary incisors will be retracted the same amount (Figure 3.88a, right). On the other hand, if *interarch* mechanics (Class II elastics, Jasper Jumpers, Forsus, etc.) are used, then tooth movements occur in both arches (Figure 3.88b), and the distance maxillary teeth are retracted will be reduced by the amount the mandibular teeth move mesially.

Q: Will masking Megan's Class II relationship improve her smile? Will a mandibular advancement surgery improve her smile?

A: Masking her Class II relationship will have minimal impact on her smile. In fact, if the maxillary arch is leveled, then the stepped down maxillary incisors could be intruded, decreasing incisal display and worsening her smile. A mandibular advancement procedure could increase her vertical dimension, if the mandible is moved downward as well as forward (say, with a tripod advancement). However, a mandibular advancement osteotomy alone will not improve her incisal display (a concurrent maxillary downgraft would be needed to do that).

Q: What are the general ways to correct Megan's vertical apical base discrepancy? List specific treatments for each of these.

A: *Orthopedics* (enhancing downward maxillary corpus growth, increasing maxillary molar eruption, and increasing mandibular molar eruption—all of which would tend to lengthen her LAFH, increase her MPA, open her deep bite—but rotate her mandible down and back worsening her Class II molar relationship.) Considerations include the following:

- Megan has finished growing. Even if we could rotate her anterior palatal plane down and back with a cervical-pull headgear (potentially increasing lower anterior facial height and incisal display) [24–26], increase her SN–MP angle (1°) using straight-pull headgear [28], increase her mandibular plane angle (1.3°) with a headgear/biteplate combination [31], or increase her SN–MP/vertical dimension slightly with a functional appliance [27, 28], the stability of such movements in an adult is questionable.
- Leveling the COS with archwires (with or without an anterior biteplate and posterior vertical elastics) will occur primarily through premolar eruption [23] plus mandibular molars tipping distally and erupting—potentially increasing her LAFH. But again, the stability of posterior tooth eruption in an adult skeletal deep bite patient is questionable.

Masking or camouflage (reducing/correcting Megan's overbite without addressing her vertical skeletal discrepancy—equivalent to treatment of a *dental* deep bite). Options include the following:

- Intruding maxillary and mandibular anterior teeth by leveling her stepped down maxillary incisors and/or leveling her stepped up mandibular incisors with fixed orthodontic appliances, enhancing this incisor intrusion by bonding maxillary and mandibular incisors more incisally than routinely positioned, and enhancing this incisor intrusion by placing

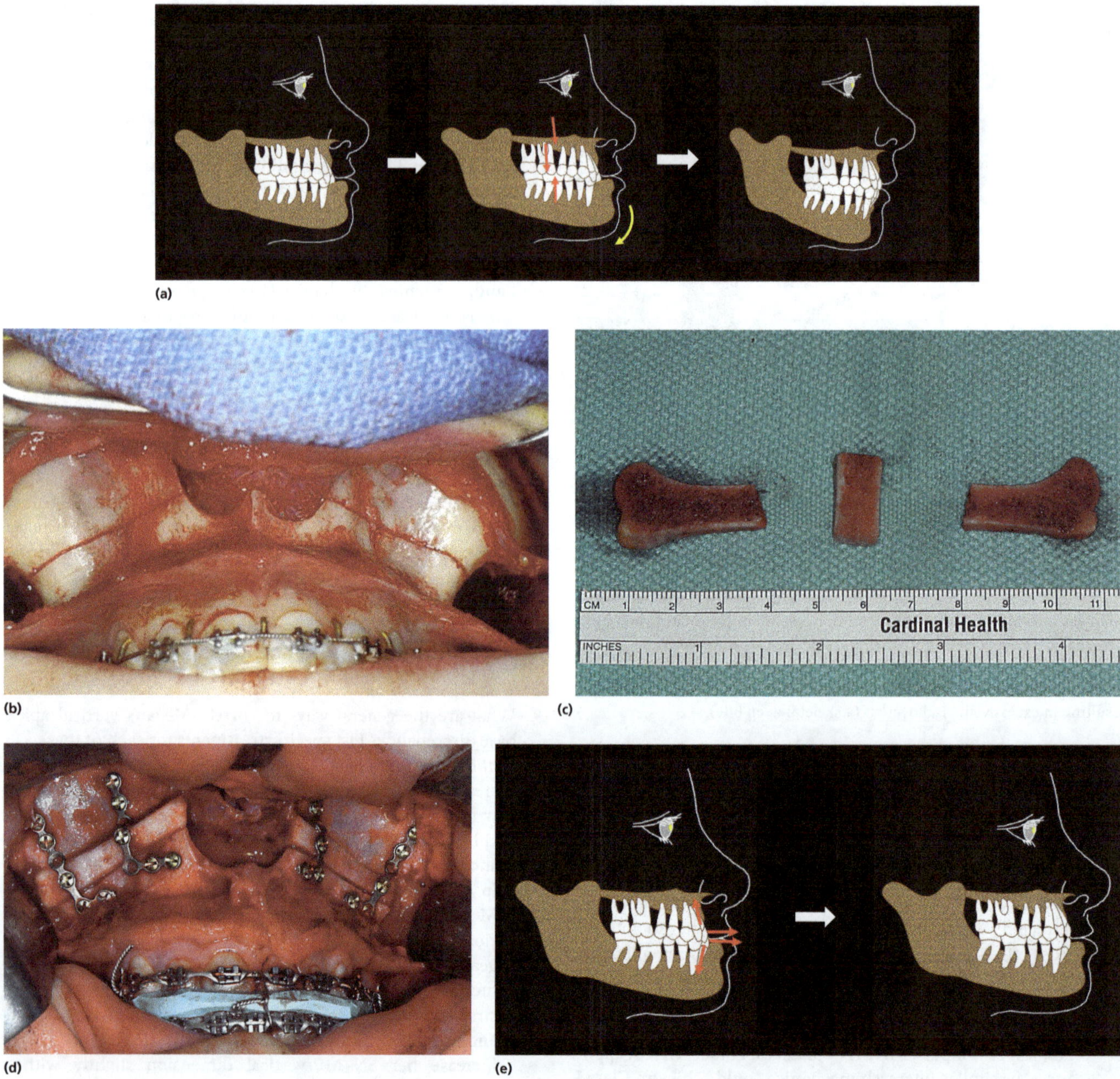

Figure 3.87 Two general approaches to correcting deep bites: (a) *erupting posterior teeth* opens the bite by increasing LAFH, and is performed either orthodontically or surgically (with a Le Fort I maxillary downgraft, b–d); (e) *Intruding/proclining anterior teeth* does not affect the LAFH.

Table 3.9 **Primary problems list for Megan** *(apical base/skeletal discrepancies italicized).*

AP	II (4–5) II (4–5) II (5–6) II (5–6) skeletal relationships WRN
Vertical	*Skeletal* and dental deep bite
Transverse	Left unilateral cross bite secondary to a *maxillary skeletal transverse deficiency*
Other	—

archwire steps to intrude anterior teeth. However, the result of maxillary incisor intrusion will be even less incisor display—adversely impacting smile esthetics.

- Proclining Megan's very upright incisors.
- Leveling her COS by eruption of mandibular premolars [7] or by distally tipping/erupting mandibular molars that are mesially tipped. Since alveolar process bone is grown during tooth eruption, and the LAFH can increase as the mandible is rotated down and back, it could be argued that this is orthopedic treatment.
- Treating Megan with prosthodontics to increase her vertical dimension would not be reasonable.

Surgery (increasing Megan's vertical facial dimension by grafting bone to vertically lengthen her maxilla) would be an ideal treatment alternative. Remember, if the maxilla is moved downward, then the mandible will rotate downward and backward—worsening Megan's Class II relationship.

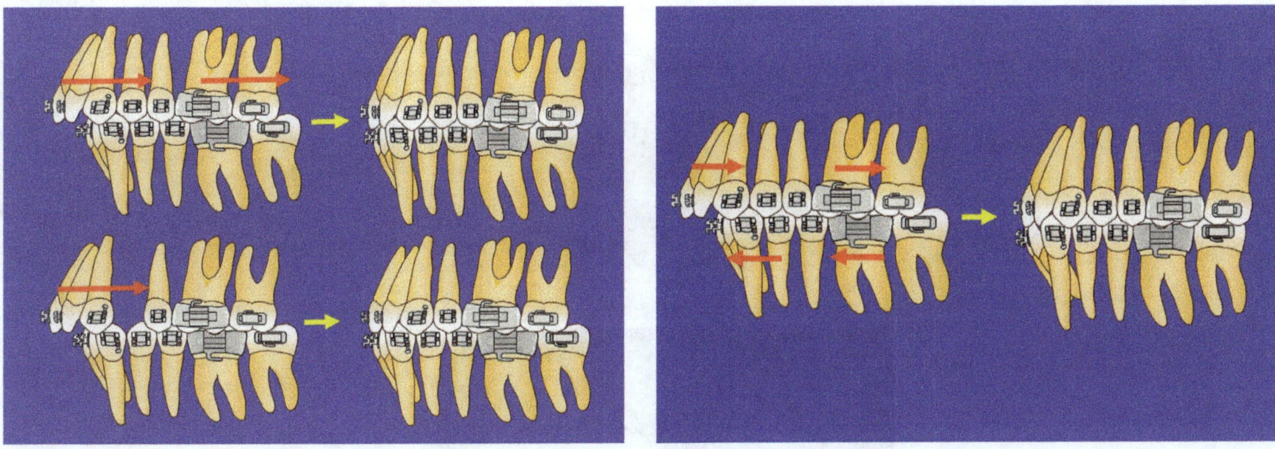

(a) (b)

Figure 3.88 Maxillary *intra-arch* mechanics (a) to correct Megan's Class II canine and molar relationship results in identical maxillary canine retraction/maxillary incisor retraction, regardless of the specific technique used (headgear, TADs, premolar extractions). Why? Because there is no movement of mandibular teeth. *Inter-arch* mechanics, on the other hand (b), results in dental movement in both arches. With interarch mechanics, the distance maxillary canines and maxillary incisors retract is reduced by the amount the mandibular teeth move forward.

A mandibular advancement (plus setback genioplasty) may also be required.

Q: What are the general ways that you can correct Megan's transverse apical base discrepancy? List specific treatments for each.

A: *Orthopedics* (expanding the maxillary arch by separating the hemi-maxillae at the midpalatal suture).

RME could result in both skeletal and dental expansion. As her maxilla is expanded, the maxillary molars would be tipped buccally (Megan's maxillary posterior lingual crown torque eliminated), her left posterior cross bite corrected, and the increased posterior overjet could be used to upright the lingually torqued mandibular posterior teeth. *Pearl: even when a young patient presents with a very severe AP or vertical apical base discrepancy, and you choose to delay treatment for future surgical correction, at least consider performing RME while the patient is young if maxillary skeletal expansion will be needed later*. Why? By performing RME at a young age, when you can maximize skeletal expansion, you can obviate a later need for SARME or for a multiple-piece maxillary osteotomy.

Masking or camouflage (correcting Megan's cross bite by increasing molar transverse compensations—adding maxillary buccal torque/adding mandibular lingual torque—and not by addressing the underlying transverse skeletal discrepancy). Even though Megan could benefit from removal of her maxillary posterior lingual crown torque, the magnitude of her transverse discrepancy is so large (7 mm of maxillary transverse expansion is needed to seat the maxillary first molar lingual cusps in the mandibular first molar central fossa), that trying to achieve the transverse correction with dental compensations alone is *not* recommended.

Surgery options include the following:

- SARME—would achieve adequate maxillary expansion. However, a SARME would be advised only if RME treatment failed to achieve a midpalatal split.
- MPMO—if a maxillary downgraft osteotomy was performed to correct Megan's vertical skeletal deficiency, then a simultaneous multiple-piece maxillary osteotomy would be a viable alternative to expand her maxillary transverse dimension. But remember, unlike a SARME (which grows transverse bone and soft tissue), the magnitude of MPMO maxillary transverse expansion is limited by the stretch of the palatal soft tissue, instantly. The limit of maxillary transverse expansion with an MPMO is approximately 8 mm, depending on the depth of the palatal vault. Stretching the palatal soft tissues can compromise the palatal blood supply.

Q: Will broadening Megan's maxillary arch (decreasing her buccal corridors) improve her smile?

A: Megan's buccal corridors are not noticeable in her posed smile (Figure 3.76b), but she may not be smiling very broadly because she is self-conscience of her smile esthetics. She has such a narrow maxilla that widening her maxillary arch with orthopedics or surgery could enhance her smile. Why? When evaluated over a *wide* range of buccal corridor/maxillary arch sizes, lay persons were found to prefer broader maxillary arches/broader smiles (narrower buccal corridors) [118].

Q: What is a potential problem in attempting RME in Megan?

A: Megan has finished growing. The most marked skeletal effect of RME is before, or during, the pubertal growth spurt [62]. RME expansion after the pubertal growth spurt consists mainly of dentoalveolar, and not skeletal, change [112]. There is little orthopedic change with RME in older patients [113]. In fact, skeletal expansion accounts for nearly 1/2 of RME maxillary arch width increase in 8- to 12-year-olds, but only 1/3 of width increase in 13- to 19-year-olds [109–111]. On the other hand, *you have nothing to lose in attempting RME expansion* in Megan, and you may actually be able to achieve a midpalatal split. If you decide to attempt RME, then do so at the rate of 0.25 mm per day or 0.25 mm every other day when beginning, and closely monitor whether the midpalatal suture separates (as seen by the formation of a midline diastema or appearance of a midpalatal split on an occlusal radiograph).

Q: What are the signs that a midpalatal split is *not occurring* with RME?

A: Signs include the following:

- *Absence* of the formation of a maxillary midline diastema. Soon after you attempt RME expansion (0.25–0.5 mm/day),

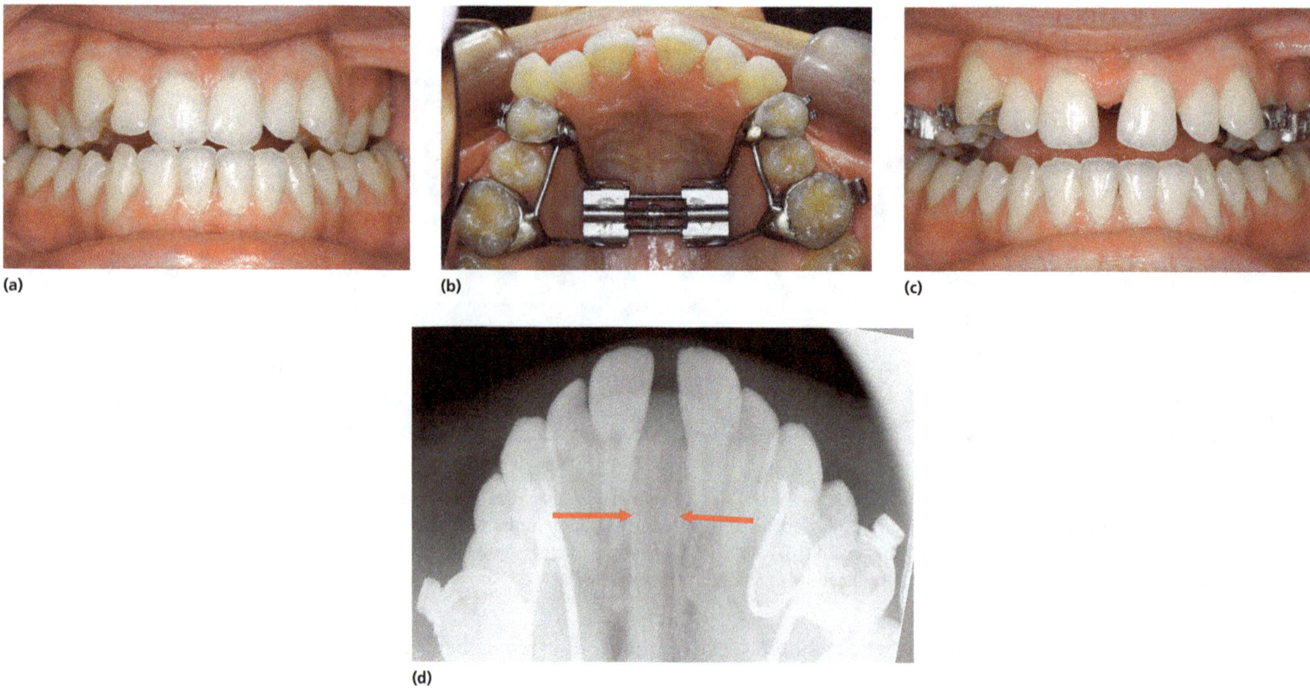

Figure 3.89 Signs of successful maxillary skeletal expansion with RME include (a–c) the formation of a midline diastema and/or (d) presence of a clear widening of the midpalatal suture on an occlusal radiograph.

you should observe the formation of a midline diastema as the two hemi-maxillae separate (Figure 3.89). If you do not observe a diastema, then you may only be achieving dental expansion and not midpalatal (skeletal) expansion. However, in some patients you may be achieving a midpalatal expansion, but the incisors could be pulled together by the stretched periodontal fibers so quickly that you never observe a diastema. If you do not observe diastema formation, make an occlusal radiograph to confirm the presence of a midpalatal split (Figure 3.89d).

- *Absence* of a clear midpalatal split on an occlusal radiograph.
- *Impingement* of the RME appliance's metal bars on the alveolar process soft tissue of the palate—a sign that the hemimaxillae are not skeletally separating, but only that the anchor teeth are moving (dentally and buccally) through the bone. Especially with an older patient, like Megan, you must carefully look for this to happen. With age, the facial skeleton, especially the zygomatic buttress, offers increasing resistance to RME.
- Complaints by the patient of *maxillary pain or of continued pressure* greater than 5–10 min after the RME screw is turned.

Q: How do you proceed if Megan's midpalatal suture does not split?

A: This depends on whether you have already achieved significant *dental expansion* of the maxillary molars with the RME appliance before you determine that she does not have a split. If only minimal expansion has occurred, then you may consider surgical intervention (SARME or multiple-piece maxillary osteotomy) or leaving her in posterior cross bite. If significant dental expansion has already occurred (and the periodontium appears robust—thick buccal bone, lots of attached keratinized gingiva), then you must make the decision either to continue dental expansion or stop and consider surgery. Thankfully, Megan does appear to have significant bone buccal to her maxillary molars, especially on her right (Figure 3.76m).

Q: Should Megan simply be left in cross bite?

A: No. In adult patients whose maxilla cannot be widened with an RME appliance, who do not wish to undergo surgery, and who cannot be treated with dental expansion to correct the transverse problem—leaving them in cross bite may be a viable alternative. This is especially true if their canines are not in cross bite (are properly coordinated) or if their canines can be brought out of cross bite. But in a young adult like Megan, you should at least *attempt* expansion with an RME appliance (informing them that a SARME or an MPMO may be necessary if a midpalatal split is not achieved). Even if you plan to downgraft her maxilla at a later age, attempting to widen Megan's maxilla now with an RME appliance is better than widening her maxilla with an MPMO later. Why? A one-piece maxillary surgery is better than a multiple-piece maxillary surgery ("the fewer the pieces, the fewer the problems").

Q: Is surgery a possible treatment option for Megan? If yes, what surgical movements do you recommend?

A: Surgery is clearly the treatment option of choice for Megan. A Le Fort I maxillary downgraft osteotomy would lengthen her LAFH and improve her incisal display. It would need to be a right-to-left maxillary *differential downgraft*—to address her right-to-left occlusal cant. Since a downgraft will rotate the mandible down and back (worsening her Class II relationship), a mandibular advancement will also be necessary. A mandibular surgery would also be necessary to correct the mandibular right-to-left occlusal cant. In addition, a setback genioplasty will be necessary to reduce her chin prominence (especially following a mandibular advancement), and the chin could also be downgrafted to lengthen her LAFH more. If your attempt to widen her maxilla with an RME appliance fails, then a maxillary differential downgraft MPMO may be the surgery of choice to widen the maxilla in addition to lengthening her LAFH.

Q: If Megan declines surgery, are other reasonable treatment options available or should you refuse to treat her?

A: If she declines surgery, you could consider *reversible* treatment options that could both help her now and still leave open the possibility of surgical treatment later. Try to avoid irreversible treatment (e.g., extraction of maxillary first premolars to retract the maxillary anterior teeth). If she declines surgery, you could attempt to expand her maxilla with an RME appliance now. If successful, that would correct her cross bite, help eliminate transverse posterior compensations, and simplify maxillary downgraft surgery (eliminate the necessity of a SARME or multiple-piece maxillary osteotomy), if she later decided to have surgery as an adult. Additionally, you could improve/correct her dental relationship with Class II elastics, Forsus, headgear, or TADs. But leveling her maxillary arch with fixed appliances will reduce her incisal display even more (because her maxillary incisors are stepped down), worsening her smile. You could consider/discuss such reversible options, but clearly the best option for Megan is surgery.

Q: Whenever surgery is an option, the orthodontist must insure that the magnitude of anticipated bony movements is within the range of the surgical envelope and stability. What are the limits for all maxillary and mandible surgical movements?

A: See Table 3.10

Q: List other guidelines that the orthodontist should follow to minimize postsurgical problems

A: See Table 3.11

Table 3.10 Limits of orthognathic surgical movements.

Maxillary surgical limits	Downgraft	5–8 mm	Note: the maxilla cannot descend straight down due to changes in the occlusal plane angle as the mandible rotates down and back.
	Impaction	6–7 mm 10 mm	In the posterior. In the anterior.
	MPMO transverse expansion	8 mm	Limit depends on the height of the palate and posterior tooth torque; a low palate permits less expansion (soft tissue stretch); ideally, the pre-surgical posterior dentition should be without transverse compensations.
	Advancement	5–7 mm	Consider distraction osteogenesis if more maxillary advancement then this is required.
	Setback	5–6 mm	The limiting factor is running into the bony pterygoid plates. If you need greater setback than this, consider extracting maxillary premolars so only the anterior segment is setback.
Mandibular surgical limits	Advancement	10 mm 14–15 mm	In high MPA cases. In low MPA cases. Note: check for impingement of maxillary second molars on the ascending ramus during advancement. You may need to extract the maxillary second molars if maxillary second molar impingement occurs.
	Setback	10 mm	Be careful to avoid airway obstruction or of creating future sleep apnea problems.

In a conversation with a colleague from the University of Iowa College of Dentistry, Department of Oral & Maxillofacial Surgery (Stein KM 2013), oral communication, September 16.

Table 3.11 Checklist to follow for surgical patients.

Presurgical tasks	• Verify relaxed lip incisal display *after leveling* to decide the magnitude of vertical maxillary surgical incisor movement. • Approve the articulated surgical occlusion (models mounted by the surgeon). • Agree on proposed surgical movements and verify that surgical movements are within surgical limits. • Schedule the patient to see you 1 week after the surgery date.
Postsurgical communication	• When should the surgeon contact the orthodontist? – Immediately after surgery (what was the surgical outcome?) – The surgeon should inform the orthodontist of problems (to better prepare for dealing with them). – **Q:** Was the bite seated during surgery? (if it was, than a later occlusal discrepancy could be due to edema / muscle spasms) • Take care what you say in front of the patient. – Seek solutions to surgical problems the cause of which may have been indeterminate/unavoidable. – Put a positive spin on intervention—"surgery helped a lot, now we are completing treatment." • Work together with the surgeon to discuss postsurgical treatment, including direction and magnitude of orthodontic forces to be applied
Postsurgical tasks	• See patient 1 week postoperatively (well within the first few months window of accelerated bony remodeling/cellular activity/possible increased tooth movement) so that you can intercede effectively, as needed. • Check for postsurgical occlusal discrepancies, including a repeatable bite at the 1 week postop appointment. • Guiding elastics—guiding elastics help the patient learn to close into the new occlusion. This is necessary since the jaw muscular length and direction have been changed with surgery, edema and muscle spasms may alter the correct closing position, proprioceptive sense may have been lost, and/or the patient may be numb. The focus of guiding elastics is on the muscles. Guiding elastics are *not* intended to move teeth. There is no specific length of time for wearing guiding elastics. Time of wear is a judgment call made between the surgeon and orthodontist. • Splints—an occlusal splint is worn by the patient for approximately 6 weeks following MPMOs to hold a transverse expansion. As soon as it is removed, a palatal splint is fabricated and worn for as long as possible through the completion of orthodontic treatment. If the maxillary archwire was sectioned at surgery, then it should be replaced with a continuous wire at the 6 week appointment.

Table 3.12 Guidelines for postsurgical biomechanics if occlusal discrepancies exist (i.e., not fully corrected or overcorrected).

General guidelines	• Use the same biomechanics that are used as for nonsurgical cases. • Discuss with your surgeon the level of forces, and direction of forces, you intend to use. • Try to stay with light forces—especially when beginning. • *Remember the direction of surgery*—do NOT immediately use mechanics that are opposite to the direction of the surgery. For example, if a mandibular advancement osteotomy overcorrected a Class II patient to a Class III relationship, do NOT begin pulling Class III elastics. You may eventually need use Class III elastics, but give the patient some months to allow edema to be eliminated and muscular function to normalize before doing so.
Mild discrepancy	• Use standard orthodontic finishing treatment.
Moderate discrepancy	• Aggressive intercession may be required, or accept a compromise result.
Severe discrepancy	• Discuss with the surgeon. • If you feel that the patient needs to go back into surgery, do it very soon so the patient has only one recovery period (if you wait a month before sending the patient to surgery, he/she will have two recovery periods).

Q: If a patient returns from surgery not fully corrected, or overcorrected, list principles of orthodontic biomechanics to get the patient back on track.

A: See Table 3.12

Q: What unknowns do you face in treating Megan? What unknowns should you try to eliminate before defining a final treatment plan for her and doing something irreversible (e.g., extractions or surgery)?

A: Unknowns for Megan include the following:

- Can her posterior cross bite be corrected with an RME appliance? Can a midpalatal split be achieved?
- Is an undetected CR–CO shift present? You should confirm Megan's AP relationship *after* you attempt RME. Why? "breaking up" the occlusion with the RME appliance may eliminate a habitual biting pattern.
- How is her cooperation and hygiene?

Q: Would you recommend a nonextraction treatment plan for Megan? Or, should anterior or posterior permanent teeth be extracted?

A: Even if you eventually decided to treat Megan with maxillary first premolar extractions, it would be prudent to *first attempt nonextraction treatment*—especially considering the uprightness of the mandibular and maxillary incisors and need for RME.

Q: After considering everything we have discussed thus far, what treatment do you recommend for Megan?

A: Following conversations with Megan and her parents about multiple treatment options, a decision was made to attempt RME followed by nonextraction orthodontic treatment and surgery. *If the RME was successful in achieving a midpalatal split*, then fixed appliances would be placed and Megan's arches leveled and aligned. Surgery would follow and consist of a Le Fort I differential downgraft osteotomy (to correct Megan's right-to-left cant and increase her LAFH), plus a BSSO mandibular advancement osteotomy, plus a genioplasty setback/downgraft). *If the RME was unsuccessful in achieving a split*, then fixed appliances would be placed, Megan's arches would be leveled and aligned, and the same surgical course followed except that the maxillary downgraft would include an MPMO to increase the width of her narrow maxilla.

Q: What are the specific objectives of treatment for the maxilla, mandible, maxillary dentition, and mandibular dentition in all three planes of space?

A: Specific objectives of treatment for Megan are as follows:

Maxilla

AP: Maintain.

Vertical: Reposition downward—differential downgraft and cant correction.

Transverse: Widen to establish normal transverse relationship.

Mandible

AP: Surgically advance mandible and set back symphysis.

Vertical: Surgically correct cant. Increase skeletal lower anterior facial height.

Transverse: Maintain.

Maxillary dentition

AP: Maintain molars and canines. Procline incisors.

Vertical: Maintain molars and intrude incisors.

Intermolar width: Widen to establish normal transverse relationship.

Mandibular dentition

AP: Maintain molars. Maintain incisors.

Vertical: Level COS. Intrude incisors. Maintain molars.

Intermolar/intercanine width: Maintain intermolar/intercanine width.

Q: How did Megan's treatment proceed?

A: Treatment began with RME, which was, surprisingly, successful in achieving a midpalatal split and maxillary skeletal expansion. Her maxilla was widened enough to

1. Correct her left cross bite.
2. Obtain posterior overjet to permit uprighting of her lingually inclined mandibular posterior teeth.
3. Provide adequate posterior overjet following a mandibular advancement osteotomy (wider part of the mandibular arch brought forward).

By this time, all second molars had erupted. Her maxillary arch was placed in fixed appliances, and leveled to create anterior OJ and room for the lower braces. Fixed appliances were then placed on her mandibular arch, and both arches were leveled and aligned.

Q: Figure 3.90 shows Megan presurgery. What do you note?

A: Her incisal display has decreased (her maxillary incisors intruded with leveling), maxillary incisors have proclined (as seen on her lateral cephalometric radiograph), overbite has decreased, and the posterior cross bite has been eliminated.

Q: Note the spaces intentionally placed presurgically between the maxillary lateral incisors and maxillary canines (Figure 3.90e and g). What is the purpose of these (Iowa) spaces?

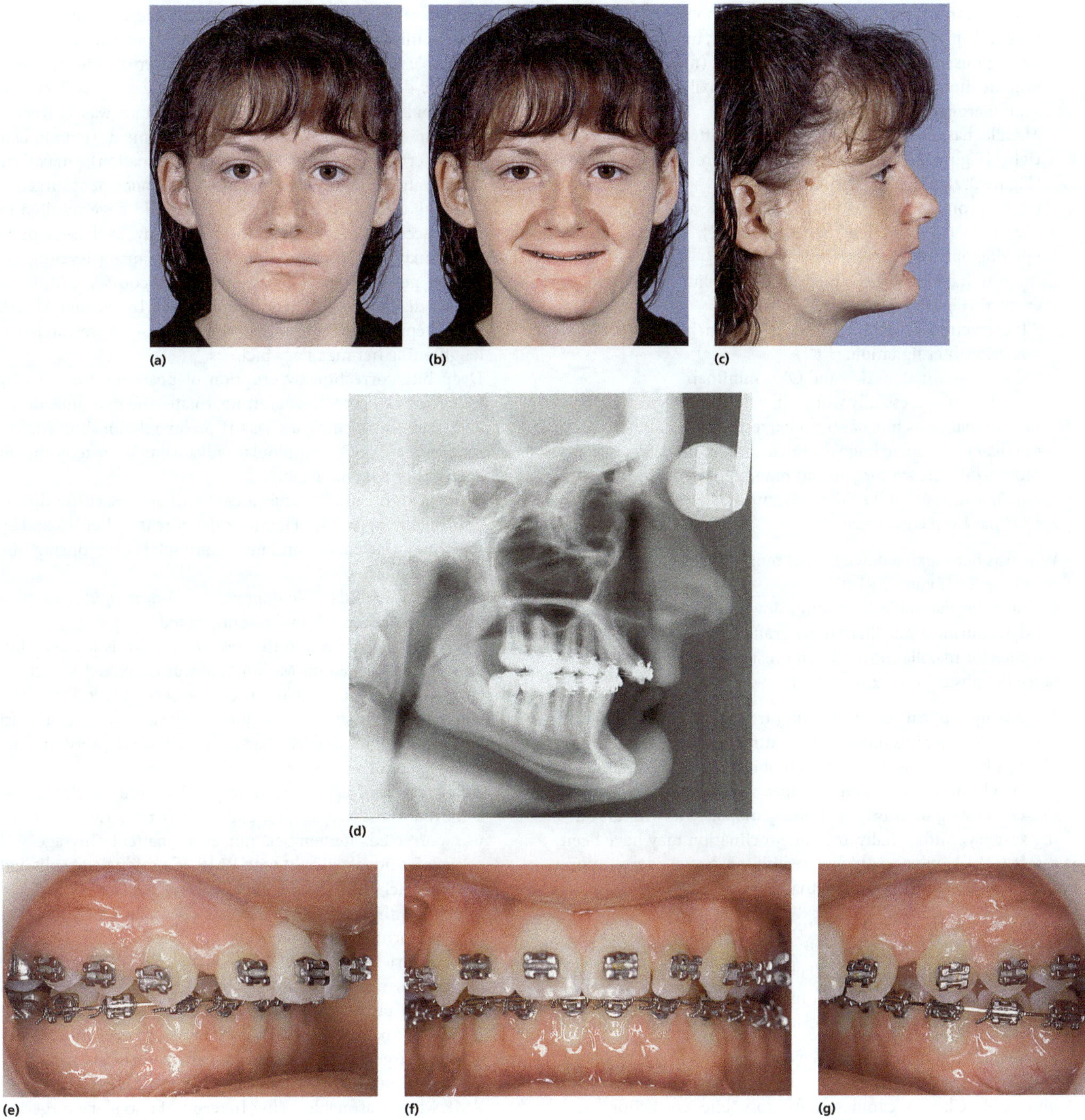

Figure 3.90 (a–g) Megan's presurgical records.

A: The purpose of creating these spaces is to advance the maxillary incisors entirely out of contact with the mandibular dentition when the mandibular canines are surgically advanced into a Class I relationship during surgery. Without these spaces, the mandibular incisors could contact the lingual surfaces of the maxillary incisors and prevent the surgeon from advancing the mandible into a perfect Class I canine relationship. The spaces are closed, postsurgically. If an anterior Bolton tooth size discrepancy (mandibular anterior excess) exists, then when the OJ is closed postsurgically there may be spaces remaining, which will require restorative treatment to close.

Q: Surgery consisted of a one-piece Le Fort I maxillary differential downgraft osteotomy, mandibular BSSO advancement osteotomy, and genioplasty downgraft/setback osteotomy. All surgical limits were well within the range of acceptable magnitude, and all of our earlier guidelines were followed to minimize postsurgical problems. Minor finishing was performed postsurgically, including maxillary incisor space closure. Figure 3.91 shows Megan at finish. What do you note?

A: Changes noted include the following:

- Treatment resulted in a beautiful smile—Megan's chief complaint has been addressed.
- Overclosed appearance has been corrected—her facial proportions are nearly ideal.
- Right-to-left facial and occlusal cants were corrected.

- Lips appear fuller with more vermillion show.
- Incisal display was improved, dramatically, but incisal display during posed smile is still less than ideal (maxillary lip vermillion should be congruent with the maxillary incisor gingival margins).
- Maxilla has been differentially downgrafted, more on her right (Figure 3.91d) than left, and more in her anterior (Figure 3.91g) than posterior.
- Chin prominence has been reduced anteroposteriorly (Figure 3.91g) and lengthened vertically, resulting in an opening of her labiomental sulcus.
- Incisors have been proclined and mandibular molars have erupted (Figure 3.91g).
- AP correction (Class I canines) has been achieved with ideal posterior interdigitation.
- OB is approximately 20% and OJ is minimal.
- Maxilla was successfully widened with RME (Figure 3.91o).
- Left lingual cross bite has been corrected (Figure 3.91n).
- Maxillary premolar lingual crown torque, maxillary second molar labial crown torque, and mandibular posterior lingual crown torque are still evident (Figure 3.91q and r).
- COS has been eliminated.

Q: Why was her maxilla downgrafted more in the anterior than in the posterior (Figure 3.91g)?

A: Because the mandible is rotating down and back around the condyle, during a maxillary downgraft osteotomy, the distance the anterior maxilla moves down must be greater than the distance the posterior maxilla moves down.

Q: Megan's lips appear fuller following treatment. How could this occur? Are fuller lips more, or less, attractive than thinner lips?

A: Her lips became fuller though a combination of maxillary V–Y closure plus nasal cinch and, possibly, as a result of her mentalis muscle moving inferiorly with the genioplasty downgraft during surgery. Additionally, incisor proclination may have been a factor. In women, a thicker vermillion is considered more attractive, and more feminine, than thinner lips [119].

Q: How was Megan's deep bite corrected?

A: Her deep bite was corrected through a combination of (Figure 3.92) downward maxillary movement, downward and backward mandibular rotation, mandibular lengthening, mandibular molar eruption, and incisor proclination/intrusion.

Q: Were your treatment goals achieved?

A: Yes. Facial balance, profile, and smile were dramatically improved. Class I canines, left cross bite correction, and improved OB were achieved.

Q: What retention protocol would you suggest?

A: Lifelong wear of maxillary and mandibular Hawley retainers when sleeping. Her maxillary retainer was designed with an anterior biteplate to disclude her posterior teeth at night and improve the chance of her maintaining deep bite correction. A fixed mandibular canine-to-canine retainer would be an acceptable alternative for the lower arch.

Q: What "take-home" messages can you draw for future practice from Megan's treatment?

A: Take-home messages include the following:

- Megan presented with a combination skeletal and dental deep bite. Her skeletal deep bite resulted from her condyles growing more vertically than normal (as opposed to posterior-superiorly), her mandible rotating forward (internally, true rotation) more excessively than normal, her maxilla descending less, and her mandibular molars erupting less than normal. As Megan's mandible rotated upward and forward, a deep overbite resulted. Megan's dental deep bite resulted from excess maxillary and mandibular incisor eruption. Her deep bite was corrected through a combination of dental movement (mandibular molar eruption, incisor intrusion/proclination), maxillary downgrafting surgery, and mandibular advancement surgery.
- Masking to address her short LAFH would have resulted in an unacceptable maxillary incisal display as her stepped down maxillary incisors were intruded during leveling (as shown postleveling, Figure 3.90b). Of course, additional incisal display could have been achieved by leaving Megan with stepped down maxillary incisors, or by restoratively lengthening her maxillary incisors.
- Deep bite correction by eruption of posterior teeth, or by maxillary Le Fort I downgrafting, rotates the mandible down and back—worsening a Class II molar relationship. Megan required a BSSO mandibular advancement osteotomy to correct her AP relationship.
- Megan's right-to-left occlusal cant was addressed by downgrafting the right side of her maxilla more than her left and by matching the corresponding mandibular cant during the BSSO osteotomy.
- Stability of maxillary downgrafts is good, *if rigid fixation is used*. Some relapse should be anticipated.
- Deep bite overcorrection (to 10% OB or less) is prudent, but was not performed on Megan (she was corrected to ~20%). Compliance with night-time retainer wear (maxillary anterior biteplate to slightly disclude posterior teeth) is a must and is being followed by Megan. Some OB relapse should be anticipated during retention.
- At 16 years of age, Megan responded well to RME. She achieved a midpalatal split, and her left posterior cross bite was corrected. Remember, not every patient this age will achieve a midpalatal split with RME. If a midpalatal split had not been achieved, then you could have considered SARME to achieve the posterior transverse correction, or you could have performed a multiple-piece maxillary osteotomy during the Le Fort I downgraft. The magnitude of the transverse correction needed (7 mm plus transverse compensation correction plus additional transverse widening in anticipation of the mandibular advancement osteotomy) was considered too large to treat with dental expansion alone.
- When facing an MPMO to widen a maxilla, first attempt an RME when reasonable. Why? In terms of maxillary surgeries, "the more pieces, the more problems."
- Widening a constricted maxilla/maxillary arch to produce a broader maxillary arch (and reducing the buccal corridor size) can enhance a patient's smile esthetics. This is true if the patient starts with very large buccal corridors and a constricted maxilla.
- Inadequate mandibular *anterior* (chin) vertical development can worsen lip overclosure and labiomental sulcus depth [1]. Genioplasty options considered for Megan included the following:
  - Genioplasty *downgraft and setback* (Figure 3.93a and b) to help increase LAFH and decrease chin prominence. This choice of genioplasty was chosen for Megan and helped flatten out the lower border of her (initially upturned) anterior mandible.
  - Genioplasty with *anteriorly tapered ostectomy* (Figure 3.93c, bony cuts shown as red lines) is indicated when normal

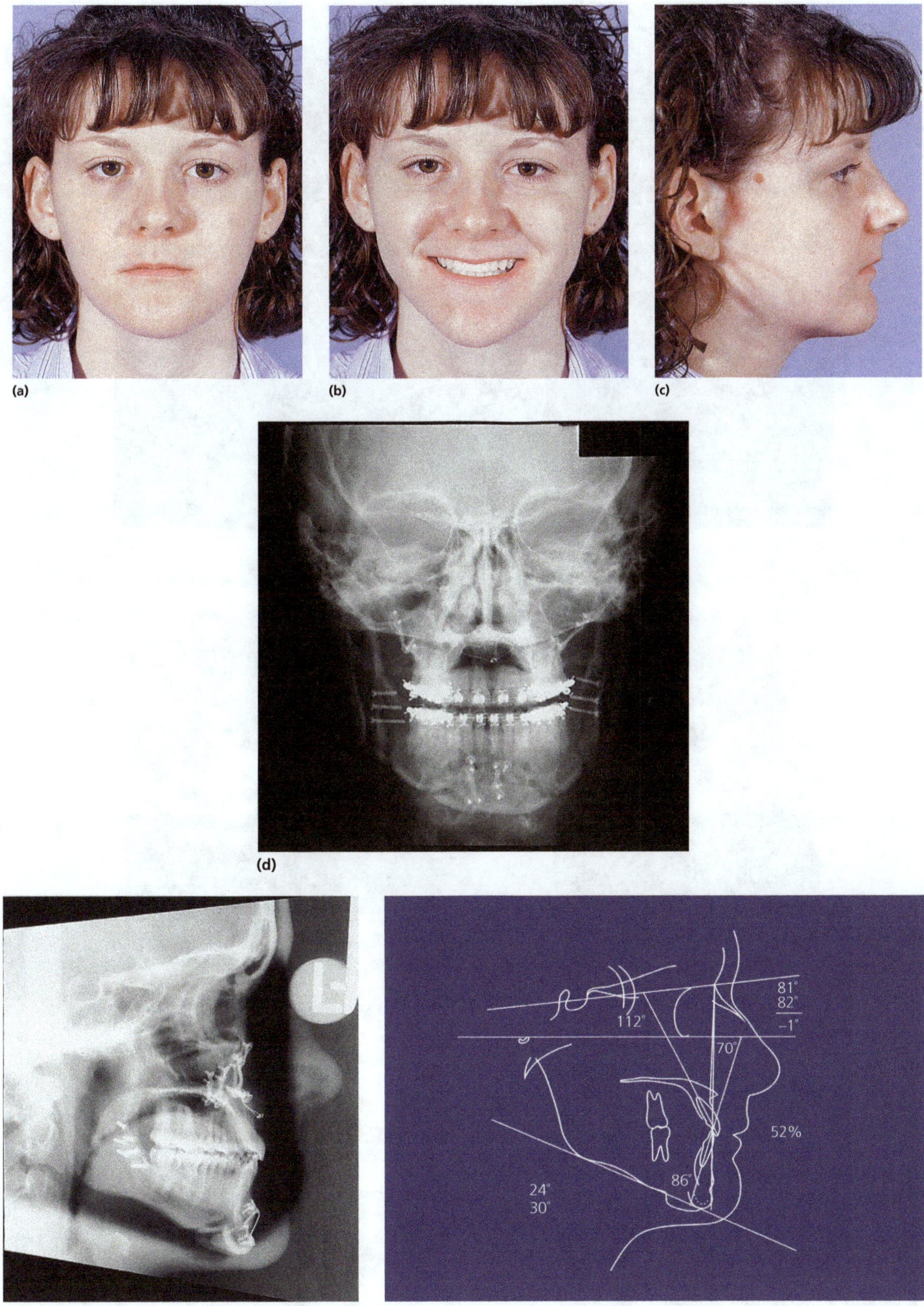

Figure 3.91 (a–s) Deband records of Megan.

mandibular anterior height exists but where bony Pogonion is overly effective. With this procedure, bony Pogonion becomes less effective while the anterior height is maintained. This procedure was not chosen for Megan since it would not have added facial height.

- *Sliding setback genioplasty* (Figure 3.93d) is indicated when minimal vertical lengthening is needed and where bony Pogonion is considered overly effective. This procedure was not chosen for Megan because more facial lengthening was desired than it would have provided. Further, a broad

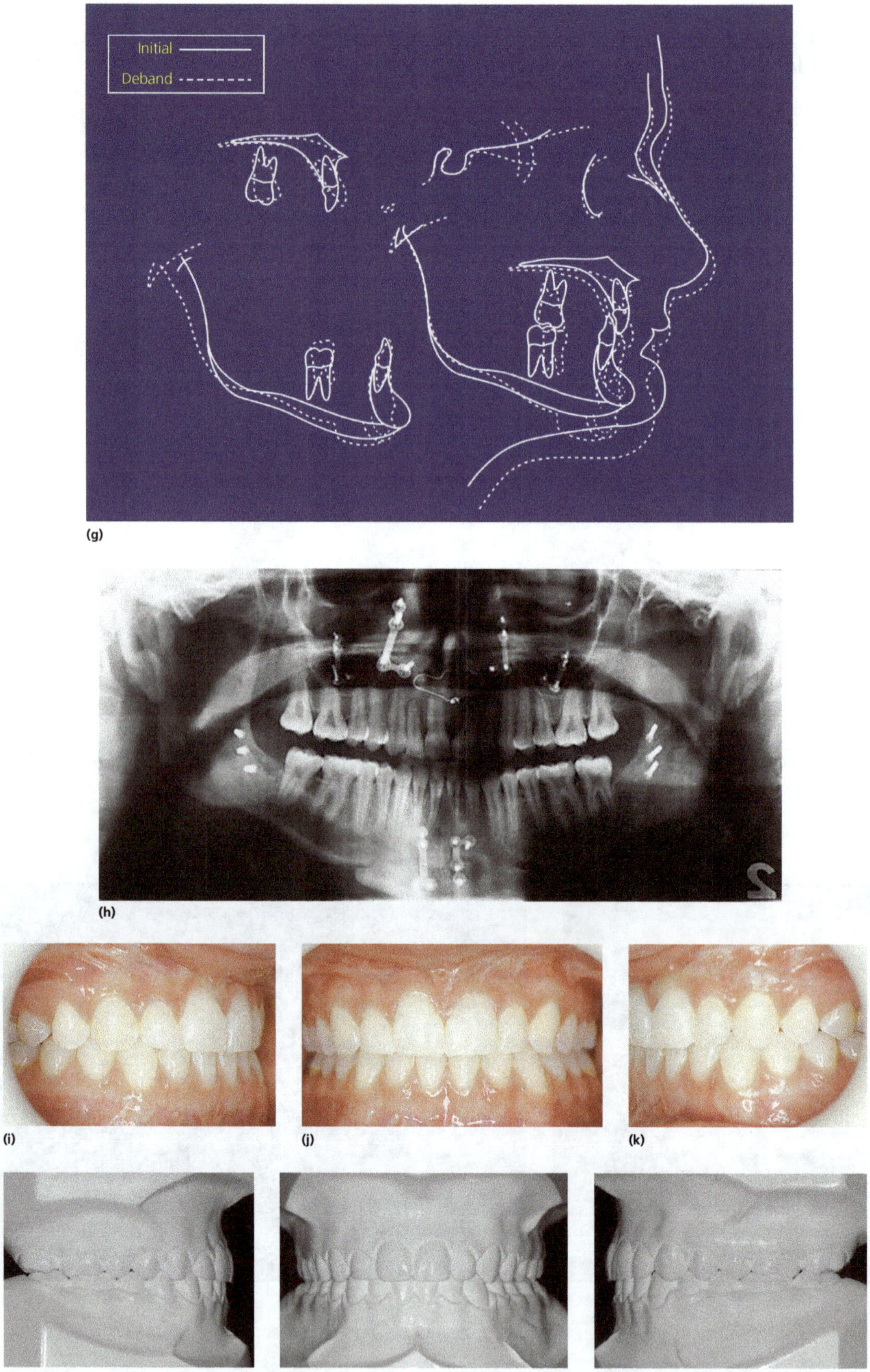

(g) (h) (i) (j) (k) (l) (m) (n)

Figure 3.91 (Continued)

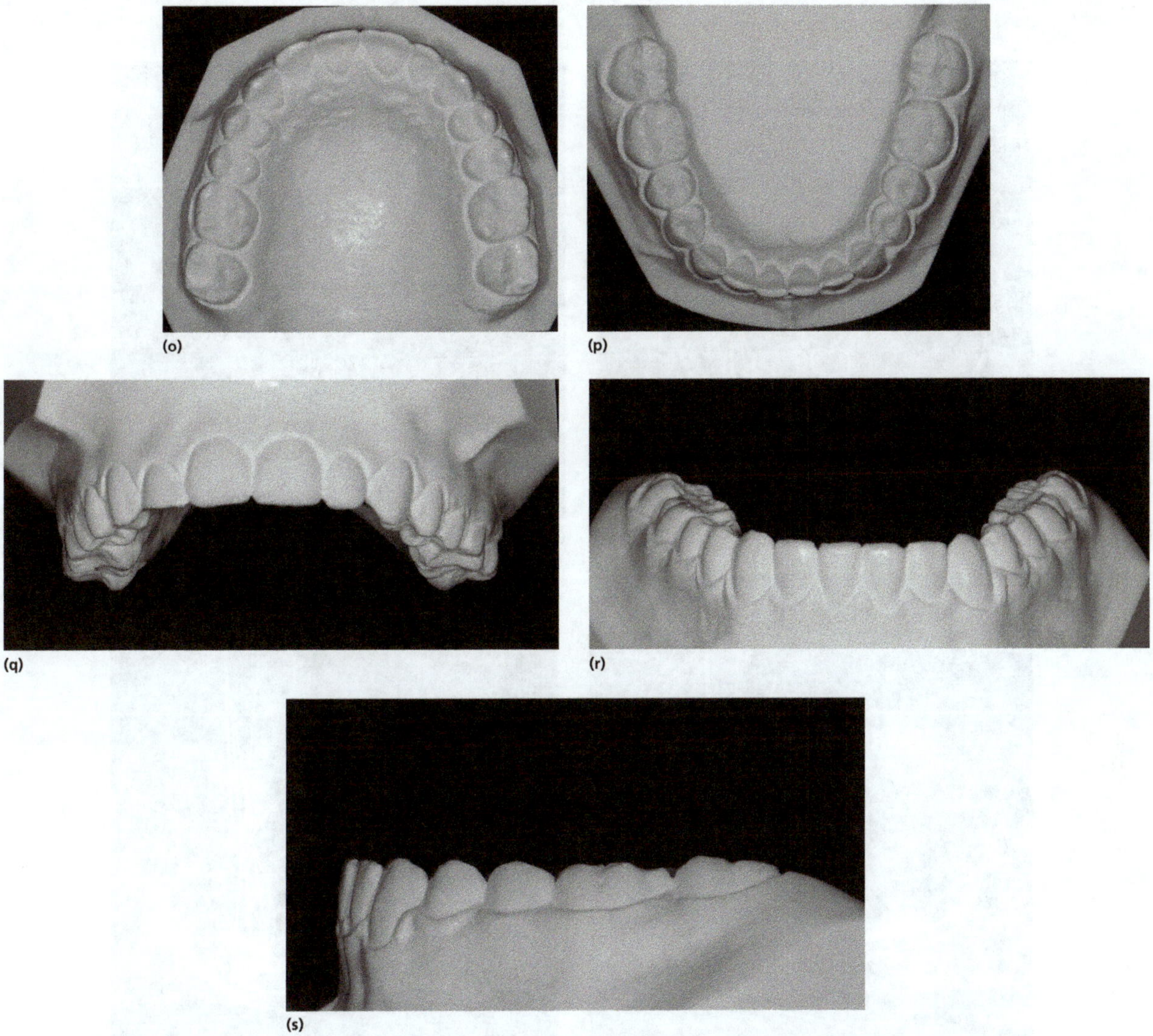

Figure 3.91 (Continued)

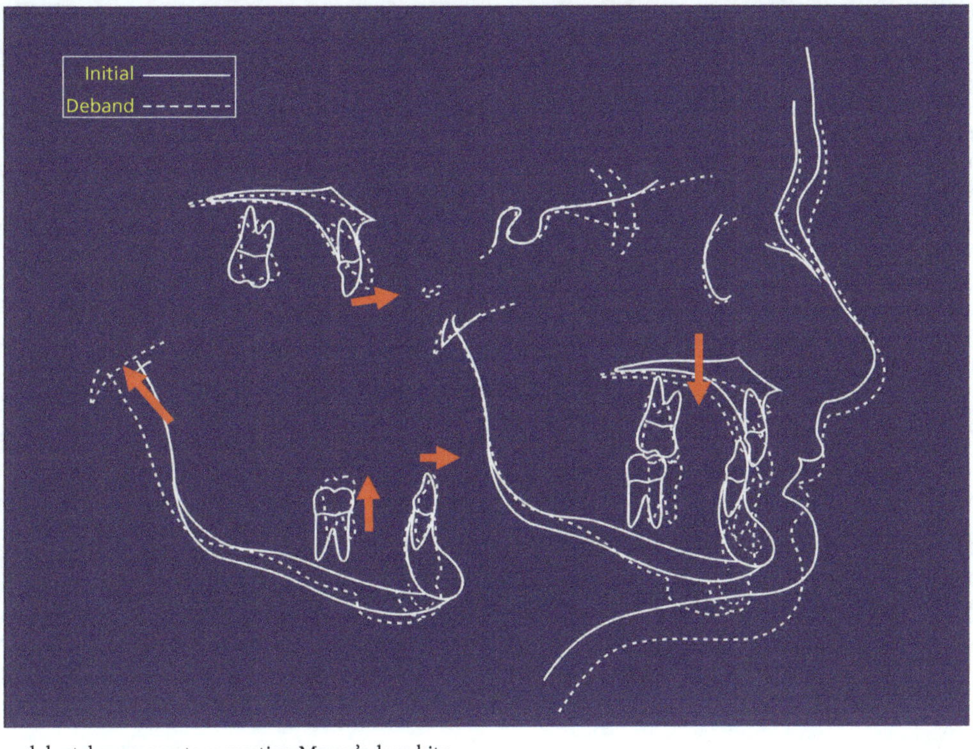

Figure 3.92 Skeletal and dental movements correcting Megan's deep bite.

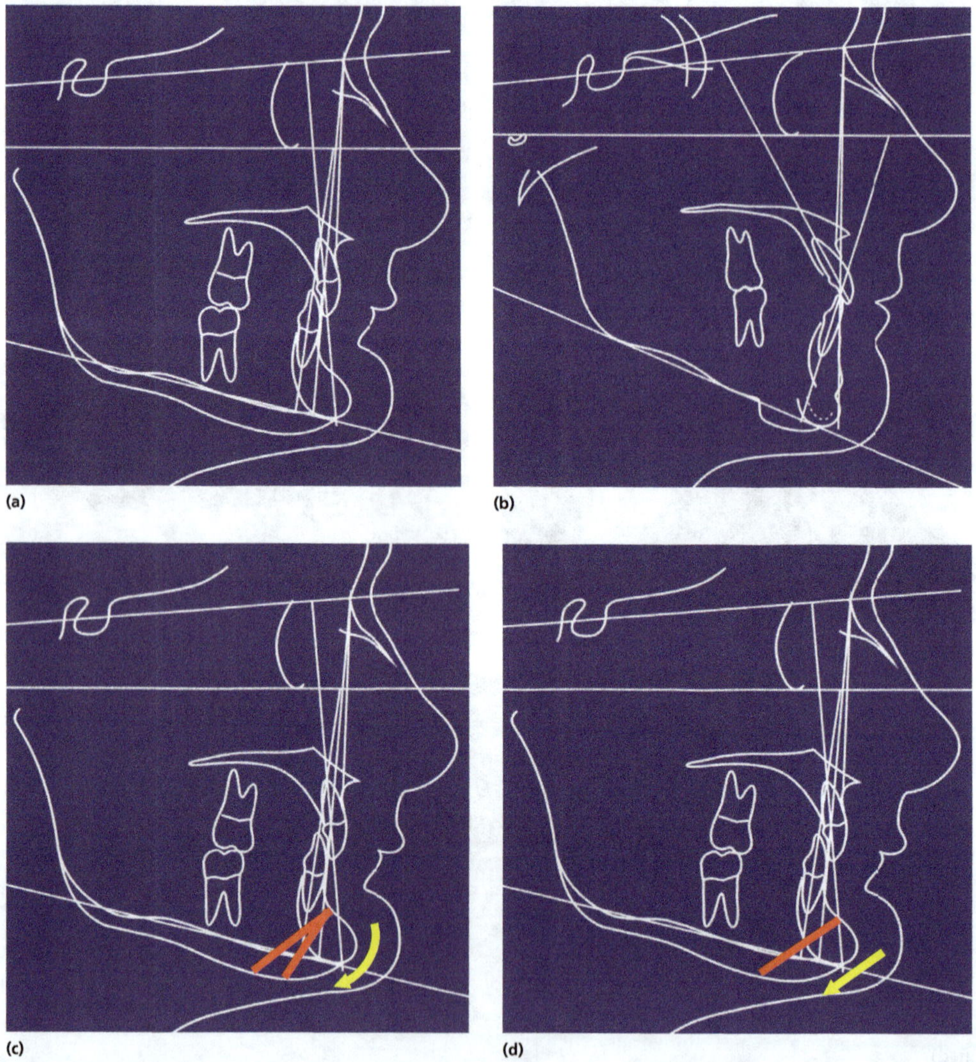

Figure 3.93 Genioplasties considered for Megan: (a and b) genioplasty downgraft and setback—actually performed on Megan, (c) genioplasty with anteriorly tapered ostectomy, and (d) sliding setback genioplasty.

frontal appearance, overlap of posterior "wings," and a fullness in the submental region can occur with a sliding setback genioplasty [120].

Case Connie

Connie (Figure 3.94) is a 25-year-old who presents to you with the chief complaint, "I am concerned with the appearance of my smile." Her PMH and PDH are WRN. She notes that previously she had suffered trauma to her maxilla and incisors, had undergone orthodontic therapy, and had her third molars extracted. CR=CO.

Q: List diagnostic findings/problems. What is your diagnosis?
A: See Table 3.13

Q: What two *critical* features were not examined/reported on Connie thus far?
A: Periodontium and TMJs—history and current status.

Q: What is the appropriate periodontal screening examination that should be performed on every orthodontic patient?
A: The consensus of a joint orthodontist/periodontist task force [121] recommended that, for every screening, the orthodontist obtain a thorough medical and dental history; examine posterior vertical bitewings and anterior periapical radiographs for disease and bone loss; request and evaluate the most recent periodontal charting from the patient's general dentist; and pay particular attention to areas of concern, including pocket depths greater than or equal to 5 mm, bleeding upon probing in several quadrants, mobile teeth, interproximal bone loss, furcation defects, lack of attached keratinized gingiva, and gingival recession.

Q: You obtain Connie's most recent periodontal charting from her general dentist. You examine her posterior vertical bitewings, anterior periapical radiographs, and her periodontal tissues using a probe. No periodontal disease is found. But if periodontal disease were found, what principles should you follow in dealing with the disease?
A: If bleeding/attachment loss/lack of attached gingiva/gingival recession is found, then you should refer the patient to a periodontist. *Control the periodontal disease first, before initiating*

orthodontic treatment. It is prudent to wait up to 6 months after periodontal treatment for healing and resolution of inflammation before beginning orthodontic tooth movement. Obtain a written approval to initiate orthodontic treatment from the periodontist before beginning orthodontic treatment, and you must document the fact that the patient is receiving regular periodontal follow-up during orthodontic treatment.

Q: Adequate width of attached keratinized gingiva is an important component of a healthy periodontium. A patient presents with mild mandibular anterior crowding and 1 mm of attached

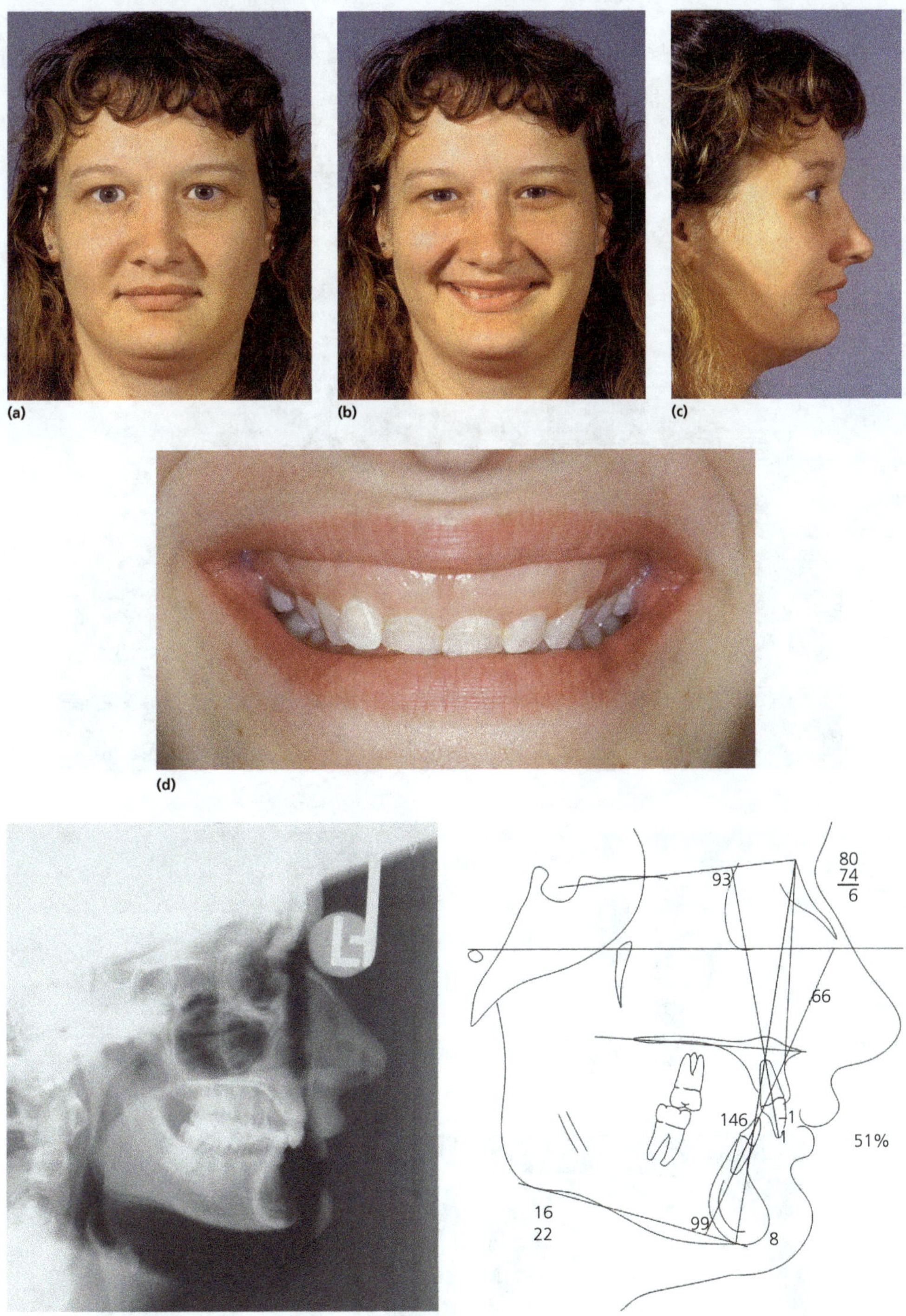

Figure 3.94 Initial records of Connie: (a–c) facial photographs, (d) posed smile, (e) lateral cephalograph, (f) cephalometric tracing, (g–k) intraoral photographs, (l) pantomograph, and (m–q) model photographs. (Low LE, Moore TE, Austin KE, Burton RG, Marshall SD, Southard KE, et al. Mandibular "tripod" advancement of a Class II Division 2 deepbite malocclusion. Am J Orthod Dentofacial Orthop. 2010;137:285–292. Reproduced with permission from Elsevier)

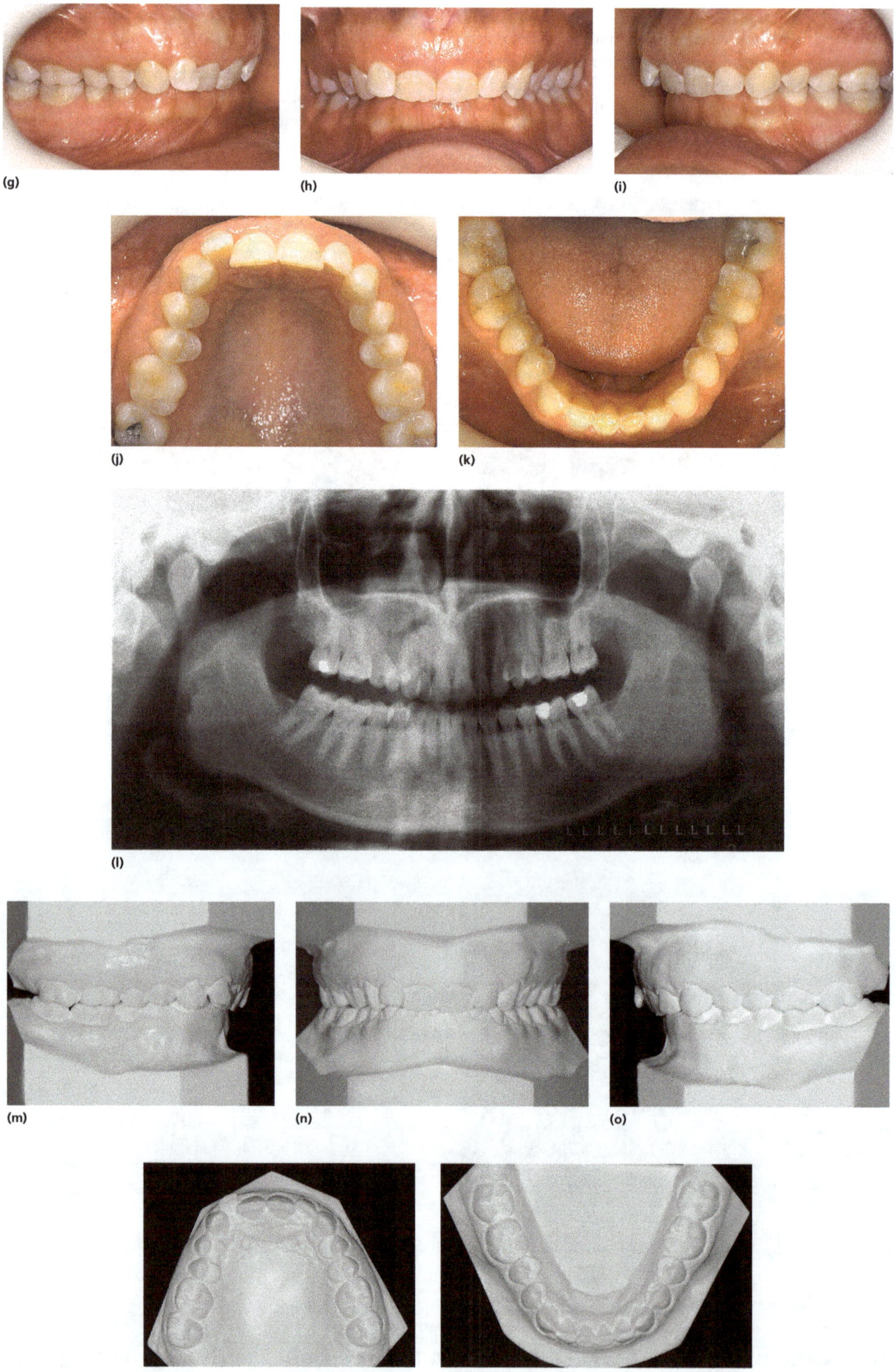

Figure 3.94 (Continued)

Table 3.13 Diagnostic findings and problem list for Connie.

Full face and profile	**Frontal view** Overclosed appearance (everted lower lip, deep labiomental sulcus) Short LAFH (Subnasale–soft tissue Menton < soft tissue Glabell—Subnasale) Excess gingival display in a posed smile Maxillary lip length 17 mm UDML 1 mm right of facial midline **Profile view** Convex profile Obtuse lip–chin–throat angle Everted lower lip Deep labiomental sulcus Retrusive mandible (soft tissue B-point) Prominent chin
Ceph analysis	**Skeletal** Maxillary AP position is slightly retrusive but WRN (A-point may retract as maxillary arch is aligned, upright maxillary incisor roots torqued to the lingual) Mandibular skeletal retrusion (ANB = 6°) Short skeletal LAFH (LAFH/TAFH = 51%; normal is 55%) Flat MPA (FMA = 16°, SNMP = 22°) FMA, SN–MP, and SN are nearly parallel Mandibular incisor angulation WRN (FMIA = 66°) Overly effective soft tissue and bony Pogonion Lip trapping **Dental** Upright maxillary incisors (upper incisor to SN = 93°)
Radiographs	Permanent dentition Wisdom teeth are missing
Intraoral Photos and Models	Angle Class II division 2 Iowa Classification: II (5) II (5) II (5) II (5) OJ: 1 mm OB: 100% Mild maxillary anterior crowding Mandibular midline 2–3 mm left of maxillary midline Maxillary and mandibular dental arches are reasonably symmetric Severe attrition of maxillary and mandibular anterior teeth
Other	—
Diagnosis	Angle Class II division 2 malocclusion Mandibular skeletal AP hypoplasia Maxillary vertical deficiency Dental and skeletal deep bite

keratinized gingiva buccal to her lower anterior teeth. You are considering treating the mandibular arch nonextraction, by proclining the anterior teeth. How much attached keratinized gingiva do you need before treating her, orthodontically?

A: *Rule of thumb: you must have some attached keratinized gingiva throughout both arches* (In a conversation with a colleague from the University of Iowa College of Dentistry, Department of Periodontics (Johnson GK 2011), oral communication, July 5). If you lack attached keratinized gingiva anywhere, seek a consultation from a periodontist. When you are in doubt as to whether you have adequate attached keratinized gingiva, seek a consultation.

Q: The other critical feature not examined/reported thus far was Connie's TMJ status. The health and function of TMJs are such important elements of orthodontic care, it is worth taking time to review very basic questions regarding temporomandibular disorders (TMDs). For instance, what questions should you ask Connie, or any patient, in screening for TMD? What TMD screening examination procedures should you perform on every patient?

A: TMD screening questions [9]:
- Do you have difficulty or pain when opening?
- Does your jaw get locked or go out?
- Do you have difficulty or pain when chewing, talking, or using your jaws?
- Do you have noises in your joints?
- Do your jaws regularly feel stiff, tight, or tired?
- Do you have pain about your ears, temples, or cheeks?
- Do you have frequent headaches or neck aches?
- Have you had a recent injury to your head, neck, or jaws?
- Are you aware of any recent changes to your bite?
- Have you been treated for jaw or joint problems?

TMD screening examination procedures:
- Measure range of motion (opening, right/left).
- Palpate for preauricular or intrameatal TMJ tenderness.
- Auscultate or palpate for TMJ sounds (clicking, crepitus).
- Palpate for tenderness of the masseter and temporalis muscles.
- Note excessive occlusal wear, excessive tooth mobility, buccal mucosal ridging.

Q: What are the six primary temporomandibular joint disorders?

A: Deviation in form, disc displacement, inflammatory conditions, dislocation, arthritides, and ankylosis [122].

Q: What is the most frequent presenting symptom of TMD?

A: Pain [9].

Q: TM joint sounds (i.e., clicking in cases of disk displacement with reduction) or deviation on mouth opening occur in what percentage of the healthy, nonpatient, population?

A: 50% [123].

Q: In cases of disc displacement *without* reduction, the patient opens by deviating to the _____ side.

A: affected [9]

Q: Myofascial pain is characterized by ______, _______, and ______.

A: regional dull pain, localized tenderness, diminished pain with muscle anesthetic injection, or vapocoolant spray [124–127]

Q: In myospasm, muscle contraction is ______ which can be verified with EMG.

A: continuous [128, 129]

Q: Osteoarthitis is characterized clinically by ______, _______, _______, and ______.

A: pain with function, tenderness on palpation, crepitus, limited range of motion, deviation to affected side on opening [9]

Q: Examples of autoimmune disorders that can affect the TM joint are _____, ______, and _____.

A: Sjogrens, systemic lupus erythematosis, scleroderma [130]

Q: Although mounted study models can be of value for the study of teeth and associated structures, do they do provide direct insight into the etiology of TMD?

A: No [9].

Q: In general, does the literature and scientific studies support the role of malocclusion as a primary etiologic factor in TMD?

A: No [11–14, 131–133].

Q: Recent retrospective clinical studies have reported _______ (greater/no greater) prevalence of TMD signs and symptoms in samples of postorthodontic subjects than in untreated subjects of similar ages.

A: no greater [134–136]

Q: Studies comparing postorthodontic patients with and without premolar extractions found ______ (no difference/a difference) in post-treatment condylar position, overbite, discrepancy between intercuspal position and retruded contact position, mandibular position, or in overall TMD symptomatology.

A: no difference [137–139]

Q: Will orthodontic treatment prevent patients from developing TMD problems later in life?

A: No [140–142].

Q: Over time, temporomandibular disorders often are _______ or _________.

A: self-limiting, remitting [143]

Q: Available research and clinical observations support ______ as an initiating and perpetuating factor in TMJ disorders.

A: parafunction [144–147]

Q: ______ factors may predispose certain individuals to TMD and may also perpetuate TMD once symptoms have been established.

A: Psychosocial [9]

Q: Chronic TMD patients have been found to have psychosocial and behavioral characteristics similar to patients with lower back pain and _____.

A: headaches [10]

Q: The articular surfaces of the TMJ (including the disc) are lined with _______ as opposed to _______ in most other synovial joints. This is important because TM joints have a greater ability to _______.

A: dense fibrous connective tissue, hyaline cartilage, repair themselves [148]

Q: As with many musculoskeletal conditions, the signs and symptoms of TMD may be ______ and _______.

A: transient, self-limiting [143, 149–151]

Q: Asymptomatic disc displacement ______ (does/does not) warrant treatment.

A: does not [152]

Q: Progression of a TM click (displaced disk with reduction) to a more serious nonreducing (locking) disk is common or uncommon?

A: Uncommon [153]

Q: With time, disc displacement w/o reduction will become ____ (less/more) painful and restriction in opening often _____ (approaches normal/becomes more restricted).

A: less, approaches normal [154, 155]

Q: In many patients with disc displacement, painless and satisfactory functions are possible although the disc remains displaced. This is because patients with disc displacement may go through a natural period of ______ and ______.

A: remodeling, healing [155–157]

Q: The majority of patients suffering with TMD achieve good relief of symptoms with ______ therapy.

A: conservative [158, 159]

Q: A successful conservative self-care program may allow healing and prevent further injury to the musculoskeletal system and is often enough to control the problem. Instruction in self-care should include what?

A: Rest through voluntary limitation of function, habit awareness and modification, and physiotherapy [159, 160]. *The hallmark of treatment for the majority of TMD patients is conservative therapy. More involved therapy, such as arthrocentisis, is used only after conservative therapy has proven unsuccessful over time and when pain or limitation of function is handicapping.*

Q: Are intraoral orthopedic appliances (interocclusal splints, orthotics, nightguards) efficacious in reducing pain in patients with temporomandibular disorders affecting muscle and joint compared to placebo control, no treatment, or other treatments?

A: Yes. A recent systematic review [161] found that hard stabilization appliances, when adjusted properly, have good evidence of modest efficacy in the treatment of TMJ pain compared to nonoccluding appliances and no treatment, although the physiologic basis has not been documented [9, 161]. Other types of appliances, including soft stabilization appliances, anterior positioning appliances, and anterior bite appliances, have some RCT evidence of efficacy in reducing TMJ pain. However, the potential for adverse events with these appliances is higher, and the need for close monitoring in their use is suggested. *Pearl: consider using a flat plane hard splint in patients who complain of symptoms (joint soreness or myalgia due to parafunction) upon waking in the morning* (clinical opinion).(In a conversation with a colleague from the University of Iowa College of Dentistry, Department of Oral Pathology, Radiology and Medicine (Vincent SD 2012), oral communication, March 28.)

Q: Occlusal adjustment as an irreversible treatment modality should _____ be considered as a primary component of TMD treatment. With regard to bruxism, there is _____ evidence that prophylactic selective grinding of occlusal surfaces is beneficial or that it eliminates bruxism. Occlusal adjustment is _____ indicated for prevention of TMD.

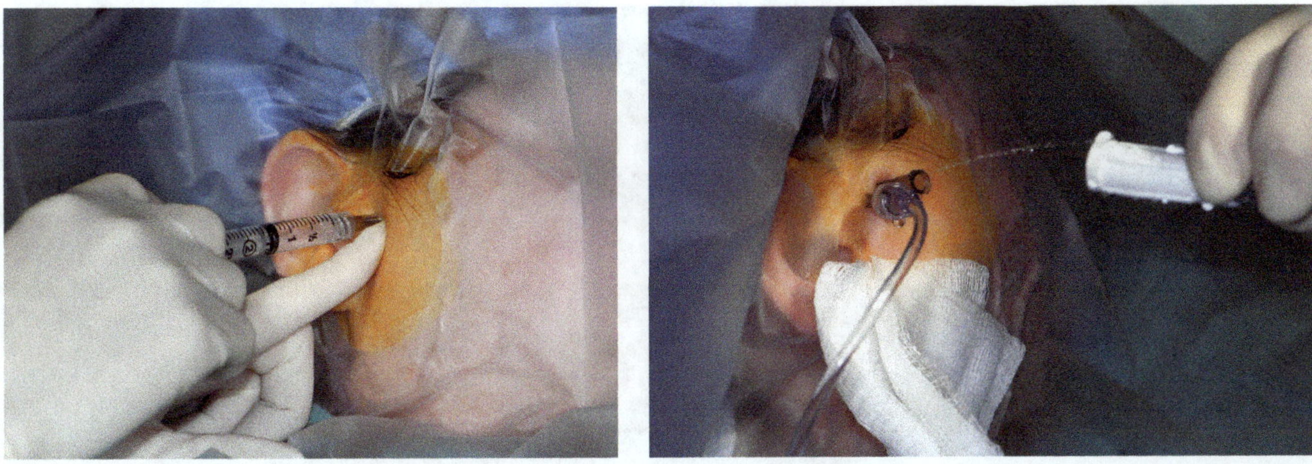

(a) (b)

Figure 3.95 (a, b) TMJ arthrocentesis (Dr. Teresa Morgan, The University of Iowa. Reproduced with permission from Dr. Teresa Morgan.).

A: rarely, no, never [149, 162, 163]

Q: Although most TM disorders appear to be mild, a significant number of patients develop a chronic pain syndrome [164], and little is known about which signs and symptoms of TMD will progress to more serious conditions. For these reasons, a special effort should be made to avoid ______.

A: nonreversible treatment procedures [165]

Q: Despite conservative care, some patients with TMD do not improve. These patients fall into two groups—those with ______ and ______.

A: major structural change, chronic pain syndrome [160]

Q: Arthrocentesis is a relatively noninvasive procedure indicated for _____. The joint may be lavaged with _____ in order to ______ (Figure 3.95) (In a conversation with a colleague from the University of Iowa College of Dentistry, Department of Oral & Maxillofacial Surgery (Morgan T. 2013), oral communication, February 19.) [166].

A: Anteriorly displaced disk without reduction that is unresponsive to conservative therapy. Lactated ringers solution, in order to break up adhesions; morphine in order to reduce pain.

Q: In cases of recurrent mandibular dislocation, a relatively noninvasive treatment may be _____ .

A: Autologous blood injection into the joint space and surrounding tissues (Figure 3.96) in order to create a hemarthrosis—a combination of an organized blood clot and loose fibrous tissue. This tissue matures and causes permanent limitation of movement [167].

Q: Open surgical intervention of the TMJ (______) may be required for bony or fibrous ankylosis, neoplasia, severe chronic dislocations, persistent painful disc derangement, and severe osteoarthrosis refractory to conservative modalities of treatment. Surgery is _______ (often/seldom) indicated in inflammatory joint disorders (synovitis or capsulitis), condylysis, and nonpainful degenerative arthritis.

A: arthrotomy, seldom [9]

Q: Total TMJ replacement may be indicated for ____, _____, and _____.

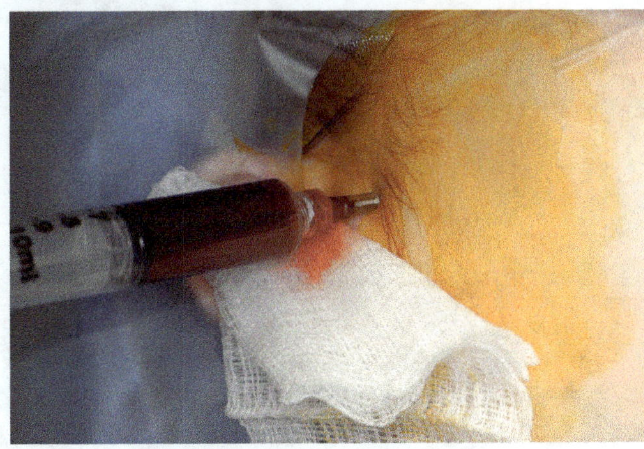

Figure 3.96 Autologous blood injection of TMJ (image courtesy of Dr. Teresa Morgan, The University of Iowa).

A: loss of a condyle, severe restriction of function with failure of other treatment, severe arthritis.

Q: Jackie (Figure 3.97) is a 54-year-old who presents to you with the CC: "I was referred for orthodontic treatment by an oral and maxillofacial surgeon." PMH includes depression and a penicillin allergy. PDH WRN. Her TMJ evaluation reveals bilateral ADD with reduction but without pain or restriction of function. She displays a significant forward and right lateral shift from CR (Figure 3.97e) to CO (Figure 3.97f). Periodontal pocketing of 4–5 mm with bleeding is noted in the maxillary right first and second molar sulci. Please evaluate her condyles using her screening panoramic image (Figure 3.97d). What recommendations do you have concerning treatment?

A: Clearly, a significant difference in form exists between her right and left condyles. The right condyle appears to have degenerated. Two immediate questions arise: what has happened to the right condyle in the past and what could happen to it in the future? To answer the first question, her general dentist should be contacted and earlier panoramic films obtained to compare with the current image. Also, any history of generalized musculoskeletal symptoms/conditions should be more thoroughly investigated. Jackie again denies any additional medical

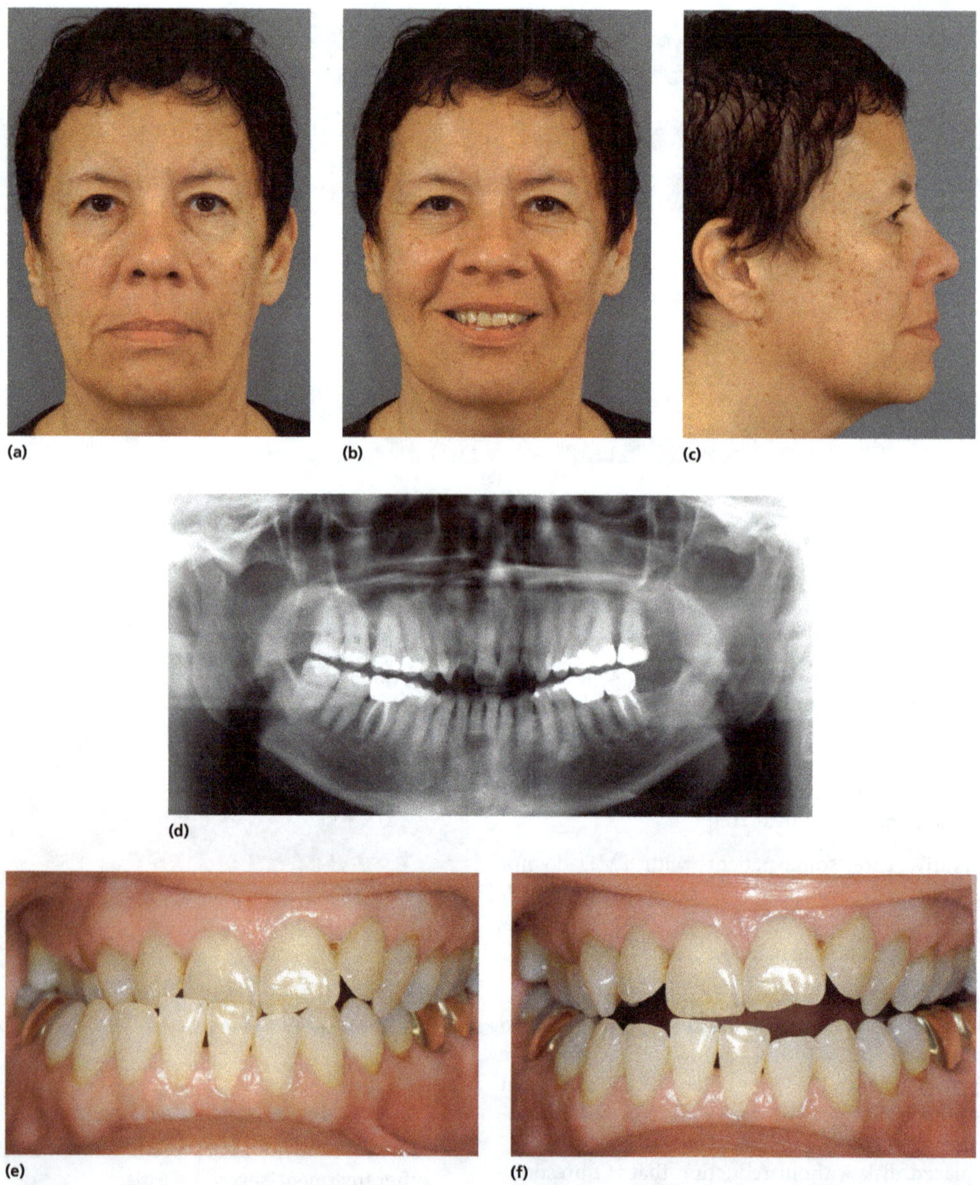

Figure 3.97 (a–f) Initial records of Jackie.

problems. In terms of the right condyles future (and future treatment), a radiologist/pathologist was contacted. He stated that the current panoramic image was suggestive of degenerative joint disease. He felt that Jackie should be informed that the joint condition may worsen, improve, or remain unchanged, independent of any planned jaw procedures, including orthodontics and surgery. But, based on the fact that she displays no other signs or symptoms of disease, orthodontic treatment could proceed.

Q: Let's speculate for a minute. What if Jackie had presented with the same condylar degeneration, but had complained of a sore jaw upon waking most mornings. What if you had identified wear facets on her teeth, right and left masseter myalgia, and limited opening (maximum incisal opening of ~ 20 mm). How would you have proceeded then?

A: First, you should strongly suspect a parafunctional habit (nocturnal bruxism), an initiating and perpetuating factor in TMJ disorders. Before beginning any orthodontic treatment, you should attempt to reduce her symptoms and, if possible, reduce her habit with rest through voluntary limitation of function, habit awareness and modification, and physiotherapy. Included in this conservative treatment would be NSAIDs to reduce her pain and wearing a hard, flat-plane interocclusal splint. Once improvement was evident, you should not immediately rush into orthodontic treatment. Instead, you should monitor Jackie for six or more months (clinical opinion). If she is clearly improved during that period of time, then consider beginning orthodontic treatment. But, first make another screening panoramic image to confirm no recent condylar changes. And, inform Jackie that her joint condition could worsen.

Q: A 17-year-old male, Julian, presents to you (Figure 3.98) for orthodontic treatment with a CC: "My chin sits back." PMH: knee discomfort and swelling with associated warmth of joints dating back to age 4 or 5. He was evaluated by a pediatric

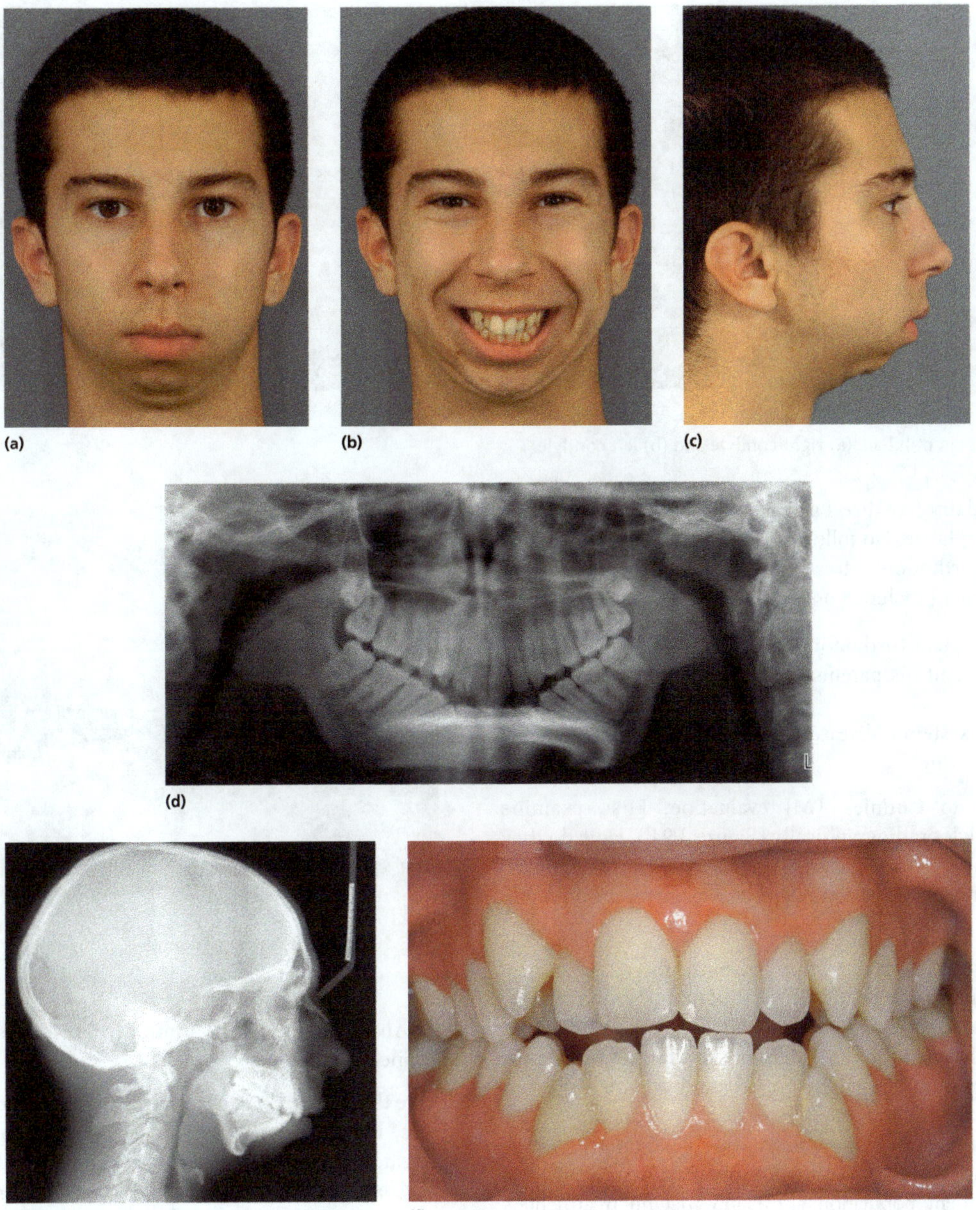

Figure 3.98 (a–f) Initial records of Julian.

orthopedic surgeon who felt that complaints were consistent with "growing pains." Later, he was evaluated by a pediatric rheumatologist who noted normal radiographs at age 8 or 9 and a low positive rheumatoid factor titer. At that time, Julian had complaints with his hands (inability to form a fist). A diagnosis of juvenile idiopathic arthritis was made and Methotrexate prescribed. Since that time, Julian has had intermittent pain and swelling in his wrist and hands, knees, and right elbow. He takes ibuprofen intermittently with improvement. His joint symptoms have not significantly impaired his activities. CR=CO. Julian is free of TMJ pain or restriction of movement. Focusing on Julian's TMJs (Figure 3.98d), should you request other imaging?

A: Yes, to better visualize the TMJs, request a CT scan.

Q: A CBCT scan was requested (Figure 3.99). What do you note regarding his condyles?

A: Julian's right and left condyles are nonexistent.

Q: How do you proceed? Should you request any consultations?

A: Both an oral surgeon and a pediatric rheumatologist were consulted. At first, the surgeon recommended a vertical ramus mandibular advancement osteotomy with a graft, so that the mandible could be advanced and rotated counterclockwise, as needed, to close the bite. Later, the surgeon modified his plan to include only orthodontics plus a large advancement genioplasty to improve Julian's chin position. Why? The surgeon said that the more he thought about it, the more concerns he had that ramus surgery would exacerbate condylar degeneration. A pediatric rheumatologist evaluated Julian and wrote: "This 17-year-old with a history of juvenile onset polyarthritis, borderline rheumatoid factor, and hypoplastic mandible has been found to be IgA deficient. I believe this patient's arthritis, which is nonerosive, likely represented intolerance to foods, and I expect the patient will do very well if he continues to adhere to

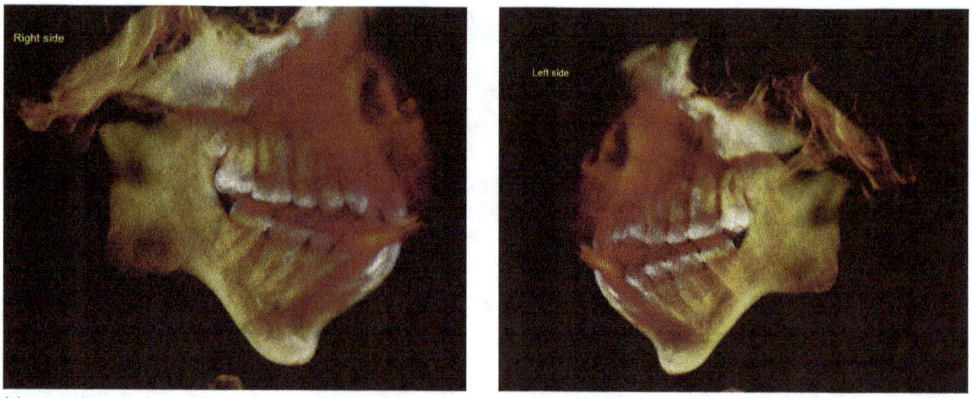

(a) (b)

Figure 3.99 CBCT scan of Julian: (a) right condyle and (b) left condyle.

a gluten and dairy free diet. I suspect that the mandible is congenitally hypoplastic. No follow-up is required." Based on this information, orthodontic treatment for Julian proceeded, but surgical treatment included only a genioplasty.

Q: With any treatment (orthodontic and/or surgical), should you inform Julian and his parents that further joint degeneration can occur?

A: Yes, this is a systemic disease and further degeneration may occur at a later time.

Q: Finally, back to Connie's TMJ evaluation. First, examine Connie's condyles radiographically (Figure 3.94l). How do they appear to you?

A: They appear normal. The condylar borders appear smooth and intact.

Q: A history and clinical examination of Connie reveals an asymptomatic anterior displaced disk *with* reduction (clicking or popping) on her left side and slight deviation to the right upon opening. She has no other TMJ signs or symptoms. Connie asks how this condition should be treated and whether she can undergo orthodontic treatment. How do you respond?

A: Lacking any other signs or symptoms, you should inform Connie that joint sounds or deviation on mouth opening occur in 50% of a healthy nonpatient population [123] and that no treatment is necessary at this time. She can proceed with orthodontic treatment. However, ask her to inform you if her condition changes.

Q: What other features must be examined on Connie's models?

A: Additional features to examine on Connie's models include the following:

- Posterior transverse compensations (Figure 3.100). Connie exhibits mild mandibular second molar lingual crown torque. But overall, her posterior transverse compensations are minimal.
- COS magnitude. Connie's COS is deep, approximately 3 mm (Figure 3.100).
- Right and left molar AP position viewed from the lingual (not shown). As anticipated from her 5 mm Class II relationship when viewed from the buccal (Figure 3.94m and o), Connie's molars are Class II when viewed from the lingual.
- Anterior occlusal steps. Her maxillary incisors are stepped down (Figure 3.100) relative to her posterior dentition and her mandibular incisors are stepped up.
- Bolton anterior tooth-size analysis. This reveals a maxillary–mandibular anterior tooth size discrepancy less than 1 mm.

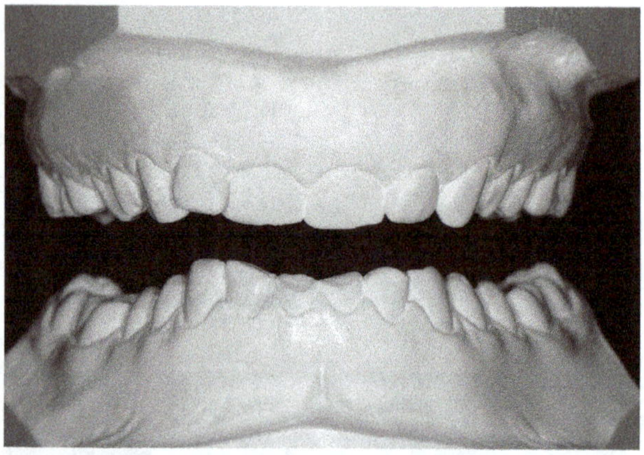

Figure 3.100 Connie's separated models.

An anterior Bolton tooth size discrepancy this small is inconsequential.

Q: Are there other images of Connie that should be made?

A: Yes, but they were not made. Other helpful images would include the following:

- *Connie with her teeth slightly separated until her lips are just touching*, because she has an overclosed appearance (with an everted lower lip). This will allow you to appreciate where her soft tissue facial drape should fall ideally (and how much her jaws need to be separated) in order to provide a balanced facial appearance.
- Connie with her teeth and lips slightly parted in order to visualize the amount of incisal display she exhibits in a relaxed lip position. This should be done now, but especially after the maxillary arch is leveled and any anterior maxillary occlusal step eliminated.
- *Photographs taken at 45°angles* (3/4 facial views) to help judge her malar (cheek) prominences.
- *A second lateral cephalometric radiograph made with her teeth just separated to where her lips are just touching.* This image can be useful in determining the amount of maxillary downward movement required to achieve an ideal facial balance (or upward mandibular molar and premolar eruption needed during COS leveling to achieve ideal facial balance). You should obtain this image for patients with low or borderline low skeletal LAFH/TAFH ratios.

- A photograph made with Connie postured forward into a Class I canine relationship—to evaluate her profile, if she underwent a nonextraction mandibular advancement osteotomy.

Q: As noted earlier, Connie displays excessive gingiva when smiling in a posed smile. What is considered to be an attractive amount of gingival display in a posed smile?
A: An attractive amount of gingival display over the maxillary central incisors is *0 mm* in a posed smile (maxillary lip vermillion congruent with the gingival margins) [168]. Lay persons consider 3–4 mm of gingival show to be unesthetic [5, 82, 168–170].

Q: What are the potential causes of excess gingival display when smiling?
A: Potential causes include the following:
- VME
- Short upper lip length
- Stepped down maxillary incisors (supraeruption)
- Hyperactive musculature when smiling
- Delayed apical migration

Q: What is delayed apical migration?
A: From childhood to adolescence, the gingival margin migrates apically until it reaches its adult position about 1–2 mm coronal to the cementoenamel junction (1 mm sulcus depth, 1 mm epithelial attachment). At this time, the cementoenamel junction should be about 1–2 mm coronal to the crest of the alveolar process bone [171]. In some patients with thick, fibrotic, and noninflamed gingival tissue, this migration occurs much more slowly (delayed apical migration). Patients with delayed apical migration will also present with a larger sulcus depth and shorter papilla height compared to crown length.

Q: What is the ideal ratio of papilla height to maxillary central incisor clinical crown length?
A: The height of the tip of the papilla is ideally *one-half* of the central incisor clinical crown lengths [171].

Q: Look at the patient in Figure 3.101. What do you notice about the gingival and periodontal architecture?
A: This patient exhibits thick, fibrotic, noninflamed gingiva, and a short papilla height compared to crown length (Figure 3.101a). Radiographically (Figure 3.101b), the crest of the alveolar process bone appears less than 1 mm from the CEJs of the maxillary incisors, and the sulcus depth is excessive (Figure 3.101c, 3 mm sulcus depth rather than a normal 1 mm depth).

Q: What do you suspect is the cause of this condition?
A: Delayed apical migration.

Q: What treatment would you recommend for this patient?
A: Gingivoplasty, in conjunction with osseous reconstructive surgery (Figure 3.102a–c), modified the periodontium into a more ideal architecture. Compared to the initial condition (Figure 3.102d), note the final improved gingiva papilla height relative to the central incisor crown length (Figure 3.102e).

Q: Connie exhibits excessive gingival display when smiling (Figure 3.94b and d). What factors contribute to *her* excessive display?
A: Let's look at our list of possible excess gingival display factors for Connie:
- *VME—No.* Connie does *not* exhibit vertical maxillary excess. In fact, she presents with LAFH *deficiency*.

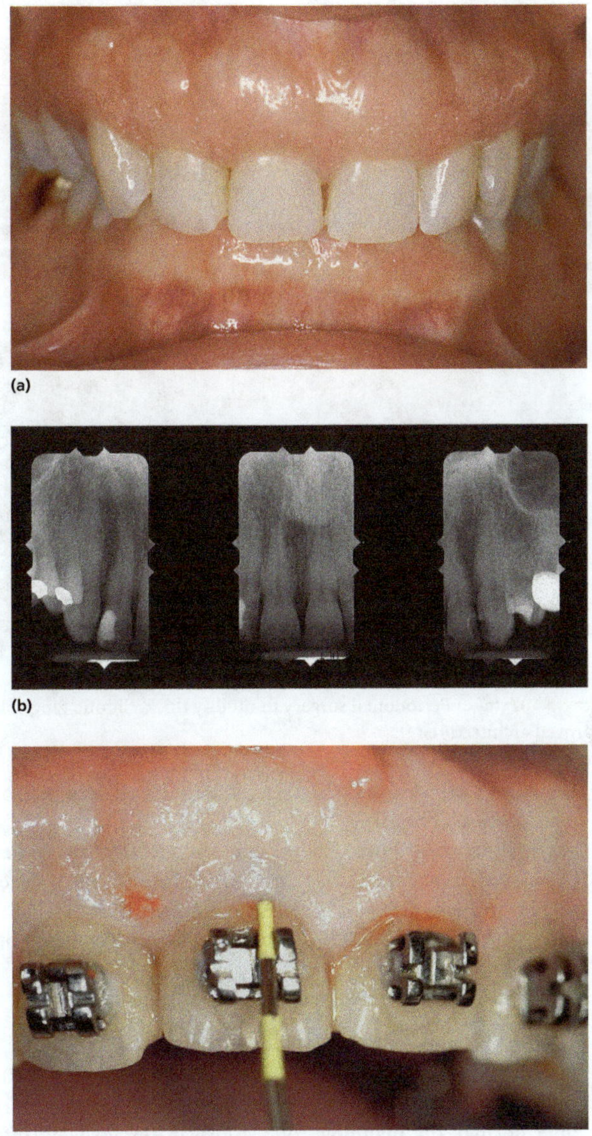
(a)
(b)
(c)

Figure 3.101 (a–c) Examination of maxillary anterior periodontal tissues.

- *Short upper lip length—No.* The normal range of maxillary lip length for adolescent girls is 17–23 mm and for adolescent boys 22–26 mm [1]. During our 20s and 30s, the maxillary lip length increases approximately 1 mm more than the maxillary incisor edge descends [172]. So, for a 25-year-old woman, Connie's maxillary lip length (17 mm) is on the low end of normal, but still reasonably normal.
- *Stepped down maxillary incisors (supraeruption)—Yes.*
- *Hyperactive musculature when smiling—Yes, possibly.* Compare Figure 3.94b–d.
- *Delayed apical migration—No.* Her maxillary incisor sulcus depths are shallow, her maxillary incisor alveolar process crest heights are greater than 1 mm from her CEJs, and the gingival tissues appear normal (not thick or fibrotic), ruling out excessive gingival display as a result of delayed apical migration.

Connie's excess gingival display when smiling results from maxillary incisor supraeruption (maxillary incisors stepped down with maxillary incisal edge wear) possibly coupled with hyperactivity of her (smiling) facial muscles.

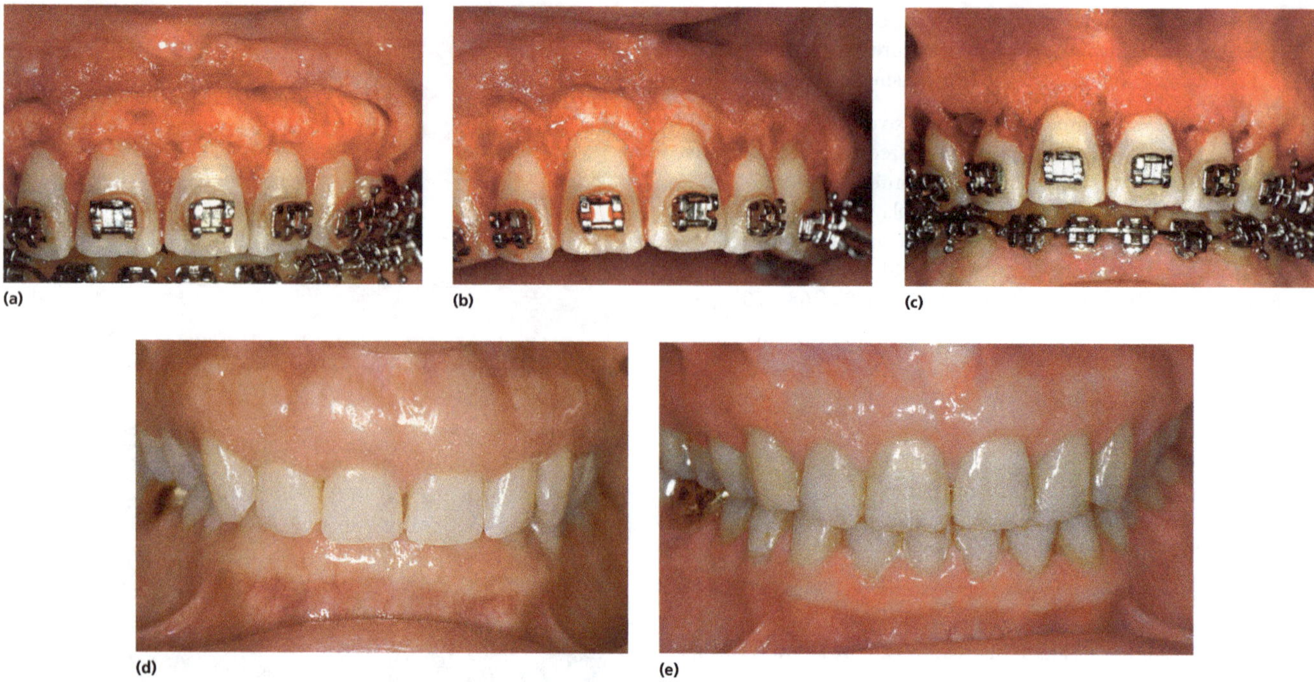

Figure 3.102 (a–c) Periodontal surgery to modify thick, fibrotic gingival tissues resulting from delayed apical migration (d) into periodontal tissue having improved architecture (e).

Q: Is Connie's deep bite a *skeletal* deep bite, a *dental* deep bite, or a combination of both?

A: A combination of both. She exhibits *skeletal deep bite features*: overclosed appearance, short soft tissue LAFH, short skeletal LAFH (LAFH/TAFH = 51%, flat MPA, and relatively parallel SN, FH, and MP lines). *Dental deep bite features* include overerupted maxillary and mandibular incisors, plus a deep COS. Connie is a combination of both moderate skeletal and dental deep bite.

Q: What is the etiology of Connie's deep bite?

A: In a skeletally short LAFH patient like Connie (Figure 3.103), the condyles grow more vertically (less posterior-superiorly) than normal, the mandible rotates forward excessively (internally, true rotation), the maxilla descends less, and/or molars erupt less than normal. A skeletal deep bite results from increased vertical overlap of the incisors as the mandible rotates upward and forward. Connie's dental deep bite resulted from supraeruption of maxillary and mandibular incisors.

Q: What are the two *general* approaches to correcting Connie's deep bite? Which would you choose?

A: The two general approaches to correct deep bites are *erupting posterior teeth* orthodontically or surgically (ideal for correcting a short soft tissue and short skeletal LAFH), and *intruding/proclining the anterior teeth* (ideal for correcting a dental deep bite with supraerupted and upright incisors). Since Connie has characteristics of both a skeletal and dental deep bite, you should consider correcting her deep bite using both approaches.

Q: In what dimensions does Connie present with apical base discrepancies?

A: AP and vertical

Q: Considering all the problems you have identified with Connie's face, jaws, and teeth, it is important to stay focused on the main, or primary, problems in each dimension (plus other). What are they?

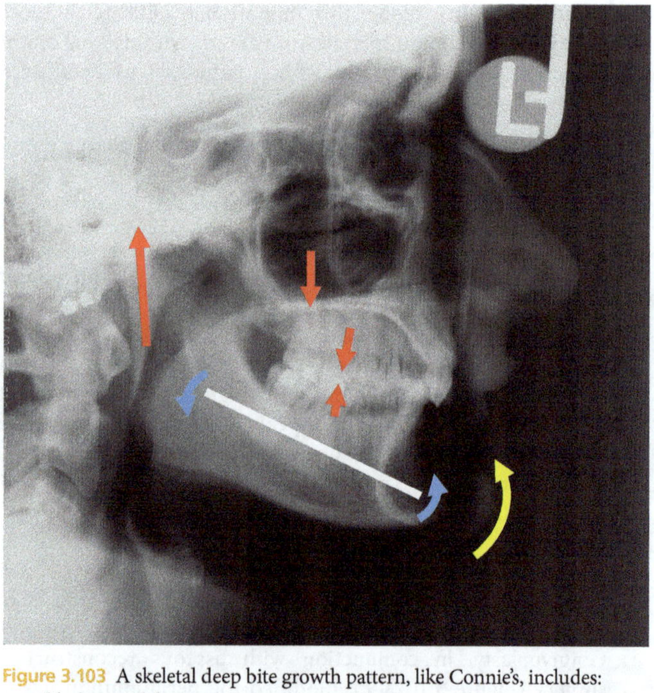

Figure 3.103 A skeletal deep bite growth pattern, like Connie's, includes: mandibular condyles growing more vertically, the maxilla descending less, the mandible rotating forward (internally, true rotation) more excessively, and/or molars erupting less than normal. As a result, the mandible rotates upward and forward increasing vertical overlap of the incisors (a skeletal deep bite).

A: See Table 3.14

Q: What are your treatment goals for Connie?

A: Facial esthetic goals: decrease facial convexity but soften chin projection, decrease labiomental sulcus depth, and increase

Table 3.14 **Primary problems list for Connie** *(apical base/skeletal discrepancies italicized).*

AP	II (5) II (5) II (5) II (5) *mandibular skeletal retrusion*
Vertical	*Skeletal* and dental deep bite
Transverse	—
Other	Severe attrition of maxillary and mandibular anterior teeth

LAFH. Dental treatment goals: correct Class II molar and canine relationship to Class I; correct deep bite to 10%; provide ideal OJ, reduce excess gingival display; and level, align, and coordinate dental arches.

Q: What are the three general ways to treat Connie's AP apical base discrepancy (Class II relationship secondary to mandibular deficiency)? Suggest specific treatments for each.

A: *Orthopedics*: Would not be considered for Connie since, as an adult, she has finished growing. From an academic perspective, the application of high-pull headgear force is capable of displacing entire maxillae posteriorly in monkeys (thereby improving Class II relationships) [173], although a similar response in humans has not been verified. Even if such posterior displacement could be achieved in humans, the stability of such orthopedic movement in adults would be questionable. The same could be true for the application of cervical headgears. Further, retracting Connie's maxilla could worsen her "dished-in" nose-to-chin profile, and would not improve her overall convex profile. Functional appliances accelerate mandibular growth in adolescents but do *not* enhance mandibular horizontal growth beyond that found in control subjects [68]. *Orthopedics should not be considered as an option for Connie.*

Masking or camouflage (correcting her dental Class II relationship without addressing the underlying skeletal discrepancy). Options include the following:

- Nonextraction interarch treatment using Class II elastics, or other Class II correctors, could achieve a Class I canine relationship through a combination of distal movement of maxillary teeth, mesial movement of mandibular teeth, and tipping of the occlusal plane. The anticipated effect of these treatments on the mandibular teeth (incisor proclination) could be tolerated as Connie has a very robust band of keratinized periodontium covering her mandibular anterior teeth, her mandibular anterior teeth currently have a good angulation (FMIA = 64°), and approximately one-half of the total AP correction (5 mm) will be made by mandibular dental movement and one-half by maxillary dental movement.
- Nonextraction treatment using HPHG, CPHG, or straight-pull headgear for purely dental movement to distalize her maxillary teeth into Class I
- Nonextraction intra-arch treatment using maxillary palatal, infrazygomatic crest, or buccal TADs to distalize the entire maxillary dental arch.
- Maxillary intra-arch noncompliance appliance treatment (e.g., using Pendulum, Distal Jet) could be used to distalize maxillary posterior teeth, but these appliances must be supported with TAD anchorage to avoid reciprocal mesial movement of anterior teeth.
- Extraction of maxillary premolars to provide space to retract her canines into a Class I position (using maxillary TADs or headgears as anchorage).

Notes: masking could improve her appearance by reducing her labiomental sulcus depth (moving her maxillary incisor edges up and back—away from pressing on her lower lip/eliminating lip trapping), but masking would not improve her overall convex profile. Further, masking could "dish in" her profile. Masking is *not* an ideal solution to correct Connie's AP relationship.

Surgery (mandibular advancement) would be the ideal treatment option since her mandible is retrusive/deficient. She has such a strong chin that if a mandibular advancement osteotomy were performed, then some form of genioplasty setback would be necessary to prevent her chin from being too prominent, post treatment.

Q: Orthopedics should not be attempted on Connie. But, will masking improve Connie's smile (address her chief complaint)? Will surgery?

A: With either masking or surgery, leveling Connie's maxillary arch should intrude her stepped down maxillary incisors—decreasing her excessive gingival display when smiling (Figure 3.94d). Of course, we need to examine her incisal display (with a relaxed lip) after her maxillary arch is leveled. In addition, post-treatment cosmetic dentistry (maxillary incisor composite or porcelain veneers) could improve her smile by addressing her worn incisors. Otherwise, correcting her anteroposterior relationship with masking would not help her smile, unless her face height increased with mandibular posterior tooth eruption (during leveling of the COS). If her maxillary incisors were erupted with masking (heavy Class II elastic wear), then her incisal display when smiling could increase. A mandibular advancement surgical procedure (with genioplasty setback) could increase her vertical dimension (improve her facial balance) if the mandible was moved downward as well as forward—but it may not improve her smile. *A final, specific, treatment plan to address her smile esthetics cannot really be made until after her maxillary arch is leveled and aligned with fixed orthodontic appliances (reduce unknowns).*

Q: Is there any evidence that Connie's profile would improve with a mandibular advancement osteotomy?

A: Yes. We found that patients initially presenting with a normally positioned maxilla plus an ANB angle equal to or greater than 6° (such as Connie) were consistently judged by laypersons to have profile improvement following mandibular advancement surgery [174]. By contrast, profiles of patients initially presenting with a normal maxilla plus ANB angle less than 6° were sometimes judged to be improved and sometimes judged not to be improved following surgery. Connie's profile should improve with a mandibular advancement, but this surgery should be performed in conjunction with a genioplasty reduction.

Q: What are the three general ways that you can treat Connie's vertical apical base discrepancy?

A: *Orthopedics* (enhance downward growth of the maxillary corpus, maxillary alveolar bone growth by erupting maxillary posterior teeth, or mandibular alveolar bone growth by erupting mandibular posterior teeth) Considerations include the following:

- The ability of cervical-pull headgears, headgears with biteplates, straight-pull headgears, activators, bionators, and Frankel regulators (FR-IIs) to produce a clinically significant increase in vertical facial proportions is equivocal in adolescents [24–33], and has not been studied in adults. Furthermore, even if a moderate vertical increase could be produced with one of these appliances, the stability of this change would be questionable.

- Leveling Connie's 3 mm COS (growing alveolar process bone by erupting premolars [23], uprighting/erupting mandibular molars) with/without anterior biteplates or posterior vertical elastics could potentially increase her LAFH, but the stability of erupting posterior teeth has been questioned, especially in adults [34].

Masking or camouflage (opening her bite dentally). Options include the following:

- Intruding Connie's stepped down maxillary incisors and stepped up mandibular incisors by banding/bonding fixed appliances and leveling her arches with archwires; banding/bonding maxillary and mandibular incisors more incisally than normally and leveling her arches; or by placing steps in her final archwires to intrude incisors additionally.
- Proclining her upright maxillary incisors, and proclining her normally inclined mandibular incisors.
- Leveling her 3 mm COS by eruption of mandibular premolars [23] and uprighting/erupting mandibular mesially tipped molars with/without anterior bite plates or posterior vertical elastics. Since alveolar process bone is grown during tooth eruption, and the LAFH can potentially increase as the mandible is rotated down and back, it could be argued that this is orthopedic treatment. The muscles of mastication play a role in determining how much her mandibular posterior teeth will erupt during COS leveling, and the stability of erupting posterior teeth has been questioned [34]. This is especially true for adult patients.
- Prosthodontic treatment (implants, crowns, or bridges) could be used to mask her skeletal deep bite by increasing the vertical facial dimension within limits dictated by the freeway space. Considering the moderate nature of Connie's vertical discrepancy and the fact that her posterior dentition is healthy, this alternative would not be reasonable.

Surgery (maxillary Le Fort I downgraft to lengthen her LAFH)—could correct Connie's overclosed appearance, but the amount of vertical LAFH increase needed is not large—so the benefits of this surgery have to be seriously weighed against the risks. If a downgraft was performed, care must be taken to not increase her LAFH to the point where an ILG occurs.

Q: Would vertical orthopedics (e.g., growing alveolar process bone by erupting posterior teeth during leveling), vertical masking (intruding/proclining incisors), or vertical surgery (maxillary downgraft osteotomy) address Connie's chief complaint and improve her smile?

A: Erupting posterior teeth (if stable) could increase her LAFH. Intruding her maxillary incisors during leveling her maxillary arch would intrude stepped down maxillary incisors/reduce gingival display during smiling (Figure 3.94d). Surgery (maxillary downgraft) would increase her LAFH, but would also increase her incisal/gingival display. Before considering a maxillary downgraft osteotomy, we need to evaluate her relaxed lip incisal display *after leveling the maxillary arch*. Note: erupting posterior teeth or maxillary downgrafting would tend to rotate her mandible down and back (worsening her Class II relationship) and increase the need for a possible mandibular advancement osteotomy.

Q: Connie does not present with a transverse discrepancy. However, if a mandibular advancement is performed, then a transverse discrepancy could result as you advance a wider part of the mandibular dental arch forward. What must you do with her models to evaluate her future transverse relationship, if she undergoes a mandibular advancement osteotomy?

A: Assuming you will treat Connie nonextraction, you must evaluate her transverse relationship as you *articulate her models with her mandibular model brought forward into a Class I canine relationship*. When her models are positioned into a Class I canine relationship, Connie's dental arches still coordinate reasonably well (transverse occlusal relationships are WRN). Furthermore, she presents with minimal posterior transverse dental compensations (correcting severe compensations worsens transverse relationships as posterior teeth are uprighted). These facts taken together, *if Connie undergoes a mandibular advancement osteotomy, you should be fine (in the transverse dimension) just leveling and aligning her arches with coordinated archwires* (no need for RME, SARME, MPMO).

Q: Should you discuss surgery with Connie? If she declines surgery, then are you willing to treat her without surgery?

A: You should discuss surgery (BSSO advancement) with Connie as her best treatment option. Should Connie (or any patient) decline your recommended treatment plan, one guiding principle is to *provide an alternative treatment plan, if it addresses the patient's chief complaint, improves function/esthetics, and is reversible (so that the option of choosing ideal treatment at a later date is not thwarted)*. In Connie's case, an alternative treatment could include leveling/aligning her arches (decreasing gingival display during smiling, possibly increasing her LAFH slightly) followed by cosmetic dentistry to address her incisal wear. You could also use an interarch Class II corrector (e.g., Class II elastics) to improve her anteroposterior dental relationship. But this option will not provide her with the best outcome.

Q: For patients presenting with mandibular anteroposterior deficiency coupled with *mild–moderate vertical deficiency and normal incisal display*, a decision may be made to advance the mandible without a maxillary downgraft osteotomy. If this is done, it may still be advantageous to maximize an increase in the LAFH as the mandible is surgically advanced. How is this done?

A: By performing a "tripod advancement." For vertically overclosed deep-bite patients, Jacobs and Sinclair [40] suggested leveling the COS *after* surgery. In this way, mandibular incisors are not intruded presurgically and, during the surgical advancement the mandibular incisors ride down the lingual surfaces of the maxillary incisors—lengthening the LAFH. As this is done, a bilateral posterior open bite is created. This open bite approximates the increase in the LAFH gained when the posterior open bite is closed postsurgically by vertical eruption of the mandibular posterior teeth. Because the COS is not leveled completely presurgically, at surgery the advanced dentition contacts only the anterior teeth and the most posterior tooth of each side—hence, the name "tripod advancement."

Q: Are there any unknowns that you can/should eliminate before defining a final treatment plan for Connie?

A: Yes: a possible undetected CR–CO shift, cooperation, hygiene, and maxillary incisal display after leveling/aligning the maxillary arch. *Always* examine each patient for a CR–CO shift at the case presentation before beginning treatment, and at every appointment thereafter. That said, there are no unknowns that should prevent you from starting Connie's treatment now, but a final treatment plan maximizing smile esthetics should not be established until after the maxillary arch is leveled and aligned.

Q: Should you treat Connie nonextraction? Should you extract anterior or posterior teeth?

A: Because the mandibular incisors have a good angulation (FMIA = 66°), with little anterior crowding, there is no need to extract mandibular premolars, if a mandibular advancement option is chosen—unless you wish to advance Connie's mandible more than 5 mm (the amount she is currently Class II at the canines). For the same reasons (good incisor angulation, little crowding), you would not extract mandibular premolars or a mandibular incisor, if a *nonsurgical option* is chosen. Even if you decided to treat her (nonsurgically) with maxillary first premolar extractions (masking), nonextraction mandibular treatment would still be prudent.

Q: Putting everything together, what treatment plan would you recommend?

A: Although a nonsurgical AP masking (headgear, TADs, extraction of maxillary first premolars, Class II interarch mechanics) option was presented to Connie as a compromised alternative, the resulting esthetic outcome was not recommended. Instead, Connie chose an orthodontic/surgical option. The final, nonextraction plan consisted of composite restoration of mandibular incisors to facilitate bracket bonding, placement of fixed orthodontic appliances, and alignment of both arches. Her maxillary arch would be leveled. Her COS would *not* be leveled in order to avoid intruding the mandibular incisors. Surgery would consist of a mandibular tripod advancement to maximize LAFH, and a genioplasty to reduce her chin projection.

Hoffman and Moloney suggest that posterior positioning of the chin is a reliable procedure to soften chin projection after mandibular advancement, particularly in Class II division 2 malocclusions [175]. Additionally, the anterior mandibular height (bony chin height) is a dimension whose contribution to the vertical dimension is often ignored [120]. A sliding setback genioplasty would soften Connie's chin projection but increase her LAFH minimally. An anteriorly tapered wedge genioplasty, while decreasing her chin projection, would likewise not increase her LAFH. Instead, a genioplasty setback/downgraft was planned which would both decrease her chin projection and increase her LAFH. Following surgery, the mandibular COS would be leveled by eruption of premolars and first molars using vertical elastics. The posterior open bite resulting from a tripod advancement would alleviate the need to overcome heavy posterior bite forces typical of a deep bite patient during COS leveling [176].

Q: What are the specific objectives of treatment for the maxilla, mandible, maxillary dentition, and mandibular dentition in all three planes of space?

A: Specific objectives of treatment for Connie are as follows:

Maxilla
- AP: Maintain.
- Vertical: Maintain.
- Transverse: Maintain.

Mandible
- AP: Lengthen mandibular body and set back symphysis.
- Vertical: Increase skeletal lower anterior facial height.
- Transverse: Maintain.

Maxillary dentition
- AP: Maintain molars and canines. Procline incisors.
- Vertical: Maintain molars and canines. Intrude incisors.
- Intermolar width: Maintain.

Mandibular dentition
- AP: Maintain molars. Minimize proclination of incisors.
- Vertical: Erupt molars, level COS post-surgically. Maintain incisors.
- Intermolar/intercanine width: Maintain intermolar and intercanine widths.

Q: How did Connie's treatment proceed?

A: The maxillary dentition was banded and bonded with edgewise appliances. The lower central incisors were restored, and the lower arch was banded and bonded—first molar to first molar. Arches were aligned and coordinated (Figure 3.104d–h). Iowa spaces were placed between the maxillary canines and lateral incisors. Resting incisor to maxillary lip position was appropriately judged *after* the upper arch was leveled and found to be approximately 2–3 mm (Figure 3.104a)—which was judged to be ideal (maxillary downgraft osteotomy not required). The COS was not leveled, and presurgical casts were mounted on an articulator to confirm the surgical movements presurgically (tripod advancement, Figure 3.104i). Surgery was performed 1 year after treatment was initiated. In addition to a mandibular advancement, a decision was made in the operating room to perform a genioplasty downgraft only (not setback, Figure 3.104j). After surgery, guiding elastics were used by the patient for 1 week.

Q: Theoretically, how much additional LAFH does a tripod mandibular advancement provide compared to a mandibular advancement where the COS is leveled before surgery?

A: Theoretically, the additional LAFH ranges up to 2.8 mm, the amount the mandibular incisors are not intruded (minus the amount molars are not erupted) by arch leveling [22]. Look at Connie's mounted presurgical models (Figure 3.104i). Because the COS was not leveled before surgery, her mandibular incisors remain stepped up. As her mandibular model was articulated forward into a Class I canine relationship, a bilateral posterior open bite remained because the posterior teeth were not erupted and the anterior teeth were not intruded with COS leveling. The *additional increase in LAFH achieved with tripod advancement equals the amount the mandibular incisor edges would have been intruded (minus the amount molars are erupted), if the COS had been leveled, presurgically.*

Q: What steps should the orthodontist take to increase the likelihood of Connie's surgical success?

A: Steps to follow that will increase the likelihood of surgical success:

- Confirm that the surgical movement is within the limits of the surgical envelope (see Appendix, Table A.4). Connie's anticipated mandibular advancement (~5 mm) was well within the 14–15 mm mandibular advancement limit for a low MPA patient
- Approve the articulated surgical occlusion (Figure 3.104i). This was done.
- Discuss with the surgeon the anticipated surgical movement(s). This was done.
- Be contacted by the surgeon immediately after surgery to discuss how the surgery went. This was done.
- See Connie one week postoperatively. This was done. At that appointment, an absence of occlusal discrepancies plus a

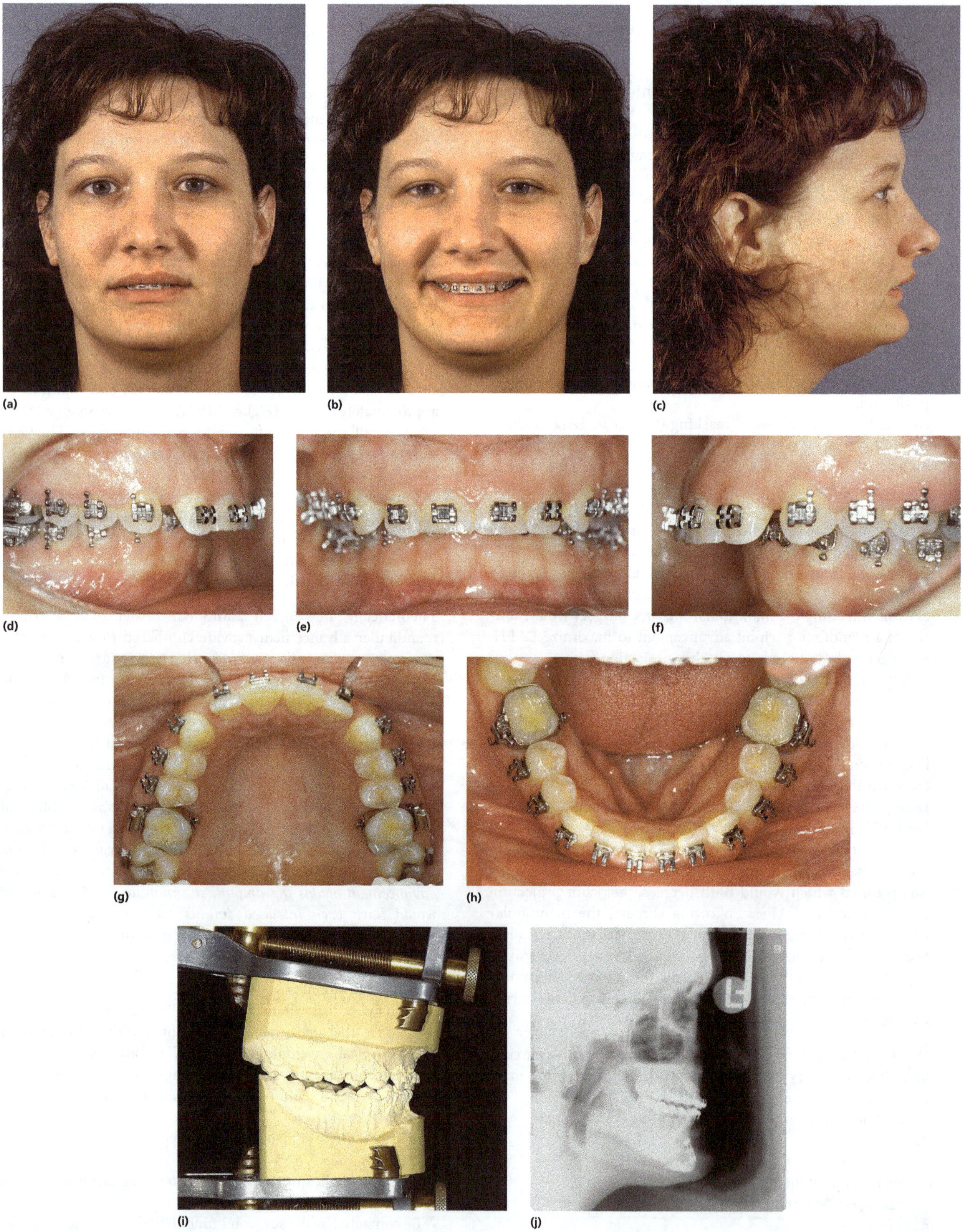

Figure 3.104 (a–i) Presurgical records and (j) postsurgical lateral cephalometric radiograph of Connie. Note that her articulated models (i) are positioned with canines Class I and contacting only at three points (anterior teeth and the most posterior tooth of each side, “tripod advancement”) and that this relationship is reflected in her immediate postsurgical radiograph (j).

repeatable bite was noted; and proper postsurgery guiding elastics wear was confirmed.

Q: What is the purpose of guiding elastics after orthognathic surgery?

A: To train the patient (the patient's muscles) to close into the new occlusion—not to move teeth. With surgery, muscles may change length or direction of pull, proprioceptive sense may be altered, and edema may be present. Guiding (usually vertical) elastics help the patient to close into the new occlusion. There is no specific length of time that they must be worn. They are worn until the patient is trained.

Q: Postsurgically, leveling of Connie's COS was initiated by adding bonded attachments to the mandibular second molars, wearing bilateral triangle elastics at the canines, and wearing box elastics posteriorly. Final orthodontic detailing proceeded; she was debanded 10 months post surgery and placed in temporary (clear, vacuum-formed) retainers. Shortly thereafter, Connie presented to our clinic carrying radiographs of her maxillary anterior teeth (Figure 3.105). She stated that she had been in a car accident two days earlier, her face had hit the steering wheel, and she had been taken to the emergency room where she was examined, observed, and released. She stated that her bite was "off," but the examining oral surgeon said this was dental (not a jaw fracture). Her maxillary incisors were palatally luxated but not avulsed. What should you do?

A: An attempt should have been made in the emergency room to gently reposition her anterior teeth back into their original location. After which, the teeth should have been stabilized for four weeks using a flexible splint, and the pulpal condition monitored. If the pulp became necrotic, root canal treatment would be indicated to prevent root resorption. In immature, developing teeth, revascularization can be confirmed radiographically by evidence of continued root formation and possibly by positive sensibility testing. In fully formed teeth, a continued lack of response to sensibility testing indicates pulp necrosis, along with periapical rarefacation and sometimes crown discoloration [177]. How do you proceed with Connie, now? Document everything she has told you regarding the trauma she suffered during the accident. Confirm lack of closed head trauma symptoms (headache, dizziness, nausea, slurred speech, visual disturbances, vomiting) and perform a complete head and neck examination. After doing this, you find that the only apparent problem is a slight misalignment of the maxillary incisors. Connie was asked if she could fit her maxillary clear retainer—which she was able to do with mild discomfort. She was asked to wear the retainer full time, to re-align the maxillary anterior teeth.

Q: Months later, composite veneers were completed on Connie's anterior teeth. Maxillary and mandibular Hawley retainers were delivered with instructions for initial full-time wear and then long-term nighttime wear. Final records are shown in Figure 3.106. What changes do you note compared to her initial records?

A: Changes noted include the following:

- Facial esthetics dramatically improved (a heightened sense of self-esteem is now projected by Connie).
- Smile esthetics were enhanced through a reduction in gingival display and the attainment of a balanced smile arc. Since her maxillary incisors were not intruded appreciably (Figure 3.106f), this reduction in smiling gingival display could be due either to her maxillary lip descending as her LAFH increased (Figure 3.106f) and/or to a diminution in activity of her smiling musculature (maybe her smile in Figure 3.94d was an unposed smile, and her smile in Figure 3.106b was a posed smile).
- Anteroposterior apical base discrepancy was reduced as the mandible was advanced. The ANB angle decreased from 6° to 1°.
- Skeletal LAFH was increased from 51 to 55% as a result of the mandibular incisors advancing downward and forward along the lingual surfaces of the maxillary incisors with the BSSO tripod advancement (Figure 3.106f) and the genioplasty downgraft.
- Labiomental sulcus was reduced and projection of the soft tissue pogonion was softened.
- Maxillary incisors were proclined and maxillary molars erupted slightly.
- Mandibular molars were erupted and incisors were proclined minimally.
- A well-interdigitated Class I molar and canine relationship was achieved.
- Final overjet was minimal.
- Final overbite was approximately 30%.
- Composite veneer buildups enhanced the patient's smile esthetics and were an integral part of the treatment plan.
- Maxillary midline was on with Connie's facial midline; mandibular midline was approximately 1 mm to the left of Connie's face.
- Canine guidance was established bilaterally during lateral excursive movements.
- Post-treatment panoramic radiograph demonstrated blunting of the maxillary central incisor roots with minimal change in root length.

Q: Was a tripod advancement the appropriate procedure to use in this patient? Would a maxillary downgraft, in conjunction with the mandibular advancement, resulted in a more favorable result?

A: A tripod advancement was the appropriate procedure. Vertically, Connie was only moderately deficient. Resting incisor to maxillary lip position was appropriately judged *after* the upper arch was leveled and found to be approximately 2–3 mm, ideal (Figure 3.104a). Further, this display would increase with cosmetic treatment of her worn incisal edges. These facts, coupled with hyperactivity of her smile musculature, led to a decision to increase Connie's lower anterior facial height only slightly with a tripod advancement and avoid a maxillary Le Fort I downgraft osteotomy.

Q: How much did the mandibular tripod advancement actually increase Connie's LAFH?

A: This is hard to quantify since her genioplasty downgraft added to her increased LAFH. But even the one or two millimeters of additional facial height estimated to be gained with a tripod advancement can help improve LAFH in a vertically deficient patient.

Q: How much did the genioplasty procedure aid in her esthetic outcome?

A: The genioplasty had a very significant impact on Connie's esthetic outcome. This is not surprising since Wessberg et al.

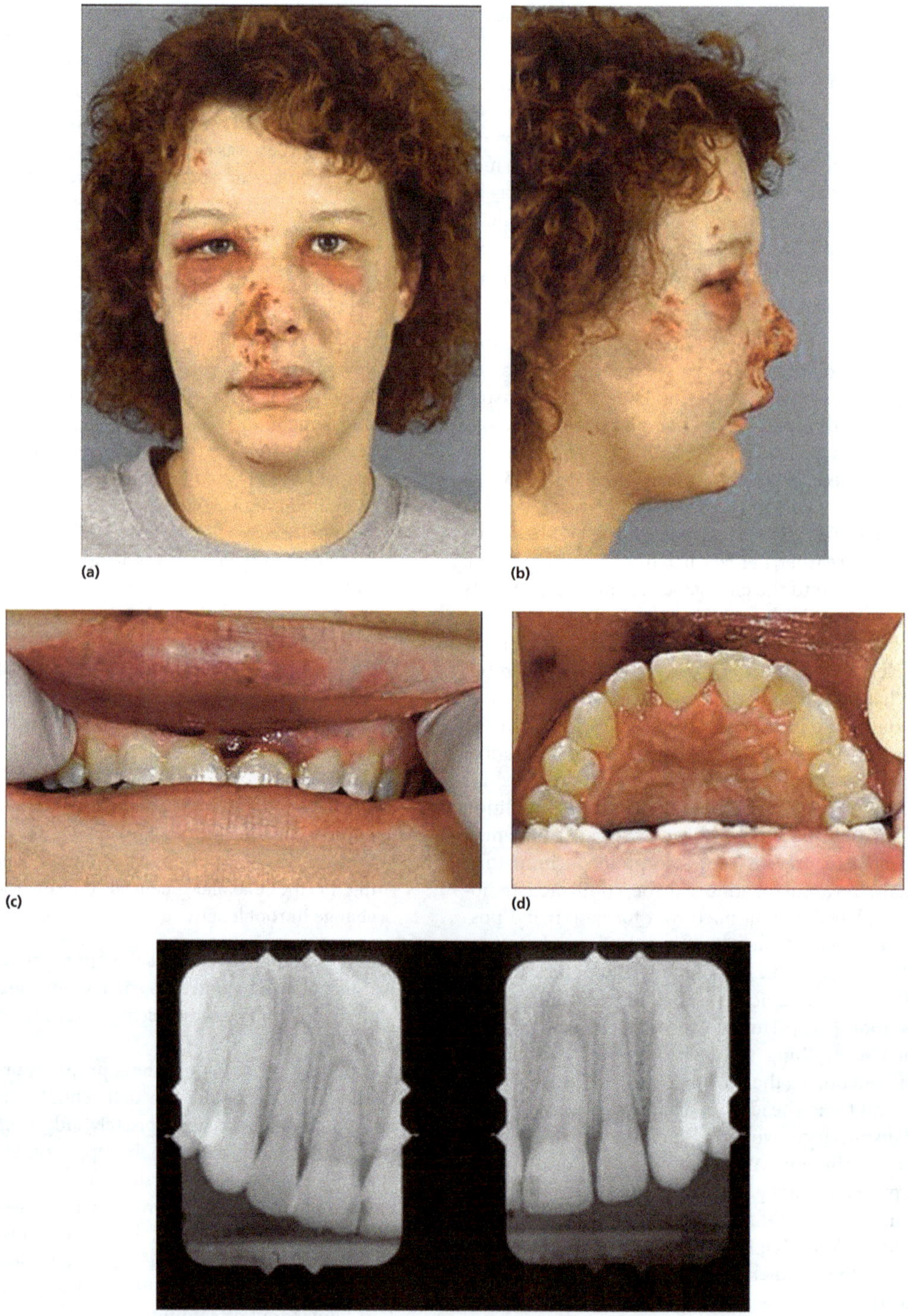

Figure 3.105 (a–e) Posttrauma records of Connie two days after her accident. She had been debanded shortly before.

noted that in the short face patient, the deformity is often located in the anterior mandible [178]. Comparing Figure 3.106c to Figure 3.94c, it is apparent that Connie still has a strong chin, post treatment. However, her profile esthetics are dramatically improved. Why? Her chin was moved down 5 mm (Figure 3.106f, mandibular superimposition), which opened up her labiomental sulcus and increased her LAFH. Should Connie's bony chin have been set back as well as brought down (as originally planned)? Perhaps, but Connie still had an excellent outcome. The total increase in her facial height with mandibular tripod advancement and genioplasty downgraft was approximately 13 mm. Overall, the vertical change was substantial and had a dramatic positive esthetic impact.

Q: How was Connie's deep bite corrected?

A: By slight eruption of her maxillary molars, eruption of her mandibular molars, proclination of her maxillary incisors, slight proclination of her mandibular incisors, and downward/forward surgical movement of her mandible (Figure 3.106f).

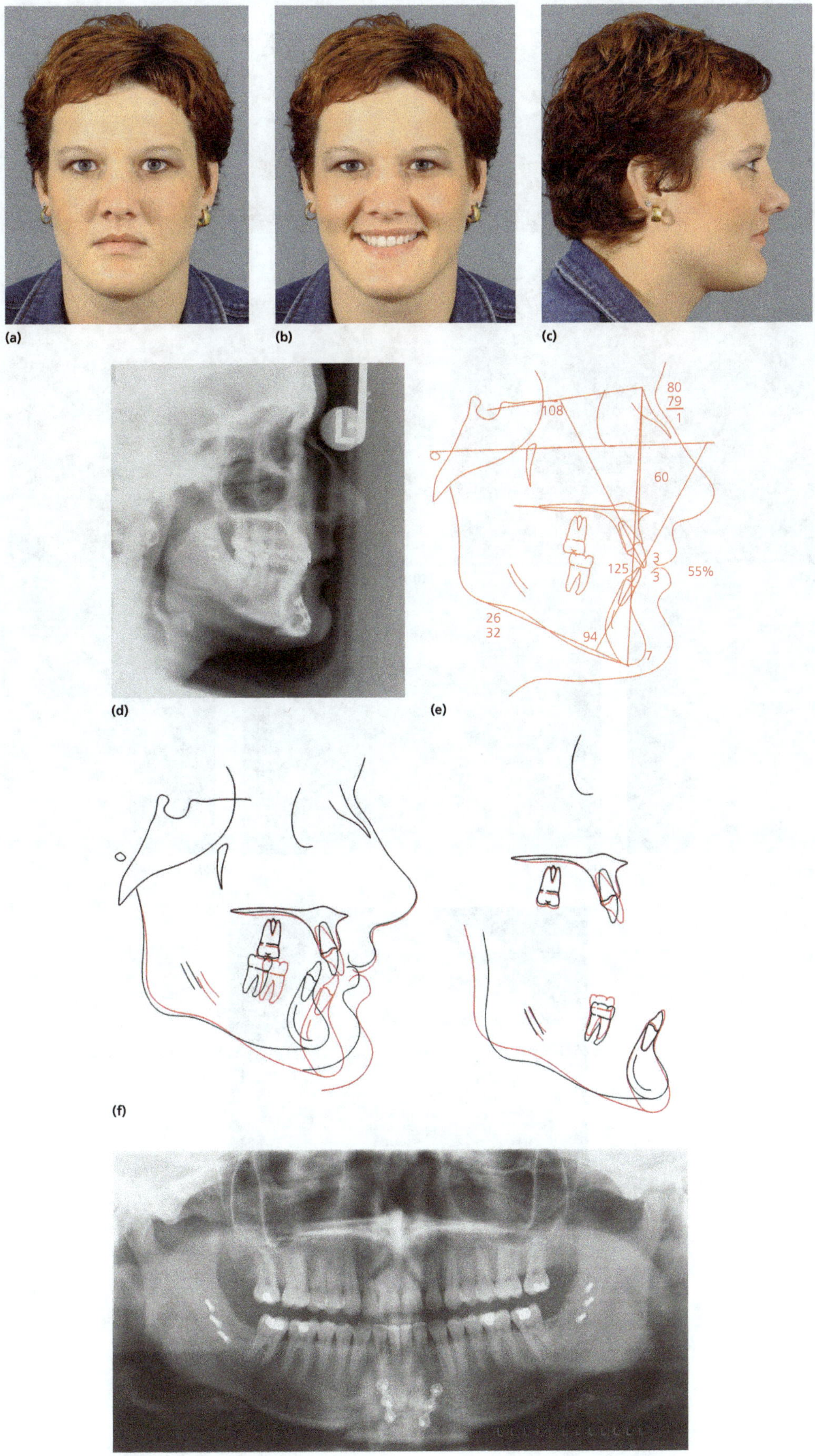

Figure 3.106 (a–p) Final records of Connie. (Low LE, Moore TE, Austin KE, Burton RG, Marshall SD, Southard KE, et al. Mandibular “tripod” advancement of a Class II Division 2 deepbite malocclusion. Am J Orthod Dentofacial Orthop. 2010;137: 285–292. Reproduced with permission from Elsevier).

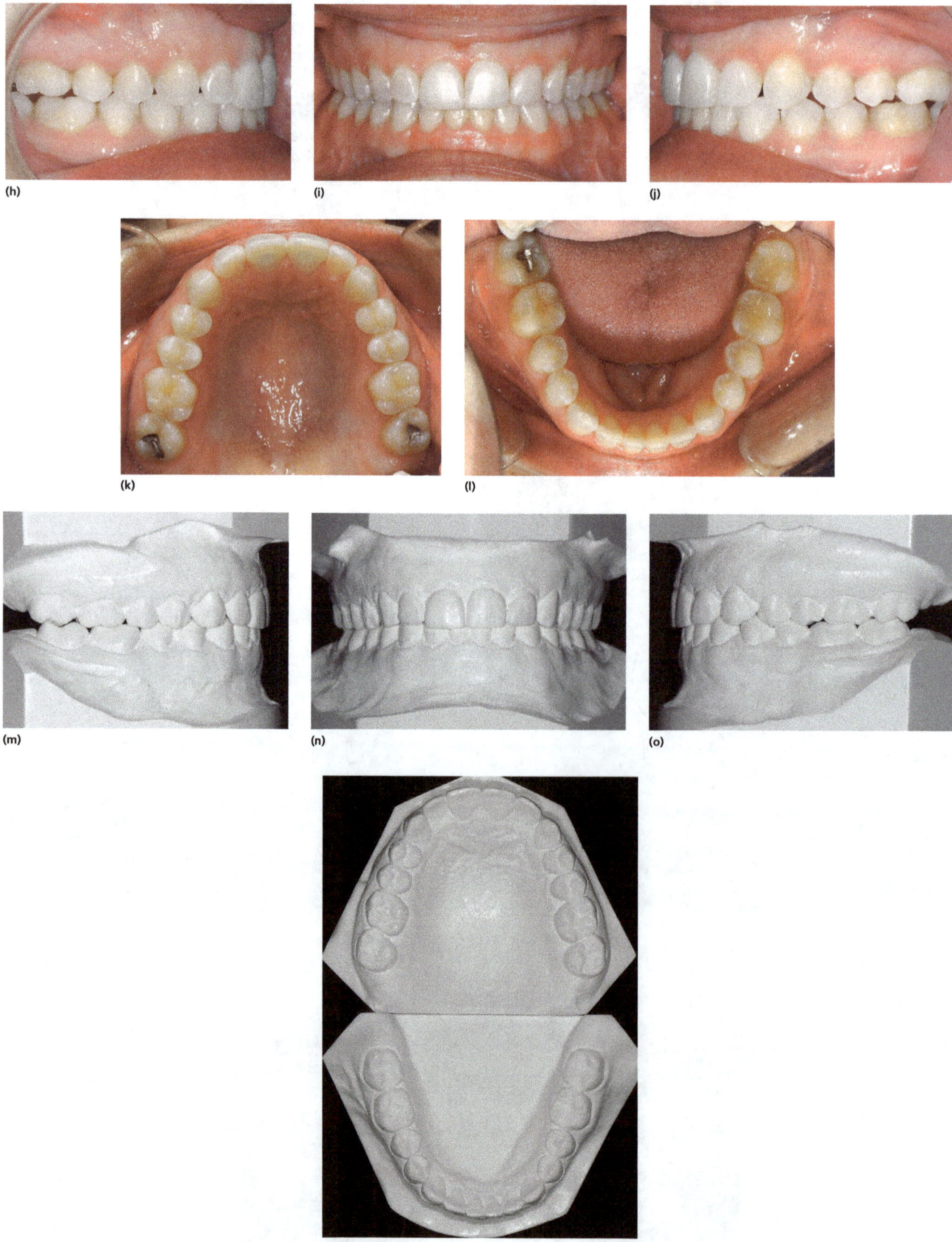

Figure 3.106 (Continued)

Q: Were your treatment goals achieved?

A: Yes. A clear improvement was seen in Connie's facial esthetics: decreased facial convexity, decreased labiomental sulcus depth, and increased LAFH. Her Class II molar/canine relationship and deep bite were corrected. Her chief complaint (concerns about her smile esthetics) was addressed.

Q: What "take-home" messages can you draw from the care of this patient?

A: Take-home messages include the following:

- Connie presented as a Class II division 2 malocclusion secondary to mandibular skeletal AP hypoplasia. Her 100% OB was a combination skeletal deep bite and dental deep bite. The etiology of her skeletal deep bite (overclosed appearance, short soft tissue LAFH, short skeletal LAFH) was a combination of more vertical condylar growth than normal, more excessive mandibular internal (true) forward rotation than normal, decreased maxillary descent, and/or less molar eruption than normal. This growth pattern resulted in increased incisor vertical overlap (deep bite) as the mandible rotated upward and forward. The etiology of her dental deep bite was over-eruption of maxillary and mandibular incisors. Connie was treated nonextraction with fixed orthodontic appliances, a mandibular tripod advancement, a downgraft genioplasty, and composite veneers.
- Every orthodontic patient should be screened for TMJ problems. If the patient presents with TMD, then these problems should be addressed, generally before orthodontic treatment is begun.
- The impact of facial attractiveness on success in all areas of life cannot be overstated [179], and orthodontists stand at the vanguard of dental teams seeking to enhance facial attractiveness.
- Improvement in this adult Class II skeletal deep bite patient occurred in much the same way as improvement in adolescent Class II skeletal deep bite patients—by significant mandibular lengthening (jaw growth in adolescents and surgical advancement in Connie). Of course, the esthetic impact of her downgraft genioplasty was significant.
- Tripod advancements can result in mild LAFH lengthening in mild-to-moderate skeletal deep bite patients needing mandibular advancement surgery (with adequate maxillary incisal display). A tripod advancement can sometimes obviate the need for a Le Fort I downgraft osteotomy.
- Some form of chin reduction should be considered when advancing a mandible with an initially prominent chin and overly effective bony pogonion. Connie underwent a genioplasty downgraft to increase her LAFH. Should a genioplasty setback have been performed as well as a downgraft? Looking at her final profile (Figure 3.106c), additional reduction in her chin projection may have been beneficial.
- In patients who will undergo surgery to move the anterior maxilla down (or up), you should evaluate maxillary incisal display *after leveling the maxillary arch, with the jaws slightly separated, and with the maxillary lip relaxed (nonsmiling)*. In Connie, following leveling of the maxillary arch (Figure 3.104a), it was clear that a maxillary downgraft was not needed.
- In mandibular advancement surgery patients, the orthodontist must decide whether to treat the mandibular arch with or without extractions. In large measure, this decision is based on the amount of advancement desired to maximize profile esthetics. (Mandibular anterior crowding and mandibular incisor proclination also influence this extraction decision.) If the amount of advancement needed approximately equals the initial amount that the mandibular canines are Class II, then a nonextraction approach to treatment should be entertained. If more advancement is needed than this, then premolars could be extracted, the canines retracted, and the surgeon forced to advance the mandible even more. In Connie's case, the decision to treat her mandibular arch nonextraction was prudent and resulted in a well-balanced facial profile (Figure 3.106c).
- She must wear her Hawley retainers (maxillary Hawley retainer incorporating an anterior biteplate to disclude her posterior teeth slightly) every night, for a lifetime.
- Connie's final OB was approximately 30% (Figure 3.106i). Connie's OB should have been reduced to 10% (even after placement of composite veneers). Despite excellent Hawley retainer wear, some vertical relapse (deepening of the bite) should be anticipated.

References

1 Burstone, C. Lip posture and its significance in treatment planning. *Am J Orthod* 1967;53:282–84.

2 Frush JP, Fisher RD. The dysesthetic interpretation of the dentogenic concept. *J Prothet Dent* 1958;8:558–81.

3 Desai S, Upadhyay M, Nanda R. Dynamic smile analysis: changes with age. *Am J Orthod Dentofacial Orthop* 2009;136:310.e1–10; discussion 310–1.

4 Tjan AH, Miller GD, The JG. Some esthetic factors in a smile. *J Prosthet Dent* 1984;51:24–8.

5 Mackley RJ. An evaluation of smiles before and after orthodontic treatment. *Angle Orthod* 1993;63:183–89; discussion 190.

6 International Headache Society. *The international classification of headache disorders*. 2nd ed. Oxford (UK): Blackwell;2004. p.160

7 Bartleson JD, Cutrer FM. Migraine update. Diagnosis and treatment. *Minn Med* 2010;93:36–41.

8 Dodick DW, Gargus JJ. Why migraines strike. *Sci Am* 2008;299:56–63.

9 American Academy of Orofacial Pain. *Temporomandibular disorders: guidelines for classification, assessment, and management*. O'Neill C, editor. Chicago (IL): Quintessence, 1993. p.141.

10 Turk DC, Rudy TE. The robustness of an empirically derived taxonomy of chronic pain patients. *Pain* 1990;43:27–35.

11 Bush FM. Malocclusion, masticatory muscle and temporomandibular joint tenderness. *J Dent Res* 1985;64:129–33.

12 De Laat A, van Steenberghe D, Lesaffre E. Occlusal relationships and TMJ dysfunction. Part II. Correlation between occlusal and articular parameters and symptoms of TMJ dysfunction by means of stepwise logistic regression. *J Prosthet Dent*. 1986;55:116–21.

13 Droukas G, Lindee C, Carlsson GE. Occlusion and mandibular dysfunction: a clinical study of patients referred for functional disturbances of the masticatory system. *J Prosthet Dent* 1985;53:402–06.

14 Duinkerke AS, Luteijn F, Bouman TK, de Jong HP. Relations between TMJ pain dysfunction syndrome (PDS) and some psychologic and biographic variables. *Community Dent Oral Epidemiol* 1985;13:185–59.

15 Schudy FF. The rotation of the mandible resulting from growth: its implications in orthodontic treatment. *Angle Orthod* 1965;35:36–50.

16 Schudy FF. The control of vertical overbite in clinical orthodontics. *Angle Orthod* 1968;38:19–39.

17 Bjork A, Skieller V. Facial development and tooth eruption. An implant study at the age of puberty. *Am J Orthod*. 1972;62:339–83.

18 Nemeth RB, Isaacson RJ. Vertical anterior relapse. *Am J Orthod* 1974;65:565–85.

19 Bjork A, Skieller V. Normal and abnormal growth of the mandible. A synthesis of longitudinal cephalometric implant studies over a period of 25 years. *Eur J Orthod*. 1983;5:1–46.

20 Bjork A, Skieller V. Contrasting mandibular growth and facial development in the long face syndrome, juvenile rheumatoid arthritis and mandibulofacial dysostosis. *J Craniofac Genet Dev Biol Suppl* 1985;1:127–38.

21 Proffit WR. Later stages of development. In: Proffit WR, Fields HW, Sarver DM, editors. *Contemporary orthodontics*. 4th ed. St. Louis: Mosby; 2007. pp. 107–29.

22 Ng J, Major PW, Heo G, Flores-Mir C. True incisor intrusion attained during orthodontic treatment: a systematic review and meta-analysis. *Am J Orthod Dentofacial Orthop* 2005;128:212–19.

23 Bernstein RL, Preston CB, Lampasso J. Leveling the curve of Spee with a continuous archwire technique: a long term cephalometric study. *Am J Orthod Dentofacial Orthop* 2007;131:363–71.

24 Baumrind S, Korn EL, Isaacson RJ, West EE, Molthen R. Quantitative analysis of the orthodontic and orthopedic effects of maxillary traction. *Am J Orthod* 1983;84:384–98.

25 Kirjavainen M, Kirjavainen T, Hurmerinta K, Haavikko K. Orthopedic cervical headgear with an expanded inner bow in Class II correction. *Angle Orthod* 2000;70:317–25.

26 Melsen B. Effects of cervical anchorage during and after treatment: an implant study. *Am J Orthod* 1978;73:526–40.

27 Jakobsson SO. Cephalometric evaluation of treatment effect on Class II, Division 1 malocclusions. *Am J Orthod* 1967;53:446–57.

28 Ghafari J, Shofer FS, Jacobsson-Hunt U, Markowitz DL, Laster LL. Headgear versus function regulator in the early treatment of Class II, division 1 malocclusion: a randomized clinical trial. *Am J Orthod Dentofacial Orthop* 1998;113:51–61.

29 Keeling SD, Wheeler TT, King GJ, Garvan CW, Cohen DA, Cabassa S, et al. Anteroposterior skeletal and dental changes after early Class II treatment with bionators and headgear. *Am J Orthod Dentofacial Orthop* 1998;113:40–50.

30 Wheeler TT, McGorray SP, Dolce C, Taylor MG, King GJ. Effectiveness of early treatment of Class II malocclusion. *Am J Orthod Dentofacial Orthop* 2002;121:9–17.

31 Dolce C, McGorray SP, Brazeau L, King GJ, Wheeler TT. Timing of Class II treatment: skeletal changes comparing 1-phase and 2-phase treatment. *Am J Orthod Dentofacial Orthop* 2007;132:481–89.

32 Southard TE, Marshall SD, Allareddy V, Moreno Uribe LM, Holton NE. An evidence-based comparison of headgear and functional appliance therapy for the correction of Class II malocclusions. *Semin Orthod* 2013;19:174–95.

33 Almeida-Pedrin RR, Almeida MR, Almeida RR, Pinzan A, Ferreira FP. Treatment effects of headgear biteplane and bionator appliances. *Am J Orthod Dentofacial Orthop* 2007;132:191–98.

34 Nanda R, Burzin, J, Kim J. Factors influencing the stability of orthodontically treated dentitions. In: Hosl E, Baldauf A, editors. *Retention and long-term stability*. Heidelberg (Germany): Huthig Verlag Gmbh;1993. pp. 41–6.

35 Huxley HE. The mechanism of muscular contraction. *Science* 1969;164:1356–66.

36 Johnson A, Wildgoose DG, Wood DJ. The determination of freeway space using two different methods. *J Oral Rehabil* 2002;29:1010–13.

37 Peterson TM, Rugh JD, McIver JE. Mandibular rest position in subjects with high and low mandibular plane angles. *Am J Orthod* 1983;83:318–20.

38 Fayz F, Eslami A. Determination of occlusal vertical dimension: a literature review. *J Prosthet Dent* 1988;59:321–23.

39 Marshall WA, Tanner JM. Puberty. In: Falkner F, Tanner J, editors. *Human growth: a comprehensive treatise*. 2nd ed. New York: Plenum Press; 1986. pp. 171–209.

40 Jacobs JD, Sinclair PM. Principles of orthodontic mechanics in orthognathic surgery cases. *Am J Orthod* 1983;84:399–407.

41 Onizawa K, Schmelzeisen R, Vogt S. Alteration of temporomandibular joint symptoms after orthognathic surgery: comparison with healthy volunteers. *J Oral Maxillofac Surg* 1995;53:117–21; discussion 122–23.

42 Panula K, Somppi M, Finne K, Oikarinen K. Effects of orthognathic surgery on temporomandibular joint dysfunction: a controlled prospective 4-year follow-up study. *Int J Oral Maxillofac Surg* 2000;29:183–87.

43 Dervis E, Tuncer E. Long-term evaluations of temporomandibular disorders in patients undergoing orthognathic surgery compared with a control group. *Oral Surg Oral Med Oral Pathol Oral Radiol Endod* 2002;94:554–60.

44 Wolford, LM. Idiopathic condylar resorption of the temporomandibular joint in teenage girls (cheerleaders syndrome). *Proc (Bayl Univ Med Cent)* 2001;14:246–52.

45 Fonseca, RJ. *Oral and maxillofacial surgery: temporomandibular disorders*. Dallas, TX: 1st ed. Vol. 4. Elsevier Health Sciences; 2000. p.426.

46 Bouwman JP, Kerstens HC, Tuinzing DB. Condylar resorption in orthognathic surgery: the role of intermaxillary fixation. *Oral Surg Oral Med Oral Pathol* 1994;78:138–41.

47 De Clercq CA, Neyt LF, Mommaerts MY, Abeloos JV, De Mot BM. Condylar resorption in orthognathic surgery: a retrospective study. *Int J Adult Orthodon Orthognath Surg*. 1994;9:233–40.

48 Simmons KE, Turvey TA, Phillips C, Proffit WR. Surgical-orthodontic correction of mandibular deficiency: five-year follow-up. *Int J Adult Orthodon Orthognath Surg* 1992:7:67–79.

49 Proffit WR, Bailey LJ, Phillips C, Turvey TA. Long-term stability of surgical openbite correction by Le Fort I osteotomy. *Angle Orthod* 2000;70:112–17.

50 Grammer FC, Meyer MW, Richter KJ. A radioisotope study of the vascular response to sagittal split osteotomy of the mandibular ramus. *J Oral Surg* 1974;32:578–82.

51 Binda SA, Kuiipers-Jagtman AM, Maertens JK, van t' Hof MA. A long-term cephalometric evaluation of treated Class II division 2 malocclusions. *Eur J Orthod* 1994;16:301–08.

52 Devreese H, De Pauw G, Van Maele G, Kuiipers-Jagtman AM, Dermaut L. Stability of upper incisor inclination changes in Class II division 2 patients. *Eur J Orthod* 2007;29:314–20.

53 Praeter J, Dermaut L, Martens G, Kuijpers-Jagtman AM. Long-term stability of the leveling of the curve of spee. *Am J Orthod Dentofacial Orthop* 2002; 121:266–72.

54 Schütz-Fransson U, Bjerklin K, Lindsten R. Long-term follow-up of orthodontically treated deep bite patients. *Eur J Orthod* 2006;28:503–12.

55 Kim TW, Little RM. Postretention assessment of deep overbite correction in Class II Division 2 malocclusion. *Angle Orthod* 1999;69:175–86.

56 Huang GJ, Bates SB, Ehlert AA, Whiting DP, Chen SS, Bollen AM. Stability of deepbite correction: a systematic review. *J World Fed Orthod* 2012;1:e89–e96.

57 Varlik SK, Alpakan OO, Turkoz C. Deepbite correction with incisor intrusion in adults: a long-term cephalometric study. *Am J Orthod Dentofacial Orthop* 2013;144:414–19.

58 Hedemark A, Freihofer HP Jr. The behaviour of the maxilla in vertical movements after Le Fort l osteotomy. *J Maxillofac Surg* 1978;6:244–49.

59 Baker DL, Stoelinga PJ, Blijdorp PA, Brouns JJ. Long-term stability after inferior maxillary repositioning by miniplate fixation. *Int J Oral Maxillofac Surg* 1992;21:320–26.

60 Quejada JG, Bell WH, Kawamura H, Zhang X. Skeletal stability after inferior maxillary repositioning. *Int J Adult Orthodon Orthognath Surg* 1987;2:67–74.

61 Bell WH, Schneideman GB. Correction of vertical maxillary deficiency: stability and soft tissue changes. *J Oral Surg* 1981;39:666–70.

62 Persson G, Hellem S, Nord PG. Bone-plates for stabilizing Le Fort I osteotomies. *J Maxillofac Surg* 1986;14:69–73.

63 Wolford LM, Hilliard FW. The surgical-orthodontic correction of vertical dentofacial deformities. *J Oral Surg* 1981;39:883–97.

64 West R. Relapse and long-term stability of orthognathic surgery: a site specific analysis. In: Hosl E, Baldauf A, editors. *Retention and long-term stability*. Heidelberg: Huthig Buch Verlag Gmbh 1993;173–186.

65 Perez MM, Sameshima GT, Sinclair PM. The long-term stability of Le Fort I maxillary downgrafts with rigid fixation to correct vertical maxillary deficiency. *Am J Orthod Dentofacial Orthop* 1997;112:104–08.

66 Proffit WR, Turvey TA, Phillips C. Orthognathic surgery: a hierarchy of stability. *Int J Adult Orthodon Orthognath Surg* 1996;11:191–204.

67 Firouz M, Zernik J, Nanda R. Dental and orthopedic effects of high-pull headgear in treatment of Class II, division 1 malocclusion. *Am J Orthod Dentofacial Orthop* 1992;102:197–205.

68 Huang G, English J, Ferguson D, Kulbersh R, Osterle L, Nah H-D, et al. Ask Us—Functional appliances and long-term effects on mandibular growth. *Am J Orthod Dentofacial Orthop* 2005;128:271–72.

69 Ghosh J, Nanda RS. Evaluation of an intraoral maxillary molar distalization technique. *Am J Orthod Dentofacial Orthop* 1999;110:639–46.

70 Chaques-Asensi J, Kalra V. Effects of the pendulum appliance on the dentofacial complex. *J Clin Orthod* 2001;35:254–57.

71 Brickman CD, Sinha PK, Nanda, RS. Evaluation of the Jones jig appliance for distal molar movement. *Am J Orthod Dentofacial Orthop* 2000;118:526–34.

72 Tulloch JF, Phillips C, Koch G, Proffit WR. The effect of early intervention on skeletal pattern in Class II malocclusion: a randomized clinical trial. *Am J Orthod Dentofacial Orthop* 1997;111:391–400.

73 Tulloch JF, Proffit WR, Phillips C. Outcomes in a 2-phase randomized clinical trial of early Class II treatment. *Am J Orthod Dentofacial Orthop* 2004;125:657–67.

74 Mitani, H, Brodie, AG. Three plane analysis of tooth movement, growth, and angular changes with cervical traction, *Angle Orthod* 1970;40:80–94.

75 Wieslander, L. The effect of force on craniofacial development. *Am J Orthod* 1974;65:531–38.

76 Proffit WR, Tulloch JF. Preadolescent Class II problems: treat now or wait? *Am J Orthod Dentofacial Orthop* 2002;121:560–62.

77 O'Brien K. Is early treatment for Class II malocclusions effective? Results of a randomized controlled trial. *Am J Orthod Dentofacial Orthop*. 2006;129(4 Suppl):S64–5.

78 O'Brien K, Wright J, Conboy F, Appelbe P, Davies L, Connolly I, et al. Early treatment for Class II division 1 malocclusion with the twin-block appliance: a multi-center, randomized, controlled trial. *Am J Orthod Dentofacial Orthop* 2009;135:573–79.

79 Pancherz H. The effects, limitations, and long-term dentofacial adaptations to treatment with the Herbst appliance. *Semin Orthod* 1997;3:232–43.

80 Sloss EA, Southard KA, Qian F, Stock SE, Mann KR, Meyer DL, et al. Comparison of soft-tissue profiles after treatment with headgear or Herbst appliance. *Am J Orthod Dentofacial Orthop* 2008;133:509–14.

81 Pinho S, Ciriaco C, Faber J, Lenza MA. Impact of dental asymmetries on the perception of smile esthetics. *Am J Orthod Dentofacial Orthop* 2007;132:748–53.

82 Kokich VO Jr, Kiyak HA, Shapiro PA. Comparing the perception of dentists and lay people to altered dental esthetics. *J Esthet Dent* 1999:11;311–24.

83 Gonzales-Ulloa M, Stevens E. The role of chin correction in profileplasty. *Plast Reconstr Surg* 1968;41:364–73.

84 Frodel JL, Sykes JM, Jones JL. Evaluation and treatment of vertical microgenia. *Arch Facial Plast Surg* 2004;6:111–19.

85 Levander E, Malmgren O. Evaluation of the risk of root resorption during orthodontic treatment: a study of upper incisors. *Eur J Orthod* 1988;10:30–8.

86 Segal GR, Schiffman PH, Tuncay OC. Meta analysis of the treatment-related factors of external apical root resorption. *Orthod Craniofac Res* 2004;7:71–8.

87 Hartsfield JL Jr, Everett ET, Al-Qawasmi RA. Genetic factors in external apical root resorption and orthodontic treatment. *Crit Rev Oral Biol Med* 2004;15:115–22.

88 Ngan P, Hagg U, Yiu C, Merwin D, Wei SH. Treatment response to maxillary expansion and protraction. *Eur J Orthod* 1996;18:151–68.

89 Ngan P. Early timely treatment of Class III malocclusions. *Sem Orthod* 2005;11:140–5.

90 Sar C, Arman-Ozcirpici A, Uckan S, Yazici AC. Comparative evaluation of maxillary protraction with and without skeletal anchorage. *Am J Orthod Dentofacial Orthop* 2011;139:636–49.

91 Cha B-K, Ngan PW. Skeletal anchorage for orthopedic correction of growing Class III patients. *Semin Orthod* 2011;17:124–37.

92 Major MP, Wong JK, Saltaji H, Major PW, Flores-Mir C. Skeletal anchored maxillary protraction for midface deficiency in children and early adolescence with Class III malocclusion: a systematic review and meta-analysis. *J World Fed Orthod* 2012;1:e47–54.

93 Vaughn G, Mason B, Moon H, Turley P. The effects of maxillary protraction therapy with and without rapid palatal expansion: a prospective, randomized clinical trial. *J Dent Res* 2001;80(Spec Iss A): p.0117.

94 Vaughn GA, Mason B, Moon HB, Turley PK. The effects of maxillary protraction therapy with and without rapid palatal expansion: a prospective, randomized clinical trial. *Am J Orthod Dentofacial Orthop* 2005;128:299–309.

95 Tortop T, Keykubat A, Yuksel S. Facemask therapy with and without expansion. *Am J Orthod Dentofacial Orthop* 2007;132:467–74.

96 Baik HS. Clinical results of the maxillary protraction in Korean children. *Am J Orthod* 1995;108:583–92.

97 Kim JH, Viana MA, Graber TM, Omerza FF, BeGole EA. The effectiveness of protraction face mask therapy: a meta-analysis. *Am J Orthod Dentofacial Orthop* 1999;115:675–85.

98 Jager A, Braumann B, Kim C, Wahner S. Skeletal and dental effects of maxillary protraction in patients with Angle Class III malocclusion: a meta-analysis. *J Orofac Orthop* 2001;62:275–84.

99 Wells AP, Sarver DM, Proffit WR. Long-term efficacy of reverse pull headgear therapy. *Angle Orthod* 2006;76:915–22.

100 Macdonald KE, Kapust AJ, Turley PK. Cephalometric changes after the correction of Class III malocclusion with maxillary expansion/facemask therapy. *Am J Orthod Dentofacial Orthop* 1999;116:13–24.

101 Turley PK. Managing the developing Class III malocclusion with palatal expansion and facemask therapy. *Am J Orthod Dentofacial Orthop* 2002;122:349–52.

102 Deguchi T, Kuroda T, Minoshima Y, Graber TM. Craniofacial features of patients with Class III abnormalities: growth-related changes and effects of short-term and long-term chincup therapy. *Am J Orthod Dentofacial Orthop* 2002;121:84–92.

103 Wendell PD, Nanda R, Sakamoto T, Nakamura S. The effects of chin cup therapy on the mandible: a longitudinal study. *Am J Orthod* 1985;87:265–74.

104 Mitani H. Early application of chincap therapy to skeletal Class III malocclusion. *Am J Orthod Dentofacial Orthop* 2002;121:584–85.

105 Barrett AA, Baccetti T, McNamara JA Jr. Treatment effects of the light-force chincup. *Am J Orthod Dentofacial Orthop* 2010;138:468–76.

106 De Clerck H, Cevidanes L, Baccetti T. Dentofacial effects of bone-anchored maxillary protraction: a controlled study of consecutively treated Class III patients. *Am J Orthod Dentofacial Orthop* 2010;138:577–81.

107 Cevidanes L, Baccetti T, Franchi L, McNamara JA Jr, De Clerck H. Comparison of two protocols for maxillary protraction: bone anchors versus face mask with rapid maxillary expansion. *Angle Orthod* 2010;80:799–806.

108 Killic N, Catal G, Kiki A, Oktay H. Soft tissue profile changes following maxillary protraction in Class III subjects. *Eur J Orthod* 2010;32:419–24.

109 Krebs A. Mid-palatal expansion studies by the implant method over a seven-year period. *Rep Congr Eur Orthod Soc* 1964;40:131–42.

110 Krebs A. Expansion of the midpalatal suture studied by means of metallic implants. *Acta Odontol Scand* 1959;17:491–501.

111 Hicks EP. Slow maxillary expansion: a clinical study of the skeletal versus dental response to low-magnitude force. *Am J Orthod* 1978;73:121–41.

112 Wertz R, Dreskin M. Midpalatal suture opening: a normative study. *Am J Orthod* 1977;71:367–81.

113 Baccetti T, Franchi L, Cameron CG, McNamara JA Jr. Treatment timing for rapid maxillary expansion. *Angle Orthod* 2001;71:343–50.

114 Isaacson RJ, Ingram AH. Forces produced by rapid maxillary expansion II. Forces present during treatment. *Angle Orthod.* 1964;34:261–70.

115 Lines PA. Adult rapid maxillary expansion with corticotomy. *Am J Orthod* 1975;67:44–56.

116 Sarnat BG. Facial and neurocranial growth after removal of the mandibular condyle in the Macaca rhesus monkey. *Am J Surg* 1957;94:19–30.

117 Benson KJ, Laskin DM. Upper lip asymmetry in adults during smiling. *J Oral Maxillofac Surg* 2001;59:396–8.

118 Moore T, Southard KA, Casko JS, Qian F, Southard TE. Buccal corridors and smile esthetics. *Am J Orthod Dentofacial Orthop* 2005;127:208–13.

119 Scott CR, Goonewardene MS, Murray K. Influence of lips on the perception of malocclusion. *Am J Orthod Dentofacial Orthop* 2006;130:152–62.

120 Fridrich KL, Casko JS. Genioplasty strategies for anterior facial vertical dysplasias. *Int J Adult Orthod Orthognath Surg* 1997;12:35–41.

121 Graber L, Kokich V, Low S, Rosen V. Periodontal screening of orthodontic patients: joint task force recommendation. *Bull Am Assoc Orthop* 2012;30:12–14.

122 American Academy of Craniomandibular Disorders. *Craniomandibular disorders: guidelines for evaluation, diagnosis, and management.* McNeill C, editor. Chicago: Quintessence, c1990. p.54.

123 Huber MA, Hall EH. A comparison of the signs of temporomandibular joint dysfunction and occlusal discrepancies in a symptom-free population of men and women. *Oral Surg Oral Med Oral Pathol* 1990;70:180–03.

124 Shiffman A. Myofascial pain associated with unilateral masseteric hypertrophy in a condylectomy patient. *J Craniomandibular Pract* 1984;2:373–76.

125 Clark GT: Muscle hyperactivity, pain and dysfunction. In: Klineberg I, Sessie BJ, editors. *Orofacial pain and neuromuscular dysfunction: mechanisms and clinical correlates.* Sydney (Australia): Pergamon Press, 1985. pp.103–11.

126 Solberg WK. Temporomandibular disorders: masticatory myalgia and its management. *Br Dent J* 1986;160:351–56.

127 Fricton JR: Myofascial pain syndrome: Characteristics and epidemiology. In: Fricton JR, Awad EA, editors. *Myofacial pain and fibromyalgia.* New York: Raven Press Ltd, 1990. pp.107–27.

128 Layzer RB. Diagnostic implications of clinical fasiculations and cramps. In: Rowlad LP, editor. *Human motor neuron diseases.* New York: Raven Press Ltd, 1982. p 23–7.

129 Roth G: The origin of fasciculations. *Ann Neurol* 1982;12:542–47.

130 Stegenga B, De Bont LG, Boering G. A proposed classification of temporomandibular disorders based on synovial joint pathology. *Cranio* 1989; 7:107–18.

131 Gesch D, Bernhardt O, Mack F, John U, Kocher T, Alte D. Association of malocclusion and functional occlusion with subjective symptoms of TMD in adults: results of the study of health in pomerania (SHIP). *Angle Orthod.* 2005;75:183–90.

132 Luther, F. TMD and occlusion part II: damned if we don't? Functional occlusal problems: TMD epidemiology in a wider context. *Br Dent J.* 2007;202:E3; discussion 38–9.

133 Greene CS. Relationship between occlusion and temporomandibular disorders: implications for the orthodontist. *Am J Orthod Dentofacial Orthop.* 2010;139:11, 13, 15.

134 Sadowsky C, BeGole EA. Long-term status of temporomandibular joint function and functional occlusion after orthodontic treatment. *Am J Orthod.* 1980;78:201–12.

135 Sadowsky C, Polson AM. Temporomandibular disorders and functional occlusion after orthodontic treatments: results of two long-term studies. *Am J Orthod.* 1984; 86: 386–90.

136 Gross A, Gale E. Mandibular dysfunction and orthodontic treatment. *J Dent Res.* (Spec Iss A) 63:1565, 1984.

137 Palla S. *Untercuchungen zur okklusionsbedingten Distraktion der Kiefergelenke nach orthodontisch indizierter Pramolaren-Extraktion [thesis].* Zurich (Switzerland): University of Zurich; 1972.

138 Kundinger KK, Austin BP, Christensen LV, Donegan SJ, Ferguson DJ. An evaluation of temporomandibular joints and jaw muscles after orthodontics treatment involving premolar extractions. *Am J Orthod Dentofacial Orthop.* 1991;100:110–5.

139 Gianelly AA, Hughes HM, Wohlgomuth P, Gildea G: Condylar position and extract treatment. *Am J Orthod Dentofacial Orthop.* 1988;93:201–05.

140 McNamara JA Jr, Seligman DA, Okeson JA. Occlusion, orthodontic treatment, and temporomandibular disorders: a review. *J Orofac Pain.* 1995;9:73–90.

141 McNamara JA Jr, Turp JC. Orthodontic treatment and temporomandibular disorders: is there a relationship? Part 1: clinical studies. *J Orofac Orthop.* 1997;58:74–89.
142 Reynders RM. Orthodontics and temporomandibular disorders: a review of the literature (1966–1988). *Am J Orthod Dentofacial Orthop.* 1990;97:463–71.
143 LeResche L, Dworkin SF, Sommers EE, Truelove EL: An epidemiologic evaluation of two diagnostic classification schemes for temporomandibular disorders. *J Prosthet Dent* 1991;65:131–37.
144 Attanasio R. Nocturnal bruxism and its clinical management. *Dent Clin North Am.* 1991;35:245–52.
145 Faulkner KD. Bruxism: a review of the literature. *Part I Aust Dent J.* 1990; 35:266–76.
146 Faulkner KD. Bruxism: a review of the literature. *Part II Aust Dent J.* 1990; 35:355–61.
147 Glaros AG, Rao SM. Effects of bruxism: a review of the literature. *J Prosthet Dent.* 1977;38:149–57.
148 Dubrul EL. The craniomandibular articulation. In: Dubrul EL, Sicher H. *Sicher's oral anatomy.* 7th ed. St Louis: CV Mosby Co; 1980. p.147–209.
149 Greene CS, Laskin DM. Long-term evaluation of treatment for myofascial pain-dysfunction syndrome: a comparative analysis. *J Am Dent Assoc.* 1983; 107:235–38.
150 Mejersjo C, Carlsson GE. Long-term results of treatment for temporomandibular pain-dysfunction. *J Prosthet Dent.* 1983;49:809–15.
151 Fricton JR. Recent advances in temporomandibular disorders and orofacial pain. *J Am Dent Assoc.* 1991;122:24–32.
152 Greene CS, Laskin DM. Long-term status of TMJ clicking in patients with myofascial pain and dysfunction. *J Am Dent Assoc.* 1988;117:461–5.
153 Pullinger AG, Seligman DA. TMJ osteoarthrosis: a differentiation of diagnostic subgroups by symptom history and demographics. *J Craniomandib Disord.* 1987;1: 251–56.
154 Eversole LR, Machado L. Temporomandibular joint internal derangements and associated neuromuscular disorders. *J Am Dent Assoc.* 1985;110:69–79.
155 Nickerson JW, Boering G. Natural course of osteoarthrosis as it relates to internal derangement of the temporomandibular joint. *Oral Maxillofac Clin North Am.* 1989; 1:27–45.
156 Helkimo E, Westling L. History, clinical findings, and outcome of treatment of patients with anterior disk displacement. *Cranio.* 1987;5:269–76.
157 Rasmussen OC. Description of population and progress of symptoms in a longitudinal study of temporomandibular arthropathy. *Scand J Dent Res.* 1981;89: 196–203.
158 Carlsson GE. Long-term effects of treatment of craniomandibular disorders. *Cranio.* 1985;3:337–42.
159 Randolph CS, Greene CS, Moretti R, Forbes D, Perry HT. Conservative management of temporomandibular disorders: a posttreatment comparison between patients from a university clinic and from private practice. *Am J Orthod Dentofacial Orthop.* 1990;98:77–82.
160 Flor H, Fydrich T, Turk DC. Efficacy of multidisciplinary pain treatment centers: a meta-analytic review. *Pain.* 1992;49:221–30.
161 Fricton J, Look JO, Wright E, Alencar FG Jr, Chen H, Lang M, et al. Systematic review and meta-analysis of randomized controlled trials evaluating intraoral orthopedic appliances for temporomandibular disorders. *J Orofac Pain.* 2010;24:237–54.
162 Clark GT, Adler RC. A critical evaluation of occlusal therapy: occlusal adjustment procedures. *J Am Dent Assoc.* 1985;110:743–50.
163 Goodman P, Greene CS, Laskin DM. Response of patients with myofascial pain-dysfunction to mock equilibration. *J Am Dent Assoc.* 1976;92:755–58.
164 Fields HL. *Pain.* New York: McGraw Hill;1987. p.354.
165 Friction JR. Clinical care for myofascial pain. *Dent Clin North Am.* 1991;35:1–28.
166 Nitzan DW, Dolwick MF, Martinez GA. Temporomandibular joint arthrocentesis: a simplified treatment for severe, limited mouth opening. *J Oral Maxillofac Surg.* 1991; 49;1163–167; discussion 1168–70.
167 Machon V, Abramowicz S, Paska J, Dolwick MF. Autologous blood injection for the treatment of chronic recurrent temporomandibular joint dislocation. *J Oral Maxillofac Surg.* 2009;67:114–19.
168 Kokich VO, Kokich VG, Kiyak HA. Perceptions of dental professionals and laypersons to altered dental esthetic: asymmetric and symmetric situations. *Am J Orthod Dentofacial Orthop.* 2006;130:141–51.
169 Hulsey, CM. An esthetic evaluation of lip-teeth relationships present in the smile. *Am J Orthod.* 1970;57:132–44.
170 Sarver DM. The importance of incisor positioning in the esthetic smile: the smile arc. *Am J Orthod Dentofacial Orthop.* 2001;120:98–111.
171 Kokich VG. Esthetics: the orthodontic-periodontic restorative connection. *Semin Orthod.* 1996;2:21–30.
172 Fudalej P. Long-term changes of the upper lip position relative to the incisal edge. *Am J Orthod Dentofacial Orthop.* 2008;133:204–09.
173 Elder JR, Tuenge RH. Cephalometric and histologic changes produced by extra-oral high-pull traction to the maxilla in Macaca mulatta. *Am J Orthod.* 1974;66:599–617.
174 Shelly AD, Southard TE, Southard KA, Casko JS, Jakobsen JR, Fridrich KL, et al. Evaluation of profile esthetic change with mandibular advancement surgery. *Am J Orthod Dentofacial Orthop.* 2000;117:630–37.
175 Hoffman GR, Moloney FB. The stability of facial osteotomies. Part 6. Chin setback. *Aust Dent J.* 1996;41:178–83.
176 Pepicelli A, Woods M, Briggs C. The mandibular muscles and their importance in orthodontics: a contemporary review. *Am J Orthod Dentofacial Orthop.* 2005; 128:774–80.
177 Flores MT, Andersson L, Andreasen JO, Bakland LK, Malmgren B, Barnett F, et al. Guidelines for the management of traumatic dental injuries. I. Fractures and luxations of permanent teeth. *Dent Traumatol.* 2007;23:66–71.
178 Wessberg GA, Fish LC, Epker BN. The short face patient: surgical-orthodontic treatment options. *J Clin Orthod.* 1982;16:668–85.
179 Cowley G. The biology of beauty. *Newsweek.* 1996;127:60–6.

CHAPTER 4

Dental Anterior Open Bites

Introduction

Connor (Figure 4.1) is an 18-year-old who presents to you with the CC, "my front teeth do not touch. I cannot bite off food." Connor's parents state that he has not grown for years.

Q: In terms of his mild anterior open bite, what features would lead you to classify Connor as having a dental open bite? A skeletal open bite?

A: Connor's *dental* open-bite features include a clinically normal LAFH (Figure 4.1a, soft-tissue Glabella–Subnasale = Subnasale–soft tissue Menton), lip competence without strain of the mentalis muscle to prevent an ILG, flat to normal MPA (Figure 4.1e; FMA=16°, SNMP=31°), anterior 1–2mm open bite with maxillary incisors stepped up relative to the maxillary posterior teeth (Figure 4.1h), and the anterior open bite including only his incisors (not extending to posterior teeth). Connor's *skeletal* open-bite features include a slightly longer skeletal LAFH (LAFH/TAFH=57%), maxillary first molar apicies erupted 3–4mm below the palatal plane (Figure 4.1d), and downward tipping of his posterior palatal plane.

Q: What other questions should you ask Connor and his parents about his open bite?

A: Ask if they have noticed his open bite, and how long has he had it. Connor and his parents respond that they have not noticed it but that he has always complained about not being able to bite off his food.

Q: Regarding Connor's open bite, what else should you look for?

A: Look for functional habits that prevent anterior teeth from erupting, including an anterior interpositional resting tongue habit or tongue sucking habit (Figure 4.2a), lip-biting habit (Figure 4.2b), or digit-sucking habit (Figure 4.2c). You observe that Connor has an anterior interpositional resting tongue habit, and he denies a digit-sucking habit. Finally, check for condylar degeneration on the screening panoramic image. With condylar degeneration, the mandible rotates down and back creating an open bite. Connor's condyles appear normal with smooth contours (Figure 4.1f).

Q: Can you suggest a good way to examine patients for anterior interpositional (resting) tongue habits?

A: Yes, the key is to *distract the patient as you pull their lip down to look for the habit*! Ask the patient to close his/her eyes for a minute, maybe while you talk to their parents. Then, prepare to reach for their lower lip—but do not touch it. Tell the patient to open their eyes (to distract them and to take their focus off of you), as you simultaneously (quickly and gently) pull their lip down and examine their tongue position.

Q: What are other possible causes of anterior open bites?

A: Other possible causes of anterior open bites include the following:

- Temporary anterior open bites occurring while permanent teeth are erupting
- Ankylosis of anterior teeth, which prevents their complete eruption into occlusion
- Lack of space for complete tooth eruption (teeth blocked out)

Q: So, does Connor have a dental open bite, a skeletal open bite, or a combination of both? What is the etiology of this open bite? Will you treat him as a dental open bite, a skeletal open bite, or a combination of both?

A: Because Connor has an interpositional tongue habit, and because his maxillary incisors are stepped up relative to his maxillary posterior teeth (his tongue has prevented his maxillary incisors from erupting), we conclude that he has a dental (functional) open bite. Determining whether Connor also has a skeletal open bite is a little more involved. On the one hand, when you look at him (Figure 4.1a), his vertical dimension looks normal (clinically normal soft tissue LAFH), and his lips are competent. This indicates that his vertical skeletal dimension is reasonably normal, and his soft tissue facial growth has kept pace with his skeletal growth. On the other hand, cephalometric measures of excess vertical skeletal growth are present (LAFH slightly > 55%, molar apicies erupted below palatal plane, and palatal plane tipped down at the posterior). So, like many patients you will treat, some features support a skeletal open bite, while other features support only a dental open bite. You must weigh the preponderance of these characteristics in making your classification and in determining your treatment plan. You must also consider the weight of these features in light of his age (18 years) and potential future growth (no potential future growth). In Connor's case, a decision was made to treat him as a dental open-bite patient with normal vertical facial growth. However, if Connor had presented with the same skeletal pattern at say, age 10, then it would have been prudent to inform his parents of a potential future problem with vertical growth and monitor his vertical facial growth very carefully for a developing skeletal open bite (or better yet, to treat Connor as if he *was* also a developing skeletal open bite).

Q: Why correct Connor's open bite?

A: Connor gave us the most important reason for correcting anterior open bite, function. Connor cannot incise food with his anterior open bite. Also, open bites can adversely impact speech and facial esthetics.

Orthodontics in the Vertical Dimension: A Case-Based Review, First Edition. Thomas E. Southard, Steven D. Marshall and Laura L. Bonner.

Q: What do the three patients in Figure 4.3 demonstrate?

A: These three patients developed open bites as a result of function: anterior interpositional tongue habit (Figure 4.3a–c), lip-biting habit (Figure 4.3d–f), and digit-sucking habit (Figure 4.3g–h).

Q: Antoine is an 8-year-old who presents to you for treatment of his open bite (Figure 4.4). As part of his examination, what etiologic factors should you check for that would contribute to his maxillary incisors not erupting completely (maxillary incisors stepped up compared to maxillary posterior teeth) and contribute to his mandibular incisors not erupting completely (mandibular incisors stepped down compared to mandibular posterior teeth)?

A: Check for a digit-sucking habit, anterior tongue interposition habit or tongue-sucking habit, and lip-biting habit. You find

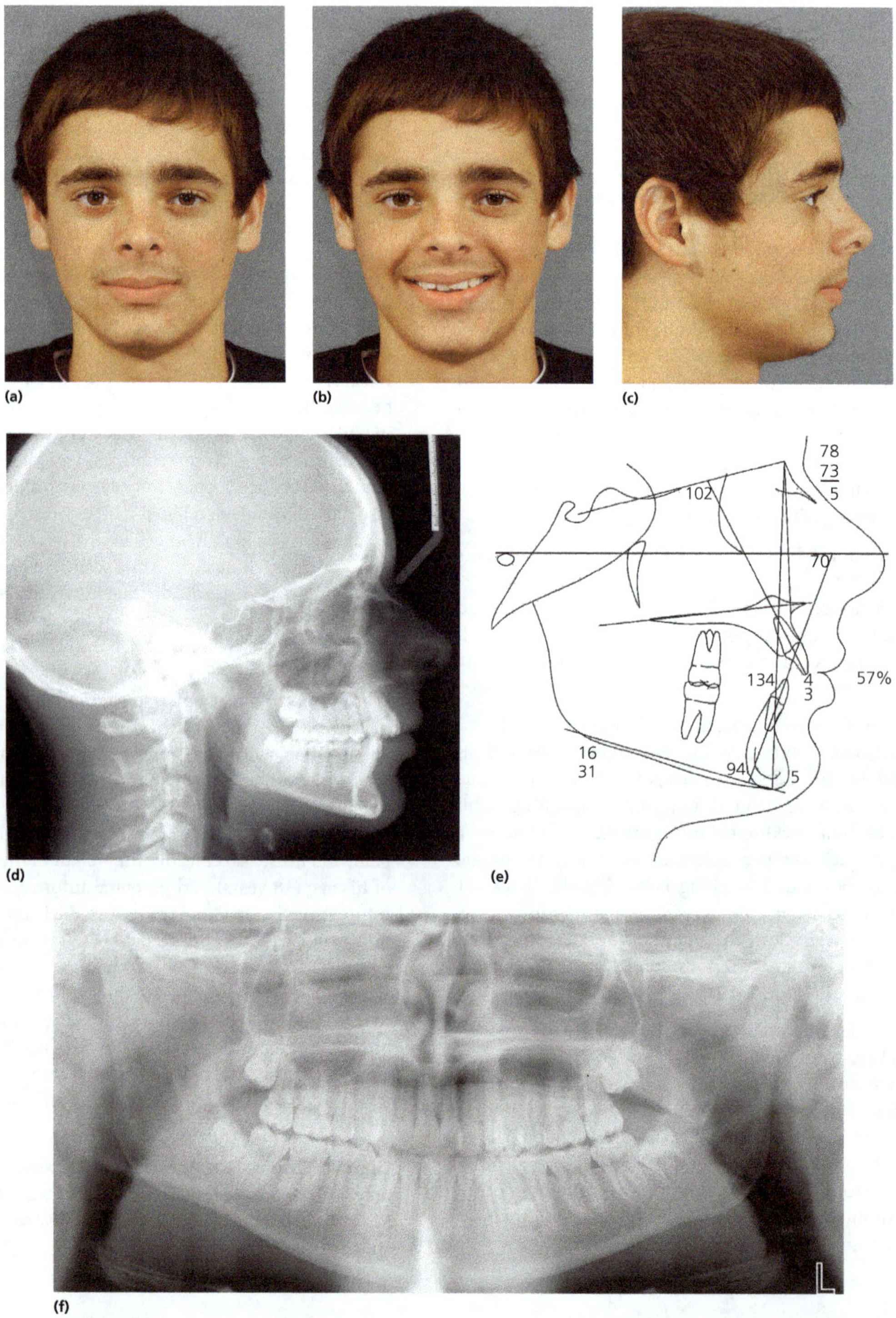

Figure 4.1 Initial records of Connor: (a–c) initial facial photographs, (d) lateral cephalograph, (e) cephalometric tracing, (f) pantomograph, and (g–k) intraoral photographs.

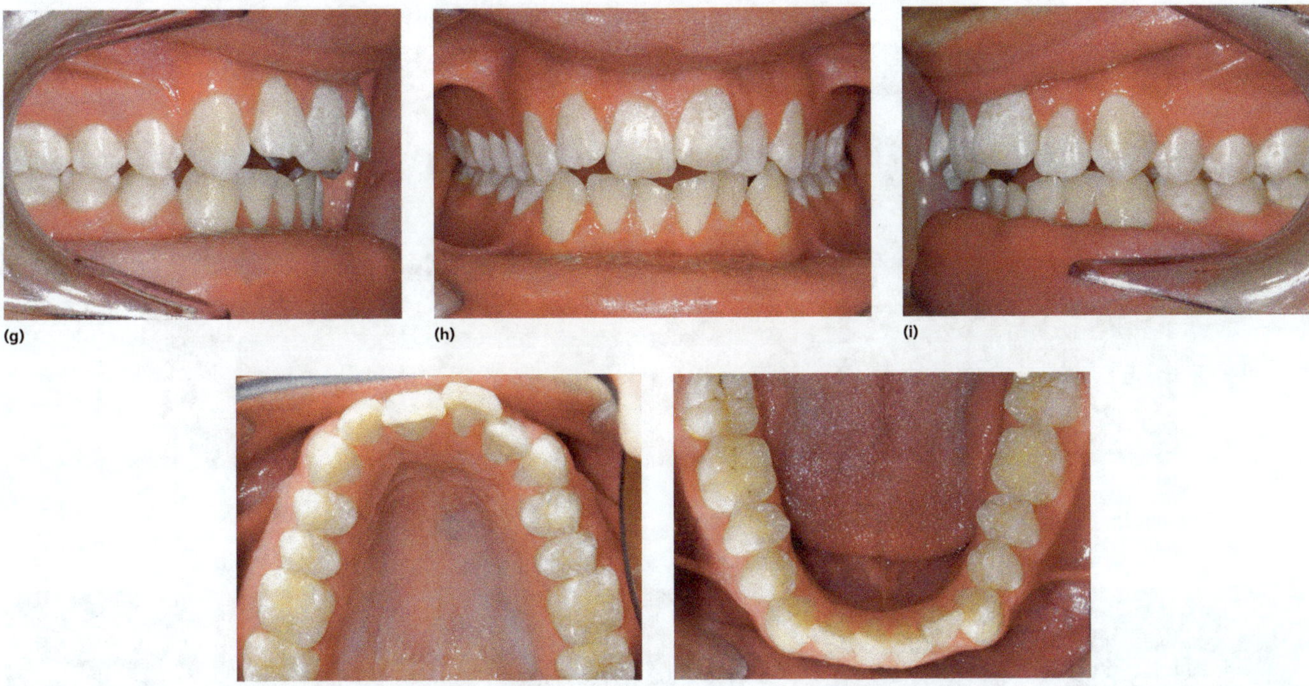

(g) (h) (i) (j) (k)

Figure 4.1 (Continued)

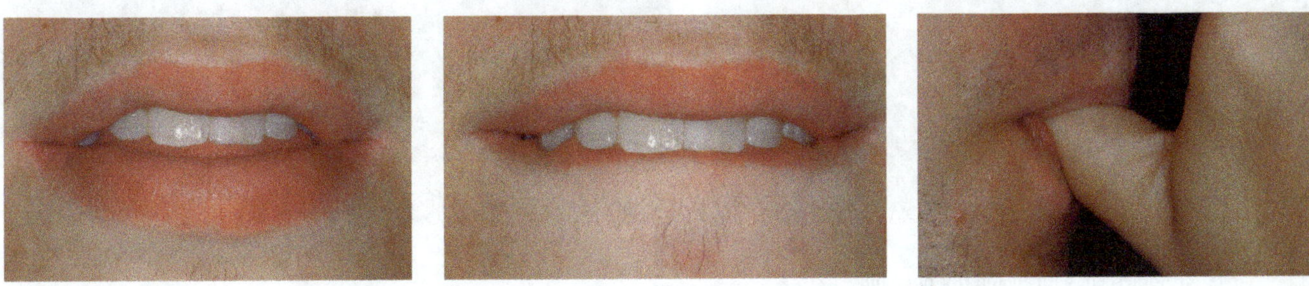

(a) (b) (c)

Figure 4.2 Habits that can cause dental (functional) open bites include (a) anterior resting tongue or tongue sucking, (b) lip biting, and (c) and digit sucking.

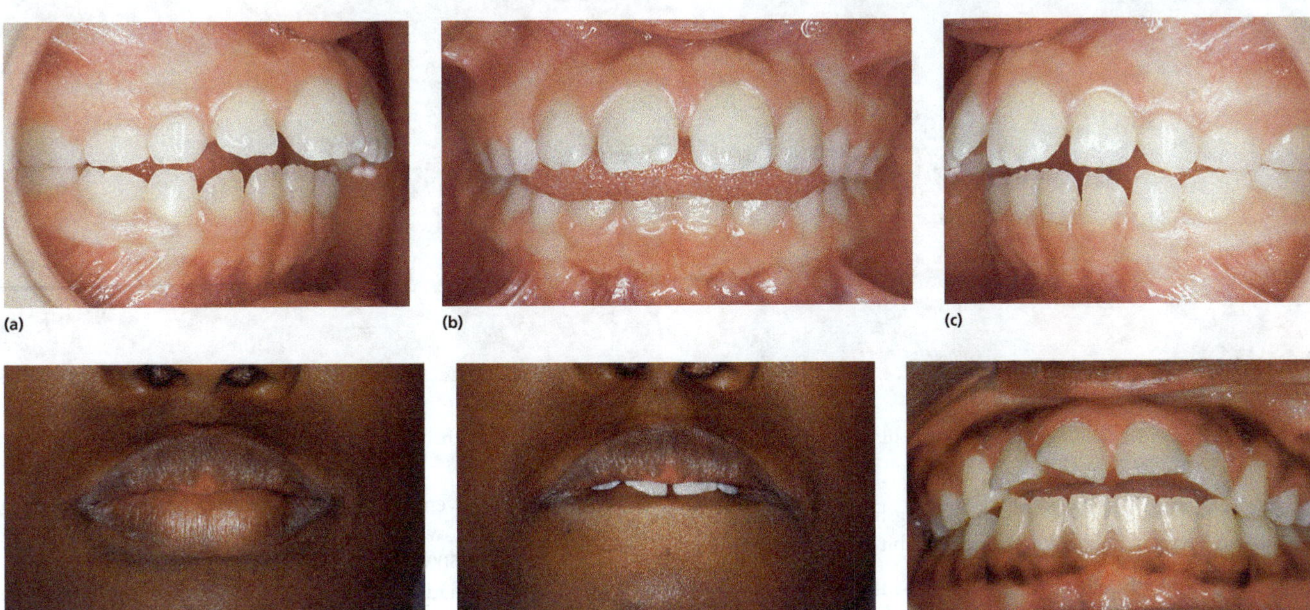

(a) (b) (c) (d) (e) (f)

Figure 4.3 Dental (functional) open bites due to a (a–c) anterior tongue interposition habit, (d–f) lip-biting habit, and (g–h) thumb-sucking habit.

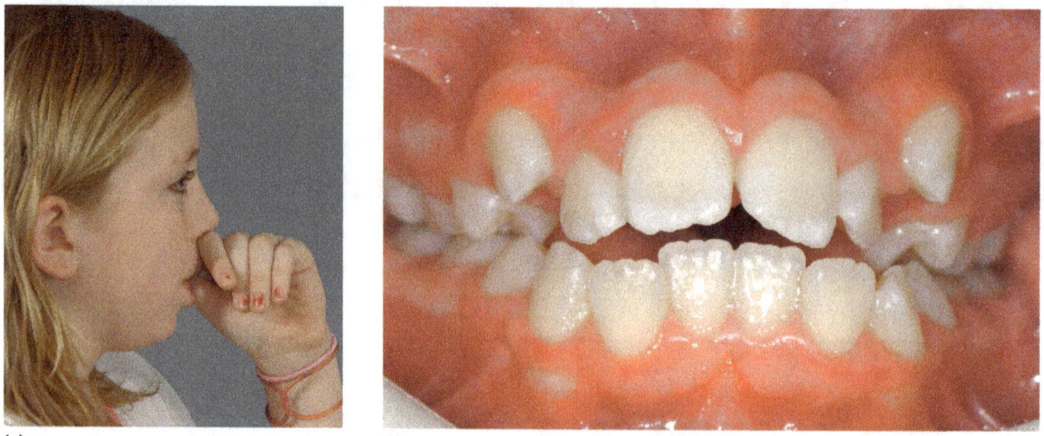

(g) (h)

Figure 4.3 (Continued)

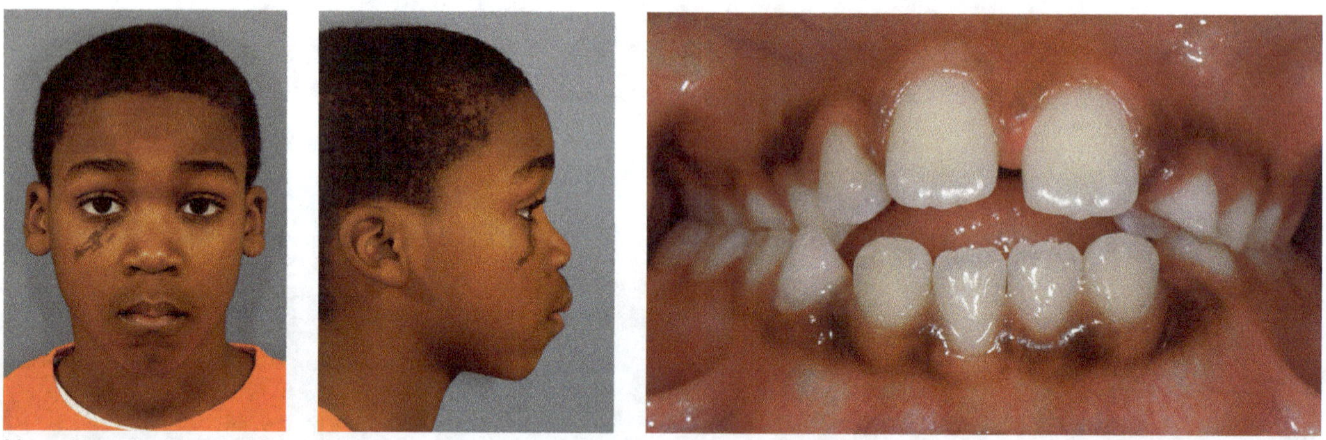

(a) (b) (c)

Figure 4.4 (a–c) Adolescent with an anterior open bite.

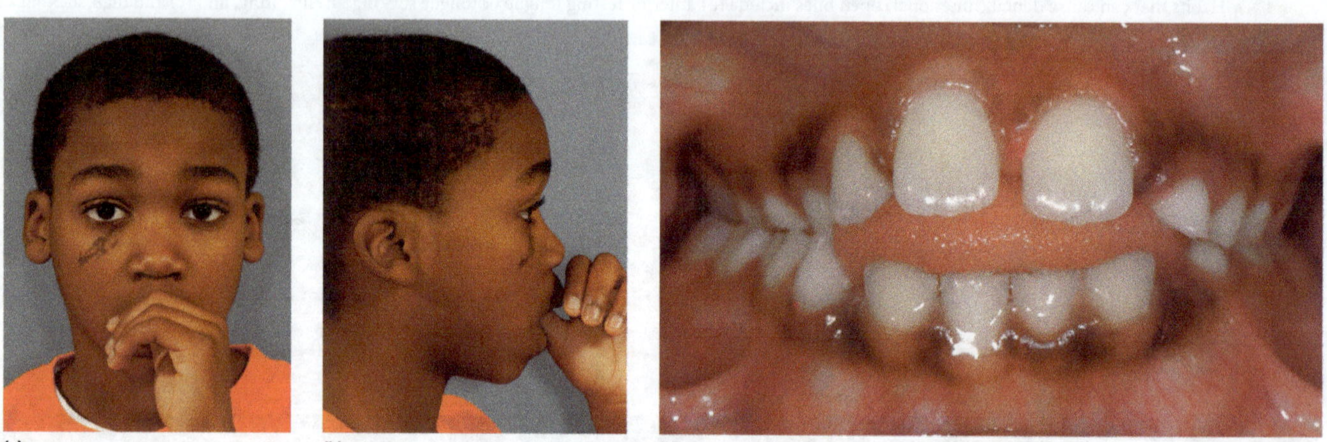

(a) (b) (c)

Figure 4.5 (a–c) Etiologic factors contributing to his anterior open bite included both a digit-sucking habit and an anterior tongue interpositional habit.

that Antoine has both a thumb-sucking habit (Figure 4.5a, b) and an anterior tongue interposition habit (Figure 4.5c).

Q: Considering thumb-sucking, tongue-interposition, or lip-biting habits—is habit *duration* or habit force *magnitude* more important in preventing teeth from erupting?

A: Duration [1]. Even light, continuous force against an erupting rodent incisors will inhibit eruption. Force applied against rabbit incisors 50% of the time had the same effect as continuous force but had more effect than a force applied 25% of the time. Force applied only 10% of the time had little or no effect on incisor eruption [2–4].

Q: What is a reasonable approach to eliminating a thumb- or digit-sucking habit?

A: Start by talking to the patient and explaining that the habit is preventing the anterior teeth from erupting and coming together. Demonstrate this to the patient with a mirror. Ask the patient if they are interested in stopping the habit. If they are not interested in stopping the habit, it may be better to wait until they are more mature to attempt stopping the habit. If they are interested in stopping the habit, ask him/her if they are performing the habit during the day (when they are conscious of it) or during the night. If they want to stop and are doing it during the day, have them try to make a conscience effort to decrease the habit over time. Tell them that if they keep trying their best, they will win over the habit, long-term. Follow them for some months to see how they do before beginning orthodontic treatment. If the patient is performing the habit while asleep, then this psychological approach may not work. However, ask them to make themselves stop the habit if they wake up to find they are sucking their digit. This approach worked well for Kolbe (Figure 4.6), who presented with a finger-sucking habit and dental open bite. After he stopped this habit, the dental open bite resolved on its own (Figure 4.6c)

Q: If the psychological approach does not work, then can you list at least two other options for correcting a digit-sucking habit?

A: A maxillary crib (Figure 4.7a, b) can be effective in discouraging digit sucking by preventing the digit from contacting the palate. But some patients may maneuver their digit around the appliance and continue the habit. A maxillary crib with soldered spurs (Figure 4.7c, d) can often discourage the habit in these patients. A thumb guard/T-guard appliance (Figure 4.7e, f) can be useful, although it requires help from the parents. Finally, for some patients who are eager to begin orthodontic treatment, simply telling them that you will not start braces until they have stopped the habit can motivate them to stop.

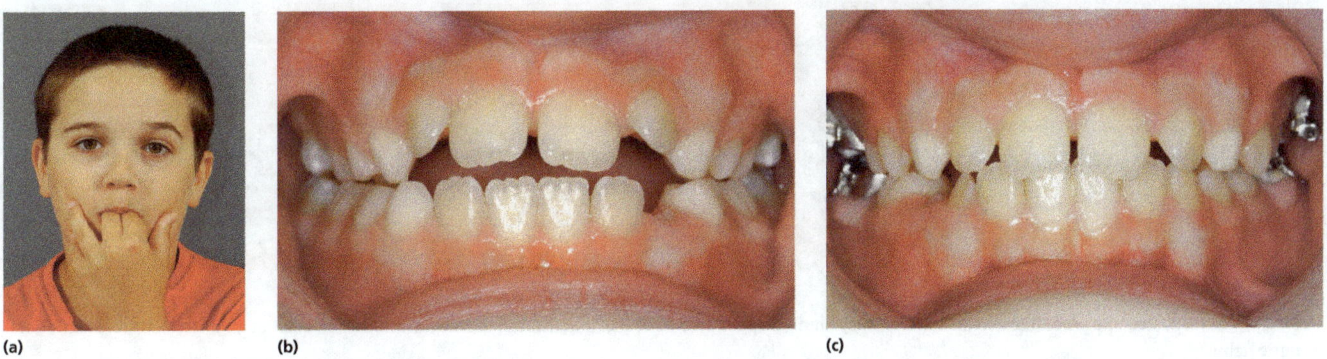

Figure 4.6 (a, b) Kolbe presented with a finger sucking habit and a corresponding dental open bite. Using the psychological approach, he stopped the habit, which allowed the dental open bite to spontaneously close (c) in 3 months.

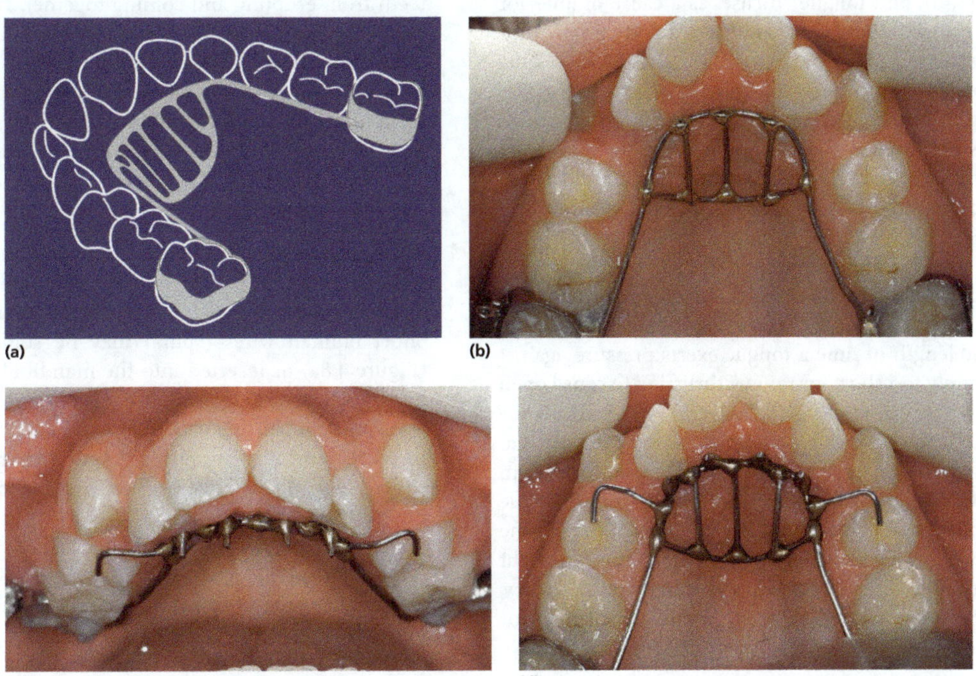

Figure 4.7 Options for correcting a digit-sucking habit: (a, b) a thumb crib appliance, (c, d) a crib with the addition of spurs, and (e, f) a thumb guard appliance.

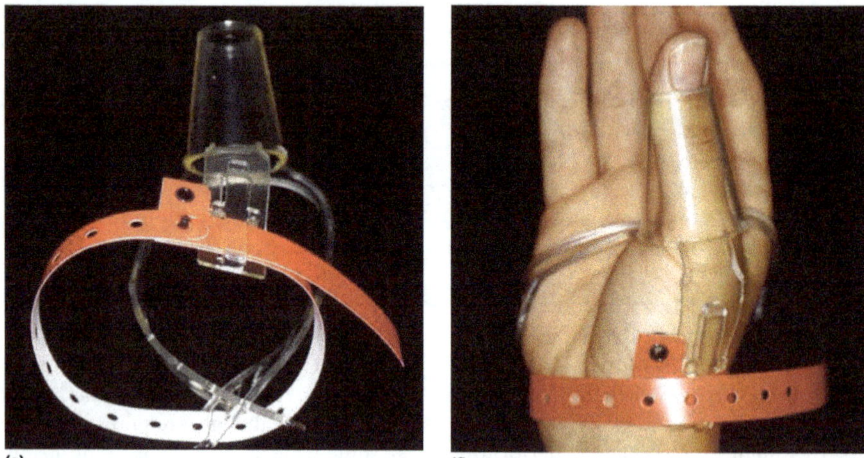

(e) (f)

Figure 4.7 (Continued)

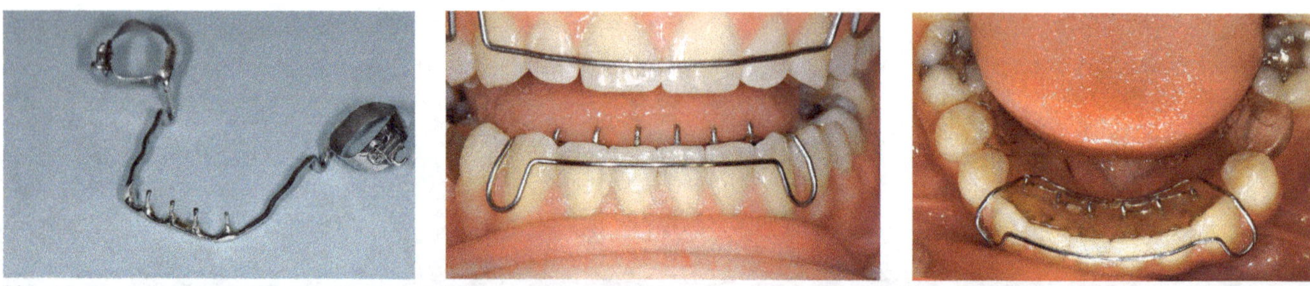

(a) (b) (c)

Figure 4.8 (a) Blunted spurs soldered to an LLHA, (b, c) blunted spurs embedded in a mandibular Hawley retainer to correct an anterior interpositional tongue habit.

Q: Does tongue *thrusting* cause anterior open bites?

A: No. The tongue's role in anterior open bites has been reported for 80 years [5, 6], and tongue "thrust" as a cause of anterior open bites gained popularity and led to treatment for retraining/restricting tongue action [7–13]. However, tongue thrust swallowing is now believed to be an adaptation to the anterior open bite and not a cause of it [14]. In other words, tongue thrusting occurs during an infantile swallow—the tongue fills the space between the gum pads to maintain a seal. During an adult swallow, teeth contact during a swallow and there is no need for the tongue to form a seal. A tongue thrust is thought to continue as an adaptation when the anterior teeth are kept apart, say, with thumb sucking or anterior tongue posturing.

Further, the length of time a tongue exerts pressure against the teeth is simply too short for tongue thrusting to cause open bites [14]. On average, swallowing lasts for 1–3 s, and people swallow 1200–1500 times per day, which leads to a potential tongue thrust pressure of less than 75 min/day, too short to move teeth. On the other hand, a long-term anterior tongue *posture* interpositional habit (including a habit of thrusting the tongue unrelated to swallowing) can exert a continuous light force, preventing anterior teeth from erupting. In summary, remember this adage regarding tongues and dental anterior open bites, "*tongue thrust NO, tongue posture YES!*"

Q: A 10-year-old presents with a dental open bite secondary to an anterior tongue interpositional habit. What is a reasonable first step to eliminate the habit?

A: As was the case with a thumb habit, start by talking to the patient and explaining that the habit is preventing the anterior teeth from erupting and coming together. Demonstrate this to the patient with a mirror. Ask the patient if he or she is interested in stopping the habit. If they are interested, ask them to try to keep their tongue off of the incisal edges of the anterior teeth—and when they swallow to have the tip of their tongue touch their anterior palate. If they are not interested in stopping the habit, it may be better to wait until they are more mature to attempt stopping it.

Q: What appliances could be placed as a "reminder" for the patient to keep his or her tongue behind the mandibular incisors—to deter an anterior tongue interpositional habit?

A: Short blunted wires (spurs) may be soldered to an LLHA (Figure 4.8a) or inserted into the mandibular Hawley retainer during retention (Figure 4.8b, c) [5, 12].

As an example, use of an LLHA appliance with spurs resulted in correction of the anterior tongue interposition habit, and subsequent open bite closure, in the patient shown in Figure 4.9.

Alternatively, the spurs could be soldered to a maxillary TPA (Figure 4.10) [15].

Bondable spurs (tongue reminders, Figure 4.11a) are commercially available, and bondable orthodontic buttons (Figure 4.11b) can be used to the same effect. Or, tongue reminders can be formed chair side by placing a small amount of composite material on the lingual surfaces of the mandibular incisors (Figure 4.11c).

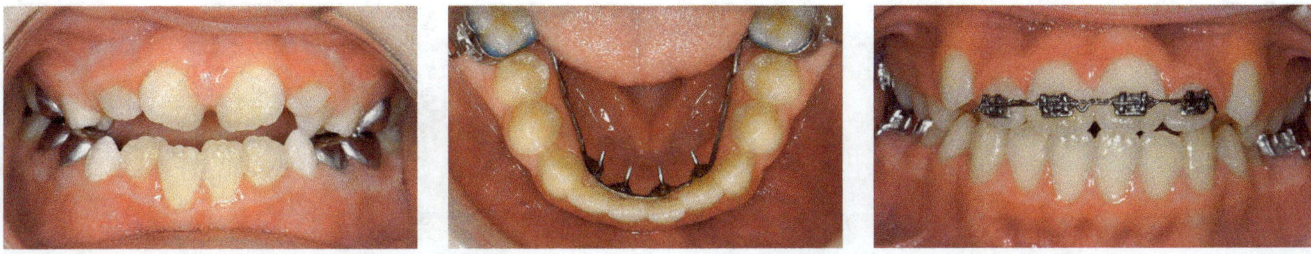

(a) (b) (c)

Figure 4.9 Interpositional tongue habit correction using blunted spurs: (a) initial open bite, (b) blunted spurs soldered to an LLHA, and (c) with tongue habit corrected, the anterior teeth erupted, and the open bite closed (brackets placed to align the maxillary incisors, only).

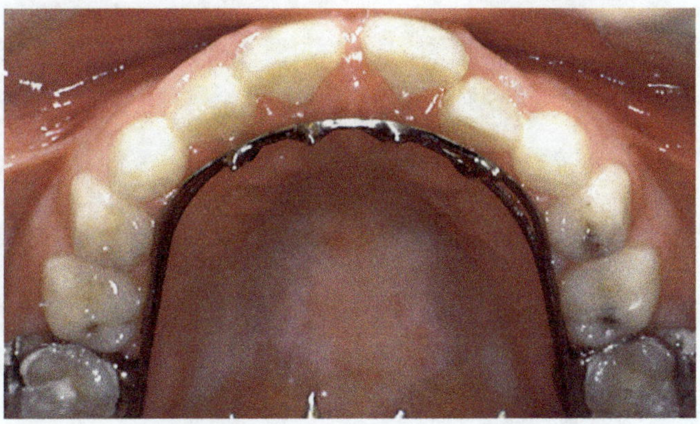

Figure 4.10 Blunted spurs soldered to a TPA to correct an anterior interpositional tongue habit.

Other commercially available appliances, such as the "Bluegrass" palatal appliance, are also useful for drawing the tongue to the anterior palate and away from the incisor edges (Figure 4.12).

At times, closing the open bite with orthodontic treatment can "train" the tongue and correct an anterior tongue interposition habit. Figure 4.13a illustrates an adult patient whose dental open bite was successfully closed during orthodontic treatment, and Figure 4.13b shows her 5 years after deband. Her tongue interposition habit was corrected by closing the open bite with braces alone. However, if the tongue interposition habit is not corrected before completion of orthodontic treatment, maintenance of bite closure is uncertain. During retention, a hole can be placed in the anterior palate of the maxillary retainer to draw the tip of the tongue away from the anterior teeth.

Q: Is myofunctional therapy helpful in training the tongue and maintaining closure of dental open bites?

A: The answer to this question is not clear. Figure 4.14 shows a young patient performing various myofunctional exercises (Figure 4.14a, button pull; Figure 4.14b, masseter isometric exercise; Figure 4.14c, d, one elastic swallow). A recent study claimed that myofunctional therapy is helpful (with orthodontic treatment) in closing and maintaining closure of dental open bites and dramatically reduces open-bite relapse in patients with forward tongue posture [16]. However, this study suffers from sample selection biases [17]. In our experience, we have found that patients willing to perform these daily myofunctional exercises are the most compliant patients. They are the patients who would probably correct their anterior tongue interposition habit by themselves once the habit was explained to them.

Q: What if no treatment is provided to an adolescent with an anterior dental (functional) open bite? Can you tell a parent that the open bite will close spontaneously?

A: No, there is no guarantee that the open bite will close spontaneously. Worms et al. [18] reported that 80% of simple anterior open bites (open from canine to canine) corrected spontaneously in the mixed dentition. But this was a cross-sectional study, so the results should be interpreted with caution. On the other hand, you can always try talking to the patient about their open bite and encourage them to eliminate the habit causing it—then *monitor* their progress for 6–12 months before treating them with habit-deterrent appliances.

Q: Partial glossectomies (Figure 4.15a, b) are procedures that have been used in cases of macroglossia to attempt to reduce tongue size and close open bites. How is the diagnosis of macroglossia made? What are the most common causes of macroglossia?

A: No objective diagnostic criteria for macroglossia exist, nor does a description of "normal" tongue size exist [19]. Possible diagnostic criteria include the following:

- Positioning of the tongue apex or border outside the dentition
- Crenations of teeth on the tongue border (Figure 4.15c, scalloping)
- Excessive labial/buccal tip of teeth
- Sleep apnea

Vascular malformations, muscular enlargement, and tumors are the most common causes of macroglossia [20].

Q: What are characteristics of a *pseudomacroglossia*?

A: In pseudomacroglossia, the tongue is of normal size but appears large due to the following: [21]

- Habitual forward posturing
- Hypertrophied tonsils/adenoidal tissue
- Low palatal vault
- Small arches that decrease oral cavity volume
- Severe mandibular deficiency, tumors, cysts, etc.

Q: Are partial glossectomies of value in treating patients with macroglossia?

A: Case reports have purported the value of these procedures in syndromic patients [22, 23] and as an adjunct in the treatment of open bites [24]. However, some surgeons consider partial glossectomies to be of little or no value (In a conversation with two colleagues from the University of Iowa College of Dentistry, Department of Oral and Maxillofacial Surgery (Fridrich KL and Burton RG 2010), oral communication, October 25).

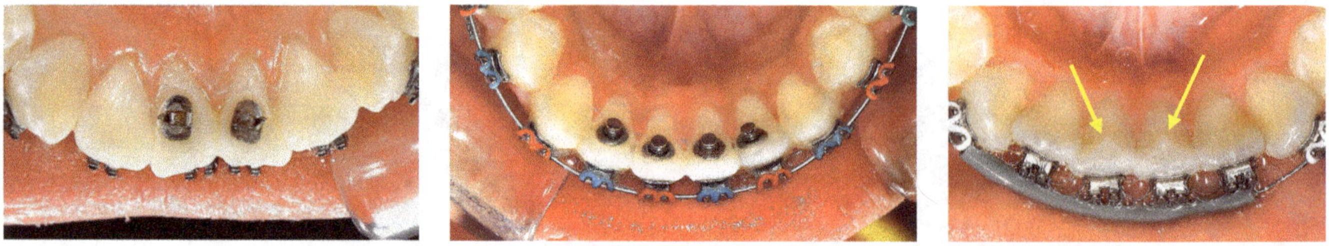

(a) (b) (c)

Figure 4.11 (a) Bondable spurs or (b) orthodontic bondable buttons can also be used to remind patients to stop their interpositional tongue habit. The "poor man's" anterior tongue habit reminder (c) is simply composite resin squirted to a point on the mandibular incisor lingual surfaces.

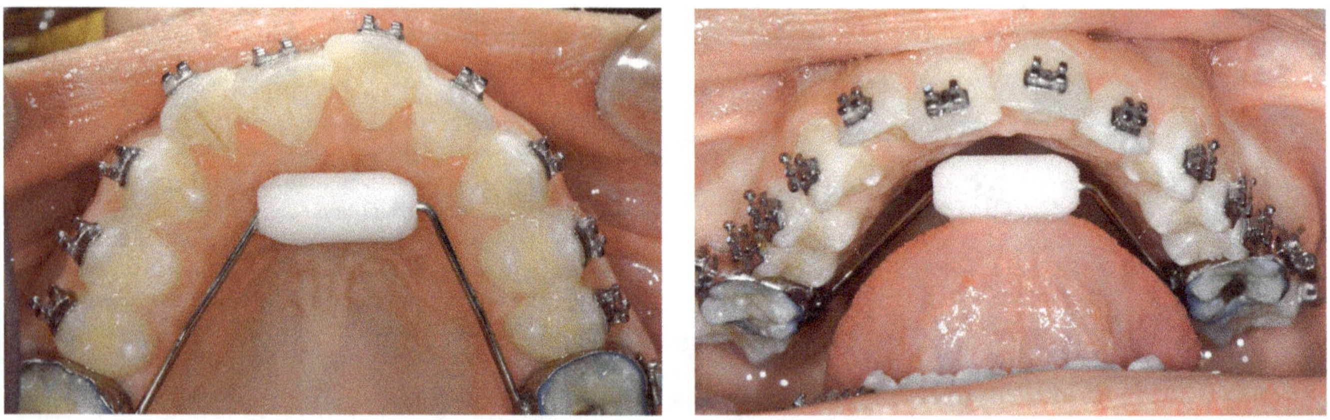

(a) (b)

Figure 4.12 (a, b) The Bluegrass appliance uses a plastic roller to draw the tongue away from anterior teeth. The same principle is employed during retention by placing a hole through the anterior palate plastic of the maxillary retainer.

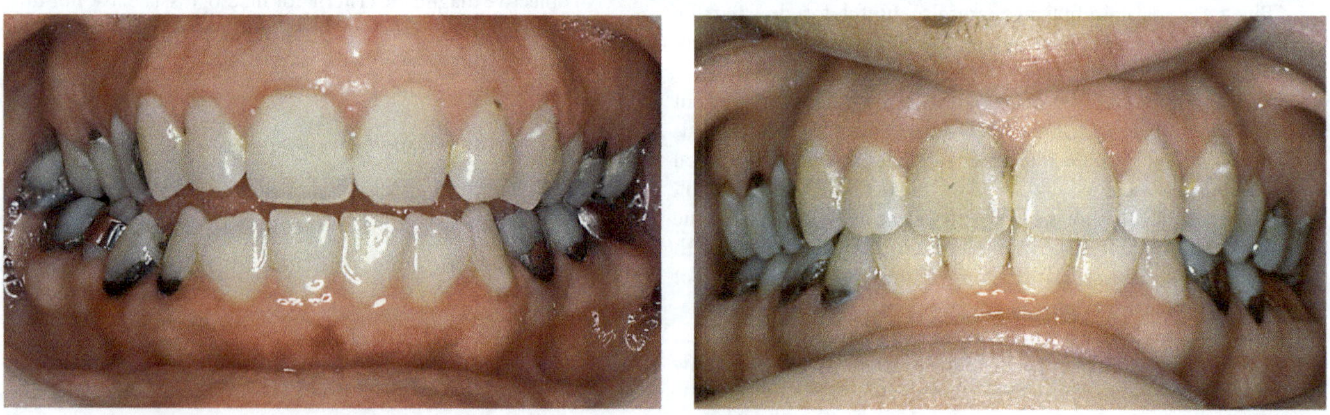

(a) (b)

Figure 4.13 (a) Example of a patient with an anterior tongue interposition habit causing a dental open bite. The open bite was closed using fixed orthodontic appliances and vertical elastics alone—without any adjunctive aides to correct her tongue habit. Fortunately, closing the open bite must have corrected her habit (trained her tongue), because the closure was stable 5 years later (b).

Q: Dental open bites result from habits which prevent anterior teeth from erupting into normal occlusion. Skeletal anterior open bites result from excessive vertical facial growth (occasionally from condylar degeneration). Dental open-bite treatment can be considered analogous to one approach (orthopedics, masking, surgery) for skeletal open-bite treatment. Can you state which one, and why?

A: Dental open-bite treatment can be considered analogous to *masking* a skeletal open bite. In other words, dental open-bite treatment consists of erupting anterior teeth into occlusion, and skeletal open-bite treatment by masking consists of erupting anterior teeth into occlusion. *Dental open-bite treatment* is performed by eliminating the functional habit (digit sucking, lip biting, tongue interposition) to permit the teeth to erupt, and by actively erupting the teeth together (Figure 4.16a, left). The vertical dimension of the face is normal in dental open bites and should not change with treatment. The patient should exhibit normal incisal display at the end of treatment, and an interlabial gap should be absent if the patient has normal lip length (Figure 4.16a, right—note lips are touching at the end of

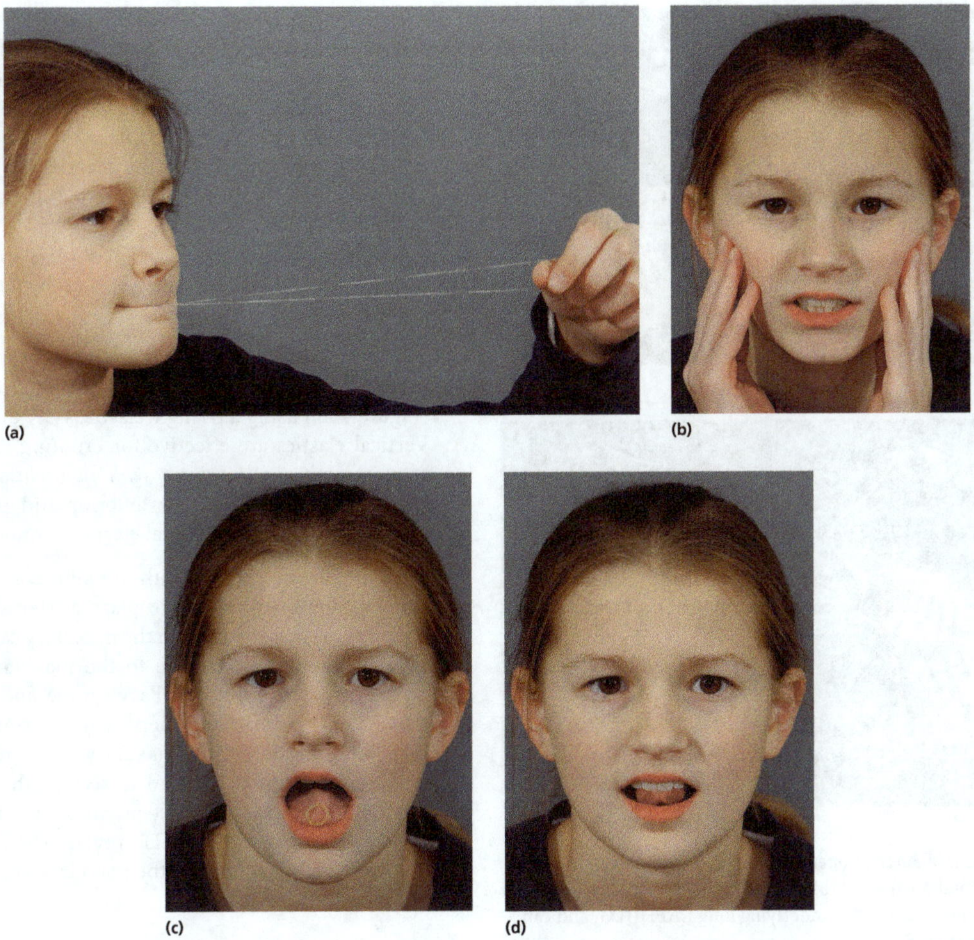

Figure 4.14 (a–d) Myofunctional exercises.

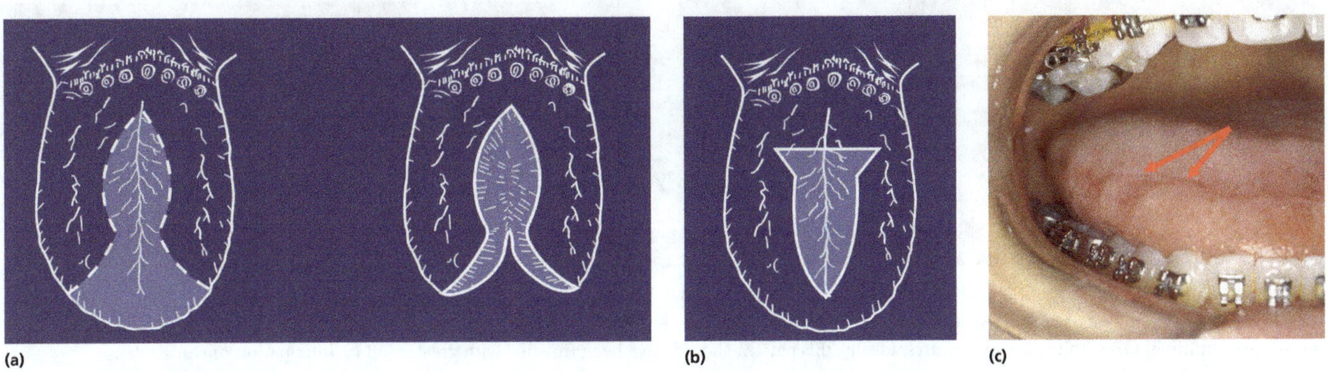

Figure 4.15 (a, b) Illustrations of partial glossectomy surgeries used to decrease tongue volume. (c) Crenations, or scalloping, of the tongue border.

treatment). The stability of this treatment is dependent on cessation of the functional habit. *Skeletal open-bite treatment by masking* likewise consists of erupting anterior teeth into occlusion (Figure 4.16b, left). The vertical dimension of the face is abnormally long (long soft tissue LAFH, ILG). Such masking (camouflage) treatment may result in excessive incisal and gingival display (Figure 4.16b, right) and be unstable.

Q: Exhaustively list (and describe) dental open-bite treatments.

A: Dental open-bite treatments include the following:

- Eliminating the functional habit. This alone can correct the open bite.
- Erupting stepped up maxillary anterior teeth or erupting stepped down mandibular anterior teeth during arch leveling using fixed orthodontic appliances (Figure 4.17). To enhance stability, *overcorrection (OB 20–40%) should be achieved and the correction should be held for some time before debanding* to allow the soft and hard tissues to remodel.
- Wearing vertical interarch elastics (Figure 4.18). *Long arch wire spans, without occlusal contacts between the maxillary and mandibular arches, must be present for vertical elastics to close open bites.* Once bite closure is achieved, elastic wear should be gradually diminished to monitor relapse.

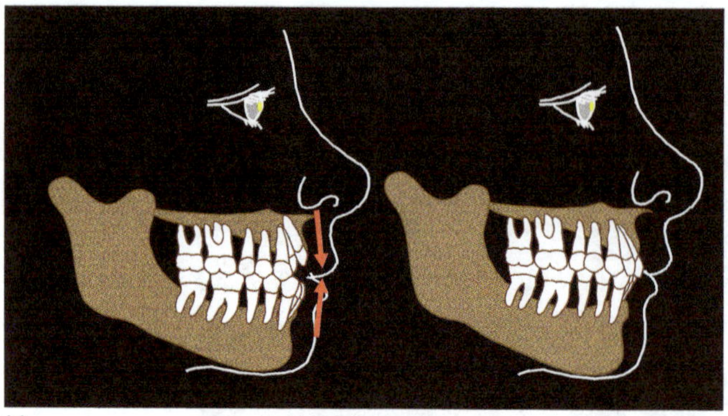

(a)

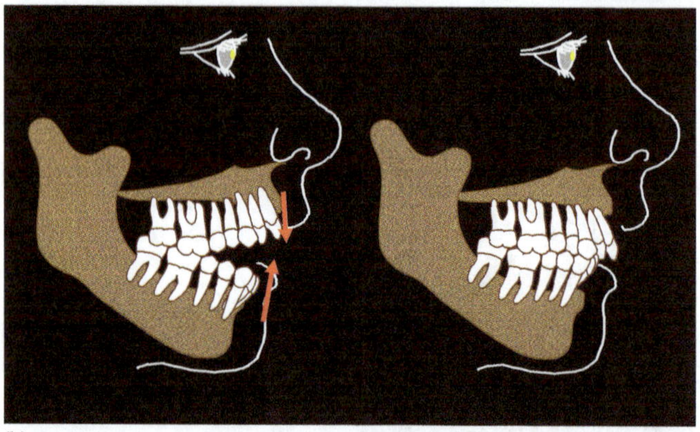

(b)

Figure 4.16 Treatment of anterior open bites by erupting anterior teeth: (a) is appropriate for dental open bites; (b) is often inappropriate for skeletal open bites as it does not address the underlying long LAFH/ILG, and can create excessive incisal display.

- Bonding maxillary and mandibular incisors more gingivally than normal (Figure 4.19, top left to right), and placing archwire "step downs" in the maxillary archwire or "step ups" in the mandibular archwire (Figure 4.19, bottom left to right), helps to erupt incisors.
- Adding curve of Spee to the mandibular archwire to erupt mandibular incisors (Figure 4.20) can aid open-bite closure.
- Retracting/uprighting proclined incisors (Figure 4.21) to rotate them about their apicies, thereby "erupting" them, and closing the open bite.

Q: An attempt was made to close an isolated open bite between the maxillary right canine and mandibular canine/first premolar (Figure 4.22) using a triangle elastic. Why did it fail?

A: Vertical elastics are effective for erupting teeth only if a *long span of archwire is present without occlusal contact* between arches. In Figure 4.22, the anterior and posterior teeth are occluding, so triangle vertical elastics cannot close the bite.

Q: How should you proceed with this situation?

A: The best option would be to place a "step-down" bend in the archwire mesial and distal to the maxillary canine. (Currently, it appears stepped up relative to the maxillary first premolar.) This would erupt the maxillary canine and close the isolated open bite. However, another solution would be to free the maxillary canine (cut the maxillary archwire mesial and distal to the maxillary canine) and to section the wire between the mandibular canine and first premolar, then to run a triangle elastic (Figure 4.23a, b). However, when using this latter method, further control of the maxillary canine is lost because the archwires are now cut.

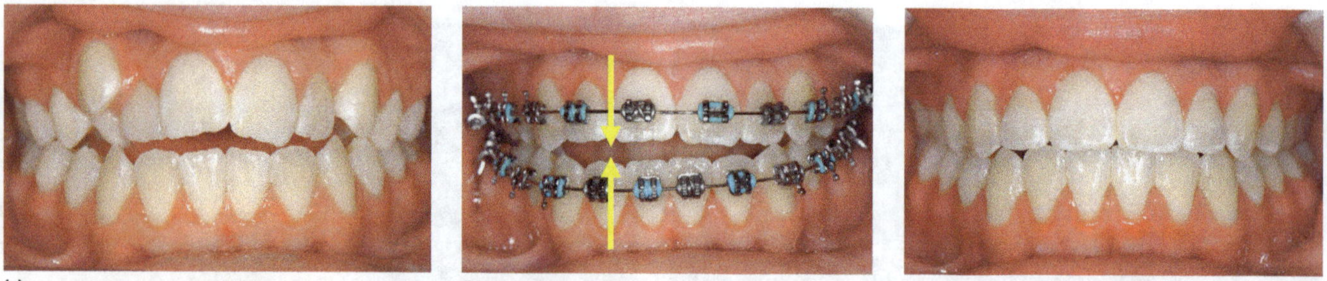

(a) (b) (c)

Figure 4.17 (a) Example of open bite (b) closure by anterior tooth eruption during arch leveling with fixed orthodontic appliances. (c) Note at deband the presence of minimal OB with incisal embrasures. Ideally, this patient should have been finished with greater OB in anticipation of some relapse.

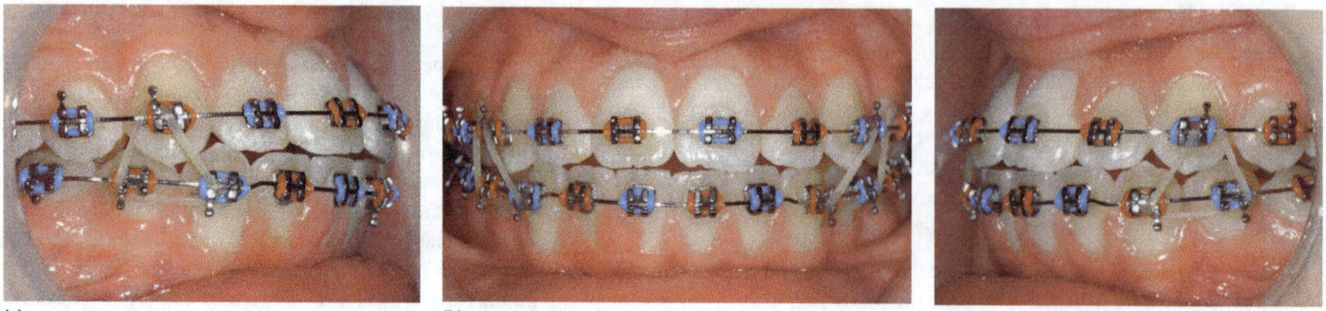

(a) (b) (c)

Figure 4.18 (a–c) Triangle vertical elastics used to close an open bite. Elastics can also be worn between maxillary and mandibular incisors.

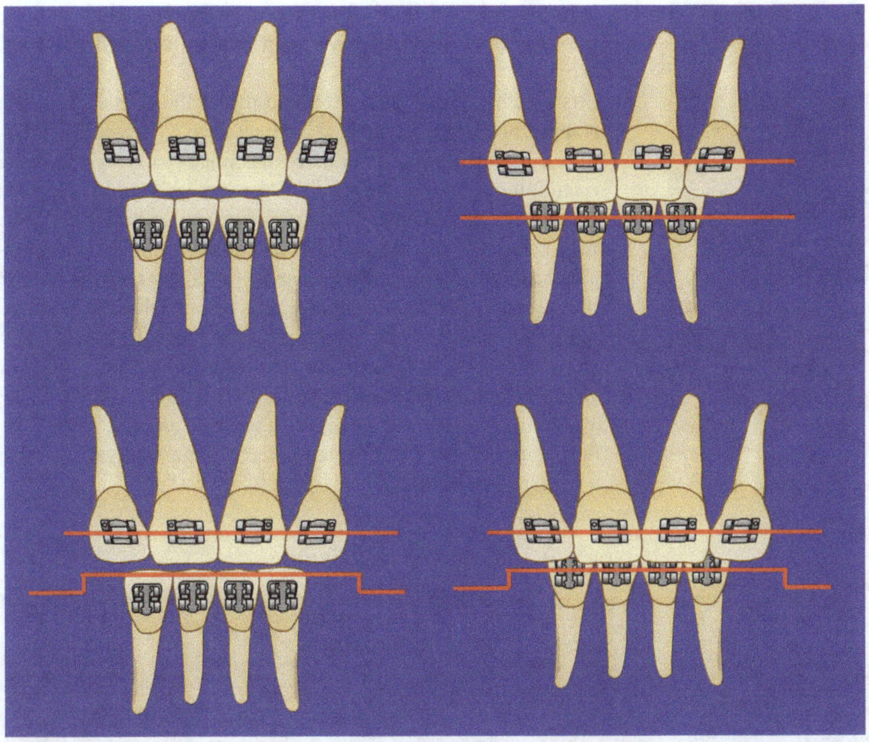

Figure 4.19 Enhancement of anterior open bite closure occurs by: (top left to right) bonding incisors more gingivally than normal and (bottom left to right) placing "steps" in the archwire ("step ups" in the mandibular archwire shown). Note that such techniques are exactly opposite to those used to open dental *deep* bites.

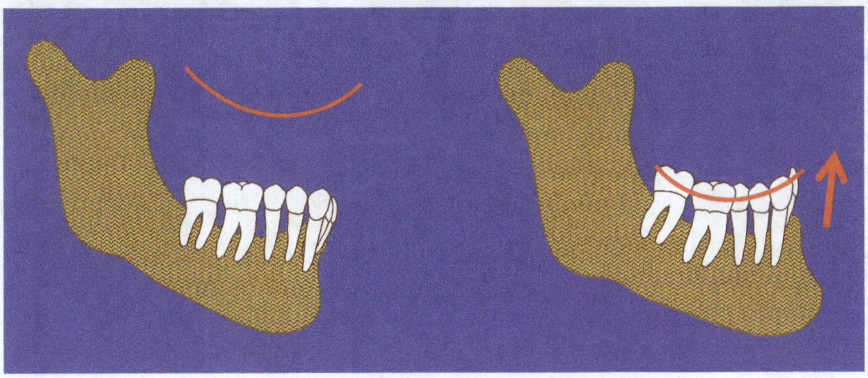

Figure 4.20 Mandibular incisors can be erupted by adding curve of Spee to the archwire.

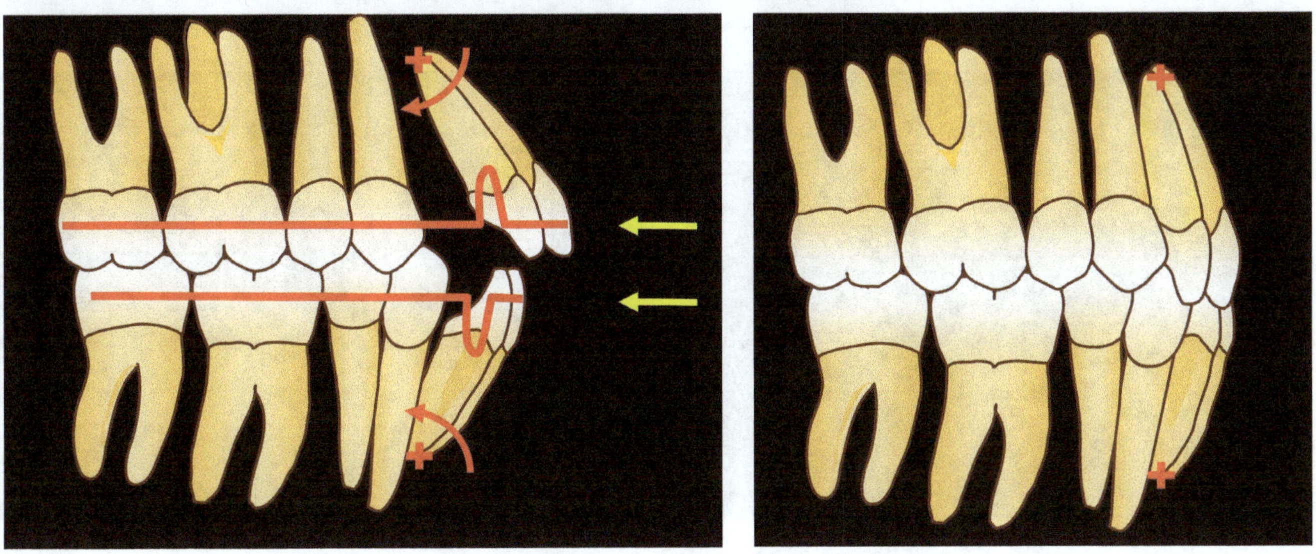

(a) (b)

Figure 4.21 (a, b) Retracting proclined incisors rotates them around their root apicies, thereby erupting them and helping to close the open bite.

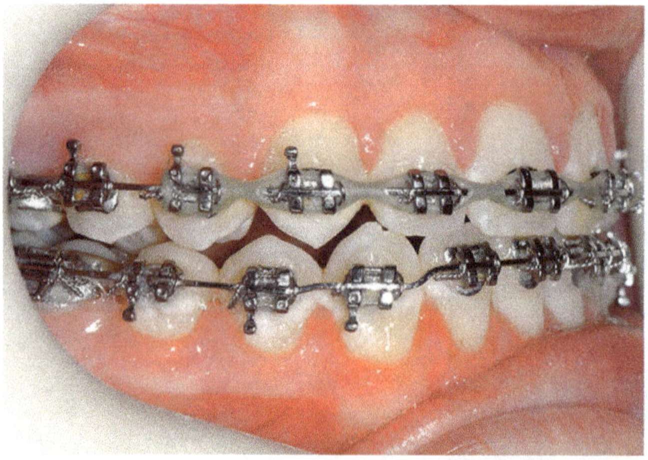

Figure 4.22 Triangle elastics failed to close this isolated open bite.

Q: What are some methods for retaining dental open-bite patients once the anterior teeth have been erupted and OB has been achieved?

A: First, realize that the underlying cause of the dental open bite (tongue posture, digit habit) must have been corrected for retention to be successful. If the habit has not been corrected, then retention of bite closure will fail. Also, realize that forced tooth eruption is probably the least stable of any orthodontic tooth movement. For this reason, *once you have obtained positive overcorrected OB (20–40%), it is important that you keep the patient in braces and the bite closed for months* before debanding. This is referred to as a period of "active retention." That is, give the new alveolar process bone and soft tissues time to form/remodel. Other retention aides can include the following:

1 Maxillary retainer with a hole in anterior palate to attract the tongue away from the anterior teeth (Figure 4.24a)—tongue interpositional habit.

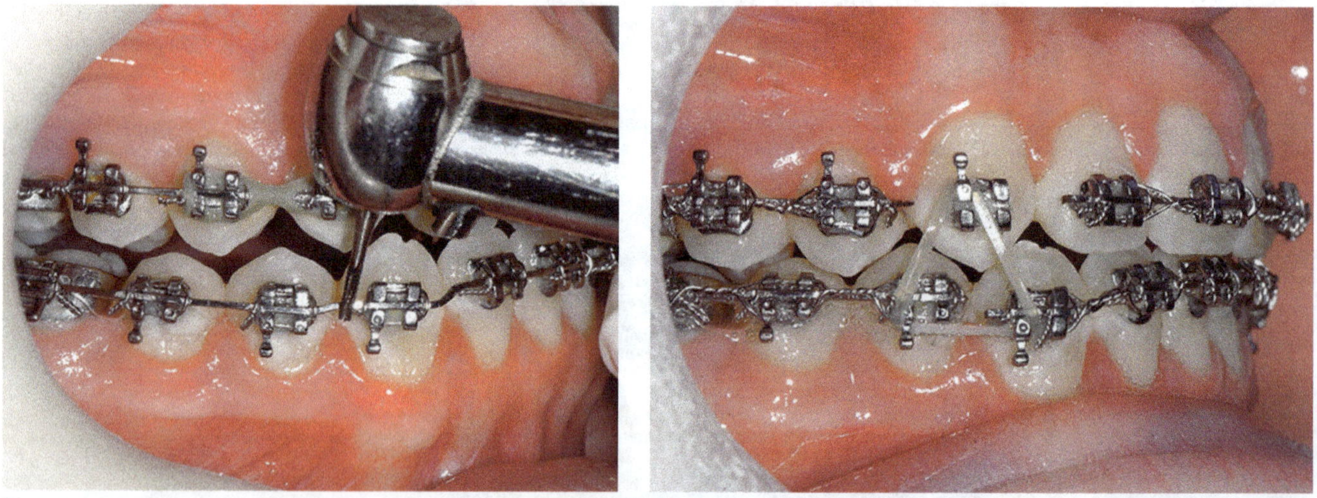

(a) (b)

Figure 4.23 (a, b) The isolated open bite was closed by sectioning the archwires plus triangle elastic wear.

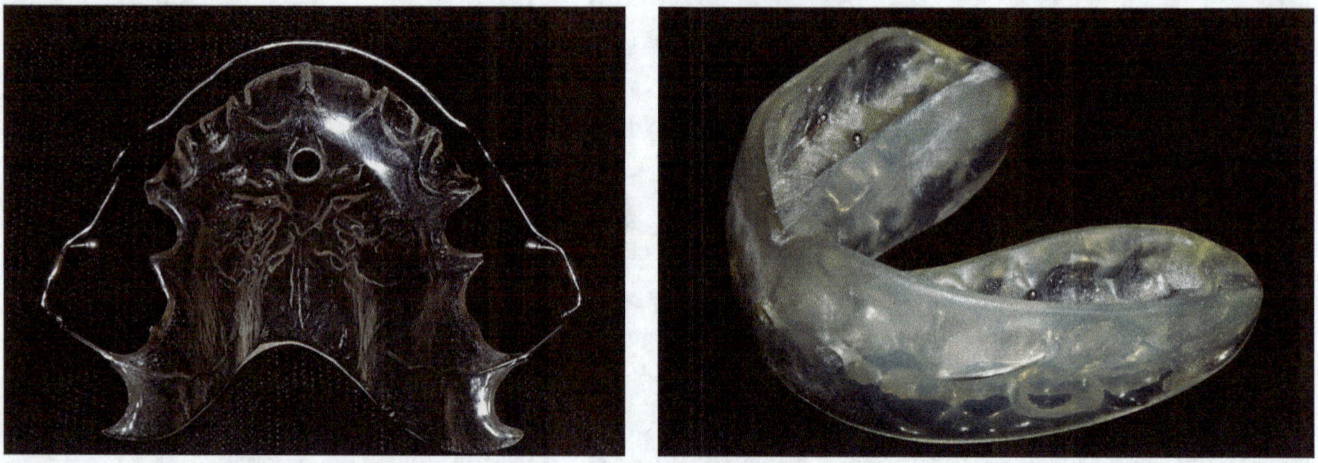

(a) (b)

Figure 4.24 In retention, aides for controlling an anterior interpositional tongue habit include (a) placing a hole in the anterior of the retainer to draw the tongue away from the teeth and (b) wearing a tooth positioner to block the tongue from the anterior teeth.

2 Mandibular retainer with lingual tongue spurs (Figure 4.8b)—tongue interpositional habit.
3 Tooth positioner (Figure 4.24b)—tongue interpositional habit.
4 Continued wear of a thumb guard (Figure 4.7e, f).
5 Placement of small "dots" of tooth-colored composite on the facials of the maxillary and mandibular incisors. The open-bite closure is held with a temporary (vacuum-formed) retainer snapping over these composite dots or with the labial wire of the Hawley retainer wire snapping over these dots. As an example, Figure 4.25a illustrates a skeletal open-bite patient who desired only alignment of her front teeth (compromised treatment—not complete bite closure). After the teeth were aligned (and the open bite slightly closed), composite dots were placed and the patient wore a vacuum-formed maxillary retainer that "snapped" into place over the composite dots to retain the aligned, and mildly erupted, maxillary teeth (Figure 4.25b, c).

Figure 4.26a illustrates an open-bite patient with Down syndrome. The same technique was used to maintain closure of the open bite—but this time with composite dots placed on both the maxillary anterior and mandibular anterior teeth (Figure 4.26b). This technique can be used with Hawley retainers by putting the small composite dots apical to the Hawley's labial bow.

Q: Is anterior open-bite treatment stable?

A: Yes, reasonably stable if the functional habit is corrected. In one long-term (minimum 9 years postretention) study, more than 35% of treated open-bite patients demonstrated a postretention open bite of 3 mm or more. Neither the magnitude of pretreatment open bite, mandibular plane angle, nor any other single parameter of dentofacial form proved to be a reliable predictor of post-treatment stability [25]. In a study of open-bite patients treated with conventional fixed edgewise appliances (plus high-pull headgear for the majority), 40% relapsed from incisor contact following treatment to horizontal incisor overlap with no incisor contact [26]. Finally, a meta-analysis study of open-bite treatment revealed that stability was reasonable (75%) in nonsurgical patients [27].

Q: In summary, what are your "take-home messages" regarding etiology, identification, treatment, and retention of dental anterior open bites?

A: Take-home messages include the following:

- Dental anterior open bites result from inadequate maxillary and mandibular anterior tooth eruption due to functional habits.
- The hallmark of a pure dental anterior bite is an anterior open bite in a patient who is otherwise normal in the vertical dimension.
- Dental anterior open bites are corrected by eliminating the habit and erupting teeth into occlusion.
- Overcorrection (OB 20–40%) should be achieved during treatment, and the correction should be held for some time, before debanding.
- Correction of dental anterior open bites is reasonably stable (if the habit is corrected), but some relapse should be expected.
- Monitor your patient, in retention, for as long as possible. Your patient should be retained for life.

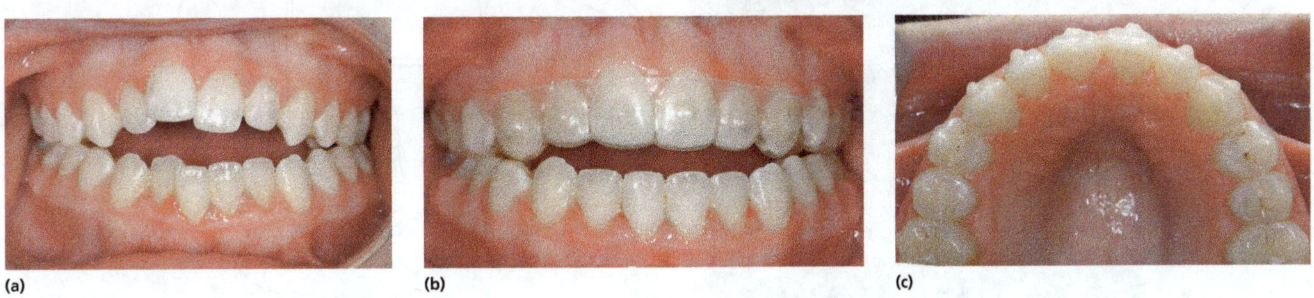

Figure 4.25 Retention aid for a skeletal open bite patient who desired only alignment of her anterior teeth: (a) initial frontal intraoral photograph; (b, c) mild eruption of her maxillary anterior teeth occurred during alignment and was retained using a vacuum-formed retainer. The retainer snapped over small composite "dots" placed on the labial surfaces of her maxillary anterior teeth.

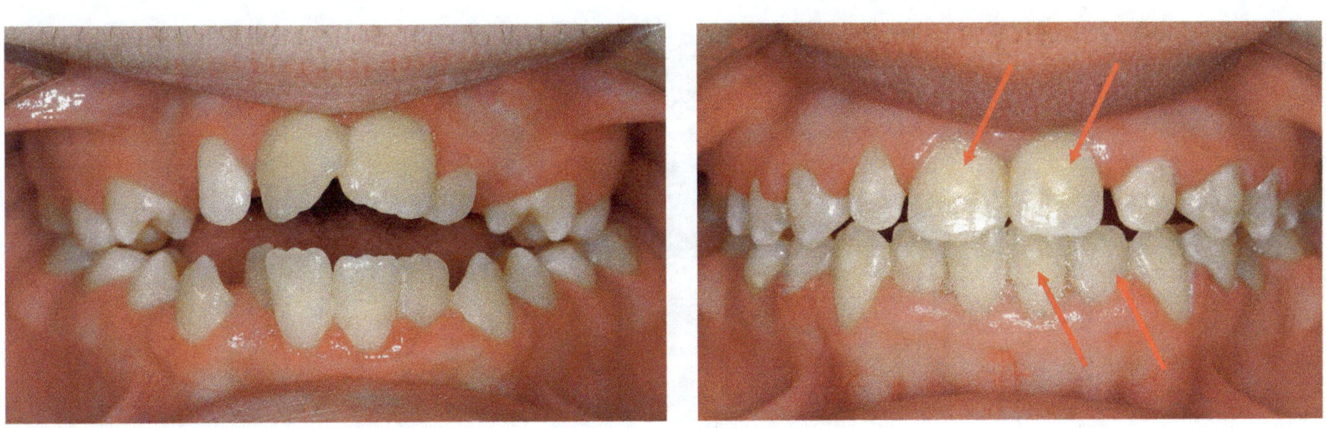

Figure 4.26 (a, b) Composite "dots" placed on the labial surfaces of maxillary and mandibular teeth to retain closure of an anterior open bite. Vacuum-formed retainers snap over these dots during wear.

Case Sasha

Sasha is 28 years old (Figure 4.27) and presents to you with the CC, "I have trouble chewing food with my front teeth—I have a large open bite." PMH: migraines, allergic to Imitrex (anaphylactic shock resulted), currently taking antibiotics for positive TB test but chest X-ray clear. PDH: WRN. TMJs: Sasha complains of pain when chewing gum, eating hard foods for a long time, or when she has her mouth open for a long time. She says symptoms are relieved if she just closes her mouth and stops chewing. You examine her and note ADD with reduction both joints and crepitus both TMJs. History and examination reveal no other signs or symptoms. She is without periodontal problems, and there is not a detectable CR–CO shift.

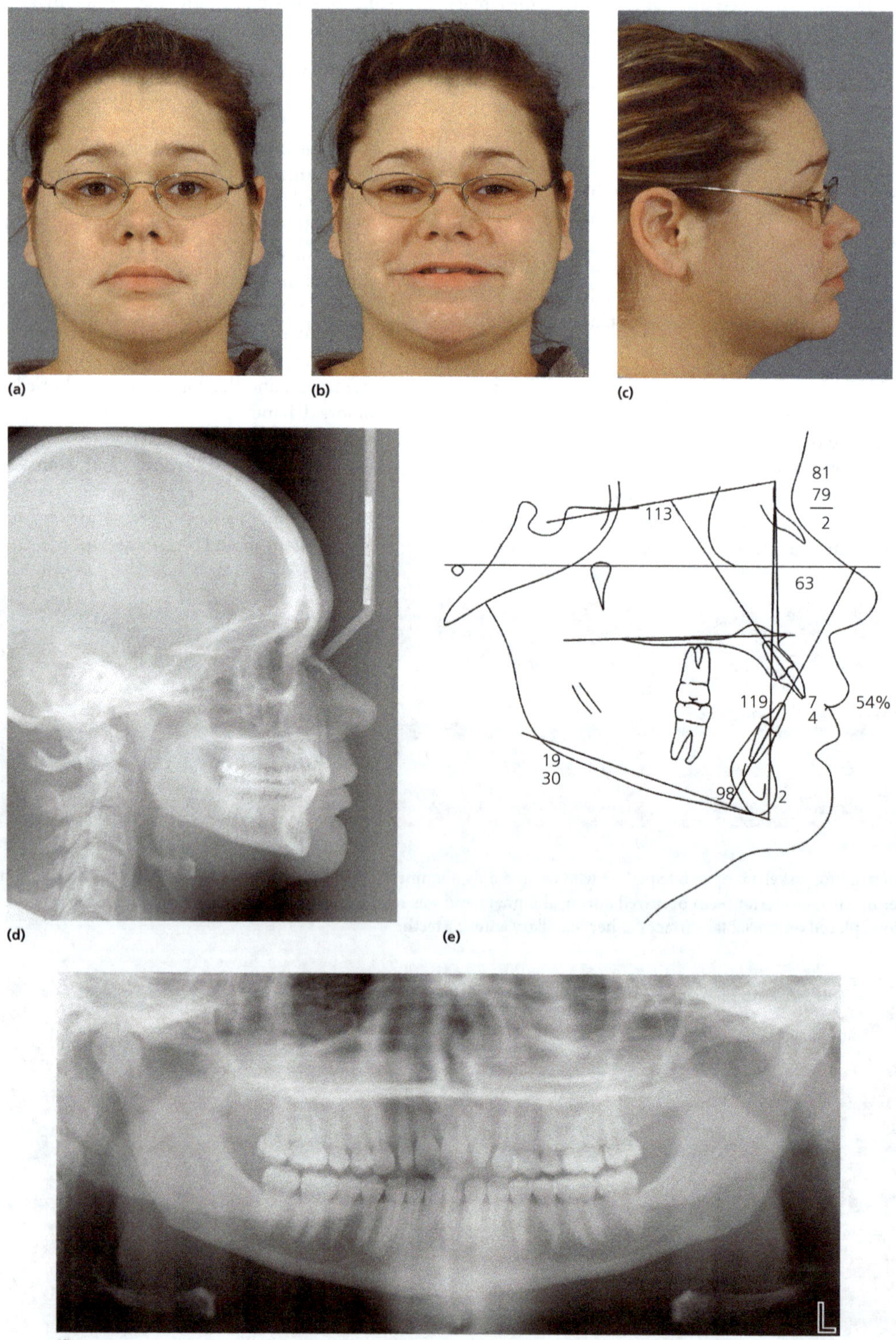

Figure 4.27 Initial records of Sasha: (a–c) initial facial photographs, (d) lateral cephalograph, (e) cephalometric tracing, (f) pantomograph, and (g–k) intraoral photographs.

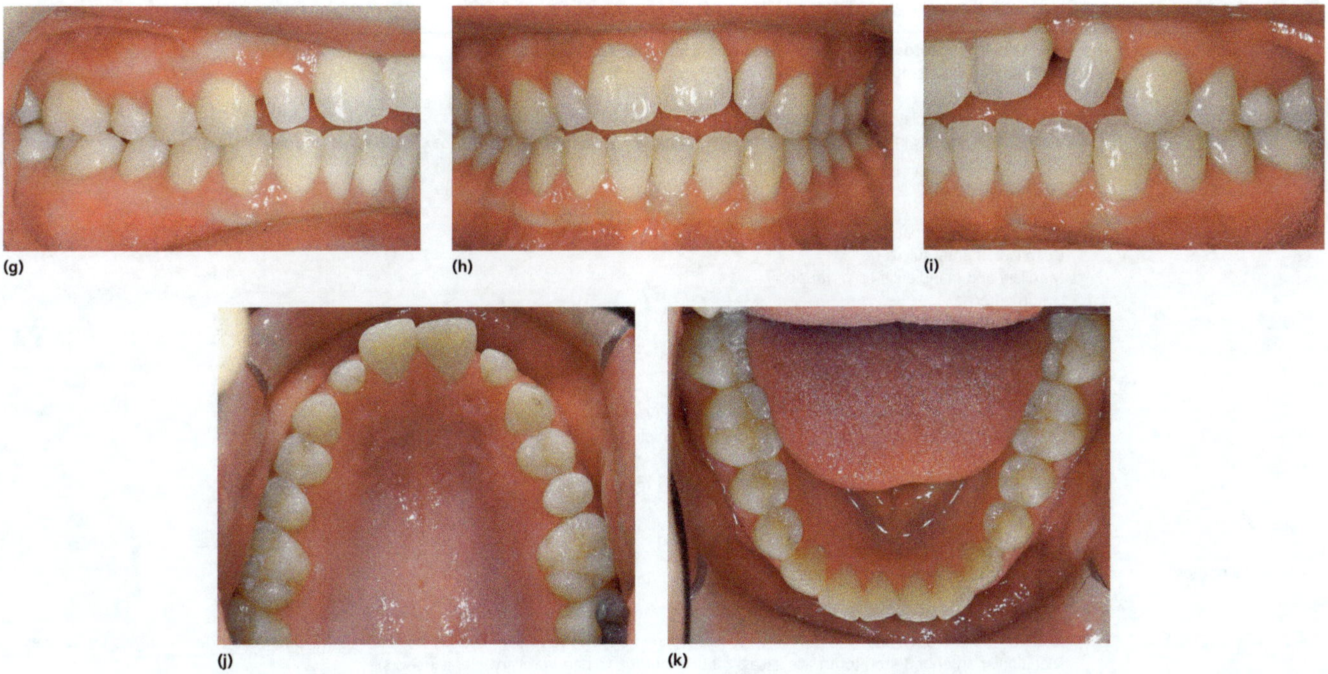

Figure 4.27 (Continued)

Q: List Sasha's diagnostic findings/problems. What is your diagnosis?

A: See Table 4.1

Q: With Sasha's TMJ signs and symptoms, would you attempt orthodontic treatment now? Or, would you monitor her for 6–12 months before starting treatment? Or, would you advise her against ever undergoing orthodontic treatment? Or, would you tell her that orthodontic treatment will alleviate her TMJ symptoms?

A: Although you can always monitor a patient with TMD, with Sasha's current signs and symptoms, *you can initiate orthodontic treatment now*. Fifty percent of the healthy, nonpatient population has joint sounds or deviation upon opening [28]. The "popping" of her TMJs is not of current concern, and progression of a TMJ click (displaced disk with reduction) to a more serious nonreducing ("locking") disk is uncommon [29]. Although nothing radiographically abnormal can be observed in her condylar heads (i.e., irregular borders, osteophytes, and degeneration), her crepitus could indicate bone-to-bone contact and should be monitored closely. You should confirm (and Sasha denies) any generalized musculoskeletal problems. You should confirm (and Sasha denies) pain in her jaw musculature, which could signify nocturnal bruxism. Recommendations are as follows:

1. Keep her appointments short so her mouth is not open for too long.
2. Advise her not to chew gum or hard foods for long periods of time (which is when she reports pain).
3. Do not advise her that orthodontic treatment will alleviate her TMJ symptoms.
4. Do advise her that her symptoms could worsen, stay the same, or improve.
5. Do have her inform you if symptoms worsen.

Q: In terms of Sasha's open bite, what else should you look for or what questions should you ask her?

A: If this is a dental (functional) open bite, identify the following:

- Does she have an interpositional tongue habit? At least from the intraoral views of Figure 4.27g–i, it would appear that she does not. But, she could have retracted her tongue for the intra-oral photos. Ask her to close her eyes while you speak with your assistant. Then, as you ask her to open her eyes (to distract her), gently and quickly pull her lower lip forward slightly. You do not observe an interpositional tongue habit.
- Does the patient have a thumb (or other digit) habit? Sasha answers affirmatively—she does. When does it occur? She responds that the habit occurs unconsciously, when sleeping at night, not consciously, during the day. She shows you her right thumb, which appears red and irritated.
- Ask her if she regularly bites her lip. She states that she does not. She denies any other habits.
- Ask Sasha how long she has had the open bite and look at her condyles on the panoramic image to confirm that the mandible is not rotating down and back following condylar degeneration, creating an open bite. In this case, Sasha says that the open bite has existed since she was young. The condylar heads appear normal (Figure 4.27f).
- Last, check for temporary anterior open bites occurring while permanent teeth are erupting (not the case here), ankylosis of anterior teeth which prevents their complete eruption into occlusion (anything is possible, but not likely here since all four maxillary incisors would be affected), and lack of space for complete tooth eruption (teeth blocked out, not the case here).

Q: What are Sasha's dental open-bite features? Skeletal open-bite features? Would you classify Sasha as a dental open bite, a skeletal open bite, or a combination of both? What is the etiology of her open bite?

A: Her *dental* open-bite features include: lip competence, skeletal LAFH WRN (LAFH/TAFH = 54%, FMA = 19°, SNMP = 29°, maxillary molar apicies appearing at or near the palatal plane), anterior 1–3 mm open bite with maxillary incisors stepped up

Table 4.1 Diagnostic findings and problem list for Sasha.

Full face and profile	**Frontal view (photos should be made without glasses, earrings, etc.)**
	LAFH slightly long (soft tissue Glabella–Subnasale < Subnasale–soft tissue Menton)
	UDML: WRN
	Maxillary incisal display absent in relaxed lip (Figure 4.27D)
	Inadequate maxillary incisal display in posed smile (maxillary vermillion is incisal to maxillary gingival margin)
	Lip competence
	Profile view
	Straight profile
	Obtuse lip–chin–throat angle
	Deep labiomental sulcus
	Maxillary and mandibular lip protrusion
	Upturned nose
Ceph analysis	**Skeletal**
	Maxilla and mandible anteroposterior positions WRN
	LAFH/TAFH = 54% (WRN)
	Flat MPA (FMA = 19°; SNMP = 30°)
	Maxillary molar apicies appear at or near palatal plane (WRN)
	Marked soft tissue thickness over effective bony Pogonion
	Dental
	Proclined maxillary incisors (maxillary incisors to SN of 113°)
	Mildly proclined mandibular incisors (FMIA = 63°)
Radiographs	Missing third molars
	Maxillary peg lateral incisors
Intraoral photos and models	Angle Class II division 1 subdivision right
	Iowa Classification: II (2) II (1) II (1) I
	OJ = 5 mm
	Anterior 1–3 mm open bite with maxillary incisors stepped up relative to the maxillary posterior teeth. Open bite extends only to the canines
	Mandibular anterior Bolton tooth size excess = 3.06 mm (due to peg maxillary lateral incisors)
	UTSALD: spacing due to peg laterals
	LTSALD: ~ −3 mm mild mandibular anterior crowding
	Dental arches appear symmetric
	Maxillary left second premolar has a small crown
Other	Thin attached tissue maxillary left first premolar
	Small maxillary lateral incisors
	ADD with reduction bilateral TMJs; crepitus bilateral TMJs
Diagnosis	Angle Class II division 1 subdivision right malocclusion
	Dental anterior open bite

Table 4.2 Primary problems list for Sasha.

AP	II (2) II (1) II (1) I skeletal relationships WRN
Vertical	1–3 mm anterior dental (functional) open bite
Transverse	—
Other	Maxillary peg lateral incisors

relative to the maxillary posterior teeth, open bite extends only to the canines, and a thumb habit. Her only *skeletal* open-bite feature is a slightly long soft tissue LAFH (soft tissue Glabella–Subnasale < Subnasale–soft tissue Menton). We therefore conclude Sasha has an overall *normal* facial skeleton with an open bite resulting from a thumb habit. Sasha is a *dental* open bite.

Q: What is your diagnosis?

A: Angle Class II division 1 subdivision right malocclusion (mild) with dental anterior open bite.

Q: What are your treatment goals for Sasha?

A: Correct her thumb habit. Achieve a Class I canine/molar relationship, minimal OJ, and *overcorrection* of OB (20–40%). Do not increase her (normal) LAFH.

Q: What are Sasha's *primary* problems in each dimension that you must stay focused on throughout treatment?

A: Sasha does not have apical base (skeletal) discrepancies in any dimension. But she does have problems in two dimensions (Table 4.2).

Q: Why is a dental open bite generally less difficult to treat than a skeletal open bite?

A: Because a dental open bite is a dental problem (Figure 4.28), not a skeletal (growth) problem. This is not to say that closure of a dental open bite is easy. The habits that cause dental open bites (prevent maxillary and mandibular anterior teeth from erupting) are generally well established and can be very difficult to correct. It is just that the excessive vertical growth of a skeletal open bite can be even more difficult to treat. Furthermore, skeletal open-bite patients can present as a combination of skeletal *and* dental open bite.

Q: What principles should you follow in treating a dental open bite?

A: The habit causing the open bite must be removed before the anterior teeth can erupt into occlusion. If the anterior tongue posture habit/digit habit/lip biting habit is not eliminated, the anterior teeth will not come together or, if brought together forcefully, will not stay together. A dental open bite is corrected with orthodontics by erupting the maxillary and mandibular anterior teeth (Figure 4.29, right) into a proper OB (Figure 4.29, left). But, orthodontically closing a functional open bite without addressing the habit will likely end in relapse during retention.

Q: How can the Class II (2 mm) right molar relationship be addressed?

A: The right Class II molar relationship should be amenable to correction with Class II elastics. Since her FMIA is only mildly proclined (63°; ideal 65–68°), the slight increase in incisor proclination with unilateral Class II elastic wear should be acceptable. Other options include asymmetric right headgear wear, right Class II spring, or right maxillary TADs to make the 2 mm correction.

Q: Would you discuss surgical treatment options with Sasha?

A: No. Her open bite is a dental problem.

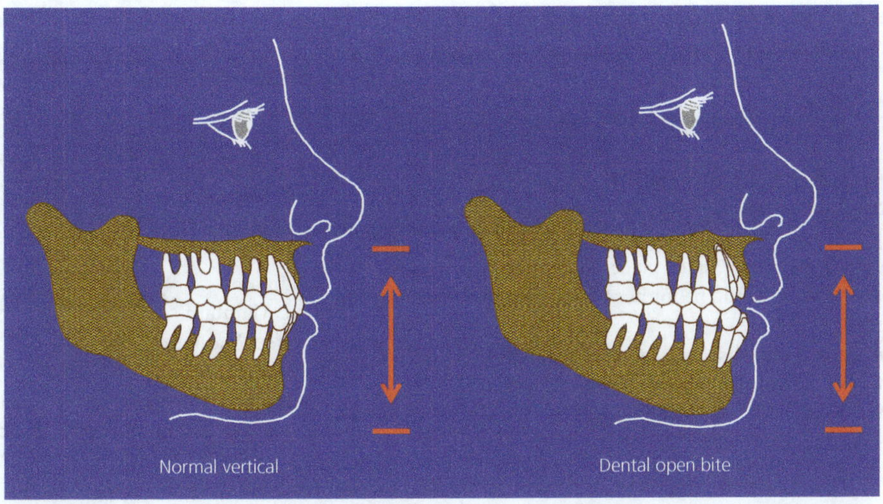

Figure 4.28 Dental open-bite patients present with normal vertical facial growth.

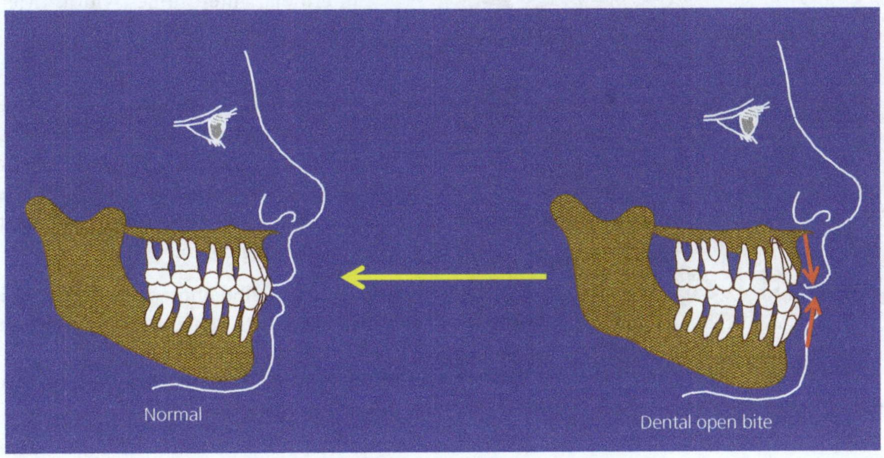

Figure 4.29 Once the habit is eliminated, the dental open bite is closed by erupting anterior teeth.

Q: What unknowns do you face during treatment? Should you reduce any unknowns before establishing your final treatment plan or doing something irreversible?

A: Cooperation, hygiene, and a possible hidden CR–CO shift are unknowns. But, the primary unknowns you face are whether her thumb-sucking habit can be eliminated and whether her TMJ symptoms will worsen. If her thumb habit can be eliminated, orthodontic treatment should be straightforward. If her thumb habit cannot be eliminated, correction and maintenance of bite closure will be problematic. So, try to *correct her thumb habit before proceeding with any other treatment*.

Q: If Sasha has a TMD flare-up during treatment, how would you handle it?

A: Words from an old scout: Be prepared. First, if she presents with heightened TMD symptoms, repeat your thorough TMJ examination of her. Be especially sure to inquire about any recent possible acute etiologies (trauma, overuse, change in medical status, etc.). The *hallmark of your treatment should be conservative therapy, conservative therapy, conservative therapy* including rest through voluntary limitation of function, habit awareness and modification, physiotherapy, and the use of nonsteroidal anti-inflammatory medications. If she is waking up in the morning with sore chewing muscles, she could be bruxing. If that is the case, consider placing her on a flat plane hard interocclusal splint (nightguard). If conservative therapy does not alleviate her symptoms, use more conservative therapy. Got the idea? If you feel the need to seek consultation with a rheumatologist or surgeon, then by all means do so. Only if she progresses to a state of debilitating pain or function would we recommend surgical intercession—and that beginning with only arthrocentisis. In fact, it has been suggested that arthrocentisis (needle puncture of the superior joint space, simple irrigation, or lavage with lactated ringer's solution, with or without intra-articular corticosteroids/morphine) may be as effective as arthroscopic lavage [30].

Q: Would you proceed with nonextraction treatment? Would you consider extraction of anterior or posterior teeth?

A: Considering the fact that Sasha's concern is her dental (functional) open bite, that she has spacing/peg laterals in the maxillary arch, and only mild crowding/mild proclination in the mandibular arch—it would be prudent to begin with nonextraction treatment. Even if you are considering extractions, you could start by leveling/aligning her arches, then re-evaluate for extractions later (reduce unknowns, see how she looks). An argument could be made for extracting a mandibular incisor. Why? Mandibular incisor extraction would permit elimination of the mandibular anterior crowding, permit uprighting of the mildly proclined mandibular incisors, and reduce the need for maxillary peg lateral incisor buildups. On the other hand, it would be difficult to formulate a compelling argument for premolar extractions.

Q: After considering all options, what specific treatment do you recommend?

A: Start by addressing Sasha's thumb habit without any other treatment. Since the habit occurs when sleeping, it is not a matter of convincing Sasha of the need to stop the habit. She wants to stop. Instead, fabricate and place a thumb crib (Figure 4.30). Another option would be for her to wear a thumb guard when sleeping.

Sasha wore the appliance for 6 months. By that time, she believed she had stopped the habit (the soft tissue of her thumb appeared normal). Also, her TMJ complaints were unchanged. A decision was made to pursue nonextraction treatment.

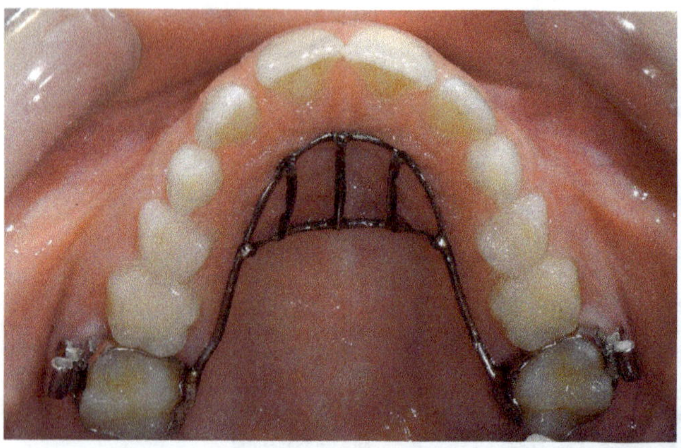

Figure 4.30 Thumb crib similar to Sasha's.

Q: What are the specific objectives of treatment for the maxilla, mandible, maxillary dentition, and mandibular dentition in all three planes of space?

A: Specific objectives of treatment for Sasha are as follows:

Maxilla
- AP: Maintain.
- Vertical: Maintain.
- Transverse: Maintain.

Mandible
- AP: Maintain.
- Vertical: Maintain.
- Transverse: Maintain.

Maxillary dentition
- AP: Retract molars and canines. Upright incisors.
- Vertical: Maintain molar. Extrude incisors.
- Intermolar width: Maintain.

Mandibular dentition
- AP: Protract molars and canines. Maintain incisor.
- Vertical: Maintain molar. Maintain incisor.
- Intermolar/Intercanine width: Maintain intermolar and intercanine widths.

Q: How did Sasha's treatment proceed?

A: Fixed orthodontic appliances were placed on all of Sasha's teeth along with light arch wires, arches were leveled and aligned, OJ eliminated, mild Class II molar relationship corrected using Class II elastics, residual maxillary anterior spaces distributed as per direction of the restorative dentist, finishing achieved, and debanding completed.

Q: Deband intraoral photos are shown in Figure 4.31. Final records after composite veneers were placed are shown in Figure 4.32. What changes do you note?

A: Observations include the following:

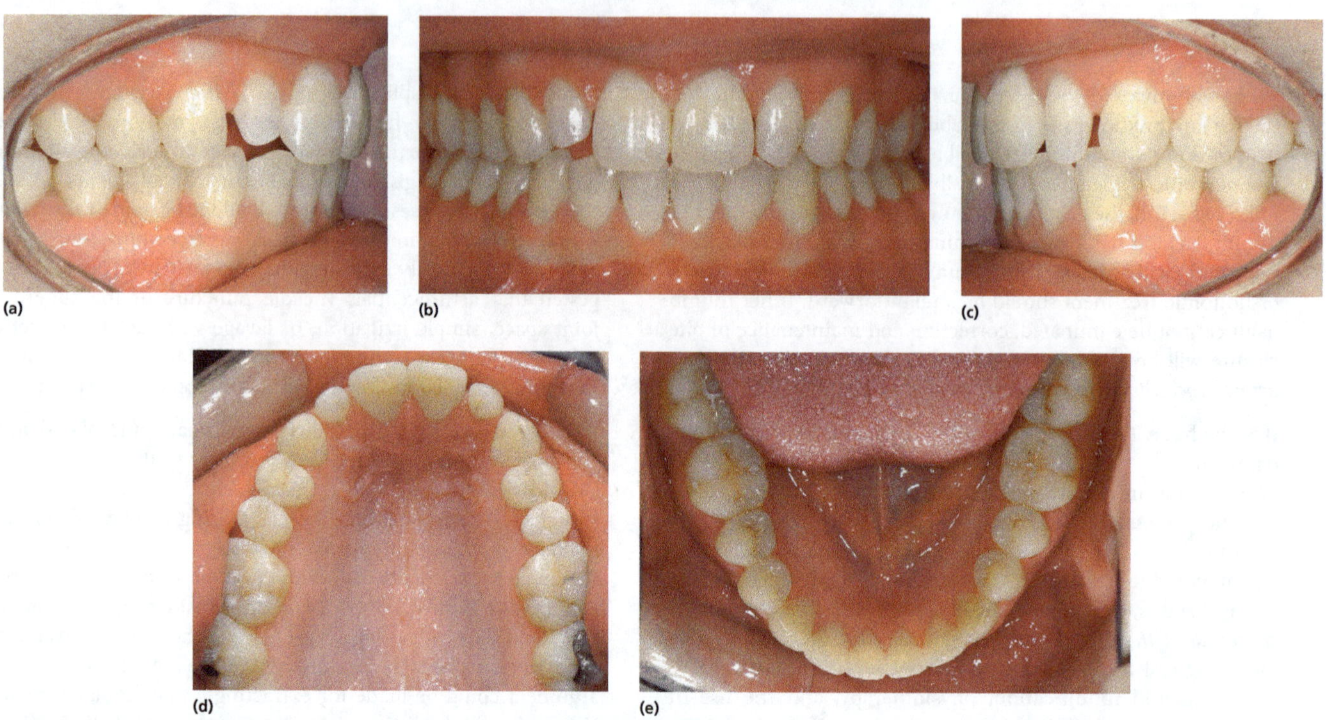

(a) (b) (c) (d) (e)

Figure 4.31 (a–e) Deband intra-oral photos of Sasha.

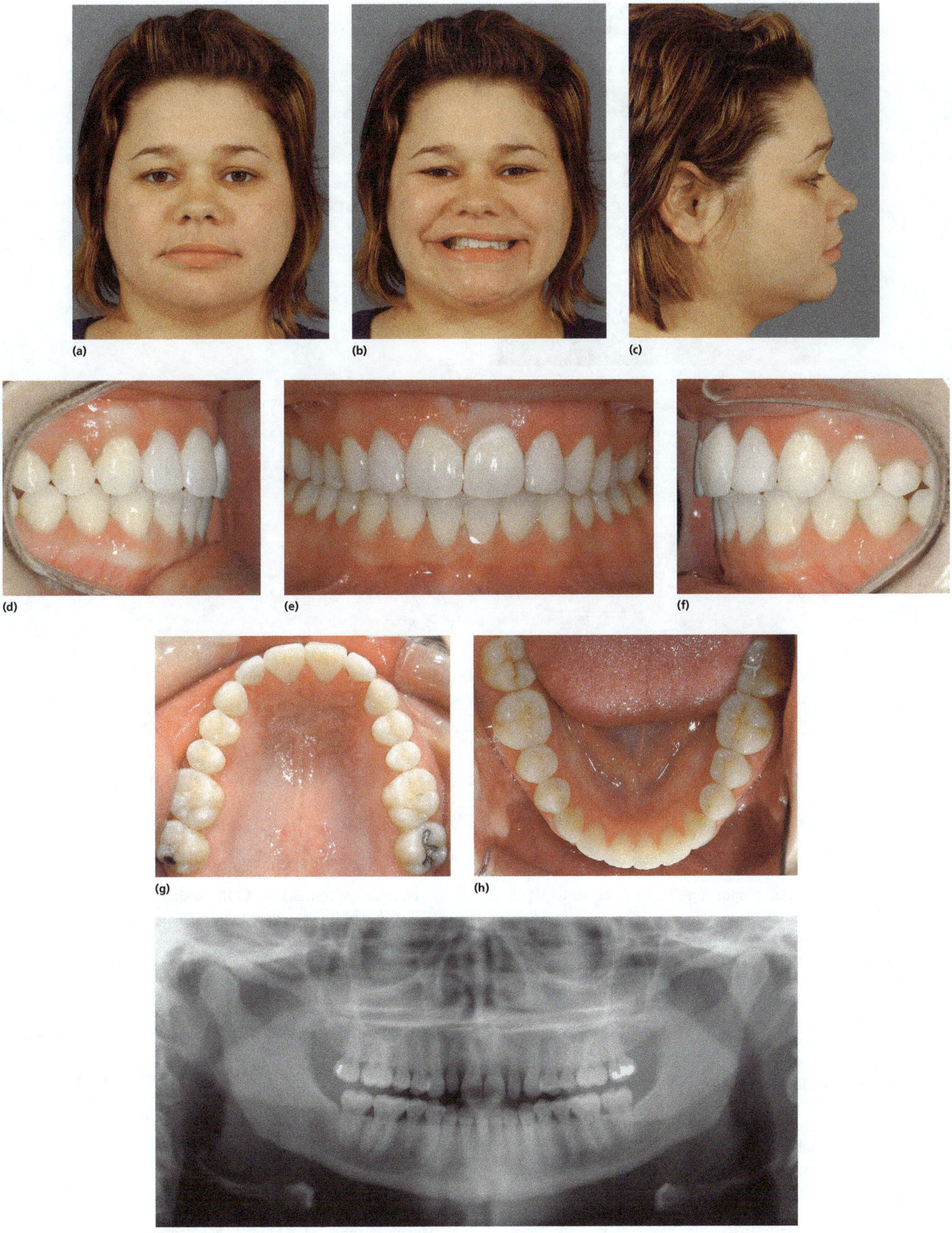

Figure 4.32 (a–l) Final records for Sasha.

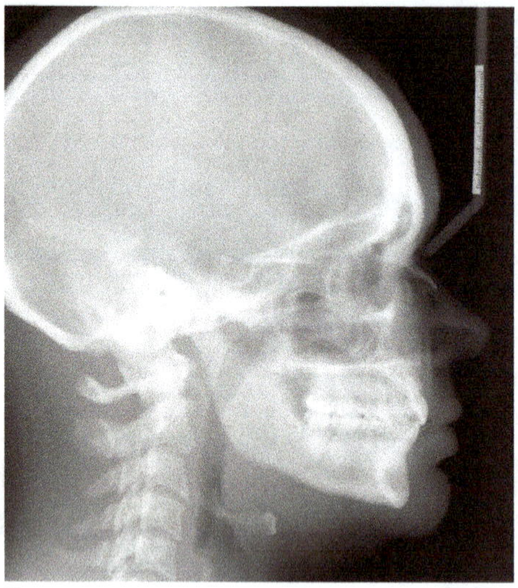

(j)

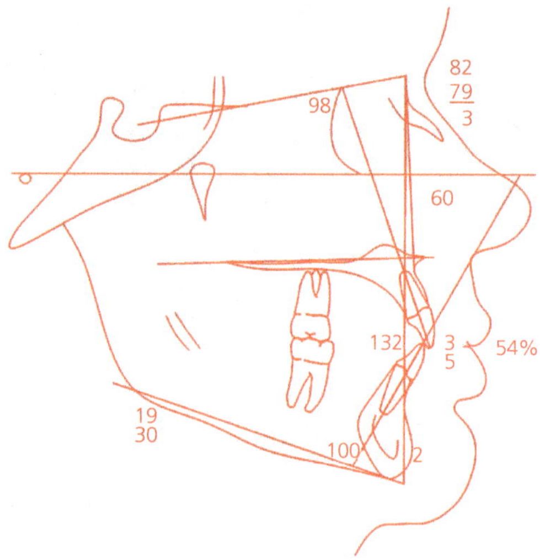

(k)

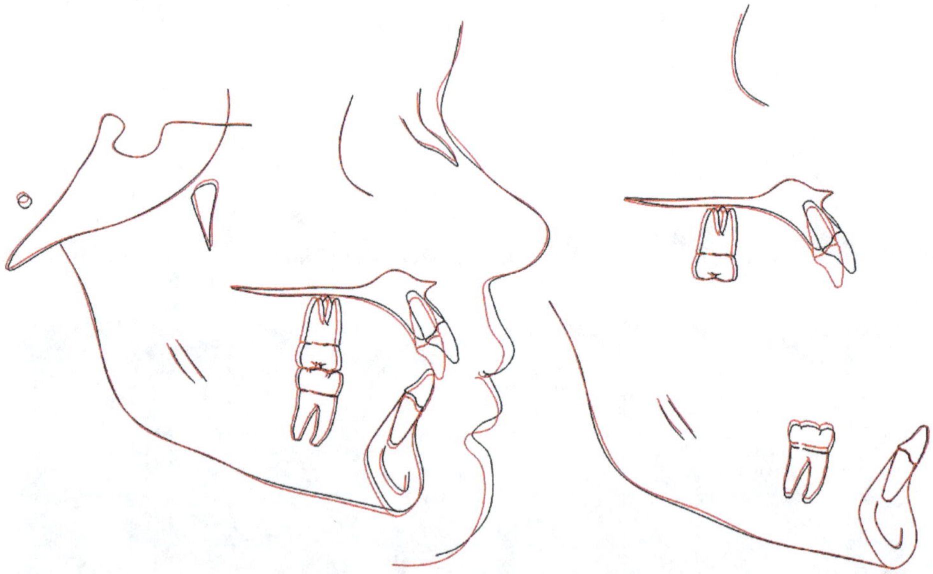

(l)

Figure 4.32 (Continued)

- No dramatic facial proportion changes—as anticipated, as desired.
- Her posed smile incisal display increased. She felt an enhanced level of self-confidence, and her smile was more animated.
- Sasha's smile is asymmetric due to heightened smiling musculature activity on the right side (Figure 4.32b).
- Cephalometrically (Figure 4.32l), the only dramatic change was Sasha's open-bite closure as a result of her maxillary incisors erupting and *retracting/rotating around their apicies*.
- Her mandibular molars erupted slightly (Class II elastic effect?), rotating her mandibular down and back very slightly. This outcome was in keeping with our goal of not changing Sasha's (normal) LAFH.
- Her maxillary lip appears to have moved backward—following her maxillary incisor retraction.
- Intraorally, her open bite was closed, but only to a minimal OB of approximately 10%.
- A Class I canine occlusion was obtained with coincident midlines.
- Following elimination of OJ, maxillary anterior spaces were distributed by centering the maxillary lateral incisors in the space between the central incisors and canines (Figure 4.31d). This was done under the guidance of the restorative dentist in preparation for composite veneers.

Q: Note that (Figure 4.32d, f) Sasha's second premolars are not ideally positioned, but demonstrate "Class II windows" at their distal. Why?

A: Her maxillary second premolars, especially the left maxillary second premolar, appear to be small (Figures 4.31d and 4.32g). In other words, with a posterior tooth size discrepancy due to small maxillary second premolars, the canines could be Class I but the maxillary second premolars and molars could be shifted forward toward Class II.

Q: How would you retain this patient?

A: Maxillary and mandibular Hawley retainers were worn. Another suggestion would be to place small "dots" of composite on the facials of the maxillary and mandibular incisors to maintain overbite—the OB would then be held with the temporary (vacuum-formed) retainers snapping over these composite dots or with the labial bows of the Hawley retainers snapping over these dots. Sasha must be mindful that her thumb habit does not return. If it does, she can wear some form of thumb guard to prevent it. Or, a thumb crib could be embedded in the maxillary Hawley retainer.

Q: What are the "take-home" messages from Sasha's treatment?
A: Take-home messages include the following:

- Sasha had an overall *normal* facial skeleton with an open bite resulting from a thumb habit. Her only skeletal open-bite feature was a slightly long soft tissue LAFH seen in the frontal photograph. But, her skeletal LAFH was normal (54%). Sasha had a pure *dental* open bite. Dental open bites result from abnormal habits preventing teeth from erupting, not from aberrant jaw growth or degeneration of the condyle.
- The dental open-bite habit must be corrected to achieve orthodontic success and to maintain the correction. Since Sasha's habit occurred while sleeping at night, a psychological approach to correcting it would not work. Instead, she was placed on a palatal thumb crib for 6 months (no additional treatment). By that time, she claimed the habit was eliminated. Her thumb habit must be monitored in retention.
- Following habit cessation, orthodontic correction of a dental open bite results from eruption of anterior teeth. In Sasha's case, her open bite was corrected by eruption of her maxillary incisors, which included uprighting them around their apicies. Sasha was a *classic* example illustrating bite closing as incisors retract/rotate around their apicies (Figure 4.32l).
- Principle: To help close an open bite, *upright*/rotate incisors about their apicies. To help open a deep bite, *procline*/rotate incisors about their apicies.
- Sasha was finished to a minimum OB (10%). Ideally, she would have been treated to an excess overbite (20–40% OB) in anticipation of some relapse.
- A screening TMJ examination must be completed on every orthodontic patient. A *thorough* examination and evaluation is warranted for those patients with a current, or past history, of joint problems. The decision if, and of when, to treat a TMD patient with orthodontics is based on this evaluation and is made in consultation with other specialists, including rheumatologists, oral surgeons, radiologists, and the referring dentist. Sasha's TMJ complaints did not change during treatment, and we were not surprised. Temporomandibular disorders are often self-limiting and remitting [31]. But, you must be prepared to deal with them, if they do worsen.

Case Derrick

Derrick is a 14-year 8-month-old male (Figure 4.33, records made in centric occlusion / maximum intercuspation) who transfers to your practice with the chief complaint, "I need braces for my open bite." He had been followed by another orthodontist who advised waiting until growth cessation and then proceeding with orthognathic surgery. Derrick and his parents declined surgery. His PMH, PDH, and TMJ evaluation are WRN. He is without periodontal problems, and there is a CR–CO shift of 2 mm anteriorly and 2.5 mm left.

Q: List diagnostic findings/problems. What is your diagnosis?
A: See Table 4.3

Q: As noted earlier, Derrick's records were made in CO. What changes do you anticipate when his CR-CO shift (2 mm anteriorly and 2.5 mm left) is removed?
A: If the magnitude of his shift is accurate, Derrick could become Class II at the molars (he is Class III by 1 mm now), and in less of a bilateral cross bite.

Q: In terms of his open bite, what else should you look for or what questions should you ask Derrick and his parents?
A: Ask Derrick if he has a thumb- or digit-sucking habit. He denies this. Look to see if he has a tongue interposition habit (Figure 4.33h–j, it appears as though he does). Your examination reveals the *presence of an anterior tongue interposition habit,* which alone could explain his anterior open bite. Ask Derrick and his parents if they have noticed his open bite. They respond that he has always had it, and it seems to have gotten worse with growth. They say this is the reason why the other orthodontist wanted him to wait until growth was complete to have surgery. Confirm on Derrick's panoramic film (Figure 4.33f) that degeneration of the mandibular condyles is not occurring. If

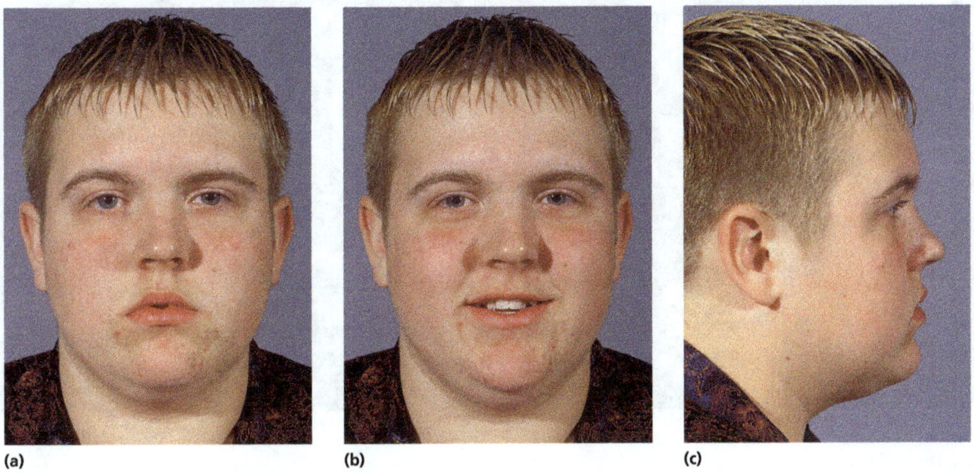

Figure 4.33 Initial records of Derrick: (a–c) initial facial photographs, (d) lateral cephalograph, (e) cephalometric tracing, (f) pantomograph, (g) complete mouth series of dental radiographs, (h–l) intraoral photographs, (m–q) model photographs, and (r, s) separated model views.

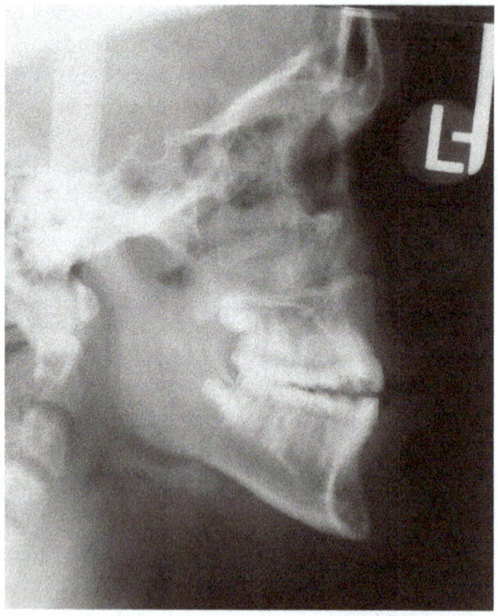

(d)

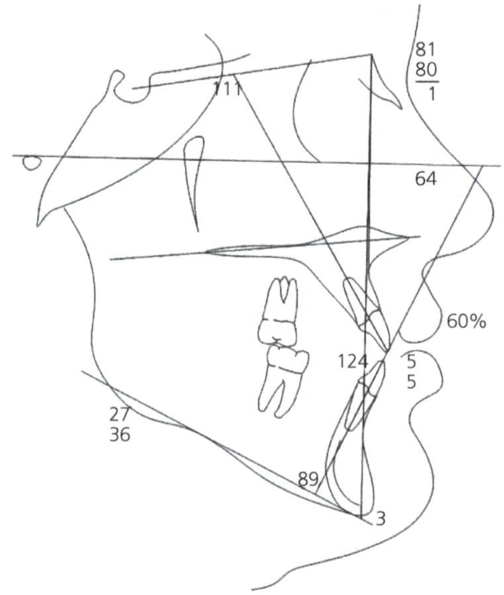

(e)

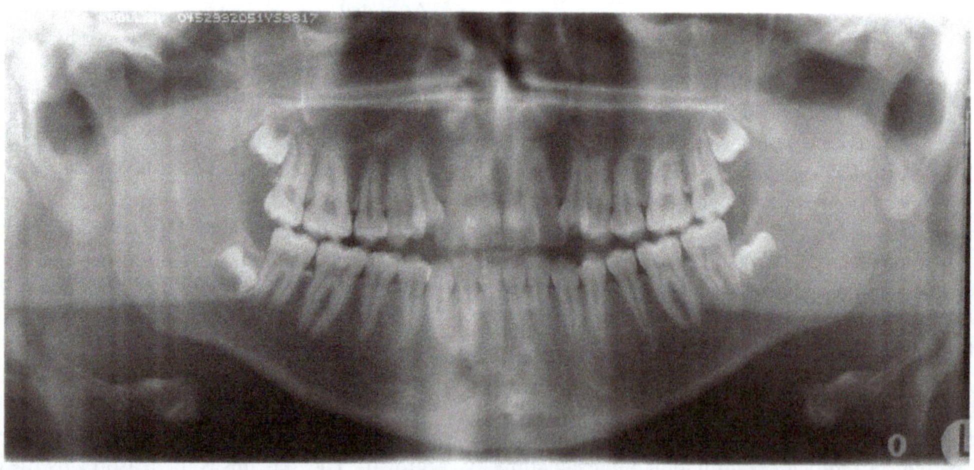

(f)

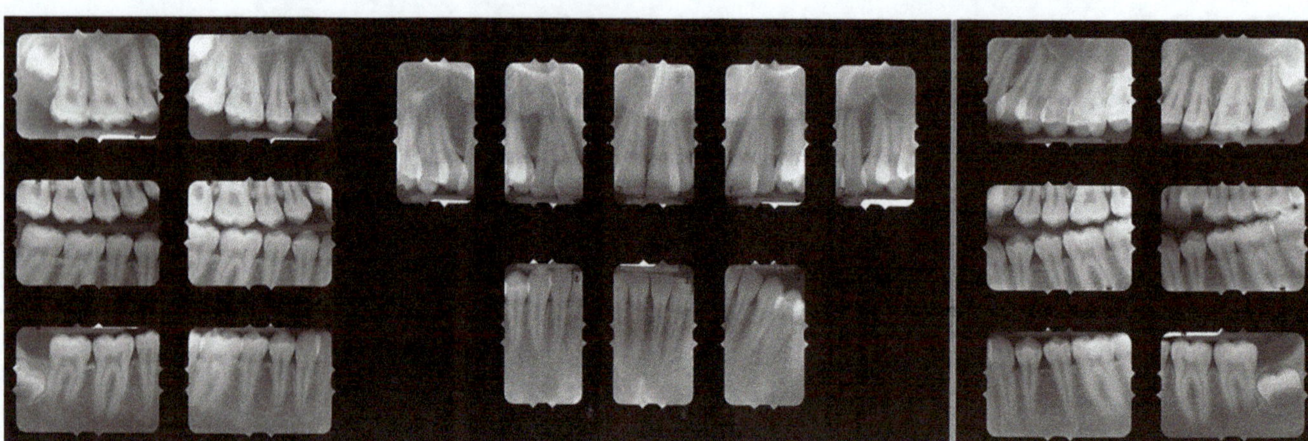

(g)

Figure 4.33 (Continued)

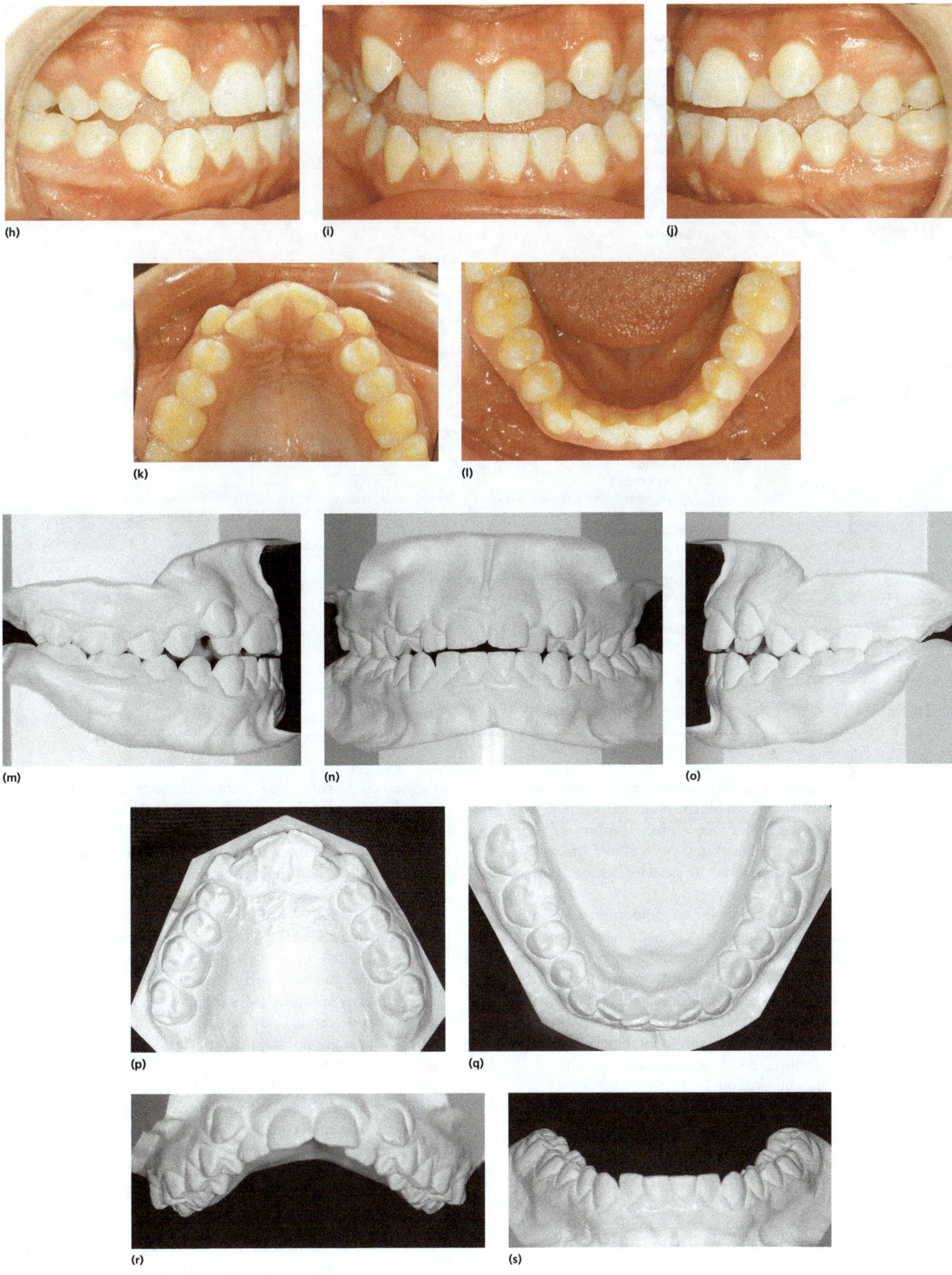

(h) (i) (j) (k) (l) (m) (n) (o) (p) (q) (r) (s)

Figure 4.33 (Continued)

Table 4.3 Diagnostic findings and problem list for Derrick.

Full face and profile	**Frontal view**
	Slight chin deviation to left
	LAFH long (soft tissue Glabella–Subnasale < Subnasale–soft tissue Menton)
	2 mm interlabial gap (limited laterally only to below the philtrum)
	Incisal display in relaxed lip position approximately 2 mm
	UDML WRN
	Profile view
	Relatively straight profile
	Tipped up nose
	Obtuse lip–chin–throat angle
	Mild paranasal flatness
	Mildly deep labiomental sulcus
Ceph analysis	**Skeletal**
	ANB = 1°
	LLAFH (LAFH/TAFH = 60%)
	FMA: WRN (27°) and SNMP: WRN (36°)
	Posterior palatal plane tipped down
	Maxillary molar apicies erupted below palatal plane
	Marked adenoid hyperplasia
	Marked soft tissue thickness over effective bony pogonion
	Dental
	Maxillary dental protrusion
Radiographs	Developing third molars
	Permanent dentition
Intraoral photos and models	Angle Class III in centric occlusion
	Iowa Classification: III (1) II (2–3) II (1–2) III (1) in centric occlusion
	OJ = 0 mm to −3 mm
	Anterior cross bite
	Anterior 2 mm open bite with maxillary incisors stepped up relative to the maxillary posterior teeth
	COS ~2 mm
	left posterior cross bite
	First molar intermolar widths: Mx 52.10 mm (between palatal cusps); Mn 56.64 mm (between central fossae)—a deficiency of 4.5 mm.
	Transverse compensations (buccal maxillary posterior crown torque, lingual mandibular posterior crown torque)
	Severe maxillary anterior crowding (UTSALD = −10 mm)
	Mild mandibular anterior crowding (LTSALD = −3)
	Maxillary canines buccally displaced
	Thin attached tissue (washboarding) over mandibular anteriors
Other	—
Diagnosis	Class III malocclusion (mild)
	Anterior open bite
	Anterior and Posterior cross bite

degeneration is occurring, the mandible could rotate down and back (and the bite open). But his condylar heads appear to have reasonable contours. Ask if Derrick has a history of snoring, sleep apnea, difficulty breathing, or repeated strep throats (marked adenoid hyperplasia). If he does have any of these problems, refer him to otolaryngology (plus sleep clinic) for an airway evaluation/evaluation for adenoidectomy. He and his parents deny any of these problems. Finally, remember to check for other possible causes for anterior open bites: temporary anterior open bites occurring while permanent teeth are erupting; ankylosis of anterior teeth, which prevents their complete eruption into occlusion; or lack of space for complete tooth eruption (teeth blocked out). Only the open bites below the maxillary canines could be attributed to one of these etiologies (canines blocked out).

Q: What dental/skeletal features differentiate a dental open bite from a skeletal open bite?

A: A *dental (functional) open bite* is just that—a dental problem—the patient's facial skeleton is normal. The dental open bite results from a habit (digit, tongue interposition, lip biting) which prevents the maxillary and mandibular anterior teeth from erupting (Figure 4.34, top right). The patient has a normal vertical skeletal dimension. The patient should appear, vertically, normal with soft tissue Glabella–Subnasale distance approximately equal to the Subnasale–soft tissue Menton distance (normal soft tissue LAFH). The cephalometric radiograph should demonstrate a normal LAFH/TAFH and normal FMA and SNMP. Intraorally, the open bite will often have the shape of a football (from the tongue or digit) and most commonly involve only the anterior teeth. A *skeletal open bite* (Figure 4.34, bottom right), on the other hand, will demonstrate excessive skeletal vertical growth: long soft tissue LAFH and an interlabial gap (lips cannot be brought together without strain because the soft tissue vertical growth could not keep pace with the skeletal vertical growth). Excess incisal and gingival display can result if the maxillary corpus has descended excessively (assuming that the maxillary anterior teeth are not stepped up relative to the posterior teeth from a concurrent functional tongue or thumb habit). Also seen are a long skeletal LAFH (LAFH/TAFH > 55%), a steep mandibular plane angle, a palatal plane tipped down in the posterior, and maxillary root apices that have erupted down and away from the palatal plane (overeruption of the maxillary posterior teeth). Because the mandible rotates downward and backward with the descent of the maxilla, the SNB angle may be small, and excessive antegonial notching may also be seen.

Q: What features would lead you to classify Derrick as a dental open bite? A skeletal open bite? What is the etiology of his open bite?

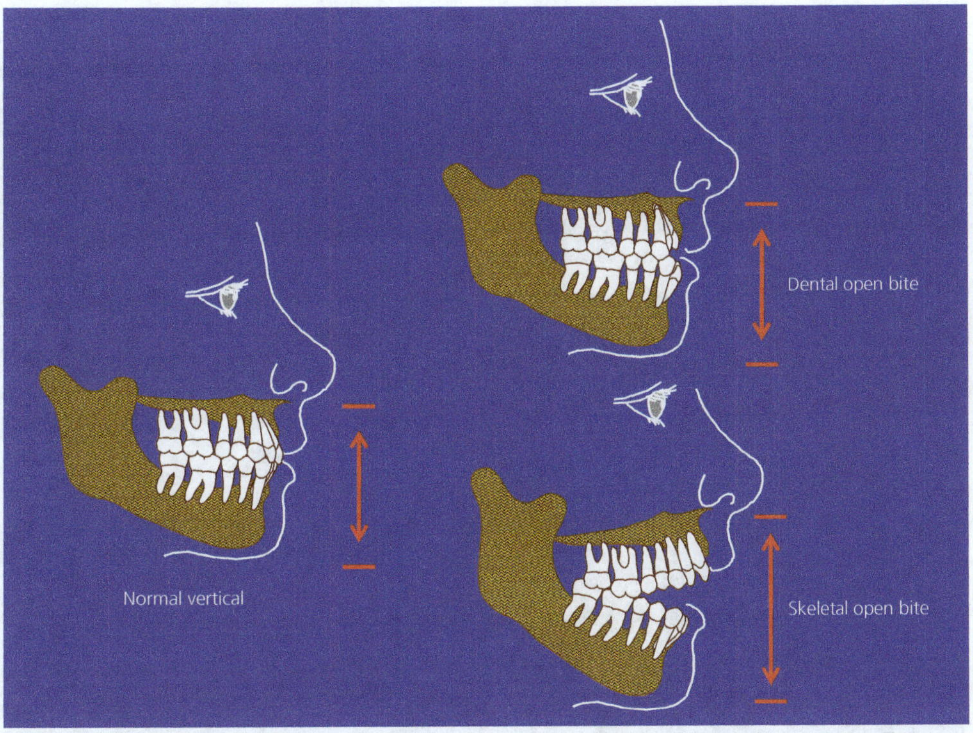

Figure 4.34 Principal difference between a dental and skeletal open bite? A dental (functional) open bite will present with a normal LAFH, while a skeletal open bite presents with a long LAFH. Of course, a skeletal open bite can also have a dental (functional) component.

A: His *dental* (functional) open-bite features include the following:
- Normal FMA (27°) and SNMP (36°) angles.
- Presence of only a very small ILG at his philtrum. An interlabial gap of up to 2 mm may be considered normal [32], and his philtrum length is much shorter than his commissure height, so part of the reason he has an ILG is short philtrum length.
- Tongue interposition habit.

His *skeletal* open bite features include the following:
- Long soft tissue LAFH
- Long skeletal LAFH (LAFH/TAFH = 60%)
- Downward posterior palatal plane cant
- Maxillary molar root apicies erupted several millimeters below his palatal plane
- Open bite extending distally from his anterior teeth to his second premolars/first molars (not limited to the anterior teeth)

The etiology of Derrick's anterior open bite is a combination of tongue habit plus excessive vertical facial growth.

Q: Based on the aforementioned features, would you classify Derrick as a skeletal open bite, a dental open bite, or a combination of both?

A: Like many (most) open-bite patients, Derrick has a combination of skeletal and dental open bite features. Derrick's skeletal open-bite features cannot be discounted. At minimum, Derrick should be considered a borderline skeletal open-bite patient. On the one hand, he has a skeletally long LAFH (LAFH/TAFH = 60%, over two standard deviations beyond a normal value of 55%). On the other hand, his FMA and SNMP are reasonably normal and his ILG is minimal (confined to the philtrum area). Further, his open bite extends past the canines, but is not so severe that it extends to the second molars. So, we will call Derrick a borderline skeletal open bite. If you treat him, you must either treat him as a skeletal open or pay very special attention to any worsening of his condition with growth. Since you do not know how he will grow in the future, it would be prudent to proceed under the assumption that the skeletal open bite will worsen, and address it with treatment. You must inform Derrick's parents that, despite your best efforts, Derrick could grow unfavorably and may require surgery at a future date to achieve an ideal result. In the same fashion, Derrick is a dental open bite. Derrick's dental open bite (interpositional tongue habit) must be addressed by discussing the habit with Derrick (make him aware of it to try to curtail the habit). Other treatments would consist of placing anterior tongue spurs or closing the open bite by leveling the arches (since the maxillary incisors are stepped up). If the open bite is closed, it may remain closed if the tongue adapts to a new position behind (instead of over) the affected teeth. In Derrick's retainers, a hole could be placed in the maxillary anterior palate for the tongue to seek instead of laying over the anterior teeth, or lingual anterior spurs could be placed in the mandibular retainer for the tongue to learn to avoid. You must inform Derrick's parents that, despite your best efforts, Derrick's tongue habit may be intractable and his open-bite correction may later relapse. In summary, *Derrick has a combination of borderline skeletal open bite and dental open bite.*

Q: Can you fault the previous orthodontist for suggesting that Derrick wait until he has completed growth to initiate treatment, including orthognathic surgery? Will you consider treating Derrick without surgery? Or should you decline treating him because he and his parents refused surgery?

A: No, you cannot fault the previous orthodontist. What he saw was an adolescent Class III skeletal open bite patient. One clear option for treatment could include jaw surgery. However, since Derrick has a borderline skeletal open bite (in addition to his

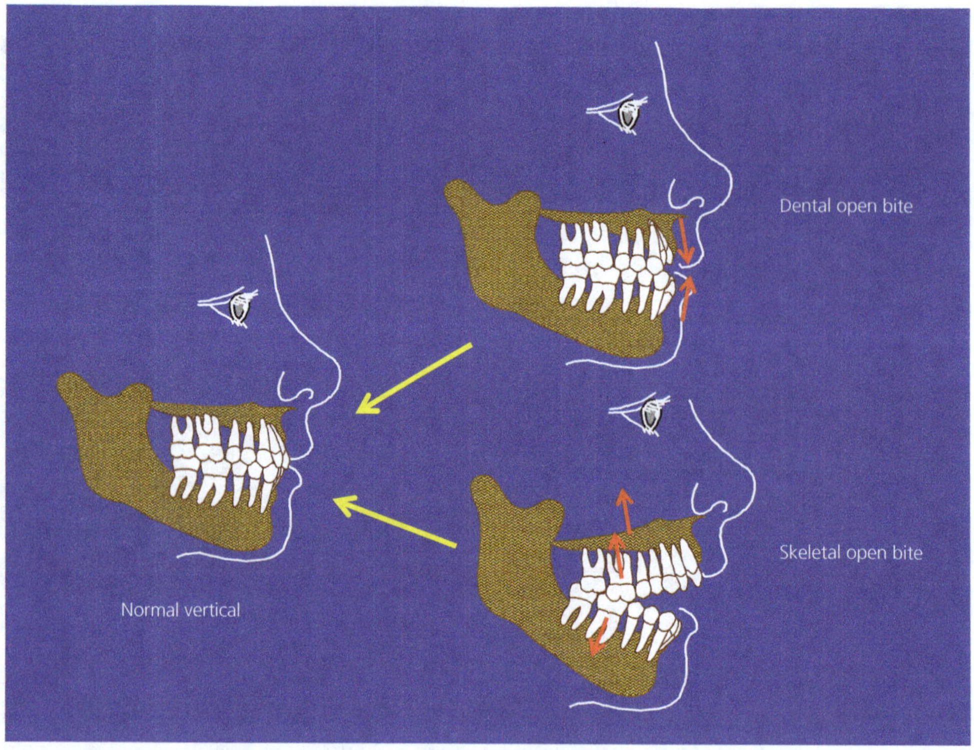

Figure 4.35 Treatment of a dental open bite consists of eliminating the habit and erupting the anterior teeth. Orthopedic or surgical treatment of a skeletal open bite consists of intruding the maxillary corpus and molars (masking a skeletal open bite consists of erupting anterior teeth).

dental open bite), and since he is nearly 15 years old, it may be worth attempting to treat him now. But, you should inform Derrick and his parents that, depending on growth, an ideal result may not be achieved without surgery.

Q: Can you describe, in general terms, the difference in how you would treat a dental open bite as opposed to a skeletal open bite?

A: Dental open bites result from habits, and the habit must be eliminated before the open bite can be corrected, or stay corrected. A dental open bite is corrected, orthodontically, by erupting the affected maxillary and mandibular teeth (Figure 4.35, top right) into proper OB (Figure 4.35, left). A skeletal open bite results from abnormal growth: condyles growing posterior-superiorly, a lack of normal forward mandibular internal (true) rotation or even a backward internal (true) rotation, the maxilla descending more than normal (palatal plane may rotate down posteriorly), and molars erupting more than normal. In rare instances, a skeletal open bite can result from condylar degeneration. As the mandible rotates backward, the mandibular plane angle steepens, the anterior face height increases, and an anterior open bite results. Treatment for skeletal open bite consists of reducing descent or even impacting the maxillary corpus and reducing eruption or even intruding molars. This will result in CCW rotation of the mandible, a normal LAFH, and normal OB (Figure 4.35, left). If a skeletal open bite exists in combination with a dental open bite, then a combination of skeletal and dental open bite treatment will be needed. Finally, masking (camouflage) of a skeletal open bite consists of ignoring the long LAFH and simply erupting anterior teeth.

Q: What is your diagnosis of Derrick?

A: Mild Angle Class III malocclusion with anterior/posterior cross bite and anterior open bite. Again, this diagnosis was based on records made in CO.

Q: Can you suggest a principle for treating patients, dentally, who present with borderline apical base discrepancies?

A: *Principle: The less severe the apical base discrepancy, and the less severe the accompanying dental compensations, the greater the likelihood you can successfully correct a malocclusion, dentally.*

Q: How does this principle apply to Derrick?

A: Derrick has a borderline skeletal open bite, and the only compensation he has for this open bite is overeruption of his mandibular incisors (Figure 4.33d). That said, we should have a reasonable chance of treating him successfully, dentally.

Q: How does the patient's age affect the above principle? How does this apply to Derrick?

A: The older the patient is, the less future growth he/she is likely to have. So, the older the patient is, the better your chances of successfully treating borderline apical base discrepancies, dentally. As a nearly 15-year-old male, we can anticipate some remaining growth with Derrick, but certainly less than if he was 10 years old.

Q: What are Derrick's *primary* problems in each dimension that you must stay focused on initially and during treatment?

A: Derrick has an apical base (skeletal) discrepancy in the transverse dimension and a borderline apical base discrepancy in the vertical (Table 4.4).

Q: What are your treatment goals for Derrick?

A: Elimination of his CR–CO shift, closure of his open bite, to 20%–40% OB correction of his cross bites, ideal arch coordination, ideal Class I canine relationship with minimal OJ.

Table 4.4 Primary problems list for Derrick *(apical base/skeletal discrepancies italicized).*

AP	III (1) II (2–3) II (1–2) III (1) in centric occlusion skeletal relationships WRN
Vertical	*Borderline skeletal* open bite and a functional open bite
Transverse	Posterior cross bite and significant compensations resulting from *the transverse skeletal discrepancy* (his cross bite would be much worse if the posterior teeth were in a corrected, upright position)
Other	Washboarding of periodontium over mandibular incisors

Q: How can the anteroposterior apical base discrepancy and Class III (1 mm) bilateral molar relationship be addressed?

A: Trick question. With a CR–CO shift of 2 mm, Derrick could end up being Class II (2 mm) in CR once the shift is eliminated, not Class III.

Q: Ok, let's rephrase the question. Hypothetically speaking, if Derrick did not have a shift, can you list at least five ways to correct a Class III (1 mm) molar relationship?

A: Class III elastics or Class III springs—could achieve correction with minimal patient compliance. Now, considering the 1 mm Class III relationship Derrick has, the following options would be overkill:

1. Class III elastics between TADs in the maxilla and mandible.
2. High-pull chin cup to restrict B-point from advancing with any remaining growth while permitting A-point to continue growing forward.
3. RPHG to possibly advance the maxilla. Then, a high-pull chin cup could maintain this correction. A drawback of RPHG treatment is that the maxillary canines are already blocked out, and the maxillary incisors are already proclined ($\underline{1}$ to SN = 111°)—an RPHG with elastics attached to the maxillary teeth could worsen these conditions by advancing the maxillary posterior teeth (RPHG could be attached to TADs in the maxilla to avoid adverse incisor proclination).
4. Extraction of mandibular first premolars. This would potentially result in too much correction—worsening a Class II canine relationship when the mandibular canines are retracted and creating a large overjet.
5. Placement of TADs in the mandibular posterior molar area to retract the mandibular posterior teeth.

Q: Of the three general approaches to addressing Derrick's borderline skeletal open bite (orthopedics, masking, and surgery), surgery was declined. List specific orthopedic or masking treatments you would consider.

A: *Orthopedics* (reduce descent of the maxillary corpus and reduce eruption of molars (or intrude molars)). The options listed will be discussed more fully in Chapter 5

- TADs placed as anchors to prevent eruption of molars or to intrude molars
- Vertical-pull chin cup
- Full posterior occlusal coverage bite plates (with and without repelling magnets)
- Transpalatal arch with acrylic button
- Lower lingual holding arch
- Chewing exercises

Masking or camouflage (achieve open-bite closure without addressing the borderline vertical apical base discrepancy). Options include the following:

- Vertical elastics (extruding the anterior teeth) that could be used during leveling of the arches to support erupting the maxillary anterior teeth incisally.

Q: How can Derrick's transverse apical base discrepancy be addressed?

A: *Orthopedics* (expanding the maxillary arch by separating the hemi-maxillae at the midpalatal suture). Options include the following:

- RME: if you achieve a midpalatal split, RME would result in both maxillary skeletal expansion and maxillary dental posterior expansion. In addition, a bonded RME appliance could reduce maxillary posterior vertical growth slightly (0.5 mm) at the posterior nasal spine (PNS) [33]. With a first molar transverse deficiency of 4.5 mm, even if you do not achieve a midpalatal split, you still may be able to correct the transverse with slow dental expansion (increasing maxillary molar compensations as the molars tip buccally). Of course, you must confirm the presence of robust periodontium buccal to the maxillary molar roots before doing this.
- A quad helix or maxillary split plate would not be the ideal treatment of choice. Although the quad helix has been shown to cause separation of the midpalatal suture in young persons [34], it may not have the force level necessary to overcome skeletal resistance in a 15-year-old. However, either appliance may provide adequate dental expansion but with increasing maxillary molar buccal tipping.

Masking or camouflage (correcting the lack of posterior overjet primarily by increasing molar transverse compensations, or torque). Options include the following:

- Cross-bite elastics—will increase posterior dental compensations (buccal tipping of maxillary molars and lingual tipping of mandibular molars) and is not the ideal solution in this patient, at least initially.
- Expanding maxillary archwires or narrowing mandibular archwires is not the ideal solution—both techniques will result in increasing transverse compensations.

Surgery (SARME) is not an option for Derrick. Furthermore, it would generally not be considered for a male at this age, especially without first attempting to gain maxillary expansion with an RME appliance.

Q: So, ideally, you would address Derrick's transverse discrepancy with RME—or, at least attempt doing so. At what age can you achieve the most transverse *skeletal* effect with an RME appliance?

A: Before or during the pubertal growth spurt [35, 36]. Expansion after the pubertal growth spurt becomes increasingly dentoalveolar instead of skeletal.

Q: Increasing skeletal resistance to expansion is the reason why the skeletal benefit of RME decreases with age. Where do we believe this resistance is focused? Is it in the midpalatal suture?

A: No, resistance to RME is thought to be focused at the zygomatic buttress, not the midpalatal suture [37, 38].

Q: What unknowns do you face with Derrick's treatment?

A: Residual growth is a major unknown. Will his borderline skeletal open bite worsen? How about his CR–CO shift? Have we measured it correctly? Can Derrick's transverse correction be achieved with an RME appliance? Or, does too much (zygomatic buttress) skeletal resistance exist to permit splitting of the midpalatal suture? Other unknowns include cooperation and hygiene. Derrick's unknowns are significant.

Q: One important principle to follow with all your patients is to try to reduce unknowns as much as possible before giving the patient/parent a *final* treatment plan or do anything irreversible. Are there any unknowns that could be eliminated?

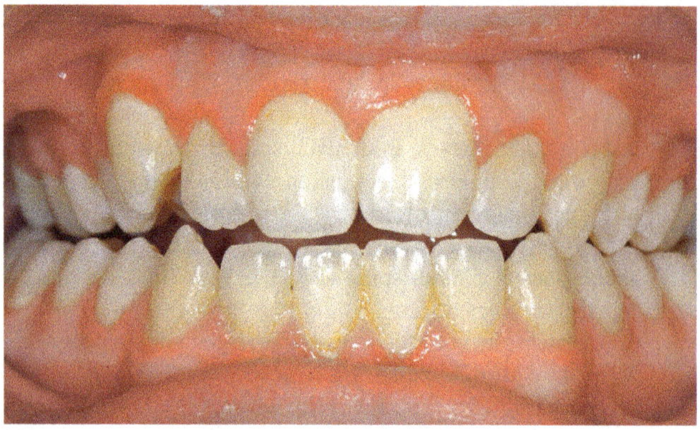
(a)

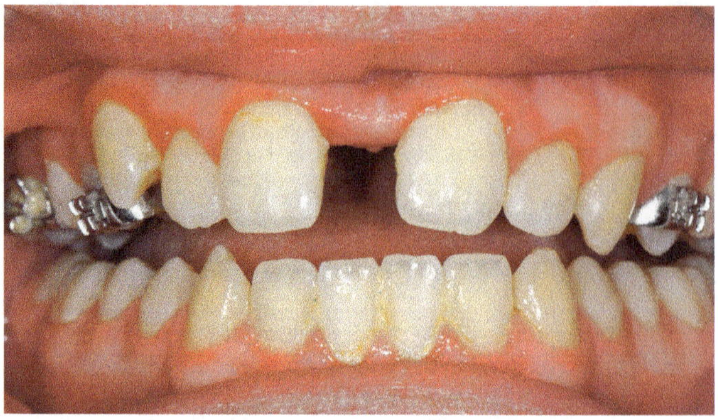
(b)

Figure 4.36 Diastema formation during RME: (a) initial maxillary posterior transverse discrepancy; (b) during RME, the formation of a midline diastema indicates that the midpalatal suture has separated.

A: Yes, you could start by attempting to split the maxillary midpalatal suture and correct the transverse discrepancy. If successful, you would then be able to better judge your AP position (CR–CO shift).

Q: Would you initially proceed with nonextraction treatment, extraction of anterior teeth, or extraction of posterior teeth?

A: Given Derrick's major unknowns, it is wise to begin with reversible procedures. Later, a final treatment plan can be defined (including extractions?). Begin nonextraction.

Q: After considering everything discussed thus far, what specific treatment option(s) do you recommend?

A: It was proposed to Derrick and his parents that we address his transverse discrepancy first by attempting RME. Depending on his response, we would reevaluate further treatment.

Q: When a patient is treated with RME (0.25–0.5 mm expansion per day), you should see a diastema forming between the maxillary central incisors when the midpalatal suture splits (Figure 4.36). Or, you will see the split on an occlusal radiograph. How do you know if you are *not* getting a midpalatal suture split?

A: No midline diastema will form, no midpalatal split will be seen on an occlusal radiograph, the palatal metal wires of the expander will impinge on the alveolar process soft tissue as the teeth move buccally, or the patient will feel unyielding pressure (pain) when the screw is activated.

Q: Be prepared: always plan ahead. What will you do if you begin RME treatment, but do not achieve a midpalatal split on any patient? How about specifically Derrick?

A: This depends on how much dental expansion you have achieved before realizing that you are not getting a midpalatal split, how much more expansion you still need, and what the maxillary buccal periodontal tissues look like. If you have not achieved a midpalatal split but have nearly the amount of expansion you need (buccal tissues look good), then you may decide to continue expanding, dentally (at the rate of 0.25–0.5 mm per week). If you think the amount of additional expansion you need is significant, or if the buccal periodontal tissues cannot support additional expansion, then stop expanding. Your options then are to leave the patient in cross bite, place compensations (maxillary buccal torque, mandibular lingual torque) to improve the transverse OJ, or to consider SARME. In Derrick's case, with only 4.5 mm of transverse maxillary expansion needed at the first molars (ignoring additional expansion needed to remove transverse compensations), if you do not achieve a midpalatal split, then you may still be able to achieve the remaining expansion, dentally.

An RME appliance was delivered to Derrick and expansion was begun at 0.25 mm per day. Thankfully, a midpalatal sutural split was achieved and maxillary expansion was completed and allowed to stabilize for 3 months. New records were made (Figure 4.37). The RME appliance was removed. A maxillary Hawley retainer was delivered. Discussions about further treatment were held.

Q: Comparing Derrick's initial (Figure 4.38a) and progress (Figure 4.38b) cephalometric radiographs, along with his initial (Figure 4.33i and 4.33n) and progress (Figure 4.37f) intraoral photographs, it appears that Derrick's open bite has worsened slightly with RME. Why would this occur?

A: As maxillary molars move buccally with RME (Figure 4.39a, horizontal red arrows), the maxillary molar cusps ride along inclined planes formed with mandibular molar cusps (green lines), forcing the mandible down (vertical red arrows). Result: molars occlude cusp-to-cusp (Figure 4.39b), and the bite is opened in the anterior.

Q: Should the slight worsening of Derrick's open bite, post-RME, concern us? What are the long-term consequences of RME in the vertical dimension?

A: The literature states that long-term RME therapy has little effect on either vertical or anteroposterior facial dimensions [39–41]. Remember, as the molars are brought into occlusion with fixed orthodontic appliances, they will no longer occlude cusp-to-cusp—so the bite should close. That said, does Derrick's slightly increased open bite concern us? Yes, we would be fools not to be concerned with any increase in Derrick's open bite. However, the increased opening is minimal, so it does not affect our overall assessment of Derrick as a borderline skeletal open bite.

Q: RME eliminated Derrick's CR–CO anterior and lateral shift. His progress records (Figure 4.37) were made in CR. What do you see?

A: No facial changes are noted, except that an ILG is absent in both the frontal photo and the lateral cephalometric radiograph. He looks Class III at the right molar, but his right premolars look well-positioned AP. His left molar looks Class III, and his left premolars look Class III by 2–3 mm. As discussed, his open bite has worsened with RME, but the open bite is not severe and he appears to exhibit minimal maxillary incisal display (Figure 4.37d).

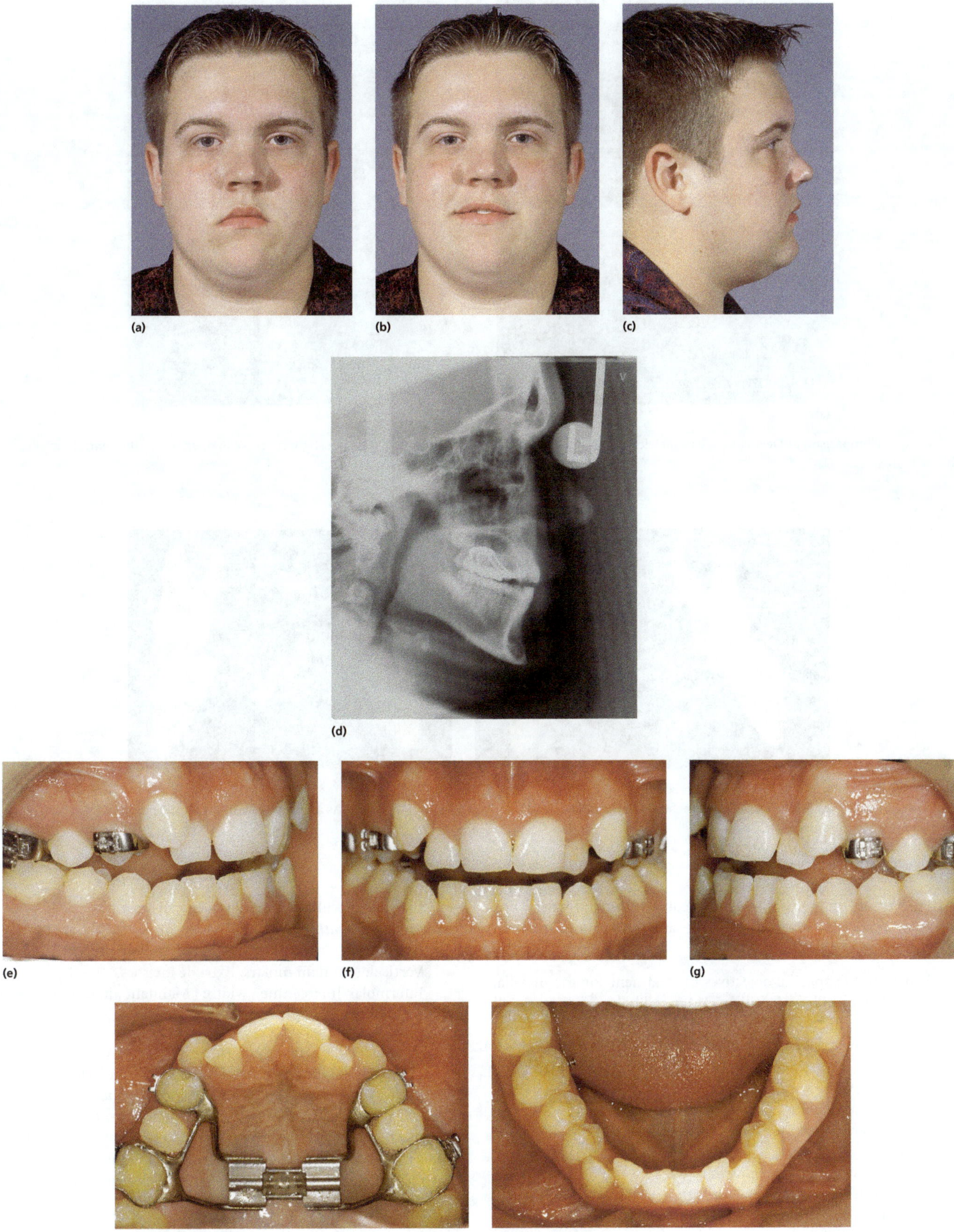

Figure 4.37 (a–i) Progress records of Derrick following RME.

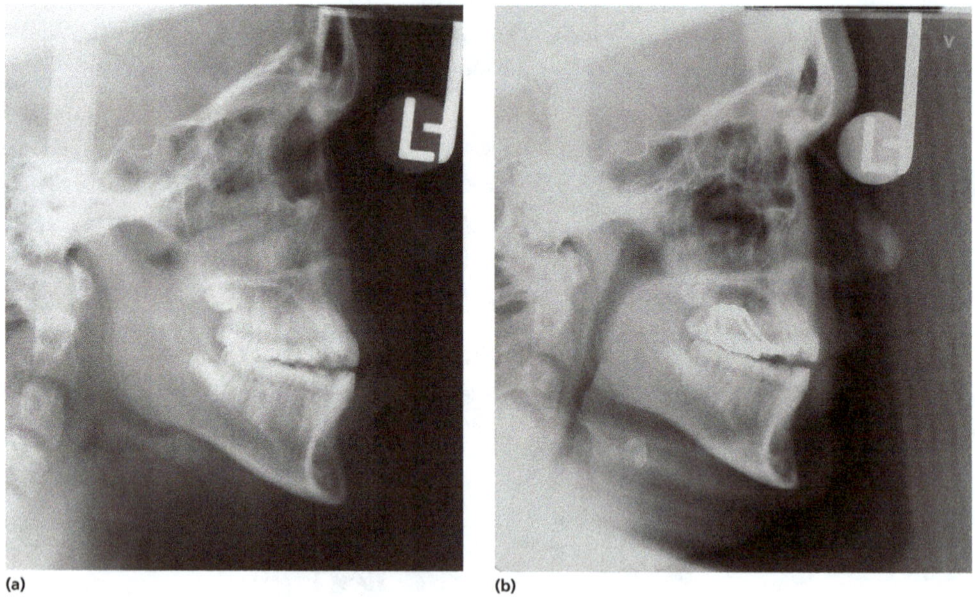

Figure 4.38 Comparison of Derrick's cephalometric radiographs: (a) initial and (b) progress. Note the slight increase in open bite at the central incisors following RME.

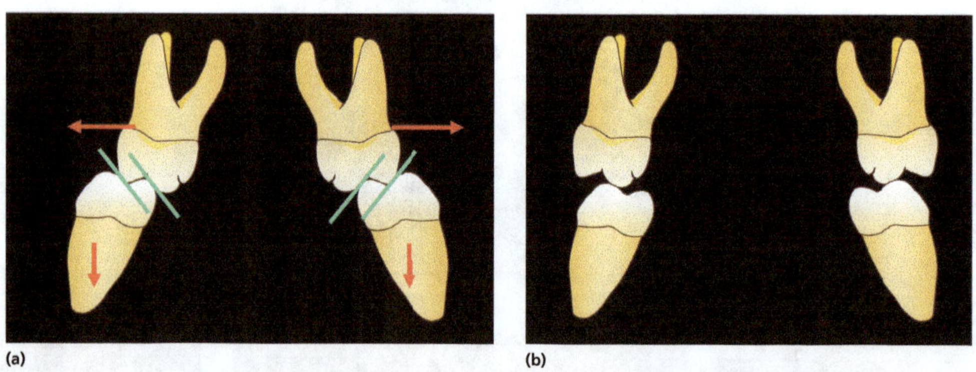

Figure 4.39 (a) During RME, buccal movement of the maxillary molars forces the mandible down. As a result, the molars occlude cusp-to-cusp (b), and the bite opens in the anterior.

Q: How would you recommend proceeding with treatment?

A: A decision was made to continue attempting nonextraction treatment.

Q: What are the specific objectives of treatment for the maxilla, mandible, maxillary dentition, and mandibular dentition in all three planes of space?

A: Specific objectives of treatment for Derrick are as follows:

Maxilla

AP: Allow for normal growth.
Vertical: Allow for normal growth.
Transverse: Increase skeletal transverse width.

Mandible

AP: Allow for normal growth.
Vertical: Allow for normal growth.
Transverse: Allow for normal growth.

Maxillary dentition

AP: Maintain molars and canines. Maintain incisors.
Vertical: Maintain molars and canines. Extrude incisors.
Intermolar width: Increase intermolar width.

Mandibular dentition

AP: Maintain molars and canines. Maintain incisors.
Vertical: Maintain molars. Extrude incisors.
Intermolar/Intercanine width: Maintain intermolar and intercanine widths.

Q: How did Derrick's treatment proceed?

A: Arches were banded/bonded, level/aligned, and Derrick wore vertical (triangle) elastics bilaterally from the maxillary canines to the mandibular canines and first premolars. Short anterior Class III elastics were worn on the left, prn. Later, the maxillary incisors were stepped down and a COS was added to the mandibular archwire to aide in open-bite closure. Artistic bends were added and finishing was performed.

Q: Deband records are shown in Figure 4.40 (initial facial photos included). What changes do you note?

A: Changes noted include the following:

- Derrick's left chin deviation was eliminated and his ILG closed (Figure 4.40a, b).
- His incisal display increased and improved (Figure 4.40c, d).
- He appears to be smiling more broadly (more self-confidence?).
- On profile (Figure 4.40e, f) his lip–chin–throat angle decreased and his labiomental sulcus softened.
- Cephalometrically, his ANB was increased to 2° (Figure 4.40h) as a result of A-point moving forward with growth plus B-point moving down and back.
- His maxillary and mandibular incisors were uprighted slightly to 105° and 67° respectively.
- His FMA and SNMP were stable.
- Looking at the cranial base superimposition (Figure 4.40i), the maxilla grew down and forward and the mandible grew downward. Some eruption of the maxillary and mandibular molars occurred, and the incisors of both arches erupted.
- The open bite was closed, but with a minimal OB of approximately 10%.
- A Class I molar and canine occlusion was achieved with coincident midlines.
- Maxillary posterior buccal crown torque and mandibular lingual crown torque remains (Figure 4.40u, v).

Q: How was Derrick's dental and borderline skeletal open bite corrected?
A: By eruption of anterior teeth (masking the borderline skeletal open bite).

Q: How would you retain this patient?
A: Maxillary and mandibular Hawley retainers were worn by Derrick. To assure maintenance of the open-bite closure, small "dots" of composite could be placed on the facials of the maxillary and mandibular incisors. The OB would then be held with the temporary (suck-down) retainer snapping over these dots or the wire of the Hawley retainer wire snapping over these dots. This was not done. Tongue posture reminders (spurs) could also be placed in the anterior of the mandibular retainer, and a hole should be placed in the anterior palate of his maxillary retainer—both as aides/reminders in keeping his tongue posture corrected. This was not done.

Q: Two year post-treatment records are shown in Figure 4.41. What changes do you note?
A: Thankfully, Derrick's tongue must have adapted to the orthodontic anterior bite closure as the bite has not reopened (in spite of the fact that no lingual spurs, hole in the maxillary retainer anterior palate, or composite "dots" on anterior facials were incorporated). His bite is very slightly opened at the left lateral incisors and canines. His midlines are no longer coincident, and he is slightly Class III on the left. Finally, his gingiva looks much healthier than at deband.

Q: What are the "take-home" messages from Derrick's treatment?
A: Take-home messages include the following:

- Derrick presented with features of a dental and *borderline* skeletal open bite. An anterior tongue interpositional habit was the cause of his dental open bite. The borderline skeletal open bite resulted from excess vertical facial growth: condyles growing more posterior-superiorly than normal, a lack of normal forward mandibular internal (true) rotation, the maxilla descending more than normal (palatal plane rotating down posteriorly), and molars erupting more than normal. Derrick was treated nonextraction with RME, fixed orthodontic appliances, and vertical elastics. His dental and borderline skeletal open bite was corrected by eruption of anterior teeth (masking the borderline skeletal open bite).
- Application of the principle of *reducing unknowns before doing any irreversible* was key to Derrick's treatment. We knew we needed to correct his transverse and eliminate his CR–CO shift, but we were not sure we could get a midpalatal

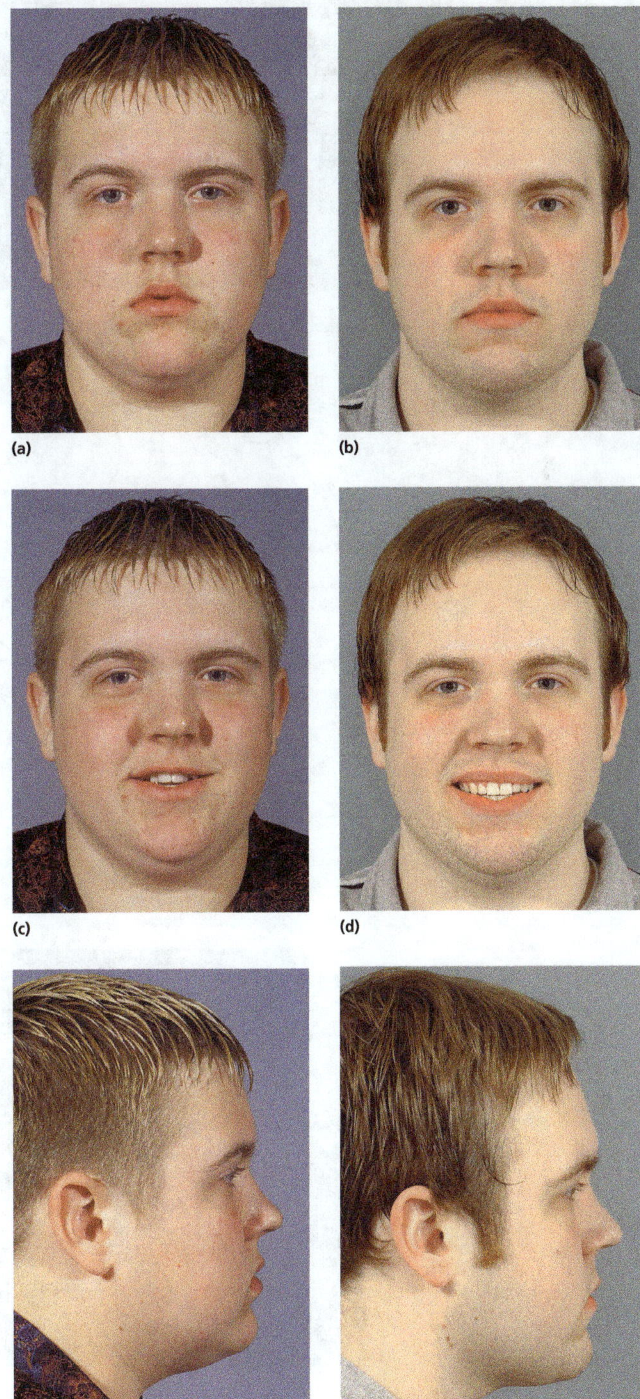

Figure 4.40 (a–v) Derrick's deband records (including juxtaposed initial facial photographs for comparison).

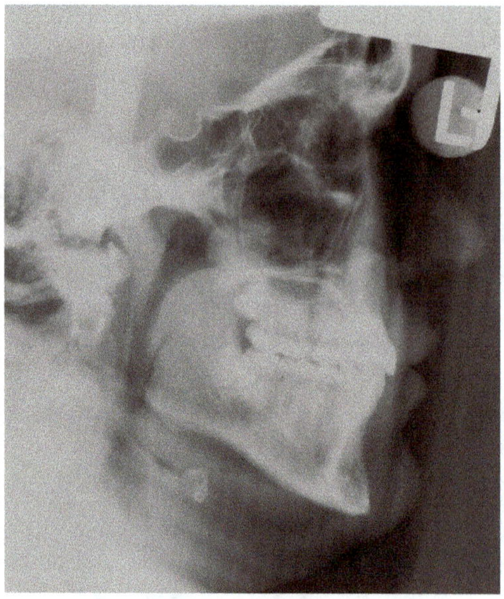

(g)

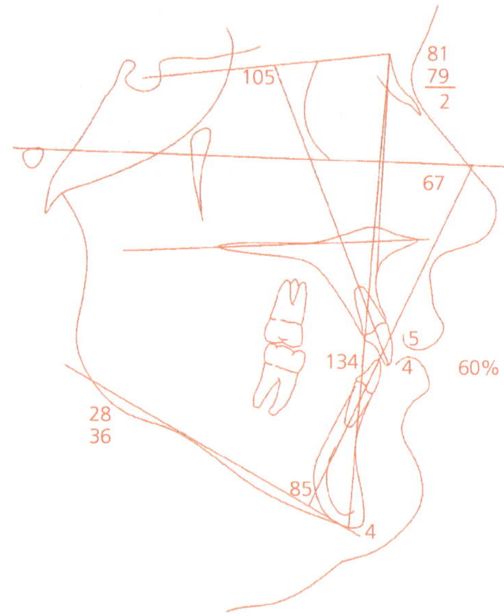

(h)

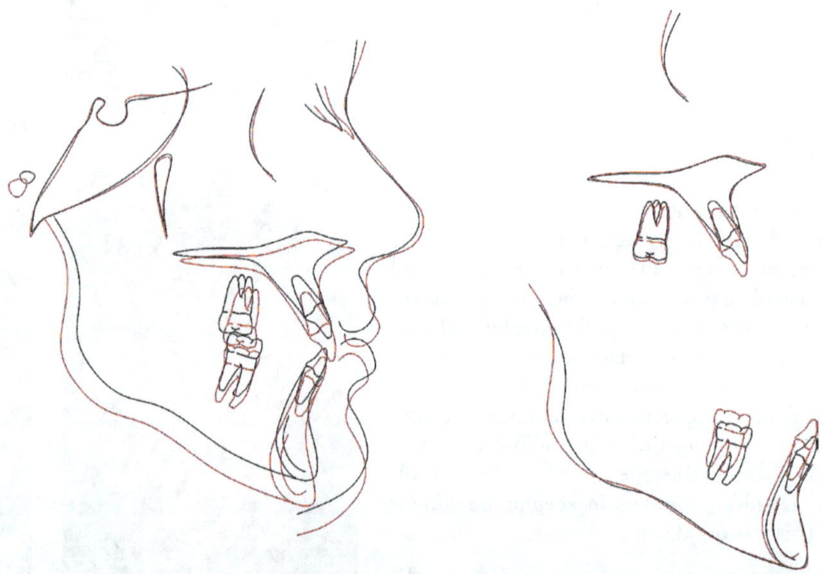

(i)

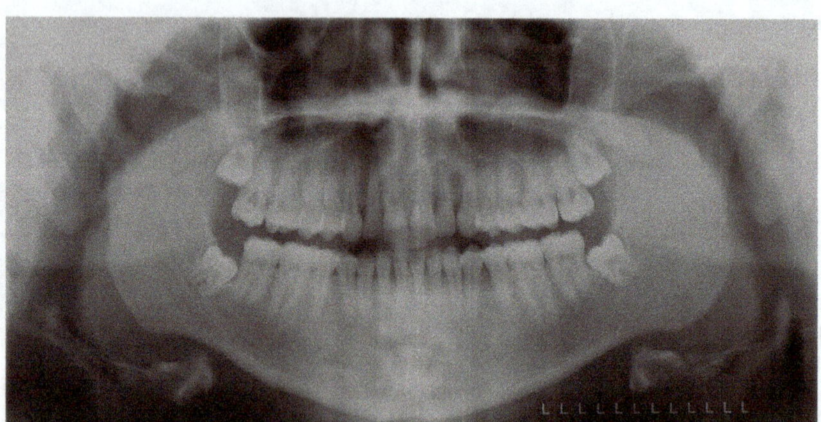

(j)

Figure 4.40 (Continued)

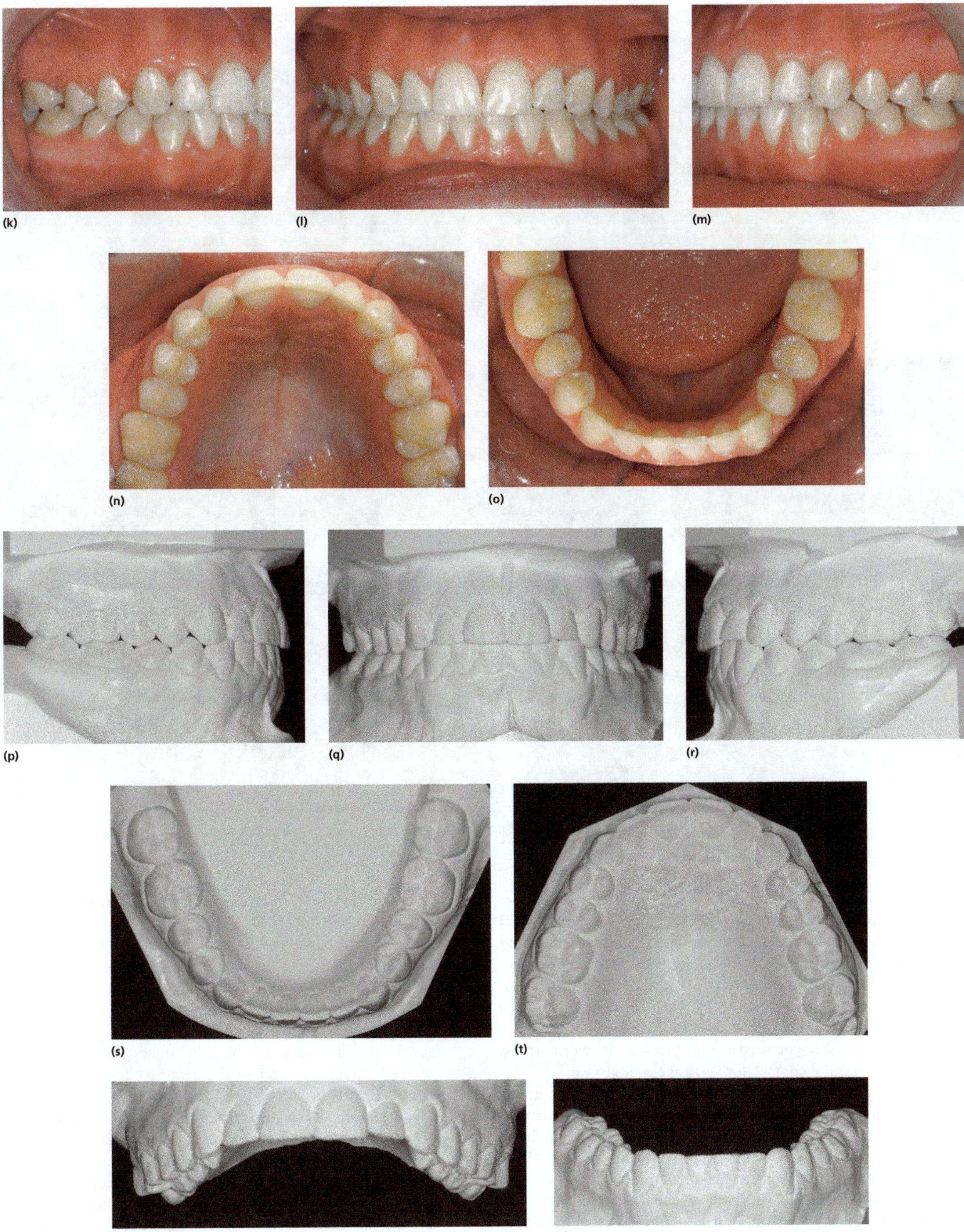

Figure 4.40 (Continued)

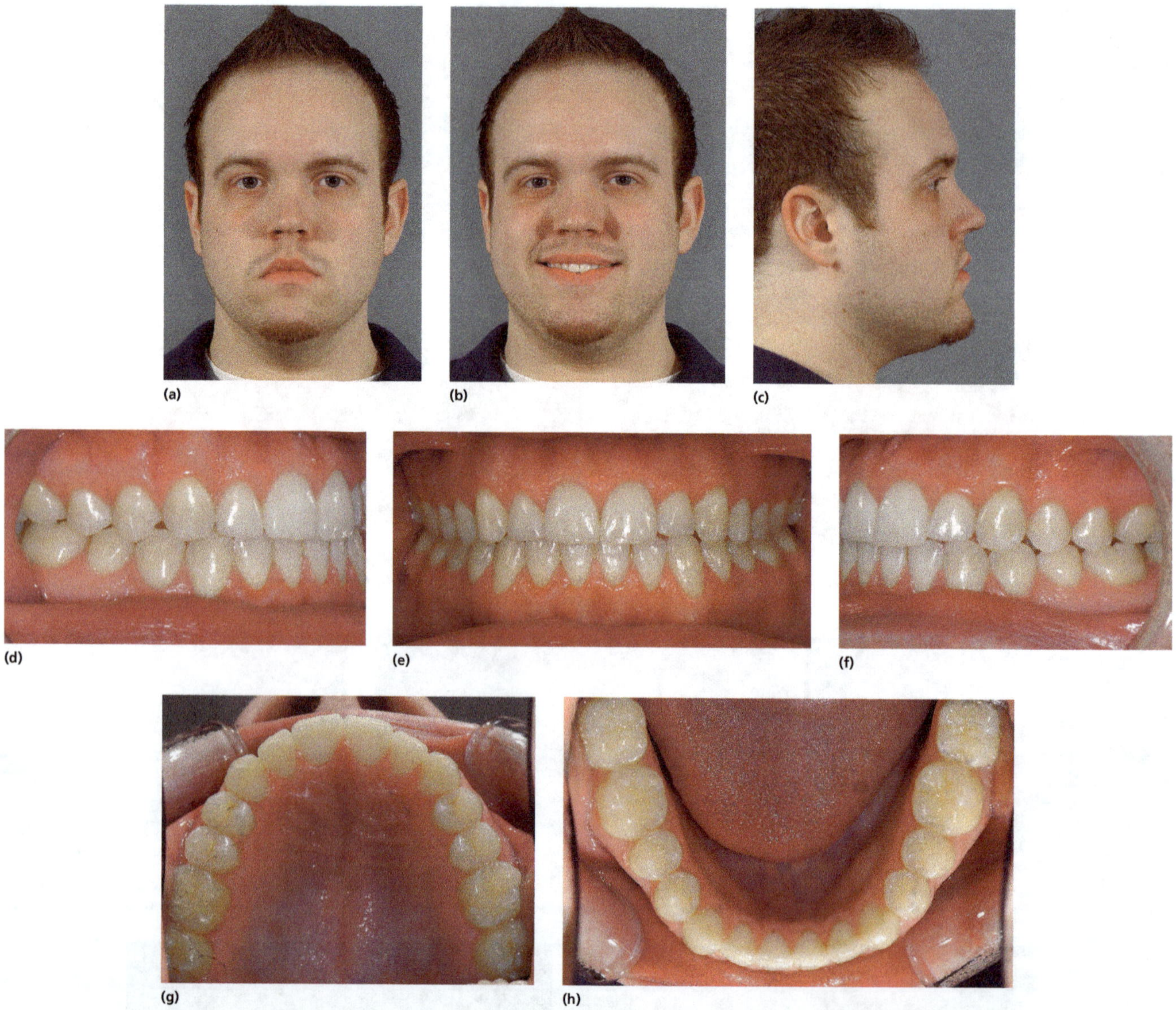

Figure 4.41 (a–h) Derrick's 2-year post-treatment records.

split with an RME appliance (due to his age). So, we attempted RME first and were rewarded: we got a midpalatal split. Next, we re-evaluated the problems we faced, including reassessing molar and canine anteroposterior positions, and decided to attempt nonextraction treatment (without chin cup to restrict mandibular forward growth). Vertical elastics successfully erupted the anterior teeth and closed the open bite. (Remember, you need a long open span between arches, without occlusal contact, for vertical elastics to work.)

- Functional habits must be eliminated to achieve and maintain correction of dental open bites. Considering Derrick's 2-year post-treatment records, it looks like his tongue habit was corrected simply by the orthodontic bite closure. *Never depend on this. Correct your habit first, before bite closure.*
- Transverse correction with an RME can be attempted in older patients. But, the patient must be informed of what to look for, if a midpalatal split does not occur: diastema between central incisors *not* forming, pressure after turning the screw *not* dissipating in a few minutes, impingement of RME bars into lateral aspects of palatal soft tissue. If a split does not occur, other options must be considered (e.g., leaving the patient in cross bite, increasing transverse dental compensations with cross-bite elastics, SARME).
- RME should have been overcorrected in Derrick to create additional OJ for uprighting molars (removing transverse dental compensations).
- RME appliance should have been converted into a TPA after maxillary expansion was complete—and the expansion held for as long as possible, while the arches were leveled and aligned. *Never trust removable retainers to hold maxillary transverse expansion.*
- Derrick's OB was corrected, but only to approximately 10%. Ideally, it should have been overcorrected to 20–40%, anticipating future relapse.
- Borderline skeletal open bites (with attendant dental open bites) can sometimes be successfully treated as dental open bites. The principle to remember is *when the skeletal discrepancy is smaller and the dental compensations are not large, you have a greater chance of successfully treating the skeletal discrepancy, dentally (by masking)*. This is true in the vertical, anteroposterior, or transverse dimensions. Also, the older the patient (less growth), the better your chances are of being successful.

Case Steven

Steven is 14 years old (Figure 4.42) and presents to you with the chief complaint, "I need orthodontic treatment." His PMH, PDH, and TMJ evaluation are WRN. He is without periodontal problems and CR=CO. He brought in a recent panoramic film (Figure 4.42f), which shows an LLHA, but it has subsequently been removed.

Q: Would any additional views, or records, be helpful?

A: Yes. It would be useful to have Steven separate his teeth, and lips, slightly to demonstrate incisal display with relaxed maxillary lip (Figure 4.43). But remember, if Steven has maxillary incisor step-up or a step-down relative to his maxillary posterior teeth, this incisal display will change once the maxillary arch is leveled.

Q: Using all the above records, list diagnostic findings/problems and make your diagnosis.

A: See Table 4.5

Q: Steven is symmetric facially. To what can you attribute him being Class II by 3 mm on the right but Class II by 4–5 mm on the left?

A: He has a mild dental asymmetry—the mandibular right posterior is ahead of the left posterior.

Q: In terms of the open bite, what other questions should you ask Steven and his parents, and what else should you check for to obtain a thorough history and determine etiology?

A: Ask if they have noticed his open bite, and if so, how long he has had it. (They respond that he has always had it.) Check for functional habits. Ask if he has a thumb habit, digit-sucking habit, or lip-biting habit. (Steven denies any such habits.) You examine him and find that *Steven does keep his tongue postured forward anteriorly (an interpositional tongue habit)*. Check the panoramic film to confirm the absence of mandibular condylar degeneration. The mandible would rotate down and back if the condyles were degenerating, possibly creating the open bite. But the condyles appear to be normal on the panoramic image (Figure 4.42f).

Q: What are other possible causes of anterior open bites?

A: Other possible causes include the following:

- Temporary anterior open bites occurring, while permanent teeth are erupting. Not the case here.
- Ankylosis of anterior teeth which prevents their complete eruption into occlusion. Highly unlikely considering the number of teeth involved in Steven's open bite.
- Lack of space for complete tooth eruption (teeth blocked out). Not the case here.

Q: What features would lead you to classify Steven as a dental open bite? A skeletal open bite?

A: Like many open-bite patients, Steven has dental *and* skeletal open-bite features. His *dental* (functional) open-bite features include the following:

- Anterior interpositional tongue posture habit.
- Absence of an ILG (his vertical facial soft tissue growth has kept pace with his vertical skeletal facial growth).
- Midface height (soft tissue Glabella—Subnasale) approximates his lower facial height (Subnasale—soft tissue Menton).
- FMA is WRN (27°—just slightly greater than an average 25°).
- Skeletal LAFH is WRN (LAFH/TAFH = 57%, within one standard deviation or 2° of average [42], 55%).

His *skeletal* open bite features include the following:

- SNMP of 43° (11° greater than an average SNMP of 32°, but this could be due to the presence of a "low" Sella).
- Maxillary first molar root apicies erupted several millimeters below his palatal plane (Figure 4.42d, a pattern often found in individuals with excessive maxillary molar eruption).
- Palatal plane is tipped down slightly in the posterior (a pattern often found in individuals with excessive vertical maxillary corpus growth).
- Open bite extends distally from his anterior teeth to his second molars (not a localized "football" shaped anterior opening formed from digit or tongue habits).

Steven is a combination borderline skeletal open bite and dental (functional) open bite.

Q: What is the etiology of his open bite?

A: The etiology of his dental open bite is an anterior tongue interposition habit. The etiology of his borderline skeletal open bite is excess vertical facial growth: condyles growing more posterior-superiorly than normal, a lack of normal forward mandibular internal (true) rotation, the maxilla descending more than normal (palatal plane rotating down posteriorly), and molars erupting more than normal. Of these, we clearly see that Steven's palatal plane is tipped down posteriorly and his maxillary first molar apicies are erupted below the palatal plane.

Q: What are the *primary* problems Steven presents with in each dimension that you must stay focused on initially and throughout treatment?

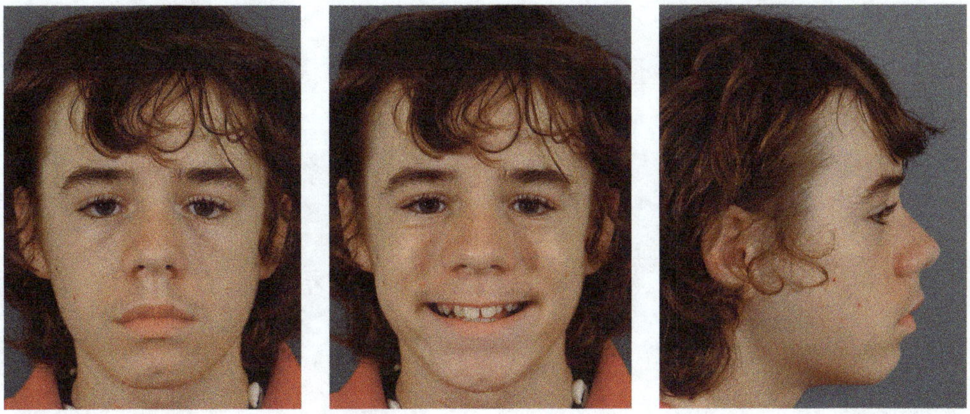

(a) (b) (c)

Figure 4.42 Initial records of Steven: (a–c) initial facial photographs, (d) lateral cephalograph, (e) cephalometric tracing, (f) pantomograph, (g–k) intraoral photographs, (l–p) model photographs, and (q–r) separated model views from front.

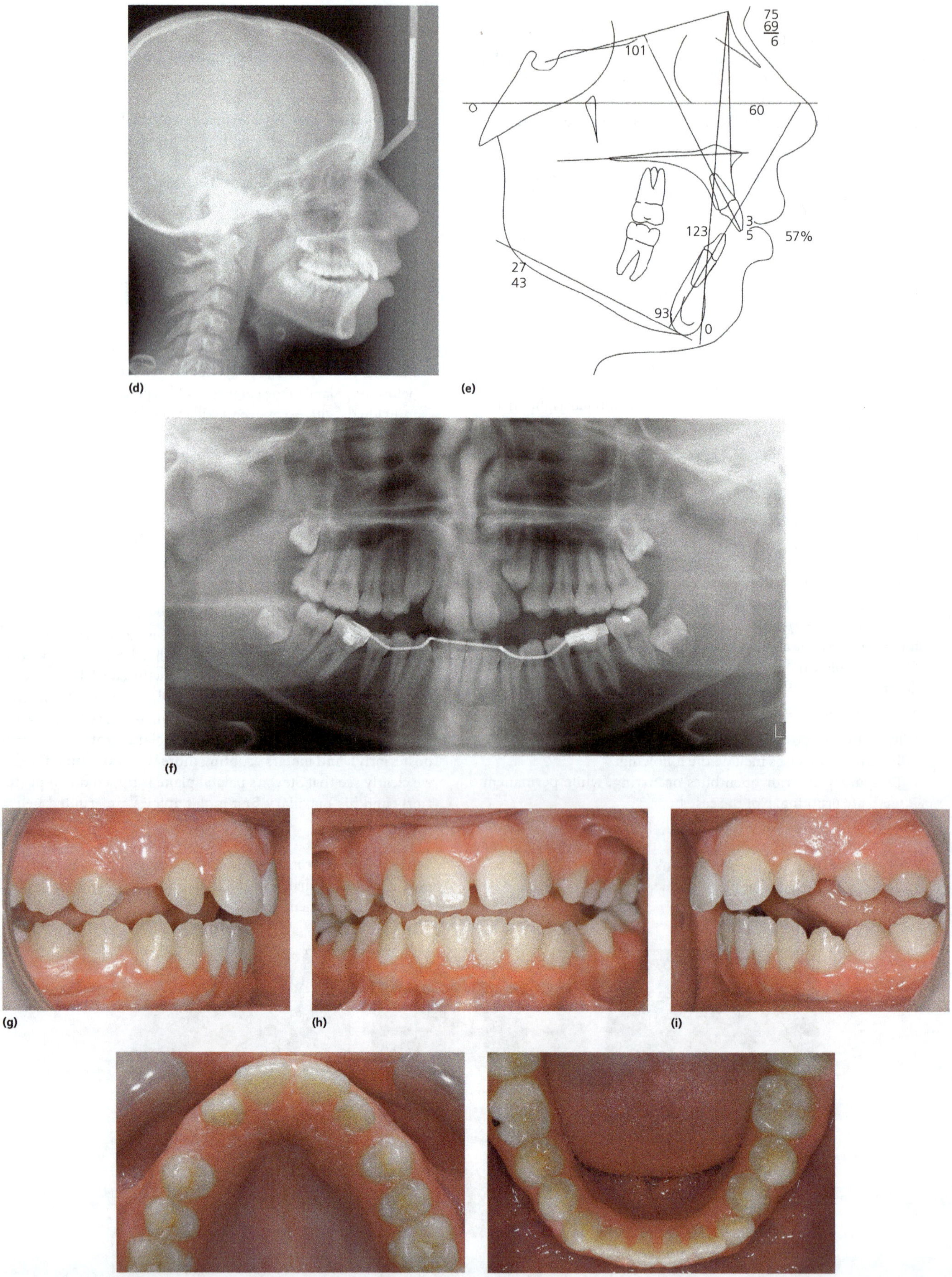

Figure 4.42 (Continued)

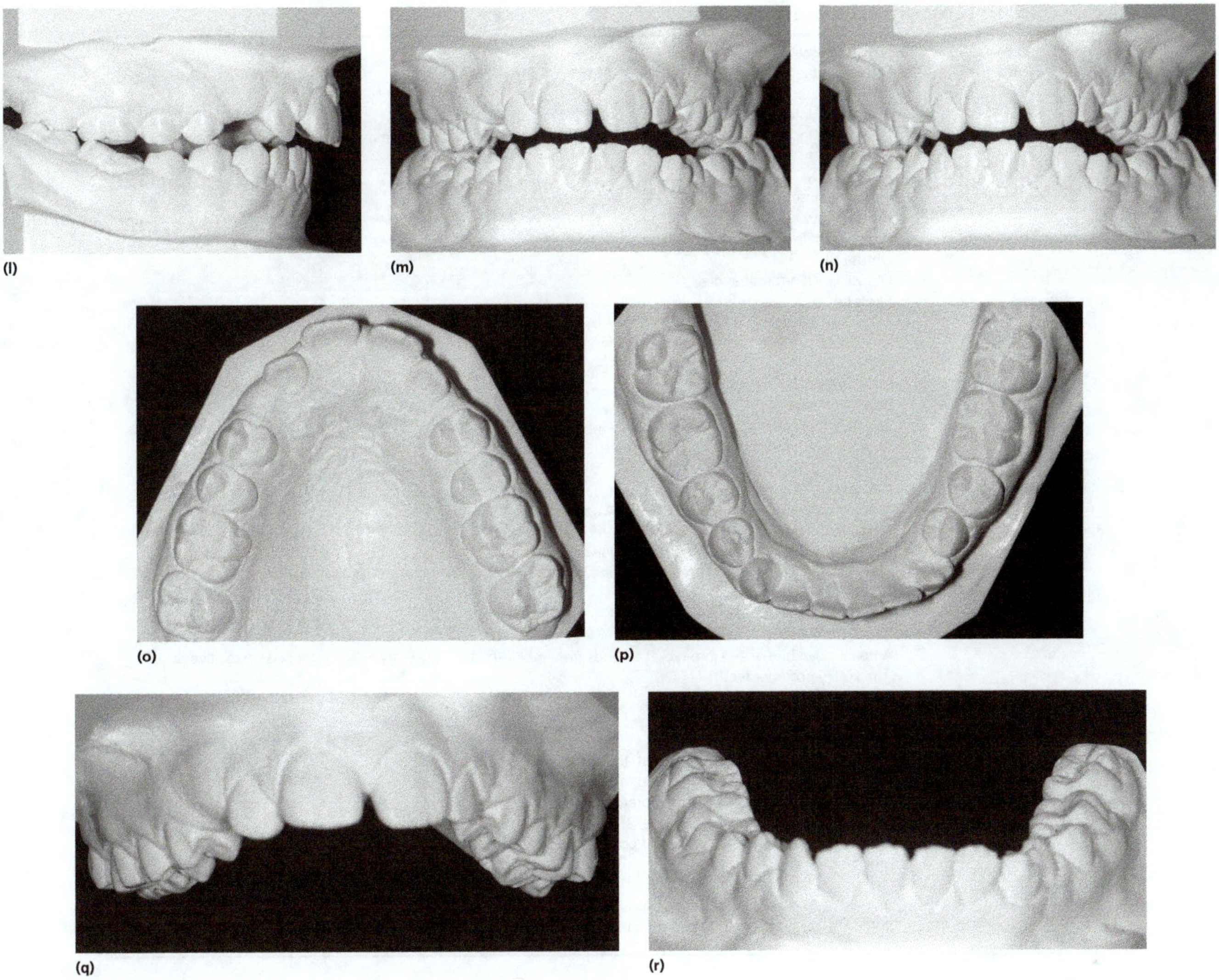

Figure 4.42 (Continued)

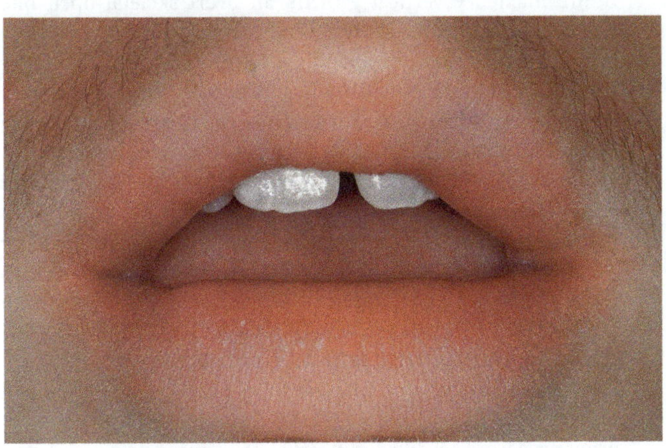

Figure 4.43 Judging maxillary incisal display with a relaxed lip.

A: Steven has apical base (skeletal) discrepancies in the AP and transverse dimensions—and a borderline apical base discrepancy in the vertical dimension (Table 4.6).

Q: Remember, there are really only two general ways to close an anterior open bite. Describe how either would be applied to Steven.

A: The two general ways to close an anterior open bite are as follows:

1. *Erupting Steven's stepped up maxillary incisors* (Figure 4.44 left, red arrow), which would be accomplished by eliminating his habitual anterior tongue posture habit and allowing the maxillary teeth to erupt; and by erupting his maxillary incisors during arch leveling with fixed orthodontic appliances. *This is the general approach used in the treatment of a dental (functional) open bite.* Note: you would not erupt Steven's mandibular anterior teeth since they are already stepped up.
2. *Intruding posterior teeth* (Figure 4.44 right, red arrows), either by surgically impacting the maxilla, possibly slowing descent of the maxillary corpus during growth, slowing eruption of molars during growth, or by intruding molars. Impacting the maxilla or intruding molars could result in a shortened LAFH as the mandible autorotates closed (Figure 4.44 right, curved yellow arrow). Even reducing maxillary descent and reducing molar eruption can result in mandibular autorotation if accompanied by adequate mandibular growth. *These are the approaches taken in the case of a skeletal open bite.* Note: masking a skeletal open bite consists of erupting anterior teeth.

Table 4.5 Diagnostic findings and problem list for Steven.

Full face and profile	**Frontal view** Face is symmetric LAFH WRN Absence of interlabial gap (lips are competent) Inadequate incisal display in posed smile (maxillary lip vermillion incisal to maxillary central incisor gingival margins) Incisal display at rest ~3 mm UDML: WRN Upturned nose **Profile view** Convex profile and retrusive chin Obtuse NLA Obtuse lip-chin-throat angle
Ceph analysis	**Skeletal** Maxilla AP WRN Mandibular anteroposterior skeletal deficiency LAFH/TAFH = 57% FMA: WRN (27°) SNMP excessive (43°) Maxillary first molar apicies erupted away (below) palatal plane Palatal plane tipped down slightly at posterior Ineffective bony Pogonion **Dental** Mildly proclined mandibular incisors (FMIA = 60°)
Radiographs	Permanent dentition Blocked out maxillary left permanent canine Unerupted maxillary right permanent canine
Intraoral photos and models	Angle Class II division 1 Iowa Classification: II (3 mm) II (3 mm) II (4–5 mm) II (4–5 mm) OJ ~3–4 mm Anterior open bite of 1–4 mm which extends from molar to molar maxillary incisors stepped up relative to maxillary posterior teeth Mandibular incisors stepped up COS ~3 mm Minimal posterior OJ Lingual crown torque mandibular first and second permanent molars Buccal crown torque maxillary second molars Lingual crown torque maxillary first premolars Moderate maxillary (impacted canine) and mild mandibular anterior crowding Dental asymmetry—mandibular right posterior slightly ahead Tapered maxillary arch form
Other	—
Diagnosis	Angle Class II division 1 malocclusion Borderline skeletal open bite and dental open bite

Table 4.6 **Primary problems list for Steven** *(apical base/skeletal discrepancies italicized).*

AP	II (3 mm) II (3 mm) II (4–5 mm) II (4–5 mm) *mandibular skeletal retrusion*
Vertical	Dental (functional) open bite and *borderline skeletal* open bite
Transverse	Minimal transverse posterior overjet with transverse dental compensations (buccal maxillary molar crown torque and lingual mandibular molar crown torque) *maxillary transverse deficiency* Note: if Steven's posterior teeth were uprighted, the maxillary molars would tip lingually while the mandibular molars would tip buccally—leaving him in posterior cross bite
Other	Blocked out maxillary left permanent canine

Q: Do you recommend treating Steven as a dental open bite or as a skeletal open bite?

A: Because he is a dental open bite and borderline skeletal open bite, *treat Steven as both a dental and skeletal open bite* (especially in view of the fact that he just turned 14 years old). If we knew Steven was a pure dental open bite, then we could assume that his vertical growth was normal (or at least not extreme) and his treatment would be greatly simplified: eliminate the tongue habit and erupt the maxillary teeth. But we cannot make this assumption. Because Steven exhibits many features of a skeletal open bite, and because he has years of potential growth ahead, we must be watchful and wary of a developing vertical skeletal problem. Steven's parents must be informed that, depending on future maxillary vertical growth, an overt skeletal open bite could develop. Note: if treatment options can be chosen to address his anteroposterior (Class II) problem while simultaneously addressing his borderline skeletal open bite problem, then that would be ideal. For instance, a HPHG would reduce forward growth of his maxilla (helping to correct his Class II), may reduce descent of his maxilla (helping to close his open bite while simultaneously helping to correct his Class II if his mandible grows), and may reduce eruption of his maxillary molars (helping to close his open bite and helping to correct his Class II). In summary, apply all of your skill and coaching to treat Steven's functional (dental) open bite *and* his borderline skeletal open bite. Looked at in a different way, if you treat Steven as a severe open bite (short of surgery), then you will only end up helping correct his AP relationship if he continues growing as only a borderline skeletal open bite. But, if you ignore his skeletal open bite; and if he starts growing as a severe skeletal open bite, then he could end up needing surgery.

Q: What principle should you follow in treating all borderline skeletal open-bite adolescent patients?

A: *Principle: Treat borderline adolescent skeletal open bite patients as if they are (can become) severe skeletal open bite patients.* The

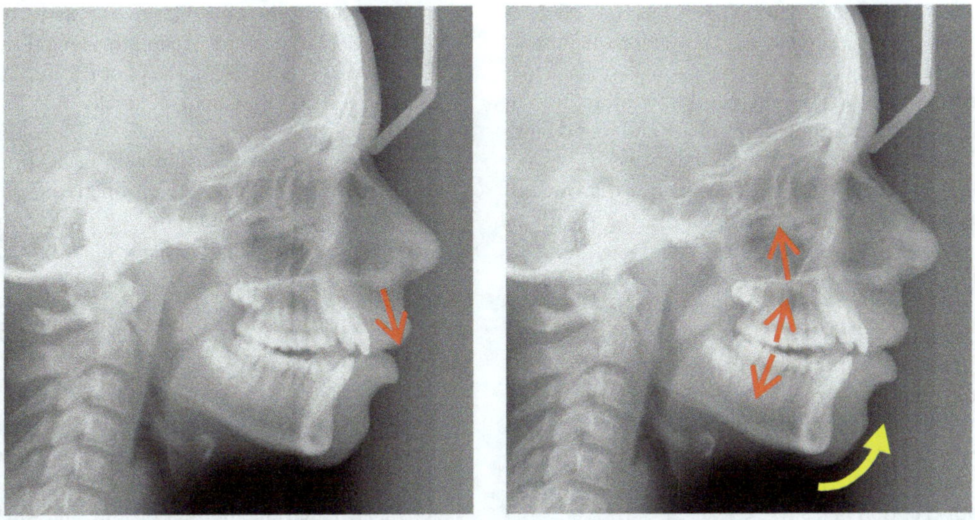

Figure 4.44 Two general approaches to consider when treating Steven's anterior open bite. (Left) treating Steven as a dental open bite (erupting "stepped up" maxillary incisors) by eliminating the tongue interposition habit and leveling the maxillary arch. (Right) treating Steven as a skeletal open bite by impacting the maxillary corpus, slowing descent of the maxillary corpus during growth, intruding (slowing eruption of) maxillary molars, and intruding (slowing eruption of) mandibular molars. As a result, the mandible autorotates closed (curved yellow arrow).

younger they are, the more potential adverse growth you could face, and the more important this principle becomes. This same principle should also be followed in excessive AP growth problems. That is, treat borderline adolescent skeletal Class III patients as if they are (can become) severe Class III skeletal patients. Do not assume they will stay borderline.

Q: What is meant by the concept of "relative" intrusion of molars during treatment of adolescent skeletal open-bite patients?

A: Molars erupt during growth. If you can do anything to reduce molar eruption, then this equates to intrusion relative to where they would have erupted. Reducing molar eruption during growth can be considered a form of "relative" intrusion. Of course, if you can actually intrude molars (e.g., with TADs), it is all the better for skeletal open-bite management.

Q: What are your treatment goals for Steven?

A: Goals include improving Steven's chin projection, increasing his incisal display at rest and when smiling, erupting maxillary canines and achieving a Class I canine AP relationship, obtaining minimal overjet, improving his transverse relationship, and *overcorrecting* his overbite (20–40% OB).

Q: How can Steven's anteroposterior apical base discrepancy be addressed? Discuss specific orthopedic, masking, and surgical options.

A: *Orthopedics* (restrict maxillary AP growth, permit the mandible to continue growing, or accelerate mandibular growth). Options include the following:

- A high-pull headgear would be ideal, if Steven would wear it. It could restrict forward growth of the maxilla while allowing the mandible to continue growing forward [43, 44]. A high-pull headgear may also reduce the downward growth of the maxillary corpus and reduce eruption of maxillary molars, which is especially important in Steven with his potentially worsening skeletal open bite. Distalizing maxillary molars with the HPHG would also make room for the maxillary left canine to erupt.
- A CPHG would not be ideal. Although it could potentially rotate Steven's anterior palatal plane downward (helping to increase his incisal display), restrict forward maxillary growth, and retract maxillary first molars [44, 45], any tendency for a CPHG to erupt maxillary molars could worsen Steven's open bite.
- Steven is not an ideal candidate for a functional appliance due to his mildly proclined mandibular incisors, steep SNMP, and open bite. For instance, during treatment with a Herbst appliance, lower incisors procline an average of 11° and the incisal edges move anteriorly by 3.2 mm. (During the first 6 months post treatment, lower incisors upright an average of 8° and the incisal edges move posteriorly by 2.5 mm.) [46]
- TADs could be used in conjunction with a TPA and an LLHA to prevent eruption of the maxillary and mandibular molars (or even intrude molars), especially if the skeletal open bite features worsen with time. Halting eruption of the maxillary and mandibular first permanent molars (or intrusion of the molars) would help decrease vertical growth and potentially favor AP correction (B-point and chin coming forward as the mandible rotates forward).

Masking or camouflage (achieve Class I canine relationship without addressing the underlying apical base discrepancy). Options include the following:

- High-pull headgear for dental movement only to distalize the maxillary molars and correct the distocclusion, even if future mandibular growth is minimal. Distalizing the maxillary molars would also make room for the maxillary left permanent canine to erupt.
- Extraction of maxillary first premolars.
- Extraction of the maxillary left first premolar to permit eruption/retraction of the maxillary left canine (leaving left molars Class II). Class II elastics or Class II springs on the right side to correct the right canine to Class I (since the Class II relationship on the right side is not as severe).
- Use of buccal, palatal, or infrazyomatic crest TADs as anchorage to distalize the entire maxillary arch.

Surgery (mandibular advancement) would generally not be considered at this age. However, Steven's parents should be informed that, depending on growth and cooperation, an ideal result may require surgery.

Q: How can Steven's borderline skeletal open bite (apical base discrepancy) be addressed? Discuss specific orthopedic, masking, and surgical options.

A: *Orthopedics* (any treatment that would reduce downward descent of the maxilla and reduce eruption of maxillary and mandibular molars would help maintain Steven's vertical dimension)

- A high-pull headgear may reduce the downward growth of the maxillary corpus and reduce eruption of the maxillary molars [43, 44].
- TADs could be used in conjunction with a TPA and an LLHA to orthopedically prevent eruption of the maxillary and mandibular first molars [47].
- Exercising (chewing gum) has been shown to reduce MPAs (compared to controls) in growing patients [48].
- Posterior bite plates (which stretch the masseteric sling causing an intrusive force against the posterior teeth) and active vertical correctors (posterior repelling magnets) can help decrease tooth eruption [49, 50].
- TPAs with an acrylic button several millimeters off the palate can reduce maxillary molar eruption through tongue pressure [51].
- LLHAs have been shown to reduce eruption of mandibular molars by approximately 1 mm compared to controls [52].

Masking or camouflage (achieve open bite closure without addressing the underlying apical base discrepancy). Options could include the following:

- Vertical elastics (e.g., triangle elastics from the maxillary canines to the mandibular canines/first premolars).
- Leveling the stepped up maxillary incisors with fixed orthodontic appliances and archwires.

Surgery (maxillary impaction osteotomy) would not be considered at this age. Why? Vertical maxillary growth during adolescence will continue after the maxillary impaction osteotomy, resulting in relapse. Furthermore, since Steven has lip competence now, you must be careful never to overimpact his maxilla (giving him an overclosed, aged appearance), if he later undergoes surgery. However, his parents should be informed that, depending on growth and cooperation, an ideal result may require surgery later.

Q: How can his transverse apical base discrepancy be addressed?

A: *Orthopedics* (expanding the maxillary arch by separating the hemi-maxillae at the midpalatal suture).

- RME—would expand the maxilla skeletally and dentally, if midpalatal suture separation is attained. *Since RME skeletal expansion (sutural separation) is greatest in the maxillary anterior* [53], *this treatment could also improve Steven's tapered maxillary arch form.* In addition, a bonded RME appliance could reduce maxillary posterior vertical growth slightly (0.5 mm) at the posterior nasal spine [33]. If a midpalatal split does not occur while attempting RME, then it is possible that enough *dental* expansion may be attained to provide adequate transverse OJ.
- A quad helix or maxillary split plate would not be the treatment of choice. Although the quad helix has been shown to cause separation of the midpalatal suture in young persons [34], it may not have the force level necessary to overcome skeletal resistance in a 14-year-old.

Masking or camouflage (correcting minimum posterior overjet by increasing molar transverse compensations—increasing maxillary molar buccal crown torque/increasing mandibular molar lingual crown torque):

- Cross-bite elastics. These would work, but increasing posterior dental compensations is not the ideal solution in this patient.
- Expanding the maxillary archwire or narrowing the mandibular archwire. Again, this would work, but increasing transverse compensations is not the ideal solution.

Surgery (SARME) would generally not be considered for a patient at this age—especially without first attempting to achieve maxillary expansion with an RME appliance. Further, the limited amount of expansion he needs may not warrant surgery, unless the expansion was in the form of an MPMO if Steven eventually required a maxillary impaction osteotomy.

Q: Is surgery an option for Steven?

A: Not at this time. But, you must inform Steven's parents that, depending on growth and cooperation, an ideal result may later require surgery.

Q: What unknowns do you face?

A: Steven's future vertical maxillary growth and mandibular forward growth are the greatest unknowns. Also, cooperation, hygiene, a possible hidden anteroposterior shift, and whether he will achieve a midpalatal suture separation with RME are all unknowns.

Q: What principle should you always follow when dealing with unknowns?

A: *Reduce significant unknowns*, whenever possible, before committing to either a final treatment plan or to irreversible treatment such as tooth extractions. In Steven's case, growth is the most significant unknown you would like to reduce.

Q: Would you proceed with nonextraction treatment? With extraction of anterior teeth? With extraction of some combination of posterior teeth? Finally, what specific treatment options would you give to Steven and his parents?

A: Considerations include the following:

- With the above unknowns, especially with growth being such a major unknown, it would be prudent to initially attempt nonextraction treatment (reversible treatment). This could include RME and a set trial period of headgear (9–12 months if he cooperates), followed by re-evaluation of growth. In other words, we did not know if Steven will cooperate. And if he does cooperate, we are unsure how much growth he will have and whether that growth would be favorable or unfavorable. Starting with reversible, initial, treatments makes sense.
- His mild mandibular anterior crowding and mild mandibular anterior proclination does not warrant extraction of a mandibular incisor.
- It does not make sense to initially extract maxillary premolars, if Steven is willing to wear a headgear. If he wears it, he may distalize his maxillary posterior teeth enough to make room for the maxillary canines to erupt/align. If he does not wear it, we may later decide to extract the maxillary first premolars to mask the AP skeletal discrepancy and correct the canine relationship to Class I. Or, we may wish to treat the maxillary arch nonextraction, if he grows into a severe skeletal open bite, and a maxillary impaction osteotomy is required.
- It does not make sense to initially extract mandibular first premolars (due to mild mandibular anterior crowding and proclination) in addition to maxillary first premolars, because doing so could result in the mandibular canines being retracted distally and the canine Class II relationship worsening. A combination of maxillary first premolars and mandibular second premolars could be considered, but at a later date.
- We may choose to extract mandibular premolars later, if we find a mandibular advancement osteotomy necessary, to retract canines and force a larger surgical advancement.

Three specific options were presented to Steven and his parents:

1 RME to correct the transverse relationship followed by TPA to maintain the transverse correction or a headgear with expanded inner bow to maintain the correction; HPHG to correct the AP relationship and control vertical growth; band and bond the arches to level and align (staying off of the second molars to avoid worsening the open bite); open spaces for the maxillary canines; and vertical elastics to close the dental open bite. Some COS would be placed in the mandibular archwire to maintain eruption of the mandibular incisors and close the bite.
2 RME, band and bond, level and align, evaluate for extraction of maxillary first premolars, leave some COS, do not bond the permanent second molars.
3 RME, band and bond, level and align, evaluate for mandibular premolar extractions/orthognathic surgery.

With any of these three options, Steven and his parents were informed that the open bite will probably not be closed entirely, or remain closed, unless he can learn to keep his tongue postured behind his teeth. They were also informed that the maxilla may not widen with the RME appliance due to transverse skeletal resistance at his age. Finally, posterior occlusal adjustment (enameloplasty) could be used to help close the open bite.

Q: Taking all of our discussions into account, what treatment option do you recommend?

A: Option number one, above, was recommended and was the option Steven chose. The dental etiology of his functional open bite was explained to him, and Steven was asked to be aware of his habit and to keep his tongue away from between his front teeth. He agreed to do so.

Q: What are the specific objectives of treatment for the maxilla, mandible, maxillary dentition, and mandibular dentition in all three planes of space?

A: Specific objectives of treatment for Steven are as follows:

Maxilla

AP: Restrict normal growth.
Vertical: Restrict normal growth.
Transverse: Increase skeletal transverse width.

Mandible

AP: Allow for normal growth.
Vertical: Allow for normal growth.
Transverse: Allow for normal growth.

Maxillary dentition

AP: Distalize molars and canines. Maintain incisor angulation.
Vertical: Level occlusal plane by molar intrusion and incisor extrusion.
Intermolar width: Increase intermolar width.

Mandibular dentition

AP: Maintain molars and canines. Maintain incisors.
Vertical: Maintain mild curve of Spee.
Intermolar/Intercanine width: Maintain intermolar and intercanine widths.

Q: How did Steven's treatment proceed?

A: The maxilla was successfully expanded with an RME appliance (midpalatal suture separation achieved), and he began wearing a HPHG. He was compliant. Later, the maxillary arch was bonded (except for the second molars) and space was created for the left canine (Figure 4.45a–c). After Steven overcorrected his anteroposterior relationship with HPHG, the headgear wear was gradually reduced (over 6 months) and then discontinued. The RME appliance was removed. At that time, a 0.032 inch stainless steel overlay wire (slightly over expanded) was placed through the headgear tubes, and ligated to maxillary brackets (Figure 4.45a, b) to maintain the transverse expansion. When the left canine appeared to have difficulty piercing the gingiva, it was exposed using a laser (Figure 4.45d). The mandibular arch was bonded (except for the second molars), and vertical elastics were worn (Figure 4.45e). The arches were aligned, and the maxillary arch was leveled. A curve of Spee was intentionally left in the mandibular archwire. Finishing was completed, and Steven was debanded.

Q: Treatment lasted 2 years and 3 months. Final records are shown in Figure 4.46 (with initial facial photographs, and initial cephalometric tracing for comparison). What changes do you note?

A: Changes noted include the following:

- No change is observed in his relaxed frontal view (Figure 4.46a, b).
- A dramatic improvement in his smile is seen (Figure 4.46c, d), with improved dental alignment and increased incisal display.
- Steven's buccal corridors remained relatively unchanged.
- His profile improved (Figure 4.46e, f) through downward tipping of his nose and improved soft tissue chin projection.
- Compared with his initial cephalometric radiograph (Figure 4.46h), his ANB angle was reduced dramatically (Figure 4.46i), from 6°to 2°.
- MPA was flattened (FMA from 27°to 20°, SNMP from 43°to 34°).
- Maxillary incisor to SN angle has reduced from 101°to 98°and lower incisor to MP increased by 2° (from 93°to 95°). However, lower FMIA increased quite nicely (from 60°to 66°) with the flattening of the MP.
- Looking at the cranial base superimposition (Figure 4.46j, left), Steven's soft tissue profile improved with soft tissue B-point coming forward much more than soft tissue A-point. His NLA closed a small amount. Comparing the maxilla to the mandible, A-point grew forward a small amount, but B-point grew forward substantially, and the mandibular plane rotated counterclockwise. The maxilla descended slightly, particularly at PNS. This rotated the maxillary incisors down and forward. Looking at the maxillary superimposition (Figure 4.46j, top right), the maxillary molars erupted slightly and came mesially. The mandibular superimposition demonstrates substantial growth at the ramus/condyle, and eruption of the molars/incisors. The key point is that, even though the maxilla descended in the posterior and the mandibular and maxillary molars erupted, Steven had so much favorable condylar/ramal growth that his mandible rotated counterclockwise and forward. This growth was the key to his successful treatment.
- Intraorally (deband photos Figure 4.46l–p), the open bite was closed (OB of ~10%), and the AP relationship corrected to Class I. The distal aspect of both maxillary canines appear to be rotated out slightly (Figure 4.46m, o)—these could have been "tucked in" by slight interproximal reduction of the distal of the maxillary canines and then inserting a rotation barrel on the distal tie wing of the canine bracket.
- Malalignment was noted between the contact of the lower left lateral and central incisors (Figure 4.46p), and the mandibular first molars were rotated mesially (Figure 4.46u).
- Third molars will be monitored for eruption (Figure 4.46k).

Q: How was Steven's open bite closed?

A: *Favorable mandibular growth* (substantial vertical condylar growth, Figure 4.46j) played the greatest role in correcting

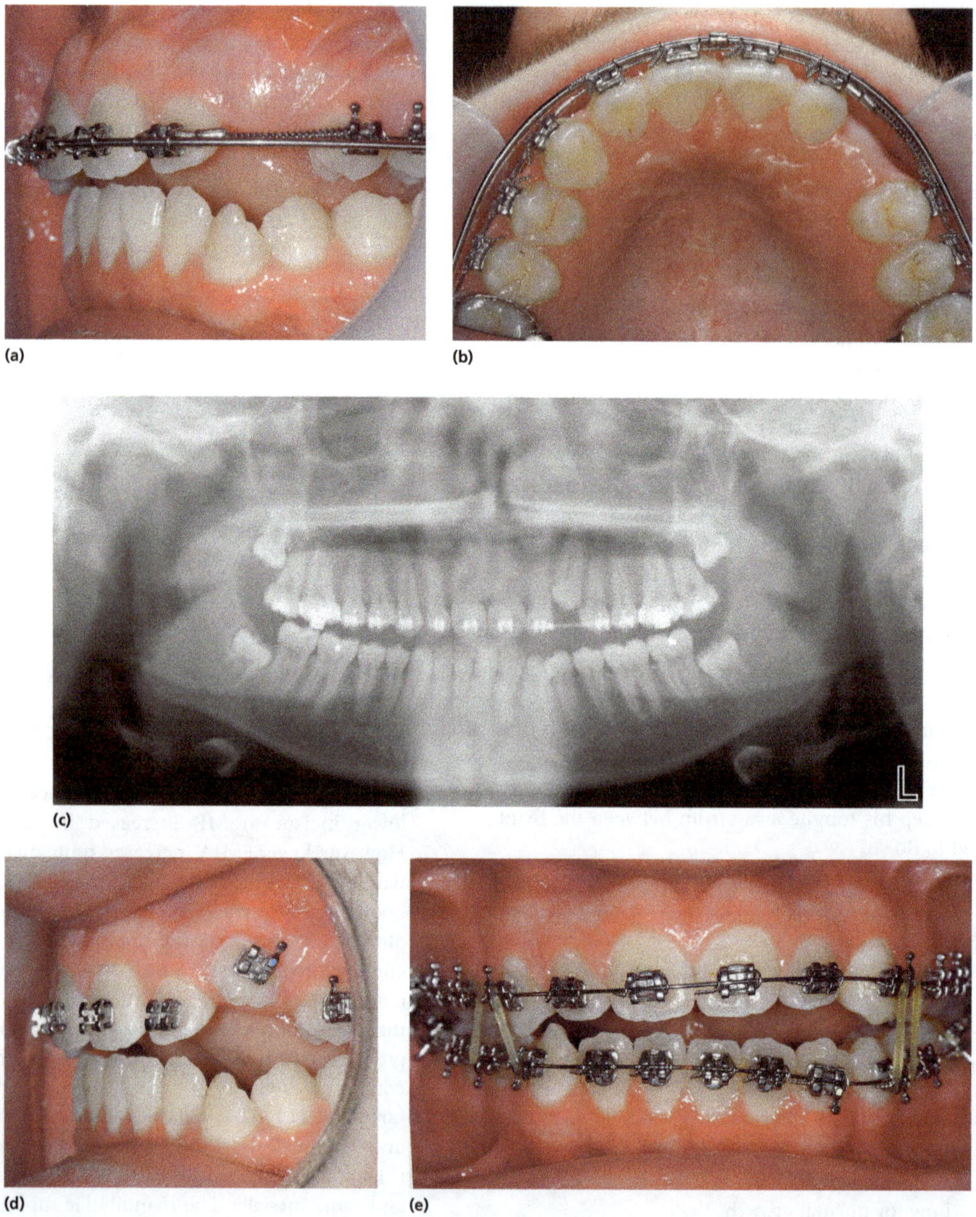

Figure 4.45 (a–e) Steven's progress records.

Steven's open bite and in correcting his Class II relationship. Yes, he did have eruption of the mandibular incisors, which helped close the bite (we had anticipated maxillary incisor eruption). And yes, the maxillary incisors were effectively erupted (rotated down and forward) as PNS descended. But, it was the magnitude and direction of favorable mandibular growth that rotated Steven's mandible upward and forward (CCW) and closed his bite, despite continued downward growth of the maxilla and continued molar eruption.

Q: Were Steven's goals achieved?

A: Almost. Treatment improved Steven's chin projection, increased his incisal display, erupted maxillary canines, achieved a Class I canine AP relationship, resulted in minimal overjet, and improved his transverse relationship. However, his OB should have been *overcorrected* to 20–40% OB, instead of only 10%.

Q: How would you retain this open-bite patient? What will you watch for?

A: Tongue posture reminders (spurs) should be placed in the anterior of the mandibular retainer, and a hole should be placed in the anterior palate of his maxillary retainer—both as aides/reminders in keeping his tongue posture corrected. Small composite "buttons" could be placed on the labial of his incisors (a vacuum-formed retainer could snap over these buttons to hold the teeth in place). The maxillary Hawley retainer could likewise snap over these composite buttons. A tooth positioner could be used as a retainer—helping to keep the tongue lingual to the teeth. His facial growth should be monitored closely until complete. One final suggestion: to help maintain the corrected interdigitation and bite, have Steven exercise daily by chewing gum.

Q: What are your "take-home" messages from Steven's treatment?

A: Take-home messages include the following:

- Steven presented with a borderline skeletal open bite combined with a dental (functional) open bite. The skeletal component of his open bite was due to excessive eruption of his maxillary

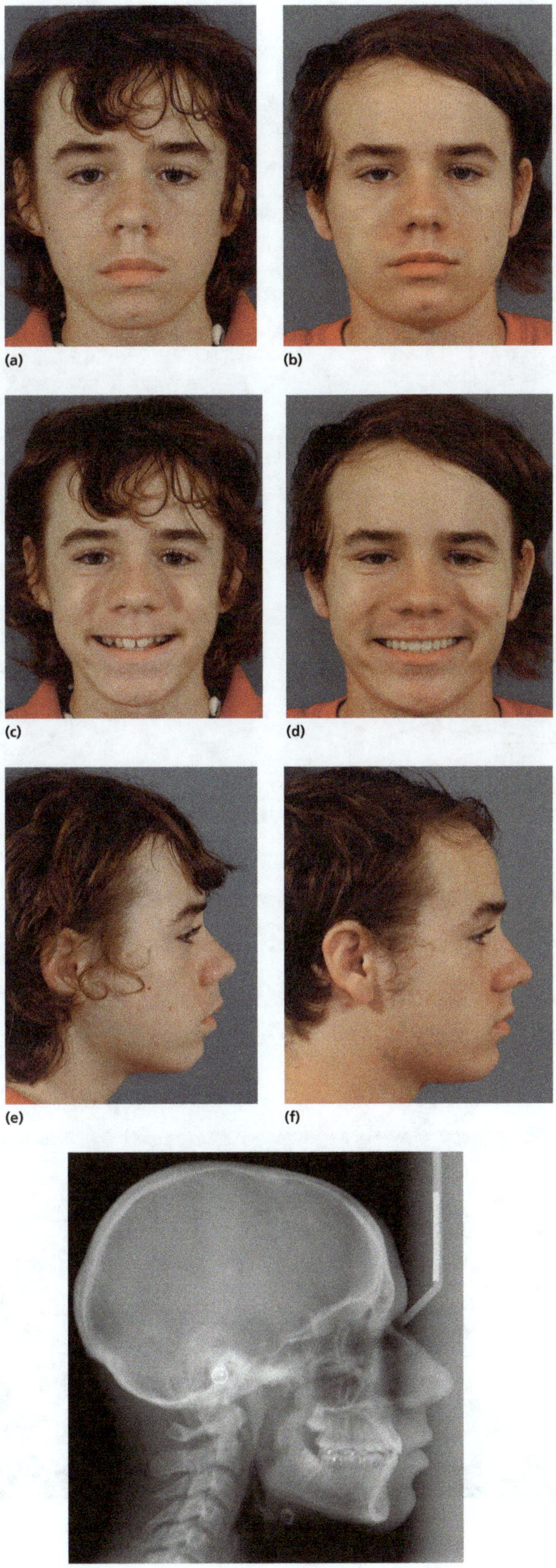

Figure 4.46 (a–u) Steven's final records (including juxtaposed initial facial photographs and initial cephalometric tracing for comparison).

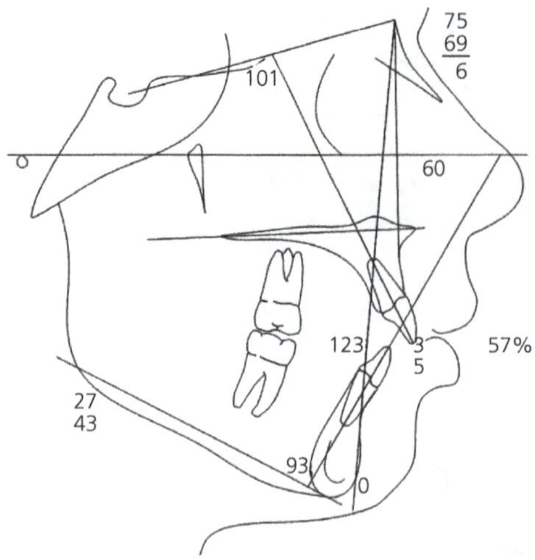

(h)

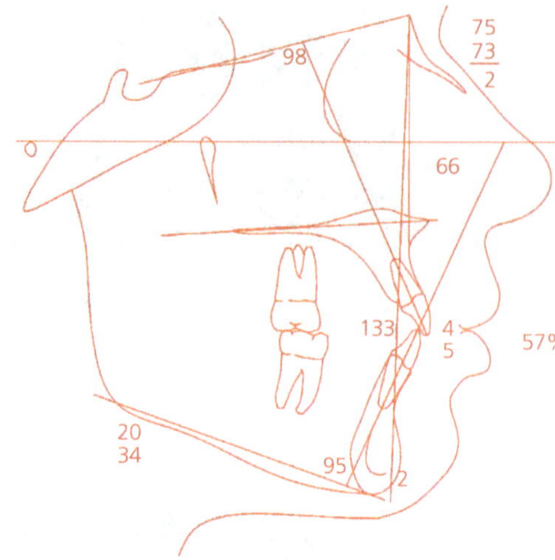

(i)

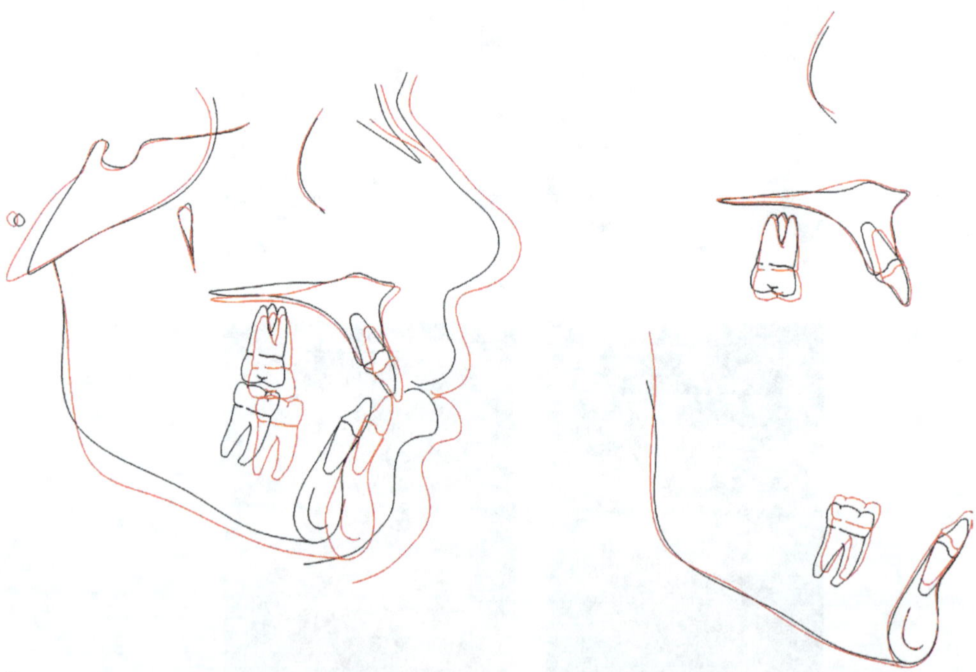

(j)

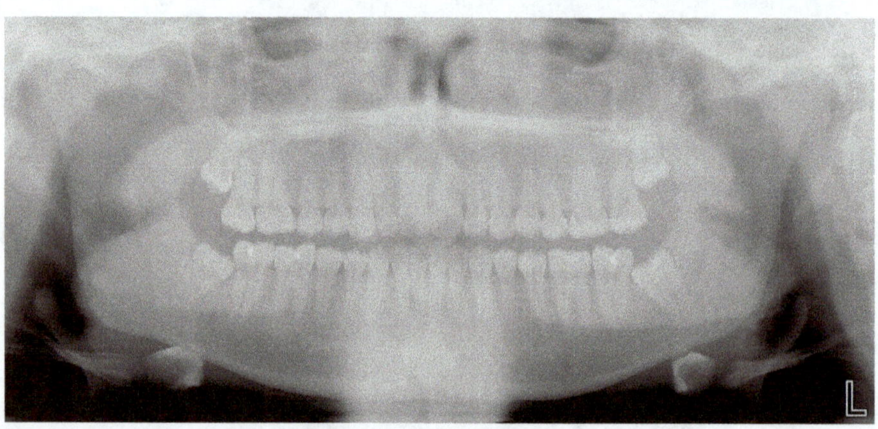

(k)

Figure 4.46 (Continued)

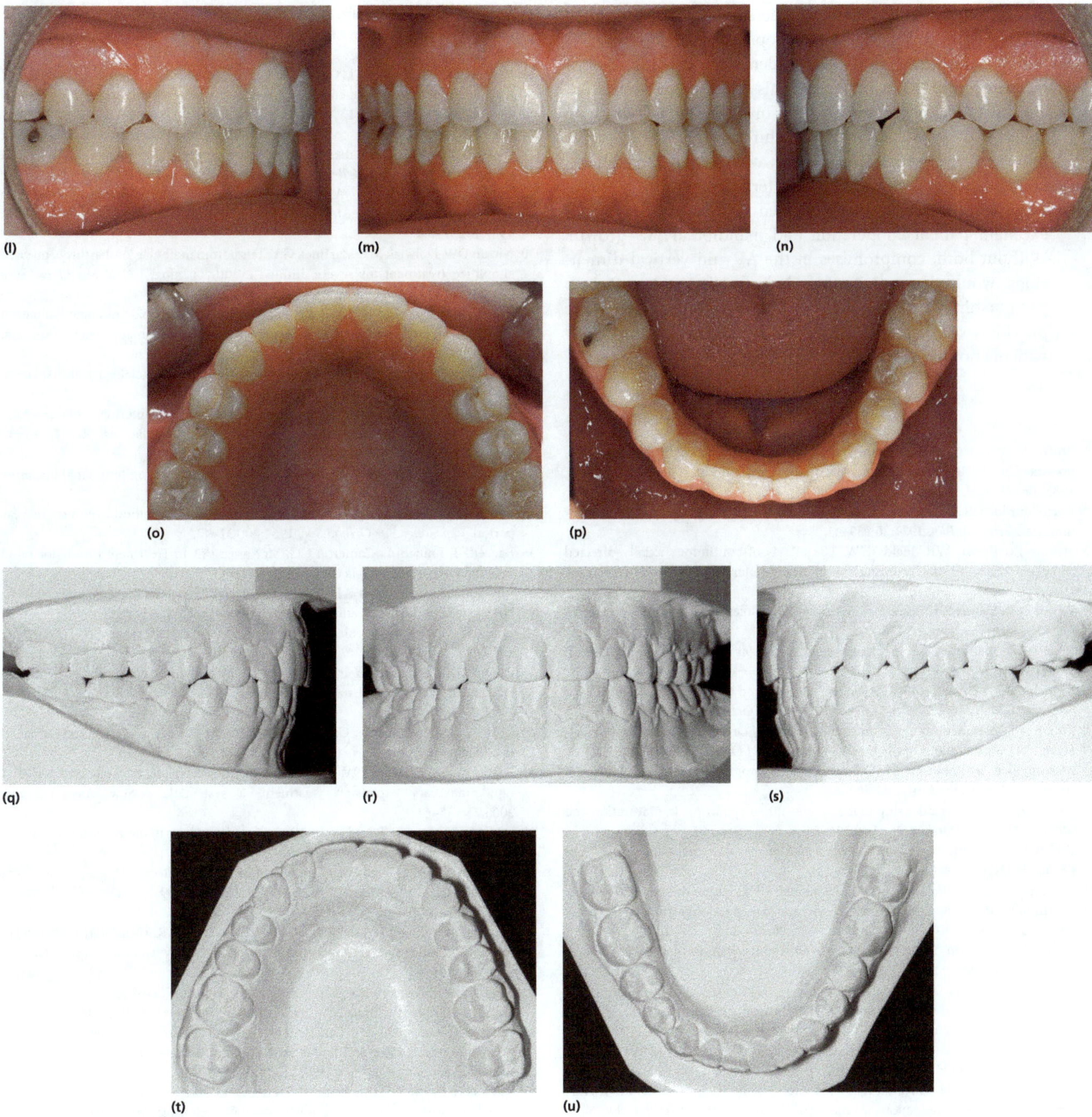

Figure 4.46 (Continued)

molars (first molar apicies erupted several millimeters below the palatal plane) and excessive vertical maxillary corpus descent (palatal plane tipped down at PNS). Additionally, his condyles may have grown more posterior-superiorly than normal, and he could have lacked normal forward mandibular internal (true) rotation. The dental component of his open bite was due to an interpositional tongue habit.

- Steven was treated nonextraction with RME, HPHG, fixed orthodontic appliances, and anterior vertical elastics. Although mandibular incisor eruption contributed to his open-bite closure, as did maxillary incisor downward and forward movement as the maxilla grew down at PNS (rotating about ANS), it was the magnitude and direction of favorable mandibular growth that rotated Steven's mandible upward and forward (CCW), closing his bite and correcting his Class II relationship.
- In dental anterior open-bite adolescent patients who are also borderline skeletal open bites, *treat them (biomechanically) as if you are fighting to prevent them from becoming severe skeletal open-bite cases*. In Steven's case, the HPHG may have helped reduce vertical facial development, permitting mandibular growth to rotate the mandible upward and forward.
- To close the dental anterior open bite, Steven wore vertical elastics, and a curve of Spee was intentionally left in the mandibular archwire.
- Ideally, his OB would have been overcorrected to 20–40% (anticipating some future relapse).

- The functional habit must be corrected to achieve correction and maintain correction of dental open bites.
- Steven did not have tongue reminders placed on his anterior teeth to correct his habit; maybe this should have been done. He did not undergo any form of myofunctional therapy to attempt to correct his tongue posture habit. He was simply asked to try to keep the tongue back away from the front teeth. Did he learn to do this? Only long-term follow-up will tell.
- This was a challenging case treated successfully because of excellent patient cooperation and mandibular jaw growth. Without both, compromises in the AP and vertical dimensions would be anticipated. Orthodontic treatment is a partnership between you and your patients. You will strive to provide excellent care—it is equally important that your patients do the same.

References

1 Proffit WR. On the aetiology of malocclusion. The Northcroft lecture, 1985, presented to the British Society for the study of orthodontics, Oxford, April 18, 1985. *Br J Orthod.* 1986;**13**:1–11.
2 Burn-Murdoch R. The effect of applied forces on the eruption of rat maxillary incisors. *Arch Oral Biol.* 1981;**26**:939–43.
3 Steedle JR, Proffit WR, Fields HW. The effects of continuous axially-directed intrusive loads on the erupting rabbit mandibular incisor. *Arch Oral Biol.* 1983;**28**:1149–53.
4 Proffit WR, Sellers KT. The effect of intermittent forces on eruption of the rabbit incisor. *J Dent Res.* 1986;**65**:118–22.
5 Rogers AP. Open-bite cases involving tongue habits. *Int J Orthod Oral Surg Radiogr.* 1927;**13**:837–44.
6 Swinehart E. A clinical study of openbite. *Am J Orthod Oral Surg.* 1942;**28**:18–34.
7 Straub WJ. Malfunctions of the tongue. Part I. *Am J Orthod.* 1960;**46**:404–24.
8 Straub WJ. Malfunctions of the tongue. Part II. *Am J Orthod.* 1961;**47**:596–617.
9 Straub WJ. Malfunctions of the tongue. Part III. *Am J Orthod.* 1962;**48**;486–503.
10 Massengill R Jr, Robinson M, Quinn G. Cinefluorographic analysis of tongue-thrusting. *Am J Orthod.* 1972;**61**:402–6.
11 Anderson WS. The relationship of the tongue-thrust syndrome to maturation and other factors. *Am J Orthod.* 1963;**49**:264–75.
12 Parker JH. The interception of the open bite in the early growth period. *Angle Orthod.* 1971;**41**:24–44.
13 Garliner D. *Myofunctional therapy*. Philadelphia: W. B. Saunders Co.; 1976. p. 443
14 Proffit WR, Mason RM. Myofunctional therapy for tongue-thrusting: background and recommendations. *J Am Dent Assoc.* 1975;**90**:403–11.
15 Justus R. Correction of anterior open bite with spurs: long-term stability. *World J Orthod.* 2001;**2**:219–31.
16 Smithpeter J, Covell D Jr. Relapse of anterior open bites treated with orthodontic appliances with and without orofacial myofunctional therapy. *Am J Orthod Dentofacial Orthop.* 2010;**137**:605–14.
17 Turpin DL. Editor's choice. *Am J Orthod Dentofacial Orthop.* 2010;**137**:11A–12A.
18 Worms FW, Meskin H, Isaacson RJ. Open-bite. *Am J Orthod.* 1971;**59**:589–95.
19 Ueyama Y, Mano T, Nishiyama A, Tsukamoto G, Shintani S, Matsumura T, et al. Effects of surgical reduction of the tongue. *Br J Oral Maxillofacial Surg.* 1999;**37**:490–5.
20 Vogel JE, Mulliken JB, Kaban LB. Macroglossia: a review of the condition and a new classification. *Plast Reconstr Surg.* 1986;**78**:715–23.
21 Wolford LM, Cottrell DA. Diagnosis of macroglossia and indications for reduction glossectomy. *Am J Orthod Dentofacial Orthop.* 1996;**110**:170–7.
22 Miyawaki S. Long-term changes in dentoskeletal pattern in a case with Beckwith-Wiedemann syndrome following tongue reduction and orthodontic treatment. *Angle Orthod.* 2000;**70**:326–71.
23 Hotokezaka H, Matsuo T, Nakagawa M, Mizuno A, Konbayashi K. Severe dental open bite malocclusion with tongue reduction after orthodontic treatment. *Angle Orthod.* 2001;**71**:228–36.
24 Tanaka OM, Guariza-Filho O, Carlini JL, Oliveira DD, Pithon MM, Camargo ES. Glossectomy as an adjunct to correct an open-bite malocclusion with shortened maxillary central incisor roots. *Am J Orthod Dentofacial Orthop* 2013;**144**:130–40.
25 Lopez-Gavito G, Wallen TR, Little RM, Joondeph DR. Anterior open-bite malocclusion: a longitudinal 10-year postretention evaluation of orthodontically treated patients. *Am J Orthod.* 1985;**87**:175–86.
26 Zuroff JP, Chen SH, Shapiro PA, Little RM, Joondeph DR, Huang GJ. Orthodontic treatment of anterior open-bite malocclusion: stability 10 years postretention. *Am J Orthod Dentofacial Orthop.* 2010;**137**:302–3.
27 Greenlee GM, Huang GJ, Chen SS, Chen J, Koepseil T, Hujoel P. Stability of treatment for anterior open-bite malocclusion: a meta-analysis. *Am J Orthod Dentofacial Orthop.* 2011;**139**:154–69.
28 Huber MA. Hall EH. A comparison of the signs of temporomandibular joint dysfunction and occlusal discrepancies in a symptom-free population of men and women. *Oral Surg Oral Med Oral Pathol.* 1990;**70**:180–3.
29 Pullinger AG, Seligman DA. TMJ osteoarthrosis: a differentiation of diagnostic subgroups by symptom history and demographics. *J Craniomandib Disord Pain.* 1987;**1**: 251–6.
30 Nitzan DW, Dolwick MF, Martinez GA. Temporomandibular joint arthrocentesis: a simplified treatment for severe, limited mouth opening. *J Oral Maxillofac Surg* 1991;**49**: 1163–7; discussion 1168–70.
31 LeResche L, Dworkin SF, Sommers EE, Truelove EL. An epidemiologic evaluation of two diagnostic classification schemes for temporomandibular disorders. *J Prosthet Dent.* 1991;**65**:131–7.
32 Fridrich KL, Casko JS. Genioplasty strategies for anterior facial vertical dysplasias. *Int J Adult Orthod Orthognath Surg.* 1997;**12**:35–41.
33 Sarver DM, Johnston MW. Skeletal changes in vertical and anterior displacement of the maxilla with bonded rapid palatal expansion appliances. *Am J Orthod Dentofacial Orthop.* 1989;**95**:462–6.
34 Harberson VA, Myers DR. Midpalatal suture opening during functional posterior cross-bite correction. *Am J Orthod.* 1978;**74**:310–3.
35 Krebs A. Mid-palatal expansion studied by the implant method over a seven-year period. *Rep Congr Eur Orthod Soc.* 1964;**40**:131–42.
36 Baccetti T, Franchi L, Cameron CG, McNamara JA Jr. Treatment timing for rapid maxillary expansion. *Angle Orthod.* 2001;**71**:343–50.
37 Isaacson RJ and Ingram AH. Forces produced by rapid maxillary expansion II. Forces present during treatment. *Angle Orthod.* 1964;**34**:261–9.
38 Lines PA. Adult rapid maxillary expansion with corticotomy. *Am J Orthod.* 1975;**67**:44–56.
39 Chang JY, McNamara JA Jr, Herberger TA. A longitudinal study of skeletal side effects induced by rapid maxillary expansion. *Am J Orthod Dentofacial Orthop.* 1997;**112**:330–7.
40 Garib DG, Henriques JF, Carvalho PE, Gomes SC. Longitudinal effects of rapid maxillary expansion. *Angle Orthod.* 2007;**77**:442–8.
41 Lagravere MO, Major PW, Flores-Mir C. Long-term dental arch changes after rapid maxillary expansion treatment: a systematic review. *Angle Orthod.* 2005;**75**:155–61.
42 Wylie W, Johnson E. Rapid evaluation of facial dysplasia in the vertical plane. *Angle Orthod.* 1952;**22**:165–82.
43 Firouz M, Zernik J, Nanda R. Dental and orthopedic effects of high-pull headgear in treatment of Class II, division 1 malocclusion. *Am J Orthod Dentofacial Orthop.* 1992;**102**:197–205.
44 Baumrind S, Korn EL, Isaacson RJ, West EE, Molthen R. Quantitative analysis of the orthodontic and orthopedic effects of maxillary traction. *Am J Orthod.* 1983;**84**:384–98.
45 Kirjavainen M, Kirjavainen T, Hurmerinta K, Haavikko K. Orthopedic cervical head-gear with an expanded inner bow in Class II correction. *Angle Orthod.* 2000;**70**:317–25.
46 Hansen K, Koutsonas TG, Pancherz H. Long-term effects of Herbst treatment on the mandibular incisor segment: a cephalometric and biometric investigation. *Am J Orthod Dentofacial Orthop.* 1997;**112**:92–103.
47 Kuroda S, Sakai Y, Tamamura N, Deguchi T, Takano-Yamamoto T. Treatment of severe anterior open bite with skeletal anchorage in adults: comparison with orthognathic surgery outcomes. *Am J Orthod Dentofacial Orthop.* 2007;**132**:599–605.
48 Ingervall B, Bitsanis E. A pilot study of the effect of masticatory muscle training on facial growth in long-face children. *Eur J Orthod.* 1987;**9**:15–23.
49 Dellinger EL. A clinical assessment of the active vertical corrector—a non-surgical alternative for skeletal open bite treatment. *Am J Orthod.* 1986;**89**:428–36.
50 Kuster R, Ingervall B. The effect of treatment of skeletal open bite with two types of bite-blocks. *Eur J Orthod.* 1992;**14**:489–99.
51 DeBerardinis M, Stretesky T, Sinha P, Nanda RS. Evaluation of the vertical holding appliance in treatment of high-angle patients. *Am J Orthod Dentofacial Orthop.* 2000;**117**:700–5.
52 Villalobos FJ, Sinha PK, Nanda RS. Longitudinal assessment of vertical and sagittal control in the mandibular arch by the mandibular fixed lingual arch. *Am J Orthod Dentofacial Orthop.* 2000;**118**:366–70.
53 Garrett BJ, Caruso JM, Rungcharassaeng K, Farrage JR, Kim JS, Taylor GD. Skeletal effects to the maxilla after rapid maxillary expansion assessed with cone-beam computed tomography. *Am J Orthod Dentofacial Orthop.* 2008;**134**:8–9.

CHAPTER 5

Skeletal Anterior Open Bites

Introduction

Allison (Figure 5.1) is a 15-year-old who presents to you with the CC, "I have an open bite, my lips are apart, and my teeth are crooked."

Q: What features would lead you to classify her as a dental open bite? A skeletal open bite?

A: *Dental* open bite features include the following:

- Maxillary incisors stepped up relative to the maxillary posterior teeth and mandibular incisors stepped down relative to the mandibular posterior teeth (Figure 5.1g and i).

Skeletal open bite features include the following:

- Slightly long LAFH (Figure 5.1a, Subnasale–soft tissue Menton slightly longer than soft tissue Glabella–Subnasale).
- 8 mm ILG with a normal maxillary lip length of 19 mm [1].
- Slightly longer skeletal LAFH (LAFH/TAFH = 57% vs a normal value of 55%).
- Steep MPA (Figure 5.1e, FMA = 36°; SNMP = 45°) due to her short posterior facial height development.
- Maxillary first molar apicies erupted 5 mm below the palatal plane (Figure 5.1d).
- Open bite that extends posteriorly past the canines.

Q: What questions should you ask Allison and her parents about her open bite, and what else should you check for?

A: Check for or ask the following questions:

- How long has she had the open bite? Allison and her parents respond that they remember her always having the open bite.
- Does she have a lip biting or digit sucking habit that could prevent her anterior teeth from erupting? She denies any such habits.
- Ask her to close her eyes while you talk to her parents. Then, ask Allison to open her eyes (to distract her) while you gently/quickly retract her lips to see if she exhibits an anterior tongue interposition habit. You do not observe an interpositional tongue habit. However, *due to the stepped up maxillary incisors and stepped down mandibular incisors, you strongly suspect an interpositional tongue habit.*
- Inquire whether Allison suffered jaw trauma or has a history of generalized musculoskeletal problems? Her parents deny a history of trauma, generalized musculoskeletal problems, TMJ pain, or dysfunction. Examine the condyles on her panoramic image (Figure 5.1f) and note that the borders of her condylar heads are difficult to visualize due to anatomic noise. However, with a history of always having had her open bite, and without additional signs or symptoms of TMJ degeneration, additional imaging is not warranted.
- Check for a temporary open bite due to erupting permanent teeth, ankylosed teeth that are not fully erupted, and teeth that are not completely erupted due to lack of space. She has none of these features.

Q: Does Allison have a dental (functional) open bite, a skeletal open bite, or a combination of both?

A: Allison has a combination of skeletal and dental open bite. Skeletally, she a long LAFH to the point where growth of her soft tissue facial drape has not been able to keep pace with her skeletal facial growth, resulting in a large ILG. Her stepped up (unerupted) maxillary incisors and stepped down (unerupted) mandibular incisors contribute to her open bite as a dental component.

Q: What is the etiology of her dental open bite?

A: It is highly probable that Allison has an anterior tongue interposition habit, which has prevented her incisors from erupting.

Q: Contrast the etiology of a skeletal open bite (long face), like Allison's, with the etiology of a skeletal deep bite (short face).

A: Vertical growth of the lower anterior face depends on magnitude and direction of condylar growth, mandibular internal (true) rotation (surface apposition and resorption), maxillary corpus descent (surface apposition and resorption), and molar eruption [2–9]. In a *skeletal deep bite growth pattern* (Figure 5.2a), condyles grow more vertically than normal, a reference line (white line) drawn from the anterior contour of the chin to the contour of the mandibular canal [6] demonstrates excessive mandibular internal (true) CCW rotation (blue arrows), the maxilla descends less than normal, and molars may erupt less than normal. As the mandible rotates upward and forward (Figure 5.2a, yellow arrow), a deep bite results from increased vertical overlap of the anterior teeth. In a *skeletal anterior open bite growth pattern* like Allison (Figure 5.2b), condyles grow more posterior-superiorly than normal, there is a lack of normal forward mandibular internal (true) rotation or there is even backward CW mandibular internal (true) rotation (blue arrows), there is a lack of posterior face height development, the maxilla descends more than normal (palatal plane may rotate down posteriorly), and molars often erupt more than normal. As the mandible rotates downward and backward (Figure 5.2b, yellow arrow), the mandibular plane angle steepens, the anterior face height increases, and an anterior open bite results.

Orthodontics in the Vertical Dimension: A Case-Based Review, First Edition. Thomas E. Southard, Steven D. Marshall and Laura L. Bonner.

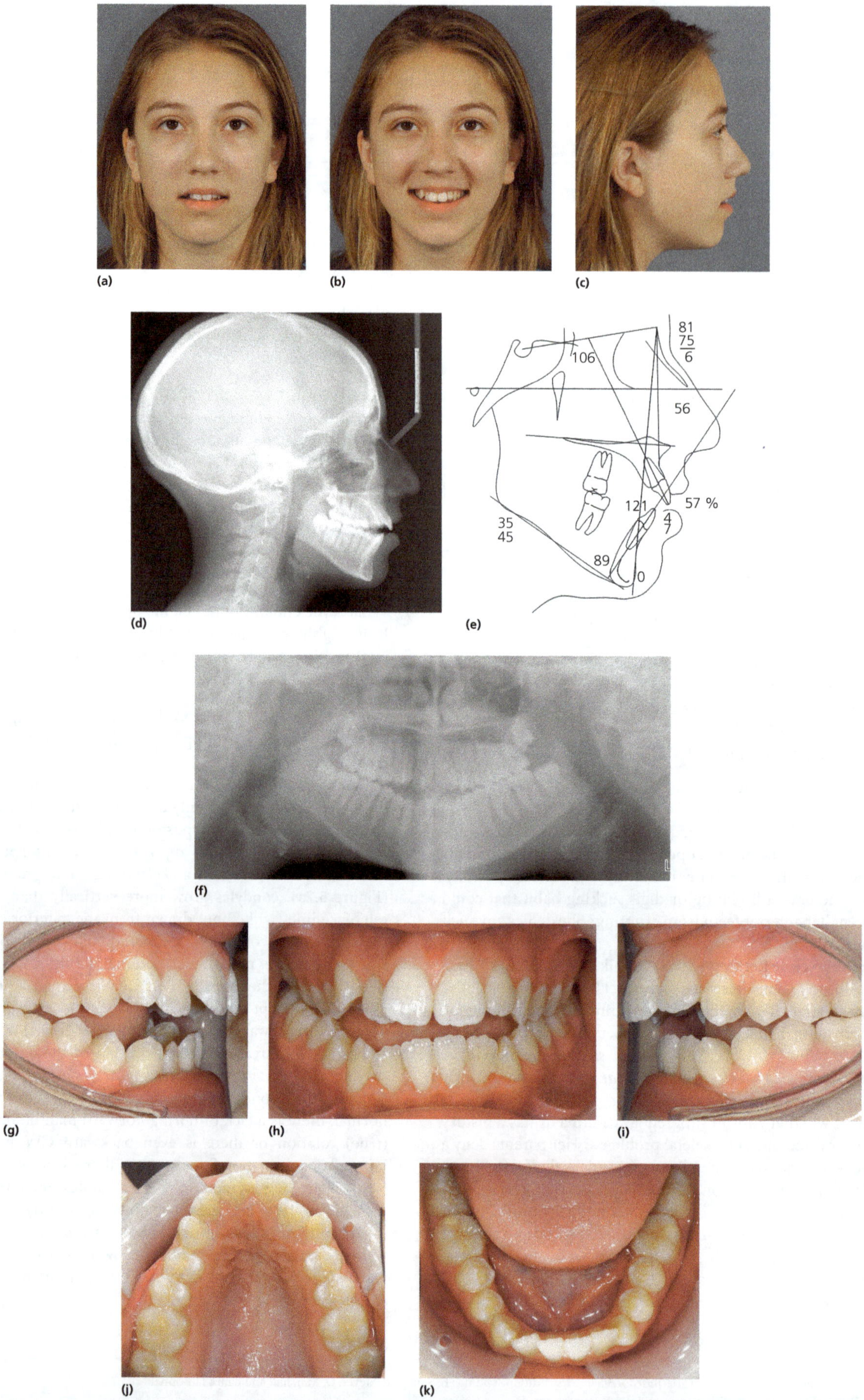

Figure 5.1 Initial records of Allison: (a–c) initial facial photographs, (d) lateral cephalograph, (e) cephalometric tracing, (f) pantomograph, and (g–k) intraoral photographs.

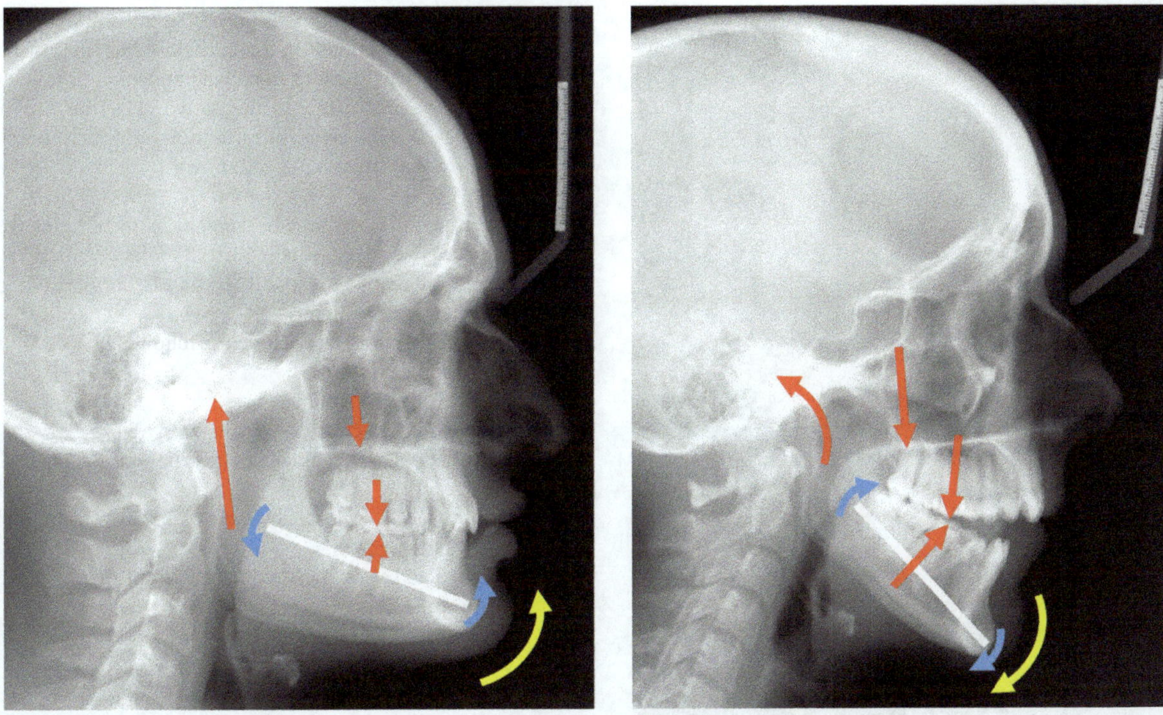

Figure 5.2 The magnitude and direction of condylar growth, mandibular internal (true) rotation, maxillary corpus descent, and molar eruption combine to create (a) a skeletal deep bite or (b) a skeletal open bite.

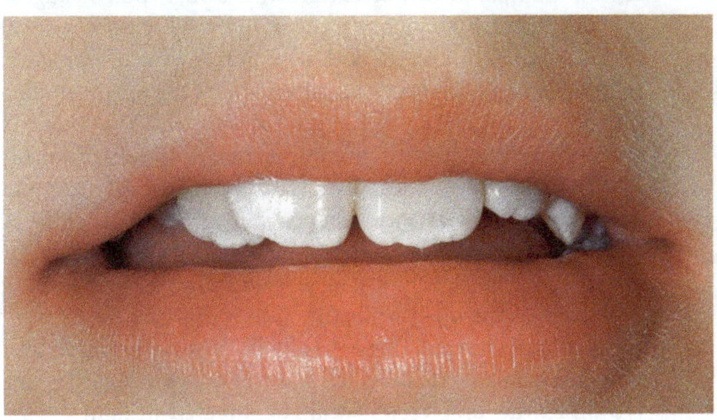

Figure 5.3 Allison's incisal display judged at rest with lips relaxed.

Q: Upon closer inspection, you notice that Allison displays 4 mm of maxillary central incisors relative to relaxed lips (Figure 5.3). Is this normal? What will happen to this amount of incisor display when her maxillary arch is leveled? What will happen as she ages?

A: On average, the amount of incisal display is 3–4 mm for adolescents, 3 mm for young women, 2 mm for young men, and 1–1.5 mm for middle-aged persons [10]. *The amount of maxillary incisor display decreases as we age and lip length increases.* So, Allison is presently at the upper limit of normal display for adolescents. Because her maxillary incisors are stepped up relative to her posterior teeth (Figure 5.1g and i), after her maxillary arch is leveled, we can anticipate a dramatic (and possibly unaesthetic) increase in incisal display/gingival display.

Q: What treatments would you consider to address Allison's *dental* open bite component?

A: The most important treatment would be *habit cessation*. Additionally, you could discuss the importance of keeping her tongue back from her anterior teeth, bond buttons or spurs on the lingual of her mandibular incisors to remind her to keep her tongue back, and place fixed appliances (with anterior vertical elastics) to level her arches and erupt her incisors—in some patients this open bite closure alone helps to re-train the tongue. But remember, although these treatments should help close her open bite, eruption of her maxillary incisors will increase maxillary incisor display and worsen her esthetics. In other words, closing Allison's open bite by erupting her maxillary incisors to the level of her posterior teeth will further display her true skeletal LAFH excess.

Q: What general treatments would you consider to address Allison's *skeletal* open bite?

A: The three general treatments for skeletal open bites are the same as for any other apical base discrepancy (vertical, transverse, or anteroposterior): *orthopedics, masking/camouflage, or surgery*. Orthopedics and surgery intrude posterior teeth (improving/correcting the vertical apical base discrepancy), while masking simply erupts anterior teeth (ignoring the vertical apical base discrepancy). Allison declined surgery.

Q: Describe the principles for treating skeletal open bites with orthopedics.

A: Orthopedic treatment of adolescent skeletal open bite patients consists of (Figure 5.4, straight red arrows) restricting downward maxillary growth, reducing molar eruption, or intruding molars. Each of these movements tends to autorotate the

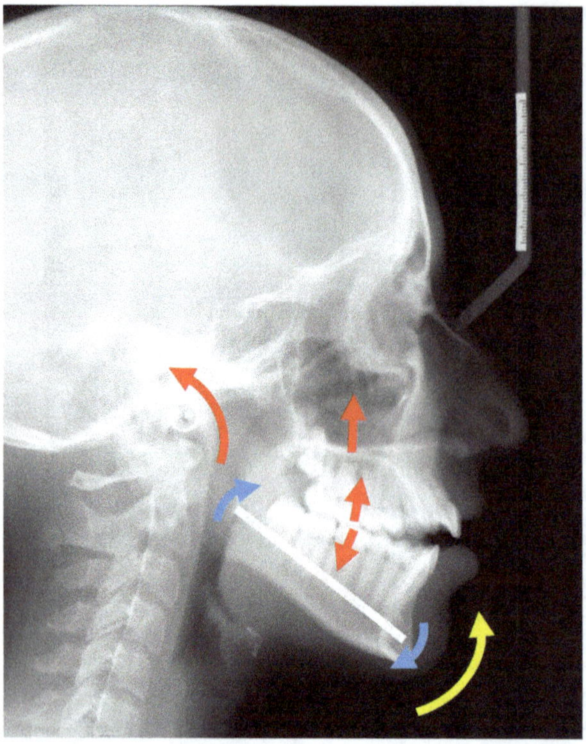

Figure 5.4 Orthopedic treatment of skeletal open bites reduces maxillary corpus descent, reduces molar eruption, or intrudes molars (resulting in mandibular autorotation and bite closure, yellow arrow). Treatment is opposed by continuing unfavorable condylar posterior–superior growth and backward mandibular internal (true) rotation.

mandible closed (Figure 5.4, curved yellow arrow), shorten the lower anterior face height, decrease the mandibular plane angle, close the anterior open bite, achieve lip competence, and improve a Class II molar relationship (or worsen a Class III molar relationship). Of course, unfavorable condyle growth posterior-superiorly (curved red arrow) or growth-related backward internal (true) mandibular rotation (curved blue arrows) can oppose these effects.

Q: You consider treating an adolescent skeletal open bite patient, orthopedically. What two factors could persuade you to attempt orthopedic treatment or dissuade you from attempting orthopedic treatment?

A: The *magnitude* of the skeletal open bite and the *time* of growth remaining. If the patient has a mild skeletal open bite and much anticipated growth, you may be successful in closing the open bite with orthopedics, if the child is compliant. If the patient has a very severe skeletal open bite and little anticipated growth, then it is foolish to attempt orthopedic treatment.

Q: Is Allison a good candidate for orthopedic treatment to correct her skeletal open bite?

A: Both the severity of her skeletal open bite and her age counsel against orthopedic treatment. Based on all of her skeletal open bite features, we judge that her open bite is more moderate than mild. Further, at age 15, little future growth is anticipated. Of course, we need to talk to her parents to ask if she is still growing, and when she achieved menarche. If you find that she has some growth potential remaining, then you can always attempt orthopedic treatment. But it would be unusual to achieve an ideal orthopedic result in Allison's case. The one "orthopedic" treatment that could close her bite would be the use of TADs to intrude maxillary and mandibular posterior teeth. A viable treatment alternative [11], the use of TADs to correct skeletal open bites, is not yet widely employed as long-term stability remains unknown.

Q: Exhaustively list orthopedic appliances/techniques to restrict downward maxillary growth, restrict molar eruption, or intrude molars. Then, discuss the specific effects of each of these appliances or techniques.

A: Appliances/techniques include the following:

- High-pull headgear
- Vertical-pull chin cup
- High-pull chin cup
- Modified Herbst appliance (acrylic splints plus high pull headgear)
- Full posterior occlusal coverage bite plates (with and without repelling magnets).
- Transpalatal arch (TPA) with acrylic button
- Lower lingual holding arch
- Temporary anchorage device
- Chewing exercises

Effects of these appliances/techniques:

- High-pull headgear (Figure 5.5a): If Allison wore a high-pull headgear, then the force vector of the headgear spring or elastic (red arrow, Figure 5.5b) is directed superiorly and posteriorly between the centers of resistance for the maxillary first molars (green cross) and the maxillary corpus (yellow cross). Compared to normal growth, a high-pull headgear reduces forward maxillary growth and may reduce vertical maxillary growth. In fact, with continuous wear in monkeys, HPHG has been shown to actually displace the maxillary corpus up and back [12]. A HPHG distalizes maxillary molars and may reduce maxillary molar eruption. Since the mandible grows forward normally, a HPHG can be ideal treatment in growing Class II skeletal open bite patients [13, 14]. A problem with HPHG use can be patient compliance. To be effective, the headgear must be worn during the early evening and through the night while the child is growing.
- Vertical-pull chin cup (Figure 5.6a): If Allison wore a vertical-pull chin cup, the use of which was first reported by Kingsley [15], then the force vector would be directed straight superiorly (Figure 5.6b). Studies have demonstrated that this force can reduce the MPA, on average, by up to 3.9° compared to controls. It does this as a result of dentoalveolar growth inhibition (inhibition of posterior tooth eruption) with 9–12 months of wear [16–18]. Vertical-pull chin cups can be challenging to fit as the frontal strap tends to slide forward down the forehead. It is important that the force vector be kept vertical and *not* directed to the posterior, which would make it a high-pull chin cup, inhibit forward mandibular growth, and thus be contraindicated in Class II patients.
- High-pull chin cup (Figure 5.7a): In a sample of 36 Class III, 5- to 10-year-old dolichofacial girls (average age, 8 years) who wore an occipital-pull or high-pull chin cup 14 h per day for 2 years with a force of 250–300 g—and then during sleep for 3 years—Deguchi et al. [19] reported: significant inhibition in ramus height, significant inhibition in mandibular body length, horizontal and vertical restriction of mandibular growth, and significant gonial angle closure. Mandibular

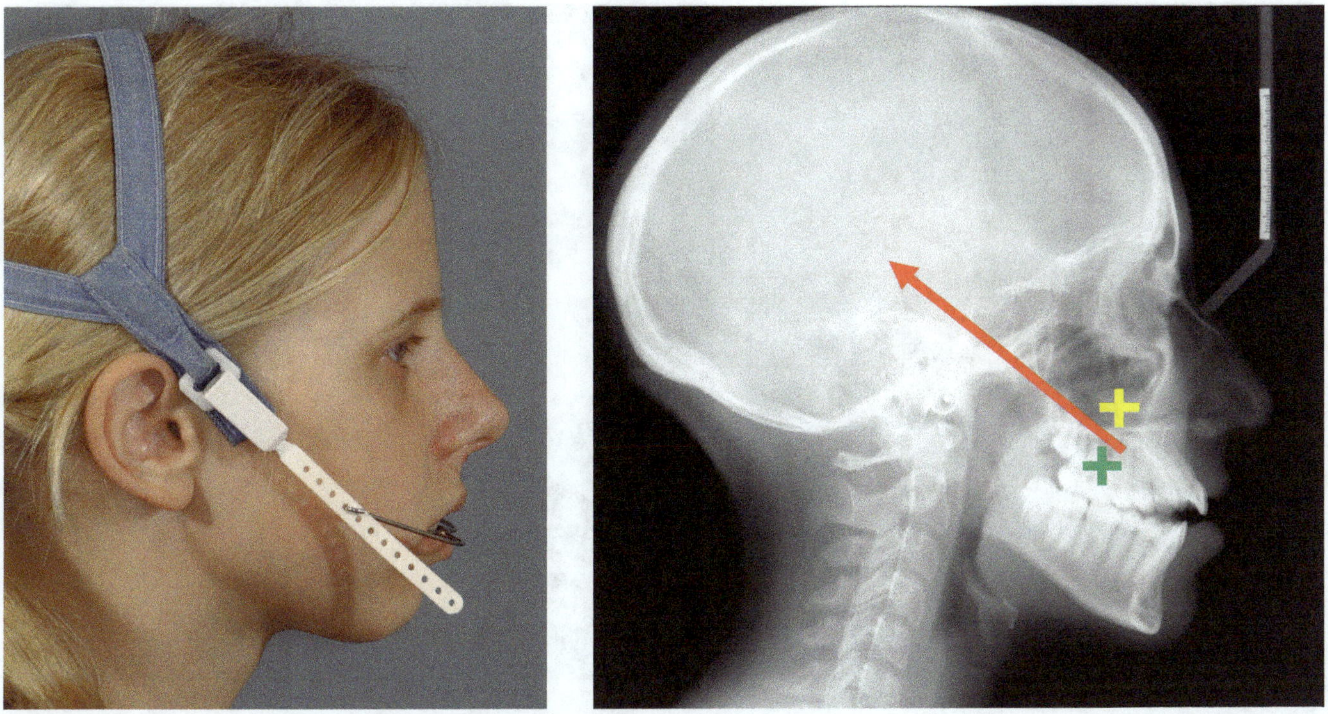

(a) (b)

Figure 5.5 (a) HPHG and (b) the resulting force vector (red arrow) in relation to the centers of resistance of the maxilla (yellow cross) and maxillary first molar (green cross). Compared to normal growth, a high-pull headgear reduces forward maxillary growth and may reduce vertical maxillary growth. A HPHG distalizes maxillary molars and may reduce maxillary molar eruption.

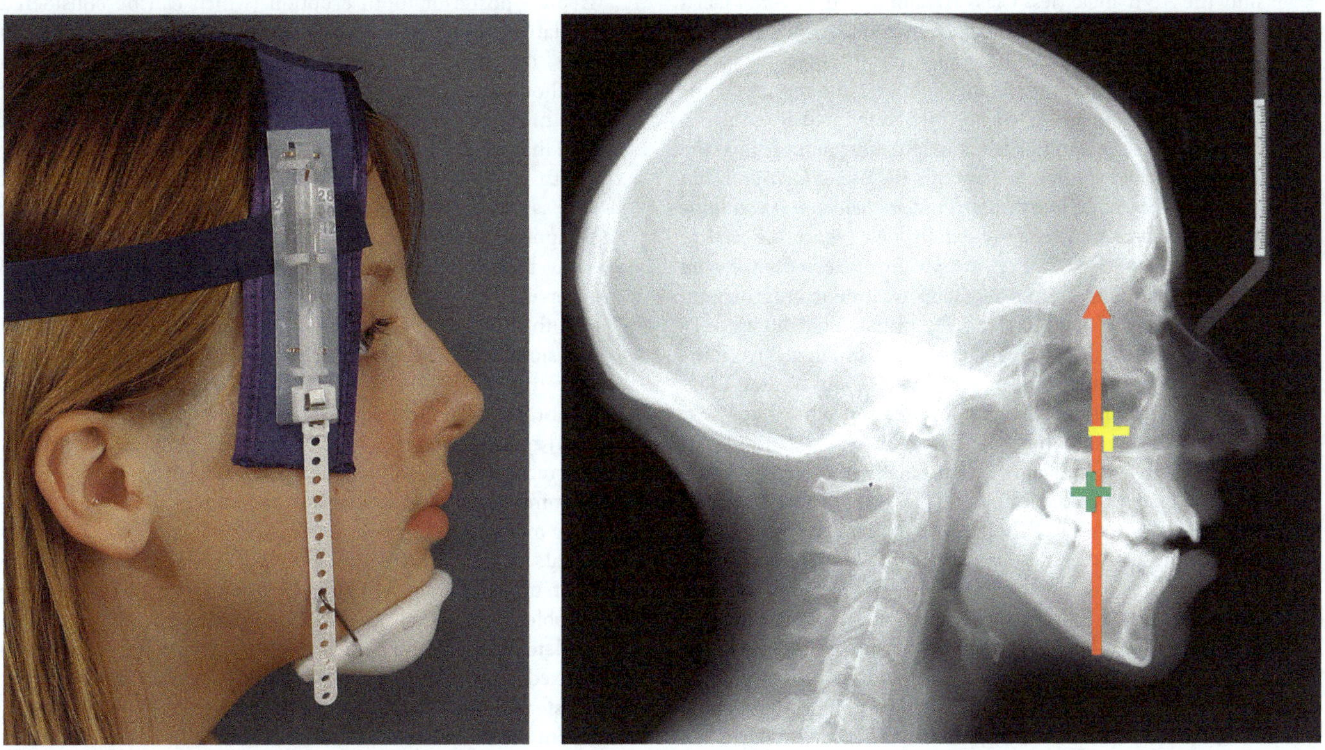

(a) (b)

Figure 5.6 (a) Vertical-pull chin cup and (b) the resulting force vector (red arrow) in relation to the centers of resistance of the maxilla (yellow cross) and maxillary first molar (green cross). Vertical-pull chin cups can reduce the MPA, compared to controls, by inhibition of posterior tooth eruption.

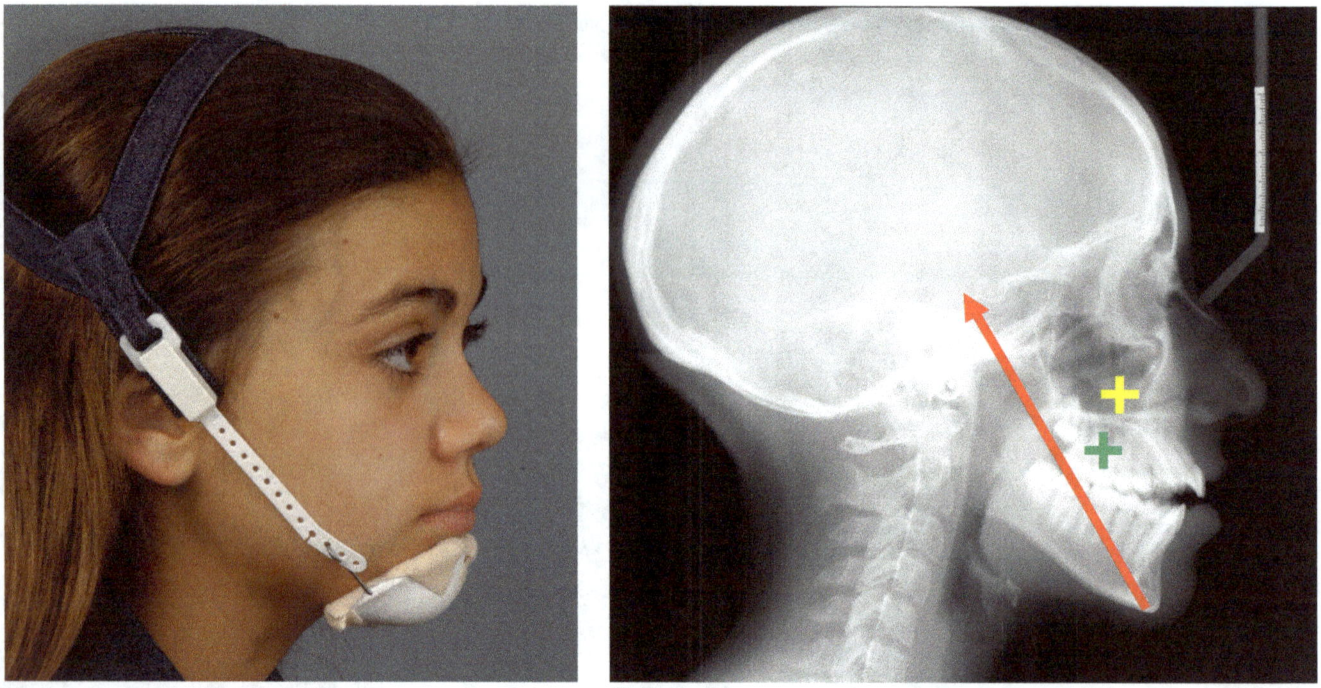

(a) (b)

Figure 5.7 (a) High-pull chin cup and (b) the resulting force vector (red arrow) in relation to the centers of resistance of the maxilla (yellow cross) and maxillary first molar (green cross). High-pull chin cups can inhibit ramus height, inhibit mandibular body length, close the gonial angle, and flatten FMA without increasing LAFH, but the force vector must be kept high.

plane angle (FMA) flattened in chin cup patients, while FMA opened in control group subjects. Treatment improved not only the ANB angle (less Class III) but also the overall facial morphology. Wendell et al. [20] examined high-pull chin cup patients treated for an average of 3 years with the force vector directed from the symphysis through Sella and reported similar improvement in skeletal profile, compared to controls, and a decrease in anterior facial height. Our point is this: the aforementioned studies indicate that the use of *high-pull chin cups do not increase lower anterior facial height, but you must keep your force vector line-of-action high (above the ear) in cases of Class III skeletal open bites.* In our experience, you should attempt high-pull chin cup treatment only in *mild* Class III skeletal open bite adolescent patients who are *very compliant* (they must wear the chin cup until they have completed growth). In fact, in patients with severe skeletal Class III malocclusions, the beneficial effects of chin cup wear often fail during retention [21].

- Modified Herbst appliance: traditionally, the Herbst appliance has been intended for patients with small MPAs/normal or reduced lower facial heights [22]. However, one study [23] reported successful use of modified Herbst appliances (acrylic splints combined with a high-pull headgear) to better control the vertical dimension in hyperdivergent adolescents (reduction in Go–Gn–SN angle of $-1°$ compared to reduction of $-0.3°$ in control group, Bolton standards). Pearl: if you decide to treat an adolescent skeletal open bite patient with a Herbst appliance, we strongly encourage you to have the patient posture forward to Class I canine, first. Only if there is no opening of the bite when you do this should, you attempt using a Herbst appliance (clinical opinion).
- Bite plates and bite plates incorporating repelling magnets (Figure 5.8a, Active Vertical Corrector): Bite plates can reduce posterior tooth eruption (which can be considered "relative" intrusion since the final tooth erupted position is less, or intruded, compared to where it would have been without treatment) and can even cause true intrusion of teeth. When worn, bite plates force the jaws apart and stretch the masseteric sling, which responds by loading the posterior teeth occlusally (Figure 5.8b). Active vertical correctors act the same as bite plates, but in addition, incorporate repelling magnets to create an additional occlusal load. Bite plates may be cemented into place, if compliance is problematic (Personal communication with Dr. Eugene Dellinger at the 100th American Association of Orthodontists Annual Session, 5th International Orthodontic Congress, and 2nd Meeting of the World Federation of Orthodontists, Chicago, IL, oral communication, May 2000). In a case series, Dellinger [24] reported posterior tooth intrusion using active vertical correctors as did Barbre and Sinclair [25] (8-month wear). In a comparison of plain acrylic bite plates to those with repelling magnets (same thickness, 18 h of wear per day), Kiliaridis et al. [26] found that the open bite was generally closed in just under 4 months in the magnet group, but transverse problems (unilateral cross-bite and scissor-bite on the contralateral side) were observed with intensive use in the early mixed dentition patients. Patients who wore plain acrylic posterior bite-blocks (no magnets) also showed improvement in the dental and skeletal vertical relationships but without transverse problems. In a follow-up of cases treated with magnetic bite-blocks, Kuster and Ingervall [27] reported a tendency for the beneficial effects of treatment to relapse.

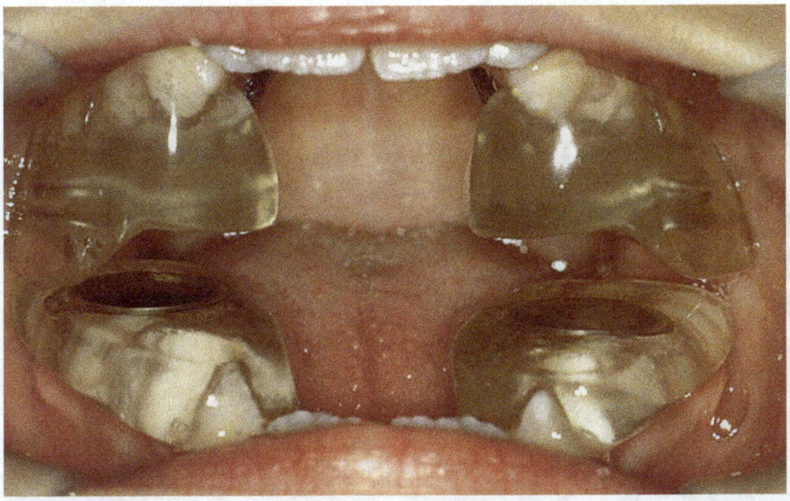

(a)

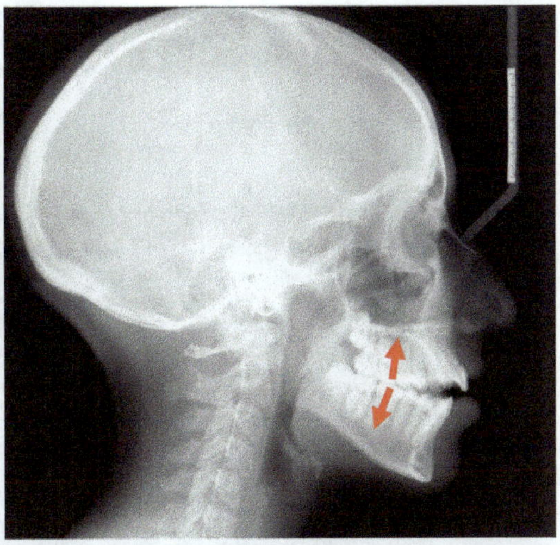

(b)

Figure 5.8 (a) Active vertical corrector bite plates incorporating repelling magnets. (b) The force vector resulting from masseter and medial pterygoid muscle stretch. Bite plates can reduce posterior tooth eruption ("relative" intrusion in a growing patient) and even achieve true molar intrusion in some patients.

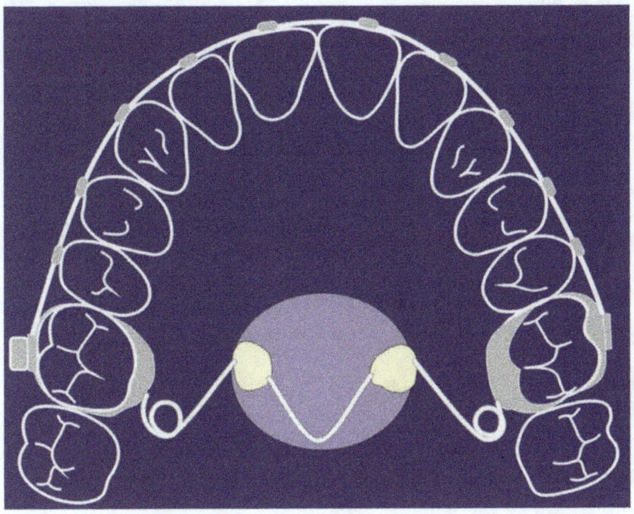

Figure 5.9 Schematic of a TPA incorporating an acrylic button. These can decrease LAFH in high angle adolescents.

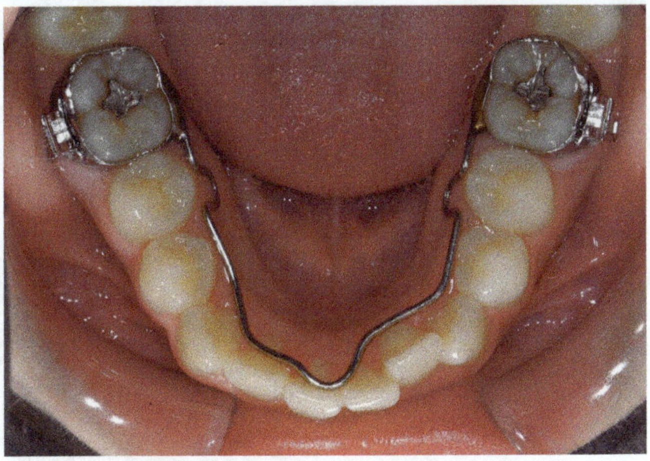

Figure 5.10 LLHAs can reduce eruption of mandibular first molars.

Bite plates with molar intrusion springs between arches have similarly been shown to intrude posterior teeth [28].

- TPA with acrylic button (Figure 5.9): By connecting maxillary first molars with a TPA (which includes a midpalatal acrylic button vertically positioned at the gingival margins of the molar bands), DeBerardinis et al. [29] found lower anterior face height increasing less (1.5 mm) in high-angle patients as compared to patients treated without it (3.4 mm, $p < 0.05$).
- Lower lingual holding arches (Figure 5.10): LLHAs are effective for reducing vertical eruption of mandibular first molars (0.3 mm of first molar eruption with a LLHA versus 1.2–2.1 mm of first molar eruption in controls over 12–24 months) [30].
- Temporary anchorage devices (TADs): Umemori et al. [31] first reported the use of miniplate anchorage to intrude posterior teeth 3–5 mm and close open bites (Figure 5.11). Later, Sherwood et al. [32] reported mean molar intrusion of 2 mm with miniplate anchorage, and others reported using screws alone to close skeletal open bites (eliminating the need for orthognathic surgery) [33, 34]. In addition to molar intrusion, we recently used miniplates to restrict maxillary corpus vertical and horizontal growth in an experimental animal model [35].

Palatal TADs were used to close our patient Allison's (Figure 5.1) skeletal open bite, as shown in Figure 5.12. Two TADs were placed in the palate (red circles, Figure 5.12a) and used to intrude the maxillary posterior teeth with elastomeric power chains. This closed the open bite (Figure 5.12b, c). If you use this technique to intrude posterior teeth, you should anticipate approximately 30% relapse (molar eruption). Therefore, consider overintruding and holding the overintruded molars for months before removing the TADS.

Another example of skeletal open bite closure using *buccal* TADs to intrude maxillary molars, with a 5-year post-treatment frontal photograph to illustrate treatment stability, is shown in Figure 5.13. Note in the superimposed lateral

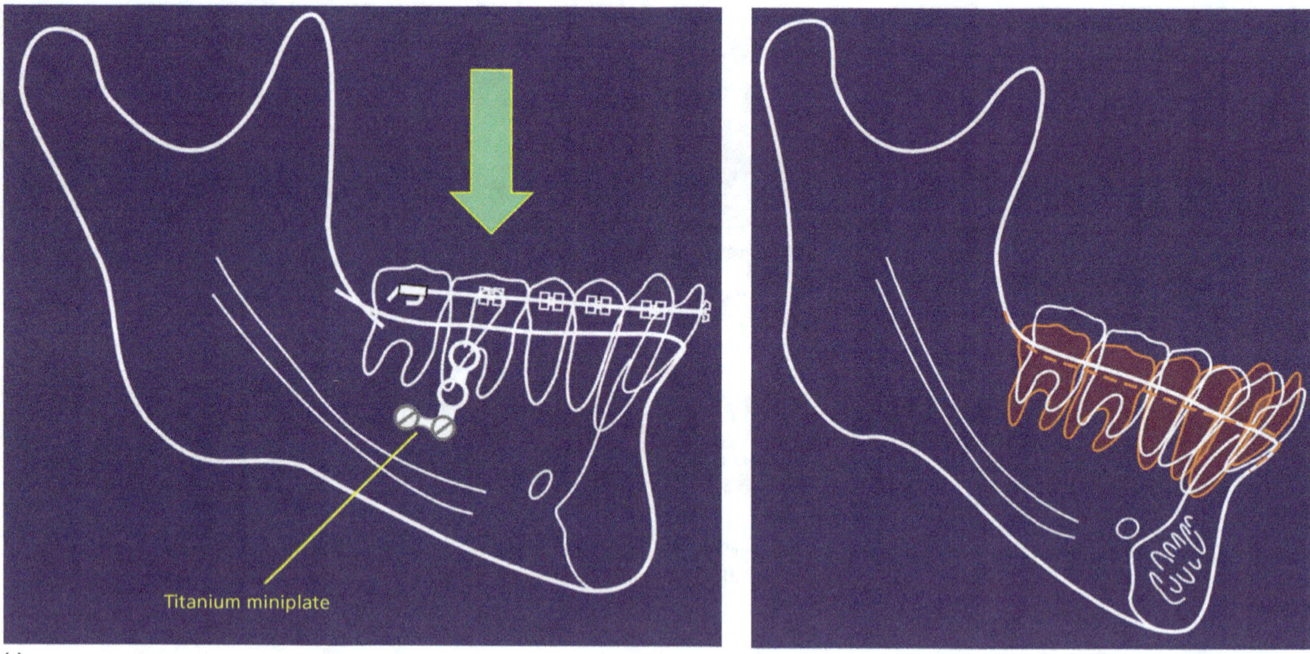

(a) (b)

Figure 5.11 (a, b) Closure of skeletal open bites by intrusion of mandibular posterior teeth using titanium miniplates [31]. (Umemori M, Sugawara J, Mitani H, Nagasaka H, Kawamura H. Skeletal anchorage system for open-bite correction. Am J Orthod Dentofacial Orthop. 1999;115:166–74. Reproduced with permission from Elsevier.)

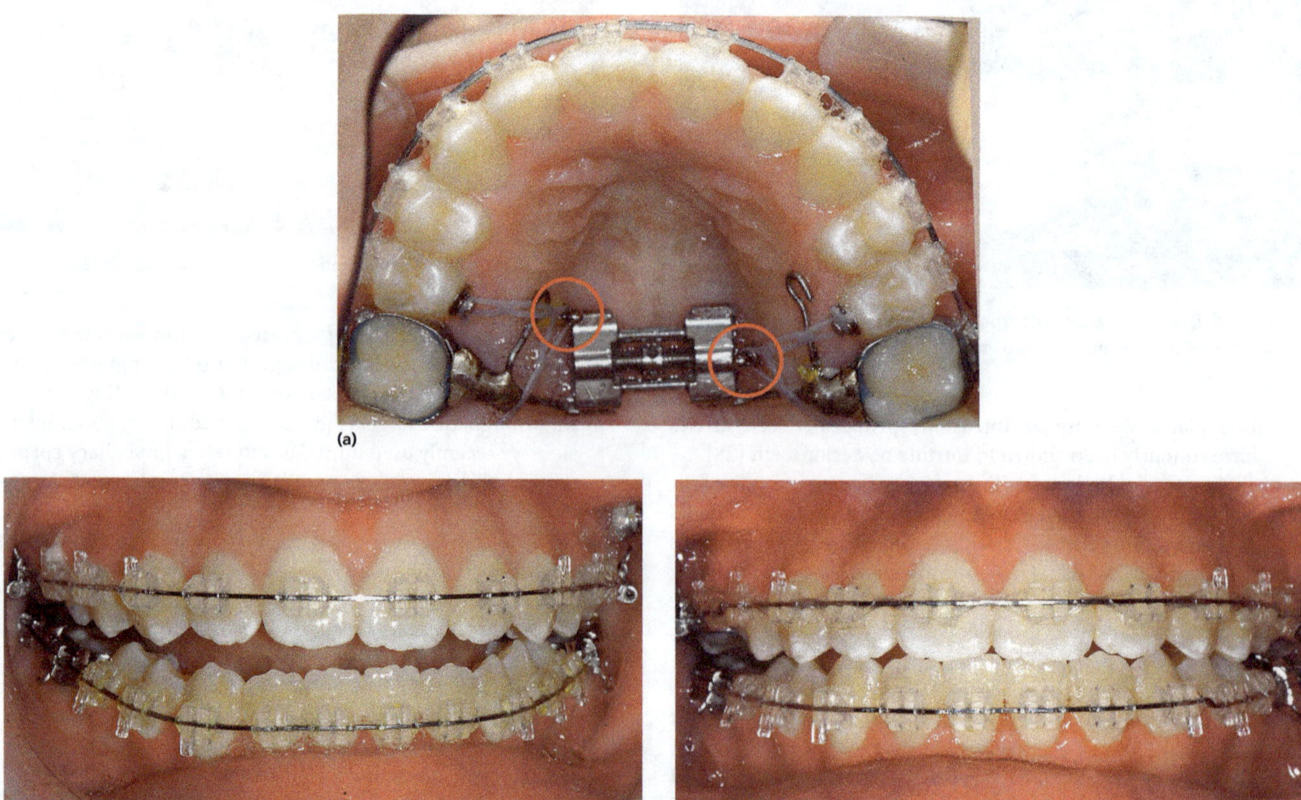

(a) (b) (c)

Figure 5.12 (a) Closure of Allison's (Figure 5.1) skeletal open bite by intrusion of maxillary molars using TADs secured in the palate. (b) Open bite after arch leveling but prior to molar intrusion. (c) Resulting open bite closure.

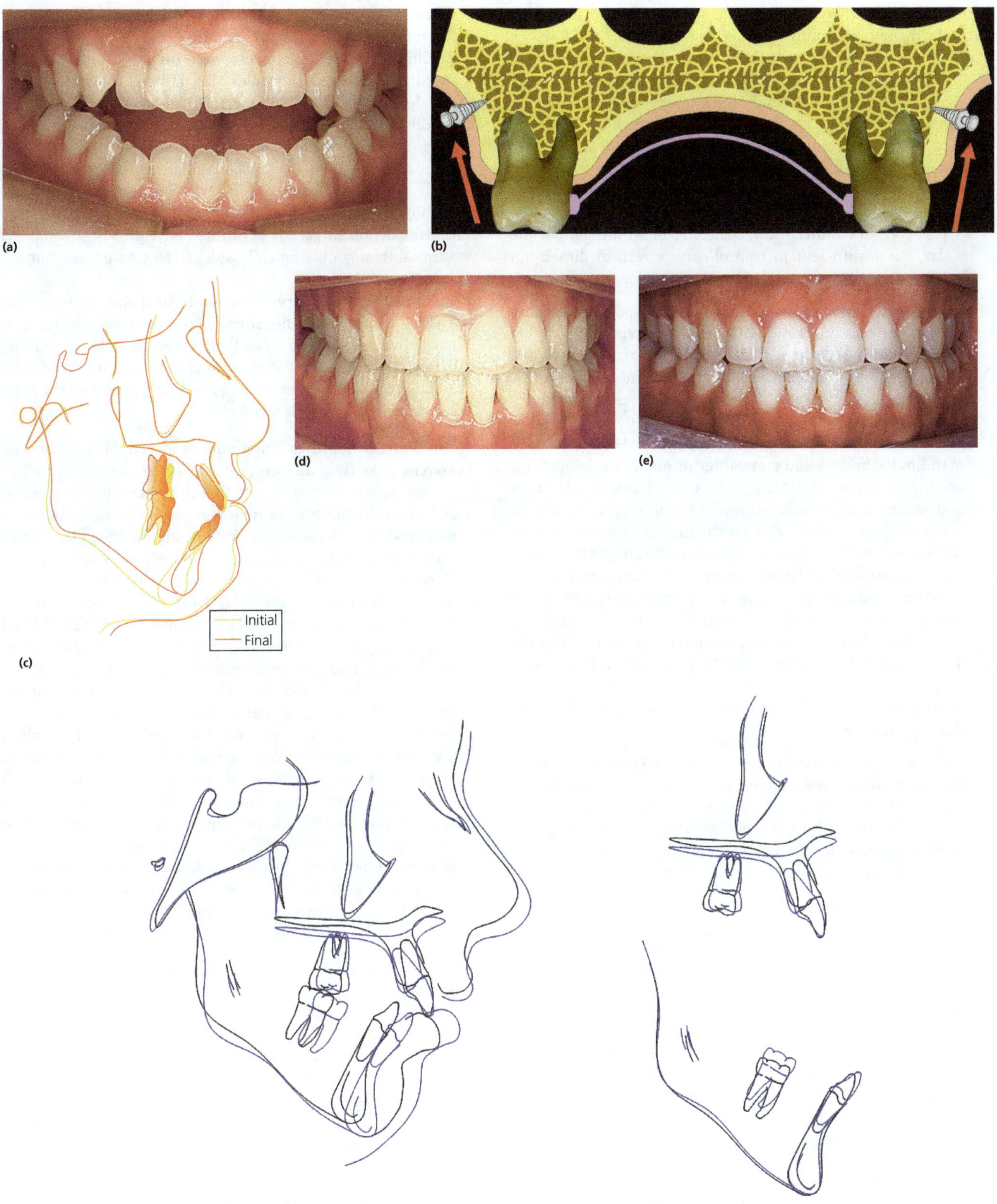

Figure 5.13 Closure of a skeletal open bite by intrusion of posterior teeth using TADs: (a) initial open bite, (b) illustration of maxillary molars intrusion using buccal TADs, (c) initial-deband cephalometric superimposition, (d) deband intraoral photograph, (e) 5-year posttreatment intraoral photograph demonstrating the stability of the skeletal open bite closure, (f) Initial and progress superimposition of another patient with TADs that have effectively intruded the maxillary molars. However, the mandibular molars have erupted into the space created by the molar intrusion (compensatory eruption). (Dr. Young Chel Park, DDS, PhD. Reproduced with permission from Dr. Young Chel Park).

cephalometric tracing that with maxillary molar intrusion, the mandible autorotated CCW and closed the open bite.

- Chewing exercises: Daily chewing exercises for one year in 13 children aged 7–12 years with long-face morphology (average SNMP angle of 42.4°) resulted in a significant decrease in the mandibular plane angle [36]. Incorporating light clenching exercises (clenching a soft bite-wafer 1–5 min, five times per day), combined with HPHG, resulted in a reduced ANB, reduced Gonial angle, and reduced MPA (average decrease of 2.2°) in a group of hyperdivergent open bite patients [37]. However, in another study, clenching 1 min throughout the day was insufficient to control/correct vertical dimension (although OB increased) [38].

Q: What is the reported stability of anterior open bite closure by TAD molar intrusion? How will this reported stability impact your future treatment decisions?

A: Using TADS to intrude maxillary molars and close anterior open bites, Lee and Park [39] reported an average maxillary molar intrusion of 2.2 mm with relapse of 10% at the end of a 17-month retention period. Using TADs to intrude mandibular molars and close anterior open bites, Sugawara et al. [40] reported average intrusion of mandibular first and second molars to be 1.7 and 2.8 mm, respectively, with average relapse rates of 27% for the first molars and 30% for the second molars. How should these findings affect your future treatment decisions? Using TADs to intrude posterior teeth and correct anterior open bites is effective. Once the open bite is closed, it is probably prudent to hold the intruded molars in their new intruded positions using the TADs until the end of orthodontic treatment, if possible. It may also be prudent to overcorrect the patient's overbite during treatment (20–40% OB)—anticipating some relapse during retention.

Q: Let's assume that you are using maxillary TADs as anchorage to intrude maxillary molars. What can happen to the mandibular posterior teeth as the maxillary molars are intruded?

A: As seen in Figure 5.13(f), mandibular molars may begin to erupt into any space created by the maxillary molar intrusion (compensatory eruption).

Q: How can you prevent compensatory mandibular molar eruption?

A: Place additional TADs in the mandibular posterior for use as anchorage to halt mandibular molar eruption (or even intrude mandibular molars in addition to maxillary molars). [41]

Q: Can excessive incisal display be reduced during adolescent orthopedic treatment?

A: Yes, if during treatment there is more vertical descent of the maxillary lip, then there is vertical descent of the maxillary incisor edges. Look at the before and after treatment frontal views of Jeff (Figure 5.14a, b, respectively) and Andrew (Figure 5.14d, e, respectively). Notice a significant decrease in their incisal display at rest following treatment. How did this happen? Look at their respective superimpositions (Figure 5.14c, f). During treatment, their maxillary lips descended more than their maxillary incisors edges descended. Maxillary lips can descend with vertical growth and with maxillary incisor retraction [42]. Decreased maxillary incisor edge decent can occur with decreased descent of the maxilla, decreased eruption of maxillary teeth, or with absolute intrusion of maxillary incisors.

Q: Compare and contrast orthopedic skeletal open bite treatment to surgical skeletal open bite treatment.

A: Traditionally, both treatments were directed at the maxilla/maxillary molars. Orthopedics (e.g., HPHG) sought to reduce the downward growth of the maxillary corpus (reduce/halt maxillary molar eruption), while Le Fort I impaction osteotomies moved the maxilla superiorly. Orthopedics was generally successful only in mild (possibly moderate) skeletal open bites, while surgery was successful in very severe skeletal open bites. Orthopedics is used while the patient is growing, while maxillary impaction surgery is performed after growth is complete. Surgical treatment is much less dependent on patient compliance than orthopedics.

Currently, if maxillary and mandibular molar intrusion with TADs is considered orthopedics, then even severe skeletal open bites can now be closed using them (growing and non-growing patients). Finally, some skeletal open bites can be closed with mandibular osteotomies alone, especially if stretch of the masseteric muscular sling is avoided.

Q: You start orthopedics (high-pull headgear, LLHA, chewing exercises) to treat an adolescent Class II skeletal open bite patient. A year later, you note that the patient has cooperated and the treatment is working (open bite is closing and Class II relationship is improving). When should you place fixed orthodontic appliances and begin comprehensive treatment?

A: *Principle: if you are having success in your treatment approach, then continue what you are doing.* Don't change your approach. Instead, continue your current treatment until full skeletal correction, or overcorrection, is achieved. And even then, slowly discontinue the treatment as you monitor stability. It is only at this point that you should place fixed appliances. However, if your cooperative patient is pleading to begin "braces," then consider placing fixed appliances—but only if they firmly commit to continue with their treatment efforts. The entire problem with facial growth is "It ain't over 'til it's over" (Yogi Berra). Even though you are seeing improvement this first year, skeletal relationships can change dramatically, if the growth rate, or growth direction, or patient cooperation changes. One final pearl: consider delaying irreversible treatment (e.g., tooth extractions) until growth is complete, or you are absolutely sure you can achieve your treatment goals in spite of any residual growth or future lack of cooperation.

Q: Should bonded RME appliances (Figure 5.15) be the appliance of choice for maxillary expansion in patients with excessive vertical development?

A: A bonded RME appliance can provide a *slight* decrease in the descent of PNS (~0.5 mm) compared to a banded RME appliance [43]. On the other hand, Haas-type RME therapy has little long-term (>6 years) adverse effects on either the vertical or anteroposterior dimension [44, 45]. So, it would be misleading to state that bonded RME appliances should always be used for expansion in skeletal open bite patients.

Q: What is masking (camouflage) of a skeletal open bite? Allison was treated with TAD molar intrusion. But, would masking have been a better treatment for Allison? Why or why not?

A: Masking a skeletal open bite is treatment to close the bite without addressing the underlying excess LAFH. For Allison's open bite, this would involve erupting her stepped up maxillary incisors and erupting her stepped down mandibular incisors

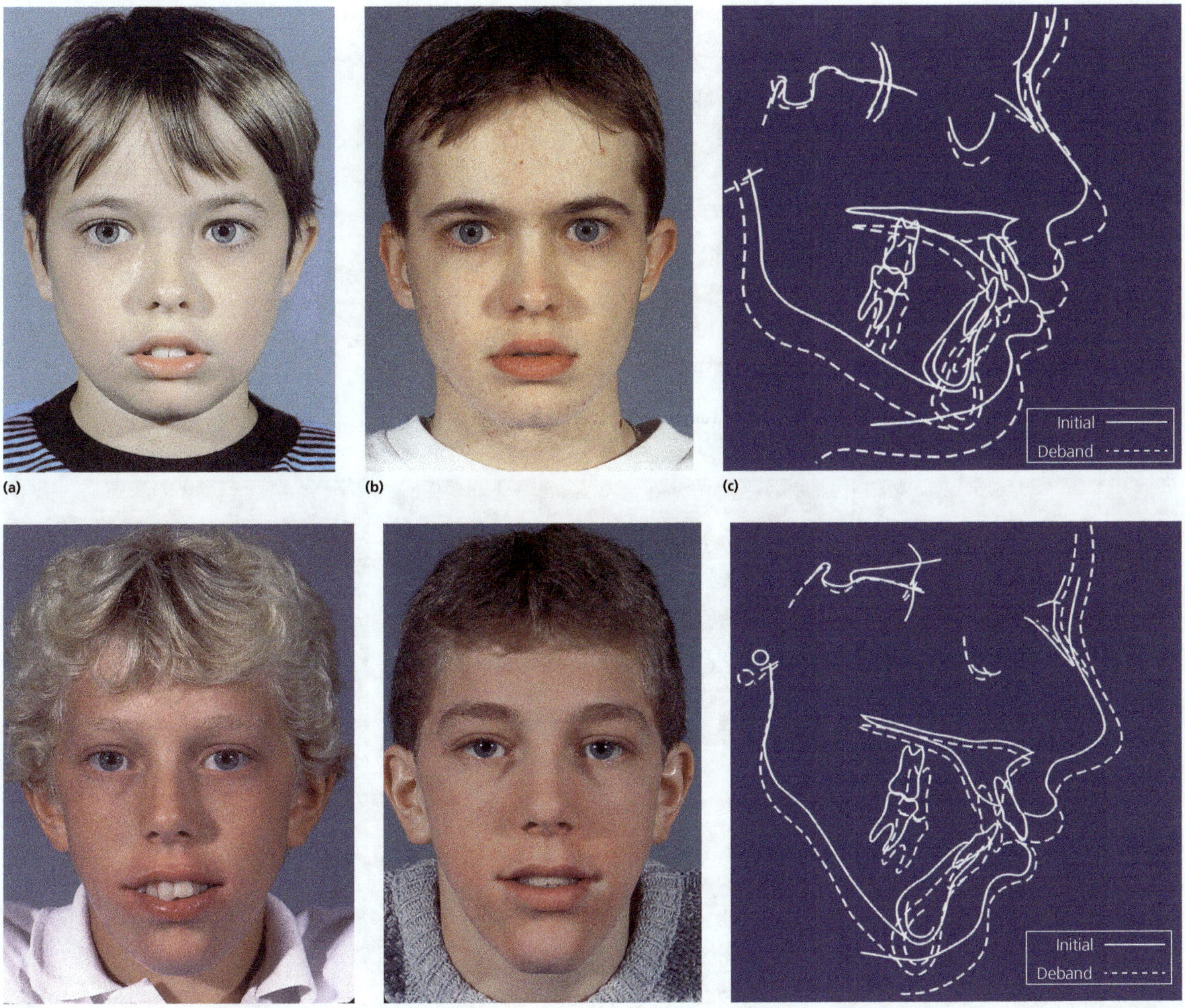

Figure 5.14 Decreased maxillary incisal display can result if there is greater vertical descent of the maxillary lip during treatment than vertical descent of the maxillary incisor edges: Initial and final records of Jeff (a–c) and Andrew (d–f) who demonstrate this concept.

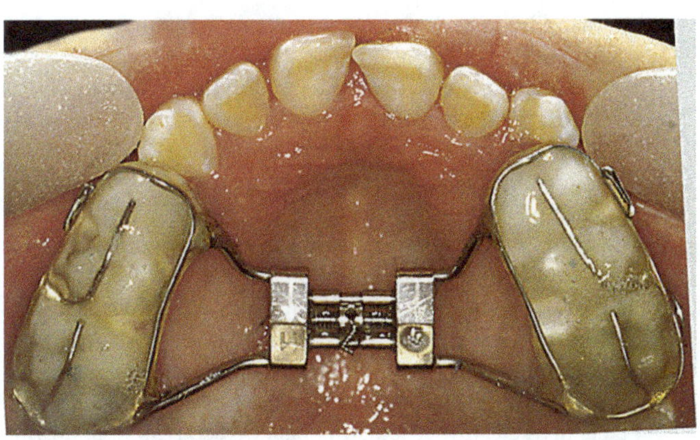

Figure 5.15 On average, PNS descends 0.5 mm less with a bonded RME (vs a banded RME).

(Figure 5.1g, i). Masking would *not* have been the best treatment for Allison because she already exhibits 4 mm of maxillary incisal display (Figure 5.3), which will only increase to an unacceptable amount as her maxillary incisors are erupted. More importantly, masking would not address her concern ("My lips are apart").

Q: Exhaustively list (and describe) skeletal open bite masking techniques.

A: Skeletal open bite masking techniques include the following:

- Erupting maxillary and mandibular anterior teeth by
  1. Leveling stepped up maxillary incisors or stepped down mandibular incisors with fixed orthodontic appliances and increasingly stiffer archwires (Figure 5.16 illustrates leveling/erupting stepped up maxillary incisors).
  2. Wearing vertical interarch elastics (Figure 5.17). *Long arch wire spans, without occlusal contacts between the*

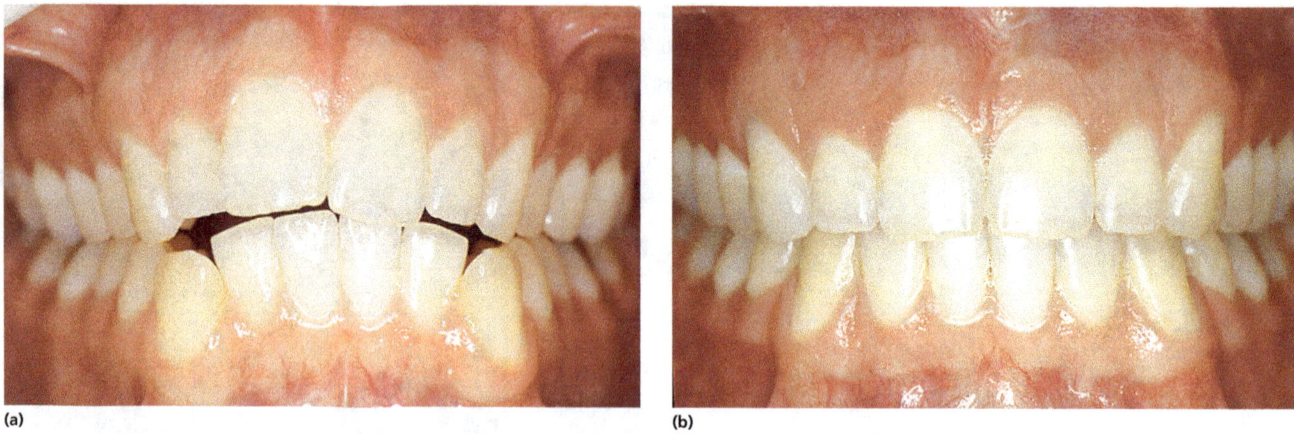

Figure 5.16 (a, b) Stepped up maxillary incisors were erupted as the arch was leveled.

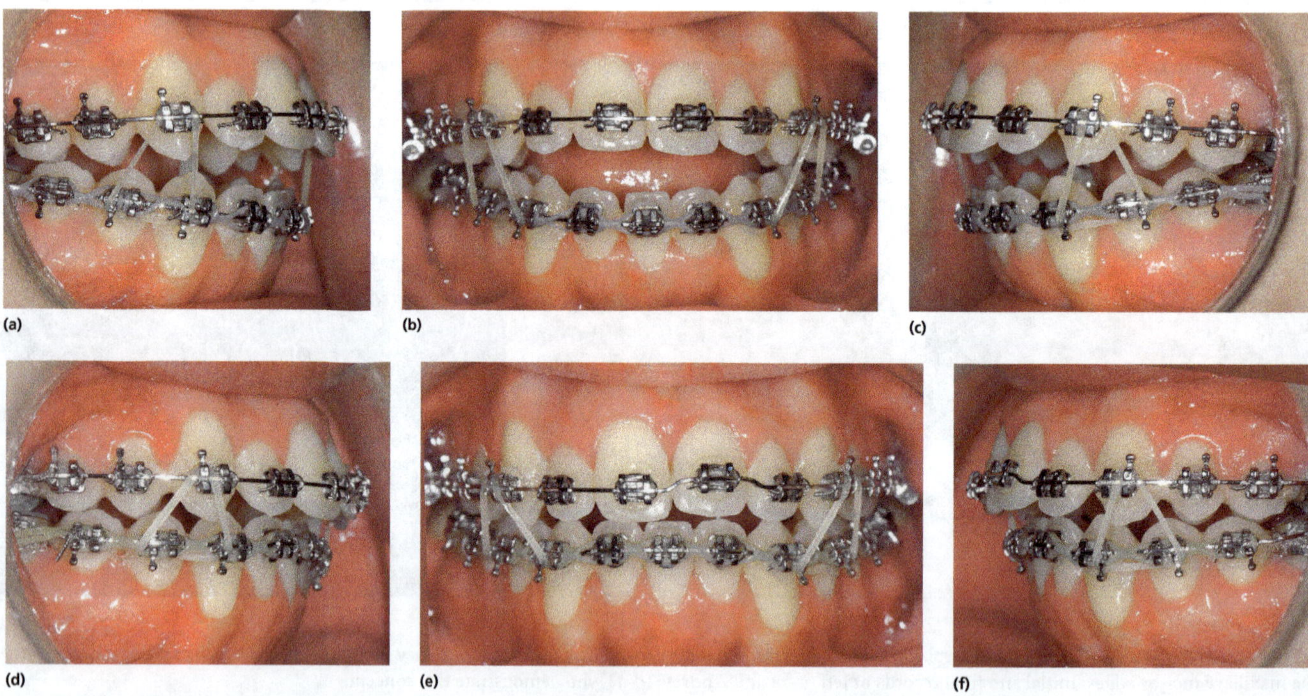

Figure 5.17 (a–f) Vertical interarch elastics can erupt teeth and mask (close) skeletal open bites only if long arch wire spans, without occlusal contacts, are present. The stability of this treatment, for moderate to severe open bites, can be poor.

arches, must be present for vertical elastics to close open bites. Notes: stability may be poor because eruption can be an unstable tooth movement; to enhance stability, the correction should be held for some time before debanding to allow the soft and hard tissues to remodel; once bite closure is achieved, elastic wear should be gradually diminished to monitor relapse; care must be taken not to create excessive incisal display.

3 Bonding maxillary and mandibular incisors more gingivally than posterior teeth—Figure 5.18 (left) illustrates bonding maxillary and mandibular incisors more gingivally than usual in an open bite patient. When archwires are engaged, the incisors erupt and the open bite closes (Figure 5.18, right).
4 Placing archwire step down artistic bends in the maxillary archwire (Figure 5.19a, left) or step up artistic bends in the mandibular archwire (Figure 5.19b, left) to force incisor eruption.
5 Adding curve of Spee to the mandibular archwire to erupt incisors (Figure 5.20).
6 Retracting/uprighting proclined incisors (Figure 5.21) erupts them as they rotate about their apicies—closing the open bite/deepening the bite.

- Extracting second molars (if the second molars are the only teeth in occlusion). The mandible will autorotate upward and forward closing the open bite until the first molars contact.
- Performing an occlusal adjustment/enameloplasty on posterior teeth. Figures 5.22a and b illustrate a mild open bite, and Figure 5.22c illustrates the maxillary posterior occlusal contacts marked with articulating paper (red arrows). Following enameloplasty of those occlusal marks, the bite closed (Figure 5.22d, e). Since the mandible pivots around the

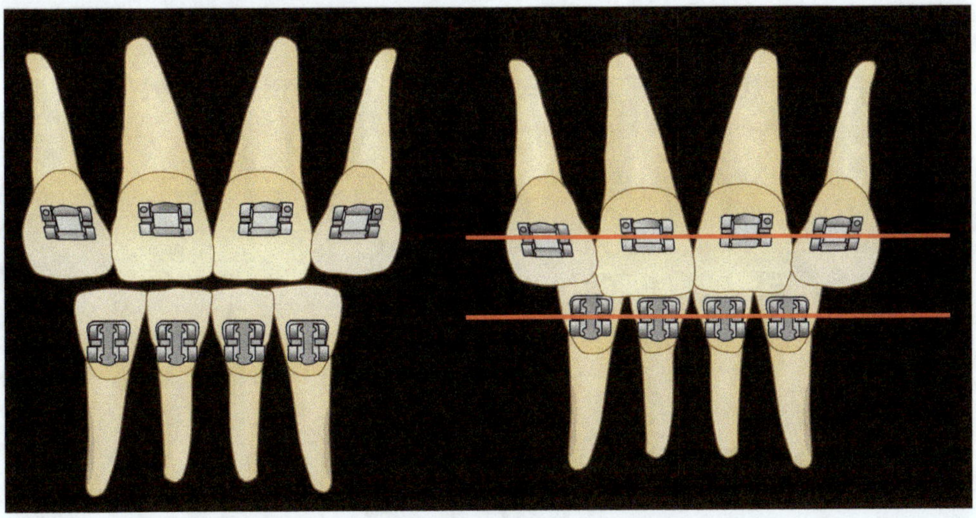

Figure 5.18 Closing an anterior open bite by leveling the arches with very gingivally bonded incisors.

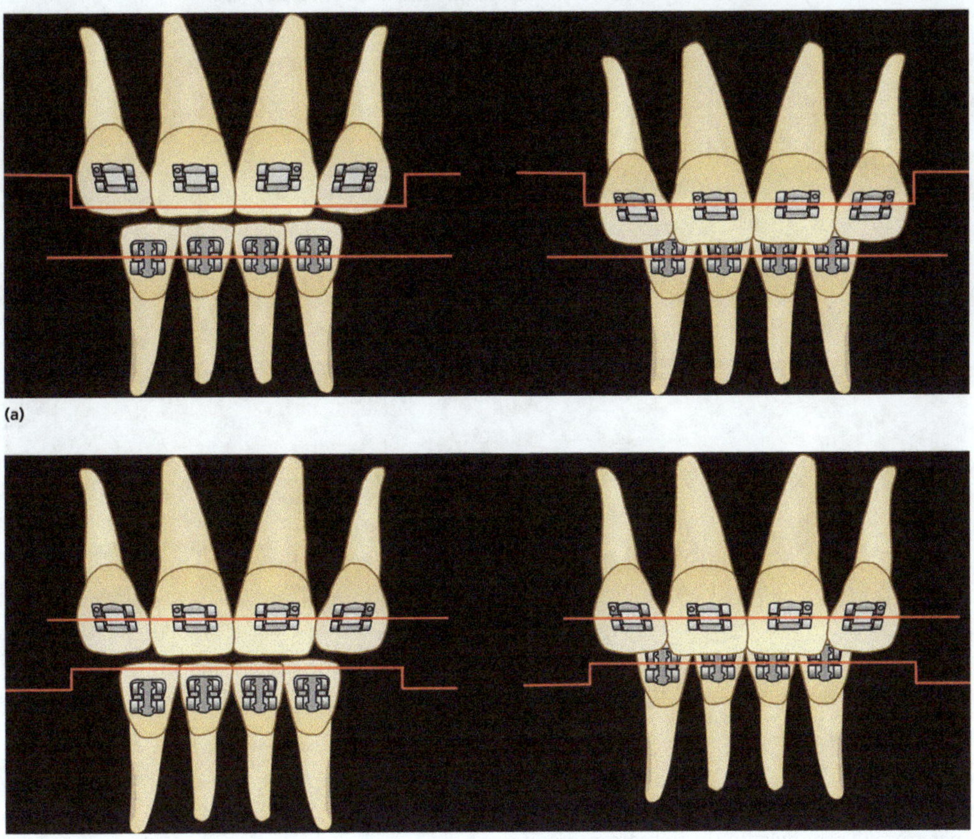

Figure 5.19 Closing an anterior open bite by placing (a) "step down" artistic bends in the maxillary archwire anterior and (b) "step up" artistic bends in the mandibular archwire.

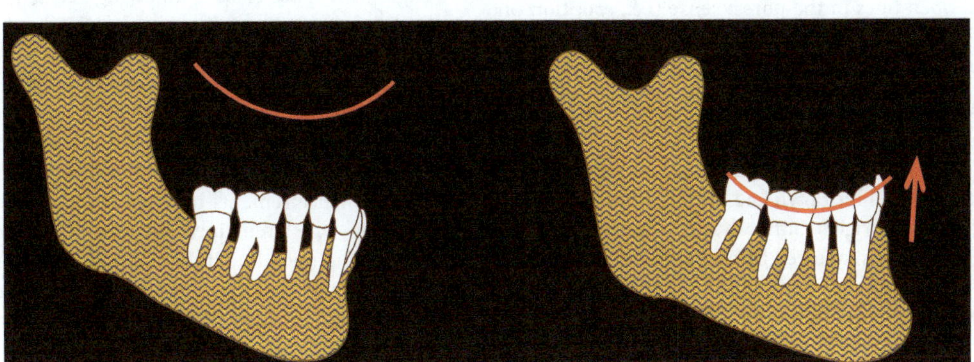

Figure 5.20 Adding curve of Spee to the mandibular archwire can erupt the incisors to help close an open bite. *Principle: adding curve of Spee to close an open bite is the opposite of removing curve of Spee to open a deep bite.*

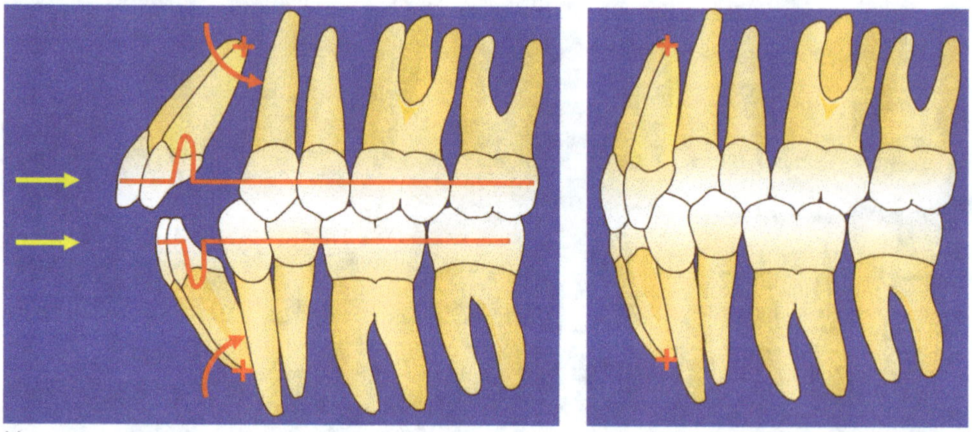

(a) (b)

Figure 5.21 (a) Retracting proclined incisors rotates them around their root apicies, deepening the bite, and eliminating the open bite (b). *Principle: retracting proclined incisors to close an open bite is the opposite of proclining upright incisors to open a deep bite.*

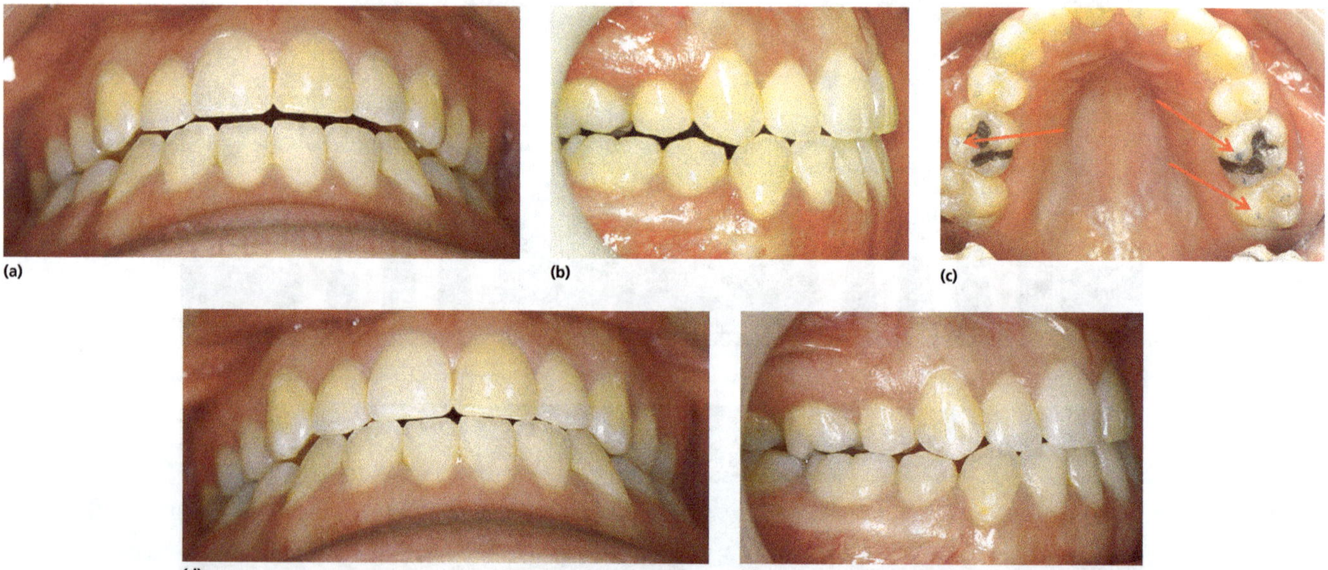

(a) (b) (c) (d) (e)

Figure 5.22 (a, b) In the case of a mild anterior open bite, (c) the posterior occlusal contacts can be marked with articulating paper, and (d, e) enameloplasty (occlusal adjustment) performed at the marks to close the open bite.

condyle during jaw closure, and the molars are about one-half the distance from the condyles to the incisors, removing 1 mm of enamel from the molars closes the open bite by about twice that amount, or 2 mm.

Note: molar extraction and molar enameloplasty are not "masking" of skeletal open bites in the purest sense (i.e., eruption of anterior teeth). We have included these treatments here since they are neither orthopedics nor orthognathic surgery.

Q: What is the "wedge effect"?

A: Some orthodontists suggest that distalizing maxillary molars (Figure 5.23a, left) drives the molars like a wedge between the jaws—rotating the mandible down and back and worsening an open bite (Figure 5.23a, right). Similarly, it has been suggested that premolar extractions followed by mesial molar movement (Figure 5.23b, left) allows the mandible to rotate up and forward—closing an open bite (Figure 5.23b, right).

Q: Is there evidence for the "wedge" effect?

A: Yes and no. On the one hand, little evidence exists to support the wedge effect during mesial molar movement (Figure 5.23b). Al-Nimri [46] reported no change in the mandibular plane angle with space closure following extraction of four first premolars or four second premolars. Comparing a group of four first premolar extraction hyperdivergent patients (mesial molar movement, intrusive mechanics, high-pull headgear) to a group of nonextraction hyperdivergent patients (distal molar movement, cervical headgear, Class II elastics), Gkantidis et al. [47] found no significant differences in the post-treatment skeletal measurements between the groups, including vertical variables, which remained unaltered. On the other hand, look at the skeletal open bite in Figure 5.24, which extends to the second molar on the right and the first molar on the left. If, during orthodontic treatment, the second molars are banded, the

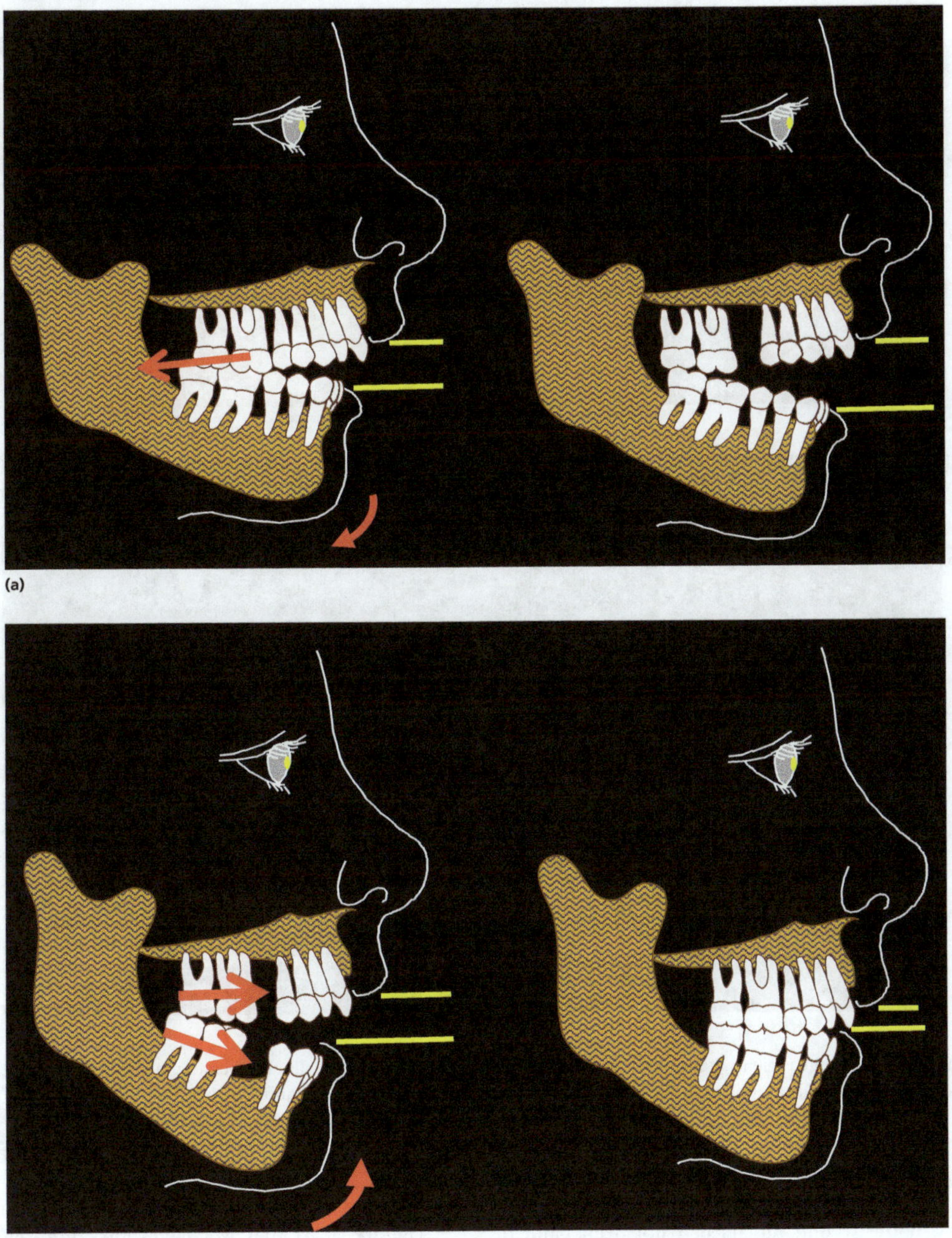

(a)

(b)

Figure 5.23 (a) It is suggested that retracting maxillary molars drives them between the jaws like a "wedge," forcing the mandible down and back—worsening an open bite. (b) In a similar fashion, it is suggested that moving molars mesially through extraction spaces reduces the "wedge" and closes an open bite.

arches leveled, and the curve of Spee flattened, then the second molars will be uprighted, tipped distally, rotated around their distal root apicies, and erupted (Figure 5.24c, left). The uprighting mandible second molars will act as a "wedge" between the jaws, forcing the mandible down and back, and worsening the open bite (Figure 5.24c, right).

This is exactly what happened in the patient in Figure 5.24a, b. After the skeletal open bite worsened because the second molars were bonded and leveled, a decision was subsequently made to extract the maxillary second molars (Figure 5.25a), which closed the bite (Figure 5.25b).

Our point is that banding second molars (leveling the curve of Spee) during nonsurgical orthodontic treatment of skeletal open bites can worsen the open bite. This is the reason *why you should* not *band second molars when masking a skeletal open bite*. Likewise, you *should* band second molars to aid in opening a deep bite. If the second molars must be banded in a skeletal open bite because of very poor alignment, you could consider aligning them later in treatment with light overlay wires while carefully monitoring the open bite. In surgical open bite treatment, the second molars should be banded/bonded, the open bite made worse prior to surgery, and the surgeon forced

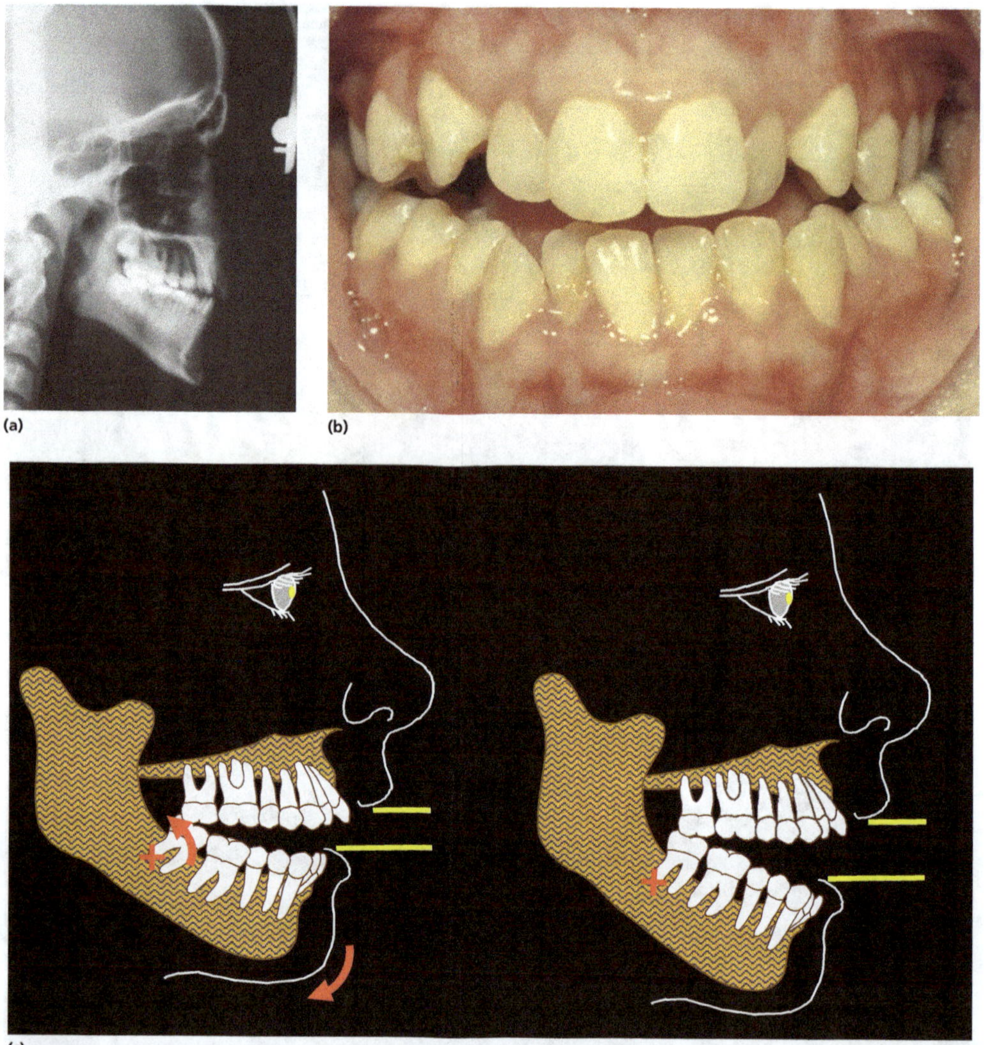

(a) (b) (c)

Figure 5.24 (a, b) In skeletal open bite patients, it is often prudent to avoid banding/leveling mandibular second molars. Why? (c) As the mandibular arch is leveled, the second molars tip distally around their distal root tip, they erupt at their mesial root, and the open bite worsens. *Principle: for (nonsurgical) treatment of skeletal open bites, avoid banding/bonding second molars to prevent worsening of the open bite; for treatment of skeletal deep bites, always band/bond second molars to help open the bite.*

to impact the posterior maxilla even more than would have been necessary, if the second molars had not been banded/bonded. In this way, any postsurgical relapse (return of the curve of Spee) will only help to keep the bite closed. To answer our original question, evidence does not exist to support the concept of the "wedge effect" in terms of mesial molar movement, but some evidence does exist to support the concept of the wedge effect during second molar distal movement, at least during curve of Spee leveling.

Q: Michael (Figure 5.26) presents with excess incisal display and *stepped up* maxillary incisors. If you treat Michael nonsurgically, is there anything you can do to prevent his incisal display from increasing?

A: Yes—avoid erupting his maxillary incisors with leveling. You can do this by leaving compensating curve in the maxillary archwire (Figure 5.27, curved red line) to maintain the maxillary incisor vertical position, and leaving curve of Spee in the mandibular archwire to maintain overbite (Figure 5.27, curved yellow line).

This was done for Michael. Note in his 2-year retention photos (Figure 5.28) that Michael shows improved incisal/gingival display when smiling and that his maxillary incisors and mandibular incisors remain stepped up relative to his maxillary and mandibular posterior teeth.

Q: Anterior vertical elastics can be used to erupt anterior teeth and close dental open bites. They can also be used in skeletal open bites where masking is appropriate and where increasing the maxillary incisal display (through maxillary tooth eruption) is an acceptable compromise. Recently, a technique termed "multiloop edgewise archwire therapy" (MEAW)—has been suggested for open bite correction [48]. Drawings of possible archwire loop conformations used in this technique, before and after anterior open bite closure using with vertical elastics, are shown in Figure 5.29. What is the biomechanical basis for this technique?

A: *The multiple loops increase the archwire flexibility. The vertical elastics close the open bite.* For decades, interarch vertical elastics have been used to close open bites and correct anteroposterior

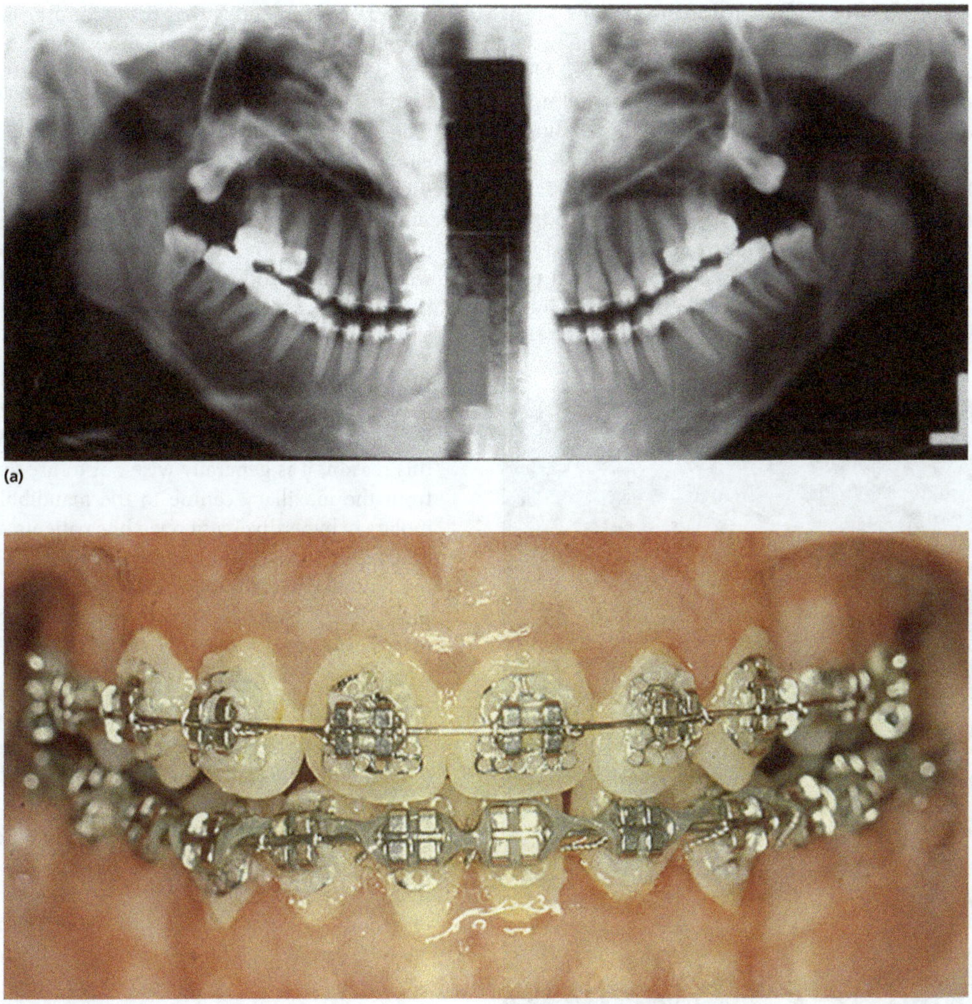

(a) (b)

Figure 5.25 (a) Mandibular second molars were banded in the skeletal open bite patient shown in Figure 5.24, arches were leveled, and the open bite worsened (only the second molars were contacting). (b) A decision was made to extract the maxillary second molars and the open bite closed.

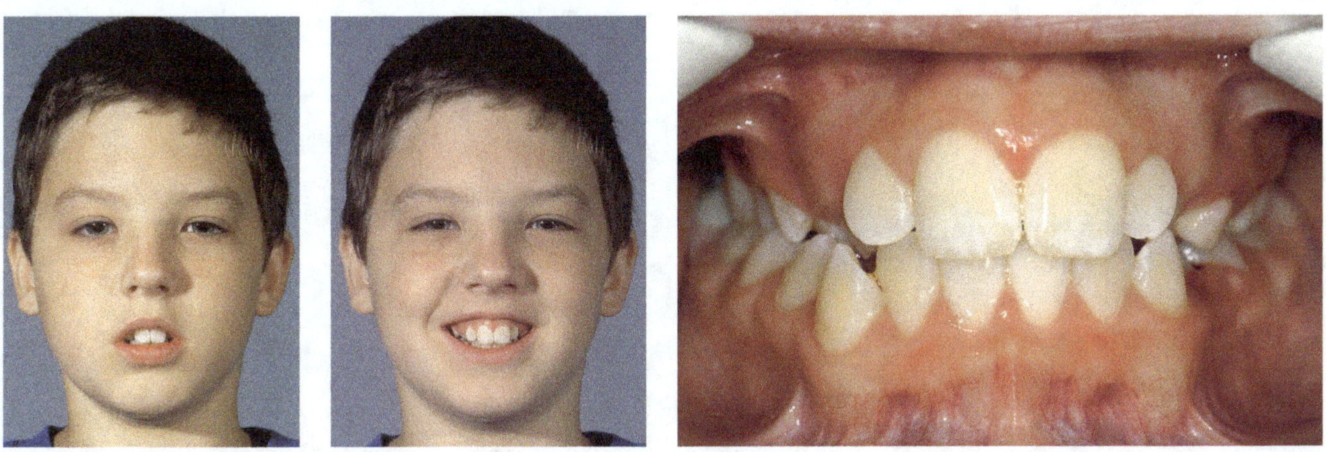

(a) (b) (c)

Figure 5.26 (a) Michael presents with excess incisal display and (b) stepped up maxillary incisors (he has a short philtrum length).

dental relationships. Renfroe [49] offered many illustrations of vertical elastics to correct open bites and Strang and Thompson [50] illustrated the use of Class II and Class III elastics. More recently, Alexander [51] and Steffen [52] even suggested using Class II, Class III, or vertical elastics without archwires during the finishing stage of orthodontic treatment. Further, for decades, multiple loops have been placed in archwires to increase their flexibility. The MEAW is a 0.016×0.022 rectangular archwire with a series of horizontal loops used in a standard edgewise appliance [53]. From a biomechanical perspective, the MEAW appliance does not offer a technical innovation. The "L-shaped loops" described in this technique are the same horizontal loops that orthodontists such as Jarabak and Fizzell [54], Thurow [55], and others described many years ago. The claim that the loops in the MEAW archwire allow the teeth to move independently is a misconception. Although more wire is incorporated between each tooth with loop placement, and although flexibility is increased, the teeth are still connected to each other by the archwire and do not move independently. In summary, the MEAW concept does not offer an improvement in open bite closure over wearing interarch vertical elastics between maxillary and mandibular arches with flexible archwires.

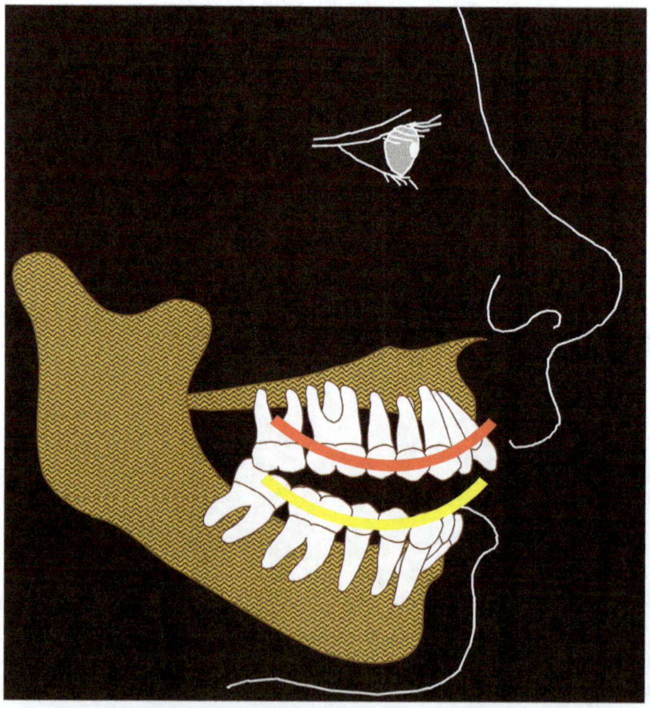

Figure 5.27 To avoid worsening Michael's maxillary incisal display, consider leaving compensating curve in the maxillary arch (curved red line) and curve of Spee in the mandibular arch (curved yellow line) during arch alignment.

Q: Explain the use of "long" Class II elastics (Figure 5.30a) versus "short" Class II elastics (Figure 5.30b) in skeletal open bite patients requiring minor Class II correction.

A: A vertical component of force results with any interarch elastic wear. Therefore, all interarch elastics tend to erupt teeth. For this reason, it is generally wise not to use *long* Class II elastics from the maxillary canine to the mandibular first or second molars in hyperdivergent open bite patients. Why? If the molars erupt even a small amount, their eruption will be magnified in the anterior, and the open bite will worsen [56]. Instead, use *short* Class II elastics from the maxillary canine to the lower premolars, which will help correct the AP relationship and close, or keep closed, the anterior open bite.

Q: Masking, or camouflage, consists of correcting a dental relationship while ignoring the underlying skeletal discrepancy that caused the dental relationship. This is true whether we are discussing the vertical, anteroposterior, or transverse dimension. Can you state a principle to describe the probable success of masking in terms of the severity of the underlying skeletal discrepancy?

A: *Principle: The success of masking a skeletal discrepancy is inversely related to the severity of the discrepancy and to the severity of the associated dental compensations.* In other words, the milder the skeletal discrepancy (the more normal the patient), the better your chances of success with masking. The more severe the skeletal discrepancy, the less successful you will be with masking.

Q: Briefly describe the surgical correction of skeletal open bites.

A: Unlike orthopedics, the goal of which is to achieve a normal LAFH by reducing vertical facial growth, or masking, the goal

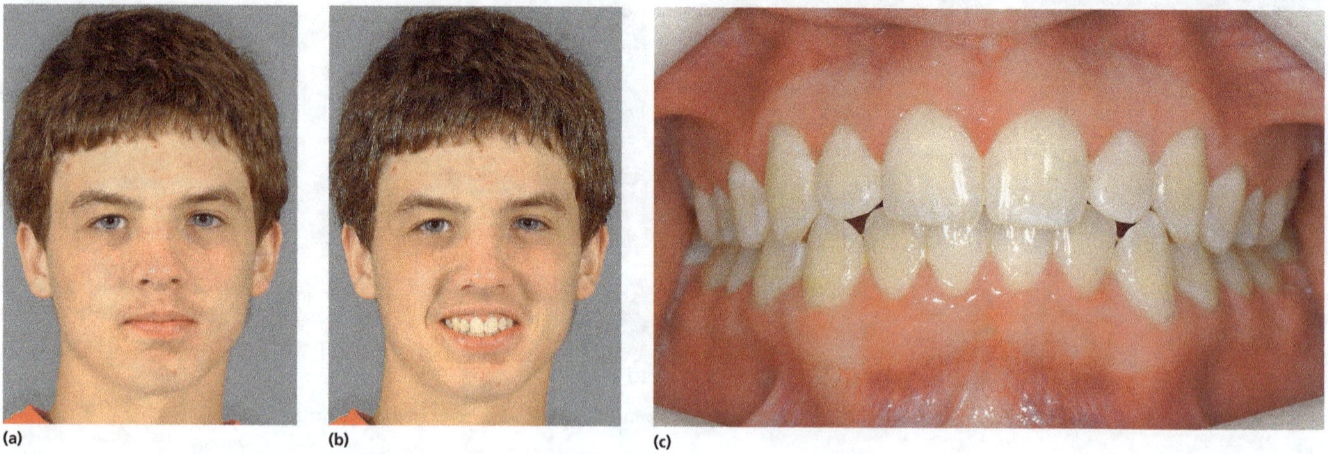

(a) (b) (c)

Figure 5.28 Michael's 2-year retention photos. (a, b) Michael's incisal display did not worsen. (c) Compensating curve was placed in his maxillary archwire, along with curve of Spee in his mandibular archwire, during leveling.

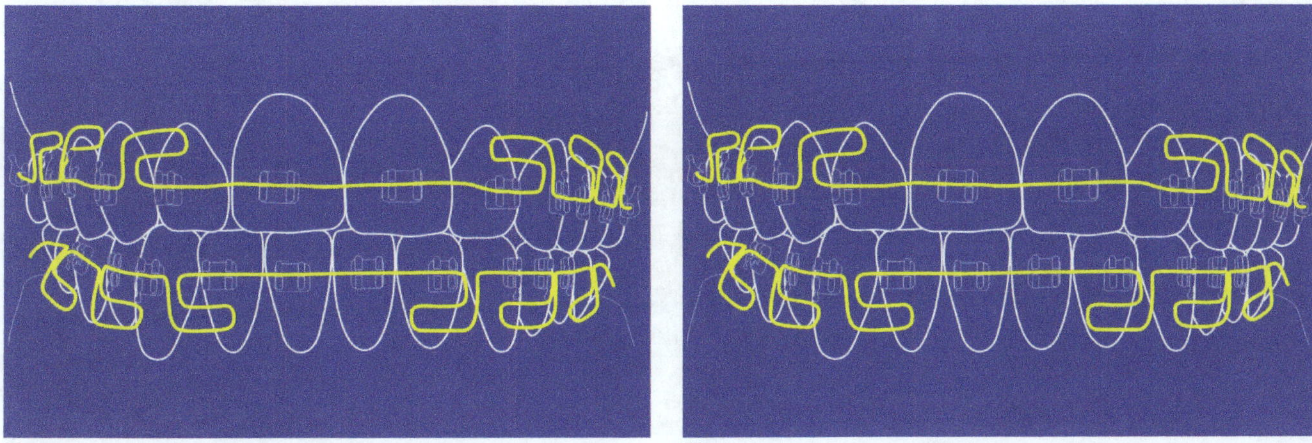

Figure 5.29 (a, b) Multiloop edgewise archwire therapy (MEAW) consists of archwires incorporating many loops, plus vertical elastics, to close anterior open bites.

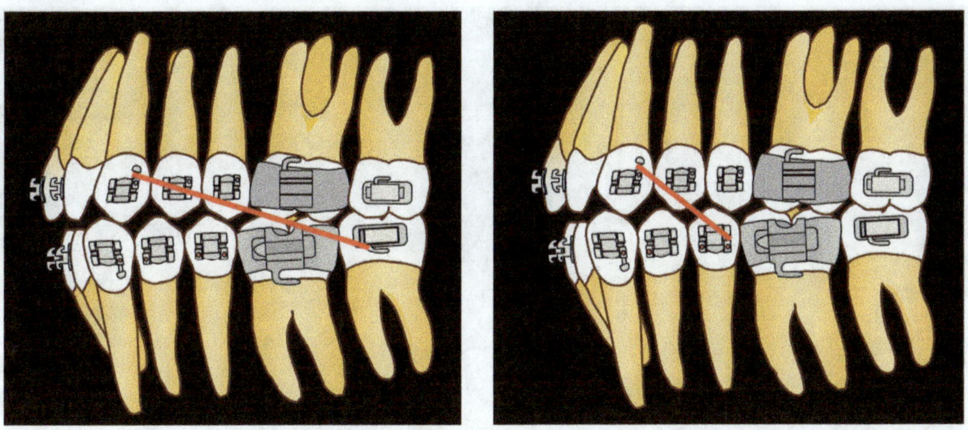

Figure 5.30 All interarch elastics include a vertical component of force which tends to erupt teeth. For this reason, if you need to use Class II (or Class III) elastics in skeletal open bite patients, (a) avoid using "long" elastics which will tend to erupt molars and worsen the open bite. (b) Instead, use "short" elastics which will tend to erupt more anterior teeth (premolars) and close the open bite.

of which is to close the open bite while ignoring the excess LAFH, the goal of surgery is achieve a normal LAFH by removing excess maxillary bone that has already formed. During surgery, the maxilla is moved superiorly, the long LAFH is shortened and normal vertical dimension restored, lip competence is achieved, and the open bite is closed. A LeFort I osteotomy is the surgical procedure used to do this. See Figure 5.31a, a skeletal open bite before surgery. A horizontal maxillary osteotomy is made above the bony palate and at a safe distance from the teeth apices, the nasal septum and lateral nasal wall are separated from the palate, the maxilla is downfractured, the nasal septum is trimmed to prevent a buckling nasal deviation, and an ostectomy is performed to remove the exact amount of maxillary bone to permit moving the maxilla superiorly and restoring a normal vertical facial dimension (Figure 5.31b). The maxilla is then fixated (Figure 5.31c). As the maxilla is moved superiorly, the mandible will autorotate upward and forward around the condyles. Depending on the anteroposterior position of the mandible following this rotation, a mandibular advancement, mandibular setback, or genioplasty osteotomy may be required to correctly relate the dental arches and provide the ideal amount of chin projection.

Q: What is meant by a "differential maxillary impaction"?

A: Depending on the magnitude of the anterior open bite and amount of incisal display, the surgeon and orthodontist can choose to move the maxilla:

- Up at the posterior and anterior, equally (Figure 5.32, left)
- Up at the posterior only if the incisor display is acceptable—a differential maxillary impaction (Figure 5.32, center)
- Up at the posterior and down at the anterior, if more incisal display is desired—a differential maxillary impaction (Figure 5.32, right)

Q: Why can it be beneficial for the surgeon to advance the maxilla when it is impacted?

A: When impacting the maxilla, it can be challenging for the surgeon to deal with the bone and neurovascular structures

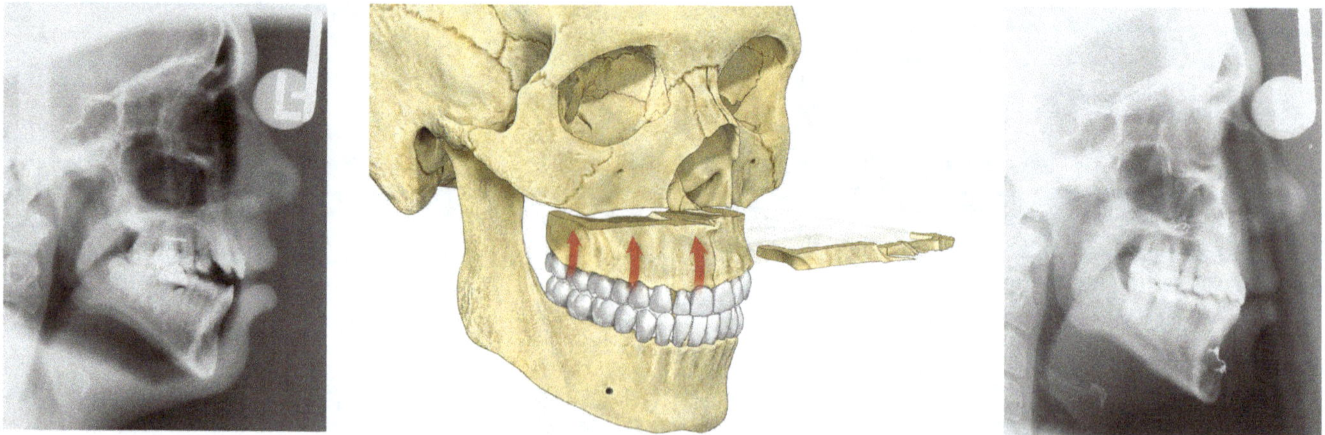

(a) (b) (c)

Figure 5.31 (a) Conventional surgical treatment of a skeletal open bite includes a LeFort I impaction osteotomy. The maxilla is downfractured, a precise wedge of maxillary bone is removed (b), and the maxilla is repositioned superiorly, or impacted. As a result (c), the LAFH is shortened to a normal vertical dimension, lip competence is achieved, and the open bite is closed.

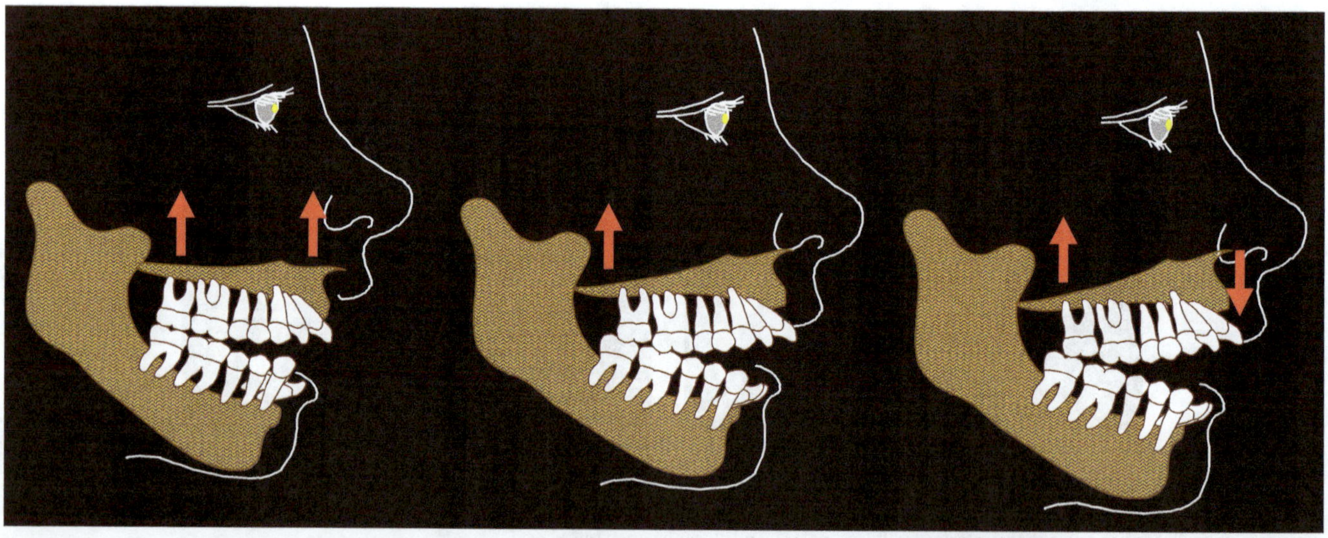

Figure 5.32 During a LeFort I osteotomy, the maxilla can be moved: (left) up equally at PNS and ANS, (center) up entirely at PNS, or (right) up at PNS and down at ANS—depending on the magnitude of the skeletal open bite and the desired incisal display change.

in the pterygoid plate region. By moving the maxilla slightly forward during surgery, the impaction osteotomy can be much easier.

Q: In terms of result stability, at what age is it safe to perform a maxillary impaction osteotomy? Why?

A: *After facial growth is complete* (as demonstrated using serial cephalometric radiographs made at least 9 months apart). Why? Patients who undergo maxillary impaction surgery before growth is complete will continue to have vertical maxillary growth postsurgically, and a second surgery may be necessary later if the open bite returns [57].

Q: What typically happens to the nasal tip and nasal alar base during maxillary impaction surgery?

A: The nasal tip follows the anterior nasal spine and moves upward. The alar base broadens when the surgeon releases the compressor naris muscle (transverse nasalis muscle), a muscle that draws ala of the nose toward the septum.

Q: The upward movement of the nasal tip can result in poor esthetics in maxillary impaction patients with obtuse nasolabial angles and upturned noses. Broadening of the alar base can result in poor esthetics in maxillary impaction patients with initially broad noses. How are the undesirable effects of maxillary impaction on nasal form controlled?

A: The upward movement of the nasal tip during surgery can be controlled by surgically reducing the anterior nasal spine and by performing an inferior-based septoplasty, including the cartilaginous septum and bony vomer. Broadening of the alar base can be prevented with a nasal cinch that re-approximates the released transverse nasalis muscle. Note: if the patient initially presents with a broad nasal tip but a narrow alar base, then some broadening of the alar base may be desirable; in this instance, the alar cinch should not be tightened too much.

Q: What is a V–Y closure and why does the surgeon place one following a maxillary LeFort I osteotomy?

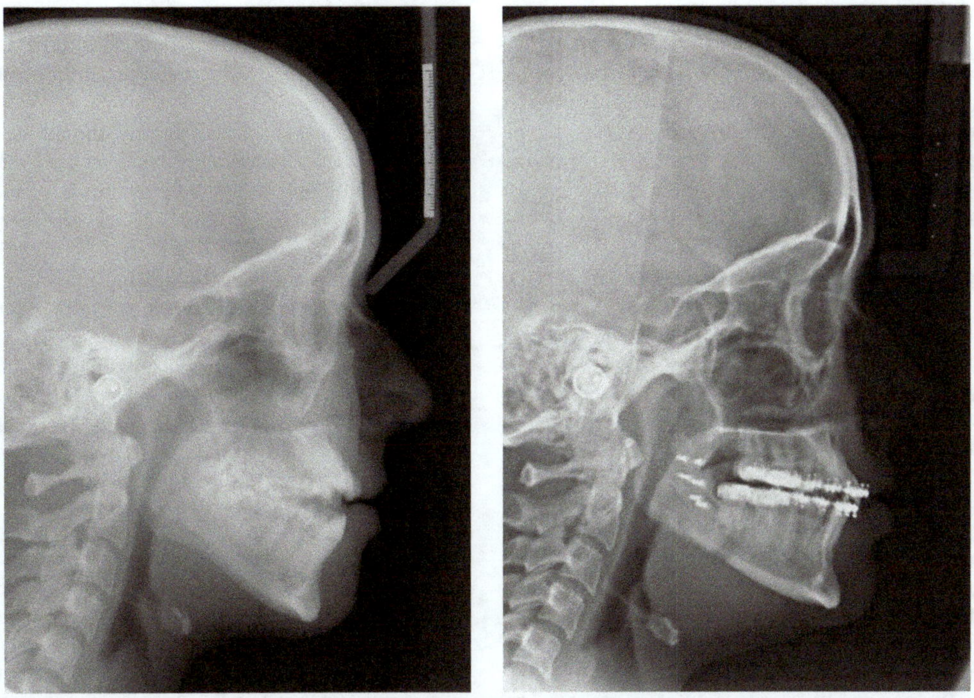

(a) (b)

Figure 5.33 Skeletal open bite closure via upward mandibular rotation only (a) initial and (b) postsurgery radiographs.

A: The V–Y closure consists of suturing the V-shaped vestibular soft tissue maxillary wound into a "Y", with the base of the "Y" in the midline of the maxillary lip [58]. Thinning and lateral retraction of the maxillary lip with reduced vermilion exposure can occur with wound healing following a LeFort I osteotomy, which a V–Y closure prevents. The V–Y closure must be accompanied by an alar cinch to be effective.

Q: Skeletal open bite closure via mandibular bilateral sagittal split osteotomy with upward rotation of the mandible (followed by rigid fixation) has been advocated as a technique to avoid the potential adverse soft tissue effects of maxillary impaction. An example of this technique in a skeletal open bite patient is shown in Figure 5.33. After leveling and aligning her arches (which erupted her maxillary incisors to a reasonable incisal display), the following observations were made which led to a mandibular-only procedure: the patient's open bite was relatively small, her maxilla was in a good position without much maxillary posterior vertical excess, her mandibular ramus was short, and she had a flat (ineffective) chin. A differential impaction of the maxilla would have rotated her mandible even more CW, making her chin even more ineffective with poorer esthetics and a higher long-term risk of obstructive sleep apnea. Closing her open bite with mandibular-only surgery created a CCW mandibular movement with a better final profile, and it opened her airway. However, what are the long-term outcomes of skeletal open bite closure via mandibular-only surgery?

A: After an average of 4.5 years following treatment, 60% of the mandibular surgical open bite closing rotation was lost—but only 10% of the patients relapsed to a point of no incisor overbite [59].

Q: Briefly describe the purpose of presurgical orthodontic treatment.

A: To position the teeth so that ideal occlusion and facial proportions are achieved with surgery. This typically includes removing anteroposterior, vertical, or transverse dental compensations that have occurred as a result of maxillary and mandibular growth deficiencies or excesses. As a result of orthodontic treatment, presurgical models of the patient should articulate ideally in all three planes of space when the canines are positioned into a Class I relationship.

Q: Now, back to our patient, Allison. She declined surgery, and her open bite was successfully closed with TADs (Figure 5.12). But what factors would have made her a good candidate for surgical open bite correction?

A: Favorable factors include the following:

- Her lower anterior facial height (Subnasale to soft tissue Menton) was slightly longer than her middle facial height (soft tissue Glabella to Subnasale). Impaction of her maxilla would result in her mandible autorotating closed and her LAFH being brought closer to ideal.
- She had an 8 mm ILG with a normal maxillary lip length of 19 mm. Impaction of her maxilla would result in her mandible autorotating closed and bringing her lips closer into contact. Note: In open bite patients whose relaxed lips are initially in contact (competent), maxillary impaction surgery can bring the lips even closer together and create an overclosed (aged) appearance. *Avoid overimpacting the maxilla.*
- Her maxillary incisors are stepped up relative to her posterior occlusion with an incisal display of 4 mm when lips are at rest (ideal incisal display range 2–4 mm). With arch leveling, her incisors would be erupted and incisal display would be increased and excessive. Following maxillary impaction, her incisal display could be returned to ideal.

- Her age—at 15 years, she is probably finished growing or close to being finished. However, age alone is no guarantee that Allison has completed growth. You should talk to her and her parents to ask if she is finished growing. If there is any question of whether she has finished growing, it would be wise to wait to begin treatment (or at least to perform surgery) until superimposition of cephalometric radiographs taken at least 9–12 months apart confirms that jaw growth is complete. As a rule of thumb, excessive growers continue to grow longer, whether in the anteroposterior or vertical dimension. If her dentofacial deformity was so severe that psychosocial pressures justified surgery before growth was completed, then Allison could grow out of the surgical correction and require a second surgery later.

Q: What important factor has been left out of the previous list factors?

A: Allison's chief complaint. She wanted to have her anterior open bite closed and her lips brought together. Occasionally, adults with severe dentofacial deformities, including skeletal open bites, will desire alignment of teeth only. They may not desire surgery. If alignment offers some improvement in the patient's condition, then the orthodontist is justified in proceeding with alignment only. However, the burden is still on the orthodontist to at least discuss the benefits of surgical correction with the patient (or the possible use of TADs to, nonsurgically, intrude posterior teeth).

Q: The amount of incisal display is important in determining how much the maxilla should be impacted. Should incisal display be judged using the relaxed lip position or smiling lip position?

A: The amount of incisal display should be judged based on *relaxed lip position after the incisors are leveled* with the posterior teeth. Look at Figure 5.34a (initial, relaxed lip), 5.34b (presurgery, relaxed lip), and 5.34c (postsurgery, relaxed lip). By basing the amount of maxillary anterior impaction upon this patient's incisal display following maxillary arch leveling, the influence of maxillary anterior teeth being initially stepped up or stepped down (relative to the maxillary posterior teeth) is eliminated and a balanced postsurgery facial proportion was achieved. Following this rule led to improved posed smile esthetics after surgery for this patient: compare the excess gingival display seen in the initial posed smile (Figure 5.34d) and presurgery posed smile (Figure 5.34e) to the improved postsurgery posed smile (Figure 5.34f).

Q: *Why* should (anterior) maxillary impaction magnitude be based on incisal display in a relaxed lip position and not based on a posed (sustainable) or unposed (nonsustainable) smiling lip position?

A: The structural relationship between the skeleton, lips, and teeth is accurately defined in the relaxed lip position. Activity, or hyperactivity, of the smiling muscles (Figure 5.35a–d: zygomaticus, levator

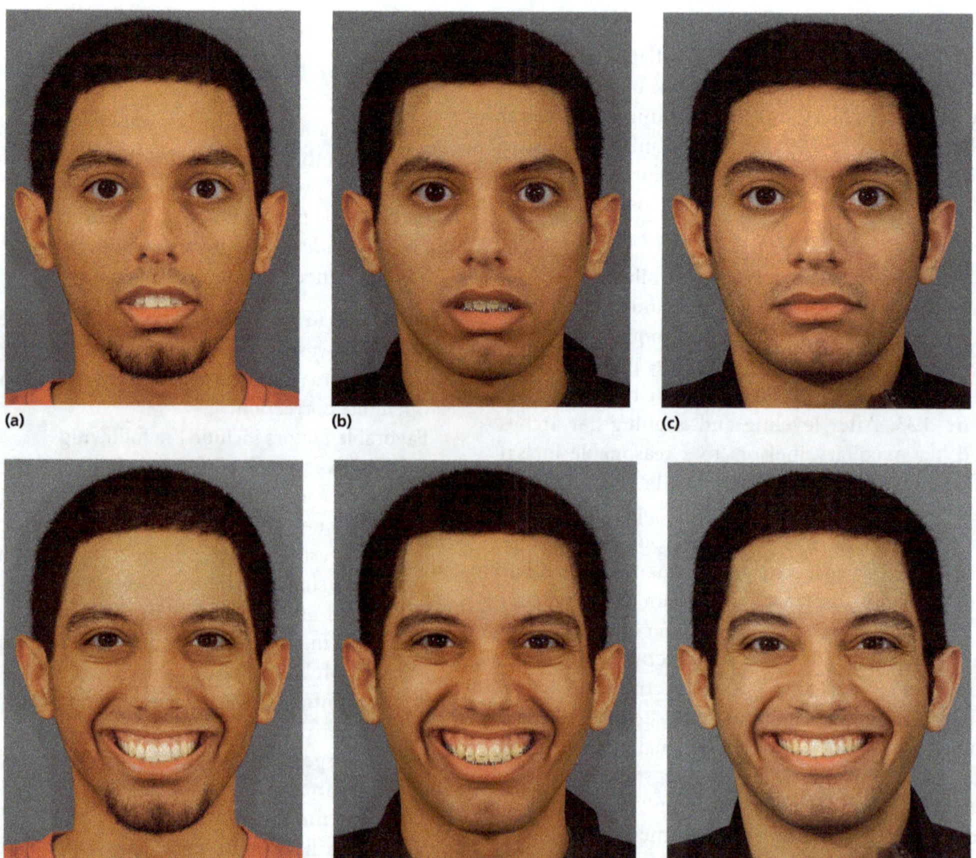

(a) (b) (c) (d) (e) (f)

Figure 5.34 As a guide to how much the anterior maxilla should be impacted during surgery, the amount of incisal display should be judged based on relaxed lip position after the incisors are leveled with the posterior teeth: (a) Initial relaxed lip position, (b) relaxed lip position following arch leveling, (c) relaxed lip position following maxillary impaction surgery, (d) initial posed smile, (e) posed smile following leveling, and (f) posed smile following surgery.

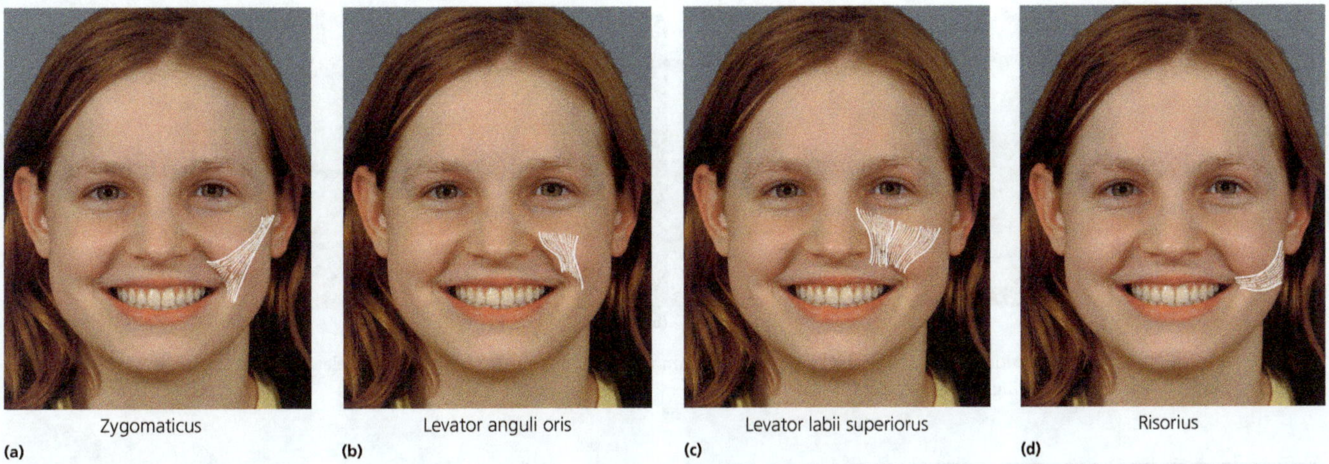

Figure 5.35 Smiling muscles: (a) zygomaticus, (b) levator anguli oris, (c) levator labii superiorus, and (d) risorius.

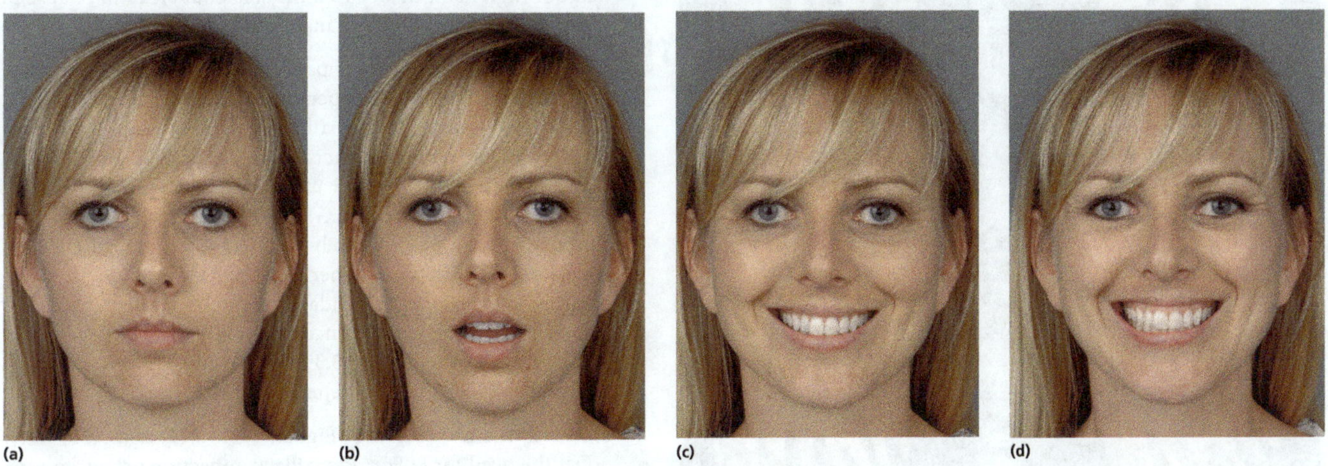

Figure 5.36 (a) Patient with normal vertical dimension, (b) at rest with teeth separated in relaxed lip position showing ideal amount of incisal display, (c) during posed smile, and (d) during an unposed smile. Decisions regarding structure (e.g., orthognathic surgery) should be based upon relaxed lip position views (a, b) and not functional views (c, d).

anguli oris, levator labii superiorus, and risorius) is a neuromuscular function, not structure, and can mislead the doctor into a false impression of excess tooth/gingival display during smiling. For example, look at the patient in Figure 5.36. She presents with a normal vertical dimension (Figure 5.36a), normal incisal display in a relaxed lip position (Figure 5.36b), and ideal incisal display in a posed smile (Figure 5.36c). But in an unposed (nonsustainable, hearty) smile (Figure 5.36d), her hyperactive smile musculature gives the false impression of excess incisal gingival display and possible need for a maxillary impaction surgery.

Q: Once a maxillary arch is leveled presurgically, would you advise the surgeon to impact a patient's anterior maxilla to achieve an *ideal* amount of incisal display (2–4 mm), to achieve the *low end* of this amount of display (<2 mm), or to achieve the *high end* of this amount of display (4+ mm)? Why?

A: As a rule of thumb—*leave the patient with slightly more incisal display than ideal postsurgically (4–5 mm).* Why? If the patient is left with slightly more incisal display than ideal postsurgically, then the patient will have a more youthful appearance as they age (as their maxillary lip lengthens). If the maxilla is overimpacted, the patient could look older as they age (less incisal display).

Q: An example of maxillary incisor presurgical arch leveling in a skeletal open bite patient is shown in Figure 5.37. Is this presurgical leveling (eruption of maxillary incisors) stable—or will it contribute to open bite relapse later?

A: *Presurgical leveling of maxillary incisors is stable up to 2 mm. Beyond 2 mm, evidence is lacking.* In a group of patients who had moderate presurgical maxillary incisor eruption during leveling (at least 1.5 mm, mean eruption = 2.1 mm, SD = 1.6 mm), the maxillary incisors were generally stable long term, and the extrusion had little influence on posttreatment stability of the open bite [60]. However, studies have not been conducted examining the maximum anterior step that can be leveled and yet remain stable. It is a fair assumption that the larger the initial step between the posterior teeth and the anterior teeth, the more likely the possibility of relapse. It is also a fair assumption that the shorter the period of time that the leveled anterior teeth are held, the more likely the possibility of relapse. Take a look at Figure 5.38. The top left figure illustrates a skeletal open bite where the anterior teeth are stepped up only a few millimeters relative to the posterior teeth. In this situation, it is reasonable to level/extrude the anterior teeth and impact the maxilla in one piece (bottom left, yellow bracket includes impaction of

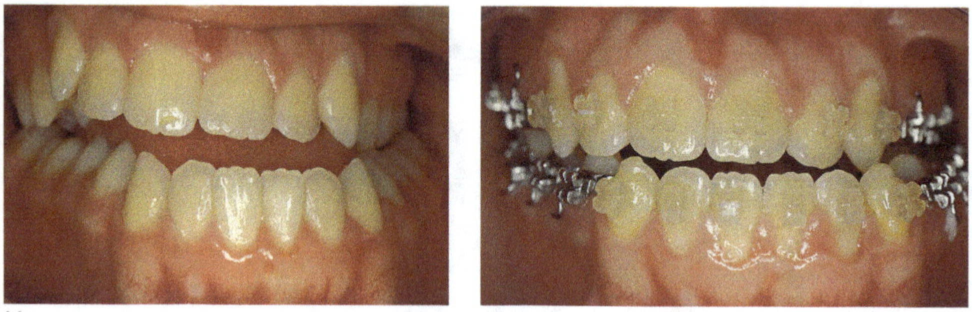

Figure 5.37 (a) Maxillary incisors initially stepped up by approximately 2 mm relative to the posterior teeth in a skeletal open bite patient. (b) The maxillary incisors were erupted during arch leveling.

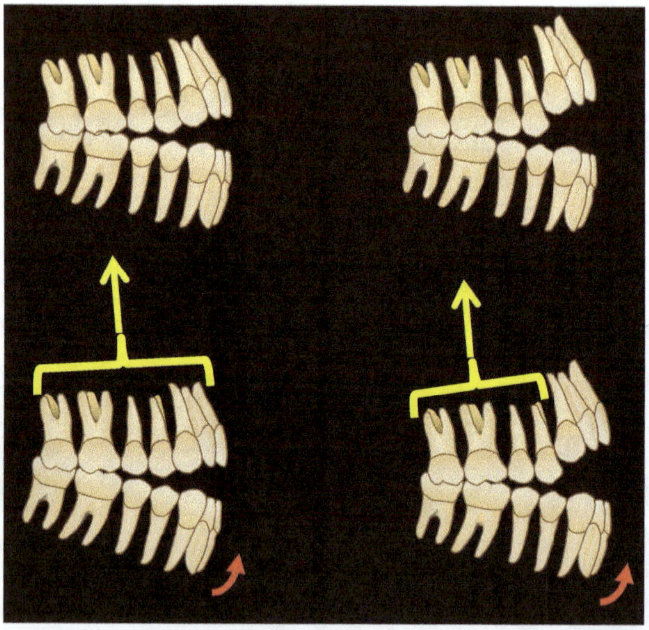

Figure 5.38 Part of the decision to impact the maxilla in one piece, or in multiple pieces, is based on the presence and magnitude of an anterior step: (top left); if an occlusal step of only 1–2 mm exists between the anterior and posterior teeth, then the maxillary arch can be leveled presurgically and the maxilla impacted as one piece (bottom left). However, if an occlusal step of 5–6+ mm exists between the anterior and posterior teeth (top right), then it may be prudent not to level the maxillary arch presurgically. Instead, the surgeon may be better able to level the maxillary arch with a multiple-piece maxillary osteotomy, impacting only the posterior teeth (bottom right) and leaving the anterior segment at the same level.

entire arch), allowing the mandible to rotate CCW (red arrow) and close the bite. The top right figure illustrates a skeletal open bite occlusion where the anterior teeth are stepped up greatly (5–6+ mm) relative to the posterior teeth. In this case, the orthodontist should consider leaving the step and having the surgeon level the maxillary arch with a multiple-piece maxillary osteotomy to impact only the posterior teeth (bottom right, yellow bracket includes impacting only posterior teeth), allowing the mandible to rotate CCW and close the bite, leaving the anterior segment at the same level.

Finally, it is important for the orthodontist to remember that an anterior open bite can be a combination of a skeletal and dental (functional) open bite. This could be the etiology of an anterior step. Failure to address a functional tongue posture habit or digit habit that caused the step could lead to relapse of the corrected open bite—no matter the surgery.

Q: Are LeFort I maxillary impaction osteotomies appropriate treatment *only* for skeletal open bites?

A: No. Stacy (Figure 5.39) has a long LAFH, but her chief complaint was her excessive incisal display at rest and gingival display when smiling (short upper lip/short philtrum length/accentuated cupid's bow/ILG). Her maxillary incisors were slightly *stepped up* relative to her posterior teeth (Figure 5.39c). Also, note the difference in her facial fullness from left to right. She was an appropriate candidate for, and underwent, maxillary impaction, mandibular advancement, and genioplasty advancement osteotomies (Figure 5.39d–f). A clear improvement in incisal display and lip competence resulted.

Q: How will the use of TADs (Figures 5.11, 5.12, and 5.13) likely affect the need for LeFort I maxillary impaction osteotomies?

A: TADs have the potential to dramatically reduce the need for maxillary impaction osteotomies.

Q: Because the maxillary lip lengthens with age (decreasing incisal display), it is important not to overimpact the maxilla during skeletal open bite closure [57]. This restriction limits the amount you can reduce LAFH. Additionally, the technical limit for impaction of the anterior maxilla is about 10 mm (6–7 mm for the posterior maxilla). Because excess *mandibular anterior* vertical development can contribute to an interlabial gap or mentalis strain, what other adjunctive surgical procedure can help close an interlabial gap, eliminate mentalis strain, and reduce LAFH?

A: An impaction genioplasty osteotomy. By removing a wedge of bone from the chin (Figure 5.40a, b), the mentalis muscle and lower lip can be moved superiorly, the LAFH reduced, and an ILG reduced or eliminated. Options include [61] the following:

- Genioplasty with parallel ostectomy (Figure 5.40c, red lines are bony cuts). This is indicated when excess mandibular anterior height is present (mentalis strain and ILG) but when chin projection is effective. Bony Pogonion is shortened, vertically (yellow arrow).
- Sliding advancement genioplasty (Figure 5.40d) with posteriorly tapered ostectomy. This is indicated when excess mandibular anterior height is present but bony Pogonion is ineffective (Figure 5.40d). Bony Pogonion is shortened *and* brought forward—becoming more effective.

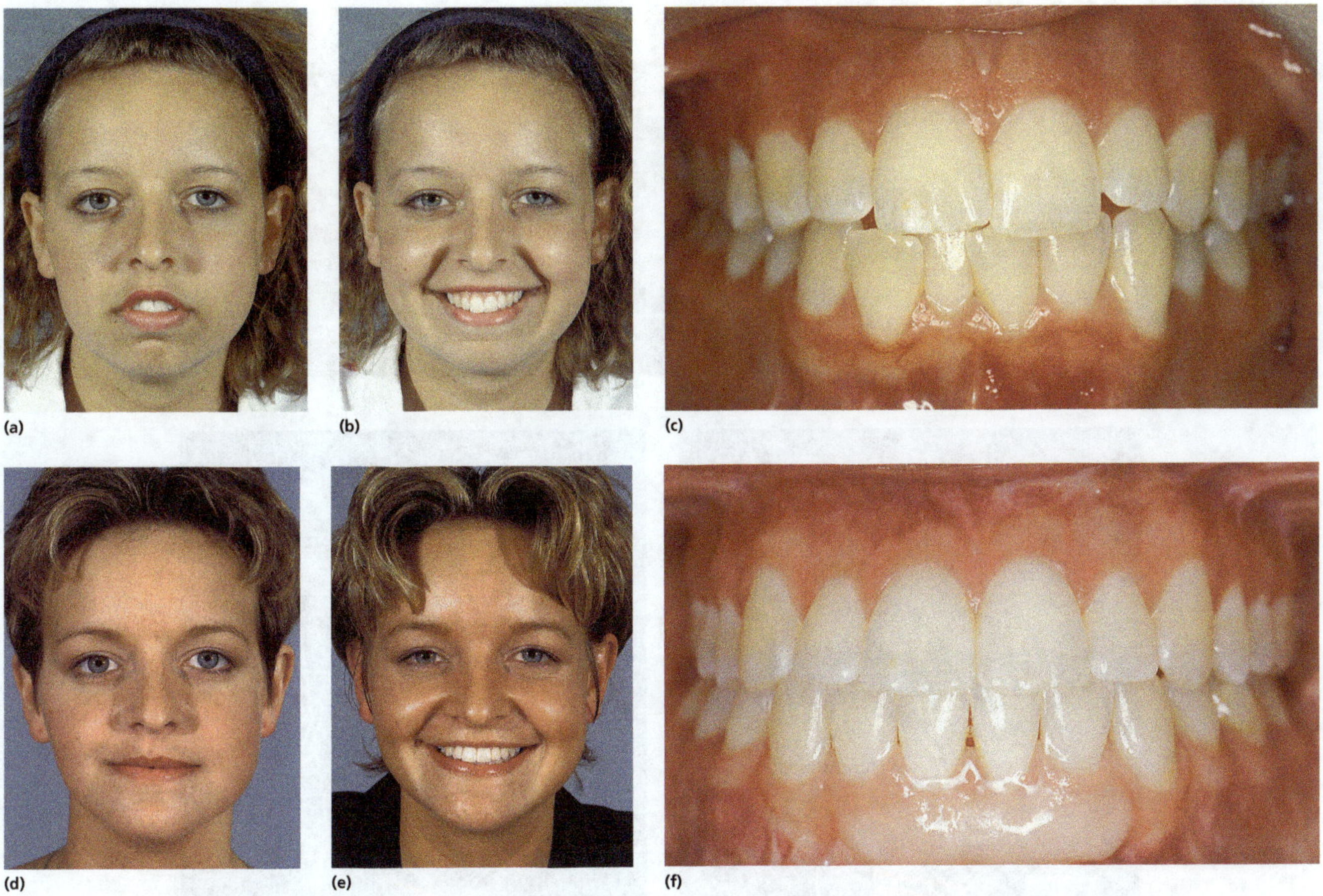

Figure 5.39 (a–c) A patient with an LLAFH and ILG but lacking an open bite. (d–f) She underwent a LeFort I maxillary impaction osteotomy to reduce her incisal and gingival display.

Q: How does relapse of dental (functional) anterior open bites differ from relapse of skeletal anterior open bites?

A: Relapse of *dental* open bites occurs when the habit has not been corrected, or, if the initially undererupted anterior teeth were erupted into occlusion, but not held long enough for the supporting tissues to remodel (resulting in incisor intrusion). Relapse of *skeletal* open bites occurs with either continued excess vertical facial growth or adverse bony remodeling following surgery. Of course, patients presenting with a combination of skeletal and dental open bite can relapse both ways.

Q: Conventional wisdom [62, 63] suggests that the vertical dimension of the face is the last to complete growth. This notion, if true, could impact concerns of adolescent skeletal open bite treatment stability. Is this notion correct? Is the vertical dimension of the face the last to complete growth?

A: *No, this notion is an oversimplification of human biology.* While concern about posttreatment vertical growth is warranted in adolescent skeletal open bite patients, the relationship between transverse, anteroposterior, and vertical growth is far more complicated than the simple belief that vertical is the last dimension to finish growing. In a recent study [64], an overlap was found to exist at any age in the amount of growth completed for different measures in the transverse, anteroposterior, and vertical dimensions. While some transverse measures (cranial width and interjugal width) attain adult size before any anteroposterior or vertical measures, there is evidence of continued growth for other transverse parameters (interzygomatic width and intergonial width). A similar overlap is seen in the anteroposterior and vertical dimensions. A distinct separation, by time and dimension, is not seen in the amount of facial growth completed during development.

Q: Assuming that all your treatment goals have been achieved, when can you safely deband a skeletal open bite patient and begin retention?

A: In adolescents, discontinuing orthopedic treatment before growth is complete is a stability gamble in any patient. Discontinuing orthopedic treatment before growth is complete in a skeletal open bite patient is a sure bet on failure. *Do not deband until growth is complete.* If growth has slowed dramatically and you decide to deband, then monitor the patient carefully for signs of open bite relapse. In a surgically treated adult skeletal open bite patient, or any surgery patient for that matter, *keep them in fixed orthodontic appliances at least 4–6 months post surgery*. This time is needed for postsurgery bony remodeling.

Q: Compare the continued growth pattern in patients exhibiting skeletal *open bite relapse* to the continued growth pattern in patients exhibiting skeletal *deep bite relapse*.

A: Patients exhibiting skeletal open-bite relapse show greater combined sutural and alveolar growth of the maxilla and alveolar growth of the mandible than posterior facial height

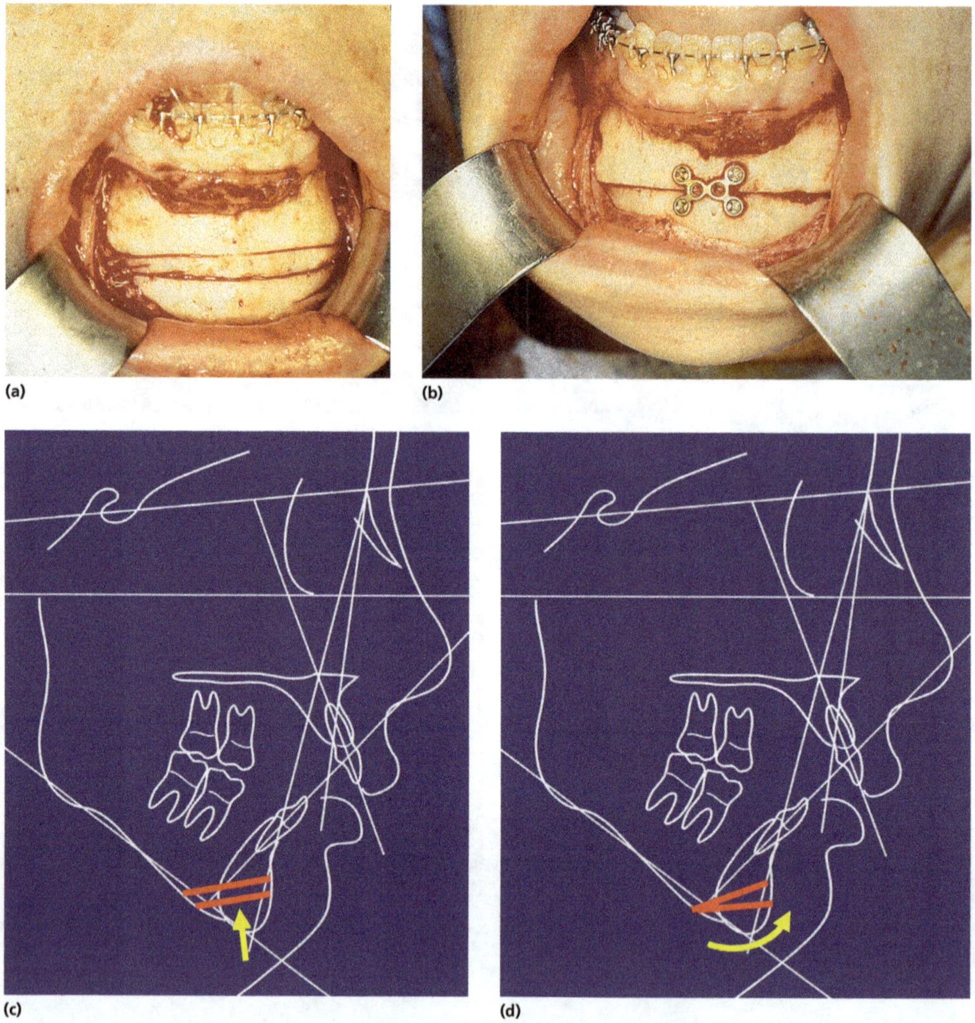

Figure 5.40 Genioplasties to reduce LAFH: (a, b) bony wedge being removed from the chin to shorten LAFH, (c) genioplasty with parallel ostectomy, (d) sliding advancement genioplasty with posteriorly tapered wedge.

increase. In other words, their maxilla descends more, and their molars erupt more, than their posterior face height increases. Patients exhibiting skeletal deep-overbite relapse show greater posterior facial height increase than combined sutural and alveolar growth of the maxilla and alveolar growth of the mandible [5]. In other words, their maxilla descends less, and their molars erupt less, than their posterior face height increases.

Q: You successfully complete orthopedic treatment of an adolescent skeletal open bite patient (Figure 5.41a). Three years later, the patient returns. He has faithfully worn his retainers, but his open bite has relapsed (Figure 5.41b). You take a cephalometric radiograph and superimpose it on his deband radiograph (Figure 5.41c, red is at deband and green is at 3-year post deband). What do you see? Why did his open bite relapse?

A: His open bite relapsed due to continued vertical growth. Vertical descent of the maxilla, coupled with molar eruption, overwhelmed any increase in posterior facial height, and resulted in return of his open bite.

Q: In terms of stability, what should you always tell parents before beginning treatment of adolescent skeletal open bite patients?

A: Despite your best efforts and the best efforts of the patient, continued and excessive vertical growth could eventually result in the need for orthognathic surgery to achieve an ideal result.

Q: What are your retention options for skeletal open bite patients?

A: Retention options for dental anterior open bites were presented in the introductory section to Chapter 4 and should be used, if the skeletal open bite included a dental open bite component. In skeletal open bite cases where growth is complete or postsurgical treatment is stable, night wear of Hawley retainers (or vacuum-formed retainers) should be adequate. If there is concern about residual vertical growth, then Hawley retainers with posterior occlusal coverage (bite blocks), tooth positioners, or retainers/tooth positioners used in conjunction with a vertical-pull chin cup could be considered (high pull chin cup if the patient tends toward Class III).

Q: Assume that a skeletal open bite patient you treated begins to relapse. What can you do?

A: Depending on the magnitude of the relapse, and its cause (continued growth or post-surgical changes), *consider all of the options we have previously discussed under orthopedic,*

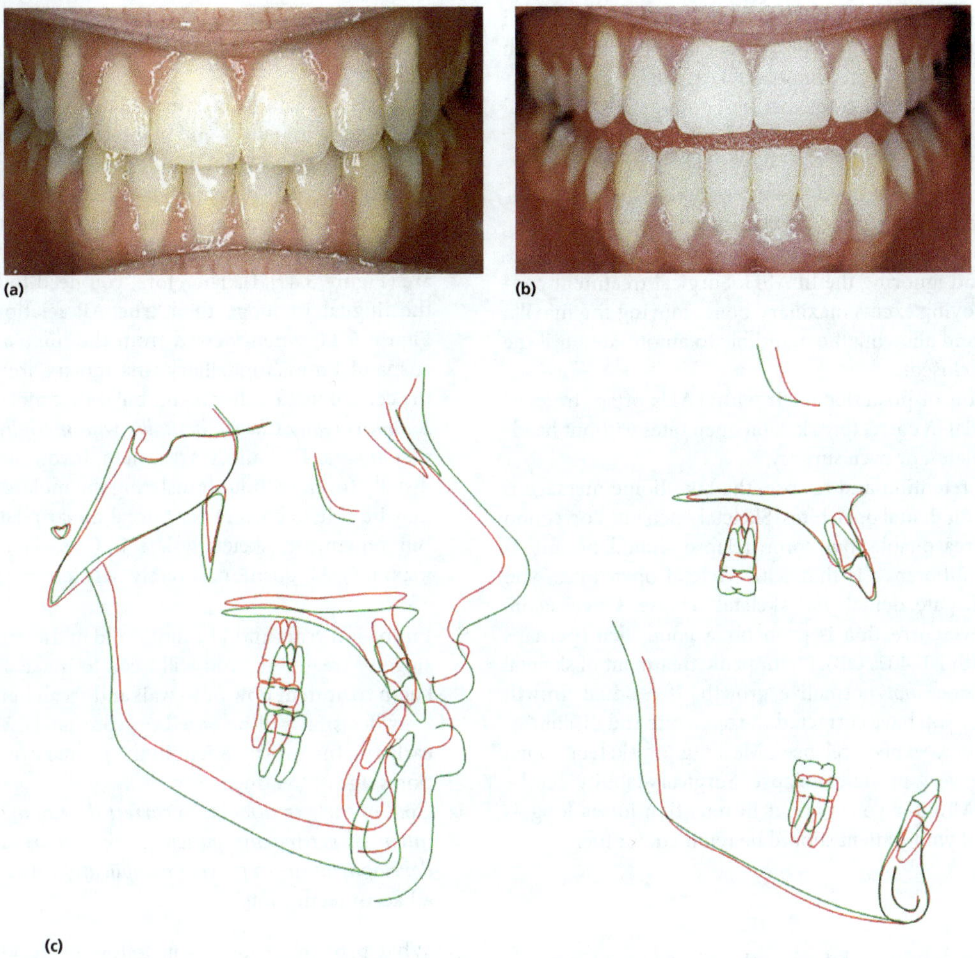

Figure 5.41 Relapse of a successfully treated adolescent skeletal open bite patient: (a) frontal intraoral photograph at the time of deband, (b) frontal intraoral photograph 3 years post deband shows open bite returning in spite of good retainer wear. (c) Superimposition of deband (red) and 3 years post deband (green) cephalometric radiographs.

masking, or surgical treatment of skeletal open bites. Discuss the appropriate option(s) with the patient, define your treatment plan, and start.

Q: Is anterior open-bite treatment stable (surgical and nonsurgical)?

A: In a recent meta-analysis, both surgical and nonsurgical open-bite treatment stability was reported to be reasonable. In a surgical treatment group, stability was found to be 82%, and in a nonsurgical group, 75% [65].

Q: Is anterior open bite *treatment with occlusal adjustment* stable?

A: Yes and no. In a study of 17 open-bite patients treated with occlusal adjustment, 67% remained stable an average of 3.4 years after treatment. To the contrary, 33% demonstrated some degree of relapse [66].

Q: Which is a more stable surgery: open bite closure with LeFort I maxillary impaction alone or, open bite closure with bimaxillary surgery (mandibular osteotomy in addition to the maxillary surgery)?

A: A one-piece LeFort I impaction osteotomy is more stable, overall [67, 68]. A higher relapse tendency is seen with bimaxillary surgery, especially in patients with high ANB angles and steep mandibular plane angles [69]. Long-term *dental* relapse is more common in patients after LeFort I osteotomy correction alone. Long-term *skeletal* relapse is more common after bimaxillary surgery [70].

Q: In summary, what are your "take-home" messages regarding etiology, identifying, treating, and retaining skeletal anterior open bite patients?

A: Take-home messages include the following:

- Skeletal anterior open bites result from a pattern of growth including: posterior–superior condylar growth, lack of normal forward mandibular internal (true) rotation or even backward internal (true) rotation, excess maxillary corpus descent (palatal plane may rotate down posteriorly), and/or excess molar eruption. As the mandible rotates downward and backward, the mandibular plane angle steepens, the anterior face height increases, and an anterior open bite results. When facial soft tissue growth does not keep pace with vertical skeletal growth, an ILG results. Rarely, skeletal open bites can result from condylar degeneration.
- Contrasted with dental open bites (usually limited from canine to canine and identified by stepped up maxillary and/or stepped down mandibular anterior teeth), the identifying features of skeletal open bites include an LLAFH (soft tissue and skeletal), an ILG (even in the presence of a normal maxillary lip length), a steep MPA, a palatal plane tipped down at

PNS, maxillary first molar apicies erupted below the palatal plane, a short posterior face height, and an open bite, which extends posteriorly to the premolars or molars.

- Skeletal anterior open bites can be combined with dental anterior open bites, which result from habits preventing incisor eruption.
- Orthopedic treatment of adolescent skeletal open bites consists of restricting downward maxillary growth plus reducing molar eruption. Masking treatment consists of erupting anterior teeth and ignoring the LLAFH. Surgical treatment consists of removing excess maxillary bone, moving the maxilla superiorly, and allowing the mandible to autorotate until the open bite is closed.
- The intrusion of posterior teeth with TADs offers tremendous potential in correcting skeletal open bites without headgears, bite plates, or even surgery.
- In terms of retention and relapse, the take-home message is the same as for dental open bites. Skeletal open bite correction stability is reasonable, but some relapse should be anticipated. The difference is that with skeletal open bites, you should anticipate dental *and* skeletal relapse. Once again, open bite overcorrection is probably a good idea (perhaps finishing with 20–40% OB). Orthopedic treatment of skeletal open bites does *not* normalize growth. If residual growth remains after you have corrected the open bite and discontinued treatment, expect relapse. Masking of skeletal open bites can be very prone to relapse. Surgical stability can be very good. Monitor your patient in retention for as long as possible, and your patient should be retained, for life.

Case Emma

Emma (Figure 5.42) is an 8-year, 11-month-old who presents to you with the parent's CC, "Emma needs braces." Her PMH, TMJ, and periodontal evaluations are WRN. CR=CO.

Q: List diagnostic findings/problems. What is your diagnosis?
A: See Table 5.1.

Q: Emma does not have a posterior cross bite, but what else should you check in the transverse dimension?
A: Look at her separated models from the front to check torques of her posterior teeth (Figure 5.43). Note that she has mild *labial crown torque of her maxillary first molars* and mild *lingual crown torque of her mandibular first molars.*

Q: Is this how you want her posterior teeth to remain? If not, how will these torques affect your treatment plan?
A: Ideally, you will want to upright these teeth with treatment. However, uprighting her maxillary molars will tend to bring the crowns lingually, while uprighting her mandibular molars will tend to bring the crowns buccally, which could put her into posterior cross bite. These movements must be anticipated before treatment. If such transverse compensations (torques) are small (which is the case with Emma), then you may be able to upright the posterior teeth and maintain posterior arch coordination using archwires only. However, if transverse compensations are large, and the initial posterior buccal overjet minimal, then it may be prudent to expand the maxilla with an RME appliance, so that you create enough buccal overjet to permit uprighting the posterior teeth. In some (adult) patients with severe transverse compensations, you may even choose to leave the compensations—as opposed to requiring the adult patient to undergo a SARME in order to achieve adequate posterior overjet.

Q: Why should you look at articulated models from the *lingual*? Specifically, maxillary and mandibular first molar relationships from the lingual? What do you see with Emma's models viewed from the lingual (Figure 5.44)? What does this mean to you?
A: When maxillary first molars are rotated mesially (Figure 5.42m), they appear more Class II in the buccal view than they really are (Figure 5.42j, l). Therefore, you need to look at them from the lingual to judge their true AP relationship. As seen in Figure 5.44, when viewed from the lingual, the mesiolingual cusps of Emma's maxillary first molars are seated squarely in the central fossa of her mandibular first molars. In other words, *Emma is really Class I, dentally, with mesially rotated maxillary first molars.* This affects treatment. If you can rotate her molars distally (even without translating the molars distally), then you may be able to correct her buccal molar relationship to Class I. But remember, skeletally she is Class II (slightly protrusive maxillary AP position, severely deficient mandible).

Q: Emma is 8 years and 11 months old in the early mixed dentition stage of treatment. You will need to make a decision either to begin treatment now or to wait and recall her when she is older. This decision will be based on your goals. What is the goal of early treatment (treatment in the primary or early mixed dentition stage of treatment)?
A: *Goal of early treatment: to correct developing problems with the intent of getting the patient back to normal for that stage of development; or to prevent complications* (such as resorption of adjacent teeth roots).

Q: What principle should you follow in deciding what cases to treat early?
A: *Principle: early treatment should be used to treat very specific problems with a clearly defined end-point, usually within 6–9 months.* In other words, be wary of early treatment that ends up one long protracted period of treatment, many years in length.

Q: What question should you ask yourself at every consultation for early treatment?
A: *Is it absolutely necessary that I do anything now? What harm will come from not doing anything now?*

Q: List at least three specific situations, or problems, you would address with early treatment.
A: Specific problems that should be addressed with early treatment include the following:

1. When early treatment will *significantly reduce later treatment complexity*. The patient in Figure 5.45a presents with ectopic eruption of her mandibular lateral incisors that are impacting her mandibular permanent canines and first premolars. Also, her mandibular right lateral incisor is impacted beneath her mandibular right primary first molar. Treating this patient now by moving the mandibular lateral incisors forward to their correct positions will allow her mandibular canines and first premolars to erupt—reducing later treatment complexity. Primary canines and primary first molars were extracted and fixed appliances placed to correctly position her lateral incisors (Figure 5.45b, c). Braces were removed and an LLHA delivered (with auxiliary wires soldered to hold the mandibular incisors in their corrected positions).

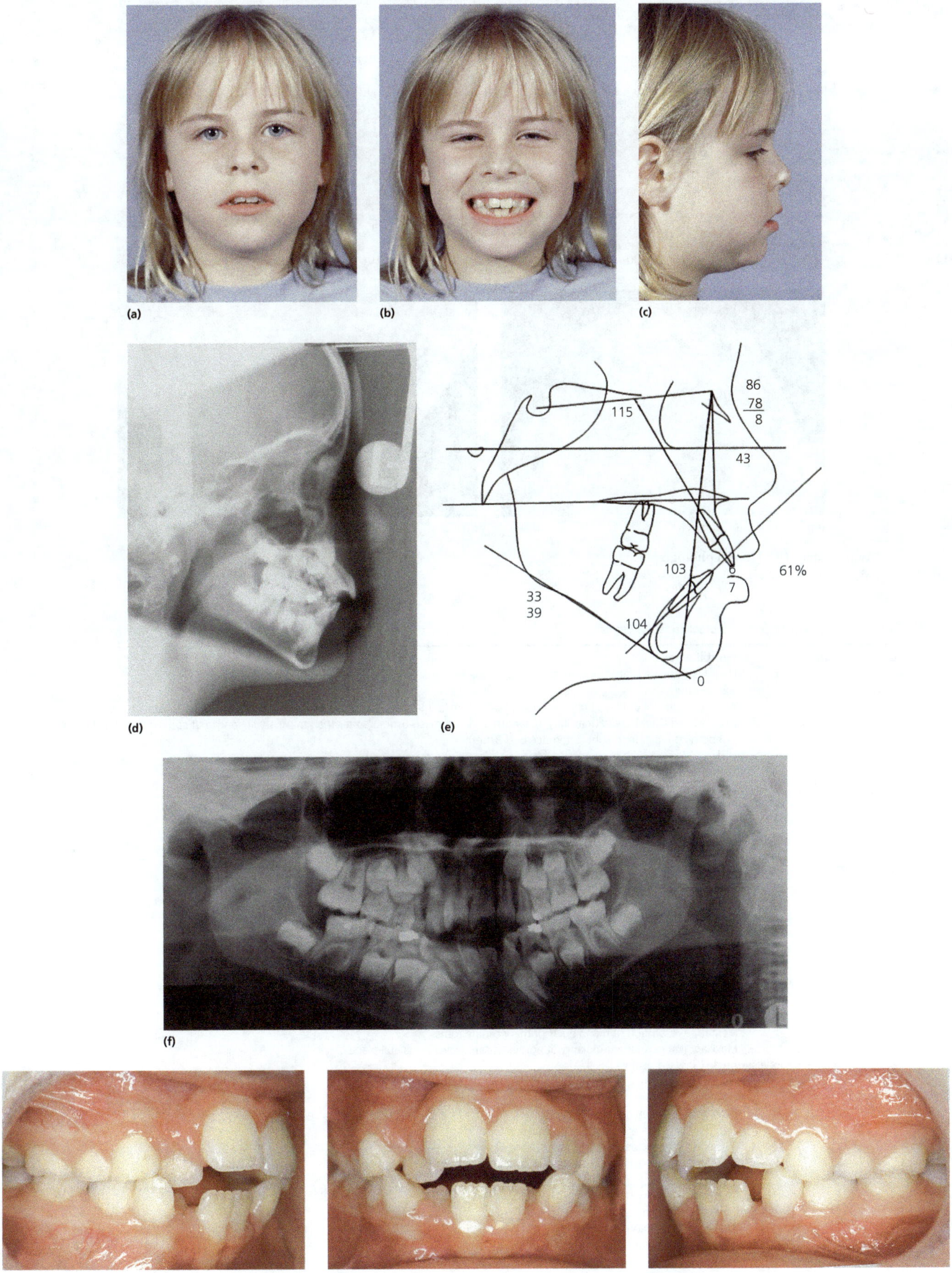

Figure 5.42 Initial records of Emma: (a–c) facial photographs, (d) lateral cephalograph, (e) cephalometric tracing, (f) pantomograph, (g–i) intraoral photographs, and

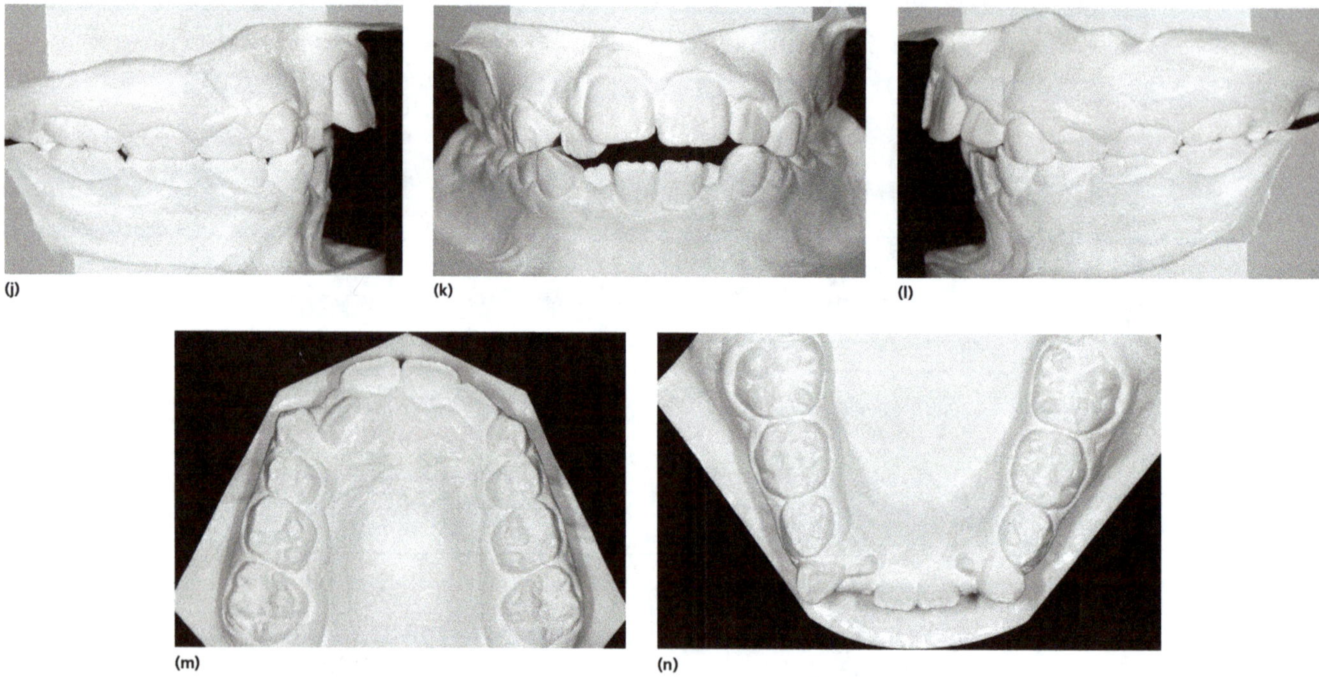

Figure 5.42 (Continued) (j–n) model photographs.

Table 5.1 Diagnostic findings and problem list for Emma.

Full face and profile	**Frontal view**
	LLAFH (soft tissue Glabella–Subnasale < Subnasale–soft tissue Menton)
	ILG: 6–7 mm
	Acceptable incisal display at rest and during posed smile (maxillary incisors are stepped *up* relative to her posterior teeth)
	Accentuated Cupid's bow (maxillary lip length at philtrum is ~6 mm shorter than maxillary lip length at commissure; ideal philtrum length-commissure height difference is 2–3 mm)
	UDML: WRN
	Face is symmetric
	Upturned nose
	Profile view
	Convex profile and retrusive chin
	Obtuse NLA
	Obtuse lip–chin–throat angle
Ceph analysis	**Skeletal**
	Maxilla slightly protrusive (A-point slightly forward of Nasion-perpendicular line)
	Mandible retrusive (ANB = 8°)
	LLAFH (LAFH/TAFH = 61%, over two standard deviations greater than an average of 55%, SD = 2%)
	Steep MPA (FMA = 33°; SNMP = 39°)
	Short posterior face height
	Dental
	Very proclined of maxillary incisors (1 to SN = 115°)
	Very proclined of mandibular incisors (FMIA = 43°)
Radiographs	Early mixed dentition
	Premature resorption of mandibular primary canine roots
	Maxillary first permanent molar root apicies at same level as palatal plane
Intraoral photos and models	Angle Class II division 1
	Iowa Classification: II (1–2) X X II (1–2)
	OJ: 4 mm
	Cross-bite maxillary right lateral incisor
	Anterior open bite extending to primary canines
	Maxillary incisors stepped up relative to maxillary posterior teeth
	Mandibular incisors stepped down relative to mandibular posterior teeth
	Mild COS
	Moderate maxillary crowding
	Severe mandibular crowding
	Absence of posterior cross bites
	Maxillary first molars are rotated mesially
	Prominent mandibular central incisor roots and thin attached tissue
Other	—
Diagnosis	Angle Class II division 1 malocclusion
	Skeletal open bite

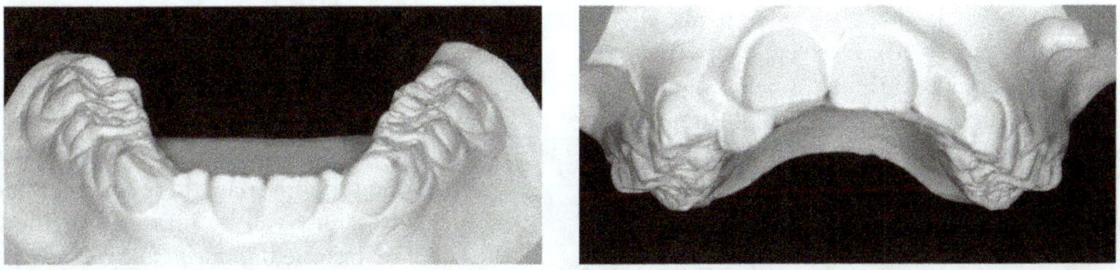

(a) (b)

Figure 5.43 (a, b) Separated model views of Emma.

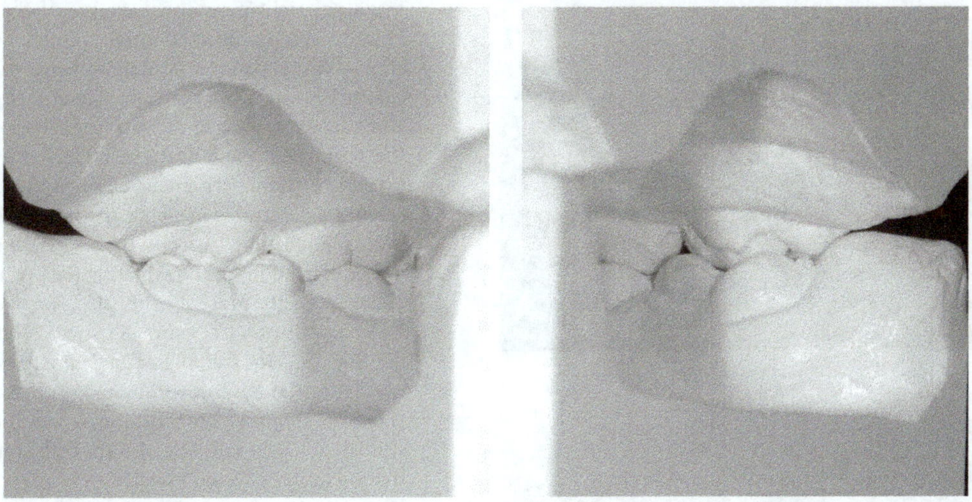

(a) (b)

Figure 5.44 Emma's models as viewed from the lingual: (a) left and (b) right.

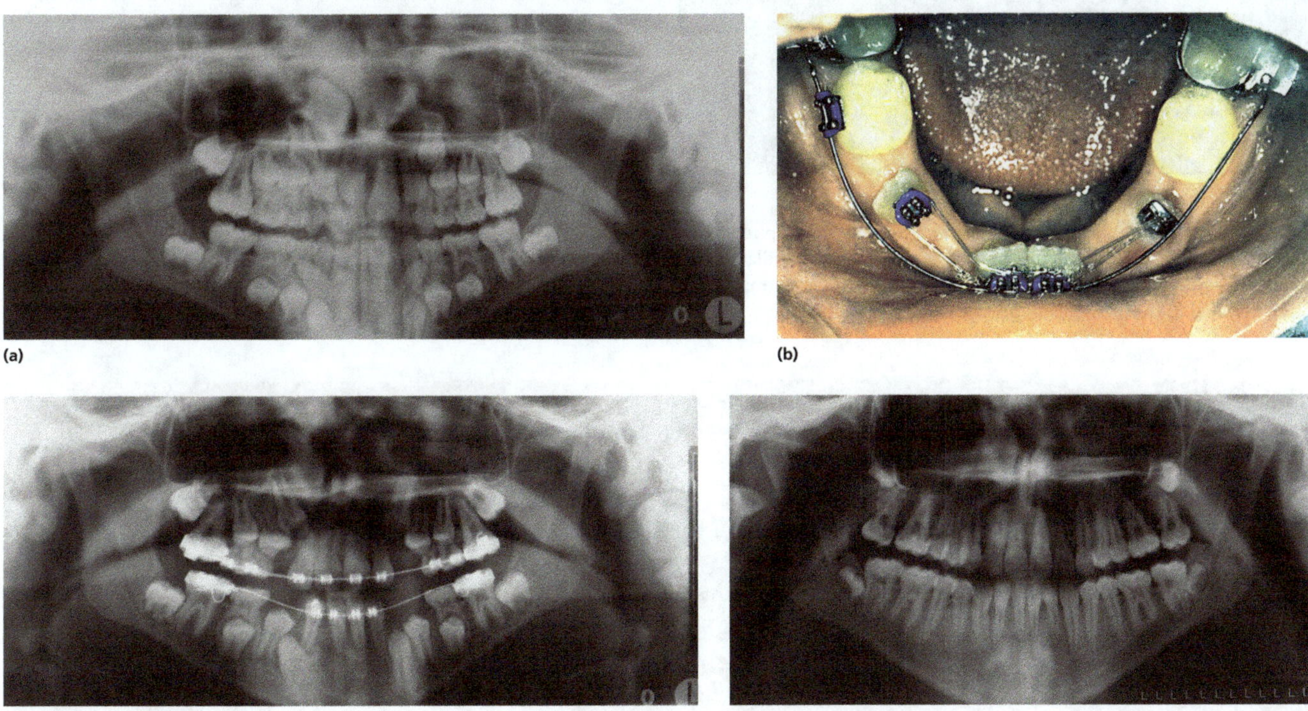

(a) (b) (c) (d)

Figure 5.45 Early treatment used to significantly reduce later treatment complexity: (a) ectopically erupting mandibular lateral incisors are impacting mandibular canines and first premolars, (b) by extracting primary mandibular teeth and advancing the ectopically erupting mandibular incisors, (c) impacted permanent mandibular canines and premolars could erupt, and (d) later treatment could be greatly simplified.

Permanent teeth erupted, fixed appliances were placed, and treatment finished (Figure 5.45d). Fixed appliance treatment was much easier, because early treatment significantly reduced later complexity. Again, this case illustrates using *early treatment to treat a very specific problem and get the patient back to normal for her stage of development. The harm that would have come from not doing anything was permanent canine and premolar impaction.* Other examples of reducing later treatment complexity by early treatment could include managing mild-to-moderate mandibular anterior crowding with an LLHA or, managing severe anterior crowding using serial extraction in Class I patients with normal vertical and normal transverse relationships.

2 When patients present with *unerupted maxillary permanent canines whose crowns overlap the permanent lateral incisor roots*—when viewed on a panoramic image. Why? With increasing root overlap, there comes an increasing likelihood that the canine will be impacted or the lateral incisor root could be resorbed. *If adequate space exists* in the arch for the permanent canines to erupt, then it can be beneficial to extract maxillary primary canines (or maxillary primary canines *plus* maxillary primary first molars) to increase the chances for spontaneous canine eruption [71–75]. As an example, the maxillary right permanent canine of the patient shown in Figure 5.46a was deemed nonerupting following serial evaluation of earlier panoramic images. As overlap of the permanent canine crown across the right lateral incisor root was noted, and adequate space in the arch for eruption was available for the permanent canine, the maxillary primary canines were extracted. Both permanent canines then erupted normally (Figure 5.46b). *If inadequate space exists* in the arch for the permanent canine to erupt, then space must be created for it to erupt, in addition to extracting the primary canine.
3 When patients present with *posterior cross bites combined with lateral CR—CO shifts.* Such cross bites with shifts can develop into morphological asymmetries of the mandible, which can largely be eliminated with maxillary expansion [76–81]. Treatment of posterior cross bites without lateral shifts can generally be postponed until comprehensive treatment in early adolescence.
4 When patients present having *anterior cross bites causing trauma to the incisors.* Incisal edge wear of both maxillary central incisors (caused by the cross bite) can be seen following cross-bite correction in Figure 5.47. Treatment of anterior cross bites *without* signs of trauma can often be postponed until comprehensive treatment in early adolescence.

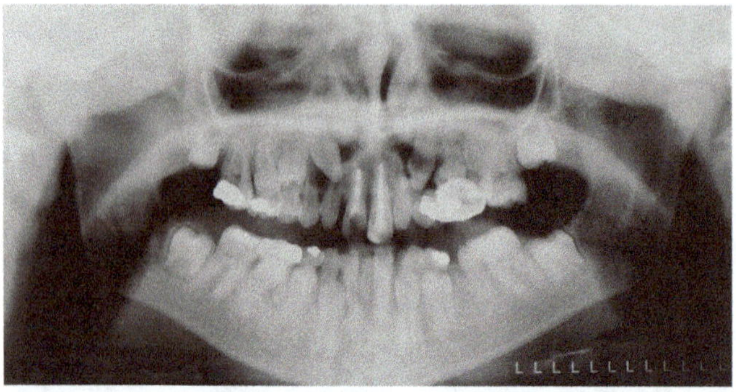

(a)

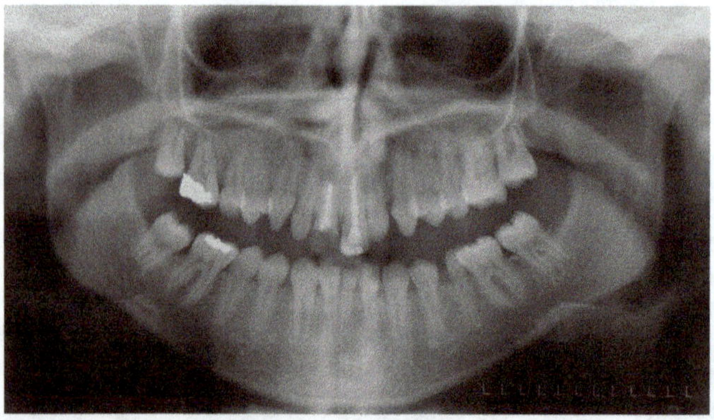

(b)

Figure 5.46 Early treatment of a patient presenting with nonerupting maxillary right permanent canine (a) which overlapped the maxillary right lateral incisor root on the panoramic image. Extraction of the primary canine resulted in (b) spontaneous permanent canine eruption.

Q: Should early treatment be started to address developing Class II malocclusions?

A: Not generally. Early mixed dentition treatment of Class II patients does not offer any advantage over Class II treatment started in early adolescence [82–87]. However, if a patient presents with a Class II malocclusion (deficient mandibular growth) in the early mixed dentition, and the parents state that the *patient is clearly entering his or her growth spurt*, then it

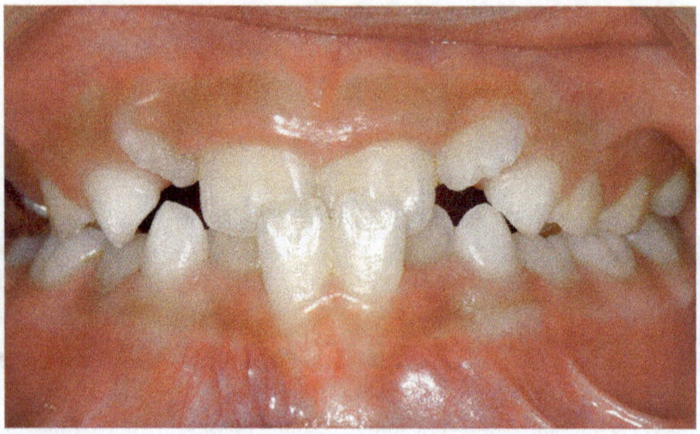

(a)

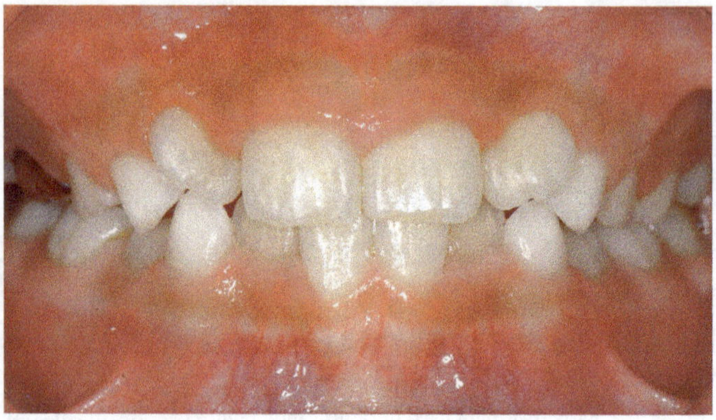

(b)

Figure 5.47 (a, b) Early treatment of a patient presenting with an anterior cross bite and trauma to the maxillary incisors.

would be wise to begin (headgear or functional appliance) orthopedic treatment and not wait for the late mixed-dentition stage of development.

Q: Should early treatment be started to address developing Class III malocclusions?

A: Unlike Class II malocclusions, we do not have the prospective clinical trials to answer this question. It is probably prudent to apply the same guidelines for patients with *excessive mandibular growth*—wait until early adolescence to begin (high-pull chin cup) orthopedic treatment, unless the parents state that the child has clearly started to grow. However, if the Class III relationship has resulted from *maxillary AP deficiency*, and the application of a reverse-pull headgear is being considered, then treatment in the early mixed-dentition stage has been reported to be more effective than treatment after the age of 10 years [88–90]. With either high-pull chin cup treatment or reverse-pull headgear treatment, please remember that you are not normalizing growth [91]. No matter how old the Class III child is when you achieve anteroposterior (molar and canine) orthopedic correction, you must *continue holding the anteroposterior correction (usually with a chin cup) until the child has finished growing.*

Q: Should early treatment be started to address developing open bites?

A: This question will be addressed, exhaustively, in the current case (Emma) we are discussing.

Q: Should early treatment be started to address issues of self-esteem?

A: Generally, self-esteem impact does not warrant early intervention [92]. However, this is a question that must be answered on a patient-by-patient basis. Your decision to treat should be based on the golden rule (what you would do if the child was your own).

Q: What specific conditions should you be cautious of when considering early treatment?

A: *Severe* AP and vertical skeletal discrepancies, unless there is a clear and overriding psychosocial benefit. Why? The probability of correcting these severe skeletal discrepancies in the early mixed dentition and maintaining their correction until adulthood is low.

Q: Finally, a member of your study club says that he used to perform a lot of early treatment but quit because all the cases evolved into very lengthy treatment that ended in the permanent dentition anyway. His patients complained that they were "in braces forever." He asks what your philosophy of early treatment is.

A: Again, early treatment should be used to treat very *specific problems—with a clearly defined end-point*, to get the patient back on the normal track. Get in, get it done, get out. Correction of most early treatment problems should begin and end within 6–9 months. Then, put the patient on recall to monitor. Confronted with an early treatment case, always ask yourself, "Is it absolutely necessary that I do anything now?" and "What harm will come from not doing anything now?"

Q: Back to Emma—she exhibits lip incompetence (ILG), an LLAFH, and an open bite. With these features, orthodontists traditionally think "mouth breather." Can you conclude that Emma is a mouth breather because she exhibits lip incompetence?

A: No. Lip incompetence alone does not signify mouth breathing [93, 94]. Lip incompetence could be due to Emma having a short upper lip or to skeletal vertical growth outpacing soft tissue vertical growth.

Q: If lip incompetence alone does not indicate mouth breathing, how would you determine whether or not to refer Emma to an otolaryngologist for an airway evaluation?

A: You could try to *observe* whether or not she breathes through her mouth. Ask her parents if Emma normally breathes through her nose or mouth. Ask Emma. In some patients, it is obvious that they can only breathe through their mouths. In others, it is unclear. If Emma is an obligatory mouth breather, has difficulty breathing, or presents with a history of sleep apnea, then refer her for an airway evaluation. If you are unsure, then ask her parents to pay close attention to Emma and let you know later what they observe. Emma's parents deny that Emma has any airway problems, and you don't observe any. Emma says that she breaths through her nose.

Q: Does it appear that Emma exhibits adenoidal hypertrophy on her lateral cephalometric radiograph (Figure 5.42d)?

A: No. Her adenoids do not appear enlarged.

Q: List at least four possible causes of airway obstruction other than adenoidal hypertrophy.

A: Allergic rhinitis, polyps, congenital nasal deformities, neoplasms, and recurrent upper respiratory infections [95].

Q: Hypothetically, if Emma had difficulty breathing through her nose, and otolaryngology corrected the airway obstruction, could you assure her parents that Emma's vertical growth pattern would change to a more normal growth pattern?

A: No. If Emma were an obligatory mouth breather, your referral for nasal obstruction treatment would be intended to help her breathe normally. You cannot guarantee a patient that nasal obstruction correction will correct their growth pattern.

Q: In terms of Emma's open bite, what should you ask her parents? What should you ask Emma? What else should you check for?

A: Show Emma and her parents that her incisors are not touching and ask them if they have noticed this before. They tell you that they remember Emma always having the open bite. Ask Emma if she has any idea why her front teeth would not have come together. She states that she sucked her thumb when she was younger (until age 5) but no longer. Even if she no longer has a digit habit, she could still be posturing her tongue anteriorly. Check for this. Tell Emma to close her eyes for a minute. Talk to her parents for a little while. Just as you are about to gently draw her lower lip forward to check for a tongue habit, ask Emma to open her eyes to distract her. As she opens her eyes, quickly and gently draw her lower lip forward and check for an anterior tongue interposition habit. You find that *Emma's tongue does appear to be interposed between her incisors*. Confirm that Emma has no other medical problems (e.g., rheumatoid arthritis) or history of trauma that could have resulted in TMJ degeneration and a resulting open bite. She has no such history, and you note that her condyles appear within the range of normal (Figure 5.42f). Finally, confirm that her anterior open bite is not due to permanent teeth still erupting, ankylosed teeth that are not fully erupted, or lack of space for complete tooth eruption. It appears that these factors are not contributing to Emma's open bite.

Q: How would you deal with her anterior tongue posturing habit?

A: The simplest thing to do is to ask Emma to move her tongue back if she notices it interposed between her front teeth and to swallow with her teeth together. If that approach is not effective, you could bond buttons on the lingual of her mandibular incisors as a "reminder" to keep her tongue back. Equally effective would be to place either an LLHA or maxillary TPA [96] (extending anteriorly) with soldered spurs (reminders) behind the anterior teeth, or to bond small amounts of composite on the lingual of her lower incisors, as reminders. In some patients, as the anterior teeth are brought together during open bite closure, the tongue may automatically learn to stay off the anterior teeth. However, there is no guarantee of habit correction with any of these techniques. Unless the anterior tongue posturing is corrected, you may not be able to close the anterior open bite or keep it closed in retention.

Q: What features would lead you to classify Emma's open bite as a dental open bite? A skeletal open bite? A combination of both? Which is she?

A: Her dental open bite features include the following:

- Presence of an anterior tongue interposition habit
- Anterior open bite extending to primary canines only
- Exaggerated Cupid's bow, which is contributing to her ILG and making her vertical excess appear worse than it is
- First molar apices have not erupted away from the palatal plane

Her skeletal open bite features include the following:

- Long soft tissue LAFH (soft tissue Glabella–Subnasale mildly $<$ Subnasale–soft tissue Menton, Figure 5.42a)
- Long skeletal LAFH (LAFH/TAFH = 61%)
- Steep MPA (FMA = 33°; SNMP = 39°)
- Short posterior face height
- Approximately 6–7 mm ILG

In summary, Emma is a combination dental *and* skeletal open bite. Note: Having a combination of dental and skeletal open bite features is not unusual. It would be unusual to have an open bite patient demonstrating *only and all* the features of either a dental open bite or skeletal open bite.

Q: Why does it matter whether Emma's open bite is of skeletal or dental (functional) origin, or a combination of both?

A: Because dental and skeletal open bites have different etiologies and require different treatments strategies.

Q: What is the etiology of Emma's dental and skeletal open bite? How does the etiology affect her treatment?

A: Her dental open bite may have started with a thumb-sucking habit when she was younger and now continues with the anterior tongue interposition habit. Emma's tongue habit must be addressed before you can either correct her open bite or keep it corrected in retention. Emma's skeletal open bite is probably due to a pattern of growth including: condyles growing posterior-superiorly (Figure 5.48, curved red arrow), lack of posterior face height development, lack of normal forward mandibular internal (true) rotation or even backward CW internal (true) rotation (curved blue arrows), her maxilla descending more than normal (palatal plane may rotate down posteriorly), and molars erupting more than normal. As her mandible rotated backward (yellow arrow), the mandibular plane angle steepened, the lower anterior face height increased, and her anterior open bite resulted. This growth pattern may continue until she is finished growing. You can attempt to treat Emma orthopedically to improve her vertical relationship (by reducing maxillary corpus descent/reducing molar eruption), but there is no guarantee that you will be successful. And *even if Emma cooperates and you are successful in controlling her vertical growth, her growth pattern will not be normalized with treatment.* To guarantee long-term success, you must treat her vertical growth pattern until she has finished growing. If you feel she is growing very little at the end of your treatment, and you decide to deband her, then you must monitor her closely until she is done growing. Note: Emma has a relatively *mild* skeletal open bite. If she had a severe open bite, then it may be wiser to let her finish growing before initiating treatment—and plan on treating her with orthognathic surgery or TAD molar intrusion.

Q: It is important to focus on the patient's *major* problems in each dimension. What are Emma's primary problems in each dimension?

A: See Table 5.2.

Q: You present Emma's records at your local study club. One orthodontist says, "I always treat open bites in children the same way—by having the child wear anterior vertical elastics." Another orthodontist says, "It is not that simple. There are really two overall approaches to treating open bites, and the specific approach should depend on whether the patient's open bite is skeletal or dental." Which orthodontist is correct?

A: The second orthodontist is correct. The two overall approaches to correcting anterior open bites are erupting

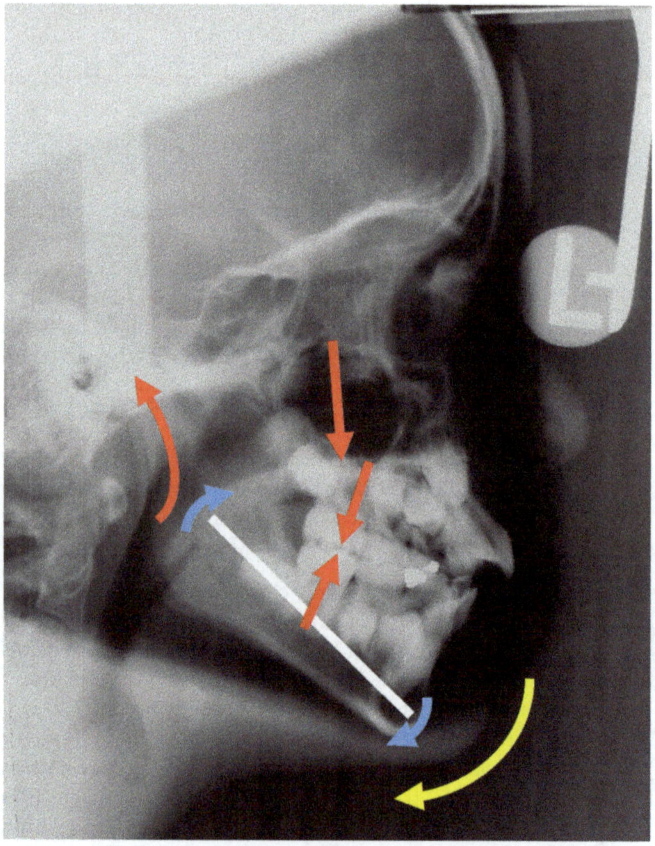

Figure 5.48 Emma's skeletal open bite probably resulted from: condylar posterior–superior growth, lack of posterior face height development, lack of normal forward mandibular internal (true) rotation or even backward internal (true) rotation (blue arrows), her maxilla descending more than normal, and molars erupting more than normal. As a result, her mandible rotated down and back, LAFH increased, and her open bite resulted.

Table 5.2 Primary problems list for Emma *(apical base/skeletal discrepancies italicized)*.

AP	II (1–2) X X II (1–2) *Mandibular skeletal retrusion*
Vertical	*Excess vertical facial growth*
Transverse	Mild transverse dental compensations
Other	Severe mandibular anterior crowding

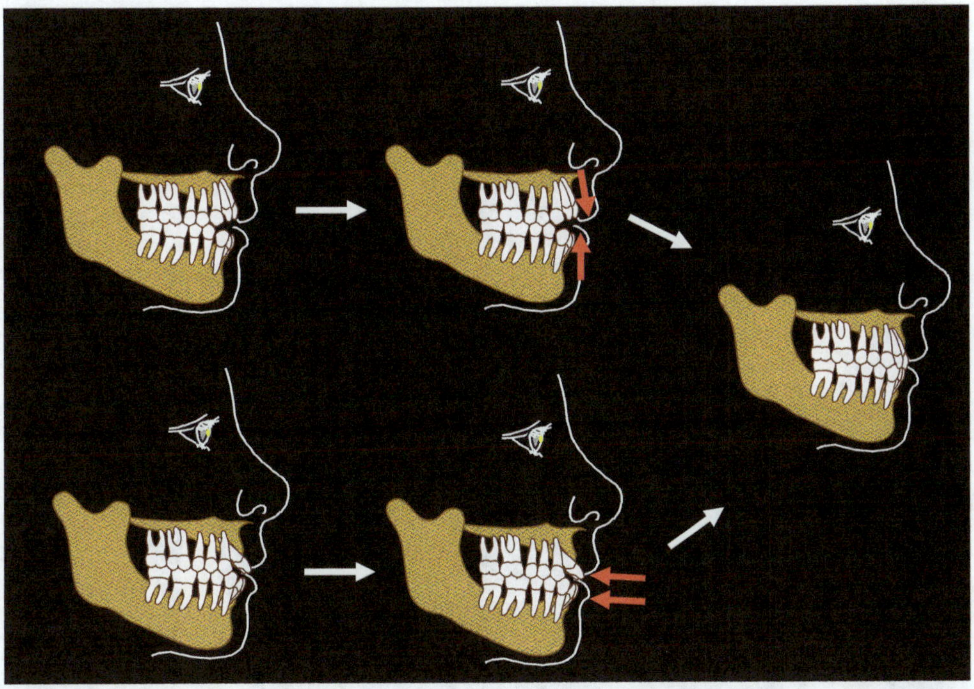

Figure 5.49 Dental open bite treatment consists of: (top) habit elimination, orthodontically erupting anterior teeth, or (bottom) orthodontically retracting proclined incisors around their apicies.

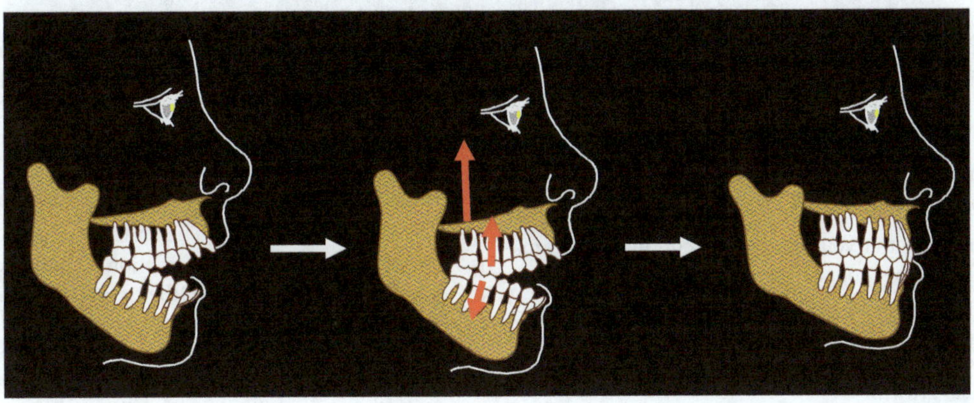

Figure 5.50 Skeletal open bite treatment consists of maxillary corpus intrusion and molar intrusion, which results in a more normal LAFH and bite closure.

anterior teeth and intruding posterior teeth. *Anterior teeth eruption* is the treatment recommended by the first orthodontist and is the treatment of choice with *dental (functional) open bites*—where the vertical skeletal dimension is normal but where a habit has interfered with anterior teeth eruption (Figure 5.49, top left). Treatment could include (Figure 5.49 top center) *elimination of the habit* (digit or anterior tongue posturing habit), which would permit the anterior teeth to erupt, erupting the anterior teeth with archwires and vertical elastics (leveling stepped down mandibular incisors or leveling stepped up maxillary incisors), or placing a curve of Spee in the lower archwire, which erupts the incisors. Each of these treatments could close the open bite (Figure 5.49, right). Or, if the patient has proclined incisors (like Emma does, Figure 5.49 bottom left), then uprighting and retracting her proclined incisors (Figure 5.49, bottom center) will result in the incisors rotating around their apices and the bite closing (Figure 5.49, right).

Posterior teeth intrusion is the treatment of choice for *skeletal open bites* (long LAFH—Figure 5.50 left), and was ignored by the first orthodontist of your study club. In Emma's case, attempting to reduce descent of her maxillary corpus (possibly with a HPHG) and reducing/preventing eruption of her posterior teeth (possibly with a HPHG, vertical-pull headgear, chewing exercises, bite blocks, LLHA, etc.) could result in *relative* maxillary corpus/molar intrusion (Figure 5.50 center) compared to where her maxillary corpus would have descended, and her molars would have erupted, without treatment. This relative molar intrusion allows the mandible to rotate forward and the bite to close (Figure 5.50 right) as mandibular ramus growth continues. Or, TADs can be used as anchors to achieve *absolute* molar intrusion, and close the open bite, even after

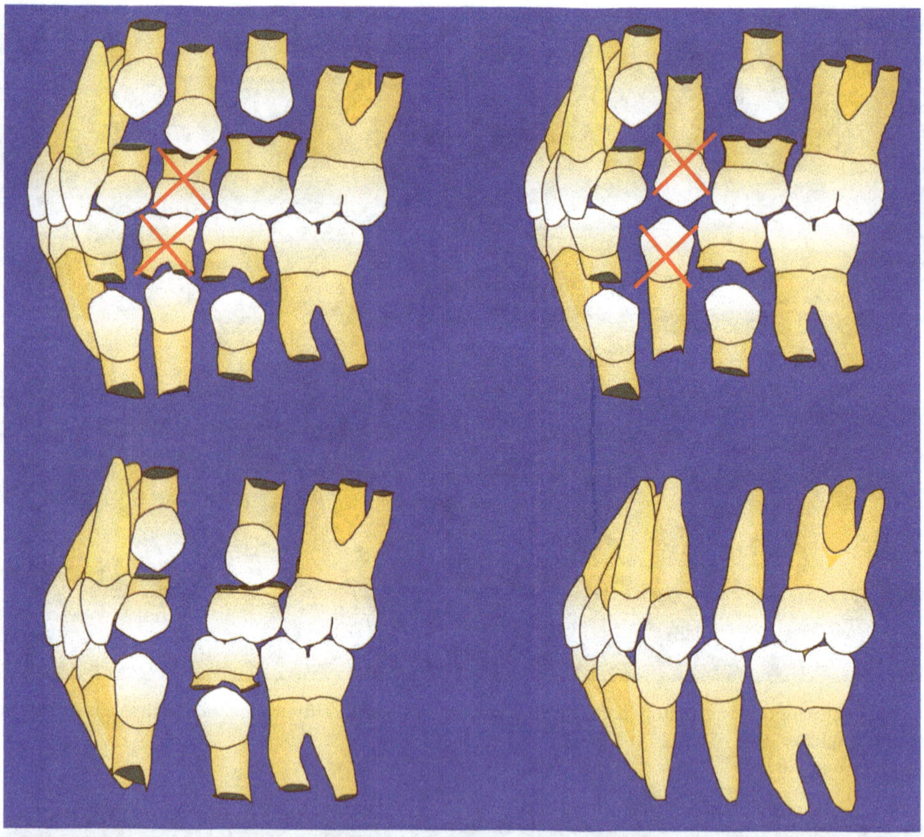

Figure 5.51 In one protocol for serial extraction, primary first molars are extracted when the roots of the first permanent premolars are 1/2 to 2/3 formed (top left). The quickly erupting permanent first premolars are extracted (top right) after they have erupted fully into the mouth (bringing alveolar process bone with them). Permanent canines erupt and drift distally (bottom left) as the second permanent premolars erupt and drift mesially (bottom right).

growth is complete. Maxillary impaction osteotomies may be viewed as another way to intrude posterior teeth.

Q: The first orthodontist at your study club continues, "Emma's open bite is due to her tongue thrusting when she swallows. When she swallows, her tongue must push her teeth forward. You agree, don't you?" How do you respond?

A: First, her skeletal open bite is not due to *any* habit. It is a result of excess vertical growth.

Even if Emma had demonstrated an obligatory mouth-breathing habit, we lack evidence at the highest level demonstrating a relationship between mouth breathing and facial morphology (discussed completely in Case Rachael). Emma's dental open bite may have originally resulted from thumb sucking, but it now appears to be maintained by anterior tongue posturing between teeth. Tongue thrusting during swallowing certainly has been considered the cause of anterior open bites for a long time. The problem with this explanation is that, at 1 second per swallow (~1200–1500 swallows per day), cumulative tongue thrusting against the teeth adds up to about 20 min of force per day. This length of time is simply too short to cause tooth movement [97]. On the other hand, light continuous forces, such as from tongue posture, can prevent tooth eruption and cause open bites. Remember, *tongue posture yes, tongue thrust no.*

Q: What are your treatment goals?

A: Focus on Emma's primary problems in all three dimensions. The KEY to her treatment will be controlling her vertical growth. Controlling her vertical growth will help close her open bite, help eliminate her interlabial gap, help reduce her LLAFH, and help correct her AP relationship (i.e., with mandibular ramus growth, B- point can rotate forward if vertical growth is controlled). The transverse goal will be to achieve ideal transverse arch coordination without increasing transverse dental compensations. Other goals include reducing incisor protrusion in both dental arches; achieving ideal smile esthetics; and obtaining a Class I canine relationship, minimal overjet, and *overcorrected* overbite. Each goal is commendable, but only if long-term stability is achieved.

Q: Emma has severe mandibular crowding, so the possibility of extractions will need to be discussed. What is serial extraction?

A: Serial extraction is the guidance of a developing dentition by sequential extraction of primary and permanent teeth (Figure 5.51).

Q: What features describe the ideal serial extraction patient?

A: The ideal serial extraction patient presents in the early mixed-dentition stage of development and is *normal in every way but with severe anterior crowding (≥10 mm per arch)*. Specifically, the patient should be as follows:

- Class I at the first molars. If the patient is initially Class II or Class III, then they should be corrected to Class I *before* serial extraction is begun. Why? A final Class I relationship will be much easier to achieve if you begin extractions with a Class I relationship.
- Vertically normal to slightly long, with minimal OB or possibly a mild open bite, but *not* a deep bite. Why? The patient's bite will deepen following extractions and incisor retraction.

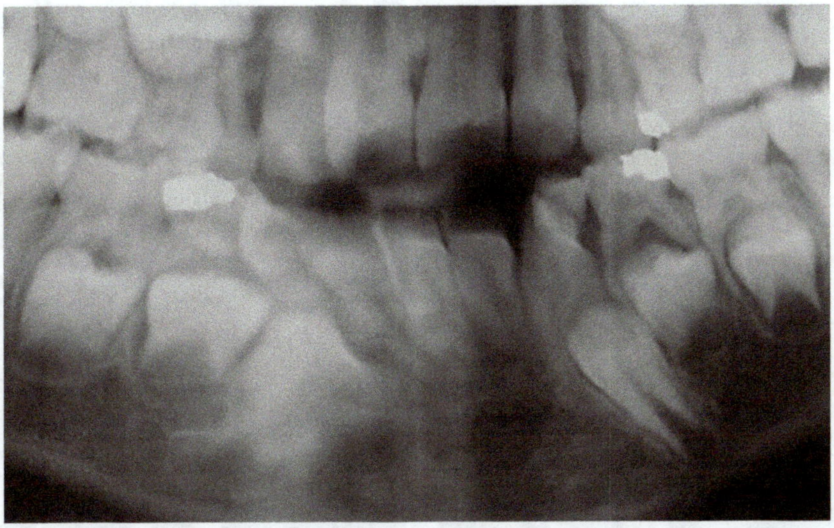

Figure 5.52 Resorption of Emma's mandibular left primary canine root by lateral incisor crown.

- Normal in the transverse (normal intermolar arch widths with good posterior interdigitation, absence of posterior cross bites, and absence of significant transverse compensations). Why? An ideal transverse relationship will be much easier to achieve if you begin with the same.
- Normal incisor angulation or proclined incisors, but *not* upright incisors. Why? Incisors will tend to upright with extractions/incisor retraction.

Q: What is the biggest error found in performing serial extraction?

A: *Poor patient selection.* If serial extraction is begun in a patient with marginal crowding, then they will be left with large extraction spaces to close after all the permanent teeth erupt. If serial extraction is begun on a Class II patient, there is a good chance they will end up Class II. If serial extraction is begun on a deep bite patient, then the deep bite will worsen during treatment. The biggest error? Poor patient selection.

Q: What should you do if you are just not sure whether a patient's mandibular arch crowding is severe enough to warrant serial extractions?

A: Place an LLHA and wait until all permanent teeth have erupted. Then decide whether you must extract permanent teeth to alleviate crowding. Do not begin serial extraction unless you are sure the mandibular arch crowding is severe.

Q: What is the *most* reliable indicator of severe developing mandibular anterior crowding? Does Emma demonstrate this feature?

A: The most reliable indicator of severe developing mandibular anterior crowding is *premature loss of primary canines* and *not* lack of interdental spacing. Emma does demonstrate (radiographically) premature resorption of mandibular primary canines (Figure 5.52).

Q: Is Emma a good candidate for serial extraction?

A: Yes, overall. Features that make Emma a good candidate for serial extraction include the following:

- Severe mandibular anterior crowding
- End-on molars when viewed from the buccal (but Class I molars as seen from the lingual, Figure 5.44a, b)
- Slightly LLAFH with open bite
- Anterior teeth are proclined (extraction space needed if you intend to upright them)
- Reasonable transverse relationship

The one feature that we find disconcerting is Emma's severely retrusive mandible. Even though she is Class I dentally at the molars, her skeletal Class II relationship is not ideal. We would feel much more comfortable with her as a serial extraction candidate if her mandible was normal, not retrusive.

Q: Let's discuss Emma's incisal display. We noted that in a relaxed lip position and during a posed smile, her incisal display was acceptable. However, this is due in part to the fact that her maxillary incisors are stepped up relative to her posterior teeth. So, if her maxillary incisors are leveled with her posterior teeth to close the open bite, then Emma's incisal and gingival display will increase, possibly to an unacceptable degree. What will tend to happen to Emma's incisal/gingival display if she is also treated with premolar extractions and her incisors are retracted?

A: If you extract premolars, retract canines through the extraction spaces, and then retract her incisors (Figure 5.53a) Emma's bite will tend to deepen, and her incisal display will tend to increase (Figure 5.53b). Why? Her incisors will tend rotate around their apices, her maxillary archwire will be deflected downward in the anterior, and her maxillary premolars will tend to erupt. However, if her chewing musculature adequately resists maxillary premolar eruption, then the premolars may not erupt, and the deflected archwire could act to intrude her maxillary incisors. Consequently, her incisal display may not increase. HPHG may also help to reduce premolar eruption, or maxillary TADs could be used to prevent maxillary premolar eruption. Of course, any maxillary vertical lip growth would also help to decrease her final incisal display.

Q: How would you address Emma's vertical excess (orthopedics, masking, or surgery)?

A: *Orthopedics* (biomechanics to reduce/prevent molar eruption and reduce downward growth of the maxilla). If we reduce/prevent molar eruption, then condylar/ramal growth will tend to rotate the mandible forward (CCW mandibular rotation) and bring her chin forward (improving Emma's chin projection and reducing her ANB angle). The same is true if we reduce her downward maxillary growth. As wonderful as these effects are,

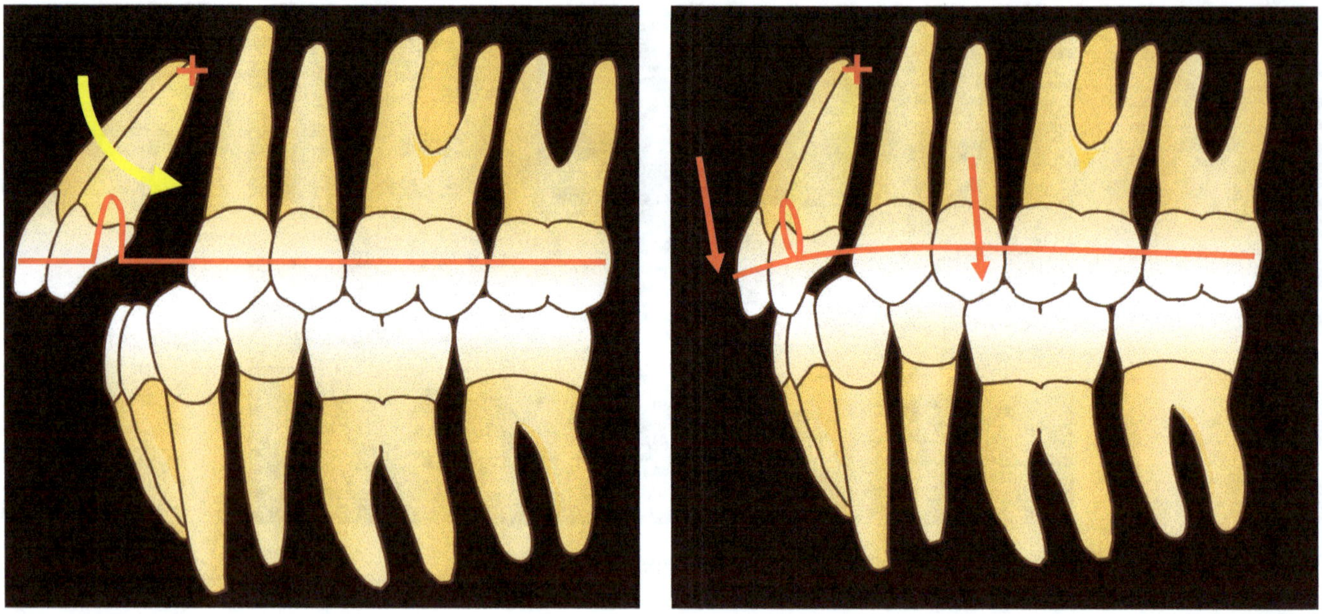

(a) (b)

Figure 5.53 (a) If Emma's premolars are extracted and her maxillary incisors are retracted following canine retraction, then (b) her bite will tend to deepen, and her incisal display will tend to increase as her incisors rotate around their apices.

they could also rotate Emma's mandible forward into a Class III molar relationship. So, what should we do? Do we try to impede vertical growth and allow mandibular forward growth to possibly make Emma Class III, or do we ignore vertical growth and leave her approximately Class I (with a retrusive mandible)? The answer lies in *focusing on Emma's worse problems—excess vertical growth and mandibular deficiency*. If treatment to control her vertical growth improves her chin projection, improves her profile, reduces her ANB angle, but makes her become dental Class III, then we could readily correct her Class III dental relationship with Class III elastics or extractions. But, if we ignore controlling/reducing her excess vertical growth, she could eventually require a maxillary impaction osteotomy to correct her skeletal open bite. Orthopedic treatments to reduce maxillary corpus descent or prevent molar eruption include the following:

- The use of high-pull headgears, which may restrict vertical and AP maxillary growth and may restrict eruption of the maxillary molars [13, 14].
- Vertical-pull headgear to inhibit dentoalveolar growth (inhibit posterior tooth eruption) [15–18].
- Temporary anchorage devices (TADs, attached to a TPA in the maxilla or an LLHA in the mandible) to halt eruption of the maxillary and mandibular first molars (or intrude molars) [31–34].
- Exercising (chewing gum) to reduce her MPA (compared to controls) [36–38].
- Posterior bite plates (stretching the masseteric sling and causing an intrusive force against the posterior teeth) or active vertical correctors (posterior repelling magnets) to reduce molar eruption [24–28].
- Tongue pressure from a TPA with an acrylic button several millimeters off the palate to reduce increases in lower face height [29].
- LLHAs to reduce eruption of mandibular molars by ~1 mm compared to controls [30].
- Modified Herbst appliance (Herbst appliance combined with acrylic splints and high-pull headgear wear) that have been reported to control the vertical dimension in hyperdivergent adolescents (reducing Go-Gn-SN angle −1° compared to a reduction of −0.3° in control group, Bolton standards) [23].

Masking or camouflage (treatment to close her open bite without addressing her excess vertical growth). Options include the following:

- Premolar extraction and retraction of anterior teeth will tend to deepen her bite as incisors upright/rotate around their apices.
- Leveling her arches with archwires will erupt her stepped up maxillary incisors and erupt her stepped down mandibular incisors—with or without vertical elastics.
- Bonding incisors gingivally (bonding for open bites) can extrude anterior teeth relative to posterior teeth to help close open bites during leveling.
- Placing steps in archwires to erupt incisors.
- Adding a curve of Spee to her mandibular archwire to erupt her mandibular incisors.
- Aggressive posterior occlusal adjustment can help close an anterior open bite.

Note: Orthopedics should at least be attempted before masking. Masking would be considered reasonable if Emma's vertical excess did not worsen, but cooperation was found to be absent.

Surgery (maxillary impaction osteotomy) could correct her skeletal open bite. It would be unreasonable to consider surgery now—she is too young. If she had surgery before growth was completed, then she would continue to grow vertically, post surgery. If orthopedics is attempted now, it will be important to inform Emma and her parents that, depending on growth and cooperation, surgery may be required to provide ideal open bite closure later.

Q: Should you guarantee Emma and her parents that you will be able to close her open bite and maintain that correction, long-term?

A: No. With orthopedics, masking, or even surgery, Emma's open bite closure will depend on variables out of your control (e.g., growth and cooperation). For instance, can she discontinue her anterior tongue posturing habit? We will not know for years to come. You should inform Emma and her parents that you will use all of your skill to care for Emma and that, with reasonable growth and cooperation; you have a good chance of providing excellent treatment for her.

Q: If you decide to attempt orthopedic treatment for Emma's excess vertical growth, should you start now or should you wait?

A: We know from extensive research that there is no advantage to beginning Class II treatment in the early mixed dentition stage [83–87, 98, 99]. Although we do not have specific guidelines suggesting when to begin vertical excess orthopedic treatment, it also seems reasonable to delay treatment for excess vertical growth until the late mixed-dentition stage. But please remember that dental age may be delayed compared to skeletal age. If you have evidence that a child is beginning their growth spurt earlier than the dental age would suggest, then it may be prudent to begin orthopedic treatment in the early mixed dentition. However, Emma's parents deny that she is growing much so you should not begin orthopedic treatment yet.

Q: What makes Emma's AP relationship so unusual?

A: The fact that from a skeletal perspective, Emma is severely Class II (convex profile, retrusive chin, mandibular AP deficiency, ANB angle = 8°). But at the same time, she is only slightly Class II (dentally) when viewed from the buccal, and actually Class I when viewed from the lingual.

Q: How should Emma's anteroposterior apical base discrepancy be treated (orthopedics, masking, or surgery)?

A: *Orthopedics* (restrict maxillary growth while permitting the mandible to continue growing—or, accelerate mandibular growth). The same question must be answered here that was answered for treating her vertical apical base discrepancy. That is, should you address her AP *skeletal* Class II relationship or should you ignore it and simply correct her mild Class II *dental* relationship (say, by rotating her mesially rotated maxillary molars distally)? And again, the answer lies in *focusing on her worse problems—excess vertical growth and a severely deficient mandible.* If treatment to address excess vertical and mandibular deficiency improves chin projection, improves profile appearance, reduces ANB angle, but at the same time creates a dental Class III relationship, then we will willingly accept this tradeoff. The dental Class III relationship can be addressed later with Class III elastics or possibly extractions. If we choose to ignore her excess vertical growth and mandibular deficiency, then she could end up needing maxillary impaction surgery and mandibular advancement surgery. Orthopedic treatments include the following:

- High-pull headgear treatment, which may tend to reduce descent of the maxillary corpus and maxillary first molars, allowing CCW mandibular rotation with condylar/ramal growth to potentially improve chin projection [13, 14, 100]. HPHG distalizes maxillary molars through the maxillary alveolar process bone, restricts maxillary forward growth, and allows the mandible to continue growing forward.
- Cervical-pull headgear treatment would *not* be ideal. Although it would restrict maxillary forward growth and distalize maxillary molars, it would *not* restrict descent of the maxillary corpus. Instead, it could create a slight clockwise rotation of Emma's palatal plane (increasing her incisal display?) and slight (<1 mm) extrusion of her maxillary first molars [14, 101]. A straight-pull headgear would produce an effect somewhere between that of a high pull and a cervical pull and would not be recommended.
- A Herbst appliance, or other functional appliance, to accelerate mandibular growth. However, since Emma has a steep MPA and severely proclined mandibular incisors (FMIA = 43°), she would not be a candidate for these. Functional appliance treatment would result in increased incisor proclination [84–87, 102–107] and the possibility of her open bite worsening as the mandibular incisors rotate forward around their apicies.
- Other orthopedic treatments that tend to help rotate the mandible up and forward (improving AP) could be considered, including: vertical-pull headgear, TADs to intrude maxillary and mandibular molars, exercises (gum chewing), bite plates (to stretch her masseteric sling/prevent molars from erupting), TPAs with acrylic buttons (reduce maxillary molar eruption), or an LLHA (reduce mandibular molar eruption).

Masking or camouflage (the goal of masking in the AP is to achieve a Class I canine relationship without addressing the underlying apical base discrepancy). Since Emma would exhibit a Class I molar relationship after her mesially rotated maxillary molars are rotated distally, there is really no need to attempt masking her AP. Masking would be considered if Emma does not cooperate with orthopedic treatment and becomes Class II as result of continued excess vertical growth (mandible rotating down and back). Although Class II elastics, or other interarch Class II correctors, can correct mild Class II relationships through dentoalveolar movement, if she becomes more Class II, these treatments would also procline Emma's mandibular incisors more [108–110].

Surgery (maxillary impaction, mandibular advancement, if Emma and her parents have concerns with chin projection) could be considered, but not at this early age. However, Emma and her parents should be warned that, depending on growth and cooperation, future surgery may be an option to achieve and ideal outcome.

Q: How would you treat Emma's transverse posterior relationship?

A: At the end of treatment, you want Emma's posterior teeth to be upright (no transverse compensations—no buccal or lingual crown torque). Because Emma's initial transverse compensations are small, you should be able to upright her posterior teeth (and maintain posterior arch coordination) using only fixed appliances and archwires. However, if you did expand Emma's maxilla with an RME appliance, you would be virtually guaranteed of being able to upright her posterior teeth.

Q: What treatment unknowns must you be prepared for? Are there any unknowns you should eliminate before finalizing your treatment plan?

A: The magnitude of Emma's future vertical maxillary growth is the principle unknown you face. If the maxilla descends significantly, then her open bite will worsen and her mandible will rotate downward and backward, worsening her convex profile and chin projection. The same will result following significant maxillary and mandibular molar eruption. Mandibular growth is another major unknown. Cooperation, hygiene, and presence of an undetected CR—CO shift are other unknowns you must be prepared for. The absence of a shift should be confirmed at the case presentation appointment. *Cooperation and growth should be reduced to some degree before finalizing your treatment plan.* The other unknowns cannot be eliminated now.

Q: When thinking about treating a child orthopedically, you must consider the *magnitude* of the child's skeletal discrepancy and the age of the child (*time* of growth remaining). Why?

A: If the magnitude of the discrepancy is mild and the child has many years of growth remaining, then you have a good chance of correcting the problem with orthopedics *if the child remains cooperative*. But remember, orthopedics does not normalize growth. After you have made the correction and stop orthopedics, the growth will revert back to its original pattern. The younger the patient, the more years of growth you will face after treatment to maintain the correction. With a severe skeletal discrepancy, or minimal years of growth remaining, you may not be able to correct the discrepancy with orthopedics. But, you may be able to improve the discrepancy with orthopedics to the point where masking (camouflage) is an option. Of course, if the discrepancy is very severe, then you may choose to wait to begin orthodontic treatment until the child has finished growing (and plan on treating with surgery).

Q: In Emma's case, how would the magnitude of the skeletal discrepancy and her age affect your decision to treat her orthopedically?

A: The magnitude of Emma's skeletal open bite is mild to moderate and she is very young. If Emma cooperates, you have a reasonable chance of treating her vertical discrepancy orthopedically. Emma's AP skeletal discrepancy is severe, but her molar relationship is Class I (from the lingual). We should attempt orthopedics in the vertical and AP, then re-evaluate her growth/cooperation after a set period of time (1 year?). We should wait to begin orthopedic treatment until her late mixed-dentition stage of development or until she begins her growth spurt. Ask her parents to begin measuring her height each month and report back to you regularly.

Q: Would a discussion of future surgery be warranted now?

A: Yes. Explain to her parents that depending on Emma's future growth and cooperation, surgery may be required at a future date to obtain an ideal result.

Q: Would nonextraction treatment be ideal for Emma?

A: No. With Emma's steep MPA, proclined incisors, open bite, and significant crowding, a nonextraction treatment would not be prudent. Why? To obtain alignment of her incisors without extraction, the incisors would be further proclined—worsening her open bite.

Q: Should you place an LLHA in Emma?

A: No. Emma has so much mandibular anterior crowding (Figure 5.42n) and incisor proclination (Figure 5.42e) that treating her nonextraction would increase her incisor proclination and open her bite to an unacceptable degree. The 4–5 mm of mandibular leeway space you may get from using an LLHA would not be enough to alleviate her severe mandibular anterior crowding/incisor proclination.

Q: Any time you are considering extracting permanent teeth, you need to consider every reasonable combination of anterior and posterior tooth extraction pattern. Why? In some cases, it will be obvious which teeth should be extracted. In other cases, it will not be obvious. *By forcing yourself to always consider* every *possible extraction pattern, you will be more likely to identify the ideal extraction pattern for that patient.* Discuss the advantages and disadvantages of each possible extraction pattern for Emma.

A: Possible extraction patterns for Emma are as follows:

- Mandibular incisor extraction. Although extraction of a lower incisor will provide ~5+ mm of space, this amount of space is simply too small to eliminate Emma's mandibular anterior crowding and proclination. Further, this will not alleviate her maxillary anterior crowding, and she will be finished with excess OJ of the incisors and canines.
- Extraction of all four first premolars. This may produce an excellent result. This would provide 14+ mm of space in both arches. The advantage of this extraction pattern is that space is created closest to where it is needed, the anterior. The disadvantage of four first premolar extractions is maintaining maxillary anchorage. That is, the maxillary anterior teeth have bigger roots than the mandibular anterior teeth—so, Emma's maxillary posterior teeth may slip forward into Class II during reciprocal space closure.
- Extraction of maxillary first premolars and mandibular second premolars. This would almost guarantee a final Class I molar relationship but lessen our ability to alleviate mandibular anterior tooth crowding (i.e., mandibular molars would move mesially more and mandibular canines would move distally less than if mandibular first premolars had been extracted). Further, since Emma is essentially a Class I now, she could end up Class III molar with this extraction pattern.

Q: We noted earlier that Emma is 8 years and 11 months old in the early mixed dentition. We also stated that *early treatment should be used to treat very specific problems with the intent of getting the patient back to normal for that stage of development. Is it absolutely necessary that you do anything now? What harm will come from not doing anything now and simply recalling Emma?*

A: The only harm of not doing anything now is possible root resorption of permanent lateral incisor roots from erupting permanent canines (Figure 5.42f). Other than that, if we do not do anything now, the crowded/impacted canines will stay that way—crowded and impacted. However, since we are sure that Emma is an extraction case (serial extraction?), it would be reasonable to begin that process now. Since Emma's parents deny that she is growing much, and since you have asked them to record her height and report back to you regularly, you do not need to institute orthopedics yet.

Q: After putting all of the above discussion together, what treatment do you recommend for Emma now (and later)?

A: Other than having a discussion of her anterior tongue positioning habit, no further treatment for the habit was given. We decided to begin serial extraction, and she was referred for extraction of primary canines. Nine months later, at her recall appointment, Emma's parents stated that her growth was beginning to increase. She was placed on an HPHG and her primary first molars were extracted when the roots of her first permanent premolars were about 1/2 to 2/3 formed. Her permanent first premolars were extracted when they fully erupted. Figure 5.54 shows Emma after her permanent canines and second premolars have erupted. She continued to wear her HPHG until her molars were slightly overcorrected.

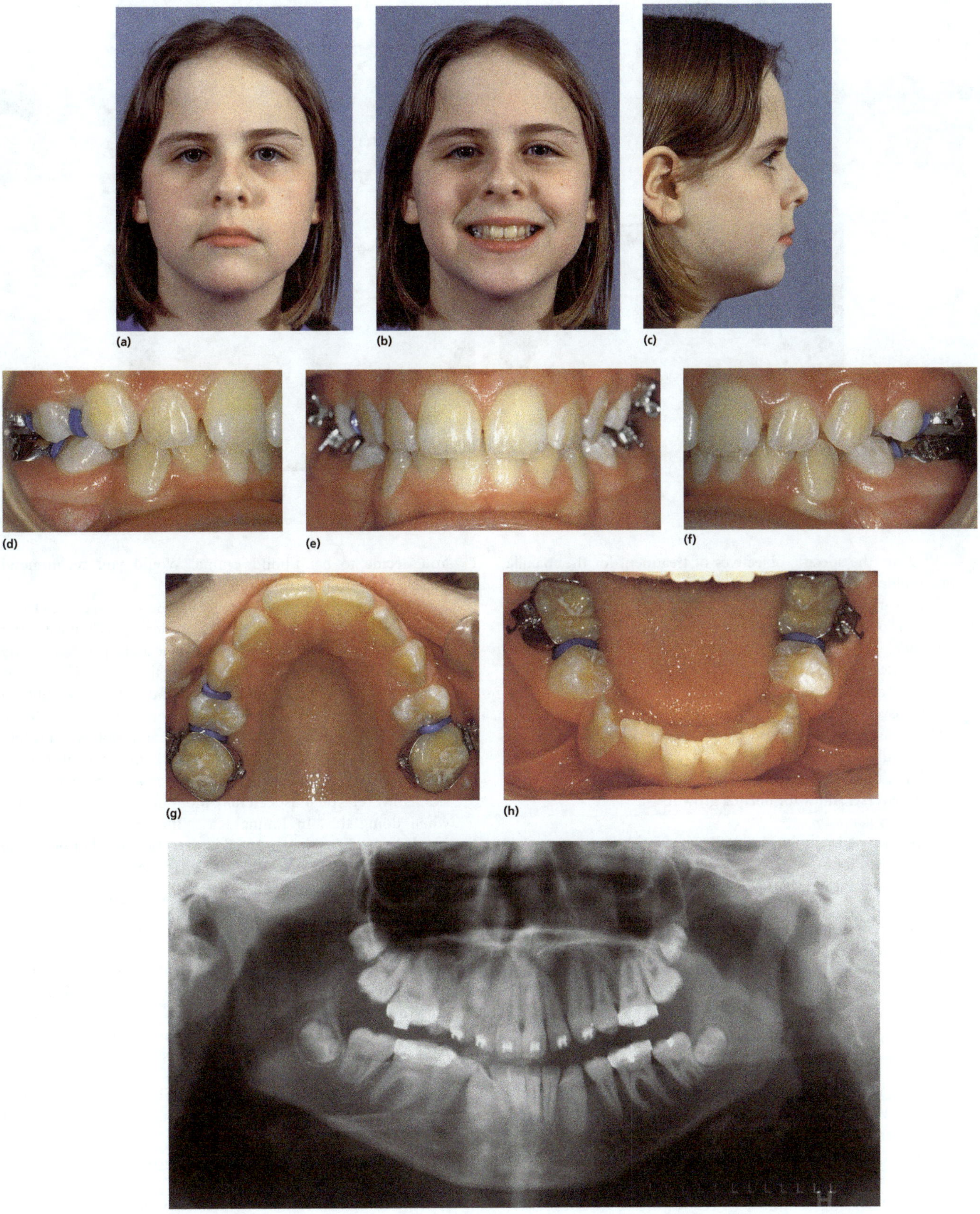

Figure 5.54 (a–n) Progress records for Emma.

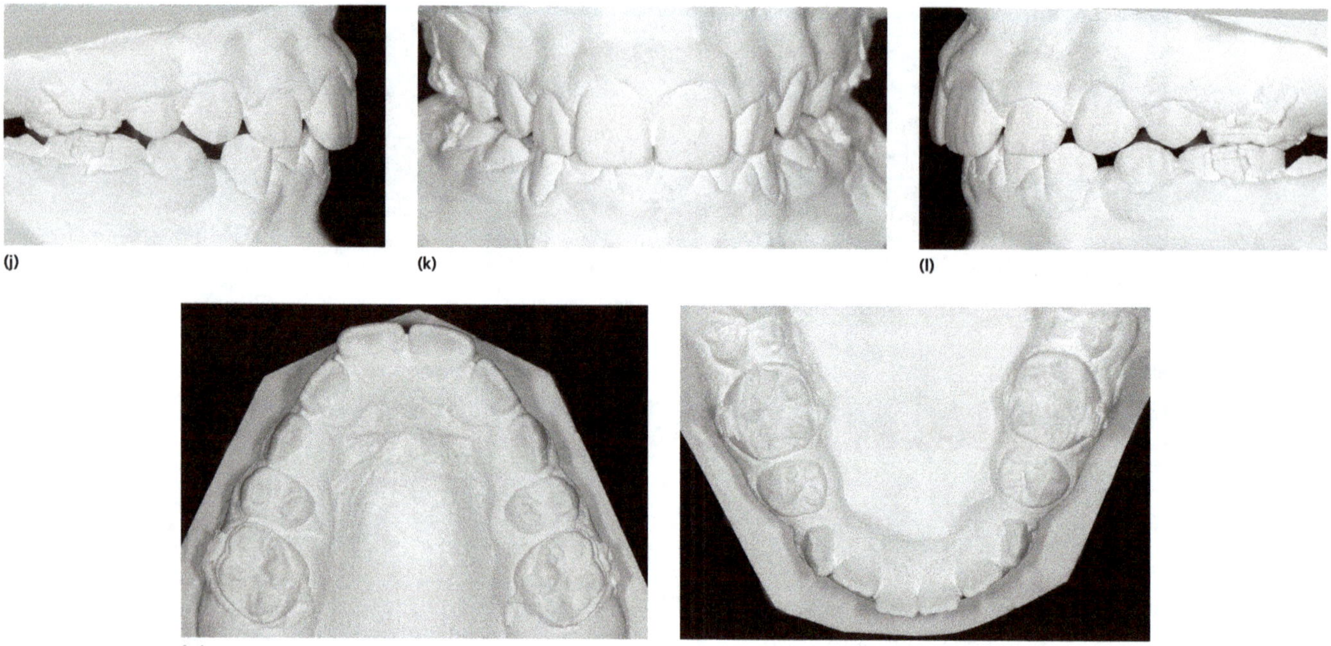

(j) (k) (l) (m) (n)

Figure 5.54 (Continued)

Q: What are the specific objectives of treatment for the maxilla, mandible, maxillary dentition, and mandibular dentition in all three planes of space?

A: Specific objectives of treatment for Emma are as follows:

Maxilla

AP: Restrict normal growth.

Vertical: Restrict normal growth.

Transverse: Maintain transverse width.

Mandible

AP: Allow for normal growth.

Vertical: Allow for normal growth.

Transverse: Allow for normal growth.

Maxillary dentition

AP: Maintain molars and distalize canines. Retract and upright incisors.

Vertical: Level occlusal plane by molar intrusion and incisor extrusion.

Intermolar width: Maintain intermolar width.

Mandibular dentition

AP: Maintain molars and retract canines. Retract and upright incisors.

Vertical: Increase curve of Spee.

Intermolar/intercanine width: Maintain intermolar and intercanine widths.

Q: Emma's maxillary molars were slightly overcorrected using HPHG. Would you have her stop wearing HPHG at this point?

A: No. Once the AP correction is made, it would be prudent to have her continue wearing her headgear at least when she goes to bed with a very light force—just to hold her correction. Remember, she is still growing, and you want to monitor the correction you have made for quite a while (months/years). If, over time, you see that her molar relationship becomes Class III, then decrease headgear wear even more (or stop it altogether). But, still monitor her closely until she has completed growth.

Q: You decide to band/bond Emma. Would you recommend banding/bonding her second molars?

A: No. Generally, you want to stay off of second molars when treating a skeletal open bite patient (nonsurgically). When you band second molars and level the mandibular arch, you tend to tip the second molars distally and upright them (eliminating the curve of Spee). As the second molars tip distally, they will tend to extrude at the mesial, which can worsen an open bite. In skeletal open bite patients where the second molars erupt into abnormal positions, consider banding them for a short while later in treatment—using an overlay wire through their bracket slot. However, you must carefully monitor the patient's overbite when doing this. In Emma's case, the second molars *were banded* as soon as they erupted and, fortunately, her open bite did not worsen. However, this was a gamble.

Q: Emma was placed in fixed appliances, her arches leveled and aligned, and treatment finished. At that point, should her braces be taken off immediately?

A: No. Remember that it will take months (or even years) for her tissues to remodel. Also, you started with some significant growth issues. So, once you think you are finished with her treatment, monitor her for a while—maintaining her in braces (active retention) for a period of months before debanding.

Q: Emma's deband records are shown in Figure 5.55 (note that a 5-year time span exists between initial and final records). What do you observe?

A: Emma had a successful, nonsurgical, correction of her skeletal open bite. Observations include the following:

- Facial proportions and her NLA do not appear to have changed.
- ILG has been eliminated.
- Emma's profile (chin projection) has improved and facial convexity reduced.
- UDML is on with her face.

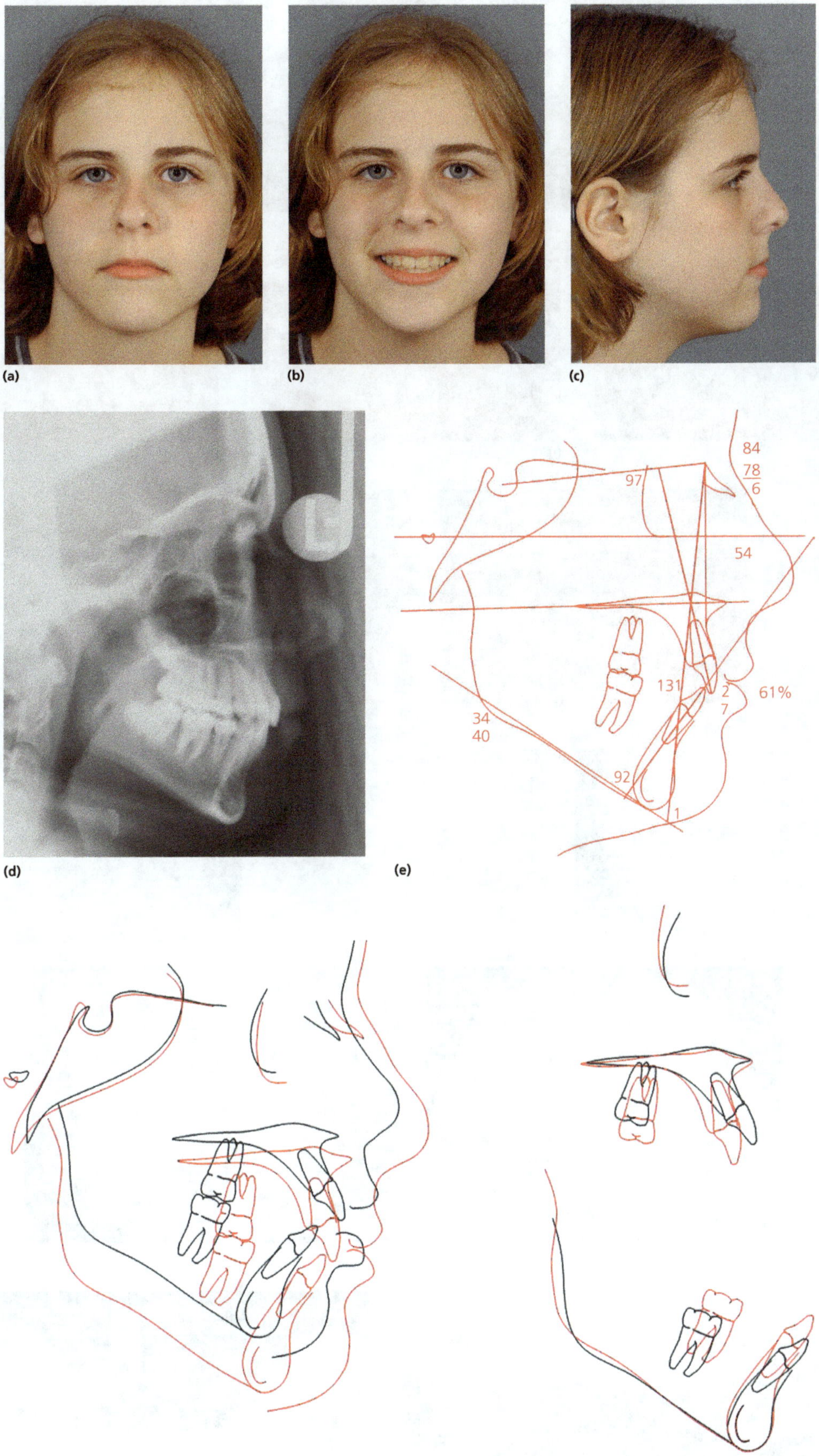

(a) (b) (c) (d) (e) (f)

Figure 5.55 (a–s) Emma's deband records.

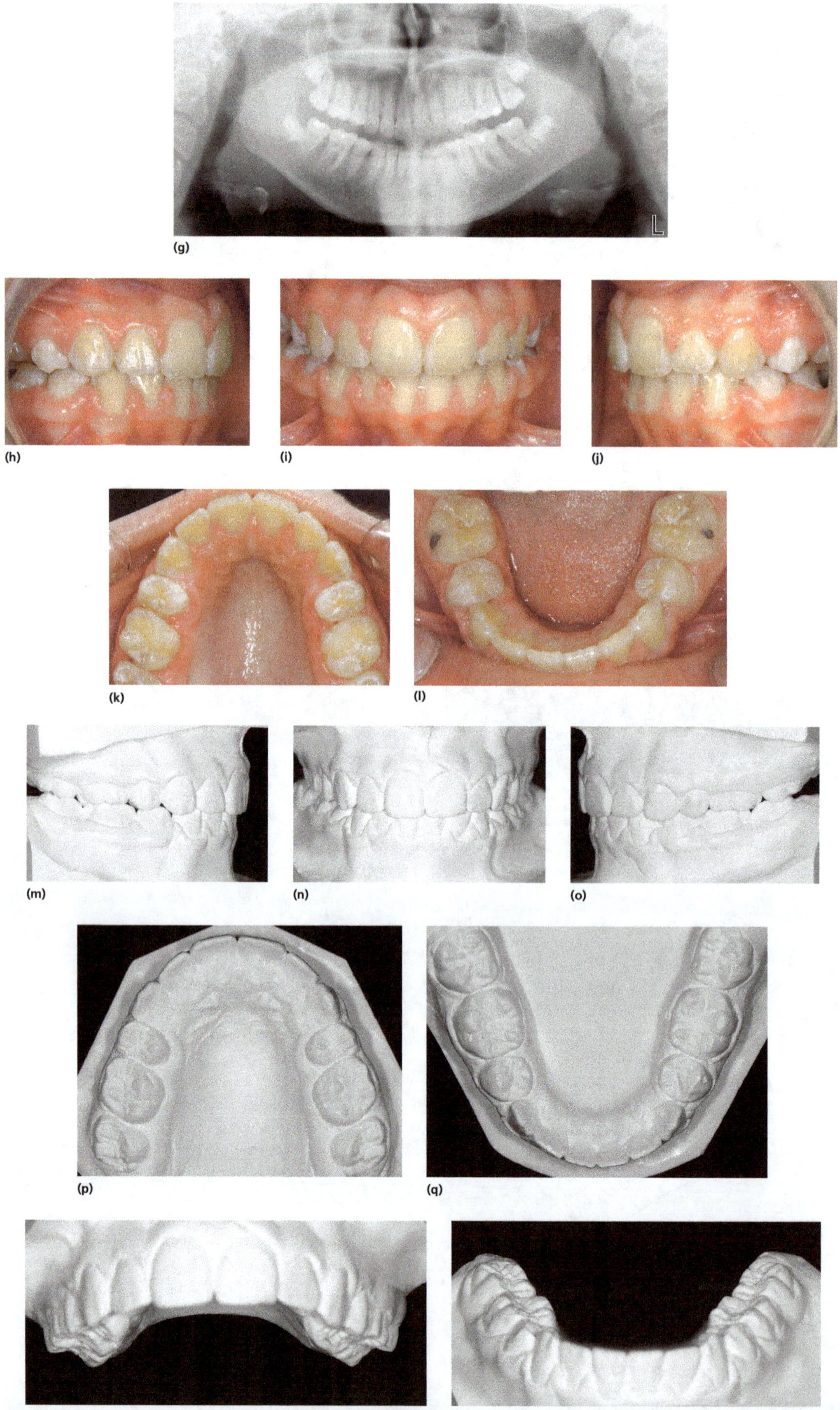

Figure 5.55 (Continued)

- ANB angle was reduced from 8° to 6° as a result of Nasion growing forward, A-point's forward growth being restricted (A-point descended vertically), and B-point descending but also growing forward.
- A-point was initially slightly protrusive but is now ideally located along a Nasion-perpendicular line.
- Her mandible descended straight down (Figure 5.55f), despite significant condylar growth, because of vertical maxillary corpus growth and molar eruption.
- The maxillary incisors were retracted to a mildly upright inclination ($\underline{1}$ to SN = 97°) with a reasonable amount of incisal display at rest (Figure 5.55e).
- Mandibular incisors were uprighted but are still protrusive (Figure 5.55e, f).
- Maxillary lip grew vertically about the same amount that her maxillary incisal tip descended vertically (a combination of incisor eruption plus maxillary anterior corpus descent).
- Amount of incisal display during posed smile is still less than ideal (gingival margin hidden above maxillary vermillion border) despite the fact that her maxillary anterior teeth were erupted during leveling.
- Open bite closure was achieved (final OB = 20–30%).
- Despite more mandibular molar mesial movement than maxillary molar mesial movement (5.55F), a mild Class II relationship is seen on the right (Figure 5.55m, "Class II windows" seen between maxillary and mandibular right posterior teeth).
- Midlines are not coincident (Figure 5.55i).
- Maxillary posterior labial crown torque and mandibular posterior lingual crown torque is still present (Figure 5.55r, s), but transverse relationships are good.
- Her smile esthetics would be greatly enhanced by referring her back to her restorative dentist for bleaching.

Q: How was Emma's open bite corrected (Figure 5.55f)?

A: Her open bite was corrected by eruption of maxillary and mandibular incisors as her arches were leveled and as her incisors were uprighted/retracted (rotated around their apicies). Significant mandibular growth, which you would expect during a 5-year period of treatment in a child of this age, did not result in CCW (up and forward) mandibular rotation. Why not? This substantial mandibular growth was just enough to keep pace with combined downward maxillary growth, maxillary molar eruption, and mandibular molar eruption. Without this mandibular growth, the mandible would have rotated CW (down and back).

Q: Emma had a slightly protrusive maxilla initially. If her maxilla had initially been normally positioned, or even retrusive, would you still have considered using a HPHG in her treatment, or would a HPHG have adversely impacted her profile esthetics?

A: In Class II adolescents with protrusive, normally positioned, or even retrusive maxillae, headgear treatment in conjunction with fixed orthodontic appliances is effective in improving facial profile esthetics; the greater the initial ANB angle, the greater the profile esthetic improvement with treatment [111].

Q: Class II elastics were not used during treatment. Should Emma have been treated with Class II elastics instead of headgear?

A: No. Class II elastics were wisely avoided in this patient. Class II elastics would tend to erupt her mandibular molars even more, rotating her mandible CW and worsening profile esthetics. Even though the maxilla descended substantially (and the maxillary molars erupted), the maxilla could have descended even more (and the maxillary molars could have erupted even more) without the vertical component of HPHG force.

Q: Are you concerned with Emma's potential future growth?

A: Yes. Orthopedics does not normalize growth, and Emma may have some growth ahead of her. (You should inquire with her parents when Emma reached menarche—this was not done.) Providing excellent care for this young lady does not mean that she will not grow out of the correction. You must monitor her closely (a good reason for keeping Emma in "active retention" for a period of months before taking her braces off after finishing is achieved).

Q: How would you retain her?

A: She was placed in, and wore, Hawley retainers full time for 4 months and every night thereafter. Unlike Hawley retainers used to retain deep bite patients, the Hawley retainers used with initially open bite patients do not include an anterior biteplate to disclude the posterior teeth (potentially allowing the posterior teeth to erupt/opening the anterior bite).

Q: What are your "take-home" messages for your practice from this case?

A: Take home-messages include the following:

- Emma presented with a combination of dental and skeletal open bite. Her dental open bite features included presence of an anterior tongue interposition habit and an anterior open bite extending to primary canines only. Her skeletal open bite features included long soft tissue LAFH, long skeletal LAFH, steep MPA, short posterior face height, and a ~6–7 mm ILG. Emma's dental open bite probably started with a thumb-sucking habit and then continued with an anterior tongue interposition habit. Her skeletal open bite was probably due to a traditional skeletal open bite growth pattern which included: condyles growing posterior-superiorly, lack of normal forward mandibular internal (true) rotation (or presence of backward internal/true rotation), lack of posterior facial height development, her maxilla descending more than normal, and molars erupting more than normal. As her mandible rotated backward from this excess vertical growth, the mandibular plane angle steepened, the anterior face height lengthened, and an anterior open bite resulted.
- Her tongue habit was successfully dealt with by discussing it with her. She was asked to discontinue the habit, but the habit should have been more closely followed. Lingual spurs should have been considered for her mandibular retainer. Placing a hole in the anterior palate of the maxillary retainer for her tongue to seek would have been prudent. We hope that Emma is one of those patients whose tongue is retrained to stay off of the anterior teeth by virtue of the orthodontic bite closure.
- Orthopedic treatment of skeletal open bites consists of biomechanics aimed at reducing maxillary corpus descent and reducing maxillary/mandibular molar eruption. Emma's treatment involved attempting to orthopedically reduce descent of the maxilla and eruption of the maxillary molars by wearing a HPHG. Treatment was successful despite a strong tendency for vertical facial growth. Ample mandibular growth was great enough to keep pace with substantial vertical descent of the maxilla and molar eruption. Vertical maxillary growth (and maxillary molar eruption) may have been much more pronounced without HPHG compliance.

- Patient compliance cannot be expected to last forever. Instead of initiating orthopedic treatment early, it was smart to wait until her parents reported that Emma was growing to begin orthopedic treatment.
- Extraction of first premolars was warranted because of crowding/incisor proclination. Her open bite was partially closed with retraction/uprighting/eruption of her maxillary and mandibular incisors as they rotated around their apicies. Her open bite was also closed with leveling of her arches (incisor eruption).
- Her final OB was 20–30%. This was excellent. Overcorrection to 20–40% OB should be a goal for your open bite cases.
- Skeletal open bites can be challenging cases to treat orthopedically. Because the vertical maxillary growth/molar eruption that causes the open bite is not normalized with orthopedic treatment, this growth must be addressed (in active treatment or retention) until it is completed. With excellent patient cooperation, mild skeletal open bites can be successfully corrected if enough growth remains. It may be heroic to attempt orthopedic treatment of severe skeletal open bites.
- Early treatment should be used to treat very specific problems with the intent of getting the patient back to normal for that stage of development. When considering early treatment, always ask yourself, "Is it absolutely necessary that I do anything now? What harm will come from not doing anything now and simply recalling the patient?"
- Emma's early treatment problem was severe anterior crowding. A risk of not initiating treatment was possible lateral incisor root resorption. Knowing that we were eventually going to extract four first premolars on her, we decided to proceed with serial extraction. She was a good candidate for serial extraction: severe mandibular anterior crowding, end-on molars when viewed from the buccal (but Class I molars as seen from the lingual), slightly LLAFH with open bite, anterior teeth proclined (extraction space needed to upright them), and reasonable transverse relationship. The one feature that we found disconcerting was Emma's severely retrusive mandible.
- A major problem with serial extraction cases is poor patient selection.
- Maxillary posterior labial crown torque and mandibular posterior lingual crown torque were still present at the end of treatment. Initial RME could have permitted uprighting these posterior teeth.

Case Rachael

Rachael (Figure 5.56) is 9 years and 4 months old and presents to you with the CC, "I want good teeth." Her PMH, TMJ evaluation, and periodontal evaluations are WRN. She fractured tooth #8 at age 8 years, and the tooth was restored with a composite buildup restoration. CR=CO.

Q: List diagnostic findings/problems. What is your diagnosis?
A: See Table 5.3.

Q: Are there other views of her models that you should examine?
A: Yes. Check the maxillary and mandibular models from the anterior (Figure 5.57) to evaluate her posterior crown torque (dental compensation for transverse apical base discrepancy).

Check the occluded models from the lingual (Figure 5.58) to evaluate first molar AP position.

Q: What do you observe in these views?
A: Figure 5.57 illustrates *mild maxillary posterior buccal crown torque and mild mandibular posterior lingual crown torque*. Why is this important? Uprighting these molars will torque the maxillary crowns lingually and torque the mandibular crown labially, tending to put Rachael into posterior crossbite. Figure 5.58 illustrates that *right and left first molar relationships are still Class II as seen from the lingual*. Why is this important? Mesially rotated molars (Figure 5.56q) appear more Class II from the buccal than from the lingual. If mesially rotated Class II molars are rotated distally around their palatal root into proper alignment, then their buccal occlusion could look much improved, in some cases approaching Class I. But this is not the case for Rachael. Since her molars are still Class II when viewed from the lingual, she will still be Class II even if her maxillary molars are rotated distally.

Q: Look at Rachael's posterior airway on her lateral cephalometric radiograph (Figure 5.56d). What do you notice?
A: Enlarged adenoids.

Q: Should you refer Rachael for adenoidectomy and tonsillectomy?
A: Not necessarily. Remember that lymphatic tissue size first increases, and then decreases, during the developmental years [1] (Figure 5.59). So, enlarged adenoids are not, by themselves, an indication for adenoidectomy.

Q: What are "adenoidal facies"? Does Rachael exhibit adenoidal facies?
A: Adenoidal facies [113] or *long-face syndrome* are terms traditionally used to describe patients who exhibit an LLAFH, narrow face, interlabial gap, narrow alar base, constricted maxillary arch (cross bite), anterior open bite, high palatal vault, and frequent self-reported mouth breathing (example, Figure 5.60). Note that this patient exhibits all features of adenoidal facies except a narrow alar base. Rachael exhibits some of these features (mild LLAFH, interlabial gap, anterior open bite), but she does not exhibit other features (narrow face, narrow alar base, high palatal vault, overt posterior crossbite). Even without knowing her mouth-breathing status, we conclude that Rachael does not exhibit traditional adenoidal facies.

Q: Why has the long-face syndrome been thought to result from nasal obstruction/mouth breathing?
A: The traditional view is that if the posterior teeth are held apart because of mouth breathing, then they will continue to erupt and the face will lengthen. An open bite/interlabial gap results, and the stretched cheeks prevent the maxilla from growing wider.

Q: What are possible causes (name at least five) of nasal obstruction?
A: Allergic rhinitis, adenoid hypertrophy, polyps, congenital nasal deformities, neoplasms, and recurrent upper respiratory infections [95].

Q: Compare airways in the four radiographs below (Figure 5.61). What do you observe?
A: The airway in Figure 5.61a appears wide open and normal. The airways in Figure 5.61b–d appear blocked/obstructed by soft tissue—hypertrophied adenoids.

Q: The lateral cephalometric radiograph in Figure 5.62a is from an 8-year-old girl. Figure 5.62b shows the same patient 2 years later. Evaluate the size of her adenoids. What is occurring? What will likely happen to this tissue in subsequent years?

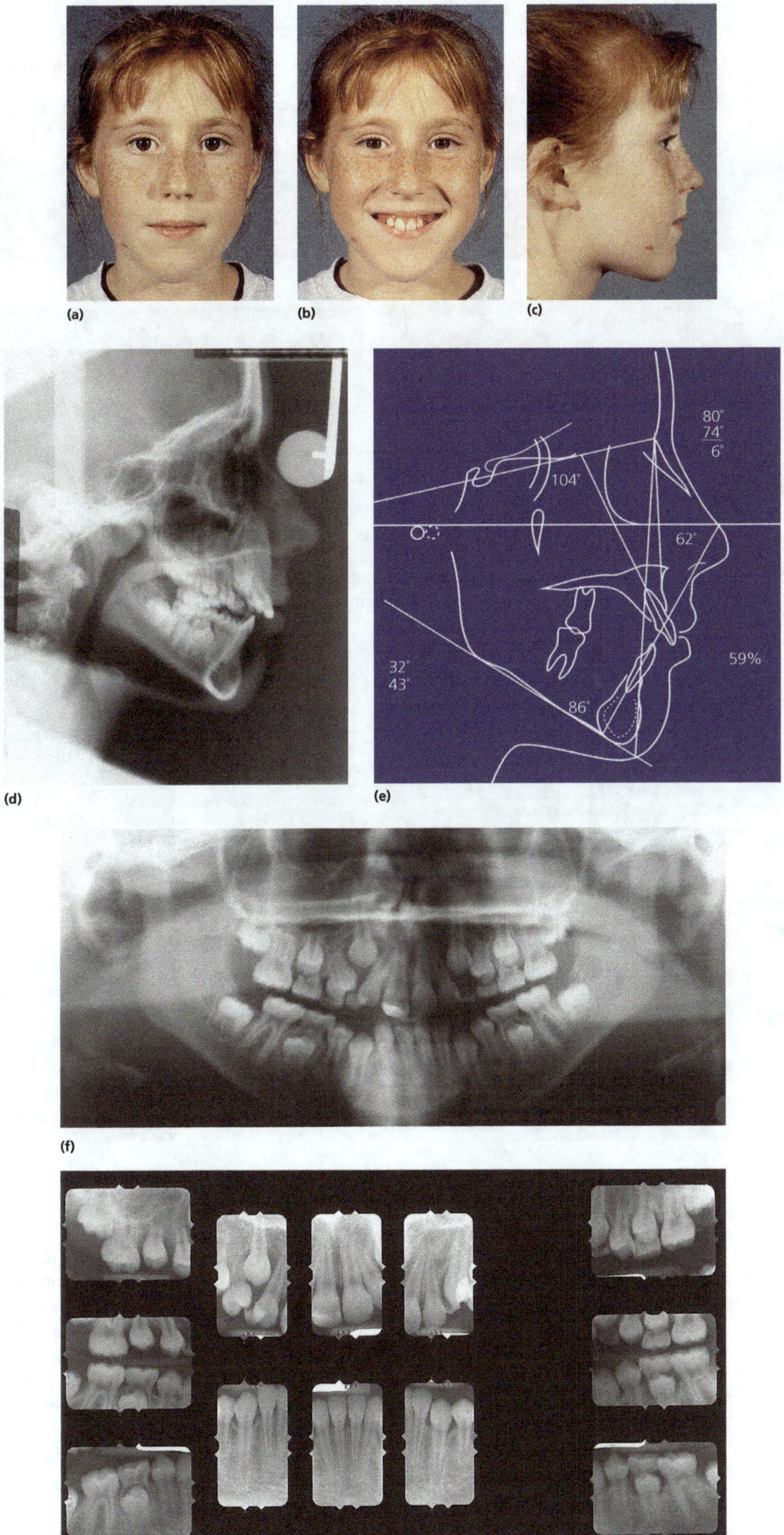

Figure 5.56 Initial records of Rachael: (a–c) initial facial photographs, (d) lateral cephalograph, (e) cephalometric tracing, (f) pantomograph, (g) complete mouth survey,

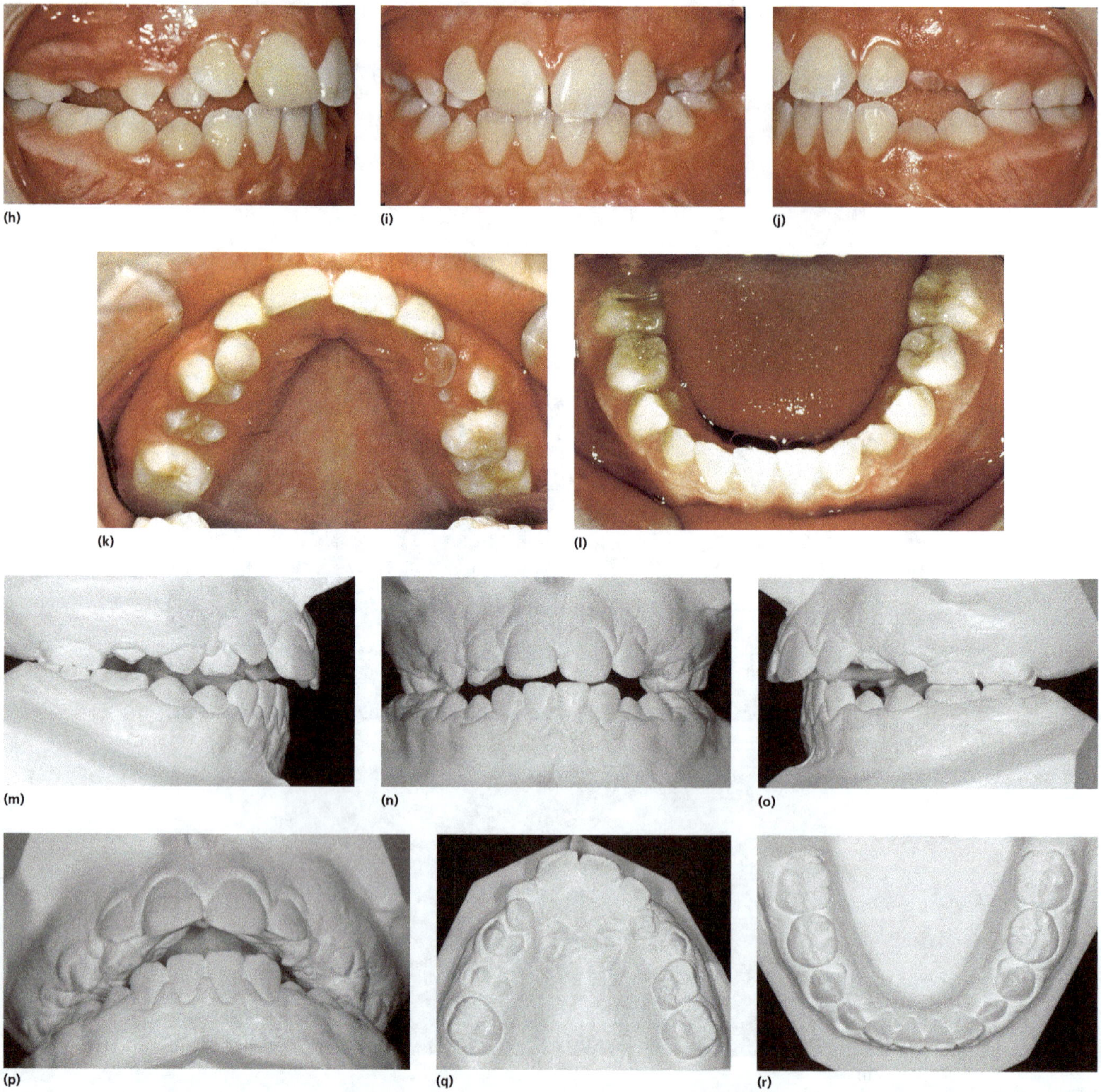

Figure 5.56 (Continued) (h–l) intraoral photographs, and (m–r) model photographs.

A: The adenoids at age 10 have enlarged, as expected (Figure 5.59), compared to the adenoids at age 8. This lymphoidal tissue should decrease in size during the latter part of her second decade.

Q: Do otolaryngologists validate the use of conventional lateral cephalometric radiographs to assess possible airway obstruction?

A: No [114, 115]. The problem in using cephalometric radiographs to assess the airway is that they are 2D representations of a 3D airway structure.

Q: What visualization techniques are used to assess nasal obstruction?

A: *Transnasal endoscopy* remains the mainstay for evaluating the cause of nasal obstruction. Anterior rhinoscopy, conveniently performed with an otoscope or with a nasal speculum and headlight, can provide limited information. Routine ordering of computed tomography (CT) scans and magnetic resonance imaging (MRI) to evaluate nasal congestion is not justified, although these modalities may be indicated rarely for difficult cases such as suspected neoplasia [116]. CBCT images, routinely made in many orthodontic practices, may find their place in airway evaluation in the future.

Q: In a review of the evidence between respiratory mode and facial morphology, Vig [117] points out problems accompanying

Table 5.3 Diagnostic findings and problem list for Rachael.

Full face and profile	**Frontal view**
	Chin may be slightly deviated to right
	Mild LLAFH (soft tissue Glabella–Subnasale < Subnasale–soft tissue Menton)
	Incisal display at rest ~2–3 mm (Figure 5.56d)
	Excess gingival display in posed smile
	UDML ~1–2 mm R
	Profile view
	Convex profile
	ILG ~2 mm
	Retrusive chin
	Obtuse NLA
Ceph analysis	**Skeletal**
	Maxilla slightly protrusive (A-point forward of Nasion-perpendicular line)
	Mandibular AP deficiency (ANB = 6° with mildly protrusive maxilla)
	LLAFH (LAFH/TAFH = 59%, two standard deviations greater than normal of 55%, SD = 2%)
	Steep cant of palatal plane (PNS much lower than ANS due to excess vertical growth of posterior maxilla compared to anterior maxilla)
	Vertical maxillary excess
	Steep MPA (FMA = 32°; SNMP = 43°)
	Short posterior face height
	Dental
	Mild proclination of mandibular incisors (FMIA = 62°)
Radiographs	Late mixed dentition
	All permanent teeth present
Intraoral photos and models	Angle Class II division 1 malocclusion
	Iowa Classification: II (4–5) X X II (3–4)
	OJ: 7 mm
	Anterior open bite extending to right first permanent molar and left primary second molar (Note: Many erupting permanent teeth are not in occlusion)
	Maxillary incisor edges are on same level as maxillary posterior teeth
	COS ~0 mm
	Mild maxillary anterior crowding (UTSALD = −3.7 mm)
	Mild mandibular anterior crowding (but LTSALD = +2 mm when 4–5 mm of leeway space included)
	First molar widths: maxillary 38 mm (mesiolingual cusp to mesiolingual cusp); mandibular 40 mm (central fossa to central fossa)
	Minimal first molar OJ ("tight" transverse relationship, but not over cross bite)
	Maxillary first molars are rotated mesially
	Thin attached keratinized gingiva mandibular anterior
Other	—
Diagnosis	Angle Class II division 1 malocclusion
	Skeletal open bite secondary to vertical maxillary excess

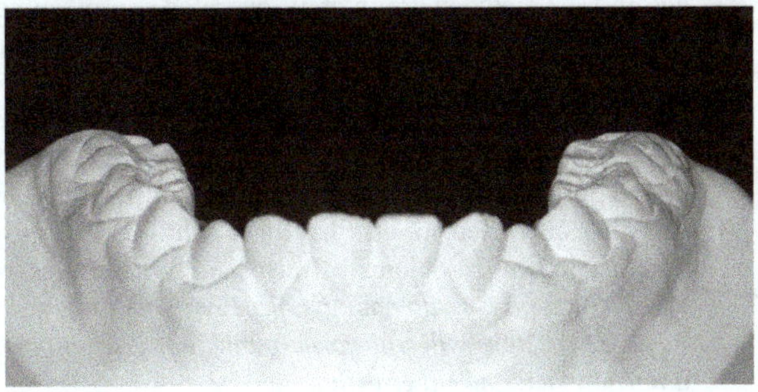

(a)

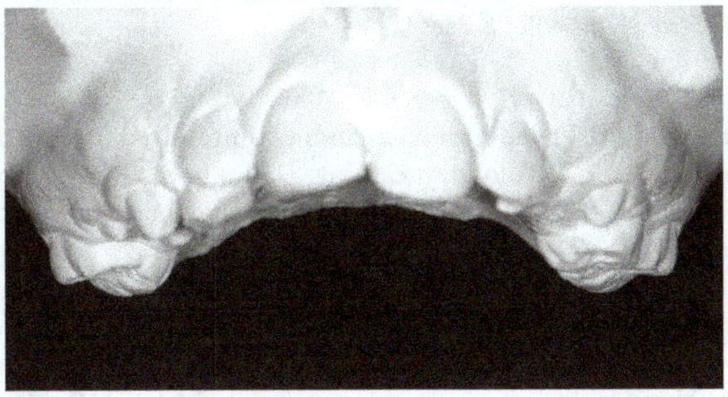

(b)

Figure 5.57 (a, b) Separated model views of Rachael.

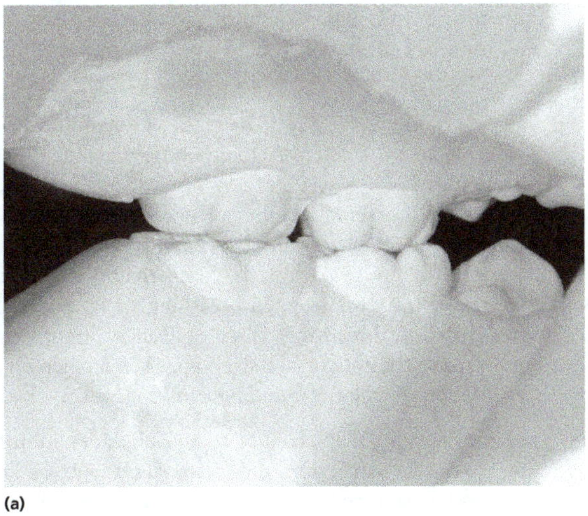

(a)

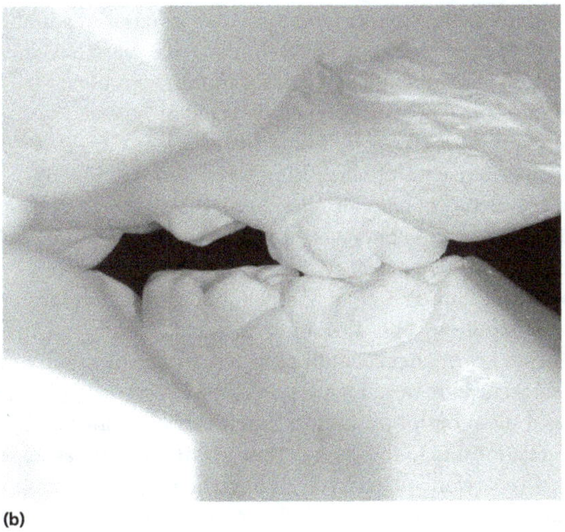

(b)

Figure 5.58 Rachael's models viewed from the lingual: (a) left and (b) right.

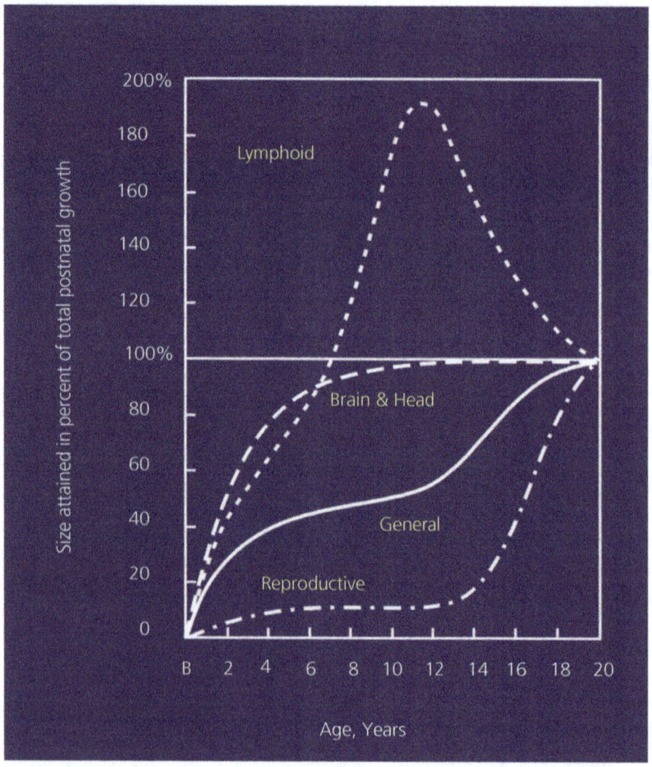

Figure 5.59 Growth curves illustrating the fact that lymphoidal tissue size increases dramatically during the developmental years and then decreases to final adult size [111]. (Tanner JM. Growth at adolescence. 2nd ed. Oxford: Blackwell Scientific Publications; 1962. Reproduced with permission from John Wiley & Sons Ltd.)

studies of this relationship, including unresolved issues of diagnostic tests for mouth breathing. *Do we have any evidence indicating a relationship between mouth breathing and facial morphology?*

A: *We have evidence, but it is not of the highest level.* Case studies have shown that children with nasal obstruction experience a downward and backward mandibular rotation, with resulting growth producing an increase lower facial height [118, 119]. Children suffering from allergic rhinitis tend to have increased total anterior face height, increased lower anterior face height, and steeper mandibular plane angles [95]. Long-faced subjects have significantly smaller components of nasal respiration [120]. In a sample [121] of 400 children, 2–12 years old (mean age 6 years) at an outpatient clinic for mouth breathers:

- Adenoid/tonsil obstruction was detected in 71.8%.
- Allergic rhinitis alone was found in 18.7%.
- Nonobstructive mouth breathing was diagnosed in 9.5%.
- The prevalence of anterior open bites, Class II malocclusions, and posterior cross bites was higher in mouth-breathing children than in the general population. Posterior cross bite was detected in almost 30% of the children during primary and mixed dentitions and 48% in permanent dentition. During mixed and permanent dentitions, anterior open bite sand Class II malocclusions were highly prevalent. However, more than 50% of the mouth breathing children carried a normal interarch relationship in the sagittal, transversal and vertical planes.

In a comparison of severely obstructed mouth-breathing and nasal-breathing children [122] mouth-breathing children had a hyperdivergent cephalometric pattern, but against all expectations, counterclockwise mandibular rotations were the average observations. Last, in a recent study of prepubertal severely obstructed mouth-breathing children and prepuberal nasal-breathing children, after adenoidectomy, the mouth-breathing children showed greater maxillary transverse development [123].

Q: What is the effect of RME in children with nasal obstruction?

A: The effects include reduction of nasal obstruction, raising of tongue posture, and enlargement of pharyngeal airway [124].

Q: Does RME have long-term positive effects on airway dimensions and breathing in growing children?

A: Yes, there is moderate evidence that RME improves conditions for nasal breathing (at least until 1 year post RME expansion) [125].

Q: What are the current pediatric indications for tonsillectomy and adenoidectomy?

A: Recurrent episodes of pharyngitis (7× strep sore throat in 1 year, or 5 each in 2 consecutive years, or 3 in 3 years with temps of 100.9°, white tonsil coverings, lymphadenopathy, and positive strep tests), or sleep apnea, or severe difficulty with respiration [126].

Q: Is there *clear* evidence showing that correction of nasal obstruction will result in normal vertical facial growth?

A: No. In a 2004 study [127], adenoidectomies were performed in a group of mouth-breathing children (nasal obstruction caused by enlarged adenoids) at age 7 years, which caused a change from mouth to nose breathing. This group was compared to an age and sex matched group of un-operated control subjects and re-examined at 12 years. Results indicated that adenoidectomy improved vertical facial growth and balance. On the other hand, the sum of upper and lower first molar height changes (amount of molar eruption) was 9.2 mm in the adenoidectomized group and 5.8 mm in the control group. This would indicate that corrected mouth breathers continued to grow more vertically. Other problems with this study have been reported [128]. *Currently, we do not have clear evidence that correction of nasal obstruction will transform a long-face growth pattern into a normal facial height growth pattern.*

Q: Does the fact that Rachael exhibits lip incompetence (ILG) indicate that she is a mouth breather?

A: No. Lip incompetence does not necessarily indicate mouth breathing [93, 94]. Furthermore, Rachael has an ILG of ~2 mm. Recall that an ILG of up to 2 mm may be considered normal [61].

Q: How would you decide if Rachael was a mouth breather and when would you refer her to an otolaryngologist for an airway evaluation?

A: First, try to *observe* whether or not she breathes through her mouth. *Ask* Rachael and her parents whether she breathes through her nose or mouth. Ask her and her parents if she snores or has ever stopped breathing while asleep. If Rachael has difficulty breathing, is an obligatory mouth breather, or presents with a history of sleep apnea, refer her for an airway evaluation. *Rachael is found to breathe nasally.*

Q: Hypothetically, if Rachael were an obligatory mouth breather due to nasal obstruction, and the nasal obstruction is corrected, can you guarantee her parents that her abnormal vertical facial

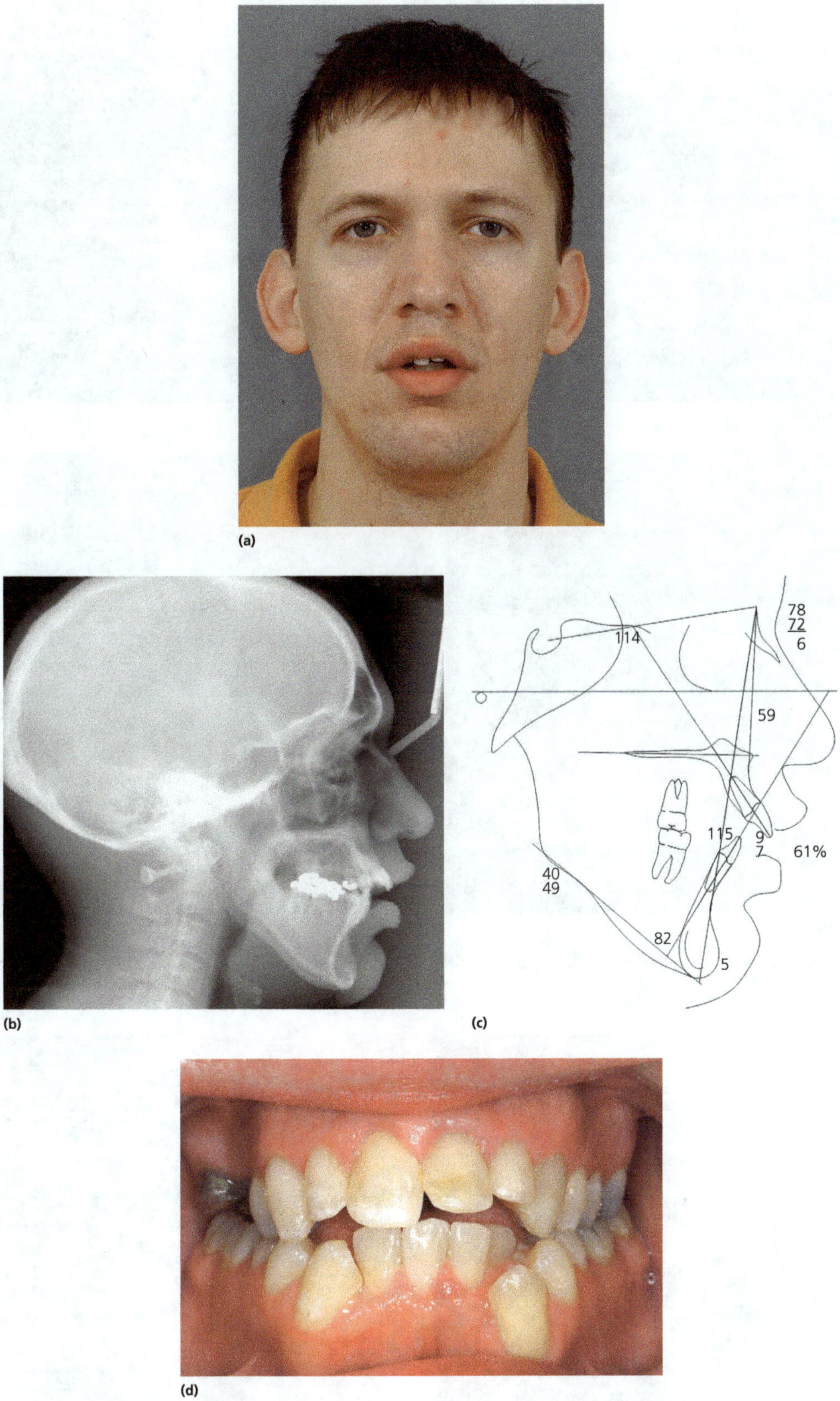

Figure 5.60 (a–d) Patient exhibiting features traditionally used to describe “adenoidal facies” or “long-face syndrome.” These features include LLAFH, narrow face, interlabial gap, constricted maxillary arch (cross bite), anterior open bite, high palatal vault, and frequent self-reported mouth breathing.

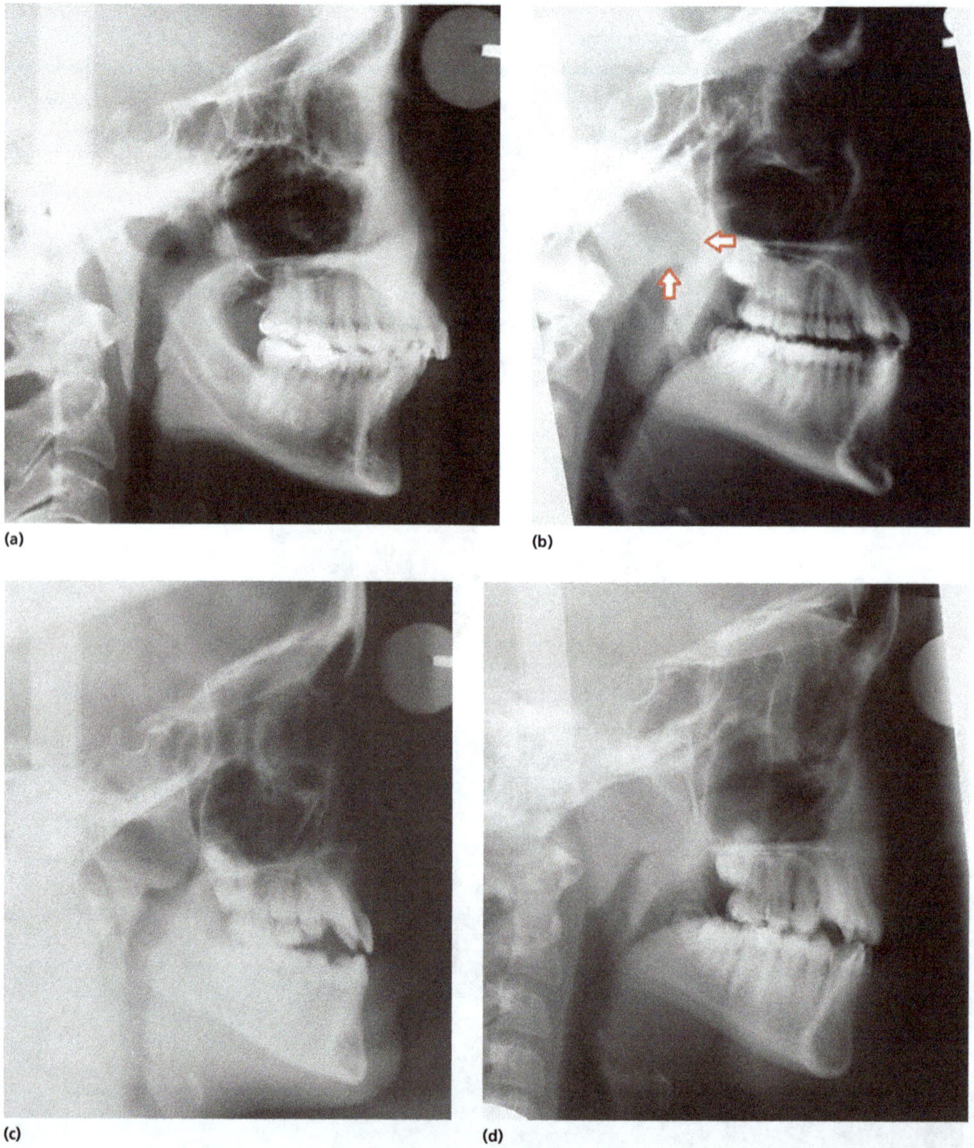

Figure 5.61 Nasopharynx viewed on cephalometric radiographs: (a) airway appears open and (b–d) airways appear obstructed by hypertrophied adenoids.

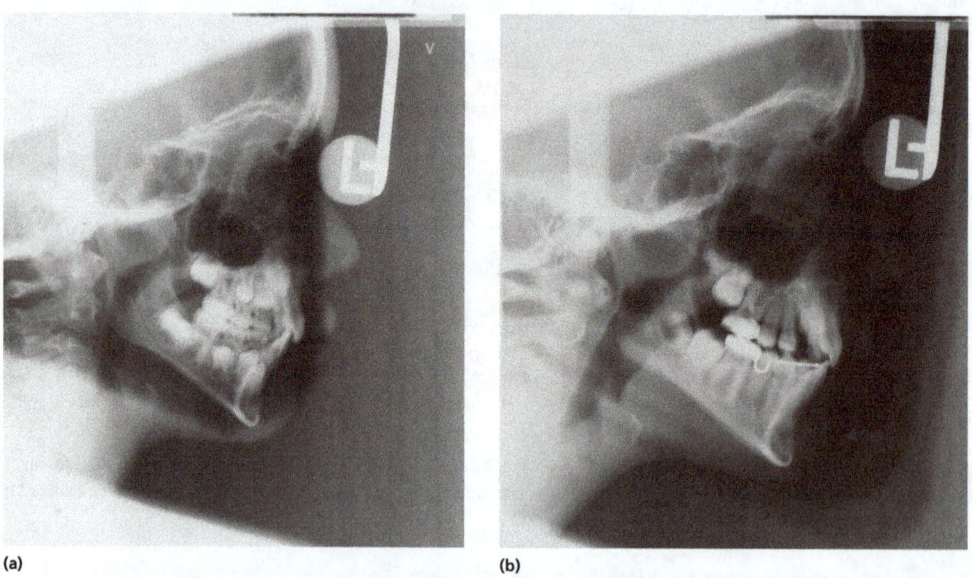

Figure 5.62 Nasopharynx of the same patient at (a) 8 years old and at (b) 10 years old. Note adenoid hypertrophy and airway reduction which has occurred in 2 years.

growth pattern would transform into a normal facial height growth pattern?

A: No. The purpose of referring her for nasal obstruction treatment is to help her breathe better. You cannot guarantee her parents that nasal obstruction treatment will change her vertical pattern of facial growth.

Q: Are there any additional questions you should ask Rachael and her parents about her open bite? Is there anything else should you check for?

A: Additional considerations include the following:

- You should show her parents the open bite and inquire how long she has had it. They respond that they have never noticed it before.
- Inquire whether Rachael has any functional habits that could have prevented her anterior teeth from erupting. She denies any thumb- or digit-sucking habits.
- Ask Rachael if she has any idea what could be preventing her front teeth from erupting into contact. Rachael states that she has no idea.
- Check for permanent teeth that are still erupting, which may cause a temporary open bite. Rachael's permanent maxillary canines and premolars are only partially erupted, which is consistent with her dental stage of development.
- Check for ankylosed teeth and blocked out teeth that are not fully erupted. There appears to be adequate space.
- Check for anterior tongue posturing. Ask Rachael to close her eyes. Talk to her parents for a minute. Then, to distract her,x ask her to open her eyes as you quickly and gently draw her lower lip forward and down. You find that her tongue is not anteriorly interposed.
- Confirm that she has not sustained jaw trauma and her condyles appear normal (Figure 5.56f). She has not sustained jaw trauma, and her condyles appear normal.

Q: Can you list Rachael's skeletal open bite features? Dental open bite features?

A: Her *skeletal* open bite features include the following:

- Mild soft tissue LLAFH (soft tissue Glabella—Subnasale mildly < Subnasale—soft tissue Menton, Figure 5.56a, c)
- Skeletal LLAFH (LAFH/TAFH = 59%)
- Steep cant of palatal plane (PNS much lower than ANS due to excess vertical growth of posterior maxilla compared to anterior maxilla)
- Steep MPA (FMA = 32°; SNMP = 43°)
- Anterior open bite extending to right permanent first molar and left primary second molar
- Approximately 2 mm ILG without an apparent short upper lip, suggesting that her soft tissue facial growth has not kept pace with her skeletal growth. But, an ILG of up to 2 mm can be WRN

Her *dental* open bite features include the following:

- None. At this time, there are no habits (or features) that would suggest Rachael has a dental open bite.

Q: Is Rachael a dental open bite, a skeletal open bite, or a combination of both?

A: Rachael is a skeletal open bite due to vertical maxillary excess (VME) growth.

Q: What is the etiology of Rachael's skeletal open bite?

A: Her skeletal open bite is due to a pattern of growth including condyles growing posterior-superiorly (Figure 5.63, curved red arrow), lack of posterior face height development, lack of normal forward mandibular internal (true) rotation or even backward internal (true) rotation (curved blue arrows), and her maxilla descending more than normal (palatal plane rotated down posteriorly). Rachael is VME. Contrasted with other skeletal open bite patients, her maxillary molars are not over-erupted (maxillary molar apicies are above the palatal plane). As a result of growth, Rachael's mandible rotated downward and backward (CW, yellow arrow), the mandibular plane angle steepened, the lower anterior face height increased, and her anterior open bite resulted.

Q: How does Rachael's skeletal open bite etiology affect treatment?

A: This vertical excess growth pattern may continue until she is finished growing. You can attempt to treat Rachael orthopedically to improve her vertical relationship (by reducing maxillary corpus descent/reducing molar eruption), but there is no guarantee that you will be successful. Even if Rachael cooperates, and you are successful in controlling her vertical growth during treatment, her growth pattern will not

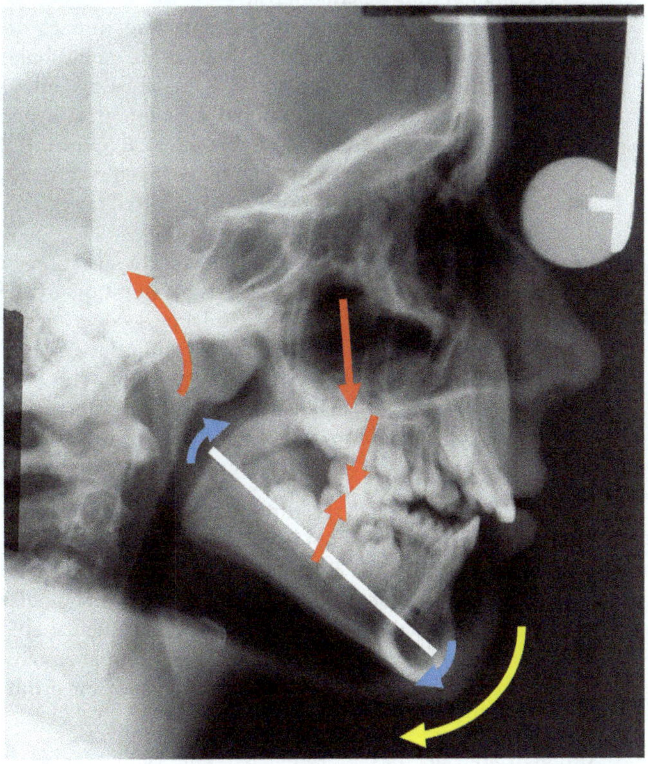

Figure 5.63 Rachael displays many of the features typical of a skeletal open bite pattern of growth: condyles growing posterior-superiorly, lack of posterior face height development, lack of normal forward mandibular internal (true) rotation or even backward internal (true) rotation (blue arrows), and her maxilla descending more than normal (palatal plane rotated down posteriorly). On the other hand, the maxillary molar root apicies are positioned above the palatal plane (the molars are not overerupted). As her mandible rotated downward and backward (yellow arrow), her mandibular plane angle steepened, her anterior face height increased, and her anterior open bite resulted.

be normalized after treatment. So, you must either treat her until she is finished growing or gamble that she only has an inconsequential amount of growth remaining after you deband. One key point—Rachael is a relatively mild skeletal open bite. If she had a severe skeletal open bite, it would be prudent to let her finish growing before initiating treatment—and plan on treating her with orthognathic surgery or TAD molar intrusion.

Q: We noted (Table 5.3) that Rachael presents with thin attached keratinized gingiva in the mandibular incisor area (Figure 5.56h–j). How much attached keratinized gingiva do you need to treat a patient, orthodontically (to prevent gingival recession)?

A: Considerations include the following:

- You must have *some* attached keratinized gingiva throughout both arches (Personal communication with a colleague from the University of Iowa College of Dentistry, GK Johnson, Department of Periodontics oral communication, July 5, 2011). One study reported that minimal widths of keratinized gingiva (fewer than 2 mm) are capable of withstanding the stresses of orthodontic mechanics [129]. If you lack attached keratinized gingiva anywhere, or are in doubt as to whether you have adequate attached keratinized gingiva, seek a consultation from a periodontist.
- Also, your planned dental movements also impact the amount you need. If you plan to procline mandibular anterior teeth significantly (stressing the labial periodontium), then more than a minimal amount of attached keratinized tissue would be desirable (clinical opinion). If you plan to retract/upright mandibular anterior teeth, then a minimal amount of attached keratinized tissue may be adequate.
- Preventing gingival recession is not only a question of attached keratinized gingiva. It is also a question of the alveolar process bone height and thickness covering the teeth roots. For example, if you are expanding the maxillary dental arch buccally, we would suggest that you have many millimeters of attached keratinized tissue plus a thick band of alveolar process bone covering the posterior teeth roots.

Q: What do the above points regarding attached keratinized gingiva mean in your treatment of Rachael?

A: Considering the fact that Rachael has no curve of Spee (no mandibular incisor proclination when leveling her mandibular arch), and actually has potential spacing in her mandibular arch when the leeway space is accounted for, her minimal amount of attached keratinized gingiva should be adequate for orthodontic treatment.

Q: Although Rachael has a "tight" left and right transverse first molar relationship (minimal OJ at the first molars), she is not in overt cross bite. How does the mesial rotation of her maxillary first molars worsen her transverse posterior relationship?

A: Mesial maxillary first molar rotation brings the mesiobuccal cusps lingually, worsening the transverse relationship (reducing first molar OJ).

Q: What are the *primary* problems in each dimension you must stay focused on for Rachael?

A: See Table 5.4.

Table 5.4 Primary problems list for Rachael *(apical base/skeletal discrepancies italicized).*

AP	II (4–5) X X II (3–4) *Mandibular skeletal retrusion* *Mild maxillary skeletal protrusion*
Vertical	*VME*
Transverse	Minimal buccal OJ due to transverse dental compensations
Other	—

Q: What are the two general approaches to close anterior open bites? Which would you chose for Rachael? Why?

A: The two general approaches for closing anterior open bites are as follows:

1. Erupting anterior teeth
2. Intruding posterior teeth

We already concluded that Rachael is a pure skeletal open bite (growth), and lacks a dental open bite component (absence of habits which could prevent anterior teeth from erupting). Her maxillary and mandibular incisor edges have erupted to be on the same plane as her posterior teeth (Figure 5.56m, o), and she shows ~2–3 mm of incisal display at rest which is normal. For these reasons, you would *not* intentionally correct her open bite by erupting her anterior teeth—as you would if her maxillary incisors were stepped up or her mandibular incisors were stepped down (Figure 5.64a). Also, she has an obtuse NLA, relatively normal maxillary incisor angulation, and only mild proclination of mandibular incisors (FMIA = 62°). For all of the aforementioned reasons, ideally you would *not* correct her open bite by retracting incisors (Figure 5.64b) to rotate the incisors around their apicies and "erupt" them.

Instead, Rachael's *skeletal* anterior open bite has resulted from excessive vertical facial growth. The treatment of choice for adolescent Class II skeletal open bite patients like Rachael (Figure 5.64c) is to reduce descent of her maxillary corpus and reduce eruption of her molars. If this can be done, then the growing mandible can autorotate upward and forward, closing the open bite. In fact, the more growth of the condyles Rachael has, or the more internal (true) closure of the mandible Rachael has, the less reduction in maxillary descent and less reduction in molar eruption you need to correct the skeletal open bite.

Q: What are your treatment goals?

A: To address her primary problems: control vertical growth and close her open bite, correct her distocclusion and improve her chin projection, and achieve ideal transverse arch coordination without increasing transverse dental compensations. Additionally, achieve ideal smile esthetics, a Class I canine relationship, minimal overjet, and overcorrected OB (20–40% OB). A final goal is to maintain this correction, long term.

Q: How can Rachael's vertical apical base discrepancy (VME) be addressed? Suggest specific treatments for orthopedics, masking, and surgery.

A: *Orthopedics* (treatments to reduce downward descent of the growing maxilla and/or reduce molar eruption). The benefit of treating Rachael's skeletal open bite with orthopedics is that she is Class II, bilaterally. Treatments

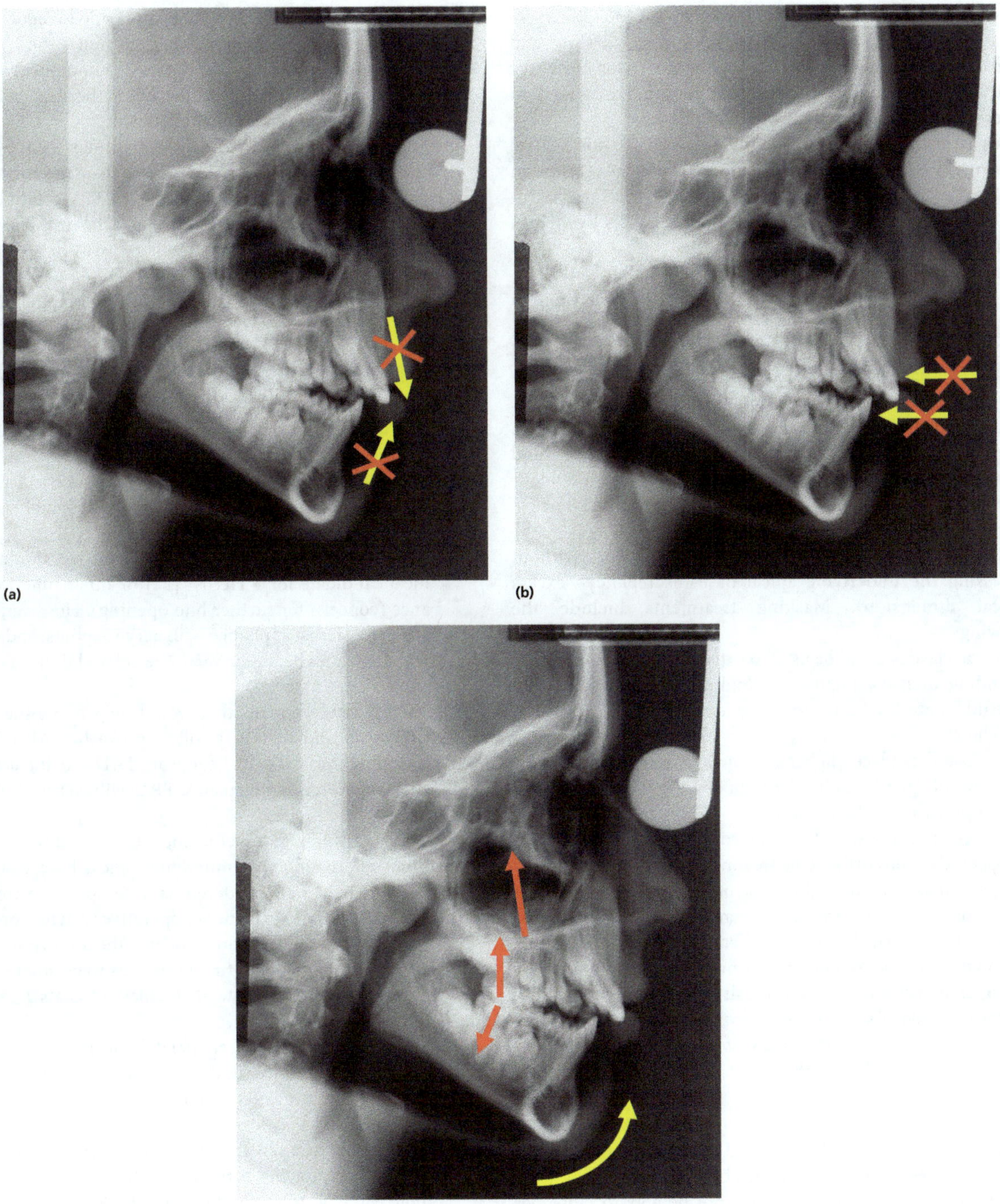

(a) (b) (c)

Figure 5.64 Because Rachael is a pure skeletal open bite with normal incisal display at rest, an obtuse NLA, relatively normal maxillary incisor angulation, and only mild proclination of mandibular incisors, she would not be a candidate for treating her like a dental open bite by (a) erupting her incisors or (b) retracting/uprighting/"erupting" her incisors. Instead, as a skeletal open bite, her treatment should be aimed at (c) attempting to reduce descent of her maxillary corpus and attempting to reduce eruption of maxillary and mandibular molars—in order to autorotate her mandible upward and forward (yellow arrow) closing her open bite.

to reduce descent of her maxillary corpus/reduce molar eruption will also tend to rotate her mandible upward and forward, improving her excess vertical dimension *and* her distocclusion/retrusive profile. Orthopedic treatments include the following:

- High-pull headgear that may restrict vertical maxillary growth and restrict eruption of maxillary molars [13, 14].
- Vertical-pull headgear that may reduce downward descent of the maxillary corpus and reduce eruption of the maxillary molars [5–18].
- Temporary anchorage devices (TADs, attached to a TPA in the maxilla or a LLHA in the mandible) to halt eruption of the maxillary and mandibular first molars [31–34] or intrude maxillary and mandibular molars.

- Exercising (chewing gum) to reduce her MPA [36–38].
- Posterior bite plates (stretching the masseteric sling and causing an intrusive force against the posterior teeth) or active vertical correctors (posterior repelling magnets) to prevent molar eruption [24–28].
- Tongue pressure from a TPA with an acrylic button several millimeters off the palate to reduce maxillary molar eruption [29].
- LLHAs to reduce eruption of mandibular molars by ~1 mm compared to controls [30].
- Herbst appliances, combined with acrylic splints and high-pull headgear wear, to control the vertical dimension in hyperdivergent adolescents such as Rachael [23].

Hypothetically speaking, if Rachael was a Class III (instead of a Class II) skeletal open bite, then any treatment to reduce maxillary descent or molar eruption would rotate her mandible forward—improving her vertical but *worsening* her Class III. In a mild Class III skeletal open bite, a *high-pull chin cup* could be used to reduce forward growth of B-point and also hold, or even reduce, LAFH [19, 20]. But the force vector must be *high*, projecting from the chin to above the ear.

Masking or camouflage (achieve open bite closure without addressing the underlying apical base discrepancy—excess vertical dimension). Masking treatments include the following:

- Vertical elastics could be used to extrude the anterior teeth.
- Bonding incisors gingivally (bonding for open bites) can extrude anterior teeth to close open bites during arch leveling.
- Steps could be placed in her archwires to erupt her incisors.
- A curve of Spee could be placed in her mandibular archwire to erupt her mandibular incisors.

At her age, masking would only be considered if Rachael were uncooperative with orthopedic treatment.

Surgery (maxillary impaction osteotomy) could correct her skeletal open bite. If orthopedics were attempted, it would be important to inform Rachael and her parents that, depending on growth and cooperation, surgery may be required to provide ideal open bite closure later. Although presurgical orthodontics (preparing Rachael's arches to coordinate at surgery) can be performed at any time, the actual *surgery should not be performed until Rachael's growth is complete* to avoid postsurgical relapse.

Q: What should you tell Rachael and her parents about the probable success of her skeletal open bite closure?

A: You should tell them that you may not be able to close her open bite or keep it closed. It will depend on her future growth, her compliance with treatment, and the presence of undetected habits. You should tell them that your goal is to correct the open bite completely, but you may only be able to improve it.

Q: How could Rachael's anteroposterior apical base discrepancy be treated?

A: *Orthopedics* (restrict her maxillary growth while permitting the mandible to continue growing—or, accelerate mandibular growth). One important point regarding Rachael's hyperdivergent growth pattern: during ages 6–12, children with steep mandibular plane angles show significantly less forward mandibular rotation than children with low mandibular plane angles [130]. Therefore, anything you can do to reduce maxillary descent or molar eruption will help minimize the CW rotation of the mandible downward and backward—a positive effect for closing her open bite *and* improving her AP relationship. Orthopedic options include the following:

- High-pull headgear treatment, which may reduce descent of the maxillary corpus, reduce descent of the maxillary first molars, permit forward mandibular CCW rotation [13, 14], distalize maxillary molars through the maxillary alveolar process bone, and restrict maxillary forward growth. Perfect for Rachael, if she will wear it.
- Cervical-pull headgear, which would *not* be the headgear of choice. Although a cervical headgear would restrict maxillary forward growth and distalize maxillary molars, it would not restrict descent of the maxillary corpus nor reduce eruption of the maxillary molars. Its use could result in slight CW rotation of Rachael's palatal plane and slight (<1 mm) extrusion of his maxillary first molars [14, 101].
- A straight-pull headgear would produce an effect somewhere between that of a high-pull and a cervical-pull headgear and would not be recommended.
- Herbst appliance: with a steep MPA, Rachael would not be an ideal candidate for a Herbst [22] or other functional appliance (concern for further bite opening). However, by modifying the Herbst appliance with acrylic splints, and combined with high-pull headgear wear, the vertical dimension may be controlled [23].
- Finally, any treatment that would help rotate the mandible CCW (up and forward) will improve her AP relationship including vertical-pull headgear, TADs to intrude molars, chewing exercises, bite plates, TPAs with acrylic buttons, and LLHAs.

Masking or camouflage (achieving a Class I canine relationship without addressing the underlying apical base discrepancy). Masking would be considered as a compromise treatment if Rachael were found to be noncooperative with orthopedics or if her growth was poor. Options include the following:

- Extraction of maxillary first premolars to permit retraction of the maxillary anterior teeth (achieving Class I canines but leaving molars Class II).
- Placing maxillary buccal, palatal, or infrazygomatic crest temporary anchorage devices to use as anchorage for distalizing the entire maxillary arch.
- Use of Class II elastics (Forsus™ appliance, or other interarch Class II correctors) would *not* be ideal because the lower incisors would procline further [23, 108–110]. Also, the mandible will tend to rotate down and back with Class II elastics as the mandibular molars erupt.
- Using a TPA to rotate Rachael's maxillary molars' buccal cusps distally could improve her molar AP relationship, at least as seen from the buccal. A complete explanation is provided in Figure 5.65. Note: the use of a TPA in this manner will *not translate* Rachael's maxillary molars distally to fully correct her Class II molar relationship as seen from both the buccal and lingual.

Surgery (mandibular advancement) could be considered in conjunction with a maxillary impaction osteotomy, but not at this age.

Q: When should Rachael's Class II correction and open bite treatment begin? Should you start now or wait?

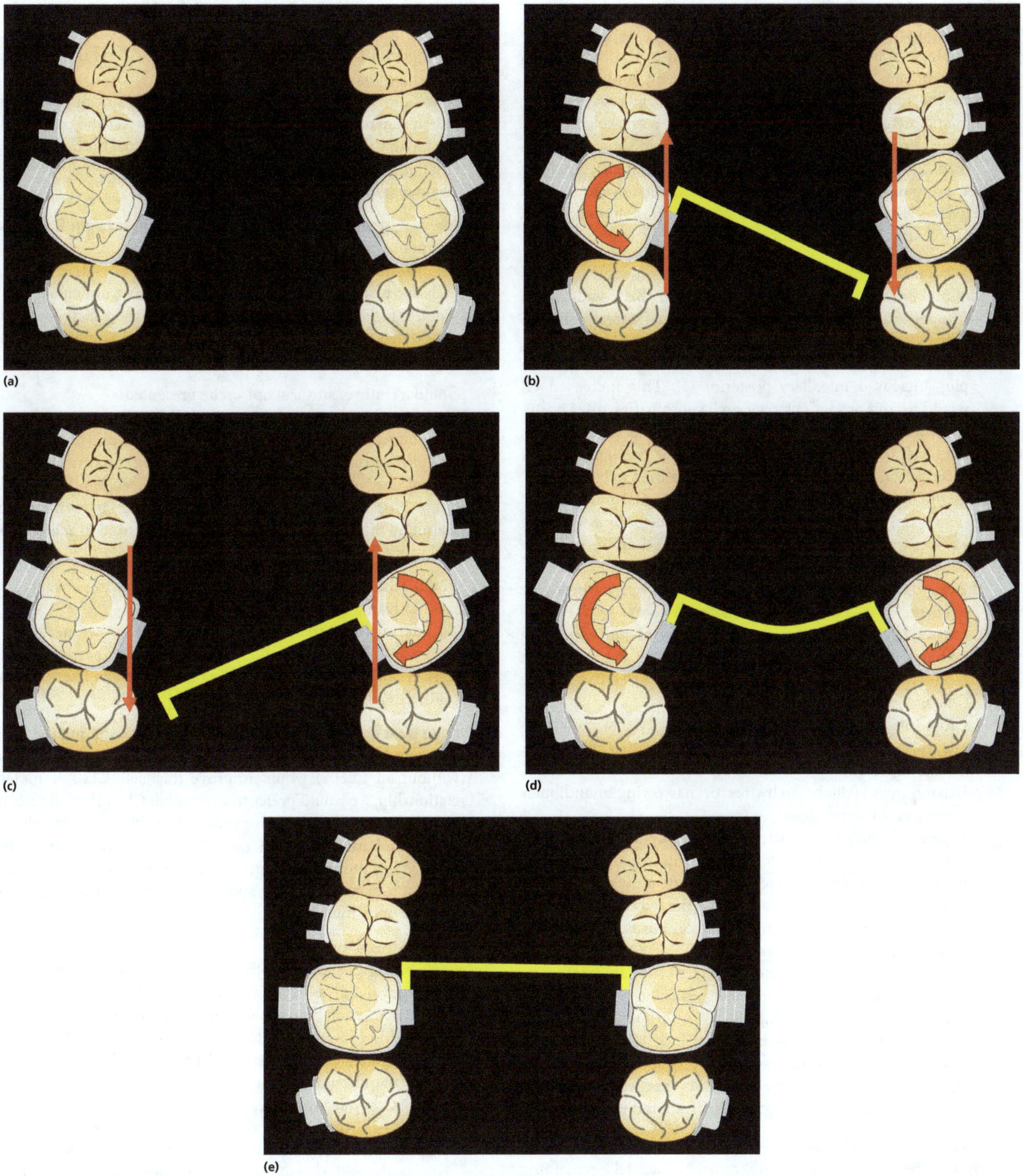
(a) (b) (c) (d) (e)

Figure 5.65 (a) Rachael has mesially rotated maxillary first molars which look more Class II when viewed from the buccal than from the lingual. A TPA can be used to rotate the facial of the molars distally (around their lingual roots). (b) If a TPA is adjusted so that when the patient's right maxillary molar TPA arm is inserted in the lingual sleeve, the left molar arm lies distal to the left molar—then when the left arm is engaged a distal force will be applied against the patient's left molar, a mesial force will be applied against the right molar, and a CCW moment will be applied against the right molar. (c) Repeating the same adjustment with the TPA inserted in the patient's left molar sleeve results in the forces and moment shown. (d) When both ends of the TPA are inserted, then the mesial and distal forces cancel each other leaving only rotation moments which rotate the molars (e). But remember, since Rachael's molars appear Class II when viewed from the lingual, full Class II correction will not be achieved by simply rotating the maxillary first molars around their palatal roots.

A: Begin *now*, while Rachael is in the late mixed-dentition stage of development. Research has demonstrated that there is no advantage to beginning Class II treatment in the early mixed dentition [83–87, 98, 99]. But, if we wait any longer, we may miss the opportunity to take advantage of growth. Further, remember that dental age may not coincide with skeletal age—so if an *early* mixed-dentition patient begins to show signs of a growth spurt, you may also wish to initiate treatment. Finally, if you are going to begin orthopedic treatment now to address Rachael's distocclusion, then you should choose biomechanics that will simultaneously address her vertical excess.

Q: Although Rachael does not have a posterior cross bite, she has minimal overjet at the molars. How should this be addressed (orthopedics, masking, or surgery)? List specific treatments.

A: *Orthopedics* (maxillary skeletal expansion) option:

- RME would provide maxillary skeletal and dental expansion plus increased maxillary posterior OJ. This increased OJ would permit proper posterior arch coordination after posterior transverse compensations are removed. At Rachael's age, her facial skeletal resistance should be small enough to permit a midpalatal sutural split and skeletal expansion to be achieved.

Masking or camouflage (increasing her minimal posterior OJ by increasing posterior compensations/torque or by attempting posterior transverse dental translation). Options include the following:

- Expanding headgear inner facebow (if she wears a headgear to correct her AP relationship, bilateral effect).
- Expanded quad Helix, which could achieve dental expansion and possibly maxillary skeletal widening, if the expansion force is great enough to overcome facial skeletal resistance (bilateral effect).
- Cross-bite elastics (worn from the maxillary first molar lingual to the mandibular first molar buccal, either bilateral or unilateral effect).
- Expanding maxillary archwires or narrowing mandibular archwires (bilateral effect).
- Expanded TPA or constricted LLHA (bilateral effect).
- Using a TPA to rotate her mesially rotated maxillary first molars distally (Figure 5.65) would not only improve her Class II molar relationship as seen on the buccal but also also rotate the maxillary first molar buccal cusps out buccally, improving her posterior transverse OJ.

Although we would expect the effect of all of these treatments to increase compensations (increasing maxillary buccal crown torque and/or mandibular lingual crown torque), some lateral dental translation would also be expected.

Surgery (SARME) would not be considered because the magnitude of the transverse correction needed is relatively small and the patient is young (i.e., RME should work).

Q: What unknowns do you face?

A: By far, the most significant unknown is Rachael's remaining growth (magnitude and direction). How much will her *maxilla descend or her posterior teeth erupt* (rotating her mandible down, worsening her open bite and Class II relationship)? How much will her *maxilla grow forward* (worsening her Class II relationship). How much will her *mandible grow*? Will her *mandible rotate forward (internally, true rotation) or will it rotate backward*? Other unknowns include her *cooperation, hygiene, and presence of an undetected CR—CO shift.*

Q: There are two important factors you should always ask yourself before initiating orthopedic treatment. What are they?

A: The *magnitude* of the apical base discrepancy and the patient's *age (remaining growth)*.

With a mild apical base discrepancy and significant potential growth remaining, you have a chance to correct the malocclusion. With a very severe discrepancy or minimal time of growth remaining, you may not be able to correct the apical base discrepancy (with orthopedics).

Q: How would these factors affect your decision to begin Rachael's treatment at the present time?

A: The magnitude of Rachael's open bite, and Class II discrepancy, is relatively mild to moderate. Given her age, we anticipate considerable facial growth remaining. Together, these factors would suggest that we have a good chance to correct her malocclusion with orthopedics, *if she is cooperative*.

Q: Should a (future) surgical option be presented?

A: Yes. Rachael and parents should be informed that you will use all of your skill to treat her, but that the amount and direction of her future growth (or lack of cooperation) may necessitate surgical intervention to achieve an ideal correction. You could phrase this as, "If Rachael is *unresponsive* to orthopedic treatment, then a surgical approach could be used to achieve an ideal result."

Q: Should you treat Rachael nonextraction? List the advantages and disadvantages.

A: Considering the mild incisor proclination and crowding, a nonextraction approach would seem reasonable, especially if Rachael can achieve AP correction orthopedically. There are no real disadvantages to a nonextraction approach.

Q: If you treat her nonextraction, should you place an LLHA?

A: Yes. Although mesial drift of the mandibular first molars (without an LLHA) would improve Rachael's Class II molar relationship, we would prefer to correct her Class II relationship by orthopedic differential growth (less forward maxillary growth and more forward mandibular growth) in order to improve her profile. Further, an LLHA would reduce mandibular first molar eruption by approximately 1–2 mm (helping to close the open bite) [30].

Q: You also need to consider every reasonable combination of anterior and posterior tooth extraction pattern. Discuss the advantages and disadvantages of each combination for Rachael.

A: Possible extraction patterns include the following:

- Extraction of a mandibular incisor. This could reduce concern of Rachael's thin attached tissue receding during the minor mandibular incisor alignment. However, the mandibular primary second molars have not been lost yet, and we will gain 4–5 mm of leeway space when they exfoliate; there is simply *not enough crowding to warrant extraction of anterior teeth*; and if you extract a mandibular incisor, then Rachael will be finished with excess OJ of the incisors and canines.
- Extraction of maxillary first premolars. This would permit correction of the Class II canine relationship (molars would remain Class II). This option is viable, especially if Rachael is not compliant with orthopedic treatment. However, her NLA may open up even more as her maxillary incisors are retracted.

- Extraction of all four first premolars. Combined with leeway space, space created by extraction of mandibular first premolars would be excessive, especially since Rachael has only mild mandibular anterior crowding and mild mandibular anterior incisor proclination. Further, reciprocally retracting mandibular and maxillary canines through those extraction spaces could result in a final Class II canine relationship (unless the patient wears a headgear for maxillary anchorage, TADs are used as maxillary anchorage, or interarch Class II correctors are used to distalize the maxillary molars and as anchorage to advance the mandibular molars).
- Extraction of maxillary first premolars and mandibular second premolars. This is a better choice than extraction of four first premolars since the mandibular canines will not retract as far during reciprocal space closure. This could be a viable treatment option, especially if Rachael would not cooperate with orthopedic treatment. However, her NLA may increase as her maxillary incisors are retracted.

Q: After considering everything, we have discussed thus far, what treatment do you recommend to Rachael and her parents?

A: We decided to begin with nonextraction treatment, *reduce unknowns* (growth/compliance), and then re-evaluate. A soldered TPA was placed and activated to rotate her maxillary molars into proper alignment (see Figure 5.65), at which time a high-pull headgear was worn until her molar relationship was corrected. Rachael was very compliant. At the same time, an LLHA was placed to slow eruption of her mandibular first molars and prevent them drifting mesially into Class I when the mandibular second primary molars were lost. Thus, a Class I molar relationship must be achieved with the headgear.

Q: What are the specific objectives of treatment for the maxilla, mandible, maxillary dentition, and mandibular dentition in all three planes of space?

A: Specific objectives of treatment for Rachael are as follows:

Maxilla

AP: Restrict normal growth.
Vertical: Restrict normal growth.
Transverse: Maintain transverse width.

Mandible

AP: Allow for normal growth.
Vertical: Allow for normal growth.
Transverse: Allow for normal growth.

Maxillary dentition

AP: Distalize molars and canines. Retract and upright incisors.
Vertical: Level occlusal plane by molar intrusion and incisor extrusion.
Intermolar width: Increase intermolar width by distal molar rotation.

Mandibular dentition

AP: Maintain molars and retract canines. Retract and upright incisors.
Vertical: Maintain curve of Spee.
Intermolar/intercanine width: Maintain intermolar and intercanine widths.

Q: Should headgear wear stop once molars are corrected to a Class I?

A: No. When a headgear is used to correct AP, it should continue to be worn after a Class I molar relationship is achieved. Have the patient wear the headgear until he/she is even slightly Class III at the molars. Then, the patient should wear the headgear less often (or with less force) to hold this corrected position during the remainder of treatment. Rachael continued to wear her headgear at a decreased force level and only while sleeping. Her AP position was carefully monitored. In addition, the inner bow of the headgear was expanded to widen her maxillary intermolar width slightly and improve her transverse relationship. Fixed appliances were placed (Figure 5.66), and eruption of the maxillary permanent canines was monitored. After the permanent canines erupted, they were bonded, arches were leveled and aligned, treatment was finished, and she was retained.

Q: Note in Figure 5.66 that the permanent second molars are not bonded (they have not erupted fully). Would you recommend, in a skeletal open bite patient, bonding second molars when they do erupt?

A: No. If a curve of Spee is present (with mandibular second molars tipped mesially to follow the curve of Spee), then the mandibular second molars could erupt as they are bonded/leveled/uprighted/tipped distally around their distal roots—worsening the open bite. So generally, it is better to stay off the second molars in skeletal open bite patients. If you do decide to bond the second molars to align them, consider doing so later in treatment with a light overlay wire while you carefully monitor the patient.

Q: What does the term "active retention" mean?

A: Maintaining the patient in fixed appliances for an extended period of time (months) after your treatment is finished. Rachael was kept in fixed appliances after all goals had been achieved for 3 months before being debanded. This is a smart thing to do—just to monitor the stability of your treatment and to give tissues time to remodel.

Q: Rachael's deband records are shown in Figure 5.67. What do you note?

A: Post-treatment observations include the following:

- Rachael's smile esthetics have improved dramatically.
- Facial proportions, profile, and NLA do not appear to have changed.
- ILG appears to be absent, although she may be exhibiting mentalis strain to achieve lip competence.
- Excess gingival display is seen in her posed smile.
- Maxillary dental midline matches the midline of her face.

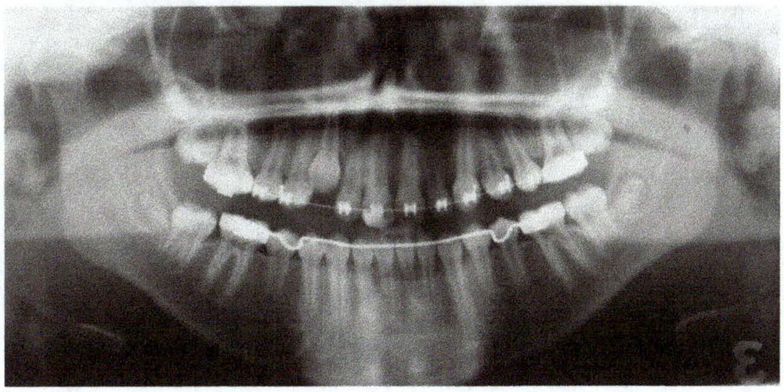

Figure 5.66 Progress panoramic image of Rachael.

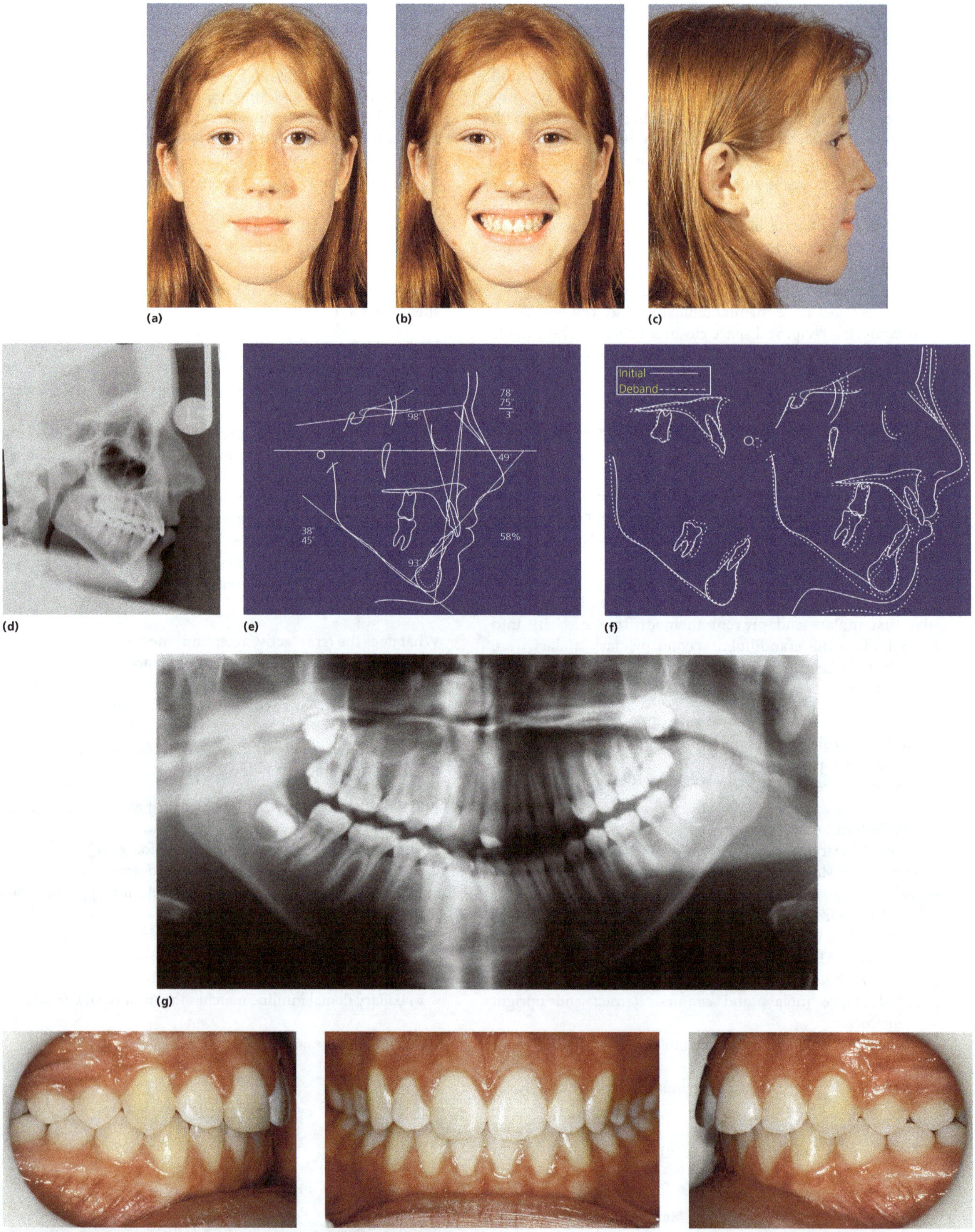

(a) (b) (c) (d) (e) (f) (g) (h) (i) (j)

Figure 5.67 (a–s) Deband records of Rachael.

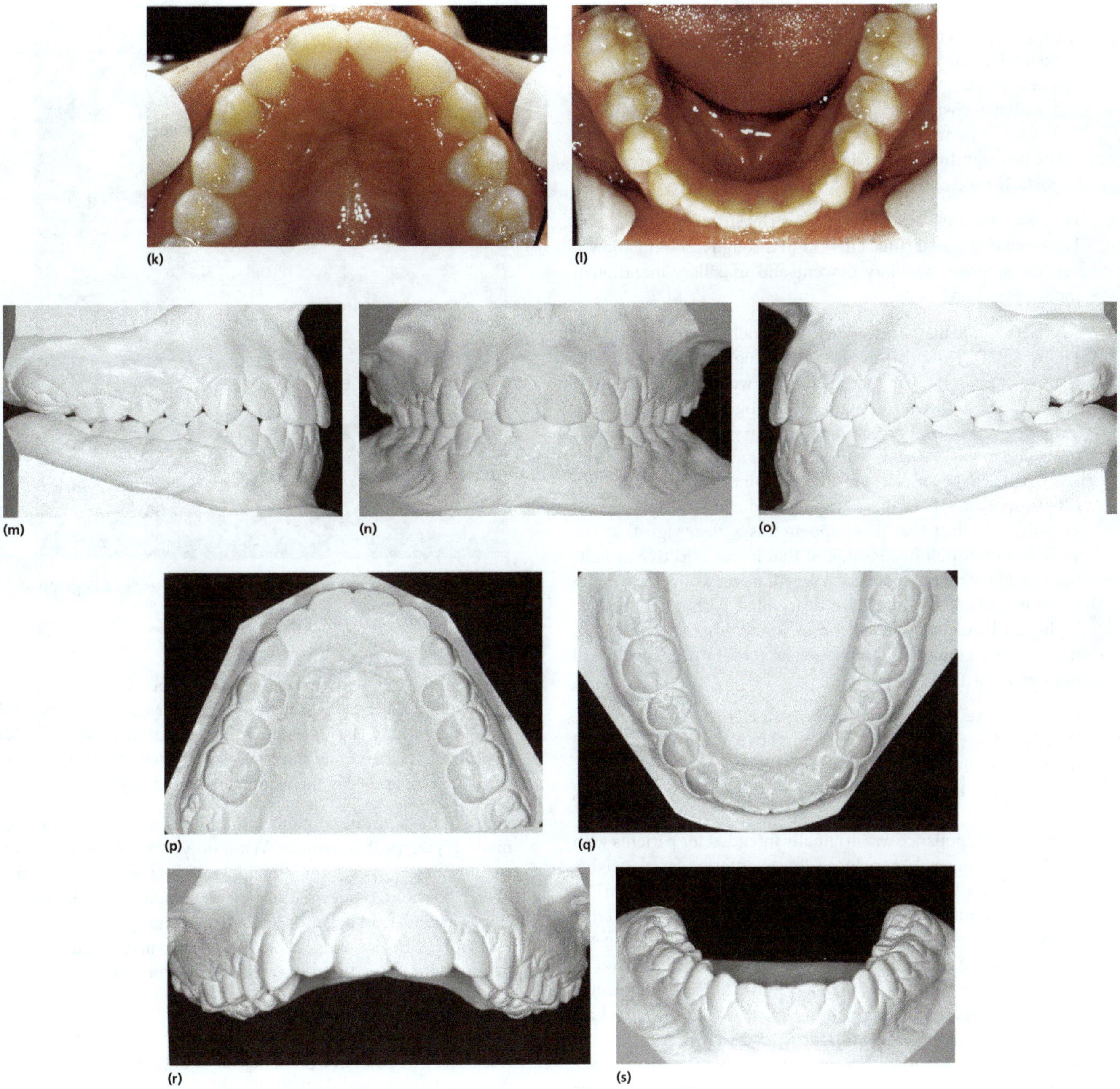

(k) (l) (m) (n) (o) (p) (q) (r) (s)

Figure 5.67 (Continued)

- She has a noticeable right-to-left occlusal cant (Figure 5.67b), which she may have had when she started treatment (Figure 5.56b).
- ANB angle was reduced from 6° to 3° by restriction of A-point forward growth and by B-point translating forward slightly (Figure 5.67f).
- Her mandible rotated down and back (Figure 5.67f) as a result of maxillary corpus descent and mandibular molar eruption. Mandibular down and back rotation would have been worse, if her maxillary molars had erupted, and if she had lacked mandibular growth.
- ANS descended much more than PNS descended.
- Maxillary and mandibular incisors erupted.
- Maxillary incisors uprights, while mandibular incisors proclined.
- Thirty percent overbite was achieved.
- Her Class II molar relationship was corrected through a combination of A-point not growing forward (maxillary growth restriction), B-point translating slightly forward (mandibular growth), maxillary molars not moving mesially, and mandibular molars moving mesially with leeway space closure (Figure 5.67f, mandibular superimposition).
- A Class I molar and canine relationship have been achieved (molars are slightly Class III on the right).
- Midlines are reasonably coincident.

- Second molars are not fully erupted and were not bonded (it was prudent to stay off of the second molars in this skeletal open bite patient to prevent the open bite from worsening).
- Maxillary posterior labial crown torque and mandibular lingual crown torque is still present (Figure 5.67r, s), and she has significant buccal corridors lateral to her maxillary posterior teeth.

Q: How was Rachael's anterior open bite closed?

A: Her open bite closed (final OB = 30%) through a combination of vertical *anterior* maxillary descent and maxillary/mandibular incisor eruption.

Q: Rachael's maxilla descended (overall superimposition, Figure 5.67f). Does this mean that the high-pull headgear did not work? Does it mean that she did not wear the headgear?

A: Neither. She did wear her high-pull headgear and it did work. How do we know? Look at her maxillary arch superimposition. The *maxillary molars did not erupt* at the same time that the mandibular molars erupted (some maxillary molar eruption would have been expected during these years of growth). The fact that this happened is a clear sign that she wore her high-pull headgear, and that it was effective in halting maxillary molar eruption. We will never know how much more her maxilla would have descended without the use of high-pull headgear. We will never know whether she would have required maxillary impaction surgery if the headgear had not been worn.

Q: Could Rachael have been treated with a Herbst appliance?

A: Possibly. Thus far, we have presented two adolescent skeletal open bite patients successfully treated with high-pull headgears. But, there are many pathways to orthodontic success.

The Herbst appliance was originally intended for patients with small MPAs/normal or reduced lower anterior facial heights [22]. The Herbst appliance was not intended for steep MPA/LLAFH patients, like Rachael. However, a modified Herbst appliance (acrylic splints combined with a high-pull headgear) has been reported to better control the vertical dimension in hyperdivergent adolescents than a traditional Herbst appliance [23]. The one problem with using a Herbst appliance on Rachael is that her mandibular incisors proclined significantly (FMIA decreased from 62° to 49°), even with headgear treatment. Her incisors would have proclined even more, on average of 3° more 6 months after treatment, if she had been treated with a Herbst appliance [131]. One final note: if you decide to treat an adolescent skeletal open bite patient with a Herbst appliance, we strongly encourage you to have the patient posture forward to Class I canine, first. *Only if there is no opening of the bite when you posture the adolescent skeletal open bite patient forward to Class I canine should you attempt using a Herbst appliance* (clinical opinion).

Q: Should Rachael's maxilla have been expanded with an RME appliance?

A: Yes. Although the amount of maxillary posterior labial crown torque and mandibular posterior lingual crown torque at deband was minimal (Figure 5.67r, s), if her maxilla had been skeletally expanded using an RME appliance, then enough posterior overjet could have been created to permit complete molar uprighting.

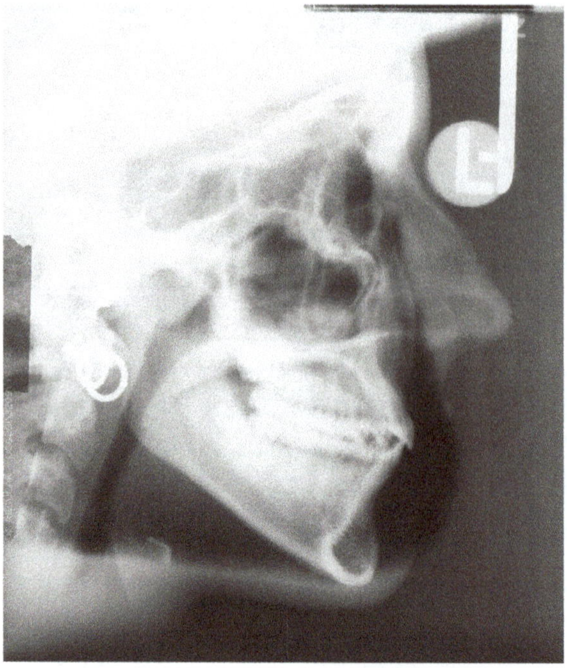

Figure 5.68 One-year posttreatment lateral cephalometric radiograph of Rachael.

Q: Why should you be concerned with Rachael's retention?

A: Because *the underlying growth pattern that caused her skeletal open bite and Class II relationship is not normalized with treatment.* Rachael may have years of growth remaining, and the open bite and Class II relationship could return.

Q: Figure 5.68 is a lateral cephalometric radiograph of Rachael made 1 year post treatment. What do you note regarding the stability of her open bite? What do you note regarding the size of her adenoid tissue in this image compared to her initial (Figure 5.56d) and deband (Figure 5.67d) images?

A: Her open bite appears stable. As anticipated (Figure 5.59), her adenoid tissue has decreased in size with age.

Q: How would you retain her?

A: Rachael was placed in maxillary and mandibular Hawley retainers. The presence (or absence) of digit sucking should be discussed again, and Rachael should be examined for anterior tongue posturing. As was true at her initial examination, neither habit appears to be present. Rachael should be encouraged to exercise (chew gum) daily to help maintain her interdigitation. She could be placed in a tooth positioner and asked to exercise with it daily. Open bite relapse should be monitored closely.

Q: What if her open bite begins to relapse? What should you do?

A: First, Rachael was kept in fixed appliances after all goals had been achieved for 3 months before being debanded (no headgear, no elastics). Keeping her in "active retention" for these months was prudent. It allowed us time to monitor Rachael and insure that severe relapse was unlikely. If mild open bite relapse occurs with minimal (or no) growth remaining, then limited fixed appliances could be placed and vertical elastics worn to close the open bite or posterior occlusal adjustment (enameloplasty) performed to close it.

Q: What are the "take-home" messages from Rachael's treatment?

A: Take home messages include the following:

- Rachael presented with a skeletal open bite due to a classic growth pattern: condyles growing posterior-superiorly, lack of posterior face height development, lack of normal forward mandibular internal (true) rotation, and her maxilla descending more than normal (palatal plane rotated down posteriorly). On the other hand, her maxillary molar root apicies were positioned above the palatal plane (the molars were not overerupted). As her mandible rotated downward and backward, her mandibular plane angle steepened, her LAFH increased, and her anterior open bite resulted. Rachael did not present with any features of a dental open bite.
- Of the three approaches to treat her skeletal open bite (orthopedics, masking, surgery), orthopedics was successfully incorporated. A high-pull headgear was employed to reduce downward descent of her maxilla, reduce forward growth of her maxilla, reduce maxillary molar eruption, and retract maxillary molars. Rachael was compliant as shown by the fact that her maxillary molar eruption was halted. An LLHA was used to reduce eruption of her mandibular molars.
- Of the three approaches to treat her AP apical base discrepancy, orthopedics was successfully incorporated. A high-pull headgear prevented A-point from advancing while allowing B-point to translate slightly forward with mandibular growth. The headgear also prevented the maxillary molars from drifting forward, while the mandibular molars came forward after the mandibular primary second molars were lost.
- Vertical and AP orthopedic correction was possible because her apical base discrepancies were mild (*magnitude*), significant remaining growth was present (*time*), and the patient was very cooperative.
- Rachael's open bite closed through a combination of vertical *anterior* maxillary descent and maxillary/mandibular incisor eruption.
- Overcorrection of her OB (final OB = 30%) was prudent in anticipation of future relapse.
- Retention is as important as orthodontic correction itself. *Growth is not normalized* once treatment is complete and the patient must be followed closely. Fortunately, Rachael's vertical and AP relationships appear stable, at least 1 year post treatment.

Case Kaylee

Kaylee (Figure 5.69) is a 14-year, 6-month-old girl who presents to your associate with the CC, "My teeth are crowded." Her PMH, TMJ evaluation, and periodontal evaluations are WRN. PDH: some years ago Kaylee wore a chin cup but stopped because it made her TMJs sore. She and her parents were told that without the chin cup, the possibility of extractions or jaw surgery increased.

Q: Your associate asks your opinion about the case. You examine Kaylee's initial records. Compile your findings and problem list. What is your diagnosis?

A: See Table 5.5.

Q: One *major* feature was completely ignored during your associate's examination of Kaylee. What did your associate fail to check Kaylee for?

A: He never checked Kaylee for a CR—CO shift. An undetected CR—CO shift can completely undermine any diagnosis you make and any treatment plan you formulate. So, you decide to bring Kaylee back to the clinic where you detect a sizable CR—CO shift. You take a CR bite, trim the models to this CR (Figure 5.70), and remind your associate to *check every patient for a CR—CO shift at every appointment.*

Q: How does Kaylee's new identified dental relationship affect her problem list and diagnosis?

A: We now see that with Kaylee shifted back in CR (Figure 5.70), she is really *Class III by only 2 mm on the right and is actually Class I on the left*; her transverse relationship is improved; and her lower dental midline is 1 mm to the left of the upper dental midline. Finally, you can see in the frontal view of her models that her maxillary incisors are stepped up relative to her maxillary posterior teeth. Undetected CR—CO shifts can be disastrous in Class II patients as shifting the mandible posteriorly to CR worsens the Class II relationship. Detecting a CR—CO shift in a Class III patient, like Kaylee, can actually improve the situation by shifting the mandible toward Class I.

Q: Do you have any suggestions for locating CR in your patient?

A: Yes. With the patient in a relaxed, supine position, ask them to hyperextend their head back slightly as they touch the tip of their tongue to their soft palate—and close slowly until their teeth just touch (Figure 5.71a). As they do this, you can "feel" them in CR, with their condyles rotating back solidly in the glenoid fossa, as you gently grasp the anterior mandible (Figure 5.71b). But, do not force the mandible back.

Q: Sometimes, when you examine a patient, you are unsure whether you have found CR (and whether the diagnostic records you made accurately represent their true AP relationship). If you are unsure whether you have located CR, then what should you do? What should you *not* do?

A: You *should* reduce your unknowns—determine CR. If you are unsure where CR is, then de-program or "break up" the patient's occlusion (de-program their biting pattern) by leveling and aligning the arches; asking them to wear a flat-plane biteplate; or, in cases of constricted maxillae, using RME. Locating CR is often much easier after you have done one of the above. You should *not* define your final treatment plan until you know the true relationship of the patient's models in CR, and you should *not* do anything irreversible (e.g., extractions) until you know where CR is. In other words, you cannot define where you want to go until you establish where you currently are.

Q: Are there other views of Kaylee's models that would be helpful?

A: Check the models from the anterior (Figure 5.72) to evaluate posterior crown torque. You should also check the articulated models from the lingual, especially if the maxillary molars are rotated, to judge the molar AP position from the lingual. This was not done.

Q: What do you see?

A: Maxillary posterior tooth labial crown torque (except for the maxillary first premolars) and mandibular lingual crown torque.

Q: What questions do you need to ask Kaylee and her parents regarding growth and breathing?

A: You need to determine if Kaylee is still growing. Have her parents kept track of her height? When did she reach menarche? Generally, females' peak rate of statural change is reached prior to the onset of menses. On average, with the onset of menses, the female rate of change in height drops to pre-pubertal levels, and decreases sharply to an adult rate of change during the subsequent 2 years [132]. Kaylee's parents report that she reached menarche (1½–2 years ago), completed her growth

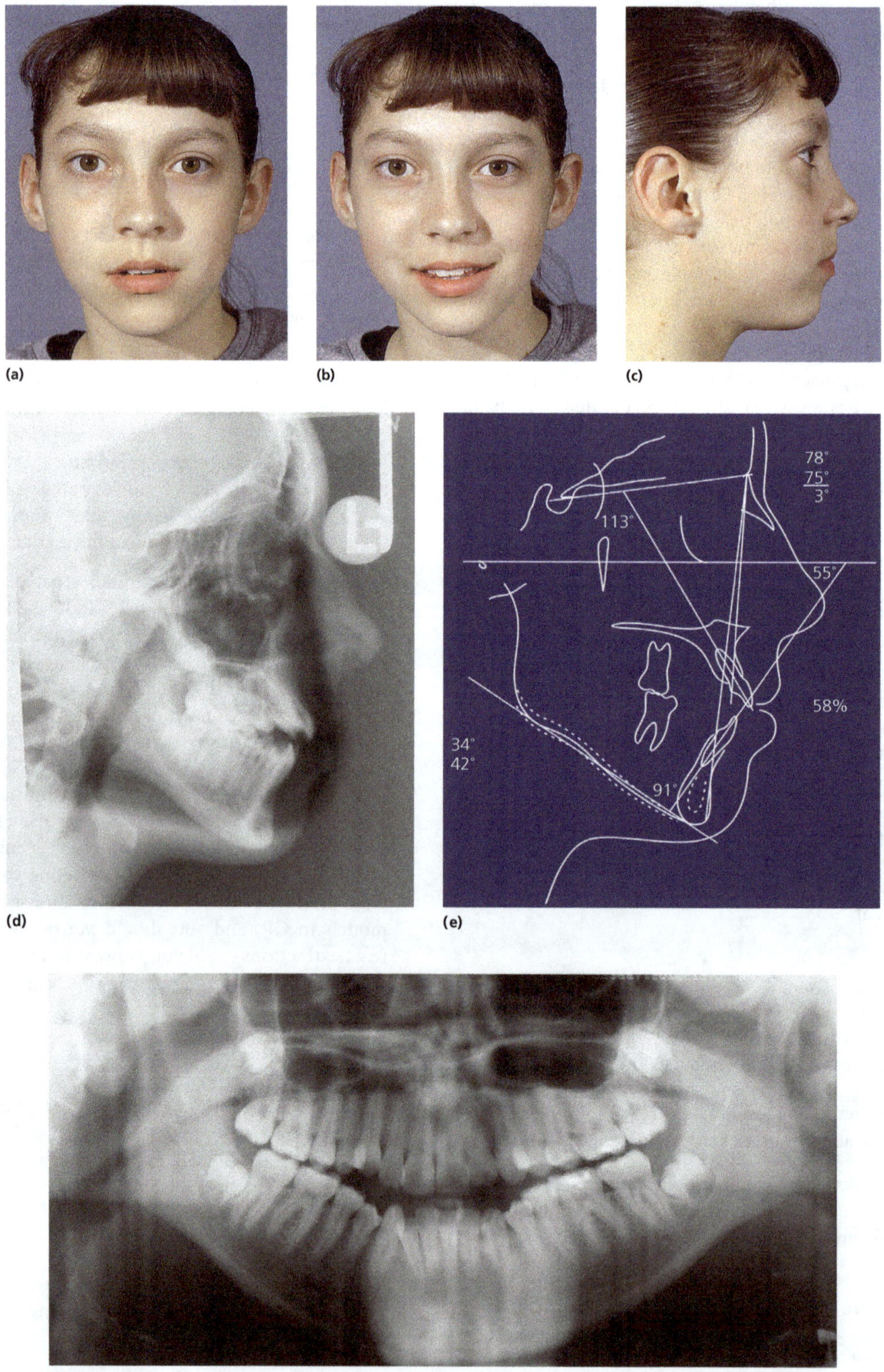

Figure 5.69 Initial records of Kaylee: (a–c) initial facial photographs, (d) lateral cephalograph, (e) cephalometric tracing, (f) pantomograph, and

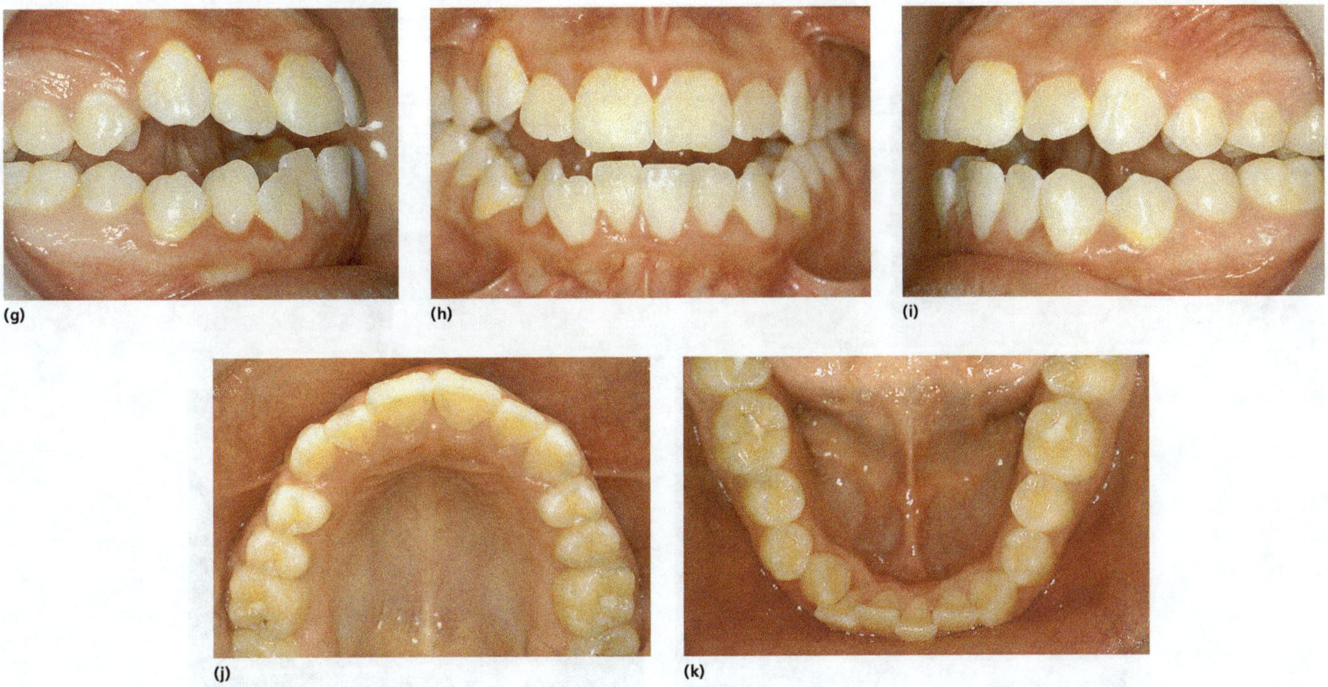

Figure 5.69 (Continued) (g–k) intraoral photographs.

Table 5.5 Diagnostic findings and problem list for Kaylee.

Full face and profile	**Frontal view**
	Soft tissue vertical proportions appear WRN (soft tissue Glabella–Subnasale = Subnasale–soft tissue Menton)
	Right side of face appears fuller, overall
	Chin appears deviated to the left
	ILG ~3 mm
	Incisal display at rest ~2 mm
	Inadequate incisal display in posed smile (but smile is minimally active)
	UDML ~1 mm right of facial midline
	LDML ~1 mm right of UDML
	Profile view
	Convex profile
	Obtuse NLA
	Retrusive chin
	Flat maxillary lip
	Short chin–throat length
Ceph analysis	**Skeletal**
	Mild maxillary AP deficiency (A-point behind Nasion-perpendicular line)
	Mandibular AP deficiency (angle formed by Nasion-perpendicular line and line Nasion-B-point is >3°)
	LLAFH (LAFH/TAFH = 58%, over one standard deviation longer than normal of 55%, SD = 2%)
	Steep MPA (FMA = 34°; SNMP = 42°)
	Maxillary molar root apices have erupted well below the palatal plane
	VME
	Short posterior face height
	Ineffective bony Pogonion
	Dental
	Proclined maxillary incisors (1 to SN = 113°)
	Proclined mandibular incisors (FMIA = 55°)
Radiographs	Permanent dentition
	Developing third molars
	Minimal adenoidal hyperplasia
Intraoral photos and models	Angle Class III malocclusion
	Iowa Classification: III (3) III (3) III (3) III (3)
	OJ: 1 mm
	Anterior open bite of ~3–4 mm
	Anterior open bite extending to first molars
	Mandibular occlusal plane curves *down* toward anterior (reverse curve of Spee)
	Posterior cross bite: maxillary left first and second premolars
	First intermolar widths: maxillary 45.7 mm (between palatal cusps); mandibular 48.5 mm (between central fossae)
	Mild maxillary anterior crowding (UTSALD = −3.6 mm) and moderate mandibular anterior crowding (LTSALD = −7.0 mm)
	Thin attached tissue and prominent lower incisor roots
Other	Poor hygiene
Diagnosis	Angle Class III malocclusion
	Skeletal open bite (vertical maxillary excess)
	Posterior cross bite

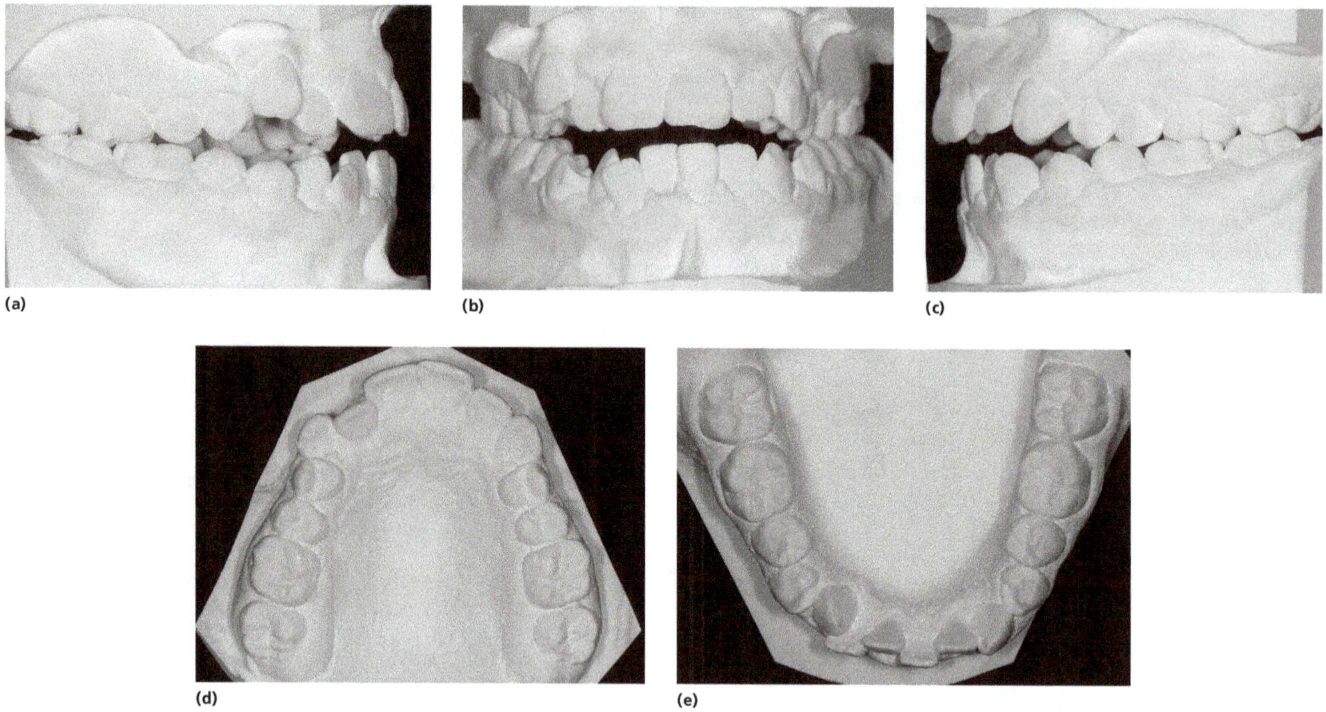

Figure 5.70 (a–e) Kaylee's initial models, trimmed to CR.

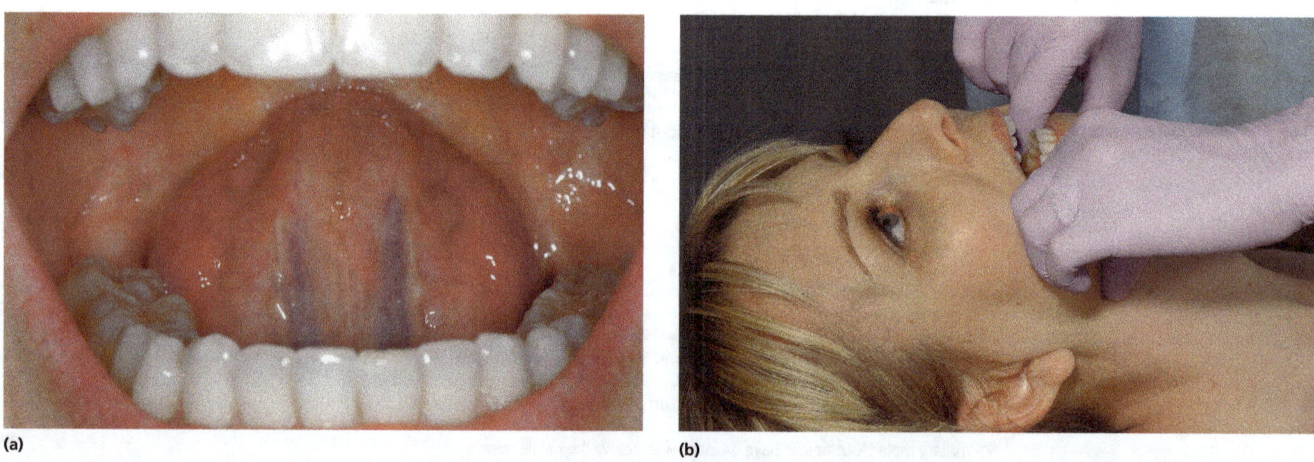

Figure 5.71 Locating centric relation: (a) With the patient in a supine position and their head slightly hyperextended, have them touch the tip of their tongue to their soft palate while closing slowly. (b) While they do this, gently grasp their anterior mandible to feel the condyles rotating in the glenoid fossa.

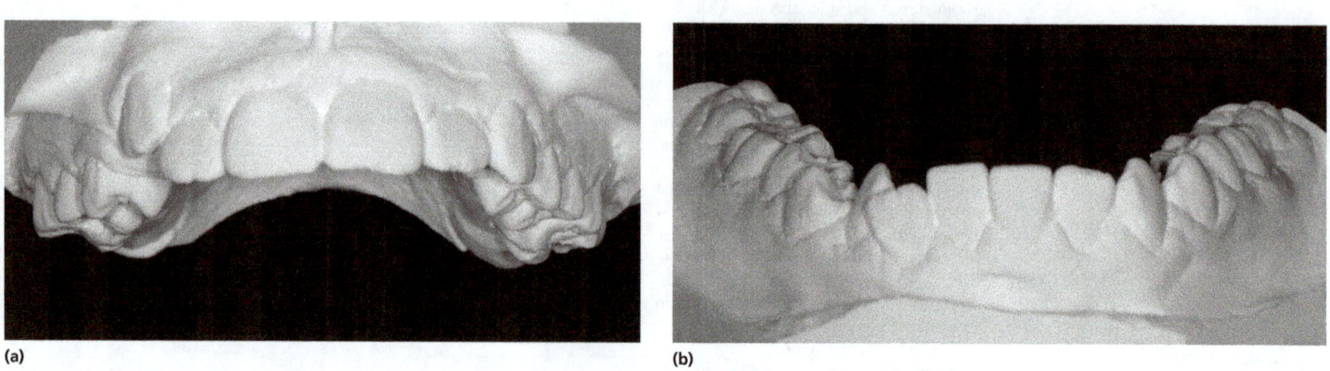

Figure 5.72 (a, b) Kaylee's separated model views.

spurt, but may still be growing a little. Also, you should observe Kaylee to determine if she is a mouth breather. Ask her and her parents if she is a mouth breather, has difficulty breathing, or suffers from sleep apnea. Kaylee breathes nasally and does not suffer from sleep apnea.

Q: Are there any specific questions you want to ask Kaylee and her parents about her open bite? Is there anything else should you check for?

A: You should ask them if they have ever noticed her open bite before. They respond that they have—she has had the open bite for as long as they can remember, but it may have become worse with age. Ask Kaylee if she has any habits that could prevent her front teeth from coming together (like thumb sucking or other digit habits). She responds that she sucked her thumb when she was much younger but not any longer. Check for anterior tongue posturing. As you slowly and gently draw her lower lip forward, you notice that the tongue is interposed between her front teeth. This is barely visible in Figure 5.69b. Also, check for ankylosed teeth that may not be fully erupted, temporary open bites due to permanent teeth not fully erupted, and lack of space for teeth to fully erupt. None of these latter conditions are present.

Q: What else should you check on her screening panoramic image?

A: Confirm the absence of mandibular condylar degeneration—which could rotate her mandible down and back creating an anterior open bite. Her condyles (Figure 5.69f) appear normal with smooth cortical outlines.

Q: What are Kaylee's skeletal open bite features? Dental open bite features?

A: Her skeletal open bite features include the following:

- ILG ~3 mm (her vertical soft tissue growth has not kept pace with her skeletal growth).
- Long skeletal LAFH (LAFH/TAFH = 58%).
- Maxillary molar root apices erupted well below the palatal plane.
- Based upon the above, Kaylee is VME.
- Steep MPA (FMA = 34°; SNMP = 42°).
- Short posterior face height.
- Anterior open bite of ~3–4 mm extending to first molars (extending well beyond an anterior open bite typically caused by a habit—canine to canine).

Dental open bite features include the following:

- Tongue anterior interpositional habit.
- Past history of thumb sucking.
- Her soft tissue vertical proportions appear WRN (soft tissue Glabella–Subnasale = Subnasale–soft tissue Menton).
- Mild reverse curve of Spee (Figure 5.70).
- Stepped up maxillary incisors.

Q: Would you classify Kaylee as a dental open bite, skeletal open bite, or a combination?

A: She is a combination skeletal and dental open bite patient.

Q: What is the etiology of Kaylee's open bite? How does that etiology affect her treatment?

A: Kaylee's *skeletal* open bite resulted from: condyles growing posterior-superiorly (Figure 5.73, curved red arrow) instead of more vertically, lack of posterior face height development, a lack of normal forward mandibular internal (true) rotation or even backward internal (true) rotation (curved blue arrows), excessive maxillary corpus descent (note the large maxillary sinuses), and molars erupting more than normal, especially her maxillary molars. As her mandible rotated downward and backward (yellow arrow), the mandibular plane angle steepened, the anterior face height lengthened, and her anterior skeletal open bite resulted. Even though Kaylee's parents state that she has completed her growth spurt, they think she may still be growing a little. The problem is that her skeletal open bite growth pattern may continue during (and after) treatment. This growth pattern could adversely impact your attempts to close her open bite, or it could cause later relapse if you are successful in closing her open bite. Kaylee's *dental* open bite is the product of her past thumb habit history and her current anterior interpositional tongue habit. An uncorrected tongue habit could adversely impact the stability of successful open bite closure even after Kaylee's facial growth is complete.

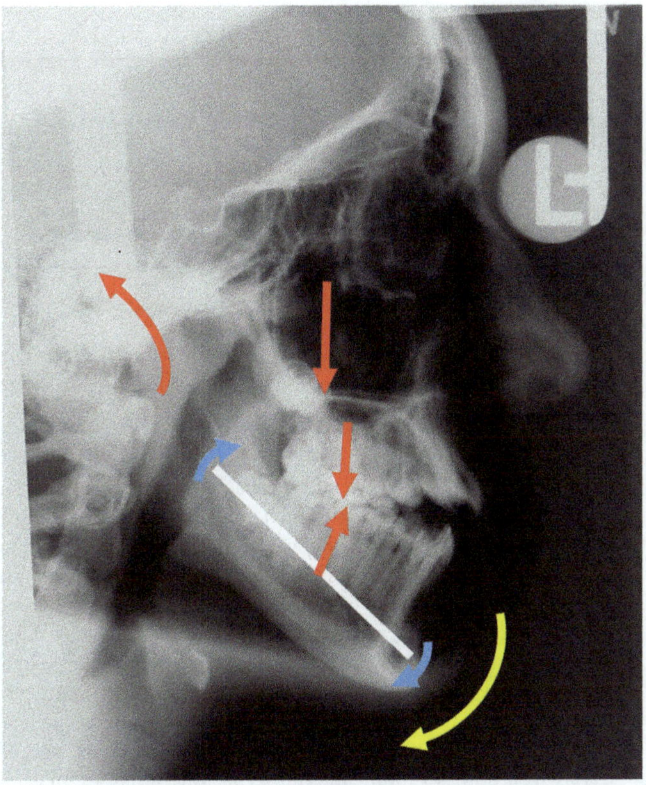

Figure 5.73 Many of the typical growth features found in developing skeletal open bites are identified in Kaylee: condyles growing posterior-superiorly, lack of posterior face height development, lack of normal forward mandibular internal (true) rotation or even backward internal (true) rotation, excessive maxillary corpus descent (note the large maxillary sinuses), and molars erupting more than usual (especially her maxillary molars whose apicies erupted below the palatal plane). As her mandible rotated down and back, her mandibular plane steepened, her skeletal LAFH lengthened, and her skeletal open bite resulted.

Q: After all the above is taken into account, what is your final diagnosis?

A: Angle Class III subdivision right skeletal open bite malocclusion.

Q: It is easy to lose sight of the most challenging problems you face, and focus on smaller problems. Don't do this. Never lose

Table 5.6 Primary problems list for Kaylee *(apical base/skeletal discrepancies italicized).*

AP	III (2) III (2) I I in CR
Vertical	*Skeletal open bite* (with minimal growth anticipated)
Transverse	Posterior cross bite at premolars (with maxillary and mandibular posterior transverse compensations)—if the posterior teeth were uprighted, a significant bilateral cross bite may be evident *Mild maxillary skeletal deficiency*
Other	Moderate mandibular anterior crowding with incisor proclination CR—CO shift

sight of the major problems you face. What are the *primary* problems in each dimension you must stay focused on when treating Kaylee?

A: See Table 5.6.

Q: There are only two, general, approaches to closing anterior open bites. What are they? Which would you choose to close Kaylee's anterior open bite? Why?

A: The two general approaches for closing anterior open bites are erupting anterior teeth (generally used to treat dental open bites) and intruding posterior teeth (generally used to treat skeletal open bites). The exception would be to close a skeletal open bite by erupting anterior teeth (masking, or camouflage). We have already identified Kaylee as a combination of skeletal and dental anterior open bite. Her treatment, therefore, should consist of both. *Erupting anterior teeth:* Kaylee has an anterior tongue interpositional habit that has prevented her maxillary (stepped up) incisors from erupting and must be corrected to insure stability of her open bite closure. Some patients with tongue habits learn to keep their tongue lingual to the teeth as the open bite is closed, orthodontically. But, it is a gamble to assume that the tongue habit will be corrected this way. Kaylee's stepped up maxillary incisors could be erupted (Figure 5.74a) with fixed orthodontic appliances and vertical elastics, especially since she currently shows only 2 mm of incisal display when relaxed. But, her mandibular incisors are *not* stepped down (Figure 5.72b)—and should not, ideally, be erupted to close her open bite (Figure 5.74a). Kaylee does have proclined maxillary and mandibular incisors. Therefore, her open bite could be closed by retracting her maxillary incisors (Figure 5.74b), which would tend to rotate the maxillary incisors around their apicies and erupt them. But again, her mandibular incisors are not stepped down—and it would not be ideal to retract them/rotate them around their apicies to erupt them (Figure 5.74b). Finally, Kaylee presents with an obtuse NLA, which could open up even more (worsen) if the maxillary lip was retracted as the maxillary incisors were retracted. So, you must take care in how much you retract her maxillary incisors. *Intruding posterior teeth*: with the current state of the art, we are not able to modify the way Kaylee's condyles grew posteriorly-superiorly (instead of more vertically), or modify her lack of posterior face height development, or modify her lack of normal forward mandibular internal (true) rotation (although maxillary molar intrusion may result in gonial angle closure). So, we are left with reducing/preventing eruption of posterior teeth (with headgears, bite blocks, LLHAs, etc., Figure 5.74c), which results in relative molar intrusion if the mandible grows. TADs can intrude posterior teeth orthodontically/orthopedically even after growth is complete. A HPHG may reduce maxillary corpus descent if Kaylee has further growth. Last, a maxillary impaction osteotomy is another way to intrude posterior teeth in adults. Such treatments can result in mandibular autorotation around the condyles, and close her open bite.

Q: Molar intrusion (including maxillary impaction) can certainly help close Kaylee's anterior open bite through CCW mandibular rotation. But, will CCW mandibular rotation (autorotation) help, or hurt, Kaylee's AP relationship?

A: Following removal of her CR—CO shift, Kaylee was found to be Class III by only 2 mm on the right and Class I on the left. Therefore, a CCW mandibular rotation will *worsen* her AP relationship—increasing her Class III relationship on the right, and making her Class III on the left. This is exactly opposite to the effect that would be observed in a *Class II* skeletal open bite patient—whose AP relationship would be helped by CCW mandibular autorotation.

Q: Kaylee had a convex profile even before her CR—CO shift was eliminated. So, she will continue to have a convex profile now (Class III by 2 mm on the right and Class I on the left). How can Kaylee have a Class III/Class I dental relationship and still be convex (instead of straight or concave)?

A: Kaylee's excess vertical growth has rotated her mandible down and back, making her less Class III (dentally) and more retrusive than if she was vertically normal.

Q: What are your treatment goals?

A: To address her chief complaint (crowded teeth), close her open bite, close her ILG, achieve ideal incisal display with relaxed lip and when smiling, obtain proper transverse coordination/interdigitation, and achieve a Class I canine relationship with minimal overjet and overcorrected overbite (20–40% OB). Finally, our goal is to maintain the correction, long term.

Q: How can Kaylee's vertical apical base discrepancy (VME) be addressed? Remember, she is Class III on the right and Class I on the left.

A: *Orthopedics* (consists of treatments that would reduce downward descent of the growing maxilla and reduce eruption of the maxillary and mandibular molars). Treatment options include the following:

- Vertical-pull headgear may reduce downward descent of the maxillary corpus and molar eruption.
- *High-pull* chin cup could reduce forward mandibular growth and increases in facial height. But with her history of TMJ pain while wearing a chin cup, you would need to be very careful in attempting this. You could have Kaylee try wearing one with a light force and see how she tolerates it. If she tolerates it, then you could gradually increase the force to >250 g, measured at the center of the chin cup [133].
- TADs could be used to prevent eruption of the maxillary and mandibular first molars.
- Exercising (chewing gum) can reduce MPAs (compared to controls) in growing patients.
- Posterior bite plates (stretching the masseteric sling and causing an intrusive force against the posterior teeth) and active vertical correctors (posterior repelling magnets) can help prevent molar eruption.
- Tongue pressure from a TPA with an acrylic button several millimeters off the palate may reduce maxillary molar eruption.
- LLHAs have been shown to reduce eruption of mandibular molars by ~1 mm compared to controls.

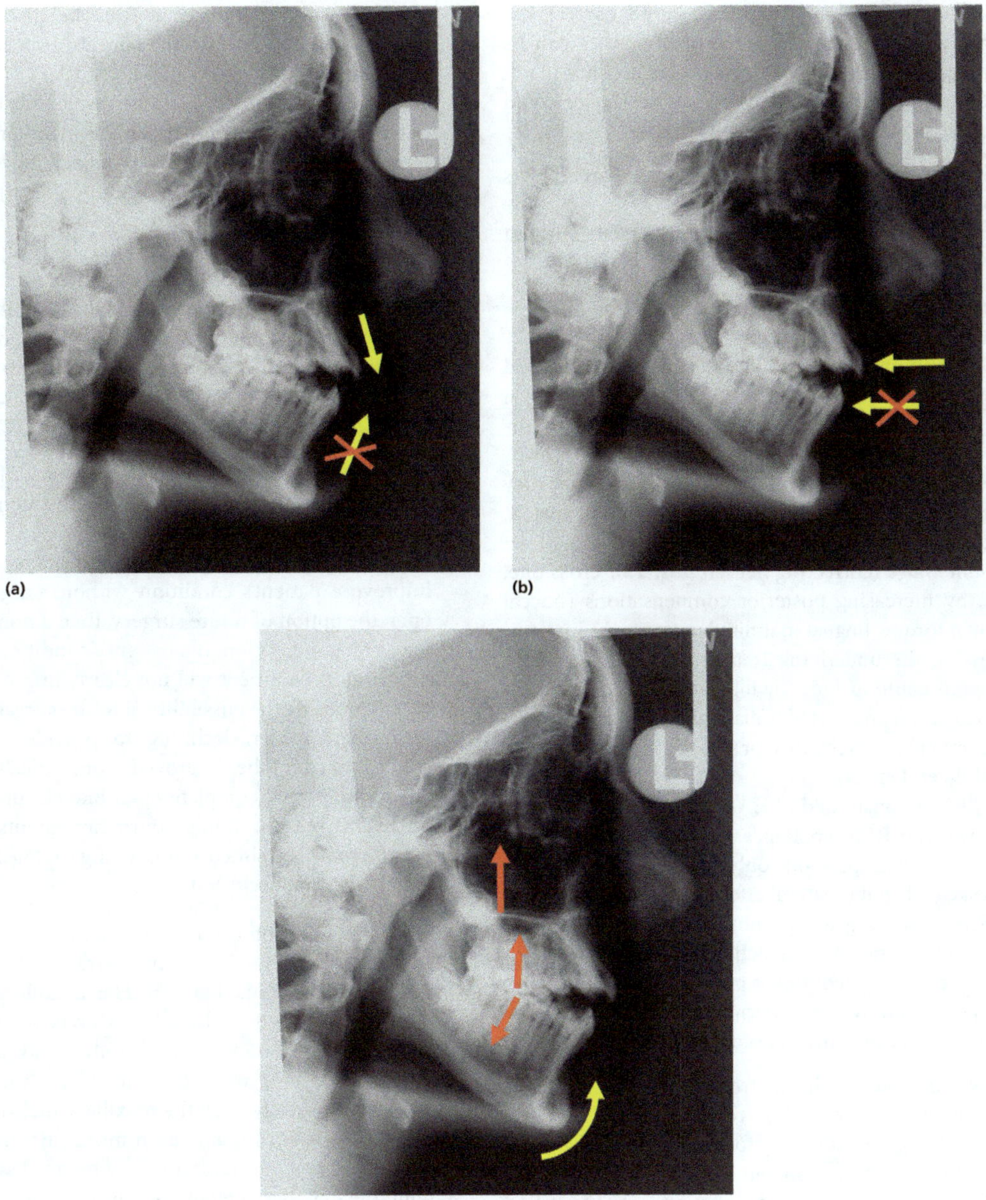

(a) (b) (c)

Figure 5.74 Because Kaylee's maxillary incisors are stepped up relative to her maxillary posterior teeth, and because she displays only 2 mm of maxillary incisor when relaxed, she would be a candidate for (a) erupting her maxillary incisors or (b) retracting/uprighting her maxillary incisors in order to help close her open bite. However, she has an obtuse NLA, so you must take care not to open this angle by retracting the maxillary incisors too far. Because her mandibular incisors are not stepped down, she is not the ideal candidate for (a) erupting her mandibular anterior teeth or (b) retracting/uprighting her mandibular anterior teeth. Additionally, as an adolescent skeletal open bite patient, her treatment should include (c) attempting to reduce descent of her maxillary corpus and reduce eruption of her maxillary and mandibular molars in order to autorotate her mandible CCW (yellow arrow) and close her open bite.

Two problems exist with any orthopedic treatment to prevent Kaylee's vertical development. First, Kaylee's parents think *she is done (or nearly done) growing*. You could start her with vertical orthopedic treatment for a defined evaluation period to rule out the chance of late growth (say, 6–9 months); TADs to intrude her maxillary and mandibular molars are the one orthopedic approach, which could close her open bite and reduce her face height even if she had finished growing. Second, *any orthopedic treatment, which will result in CCW mandibular rotation, will worsen her Class III relationship*. Of course, you would not use a high-pull headgear on her since she is Class III, but a high-pull chin cup would be ideal to address her Class III and vertical problems.

Masking or camouflage (achieve open bite closure without addressing the underlying apical base discrepancy). Options include the following:

- Fixed orthodontic appliances with vertical elastics (erupt anterior teeth)
- Bonding incisors gingivally (bonding for open bites) closes open bites during leveling
- Placing anterior steps in archwires to erupt anterior teeth

Surgery (maxillary impaction osteotomy) could correct her skeletal open bite. Although presurgical orthodontics can be performed at any time, the actual surgical procedure should not be performed until growth has ended (otherwise, Kaylee could continue to grow out of the correction).

Q: Which of the above approaches for treating skeletal open bites is used to close dental open bites?

A: Masking—since you attempt to erupt anterior teeth without attempting to change the vertical skeletal dimensions.

Q: How can her transverse relationship be addressed?

A: *Orthopedics* (maxillary skeletal expansion).

- RME could be attempted to provide maxillary skeletal and dental expansion: creating posterior OJ, permitting removal of posterior transverse compensations, and providing additional arch perimeter to eliminate maxillary anterior crowding. However, at Kaylee's age her facial skeletal resistance may be too great to permit a midpalatal split/skeletal expansion. But, you could attempt RME.

Masking or camouflage (correcting her left posterior cross bite, Figure 5.70b, by increasing posterior compensations (buccal maxillary crown torque, lingual mandibular crown torque) and *not* by addressing the underlying transverse skeletal discrepancy). Treatments could include the following:

- Cross-bite elastics (can be used unilaterally or bilaterally)
- Expanding maxillary archwires or narrowing mandibular archwires (bilateral effect)
- Expanded TPA or constricted LLHA (bilateral effect)
- Expansion with an RME appliance (at the rate of 0.25 mm per week)—dental expansion only without achieving a midpalatal skeletal split (bilateral effect)

Surgery (SARME) would generally not be considered because the magnitude of the transverse correction is not large. However, if a maxillary impaction osteotomy is pursued, then a multiple-piece maxillary osteotomy would permit impaction of the jaw in conjunction with some transverse correction.

Q: What unknowns do you face during treatment?

A: The magnitude and direction of remaining jaw growth, cooperation, and hygiene. It is very fortunate that you picked up the CR—CO shift your associate missed. An erroneous treatment plan could have resulted if you had not identified this shift.

Q: Should you begin Kaylee's treatment now, or wait?

A: This question arises because Kaylee may still be growing. If you intend to treat Kaylee *surgically,* then you could wait, take additional lateral cephalometric radiographs every 9–12 months, and superimpose them until you can confirm that she has stopped growing. Or, you could begin her treatment now (leveling/aligning) but postpone her surgery until you are sure she has completed growth. The point is that growing patients continue to grow after maxillary impaction osteotomies. Surgery should not be performed until growth is complete. If you intend to treat Kaylee *nonsurgically*, then you could begin treatment now, including orthopedic treatment to reduce/prevent further vertical jaw growth (vertical-pull chin cup, bite blocks, active vertical correctors, LLHAs, TADs, etc.). Irreversible treatment (e.g., extractions) should be performed now only with the parent's understanding that an ideal correction may not be achieved, depending on growth and compliance.

Q: Should a surgical option at least be discussed with Kaylee and her parents? If yes, what surgical procedure(s) would you recommend?

A: Yes, a surgical option should be discussed. The best treatment outcome for Kaylee may include a maxillary impaction osteotomy (possibly including a maxillary advancement). At this time, you could leave the option open for a differential maxillary impaction osteotomy (depending on the amount of maxillary incisal display present after leveling and aligning the maxillary arch), multiple-piece maxillary osteotomy to address her transverse relationship, possible mandibular procedure to correct her AP relationship (depending on the amount of mandibular autorotation which occurs with the maxillary impaction), and even a possible genioplasty advancement/impaction.

Q: If Kaylee declines surgical treatment (lack of insurance, lack of interest), then should you proceed with a nonsurgical treatment plan or decline to treat her?

A: This is a never an easy decision to make. If you can clearly improve a patient's condition without surgery, and yet leave open the option of future surgery, then a nonsurgical treatment may be a good option. If a patient's condition is so severe that a nonsurgical treatment will not clearly improve their condition, or will preclude the possibility of future surgery, then you should seriously consider declining to provide treatment. Kaylee's condition could be improved nonsurgically (elimination of crowding, partial/complete open bite closure with TAD molar intrusion), but you should inform her parents that a nonsurgical treatment will be aimed at improving (not necessarily correcting ideally) her malocclusion.

Q: If a surgical option is pursued, would you recommend extracting teeth or treating Kaylee nonextraction?

A: Let's look at her maxilla first. Her maxillary incisors *are* proclined (Figure 5.69e), but she exhibits minimal maxillary lip support (Figure 5.69c), and only mild anterior crowding (Figure 5.69j). If we extract maxillary premolars and close spaces reciprocally, then the maxillary incisors will upright and may decrease lip support even more (increasing her NLA and worsening her profile). So it may be prudent to first level and align the maxillary arch before making the decision whether or not to extract premolars. Let's look at the mandibular arch (Figures 5.69k and 5.70e). The lower incisors are proclined with moderate anterior crowding, and she has a retrusive profile (Figure 5.69e). If we do not extract teeth in the lower arch, the mandibular incisors will become even more proclined during leveling. Further, she has thin tissue covering the mandibular incisor roots. If we extract mandibular premolars and close space reciprocally, then that space could be used to alleviate the incisor crowding and bring the canines into a Class II relationship prior to surgery. With a maxillary impaction osteotomy, the mandible will autorotate forward, and a mandibular advancement may also be needed to move the canines into a Class I relationship (this could improve Kaylee's profile). So, *extraction of mandibular first premolars would be reasonable if surgery is planned. A decision regarding the maxillary first premolars could be postponed.*

Q: If Kaylee decides to undergo surgery and you extract mandibular premolars, should you close the mandibular extraction spaces reciprocally or place TADs distal to the extraction spaces and retract the mandibular canines through the entire extraction space?

A: The answer to this question lies in the magnitude of the mandibular advancement you want the surgeon to provide. If, in your opinion, Kaylee would look good with a 3–4 mm advancement, you should close the mandibular extraction spaces reciprocally. If you feel that Kaylee would benefit from 7+ mm of advancement, then you should retract mandibular canines using posterior TADs as anchorage. Looking at Kaylee's initial profile (Figure 5.69c), we recommended a mild advancement of 3–4 mm (closing the extraction space reciprocally), plus an advancement genioplasty.

Q: If a nonsurgical approach is attempted, you need to decide if the patient should be treated nonextraction. What would be the advantages and disadvantages (costs and benefits) in treating Kaylee nonextraction?

A: The advantage of a nonextraction approach is that no permanent teeth will be removed. The cost is that as the mandibular incisors are aligned they will procline, and the open bite will worsen. Another disadvantage is that the thin tissue covering the lower incisor roots will be stressed—with gingival recession being a possibility.

Q: If a nonsurgical approach is attempted, you need to consider every reasonable combination of anterior and posterior extraction pattern before you decide what to do. Can you suggest extraction patterns and the cost/benefits of each?

A: Possible extraction patterns for Kaylee include the following:

- Extraction of a mandibular incisor. The advantage is that Kaylee's crowding can be eliminated without proclining her incisors and stressing her periodontal tissues. The disadvantage is that since her maxillary lateral incisors are not small (no anterior Bolton tooth size discrepancy exists), she will be left with excess OJ of the incisors and canines (i.e., canines will not be coordinated).
- Extraction of maxillary and mandibular first premolars. The advantage is that Kaylee's bite will tend to deepen as her incisors are retracted and uprighted. Also, the mandibular anterior periodontium will not be stressed. The disadvantage is that retracting maxillary incisors could reduce maxillary lip support and make her NLA more obtuse (worsening her profile).
- Extraction of maxillary and mandibular second premolars. The advantage is that less retraction of anterior teeth will occur—so less opening of her NLA will occur. The disadvantage is the same—less retraction of anterior teeth will occur—so there will be less uprighting of her proclined incisors/less closure of her open bite with uprighting of incisors. Extraction of second premolars offers little advantage over extraction of first premolars.
- Extraction of maxillary right second premolar, maxillary left first premolar, and mandibular first premolars. The advantage is that Kaylee's bite will tend to deepen as her incisors are retracted and uprighted, the mandibular anterior periodontium will not be stressed, and the right Class III relationship will be easier to correct with extraction of the maxillary right second premolar. The disadvantage is the reduction of maxillary lip support plus the fact that the maxillary arch is fairly symmetric (extracting asymmetrically will tend to overcorrect the right side, with the right canine becoming Class II).

Q: You meet with Kaylee and her parents for a case presentation. What treatment do you recommend as the most ideal?

A: Kaylee and her parents were advised that a surgical approach to treatment would provide the most ideal result. Kaylee and her parents declined surgery and stated that they only wanted alignment of her teeth.

Q: Should you recommend a nonsurgical treatment option, or should you decline treating Kaylee because they refused surgery?

A: If you can help address Kaylee's chief complaint by aligning her teeth, especially if you can align her teeth while leaving a possible future surgical option open, then you should offer a nonsurgical treatment option. Inform her and her parents that without surgery, you will be seeking improvement but may not be able to achieve an ideal result.

Q: How can you correct Kaylee's right Class III relationship, nonsurgically?

A: Remember, once her CR—CO shift was detected, Kaylee was found to be a molar Class III by 2 mm on her right side and molar Class I on her left (Figure 5.70). The most straightforward treatment would be to use (short) Class III elastics on the right (running from maxillary right premolars to mandibular right canine and first premolar). As a rule of thumb, *treat mild dental arch asymmetries with biomechanics as opposed to asymmetric extraction patterns*. So, if you believe that Kaylee requires extractions, consider extracting four first premolars and treating the small Class III relationship on the right with short elastics, as needed. Extracting asymmetrically is reasonable with more moderate-to-severe dental asymmetries in patients requiring extractions. In such cases, extracting asymmetrically can aid in improving symmetry.

Q: Considering Kaylee's previous chin cup history, what problem could you encounter using Class III elastics? How should you approach your use of Class III elastics, if you decide to use them?

A: Chin cup treatment was terminated earlier because it caused Kaylee TMJ pain. Elastics could, potentially, do the same thing as they pull the mandible back. It would be prudent to start with a very light Class III elastic force, and see how Kaylee responds, before increasing the force. If she develops joint pain, seriously consider discontinuing Class III elastics.

Q: What should you tell Kaylee and her parents about the probable success of her nonsurgical open bite closure and stability?

A: You should tell them that you may not be able to close her open bite or keep it closed (nonsurgically). We told them that we would attempt some open bite closure but that we could not say how much. They said, and we documented, that they understood.

Q: Kaylee and her parents declined surgery. After considering everything we have discussed, what nonsurgical treatment do you recommend?

A: Kaylee was treated with extraction of her four first premolars (Figure 5.75). Note in these figures the 2 mm Class III relationship on her right side and Class I relationship on her left.

Q: What are the specific objectives of treatment for the maxilla, mandible, maxillary dentition, and mandibular dentition in all three planes of space?

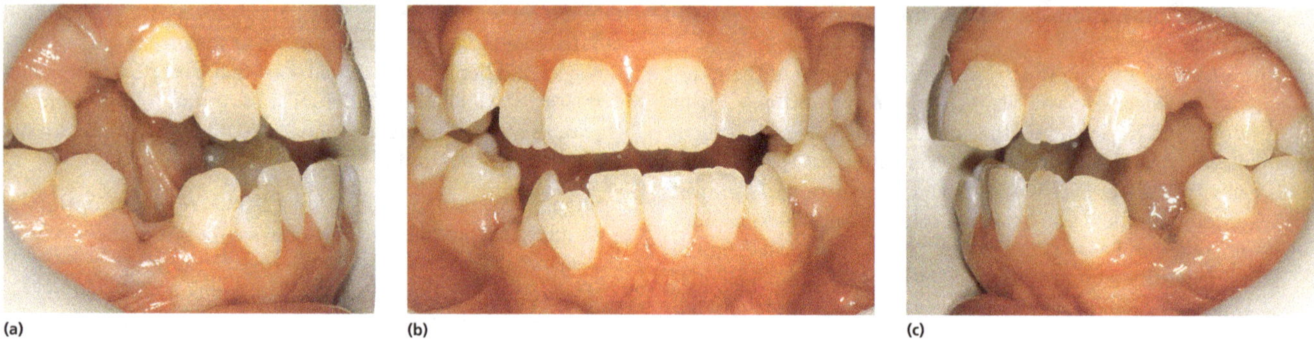

Figure 5.75 (a–c) Progress photos of Kaylee following extraction of first premolars.

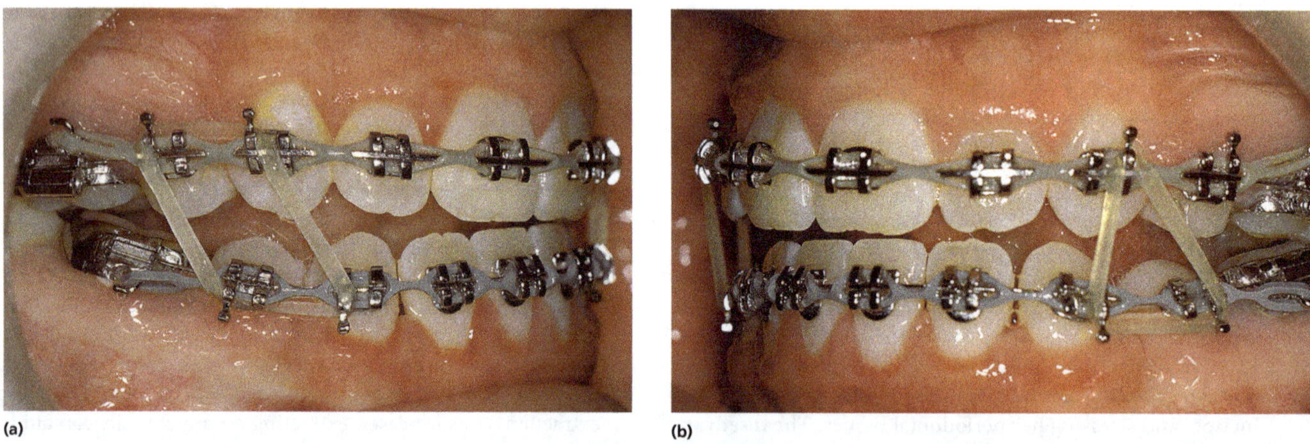

Figure 5.76 Kaylee during reciprocal space closure wearing elastics that provide an anterior vertical force: (a) short Class III parallelogram right and (b) triangle left.

A: Specific objectives of treatment for Kaylee are as follows:

Maxilla

AP: Allow for remaining growth.

Vertical: Allow for remaining growth.

Transverse: Allow for remaining growth.

Mandible

AP: Allow for remaining growth.

Vertical: Allow for remaining growth.

Transverse: Allow for remaining growth.

Maxillary dentition

AP: Protract molars and retract canines. Retract and upright incisors.

Vertical: Level occlusal plane by extruding incisors relative to molars.

Intermolar width: Decrease intermolar width by molar protraction.

Mandibular dentition

AP: Protract molars and retract canines. Retract and upright incisors.

Vertical: Eliminate reverse curve of Spee.

Intermolar/intercanine width: Decrease intermolar width by molar protraction. Increase intercanine width by canine retraction.

Q: How did Kaylee's treatment proceed?

A: Fixed appliances were placed. Her second molars were NOT bonded as a precaution to avoid distal tipping/eruption of mandibular second molars during leveling (thus worsening her open bite)—despite the fact that her mandibular second molars do not appear mesially tipped (Figure 5.70a, c). Arches were leveled and aligned. Extraction spaces were closed reciprocally. A (short) Class III parallelogram elastic on the right, and a triangle elastic on the left, were worn (Figure 5.76).

The left elastic was later changed to a Class II parallelogram (Figure 5.77). Notice that the anterior open bite is beginning to close as anterior teeth are retracted and erupted.

After obtaining a Class I canine relationship on the right, the right elastic was changed to a triangle elastic (Figure 5.78).

Q: Once Kaylee's open bite is closed and her AP corrected, should you immediately discontinue treatment and deband?

A: No. It would be prudent to keep her in "active retention" for months, gradually decreasing her elastic wear—to see how your correction holds. If she looks like she is stable, stop elastic wear and see how she responds for some months. If you find your correction holding, and only if you find your correction holding, then consider debanding. This was *not* done in Kaylee's case. She was immediately debanded when her open bite closure was achieved. This was a mistake.

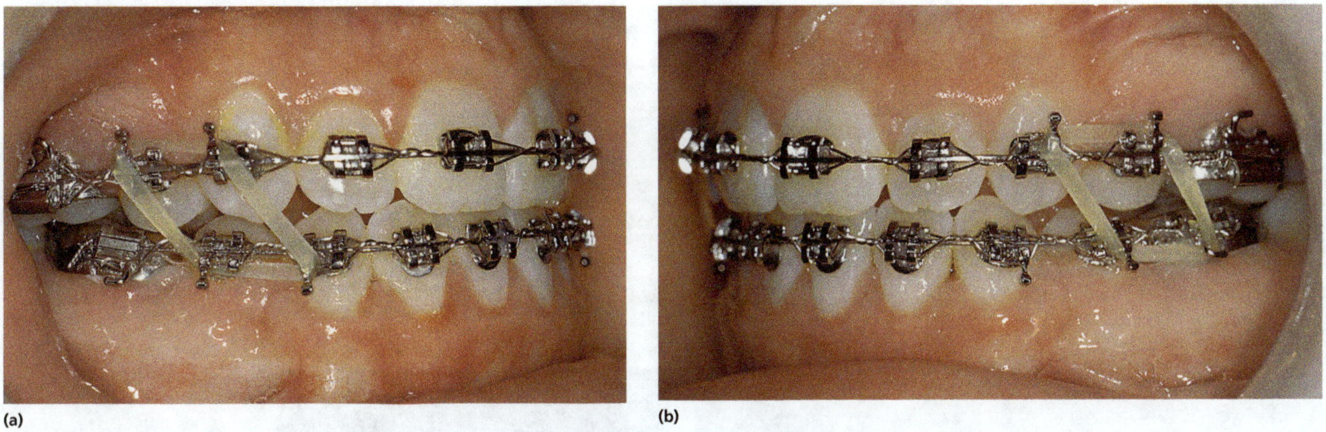

Figure 5.77 As her open bite was closing, and as her AP relationship was improving, Kaylee continued to wear elastics: (a) Class III parallelogram elastic on her right side and (b) her left elastic was changed to a Class II parallelogram.

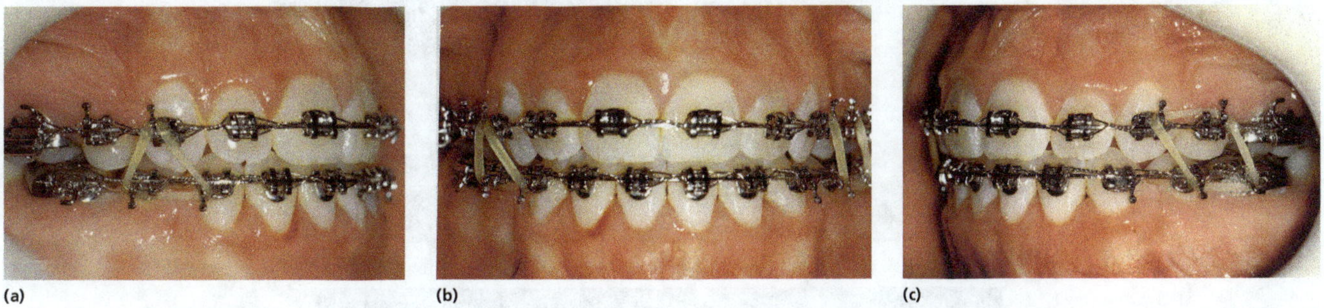

Figure 5.78 Following correction of her right Class III relationship, Kaylee's (a) right elastic was changed to a triangle elastic and (b, c) she continued to wear a Class II parallelogram elastic on her left.

Q: Kaylee's deband records are shown in Figure 5.79. What do you note?

A: Kaylee had an acceptable, nonsurgical, result. Observations include the following:

- Facial proportions, profile, and NLA appear unchanged (note that the right side of her face has always appeared fuller than her left, Figures 5.69a and 5.79a).
- ILG is still present.
- Chin is still deviated to the left.
- Maxillary midline is to the right of the facial midline and to the right of the mandibular midline (Figure 5.79b, i)
- Her mandible has rotated down and back (Figure 5.79f) due to eruption of the maxillary and mandibular molars (note that the maxillary corpus did not descend).
- Her LAFH has increased from 58% to 59% (Figures 5.69e and 5.79e) due to the mandibular downward and backward rotation.
- Maxillary and mandibular incisors were erupted and uprighted (especially maxillary incisors, Figure 5.79f).
- Approximately 10% overbite was achieved.
- Right first molars are not in occlusion on mesial.
- Class I canine and molar relationships have been achieved.
- Maxillary posterior labial crown torque has been reduced slightly (Figures 5.72a and 5.79r), but mandibular posterior lingual crown torque has remained about the same (Figures 5.72b and 5.79s).
- Hygiene improved (without improved oral hygiene, Kaylee's treatment would have been compromised).

Q: How was Kaylee's open bite corrected?

A: Her open bite was corrected by maxillary and mandibular incisor eruption (Figure 5.79f) with vertical elastics and with incisor retraction/uprighting around their apicies during space closure. The open bite was closed by incisor eruption despite the downward and backward (CW) rotation of the mandible as molars erupted.

Q: A major concern was that Kaylee's obtuse NLA would increase, adversely impacting profile esthetics, with extraction of maxillary premolars and retraction of incisors. Why would this happen?

A: Studies indicate that as maxillary incisors retract, maxillary lips retract. This is in a ratio of 1 mm of maxillary lip retraction to every 2–3 mm of incisor retraction [42, 134]. In other words, if Kaylee's incisors were retracted about 4 mm (Figure 5.79f, see maxillary superimposition) her maxillary lip would be expected to retract up to 2 mm. This is exactly what happened (Figure 5.79f, see cranial base superimposition).

Q: Even though Kaylee's maxillary lip retracted, her NLA did not increase (compare Figure 5.69c to Figure 5.79c). Why?

A: Looking at her cranial base superimposition (Figure 5.79f), we see that Kaylee's nose grew downward, keeping her NLA about the same. If Kaylee had been treated similarly after growth had ceased, then her NLA may have opened.

Q: Should an RME appliance have been used?

A: Yes, at least attempted. At Kaylee's age, her facial skeletal resistance may have been too great to permit a midpalatal sutural

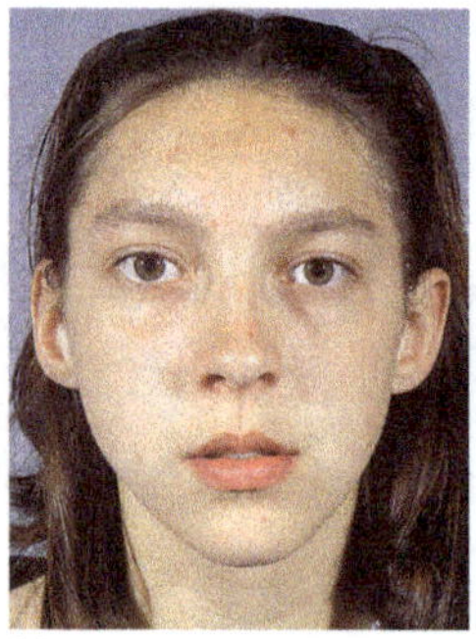
(a)

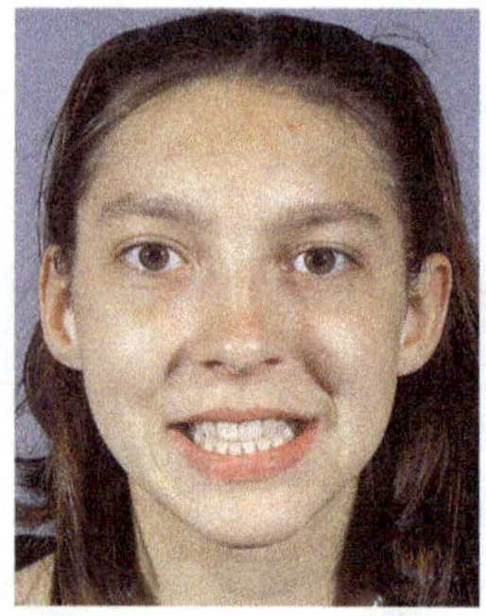
(b)

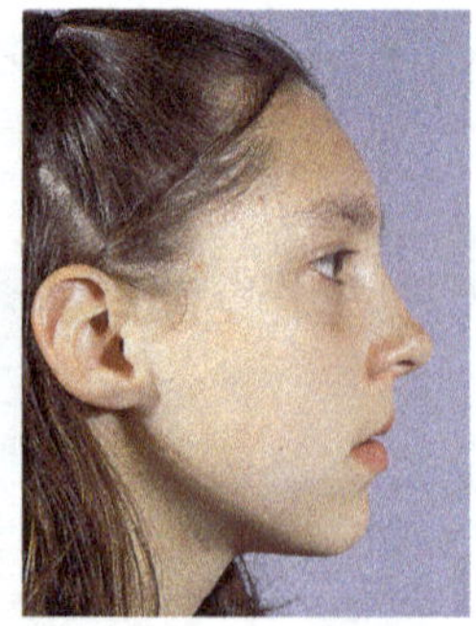
(c)

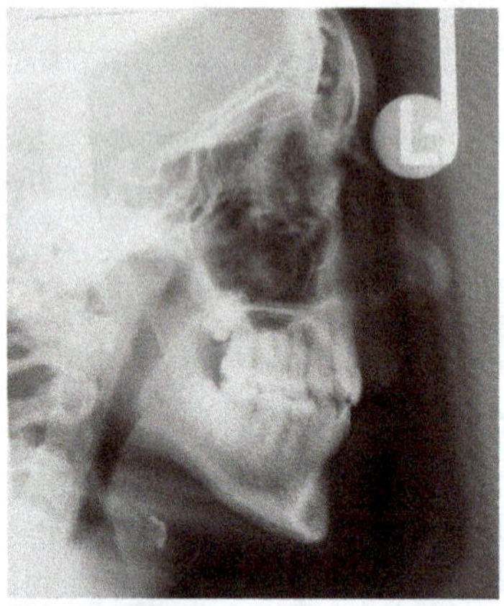
(d)

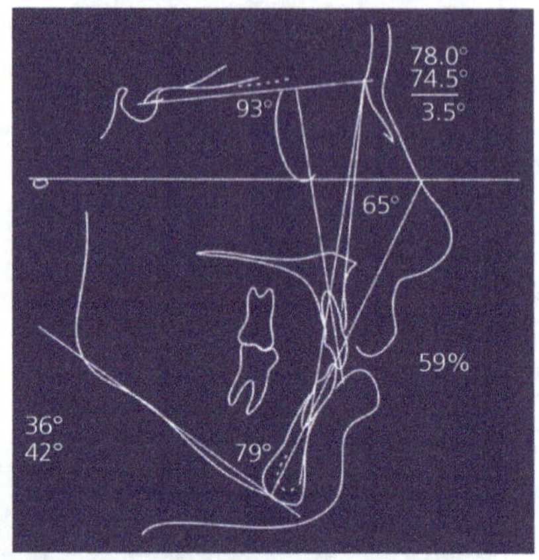

(e)

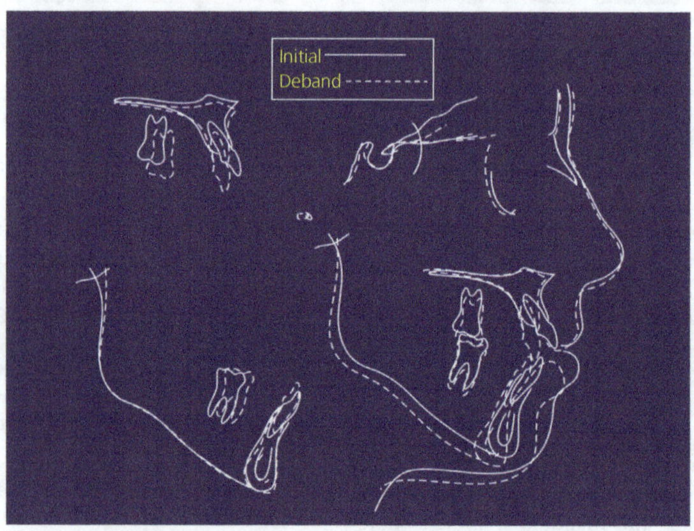

(f)

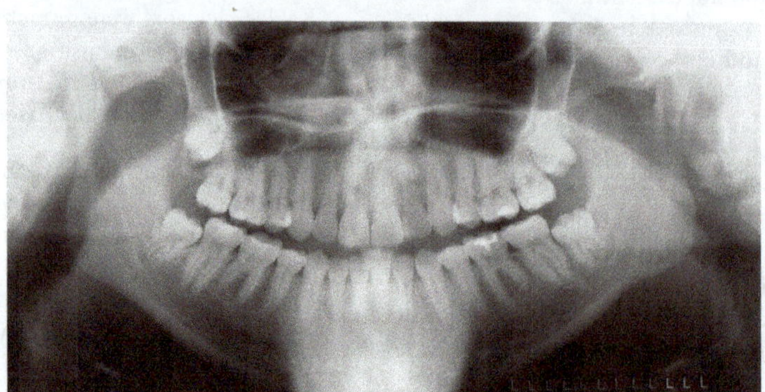
(g)

Figure 5.79 (a–s) Kaylee's deband records.

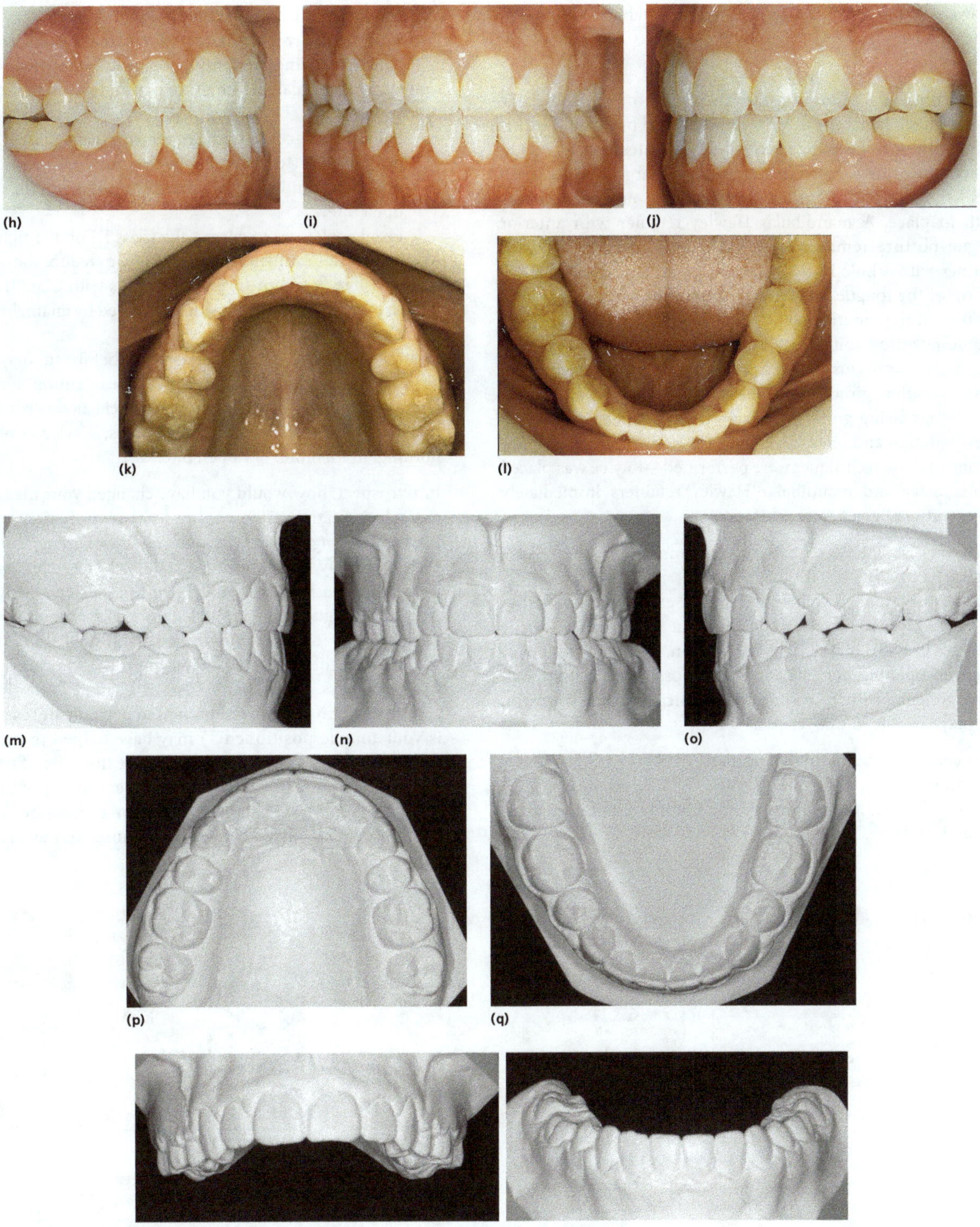

Figure 5.79 (Continued)

split/skeletal expansion using an RME appliance. But, you could have attempted RME. If you had been successful in achieving a midpalatal split, then you could have created posterior OJ, permitting removal of posterior transverse compensations, and provided additional arch perimeter. If you had been unsuccessful in achieving a midpalatal split, then you could have considered slow maxillary dental expansion using the expander to gain some OJ.

Q: What retention principles should you follow with Kaylee?

A: First, remember the direction of active tooth movement. The anterior open bite was closed by masking—eruption of the maxillary and mandibular anterior teeth. Expect the anterior teeth to intrude and the open bite to reoccur over time. Second, watch for any residual vertical skeletal growth with the maxilla descending and the mandible rotating down and back. Third, be aware of Kaylee's tongue interpositional habit in the design of her retainers and retention protocol.

Q: How would you retain her?

A: Small composite buttons could be placed on the maxillary anterior teeth labial surfaces. A Hawley labial bow could be fitted over these to keep the maxillary anterior teeth erupted. Or, a vacuum-formed clear retainer could be fabricated to "snap over" the composite buttons and hold the erupted anterior teeth in place. A mandibular Hawley retainer with anterior tongue posture reminders (spurs), and a maxillary Hawley retainer with a hole in the palate could be fabricated to draw the tip of the tongue away from the anterior teeth and toward the roof of the mouth (in anticipation of a continued anterior tongue posture habit). If a slight anterior open bite occurred later, posterior occlusal adjustment (enameloplasty) could help close it—after growth was clearly finished. Finally, daily exercise (chewing gum) could help to maintain the corrected interdigitation and bite.

None of these techniques were performed—Kaylee was placed in maxillary and mandibular Hawley retainers immediately after treatment goals were achieved.

Q: Two years later, Kaylee presents with some open bite relapse (Figure 5.80). Why has this happened?

A: This relapse probably follows the incisor eruption with elastics plus the Class III correction on the right with elastics (as she becomes Class III on the right in retention, her incisors hit edge to edge—opening her bite). It is also possible that interpositional tongue posture, or continued vertical maxillary growth, has played a role in this relapse.

Q: How could you deal with this relapse?

A: You could:

1. Do nothing, if Kaylee is happy and not interested in correcting the relapse.
2. Re-treat after a more comprehensive evaluation of Kaylee's relapse etiology is conducted (evaluation of continued tongue posturing and cephalometric evaluation of post-treatment vertical growth). Options for treatment include the following:
   - Fixed appliances in both arches with short Class III elastics on the right (to create OJ, correct midlines, and close the open bite) and vertical triangles on the left (to close the open bite).
   - Fixed appliances to correct the Class III on the right—then, occlusal adjustment (enameloplasty) to reduce the open bite.
   - Invisible (vacuum-formed) retainers with Class III elastics to buttons on her right side—followed by enameloplasty to close the open bite.

Remember, if the open bite relapsed before, it may relapse again. If you retreat, hold Kaylee in "active retention" for months after bite closure, then wean her off the elastics as you confirm that the bite is stable. Of these options, Kaylee chose to do nothing, to maintain her open bite.

Q: In retrospect, how would you have changed your management of Kaylee's treatment?

A: *First, a more aggressive approach to Kaylee's tongue interposition habit* may have improved stability. The habit (and need to correct the habit) should have been discussed with her. Adding a tongue habit appliance during treatment (lower lingual holding arch with tongue spurs soldered along the anterior segment of the arch) and attempting to increase Kaylee's self-awareness of her habit (use of a small digital timer or smart phone to prompt the patient to periodically ask "Where is your tongue positioned?") may have helped to reduce the frequency of the habit. Additionally, at the time of retention, a reinforcement of habit self-awareness along with one of the aforementioned retainer designs may have been helpful to improve stability. However, because self-awareness of

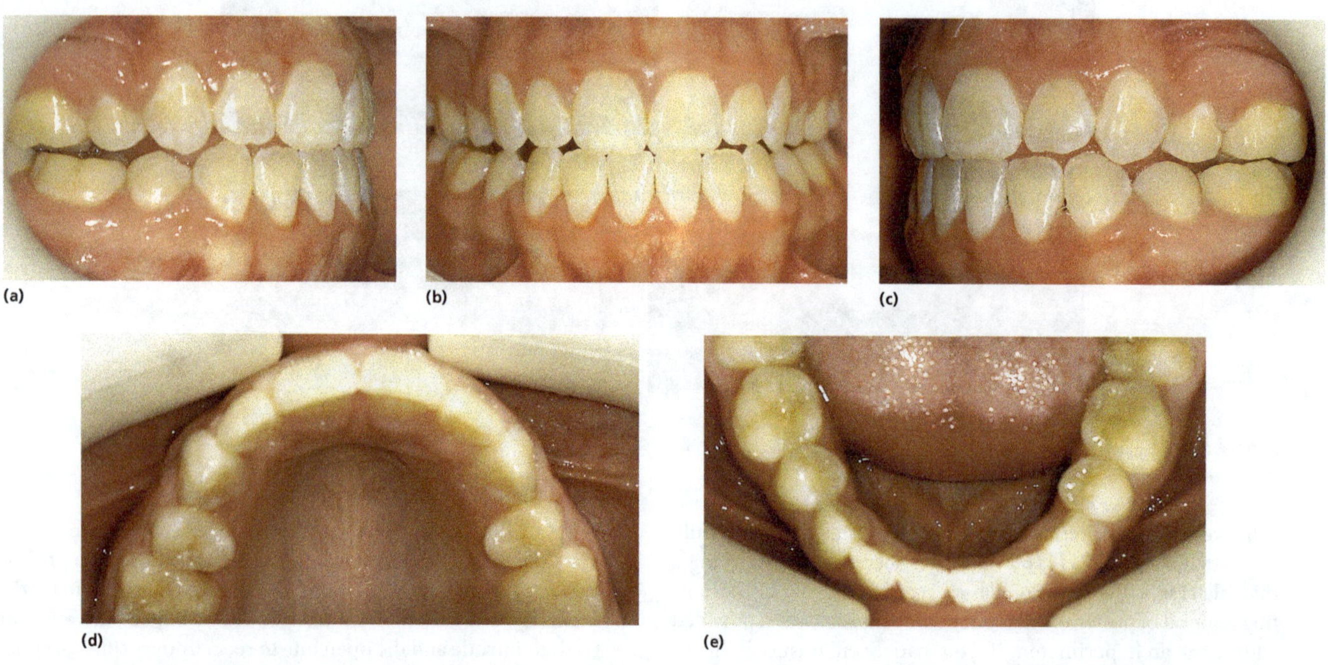

Figure 5.80 (a–e) Two-year posttreatment intraoral photographs of Kaylee. Note some relapse of her open bite and some relapse of her right Class III correction.

the habit is key to successful habit cessation, long-term stability is dependent on the individual patient, and thus the probability of long-term stability remains largely unknown. *Second, after successfully correcting her open bite and Class III relationship, you should keep Kaylee in "active retention."* Keep her in braces, slowly discontinue elastics, and maintain her in braces (without elastics) for months before debanding (to insure treatment stability). *Third, overcorrect her OB to 20–40%.*

Q: What are the "take-home" messages from this patient's treatment?

A: Take home messages include the following:

- Kaylee presented with a combination skeletal and dental open bite. Her skeletal open bite resulted from condyles growing posterior-superiorly instead of more vertically, lack of posterior face height development, a lack of normal forward mandibular internal (true) rotation, excessive maxillary corpus descent, and molars erupting more than normal (especially her maxillary molars). As her mandible rotated downward and backward, the mandibular plane angle steepened, the anterior lower face height lengthened, and her anterior skeletal open bite resulted. Her dental open bite was the product of her past thumb habit history and her current anterior interpositional tongue habit.
- Checking for (and documenting) a CR—CO shift is critical for diagnosis and treatment planning. If you are not sure whether there is a shift, do not define your final treatment plan until you have determined CR. You may not be able to do this until both arches have been leveled and aligned or, in some cases, until the maxilla has been expanded with an RME appliance. *Check for a CR—CO shift on every patient at every appointment.*
- Later detection of an (initially) undetected CR—CO shift changed Kaylee's AP relationship dramatically—from Class III by 3 mm bilaterally—to Class III by 2 mm on the right and Class I on the left.
- Orthopedic treatment was not the ideal alternative for treating Kaylee's VME since she had reached menarche (1½–2 years ago) and completed her growth spurt. However, her parents stated that she could still be growing, "a little," so you needed to monitor her growth closely. Also, most orthopedic treatments to address her VME would have tended to rotate her mandible upward and forward (CCW), worsening her Class III relationship. High-pull chin cup wear was the one orthopedic approach that could have prevented both VME and Class III from worsening. You could have used high-pull chin cup for a trial period to confirm that she was not growing. But, you would have to monitor its use closely since Kaylee had developed TMJ pain when wearing one before.
- Surgery, probably the ideal option, was declined by her and her parents. But, if surgery is an option, you must discuss it with the patient.
- Masking her skeletal open bite (forced eruption of her incisors with vertical elastics plus incisor eruption as her incisors were uprighted/retracted around their apicies) was considered reasonable since: extraction of her four first premolars would help address her chief complaint (anterior crowding); her initial incisal display at rest (~2 mm) was not excessive; her incisors were proclined; and she exhibited mild-to-moderate anterior crowding. The amount of maxillary incisor uprighting and eruption was excessive.
- *The problem with a masking approach to treating skeletal anterior open bites is relapse.* Extrusion of anterior teeth can close open bites. But this movement can be very unstable. Additionally, in many cases of skeletal open bites, eruption of anterior teeth can result in excessive incisal and gingival display. Do not erupt anterior teeth more than is acceptable esthetically.
- Kaylee's NLA would normally be expected to increase as her maxillary lip retracted during maxillary incisor retraction. This can have potentially adverse effects on the patient's profile (it did not here only because Kaylee's nose grew downward simultaneously).
- In open bite cases, let the parents and patients know that you will try your best to achieve closure, but that (depending on cooperation, growth, etc.) you may not be able to close it or keep it closed.
- Methods to improve self-awareness of an interpositional tongue habit should be part of the overall treatment plan and retention protocol. This was not done with Kaylee. Her tongue habit was ignored. Her habit should have been addressed with habit awareness aids during treatment and in her retainers.
- Final OB should have overcorrected to 20–40%, instead of only 10% (anticipating future relapse).
- Retention of an open bite correction is just as important as the correction itself. Follow the suggestions made in this case report, including the concept of "active retention" before removing appliances. Once you achieve your treatment goals, maintain the patient in active retention as you slowly diminish your mechanics (i.e., elastic wear) and monitor stability before debanding. *It was a mistake to deband Kaylee as soon as treatment goals were achieved.*

Case Greg

Greg is 39 years old and presents to you with the chief complaint, "I have problems with my overbite, my open bite, my chewing, and my breathing." His PMH includes sleep apnea (height 5′10,″ morbid obesity, weight of 310 lb, two recent polysomnography tests) for which he wears a CPAP every night. His PDH is WRN. TMJ evaluation is WRN, maximal incisal opening (MIO) is 60 mm, and CR=CO (Figure 5.81).

Q: List diagnostic findings/problems. What is your diagnosis?

A: See Table 5.7.

Q: Greg suffers from sleep apnea. What are the forms of sleep apnea?

A: Central (CSA), obstructive (OSA), and complex or mixed sleep apnea (a combination of central and obstructive). In CSA, breathing is interrupted by a lack of respiratory effort. In OSA, breathing is interrupted by a physical block to airflow despite respiratory effort [135].

Q: Name some examples of structural components that can cause a physical blockage and OSA.

A: Collapse of the alar cartilage (resulting in airflow reduction at the nasal valve), septal deviations, enlarged turbinates, narrow nasal floor, lymphoid hyperplasia (the most common cause of airway obstruction in adolescents), and mandibular retrognathia [136].

Q: What are the common signs and symptoms of sleep apnea?

A: Snoring, daytime fatigue, slower reaction time, vision problems [137], and behavioral effects including moodiness, belligerence, as well as a decrease in attentiveness and drive [138].

Q: How is sleep apnea diagnosed?

A: The diagnosis of sleep apnea is based on both evaluation of clinical symptoms (excessive daytime sleepiness and fatigue) and the results of a formal sleep study (*polysomnography*) or

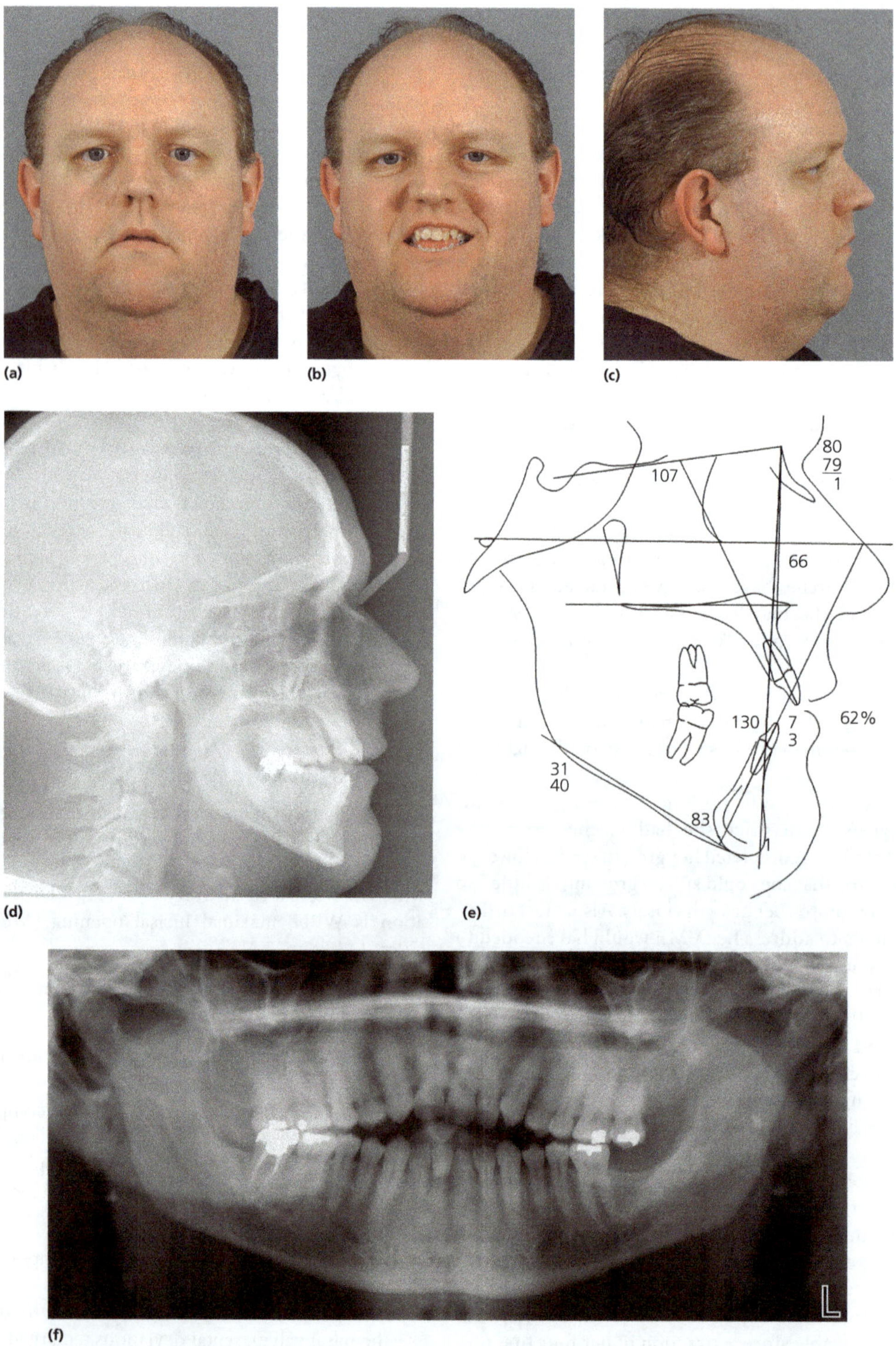

Figure 5.81 Initial records of Greg: (a–c) initial facial photographs, (d) lateral cephalograph, (e) cephalometric tracing, (f) pantomograph,

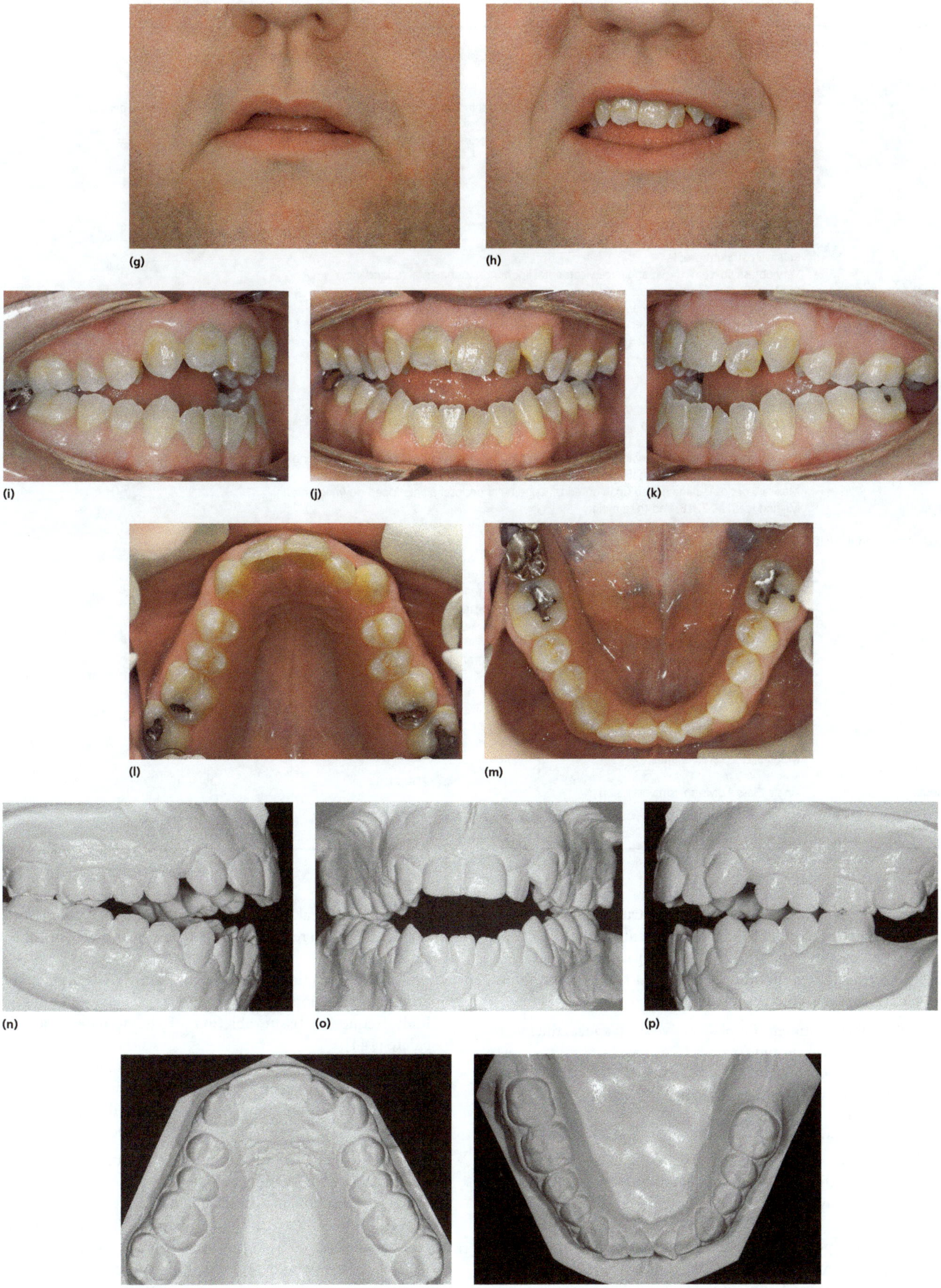

Figure 5.81 (Continued) (g) relaxed lip position, (h) posed smile, (i–m) intraoral photographs, and (n–r) model photographs.

Table 5.7 Diagnostic findings and problem list for Greg.

Full face and profile	**Frontal view** LLAFH (soft tissue Glabella–Subnasale << Subnasale–soft tissue Menton) ILG 7–8 mm Minimal incisal display at rest Ideal central incisor display in posed smile (maxillary central incisor gingival margins congruent with vermillion margin of upper lip) Upper lip length 24 mm Exaggerated cupid's bow (philtrum length exceeds commissure height by >2–3 mm) UDML 3 mm right of facial center LDML on with face Large buccal corridors Narrow nares—alar base width 36 mm **Profile view** Slightly obtuse nasolabial angle Relatively straight profile Very obtuse lip–chin–throat angle (cervicomental lipomatosis/submental redundancy)
Ceph analysis	**Skeletal** AP positions of maxilla and mandible are WRN LLAFH (LAFH/TAFH = 62%, over three standard deviations greater than an average of 55%, SD = 2%) Steep MPA (FMA = 31°; SNMP = 40°) Maxillary first molar apices are erupted well below the palatal plane VME Short posterior face height Slightly effective bony Pogonion Effective soft tissue Pogonion **Dental** Slight proclination of maxillary incisors (1 to SN = 107°, but the maxillary central incisor's long axis projects through the distal of the orbit properly) Ideal mandibular incisor inclination (FMIA = 65°) Maxillary occlusal plane tipped up in anterior; mandibular occlusal plane tipped down in anterior
Radiographs	Missing teeth #s 7, 18, and third molars Endodontic treatment tooth #31
Intraoral photos and models	Angle Class II division 1 malocclusion Iowa Classification: II (2–3) II (5) II (5) II (3) OJ: 6 mm 10 mm anterior open bite extending from right first molar to left second premolar Maxillary anterior teeth stepped up ~2–3 mm relative to posterior teeth Mandibular anterior teeth stepped down ~2–3 mm Bilateral posterior cross bite Intermolar widths (maxillary first molar palatal cups = 39 mm, mandibular first molars central fossae = 45 mm) Maxillary anterior spacing (UTSALD = +2–3 mm) Mild mandibular anterior crowding (LTSALD = −3 mm) Maxillary arch symmetric Mandibular arch asymmetrical: right posterior slightly ahead Hourglass shape of maxillary arch Mottled, discolored enamel
Other	—
Diagnosis	Angle Class II division 1 malocclusion Skeletal anterior open bite Posterior cross bite

oximetry. Typical values indicative of obstructive sleep apnea include a hypopnea index score (apnea events lasting ≥10 seconds divided by number of hours of sleep) greater than 5, a decrease in oxygen saturation (<90%), and clinical symptoms (excessive daytime sleepiness) [136].

Q: Name possible treatments for obstructive sleep apnea, the most common form of sleep apnea.

A: Possible treatments include:

- Avoiding alcohol or muscle relaxants.
- Losing weight.
- Smoking cessation.
- Sleeping with a 30° elevation of the upper body [139] or sleeping on the side (preventing gravitational collapse of the airway) as opposed to sleeping in a supine position [140–142].
- Continuous positive airway pressure (CPAP)—the most effective treatment for obstructive sleep apnea [143].
- Use of various oral appliances to keep the airway open, especially in patients who refuse CPAP or surgery.
- Soft tissue surgical procedures (uvulopalatopharyngoplasty—UPPP or UP3) to remove and tighten tissue or tracheostomy if necessary.
- Septoplasty, functional rhinoplasty, nasal valve surgery, and turbinate reduction.
- Radiofrequency tissue ablation of the tongue base and palate [144].
- Maxillomandibular advancement jaw osteotomies—to increase the pharyngeal diameter, tighten surrounding tissues, and decrease the collapsibility of the airway during sleep. A minimum of 10 mm advancement (at Pogonion) is advocated.

Q: Which oral mandibular advancement appliances (nonsurgical) are beneficial in the treatment of OSA?

A: All active mandibular advancement devices improve the apnea–hypopnea index or the respiratory disturbance index scores when compared to inactive appliances. Mandibular advancement appears to be crucial for treatment success, but oral appliances may not address all causative elements of the disorder [145].

Q: Can the long-term use of oral appliances for treating obstructive sleep apnea cause occlusal changes?

A: Yes. In a study of 70 patients—after 7 years of oral appliance wear for obstructive sleep apnea, 14% had no occlusal changes, 41% had favorable occlusal changes, and 44% had unfavorable occlusal changes changes [146].

Q: What is the success of maxillomandibular advancement in treating OSA?

A: In a recent systematic review, the reported success rates ranged from 65 to 100% [147]. In one prospective randomized controlled trial, no significant difference was found between a ventilation therapy group and a maxillomandibular advancement group at 1 year post treatment.

Q: Looking back at Greg, what else should you check for in your initial examination? What other questions should you ask?

A: Even though skeletal anterior open bites result from excessive vertical growth, a functional component (dental open bite) may also be present. If a functional habit is missed and/or not corrected, then the open bite treatment can relapse. You carefully watch Greg and notice that he interposes his tongue between his front teeth (Figure 5.82). Also, an anterior open bite can result from condylar degeneration—with the mandible rotating downward and backward. You check Greg's screening panoramic image (Figure 5.81f) and confirm that the joints appear normal. Ask Greg how long he has had the open bite (did he develop it recently following an injury?). He states that he has always had it. Finally, be sure to check for a temporary open bite resulting from permanent teeth erupting, ankylosis of anterior teeth that are not fully erupted, and lack of space for complete eruption of permanent teeth. Greg does not appear to exhibit these possible open bite etiologies.

Q: What other records would be helpful?

A: Left and right 3/4 facial images (Figure 5.83a, b) should be made to check the degree of malar projection. Greg's malar projection seems adequate. The presence of a posterior occlusal cant can be checked by having Greg hold a tongue blade between the posterior teeth (Figure 5.83c). You can see the absence of an occlusal cant—the tongue blade appears to parallel his interpupillary line.

Q: How else would you examine his models?

A: Examine the separated models to determine maxillary and mandibular posterior crown torque (Figure 5.84). Note that the maxillary first premolars exhibit lingual crown torque, while the remaining maxillary posterior teeth exhibit mild labial crown torque (transverse dental compensations). The mandibular first molars exhibit slight lingual crown torque. Models were also examined from the lingual which confirmed Greg's Class II molar relationship.

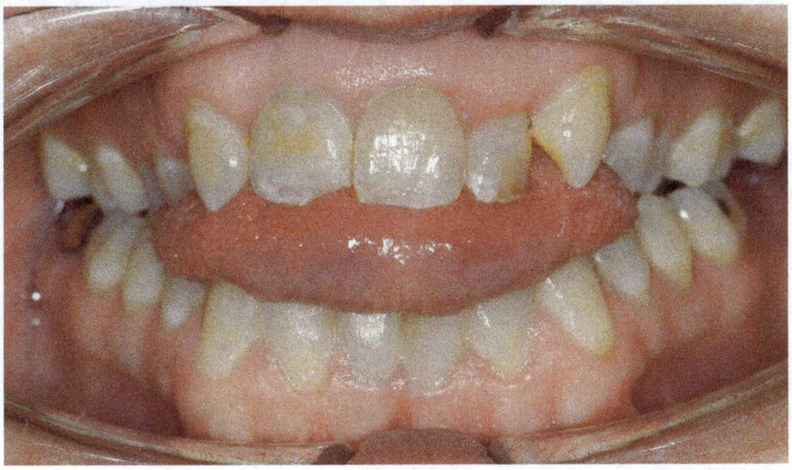

Figure 5.82 Greg's anterior tongue interposition habit.

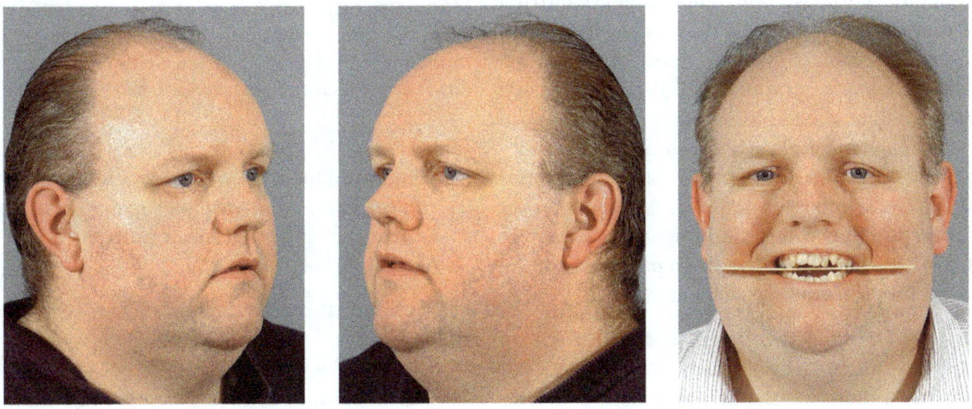

(a) (b) (c)

Figure 5.83 (a, b) Greg in 3/4 facial views and (c) with a tongue blade held between the posterior teeth to check for an occlusal cant.

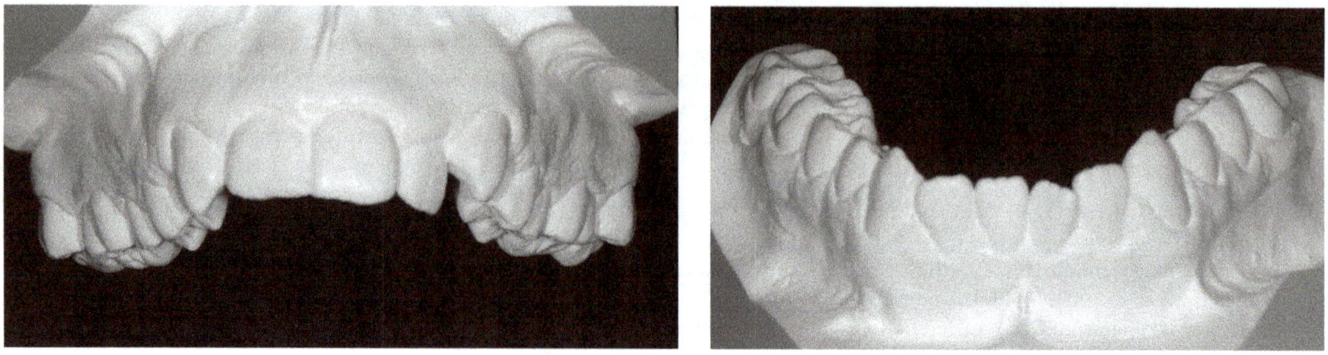

(a) (b)

Figure 5.84 (a, b) Separated model views to evaluate maxillary and mandibular posterior crown torque.

Q: In terms of his anterior open bite, does Greg exhibit features of a dental open bite? A skeletal open bite? List these features.

A: His *dental* open bite features include the following:

- Interpositional tongue habit
- Maxillary anterior teeth stepped up ~2–3 mm
- Mandibular anterior teeth stepped down ~2–3 mm

His *skeletal* open bite features include the following:

- Soft tissue LLAFH (Glabella–Subnasale << Subnasale–soft tissue Menton)
- Skeletal LLAFH (LAFH/TAFH = 62%)
- Steep MPA (FMA = 31° and SNMP = 40°)
- First molar root apicies erupted well below the palatal plane
- VME
- ILG
- Anterior open bite extending from right molar and left second premolar
- Short posterior face height

Q: Which type of open bite does he have?

A: Greg has a combination of dental and skeletal open bite.

Q: What is the etiology of Greg's anterior open bite? How will this etiology affect his treatment?

A: Greg's *dental* open bite resulted from an anterior interpositional tongue habit. His habit could adversely impact our ability to correct his open bite and to maintain stability of the correction. His *skeletal* open bite resulted from a classic skeletal open bite pattern of growth including condyles growing posterior-superiorly (Figure 5.85, curved red arrow), lack of posterior face height development, backward mandibular internal (true) rotation (curved blue arrows), maxilla descending more than normal, and maxillary molars erupting more than normal (maxillary molar root apicies erupting well below his palatal plane). As his mandible rotated downward and backward (yellow arrow), his mandibular plane angle steepened, his anterior face height increased, an ILG formed, and the anterior open bite resulted. The fact that his growth is finished removes one variable from our treatment planning, but the severe magnitude of his vertical apical base discrepancy will make treatment, and stability of treatment, challenging.

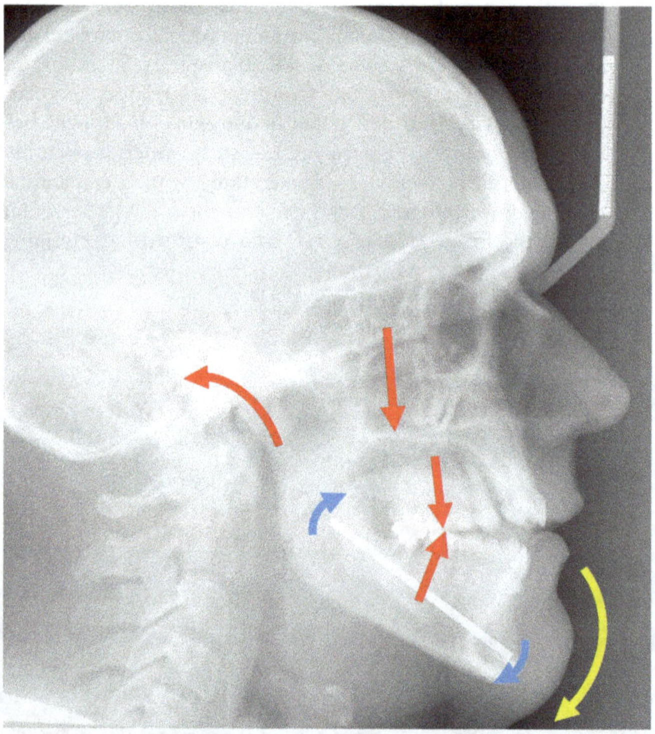

Figure 5.85 Greg illustrates a classic skeletal open bite growth pattern: condyles growing posterior-superiorly, lack of posterior face height development, backward mandibular internal (true) rotation, maxilla descending more than normal, and molars erupting more than normal (maxillary molar root apicies erupted well below his palatal plane). As his mandible rotated down and back, Greg's mandibular plane steepened, his lower anterior face height increased, and his skeletal open bite resulted.

Q: A good principle is for the orthodontist to stay focused on the *major* problems the patient presents with in the AP, vertical, and transverse dimensions, plus other major problems (e.g. impacted teeth). The idea being that once you correct the major problems, then you can move on to the smaller problems. But, if you focus on smaller problems, then you lose sight of the bigger ones. What are Greg's major (primary) problems in each dimension and other major problems?

A: See Table 5.8.

Q: Simply stated, anterior open bites can be treated in only one of two ways. Describe them. Which would you use to you treat Greg, and why?

A: The two approaches for correcting anterior open bites are erupting anterior teeth (generally used to correct dental open bites) and intruding posterior teeth (generally used to correct

Table 5.8 Primary problems list for Greg *(apical base/skeletal discrepancies italicized).*

AP	II (2–3) II (5) II (5) II (3) Skeletal relationships WRN
Vertical	*VME, skeletal open bite*
Transverse	Bilateral posterior cross bite *Mild maxillary skeletal transverse deficiency*
Other	Missing teeth #s 7, 18

skeletal open bites). Because Greg presents with a combination dental and skeletal open bite, both approaches will need to be used in his treatment. *Erupting anterior teeth:* Greg's anterior tongue interpositional habit has prevented his maxillary (stepped up) and mandibular (stepped down) incisors from erupting. If this habit were eliminated, then his incisors would erupt, his open bite would start to close, and the stability of his open bite correction would be enhanced. Although some patients with tongue interposition habits eliminate the habit as a result of orthodontic bite closure, this cannot be guaranteed. The best approach to dealing with tongue habits is to *eliminate the habit before treatment begins.* Greg's stepped up maxillary incisors, and stepped down mandibular incisors, could then be erupted using fixed orthodontic appliances and leveled with the posterior teeth (Figure 5.86a). Incisor eruption is especially viable since he currently exhibits only minimal incisal display when relaxed. Because Greg has only slight proclination of his maxillary incisors, and ideal mandibular incisor inclination, retraction/uprighting of his incisors (rotating them around their apicies/erupting them), would not be ideal and is not recommended (Figure 5.86b). *Intruding posterior teeth* (Figure 5.86c): intruding Greg's mandibular posterior teeth with TADs, intruding his maxillary posterior teeth with TADs, or intruding his maxillary posterior teeth with a LeFort I maxillary impaction osteotomy, would permit upward and forward (CCW) autorotation of his mandible around the condyles, reduction of his LLAFH, reduction or elimination of his ILG, and closure of his anterior open bite.

Q: What are your treatment goals?

A: Your highest priority should be to *avoid compromising Greg's airway* or worsening his sleep apnea. If Greg was a patient where a mandibular setback was necessary, then potential airway problems could prohibit surgery. Additional goals are to address Greg's occlusal and chewing concerns, address his postural tongue habit, correct his cross bite, align and coordinate his arches, achieve a Class I canine relationship with overcorrected overbite (20–40% OB) and minimal overjet, and deal with his missing maxillary right lateral incisor.

Q: How would you address Greg's vertical apical base discrepancy?

A: *Orthopedics* (treatment attempting to reduce downward descent of the maxilla and reduce eruption of the maxillary and mandibular molars during growth). Orthopedics (HPHG, active vertical correctors, etc.) to modify jaw growth is not an option since Greg has finished growing. However, we could consider posterior tooth intrusion with TADs as a form of orthopedics.

Let's look at an example of this approach (Figure 5.87). A 16-year, 7-month-old female with a skeletal open bite malocclusion presents for treatment (Figure 5.87a–d). She and her parents decline a surgical option, and treatment proceeds with TAD-supported maxillary molar intrusion. An intrusion arch (Figure 5.87e–h) to the maxillary molars is supported, bilaterally, by rigidly connected maxillary premolars and canines (supported themselves by TADs, indirect anchorage). Note on the cephalometric superimposition (Figure 5.87j) the significant maxillary molar intrusion which occurred and which allowed CCW rotation of the mandible/open bite closure (Figure 5.87i–m).

Now, let's go back to Greg. Intruding the maxillary and mandibular molars with TADs could permit the mandible to autorotate forward and upward (rotate CCW), reducing the interlabial gap and closing his open bite. With an anterior open bite of approximating 8 mm, you would need to intrude the molars by ~4 mm (since the mandible is rotating around a fulcrum, the condyle). This means that if you intruded the maxillary molars by 2 mm and the mandibular molars by 2 mm, then his open bite would close. TAD-supported molar intrusion to close Greg's open bite is a viable alternative.

Masking or camouflage (achieve open bite closure without addressing the underlying vertical apical base discrepancy). Erupting his anterior teeth to close his open bite would not reduce Greg's interlabial gap. Erupting his anterior teeth could increase his incisal/gingival display to an undesirable degree and may be very unstable.

Surgery: A differential maxillary impaction osteotomy (PNS intruded, ANS not intruded) could provide an ideal result. Further, if his jaws are brought forward surgically, then his sleep apnea may be improved.

Q: How would you address Greg's transverse apical base discrepancy?

A: *Orthopedics* (widening the maxillary dental arch by separating hemi-maxillae at the midpalatal suture). RME—the facial skeletal resistance of a 39-year-old would be too great to permit sutural splitting and separation of the hemi-maxillae.

Masking or camouflage (correcting the posterior cross bite by lateral dental translation, increasing maxillary labial crown torque, increasing mandibular lingual crown torque, and *not* by addressing the underlying transverse skeletal discrepancy). Is obtaining a correction with masking *possible* in Greg's case? This is a difficult question to answer. On the one hand (Figures 5.81i–k, n–p, and 5.84), the amount of current transverse correction needed at the first molars is only ~3 mm per side (total intermolar correction needed = 6 mm), the amount of maxillary posterior labial compensation currently present is not large, and the maxillary buccal periodontium appears robust. On the other hand, an AP correction must be made with the mandibular arch probably coming forward—which will necessitate even greater transverse correction, especially if the mandibular posterior compensations are removed. An argument could be made for aligning the maxillary arch and attempting some dental expansion—then re-evaluating the transverse relationship later (reducing unknowns before making a final treatment decision).

Surgery

- SARME—could achieve adequate maxillary expansion. However, since a maxillary impaction may be planned, this approach would require two separate surgeries (and two surgical recoveries, and two insurance submissions—all of which could present difficulties). We have had patients who—scheduled for a SARME and a subsequent surgical

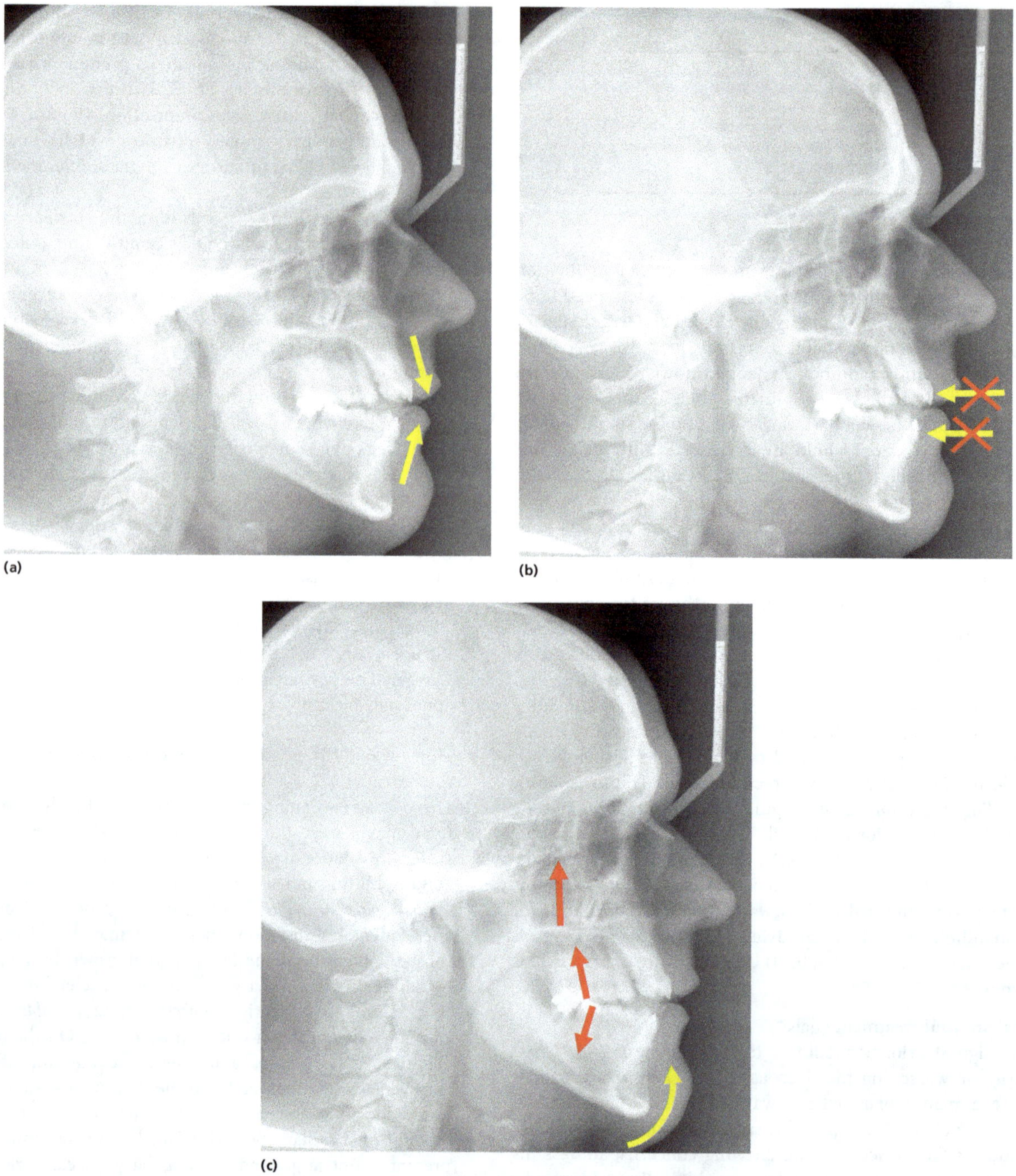

Figure 5.86 (a) Because Greg's maxillary incisors are stepped up (and his mandibular incisors are stepped down) relative to his posterior teeth, and because he displays only minimal maxillary incisor when relaxed, he is a candidate for incisor eruption. (b) Because Greg exhibits only slight maxillary incisor proclination and normal mandibular incisor inclination, he is not the ideal candidate for retracting/uprighting his incisors in order to erupt them by rotation around their apicies. (c) Intruding Greg's molars with TADs, or impacting his maxilla, would permit CCW autorotation of his mandible around the condyles, reducing his LLAFH, eliminating his ILG, and closing his anterior open bite.

procedure—opted out of the second procedure after undergoing the SARME.

- Considering the limited magnitude of the transverse expansion needed, a multiple-piece maxillary osteotomy (MPMO) to expand the transverse during maxillary impaction would seem reasonable. However, with a MPMO you are stretching the palatal soft tissue quickly and may compromise the palatal blood supply if it is stretched too much. The limit of transverse expansion with an MPMO is ~8 mm depending on the height of the palate and posterior transverse compensations.

Q: If a surgical option is selected, would you extract teeth?

A: No. There is already space in the maxillary arch, and Greg is missing the right lateral incisor. If you were considering canine substitution, then you could argue for extracting the maxillary

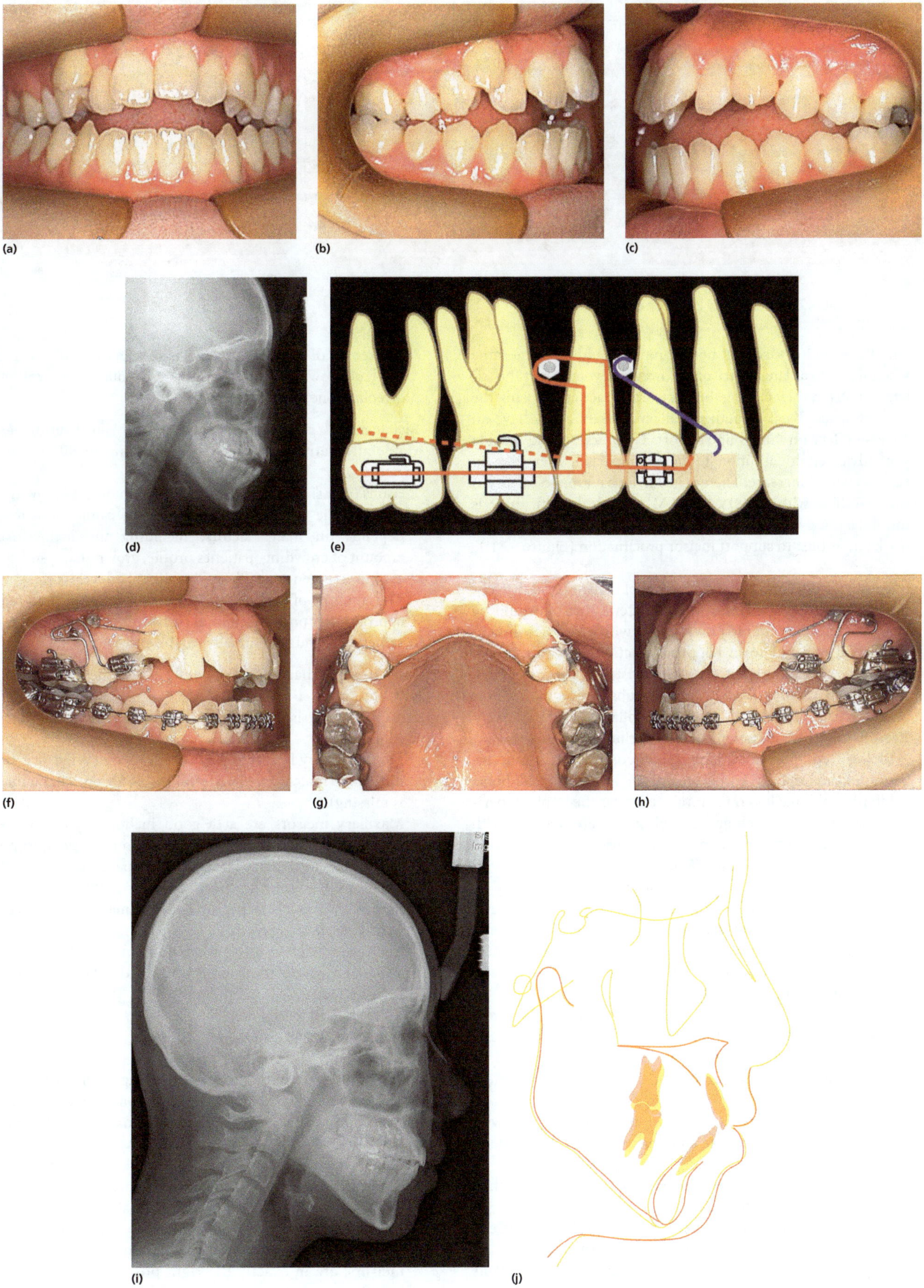

Figure 5.87 TAD supported indirect anchorage for skeletal open bite closure: (a–d) initial records, (e–h) schematic diagram and intraoral photographs illustrating TAD supported indirect anchorage with intrusion archwire to the maxillary first and second molars, and (i–m) deband records (Dr. Young Chel Park, DDS, PhD. Reproduced with permission from Dr. Young Chel Park).

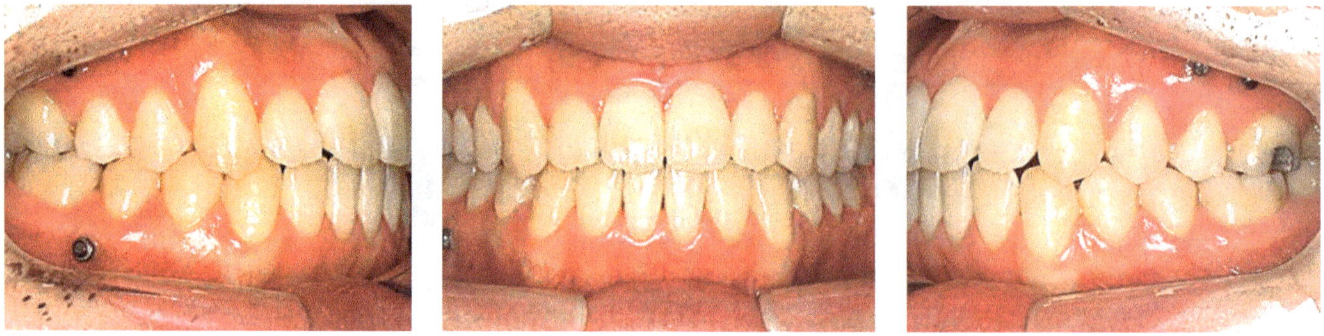

(k) (l) (m)

Figure 5.87 (Continued)

left lateral incisor—so that both canines would look the same when restored as lateral incisors. However, if you extract the left lateral incisor, then closing the left lateral space and closing the current space distal to both maxillary canines could have an adverse effect on Greg's lip support. Of course, if the maxilla was advanced in addition to being impacted, then the lip support would increase. There is no obvious reason to extract in the mandible with surgery. The FMIA is ideal (65°), there is minimal lower anterior crowding, and the periodontium is thick and robust to support incisor proclination (Figure 5.81j).

Q: Greg has a missing maxillary right lateral incisor. Traditionally, prosthetic replacement of a missing lateral incisor would be viewed as ideal in order to provide Greg with a complete maxillary dental arch and normal occlusal function. However, canine substitution is an alternative which must also be considered. List general reasons *favoring* canine substitution as a viable alternative for congenitally missing maxillary lateral incisors.

A: Reasons favoring canine substitution include the following:

- Biologic complications (gingival discoloration, infraocclusion of the implant crown, progressive loss of cortical bone, interdental bone loss on natural teeth near the implant, peri-implantitits), and technical complications are frequent with implants and implant-supported crowns—and may appear after only a few years [148–151].
- Chang et al. [152] found more mucositis and bleeding on probing (and greater probing depths) on implants compared to contralateral natural teeth.
- It is not possible to predict when, or to what degree, unesthetic changes will occur around implant supported crowns in the anterior maxilla [153–155].
- Patients with lateral incisor spaces closed are significantly healthier periodontally than those with prosthetic lateral incisors. Space closure produces results that are favored by patients and are healthier compared to prosthetic replacement [156, 157].
- No difference exists in function between patients with closed lateral incisor spaces and those with prosthetic lateral incisors [156].
- Space-closure patients are more satisfied with the results than the prosthetic patients [157].
- No difference exists in prevalence of TMJ problems between space-closure and prosthetic-replacement patients [157].
- Progressive infraocclusion can occur after years with implants because of the continuous eruption of adjacent teeth, even in adults and elderly patients [153–155].
- Darkening of the labial gingival is seen in over 50% of single-implant crowns at 4-year follow-ups (due to resorption of alveolar bone) [149].

Q: List general reasons *opposing* canine substitution as a viable alternative for congenitally missing maxillary lateral incisors.

A: Reasons opposing canine substitution include the following:

- The esthetic and functional success of canine substitution depends on many factors, including the malocclusion, amount of crowding, patient's profile, crown shape and color, canine emergence profile, and smiling lip level [158].
- The amount of crown reduction that may be required to appropriately position canines (substituted as lateral incisors) esthetically and functionally can be excessive [159].

Q: List dental characteristics describing the ideal canine substitution case.

A: Dental characteristics for an ideal canine substitution include the following:

- *Both* maxillary lateral incisors are missing (Why? It is often difficult to match right and left sides if only one lateral incisor is missing).
- Maxillary incisors are at a good inclination, and there is adequate lip support (Why? No need to increase lip support by opening a maxillary lateral incisor space.)
- Maxillary posterior teeth are already a full step Class II forward without spacing (Why? No need to protract the maxillary posterior teeth.)
- The mandibular arch is a nonextraction arch, or there exists a Class I molar relationship if two mandibular premolars are to be extracted.
- The maxillary permanent canines:
  - are already positioned ideally in the lateral incisor locations.
  - look just like lateral incisors including color, shape (flat B-Li so that the restorative dentist can build up the facial surface for color match), and gingival margin width (narrow like that of a lateral incisor, not wide).
- Maxillary first premolars look just like maxillary canines (when the first premolar lingual cusps are reduced and when the first premolars are rotated mesially slightly).
- Therefore, the ideal canine substitution case is one where the maxillary canines look exactly like the missing lateral incisors, are in exactly the right position, *plus* the maxillary first premolars look exactly like maxillary canines. In other words, *the ideal canine substitution case is one where*

there is nothing for the orthodontist or restorative dentist to do. All other cases are compromises in some way. Generally, the less ideal the patient would be for canine substitution, the more ideal the patient would be for prosthetic replacement.

- Finally, remember maxillary first premolars are generally narrower than maxillary canines. An anterior Bolton discrepancy must be anticipated and dealt with.

Q: Ahmed (Figure 5.88) presents with both maxillary lateral incisors missing (retained maxillary right primary lateral incisor is deemed hopeless, long term). He is Class I on the right and a full step Class II on the left (6 mm Class II at the left molar). Maxillary incisors are upright. Minimal maxillary lip support is evident. Using the previous question's list of dental characteristics for guidance, would you recommend treating Ahmed as a canine substitution case or as a prosthetic replacement case?

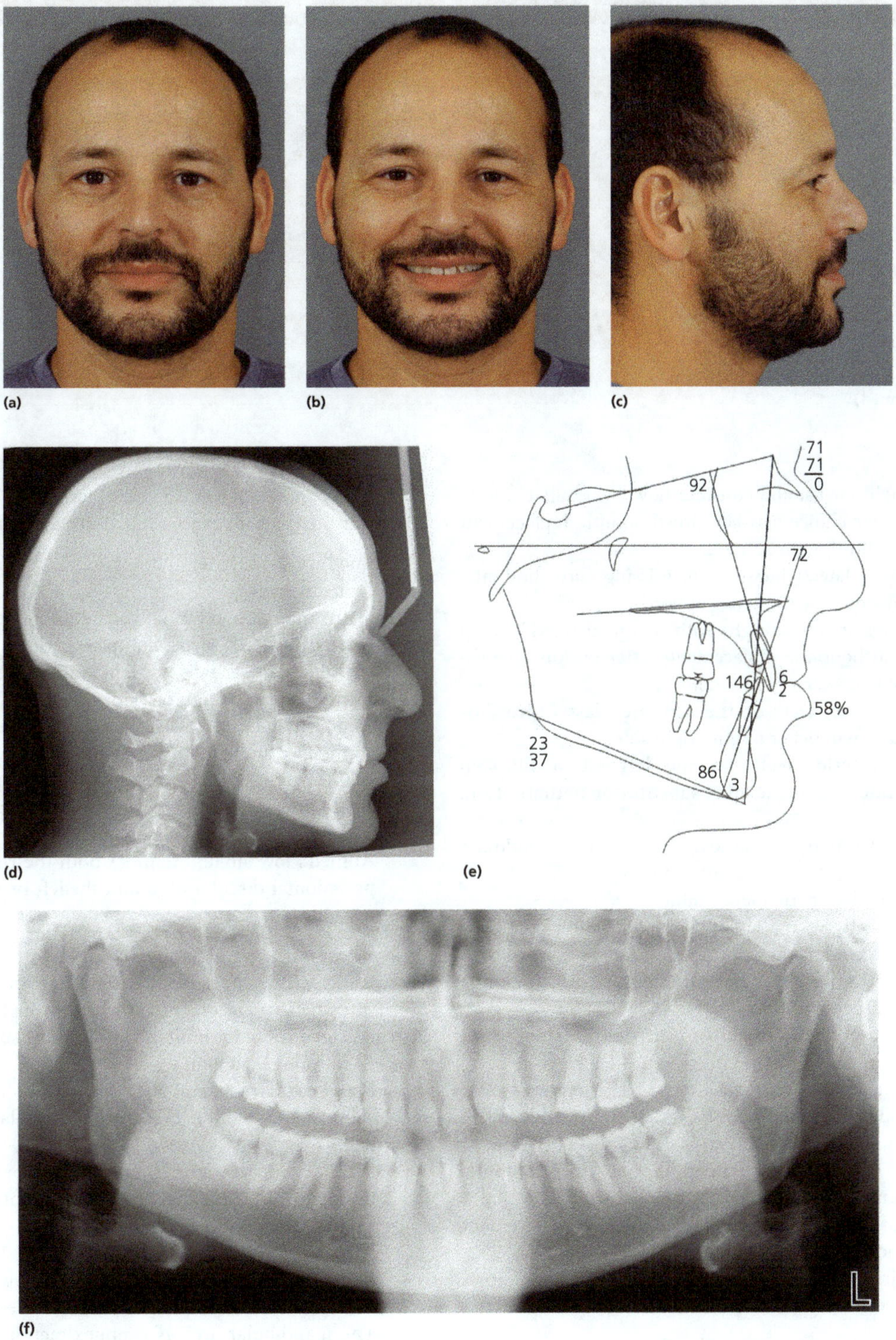

Figure 5.88 (a–k) Initial records of Ahmed, who presents with two congenitally missing permanent maxillary lateral incisors (the maxillary right lateral incisor is a primary tooth).

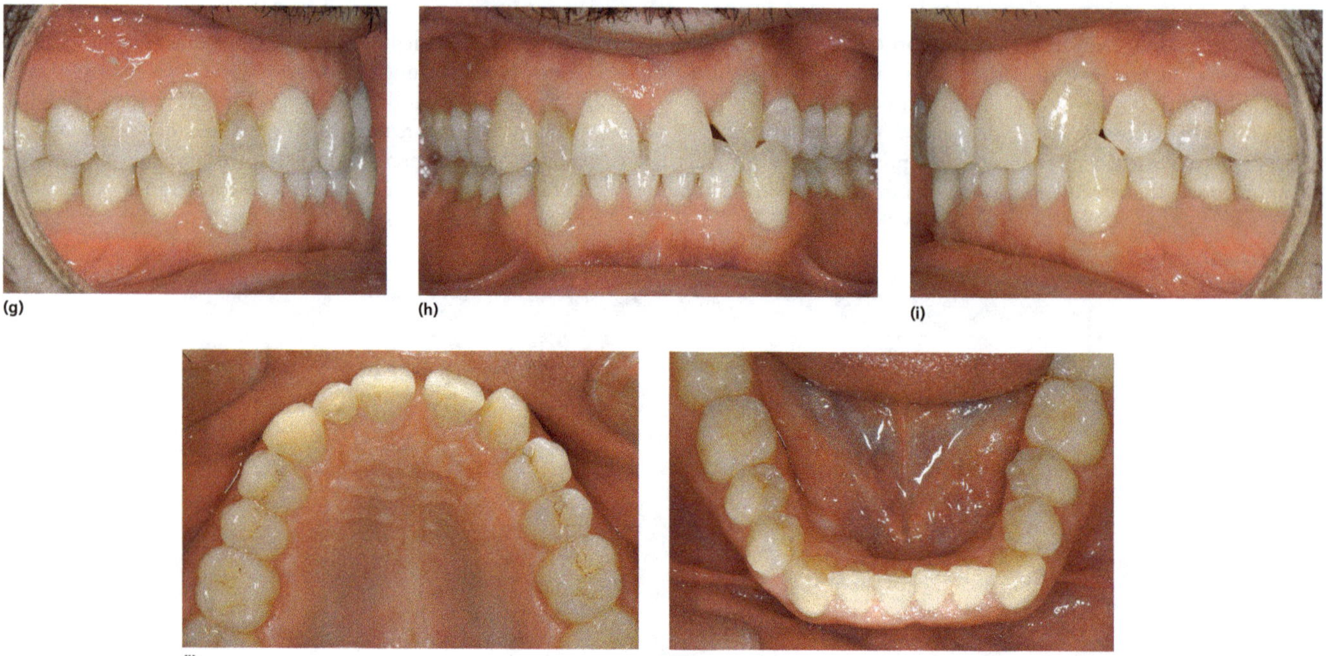

(g) (h) (i) (j) (k)

Figure 5.88 (Continued)

A: Let's go through our list and consider how each bulleted item will influence our choice between prosthodontic replacement and canine substitution for Ahmed.

- *Both* maxillary lateral incisors are missing (prosthodontic replacement would be the better option).
- Maxillary incisors are upright with marginal maxillary lip support (prosthodontic replacement better option to open space/procline maxillary incisors).
- Maxillary posterior teeth on the right are Class I (prosthodontic replacement better option, right side).
- Maxillary posterior teeth on the left are a full-step Class II without spacing (canine substitution better option, left side)
- The mandibular arch is a nonextraction arch (prosthodontic replacement right side, canine substitution left side).
- The right maxillary permanent canine
  - Is NOT already in the lateral incisor location (prosthodontic replacement better option).
  - Does NOT look like a lateral incisor (prosthodontic replacement better option).
  - Has a broad cervical margin (prosthodontic replacement option).
- The left maxillary permanent canine
  - Is already in the lateral incisor location (canine substitution better option).
  - Does NOT look like a lateral incisor (prosthodontic replacement better option).
  - Has a broad cervical margin (prosthodontic replacement better option).
- Maxillary first premolars could reasonably pass for canines when viewed from the front (canine substitution better option).

Based on these factors, we decided to open space on Ahmed's maxillary right for prosthodontic replacement (maxillary right primary lateral incisor was extracted). On his left side, Ahmed was treated as with canine substitution (Figure 5.89).

Q: Ahmed's post-treatment photos are shown in Figure 5.90. What do you observe?

A: Post-treatment observations include the following:

- An example of successful prosthetic replacement of one maxillary lateral incisor (right side) and canine substitution of one maxillary lateral incisor (left side). Ahmed has a wonderfully improved smile, and he smiles with much more confidence and enthusiasm.
- A mismatch is seen between the mesiodistal width of the right implant supported lateral incisor crown and the left canine substituted as a lateral incisor.
- Ahmed's low smile line hides both the right lateral implant periodontal discoloration and the left broad canine cervical margin.

Q: Now, back to Greg. Would you recommend treating Greg's missing permanent right lateral incisor with canine substitution or prosthetic replacement (hint: go through our list of dental characteristics describing the ideal canine substitution case).

A: Let's consider each item on the list.

- *Both* maxillary lateral incisors are not missing (maxillary right lateral incisor prosthodontic replacement would be better).
- Maxillary incisors are at a good inclination (Figure 5.81e) and lip support is adequate (either prosthodontic replacement or canine substitution would be adequate).
- Maxillary right molars are Class II by 3 mm, and there is some maxillary right spacing (either prosthodontic replacement or canine substitution would be adequate).
- The mandibular arch is a nonextraction arch (either right prosthodontic replacement or canine substitution would be adequate).

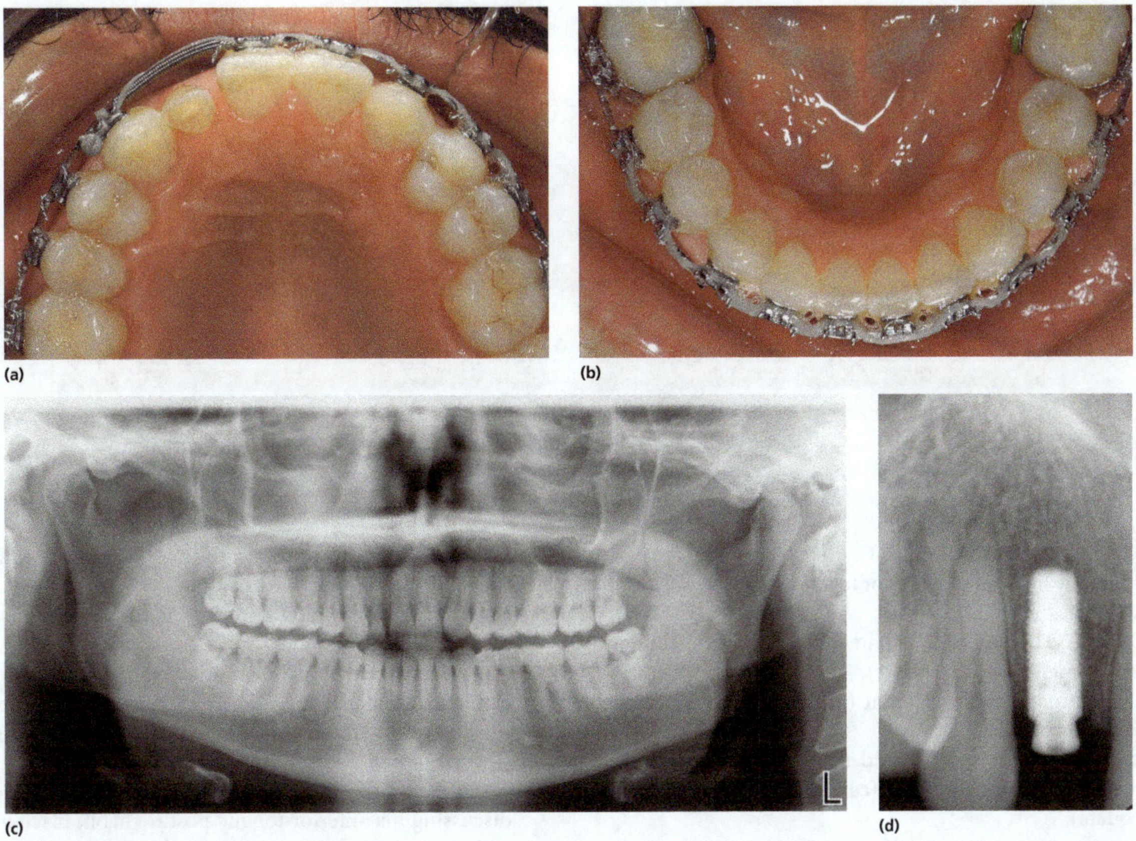

Figure 5.89 Progress records of Ahmed: (a) maxillary occlusal view illustrating space opening for maxillary right lateral incisor prosthetic replacement and left lateral canine substitution, (b) mandibular occlusal view, (c) panoramic image at deband, and (d) implant placed after extraction of the primary maxillary right lateral incisor.

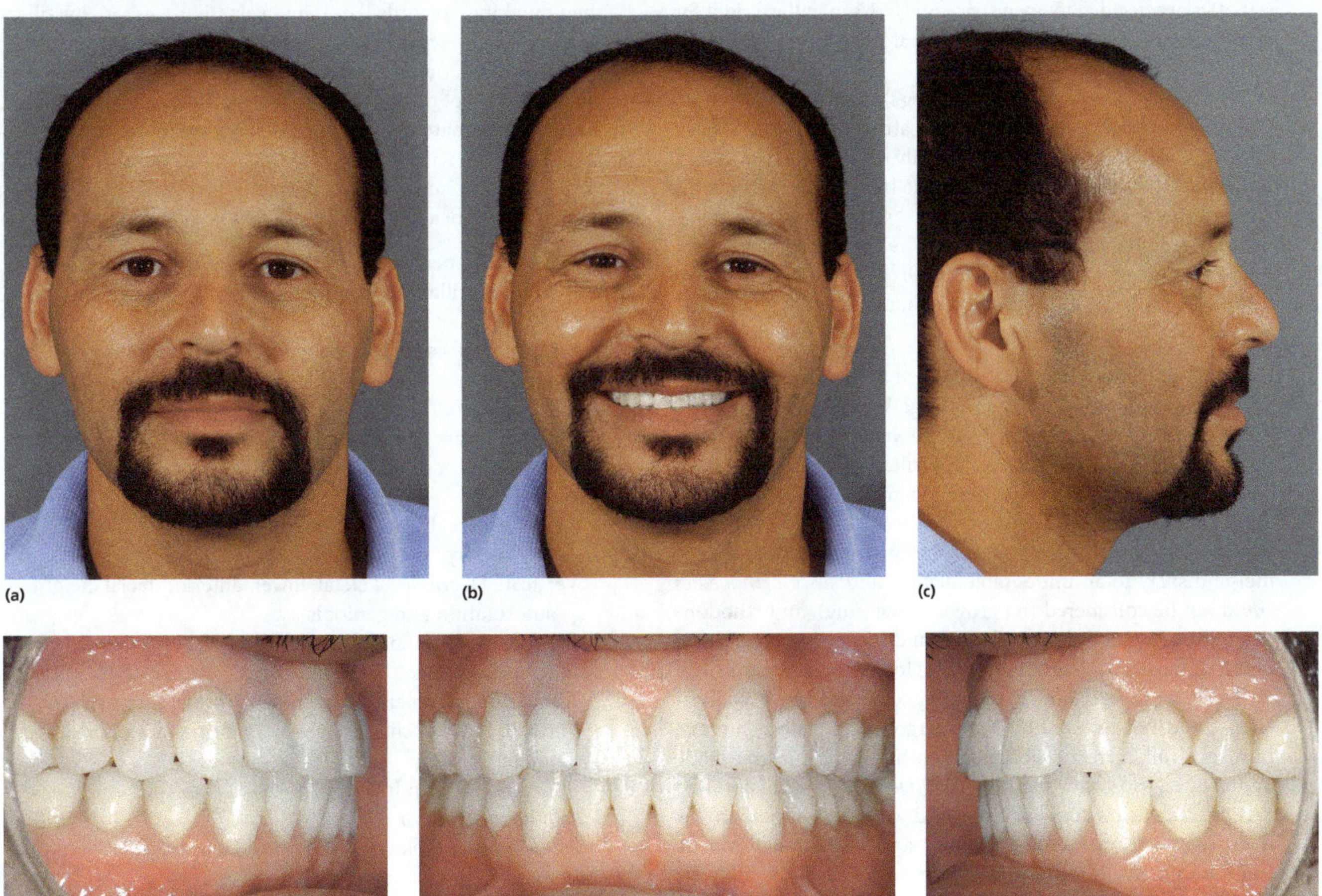

Figure 5.90 (a–h) Posttreatment photos of Ahmed.

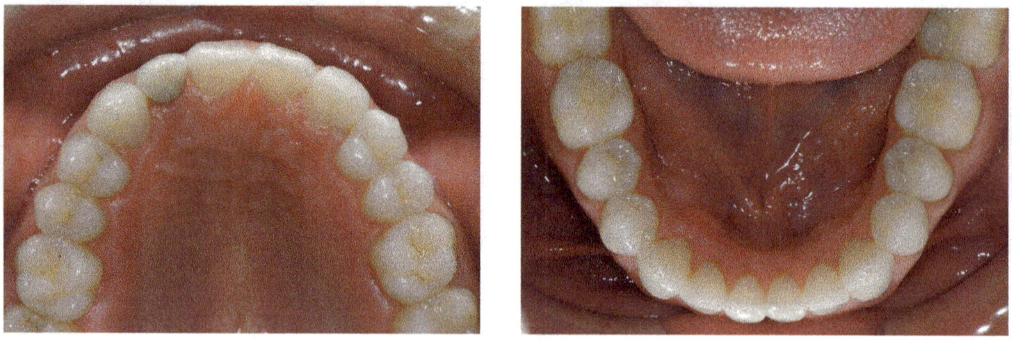

(g) (h)

Figure 5.90 (Continued)

- The right maxillary permanent canine
  - Is already in the lateral incisor location (canine substitution would be better).
  - Does NOT look like a lateral incisor (prosthodontic replacement would be better).
  - Has a broad cervical margin (prosthodontic replacement would be better).
- Maxillary first premolars could reasonably pass for canines when viewed from the front (canine substitution would be adequate).

In summary, there appear to be three factors that favor prosthodontic replacement, three factors that are neutral, and one factor that favors canine substitution. In our desire to maximize (and match) the final maxillary right and left lateral incisor esthetics, we decided to open space on Greg's maxillary right for prosthodontic replacement of the lateral incisor.

Q: What unknowns do you face with Greg's treatment?

A: Unknowns include the effect of treatment on Greg's sleep apnea. In other words, if we initially try to correct Greg's tongue habit (causing him to retract his tongue behind his anterior teeth), will that worsen his sleep apnea? Can his tongue habit be corrected, or will he have post-treatment relapse because of his habit? Does Greg have an undetected CR—CO shift? Will he be compliant with hygiene and instructions?

Q: Based on everything we have discussed so far, what treatment options would you consider for Greg? Would you consider a nonsurgical treatment option? Would you consider a surgical treatment option? Are there any consultations you would want before deciding on a final treatment plan?

A: Since *masking* Greg's skeletal open bite would likely be unstable, would not correct his ILG, and could potentially increase his incisal display to an undesirable degree, and since *orthopedics* could not be considered (no growth remaining), an orthodontics only treatment plan to close would have been considered heroic (impossible) some years ago. However, with the arrival of TADs, it should now at least be considered, especially if Greg could not or would not, undergo orthognathic surgery. Even if a full correction of the open bite could not be made by intruding posterior teeth with TADs, Greg's occlusion and vertical dimension could be improved with this approach. This is especially true if both maxillary and mandibular molars could be intruded. Further, if molars were intruded, then the mandible would autorotate up and forward—improving his Class II molar relationship. Judicious placement of TADs (on the palate) would also permit distalizing the maxillary dentition. Greg's arches could be leveled/aligned with fixed appliances (nonextraction), maxillary spaces distal to the canines closed, and space for the upper right lateral opened for prosthodontic replacement. However, an orthodontics only treatment plan was not presented to Greg.

A surgical-orthodontics treatment plan was given and included discussing his anterior tongue posture habit, placing an LLHA with spurs in an attempt to correct his tongue habit, banding and bonding both arches, attempting to correct his transverse discrepancy (dentally) with a TPA and archwires, opening space for prosthetic replacement of his missing right lateral incisor, then making records and re-evaluating for a maxillary differential impaction osteotomy (posterior maxilla impacted) with mandibular autorotation. The advantage of a surgical plan was that the open bite could be corrected, LLAFH decreased, and ILG eliminated. Surgical risks were the disadvantage. You should consult with the surgeon, the prosthodontist (maxillary right lateral incisor replacement), and the physician overseeing Greg's sleep apnea treatment to discuss your treatment plans.

Q: What are the specific objectives of treatment for the maxilla, mandible, maxillary dentition, and mandibular dentition in all three planes of space?

A: Specific objectives of treatment for Greg are as follows:

Maxilla

AP: Maintain.

Vertical: Impact posterior, maintain anterior.

Transverse: Increase skeletal width.

Mandible

AP: Advance by autorotation. Lengthen by advancement genioplasty.

Vertical: Decrease skeletal lower anterior facial height by autorotation and genioplasty.

Transverse: Maintain.

Maxillary dentition

AP: Maintain molars and canines. Protract incisors.

Vertical: Level occlusal plane by erupting incisors relative to molars.

Intermolar width: Increase intermolar width.

Mandibular dentition

AP: Maintain molars, canines, and incisors.

Vertical: Eliminate reverse curve of Spee.

Intermolar/intercanine width: Maintain intermolar and intercanine widths.

Q: Will Greg's maxillary anterior teeth, stepped up by 2–3 mm, be stable if they are leveled with the maxillary posterior teeth before surgery? Or, should the anterior step be left intact, presurgically, and Greg treated with a MPMO to bring the maxillary posterior segments up to level the arch?

A: The decision to level stepped up maxillary incisors before surgery, or to level the posterior and anterior segments independently during surgery, is a decision made based on the MAGNITUDE of the anterior step. It has been reported that, if the anterior step is only a few millimeters, then leveling before surgery will be stable [60]. Therefore, level Greg's arches before surgery.

Q: Greg elected to be treated with surgery (maxillary impaction osteotomy). How should you proceed?

A: Consultations with the surgeon, prosthodontist, and Greg's physician were obtained. A discussion of the tongue interposition habit was held with Greg. Fixed appliances were placed, including an LLHA with spurs to discourage the tongue habit, and arches were leveled and aligned. Maxillary canines were retracted, and space was opened for the maxillary right lateral incisor. Adequate space was opened (Iowa space) between the maxillary left canine and left lateral incisor to insure that the maxillary and mandibular incisors did not interfere when the canines were (surgically) positioned forward into a Class I relationship. A periodontist was consulted when inflammation and recession distal to the maxillary right central incisor was observed. Oral hygiene instructions were provided, but no further treatment was deemed necessary. A removable TPA was placed (with lingual crown torque) to increase maxillary first molar intermolar width. Later, it was noted that roots of the maxillary first molars became palpable.

Q: Presurgical records were made (Figure 5.91). What do you note?

A: Presurgical observations include the following:

- Leveling the maxillary arch has resulted in only 1 mm of maxillary incisor display in relaxed lip position (Figure 5.91g), but good incisor display during smiling (Figure 5.91b, maxillary central incisor gingival margins approximately congruent with maxillary lip vermillion). Remember, the amount of maxillary anterior impaction is based on incisal display in RELAXED LIP POSITION AFTER LEVELING THE MAXILLARY ARCH. It is not based on the amount of display when smiling—which can vary widely depending on activity of the smiling musculature.
- Maxillary midline now appears approximately on with his face.
- Maxillary dentition when smiling is clearly broader (compare Figure 5.91b to Figure 5.81b).
- ILG is approximately the same as when Greg presented initially (compare Figure 5.91a to Figure 5.81a).
- Maxillary incisors have proclined with space opening for the right lateral incisor (Figure 5.91e). This has increased his lip support.
- Left occlusion still appears Class II by 3–4 mm (Figure 5.91k), but the right side now appears Class I (Figure 5.91i, undetected shift?).
- Recession on the lingual of the maxillary right central incisor is noted (Figure 5.91l).
- Iowa space is noted (Figure 5.91l).
- LLHA with anterior tongue spurs (Figure 5.91m) is seen. It is unknown, at this point, whether the spurs have been effective in curtailing his tongue habit.
- Figure 5.91j illustrates that the left posterior buccal OJ appears inadequate.

Q: What surgical movements do you recommend for Greg? How do you use Greg's presurgical cephalometric radiograph to make vertical and sagittal surgical predictions?

A: With Greg, you want to impact his maxilla in the posterior to close his open bite but not reduce his incisal display. The maxilla is first impacted differentially in the *posterior* on the tracing (Figure 5.92, center), leaving acceptable incisal display at rest. Then the mandible is autorotated around the condyles into occlusal contact (Figure 5.92, right). Depending on the initial AP relationship of a patient's dentition, and on the amount of maxillary impaction, the autorotation of the mandible may result in the following:

- Class I canine relationship
- Class II relationship (necessitating a mandibular advancement procedure to achieve Class I canines)
- Class III relationship (necessitating a maxillary advancement or mandibular setback to achieve a Class I canine relationship)

Q: In Greg's surgical prediction, a maxillary posterior differential impaction of 6 mm was considered. This resulted in a mandibular (CCW) rotation forward of 7 mm (B-point advancing 7 mm). However, a dental Class III molar relationship was found to result (Figure 5.92, right). How would you recommend addressing this?

A: Remember that Greg suffers from sleep apnea. You would NOT want to correct a Class III relationship by setting Greg's mandible back (possibly worsening his sleep apnea). Instead, a decision was made to advance his maxilla by 3 mm to bring him into Class I occlusion. Also, to potentially help with the sleep apnea, an advancement genioplasty of 5 mm was recommended to protract the musculature attached to the mandible away from the airway and to *provide a total Pogonion advancement ≥10 mm.*

Q: How do you use Greg's presurgical models to make judgments about his transverse relationship?

A: Hold his presurgical models in a Class I canine relationship. The need for additional dental transverse correction, surgical transverse correction, addition/removal of transverse compensations, and other transverse changes is made based on the magnitude of transverse discrepancy. When you hold Greg's presurgical models together with canines in a Class I relationship (Figure 5.93), you note that his AP relationship coordinates reasonably well. But looking down on the left side (Figure 5.93c), you notice the inadequate maxillary transverse dimension (the right transverse was adequate).

Q: How do you recommend dealing with this inadequate left transverse dimension, especially recalling that Greg's maxillary first molar roots are palpable from the buccal?

A: If there are any maxillary posterior dental compensations—then remove the TPA, and reduce the posterior compensations

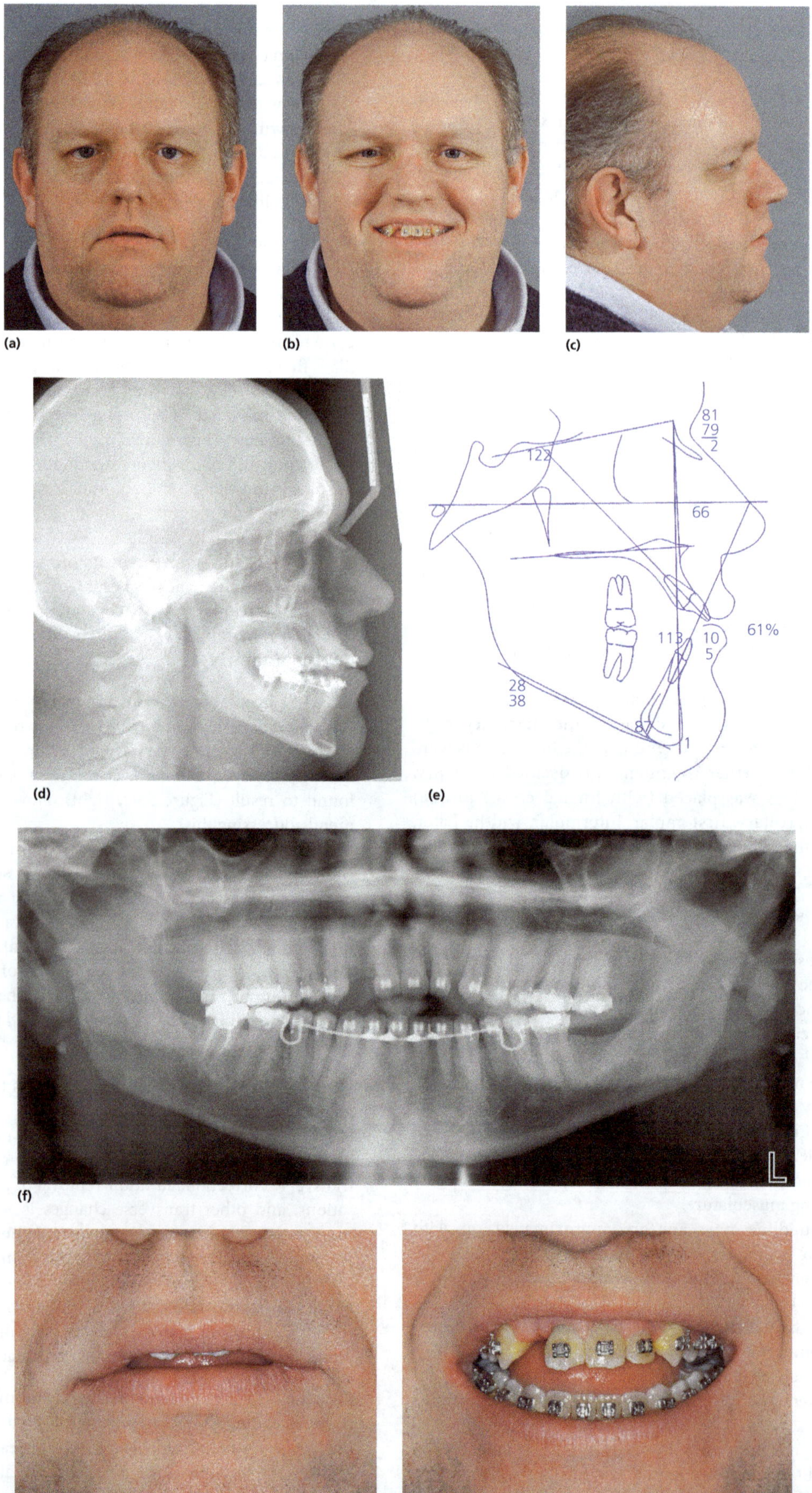

Figure 5.91 (a–p) Presurgical records of Greg.

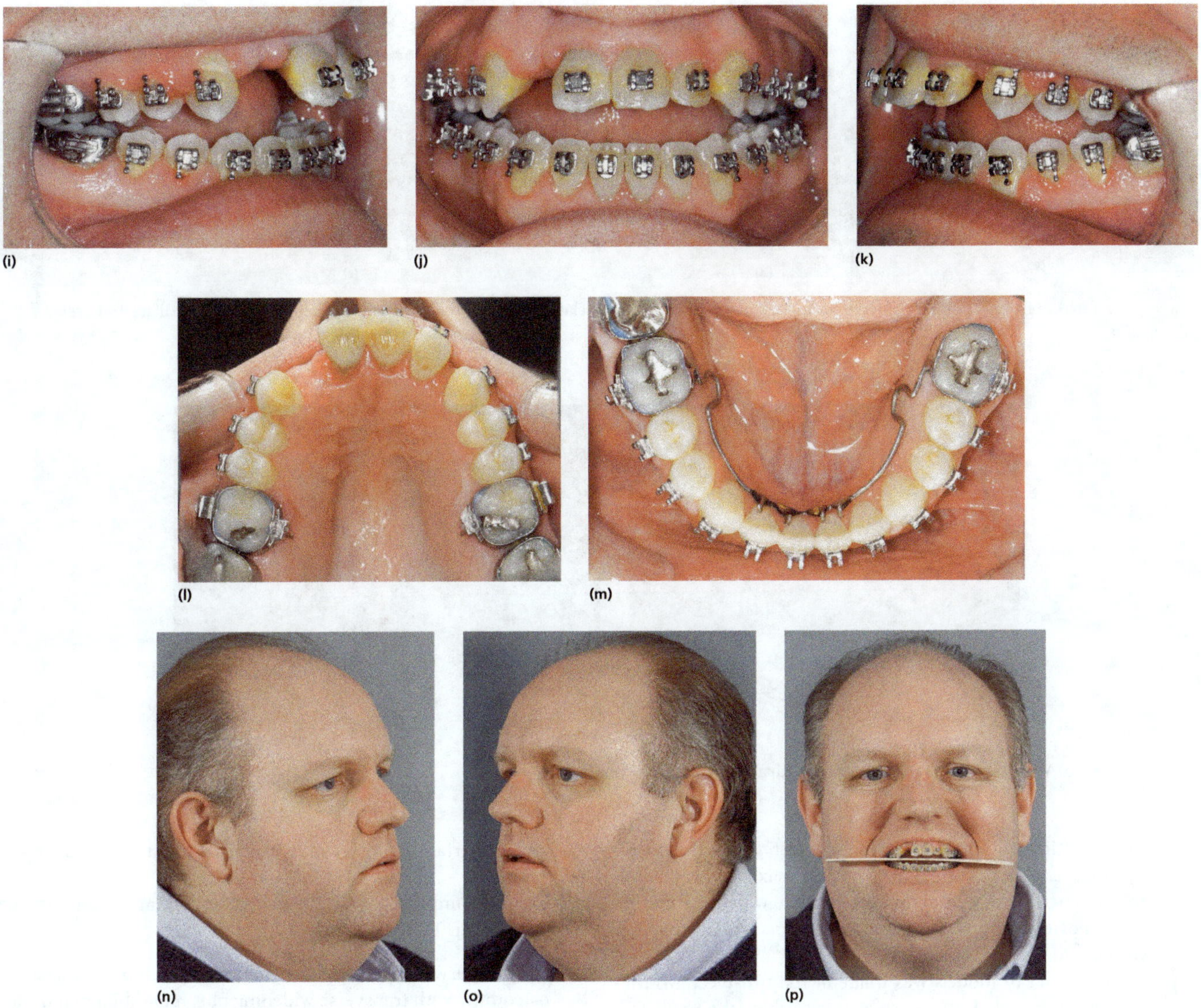

Figure 5.91 (Continued)

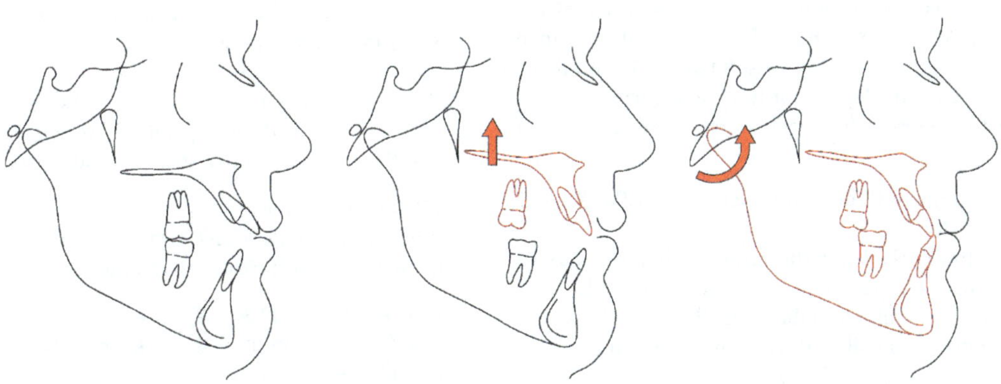

Figure 5.92 Use of a presurgical lateral cephalometric tracing in treatment planning surgery: (left) Greg's presurgical cephalometric tracing; (center) to close his anterior open bite, Greg's posterior maxilla is impacted differentially leaving adequate incisal display; (right) his mandible autorotates upward and forward (CCW) around his condyles bringing the dentition into contact, closing the open bite, and reducing his LAFH.

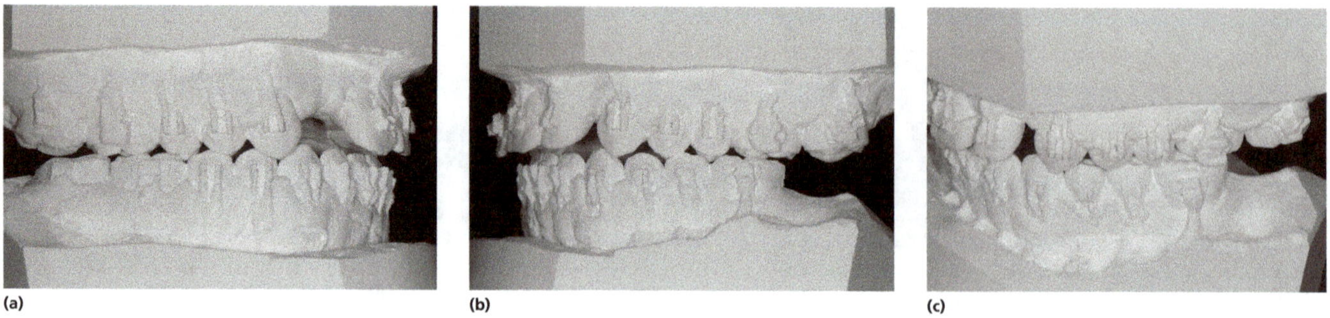

Figure 5.93 (a, b) Presurgical models of Greg positioned into a Class I canine relationship and (c) demonstrating an inadequate maxillary transverse dimension.

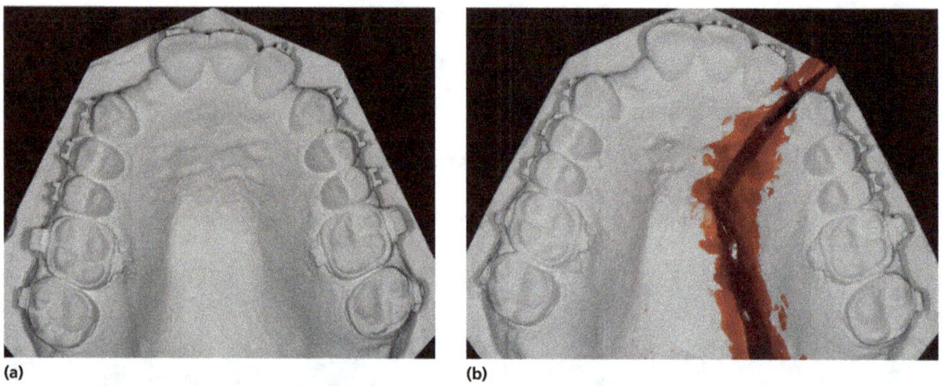

Figure 5.94 (a, b) Widening Greg's maxillary arch with a simulated two-piece MPMO.

by constricting the maxillary archwire. Later, widen the maxillary transverse with an MPMO during maxillary impaction surgery. Since the maxillary arch needs to be widened from the canines posteriorly, a decision was made to perform a maxillary two-piece MPMO (Figure 5.94).

A surgery set of models was made of the two-piece MPMO which were mounted on an articulator to show the predicted, postsurgical, occlusal relationship (Figure 5.95). The anteroposterior and transverse occlusion appear reasonable.

Q: Should the surgeon overexpand the maxilla with an MPMO? Why or why not?

A: Yes. Remember what you are doing when you are widening the maxilla with an MPMO. You are making bony cuts and then separating the bones by stretching the soft tissue. The soft tissue will pull back, trying to relapse your transverse correction. It is a good idea to overcorrect the transverse in anticipation of some relapse.

Q: Describe your protocol to help insure stability of the MPMO transverse expansion.

A: An occlusal splint is placed by the surgeon when the maxilla is widened. This is worn for 6 weeks at which time it is removed. A palatal splint is fabricated that same day and worn for as long as possible during the remaining orthodontic treatment.

Q: Should Greg be given chewing restrictions postsurgically?

A: Yes, for a multiple-piece maxillary osteotomy 2–6 weeks of chewing restrictions should be followed, depending on the surgeon's philosophy.

Q: List important factors which can help minimize postsurgery problems.

A: Factors minimizing postsurgery problems are found in the checklist in Table 5.9.

Q: Greg underwent a two-piece maxillary impaction/advancement osteotomy with transverse widening plus mandibular autorotation and genioplasty advancement. Remarkably, he felt well enough to stop by the orthodontic clinic to say hello 1 day post surgery (Figure 5.96).

At 1 week post surgery (Figure 5.97) Greg said, "I threw away my CPAP since the surgery, I am sleeping so well, my sleep apnea is cured." In addition to the ILG still present, a 2 mm open bite was noted. How do you handle the open bite?

A: Talk to the surgeon. The surgeon states that the desired occlusion was obtained intraoperatively (Greg was seated properly into the occlusal splint at the end of surgery).

Q: What does this mean?

A: It means that, most likely, his postoperative open bite is related to swelling or soft tissue interference in some way.

Q: How should you proceed?

A: Ask Greg to continue wearing his guiding elastics. He says he will.

Q: You see Greg again 1 week later (Figure 5.98). He is wearing his guiding elastics. What do you note?

A: His hygiene is poor, but the open bite has improved. His midlines are not coincident, and he appears Class III by 2–3 mm on

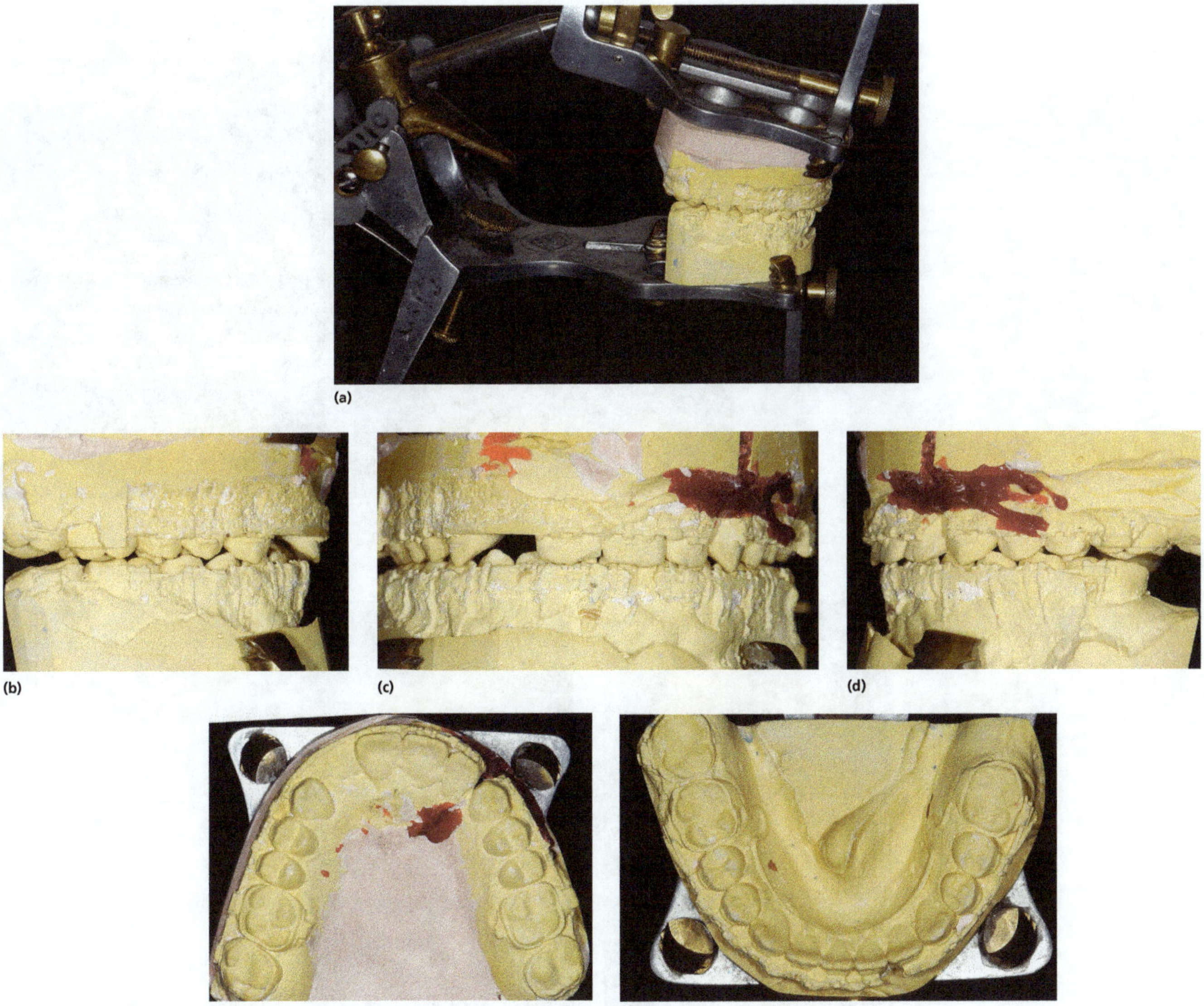

(a) (b) (c) (d) (e) (f)

Figure 5.95 (a–f) Models of the two-piece MPMO are mounted on an articulator with the predicted, postsurgical, occlusal relationship. Note that the maxillary osteotomy cut will be made between the maxillary left lateral incisor and left canine.

Table 5.9 Checklist to follow for surgical patients.

Presurgical tasks	☐ Verify relaxed lip incisal display *after leveling* to decide the magnitude of vertical maxillary surgical incisor movement
	☐ Approve the articulated surgical occlusion (models mounted by the surgeon)
	☐ Agree on proposed surgical movements and verify that surgical movements are within surgical limits
	☐ Schedule the patient to see you 1 week after the surgery date
Postsurgical communication	☐ When should the surgeon contact the orthodontist? – Immediately after surgery (what was the surgical outcome?) – The surgeon should inform the orthodontist of problems (to better prepare for dealing with them) – **Q:** Was the bite seated during surgery? (if it was, then a later occlusal discrepancy could be due to edema/muscle spasms)
	☐ Take care what you say in front of the patient – Seek solutions to surgical problems the cause of which may have been indeterminate/unavoidable – Put a positive spin on intervention—"surgery helped a lot, now we are completing treatment"
	☐ Work together with the surgeon to discuss postsurgical treatment, including direction and magnitude of forces to be applied
Postsurgical tasks	☐ See patient 1 week postoperatively (well within the first month window of accelerated bony remodeling/cellular activity/possible increased tooth movement) so that you can intercede effectively, as needed
	☐ Check for postsurgical occlusal discrepancies, including a repeatable bite at the 1 week postop appointment
	☐ Guiding elastics—guiding elastics help the patient learn to close into the new occlusion. This is necessary since the jaw muscular length and direction have been changed with surgery, edema and muscle spasms may alter the correct closing position, proprioceptive sense may have been lost, and/or the patient may be numb. The focus of guiding elastics is on the muscles. Guiding elastics are *not* intended to move teeth. There is no specific length of time for wearing guiding elastics. Time of wear is a judgment call made between the surgeon and orthodontist
	☐ Splints—an occlusal splint is worn by the patient for ~6 weeks following MPMOs to hold a transverse expansion. As soon as it is removed, a palatal splint is fabricated and worn for as long as possible through the completion of orthodontic treatment. If the maxillary archwire was sectioned at surgery, then it should be replaced with a continuous wire at the 6-week appointment

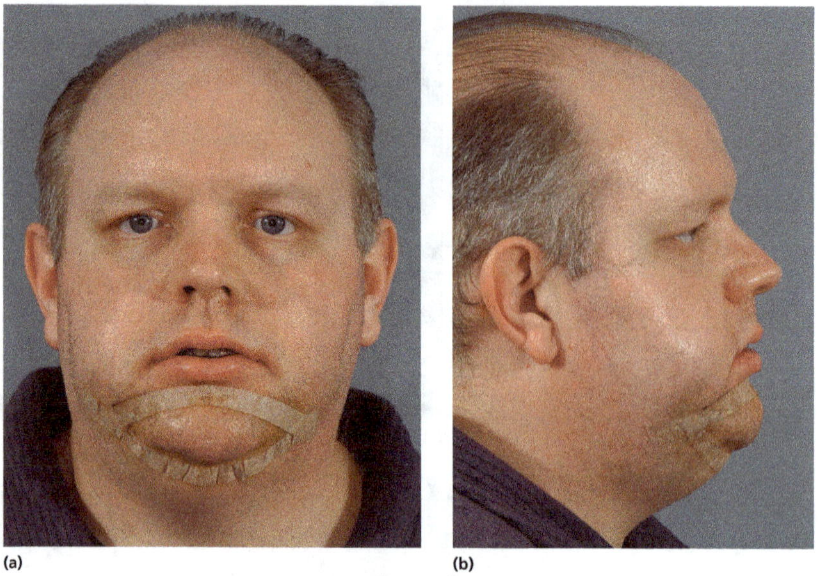

Figure 5.96 (a, b) Greg 1 day post surgery.

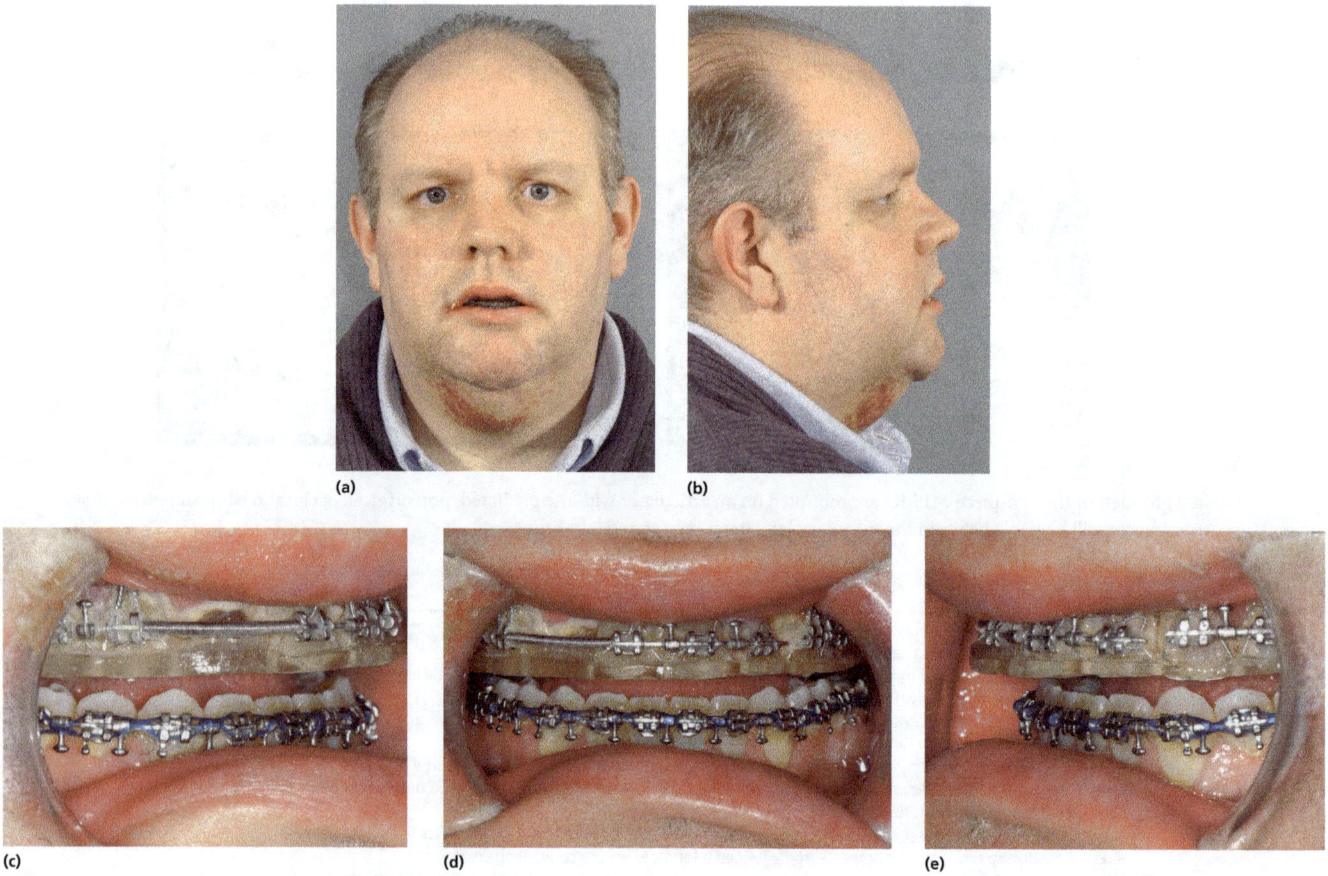

Figure 5.97 (a–e) Greg at 1 week post surgery: Note that Greg is not seating into his occlusal splint and demonstrates a 2 mm anterior open bite.

the right and Class I on the left. In addition, if you look carefully at his maxillary left canine (note the sectioned archwire where an osteotomy cut was made, Figure 5.98c), you see how inflamed the tissue looks.

Q: What should you do?

A: Since the occlusal discrepancies appear manageable—you are prudent to *focus only on Greg's poor healing for now*. Discontinue guiding elastics, and appoint Greg to see the surgeon immediately.

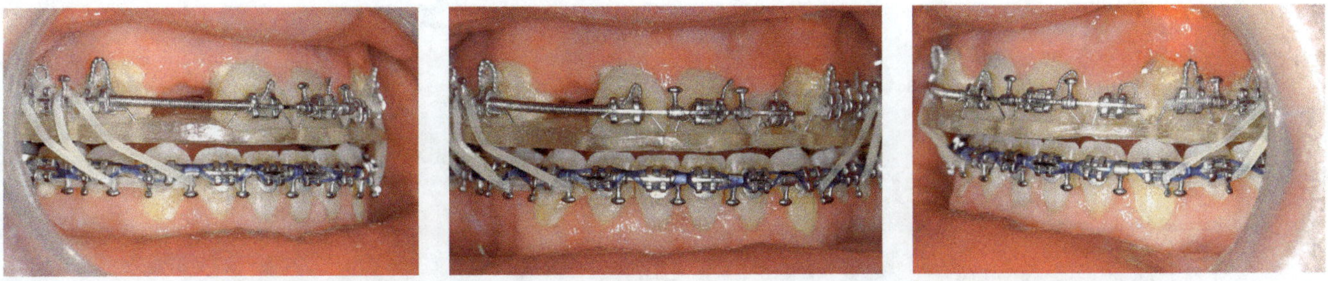

(a) (b) (c)

Figure 5.98 (a–c) Greg at 2 weeks post surgery. Note that, although his bite has improved with guiding elastic wear, Greg's hygiene is poor and very inflamed tissue is present apical to his maxillary left canine (the site of the two-piece osteotomy cut).

Later, you are told that Greg's blood perfusion during surgery was less than ideal, and now the segmented maxilla is healing poorly. Antibiotic treatment has been started, and Greg is to undergo hyperbaric oxygen treatments to facilitate healing.

Q: At 6 weeks, a palatal splint was fabricated and delivered in place of the occlusal splint. It was noted that Greg's transverse dimension was "tight." A continuous maxillary archwire was inserted to replace the surgical archwire. Greg complained of significant suborbital maxillary pain. The surgeon felt that the pain was due to nerve regeneration. At 14 weeks post op, you ask Greg to chew gum daily to help seat his posterior occlusion. The LLHA was removed. Minor posterior occlusal adjustments (enameloplasty) resulted in significant occlusal improvement. At 6 months post surgery, anterior vertical elastics were started, and a small curve of Spee placed in the lower arch, to help close a slight open bite. A second prosthodontic consultation was held. The prosthodontist felt that there is inadequate room between the maxillary right canine and central incisor roots for an implant. Other options (cantilever bridge off the canine and acid-etched bridge) were given. Finishing was completed and Greg was debanded (Figure 5.99).

A cantilever bridge was fabricated to replace the missing maxillary right lateral incisor. Final records are shown in Figure 5.100. What do you note?

A: The final records show the following:

- Greg had an excellent esthetic and functional result.
- A maxillary differential impaction brought PNS up (Figure 5.99f), rotated the maxilla (CW) around ANS, and permitted mandibular autorotation (CCW) and open bite closure.
- The maxilla was advanced by ~2 mm.
- Lip competence was achieved.
- Nasal shape (alar base) widened.
- Mandibular autorotation plus genioplasty advancement have brought bony Pogonion and soft tissue Pogonion forward ~8–10 mm.
- LAFH was reduced to near ideal proportions (contrast Figure 5.81a to Figure 5.100a).
- A much broader, more esthetic smile, is now present (Figures 5.81b and 5.100b).
- A straighter profile and more acute lip–chin–throat angle is now present (Figures 5.81c and 5.100c).
- The maxillary midline is congruent with the facial midline but 1–2 mm to the right of the mandibular midline.
- There is far more prominence to the maxillary left canine (as seen in the frontal view, Figure 5.100e) than the maxillary right canine. The maxillary left lateral incisor is positioned too far to the lingual. Also, the left canines do not coordinate.
- Greg was finished to a shallow overbite (~10% OB).

Q: How was Greg's open bite corrected?

A: By maxillary molar intrusion, entirely (Figure 5.99f). A maxillary differential impaction "intruded" Greg's maxillary molars, permitting mandibular autorotation and open bite closure. The anterior open bite was not closed by incisor eruption.

Q: The right first molars are Class I, the left first molars are slightly Class III, but the canines are Class II by ~2 mm (Figure 5.100d–f). How could the maxillary canine position have been improved?

A: The mesial inclination of the maxillary canines could have been reduced, slightly. This would have positioned the maxillary canine tips more Class I. Also, interproximal reduction (IPR) could have been used to create space between the maxillary canines and first premolars. This space could have been used to distalize the maxillary canines to an ideal Class I position. If IPR were done, and the maxillary canines retracted, space would have resulted mesial to the maxillary left canine. A composite or porcelain veneer may have been required to close the maxillary left space.

Q: Would you suggest any changes to Greg's orthodontic treatment or surgery?

A: In retrospect, a SARME would have eliminated the need for an MPMO. The maxillary impaction could then have been a one-piece impaction and may have eliminated the maxillary healing problems that occurred with the MPMO. *Hygiene should have been emphasized.* Opening more space for the maxillary right lateral incisor could have achieved midline coordination and allowed placement of an implant.

Q: How would you retain this patient? What will you watch for? Suggest treatments if Greg begins to relapse.

A: Hawley retainers were placed. If Greg begins to show (functional) open bite relapse, then composite buttons could be placed on the facial of his maxillary incisors and a vacuum-formed retained worn that "snaps" into place over the buttons to hold the incisor vertical positions. Lingual spurs could be placed in the mandibular retainer, and a hole could be placed in his maxillary Hawley retainer palate to help keep his tongue off his anterior teeth. Posterior enameloplasty could help close down minor

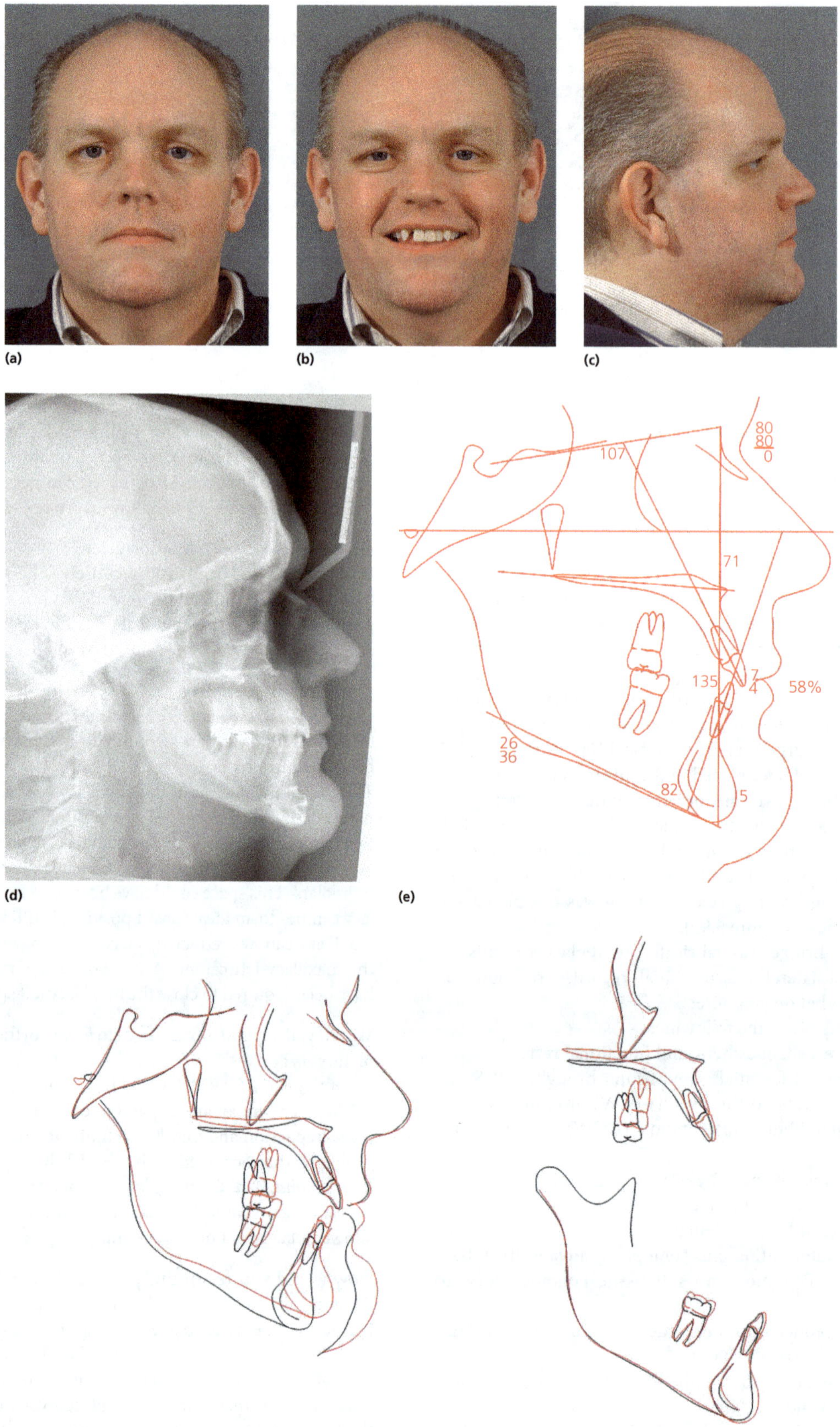

Figure 5.99 (a–l) Greg's deband records.

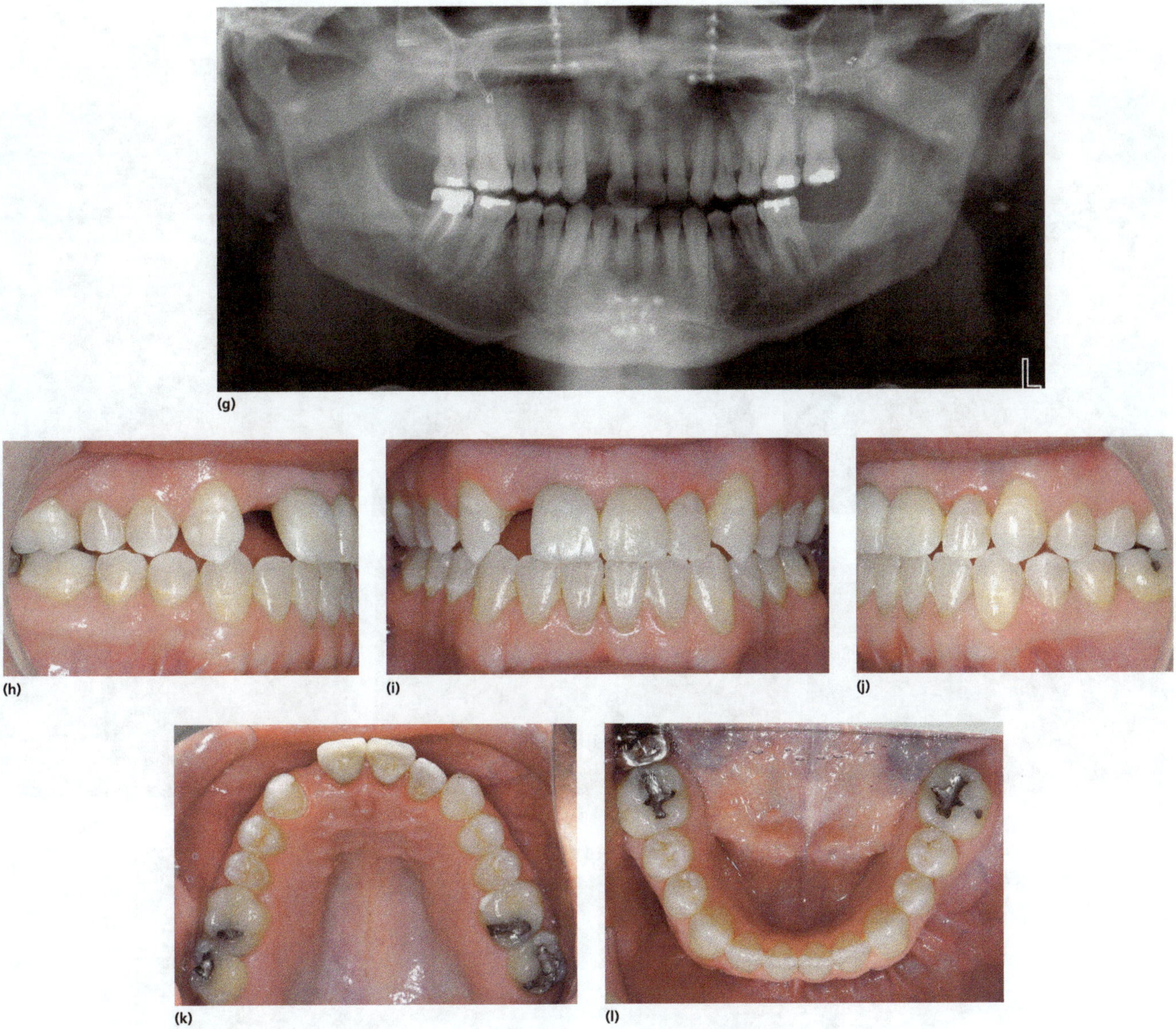

Figure 5.99 (Continued)

anterior open bite relapse. Moderate relapse could be treated with fixed orthodontic appliances and vertical elastics.

Q: What are the "take-home" messages from treatment of this patient?

A: Take-home messages include the following:

- Greg presented with an anterior open bite, a combination dental *and* skeletal anterior open bite. Greg's dental open bite resulted from an anterior interpositional tongue habit. His skeletal open bite resulted from a classic skeletal open bite growth pattern: condyles growing posterior-superiorly, lack of posterior face height development, backward mandibular internal (true) rotation, maxilla descending more than normal, and maxillary molars erupting more than normal. As his mandible rotated (CW) downward and backward, his mandibular plane angle steepened, his anterior face height increased, an ILG formed, and the anterior open bite resulted.
- Greg's tongue posture habit was discussed with him, and an LLHA with spurs was placed in an attempt to correct the habit. Sometimes, anterior tongue interposition habits will resolve on their own when orthodontic treatment closes the open bite, but this is a gamble. Greg's skeletal open bite was successfully treated with a LeFort I impaction osteotomy. We have monitored Greg for 5 years post surgery and, thankfully, his open bite (dental and skeletal) has not returned.
- The amount of maxillary anterior impaction is based on incisal display in relaxed lip position after leveling the maxillary arch. In Greg's case (Figure 5.99f), we did not want to impact his anterior maxilla and decrease his incisal display. Should we even have brought Greg's anterior maxilla down? Possibly, but his final smile looks very good with the surgery he had (Figure 5.100b).
- Greg's bilateral posterior cross bite was initially treated with dental expansion because the amount of transverse correction

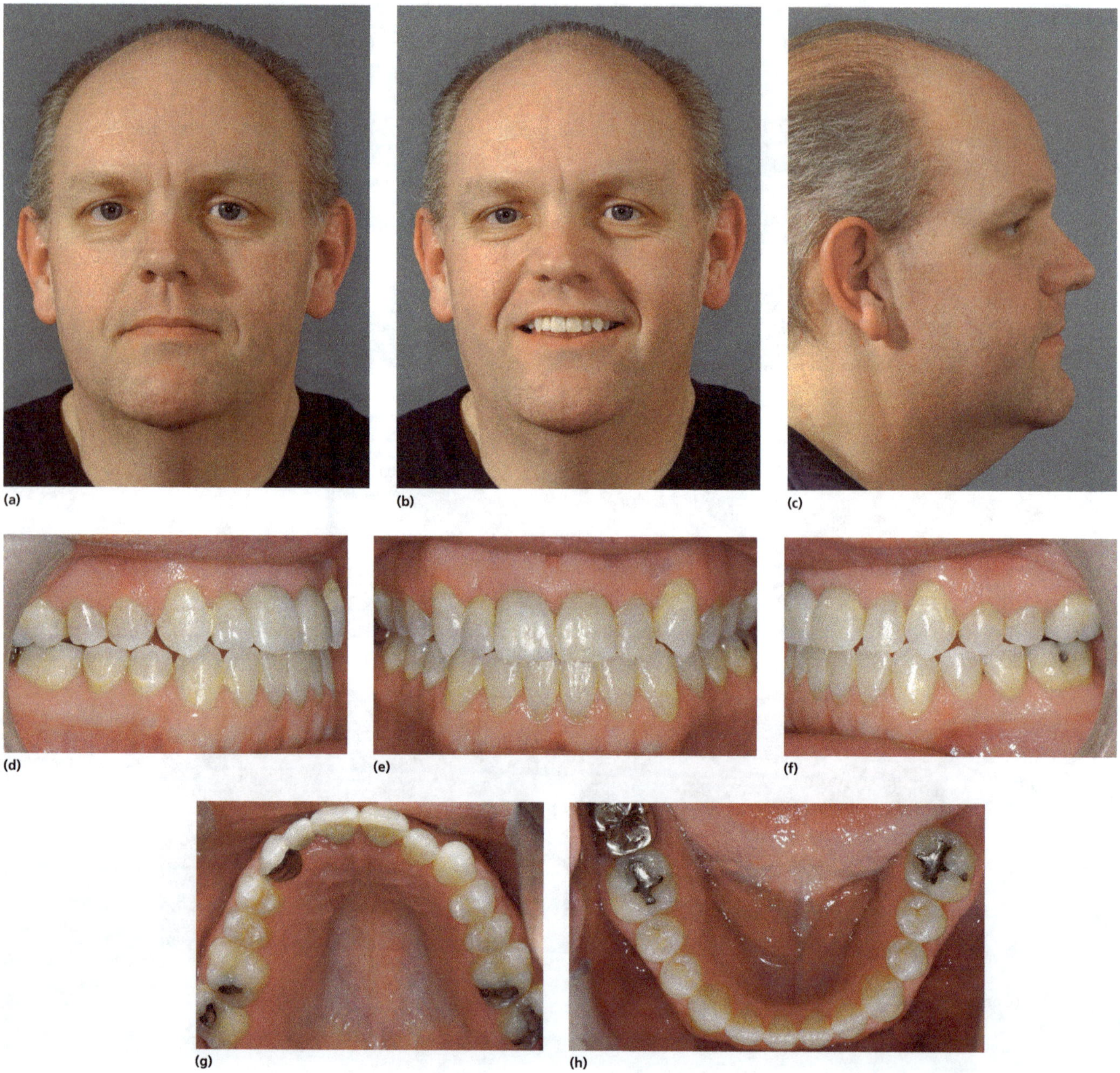

Figure 5.100 (a–h) Greg's final records.

needed (~3 mm per side) was reasonable, he exhibited only mild maxillary molar labial crown torque, and he had robust buccal periodontium. However, presurgically it was determined that this dental expansion would be inadequate when the mandible autorotated forward. Since Greg was undergoing a LeFort I osteotomy anyway, an MPMO was chosen to make the final transverse widening. Many patients can be treated successfully with a pieced maxilla. But, as a rule of thumb, "*the more pieces, the more problems*." In Greg, the problem was poor perfusion of the left osteotomy cut site. It later became infected (poor hygiene) and was cured with intense antibiotic treatment combined with hyperbaric oxygenation.

- Greg was finished to a shallow overbite (~10% OB). Ideally, his overbite should have been corrected to 20–40% OB in anticipation of some future relapse.
- Greg initially presented with a history of obstructive sleep apnea, and was wearing a CPAP every night when sleeping. This condition influenced the decision to advance the maxilla and chin following autorotation of the mandible (double-jaw surgical advancement). Immediately after surgery, Greg claimed that he could breathe, perfectly. Six months post surgery, Greg stated that his sleep apnea had returned, and he was again using a CPAP. The treatment of sleep apnea can be challenging, without guaranteed results for every patient. I saw Greg many years later and asked how he was doing. Greg replied, "I am doing very well. Sometime after the double-jaw surgery I underwent bariatric surgery and lost a lot of weight. I no longer need my CPAP. I feel that it was the combination of double-jaw surgery and weight lost that cured me, long term."

- In retrospect, Greg could have been treated successfully without jaw surgery using TADs to intrude the maxillary and mandibular molars. Since he underwent an impaction of 6 mm at PNS during surgery this would have been equivalent to intruding the maxillary molars by 3 mm and intruding the mandibular molars by 3 mm. However, the use of TADs to correct his open bite would *not* have helped cure his sleep apnea (the maxilla would not have been advanced, and he would still need an advancement genioplasty to protract the musculature away from his airway).

Case Ashley

Ashley is 16 years and 6 months old, presenting to you with the chief complaint, "I need orthodontic treatment for my crowded teeth (Figure 5.101). My lips don't come together and my lower jaw sits back." Her PMH includes a brachial cleft cyst as a child, and her PDH is WRN. TMJ evaluation includes a history of anterior disk displacement (ADD) with reduction. She is without periodontal problems and has a CR—CO shift of 2 mm AP.

Q: List diagnostic findings/problems. What is your diagnosis?

A: See Table 5.10.

Q: Your partner disagrees with your diagnosis, stating that Ashley's bite does not appear "open" when viewed from the front, and therefore cannot be diagnosed as an open bite. Is he correct?

A: No. An anterior open bite refers to the condition where mandibular anterior teeth do not contact the maxillary anterior teeth or the palate (Figure 5.102a, left). Vertical incisor overlap (Figure 5.102a right) refers to an open bite where the incisal edges of the maxillary and mandibular incisors "overlap" when viewed from the front. However, if the mandibular anterior teeth do not touch the maxillary anterior teeth or the palate, then this is still an open bite. Look at Ashley's initial models from the front again (Figure 5.102b) and the models tipped up slightly (Figure 5.102c). Her mandibular anterior teeth touch neither her maxillary anterior teeth nor her palate. *Ashley exhibits vertical incisor overlap when viewed from the front, but her maxillary and mandibular teeth do not contact. She has an anterior open bite.*

Q: Look at Ashley's cephalometric radiograph (Figure 5.101g). How has her mandibular incisor tooth eruption minimized her anterior open bite?

A: Her mandibular incisors have undergone excessive eruption. Note the long, narrow alveolus that has resulted from this eruption. If the mandibular incisors had not erupted excessively, then Ashley's anterior open bite (gap) would be *much* worse.

Q: What is this excessive mandibular incisor eruption an example of?

A: *Dental compensation for an underlying apical base discrepancy* (excessive mandibular incisor eruption compensating for a

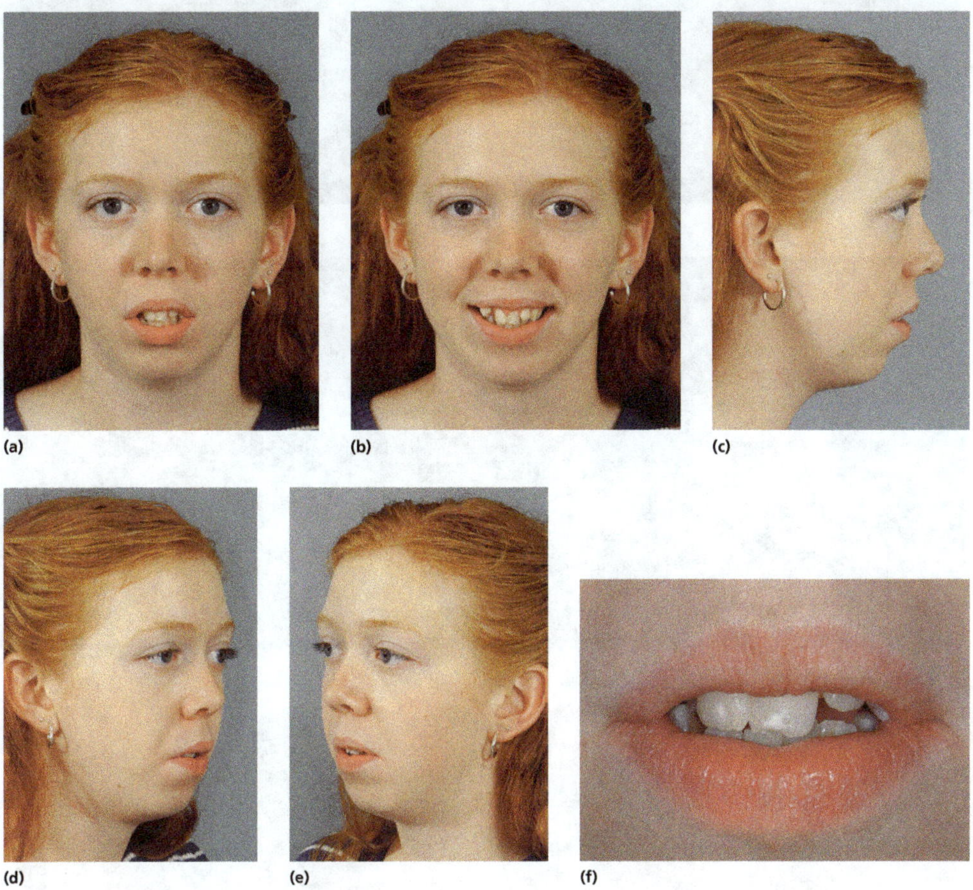

Figure 5.101 Initial records of Ashley: (a) frontal facial photograph, (b) posed smile, (c) profile, (d, e) right and left ¾ facial views, (f) close-up of relaxed lip, (g) lateral cephalograph, (h) cephalometric tracing, (i) pantomograph, (j) anterior periapical images, (k–o) intraoral photographs, (p–s) model photographs, and (t–w) separated model photographs.

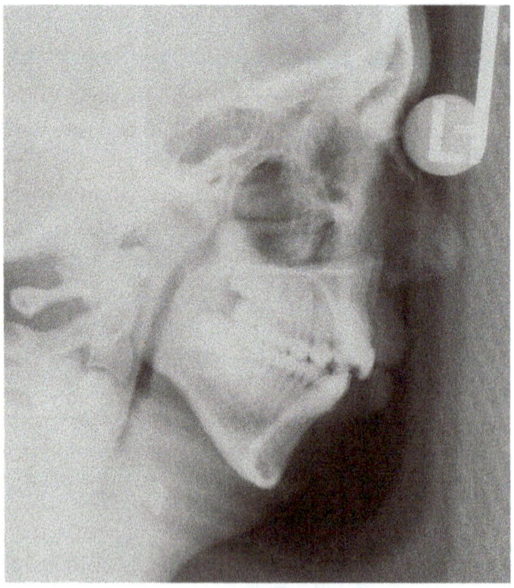

(g)

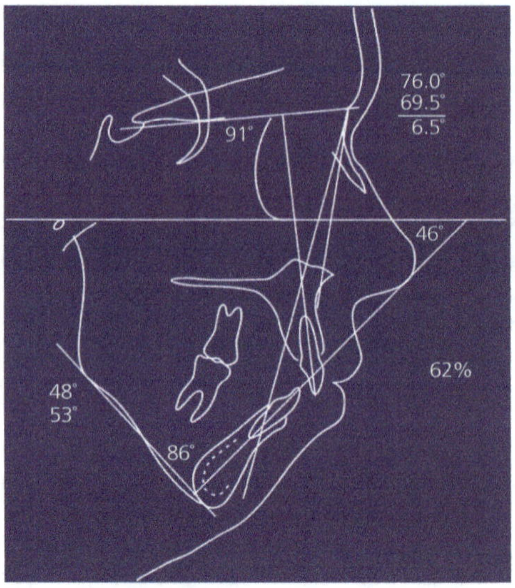

(h)

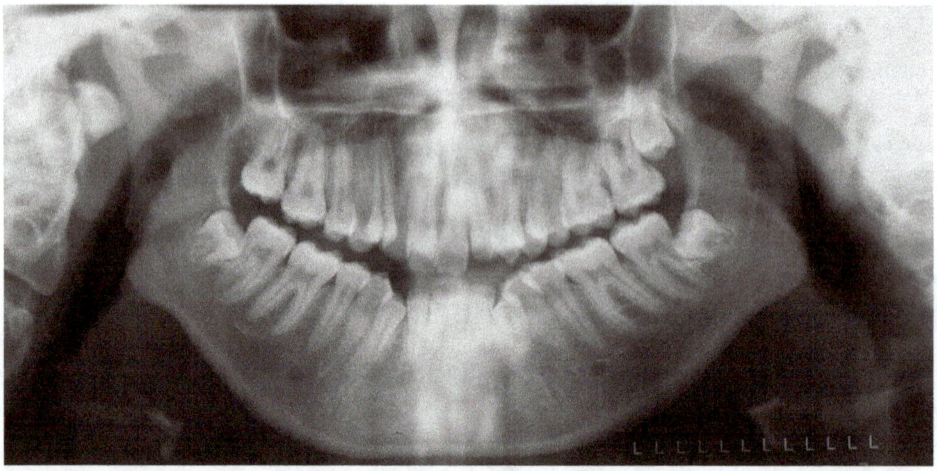

(i)

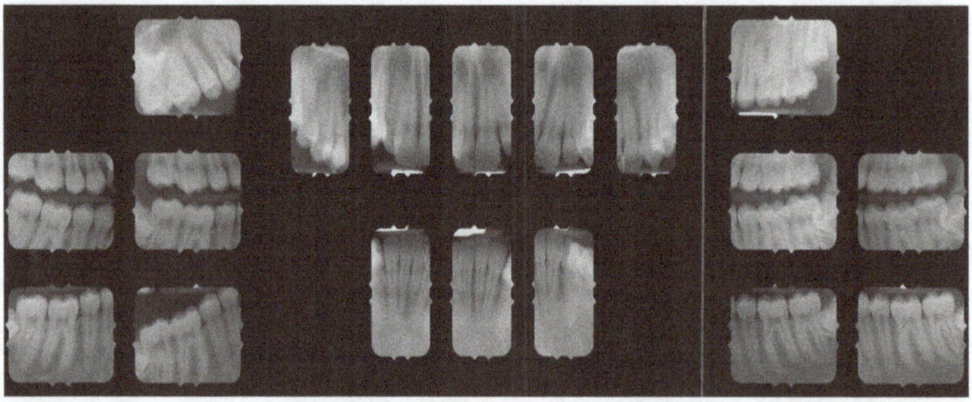

(j)

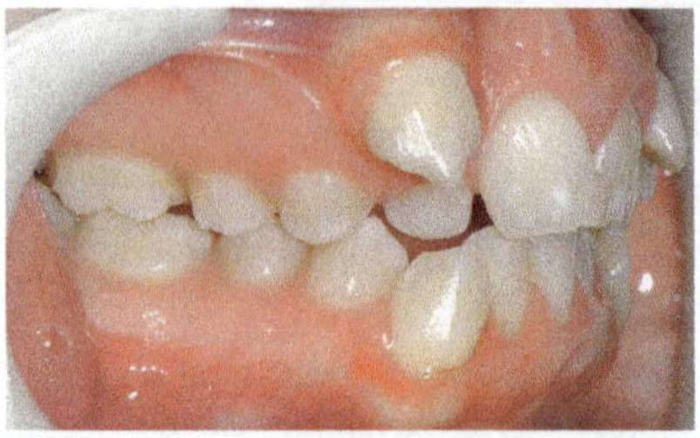

(k)

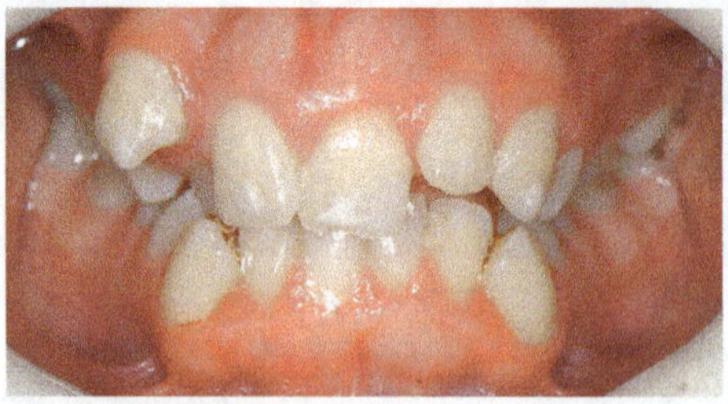

(l)

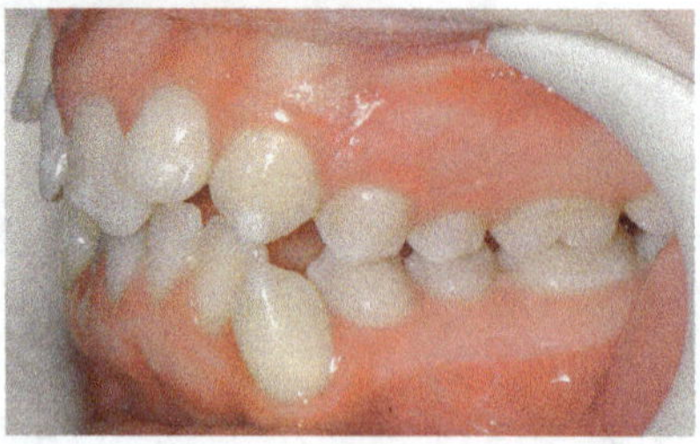

(m)

Figure 5.101 (Continued)

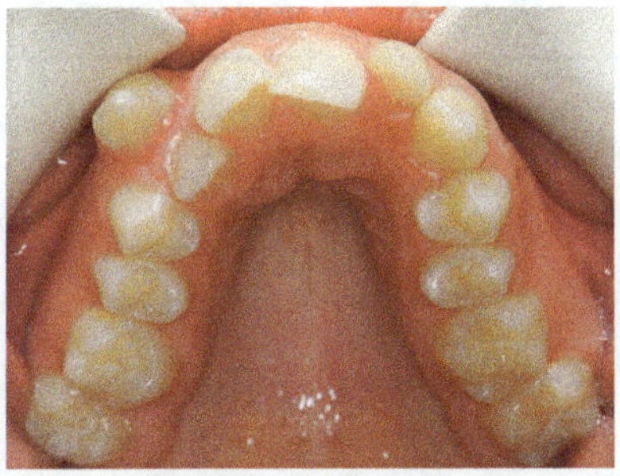
(n)

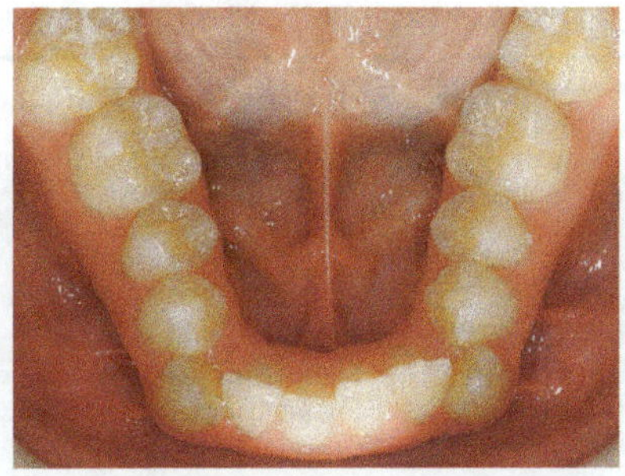
(o)

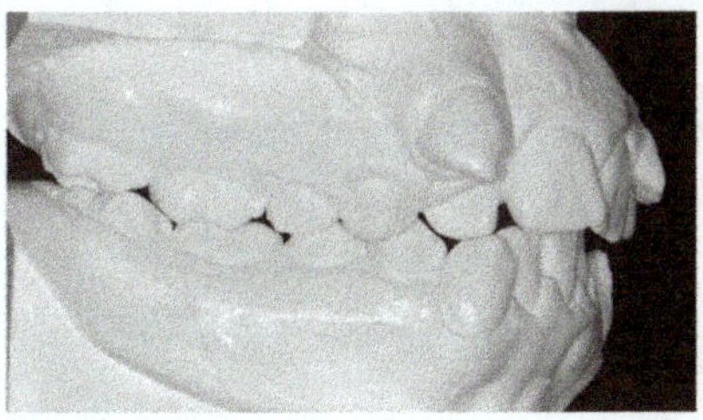
(p)

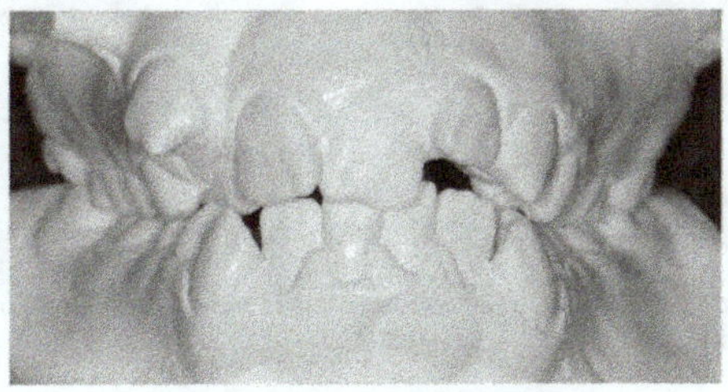
(q)

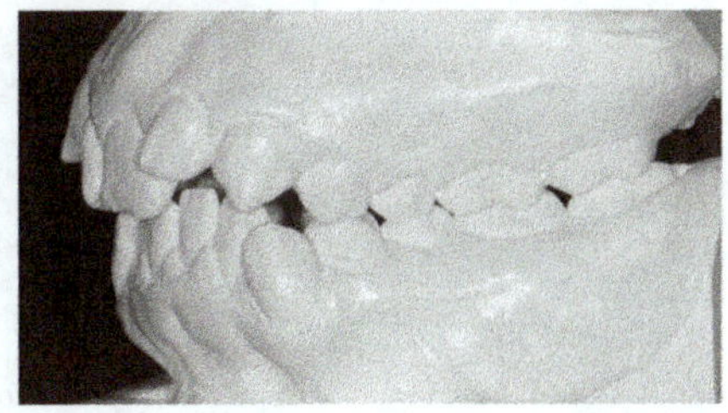
(r)

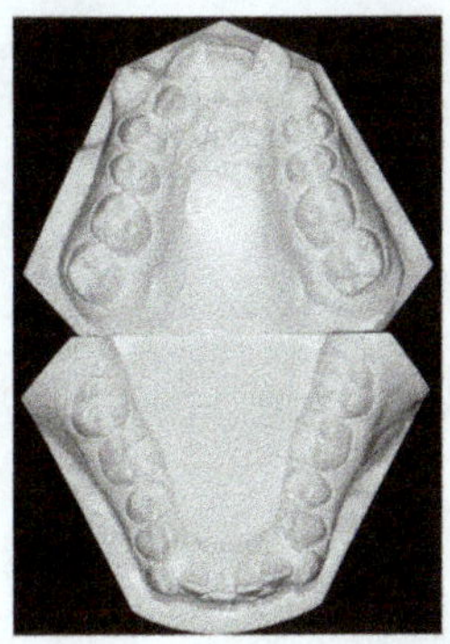
(s)

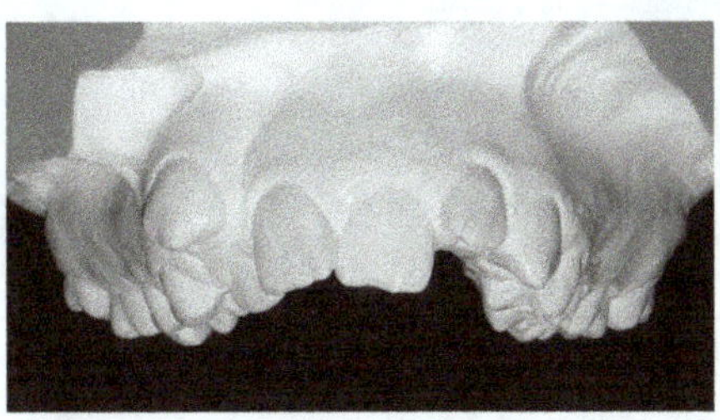
(t)

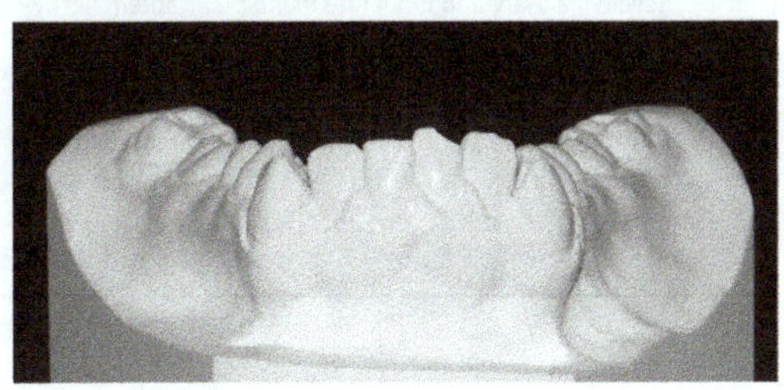
(u)

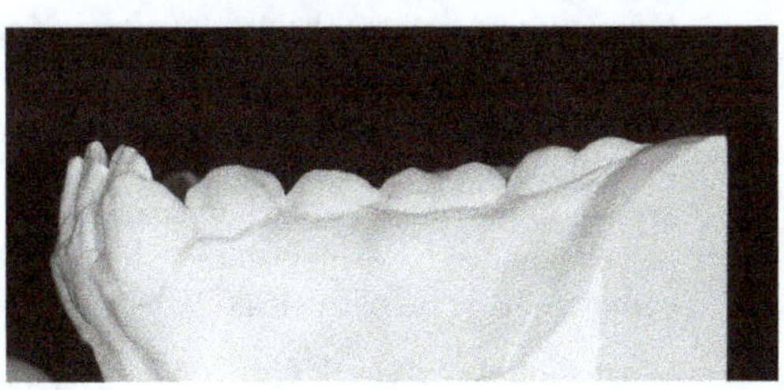
(v)

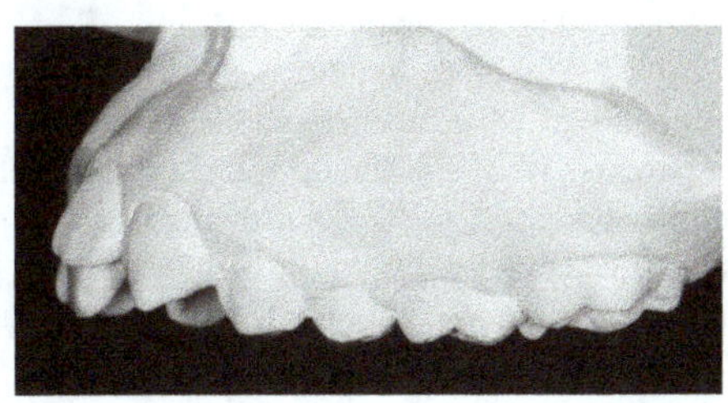
(w)

Figure 5.101 (Continued)

Table 5.10 Diagnostic findings and problem list for Ashley.

Full face and profile	**Frontal view** Symmetric face Soft tissue LLAFH (although Ashley's midface and LAFH at first appear equal in Figure 5.101A, her disproportionately long LAFH is clearly seen in Figure 5.101C) ILG 10 mm Excessive incisal display at rest: 5–6 mm UDML: 3 mm R LDML: 2–3 mm L Buccal corridors do not appear especially wide, but she may not be smiling broadly in this photograph Malar (zygomatic) projection adequate in 3/4 facial views **Profile view** Convex profile 90° nasolabial angle Upturned nose Retrusive chin Obtuse lip–chin–throat angle Short chin–throat length
Ceph analysis	**Skeletal** Maxillary skeletal AP deficiency (A-point posterior to Nasion-perpendicular line) Mandibular skeletal AP deficiency Skeletal LLAFH (LAFH/TAFH: 62%, over three standard deviations greater than an average of 55%, SD = 2%) Steep MPA (FMA = 48°; SNMP = 53°) Vertical maxillary excess, VME (LLAFH; first molar apicies erupted below palatal plane, maxillary molar template exaggerates this eruption, Figure 5.101h; palatal plane tipped down in posterior) Ineffective bony Pogonion Short ramus height Mild adenoidal hypertrophy **Dental** Upright maxillary incisors Proclined mandibular incisors
Radiographs	Permanent dentition Blocked out maxillary right canine Third molars developing
Intraoral photos and models	Angle Class II division 1 subdivision left malocclusion Iowa Classification: I II (2) II (5) II (5) OJ: ~3 mm Anterior crossbite (maxillary right lateral incisor, mandibular right canine) Anterior open bite Maxillary incisors stepped up Mandibular incisors stepped up COS 2–3 mm Minimal transverse OJ Lingual crown torque mandibular first and second molars Buccal crown torque maxillary second molars Severe maxillary and moderate mandibular anterior crowding (UTSALD = −9 mm; LTSALD = −9 mm) Maxillary right canine blocked out Mild dental arch asymmetries (Mn R ahead; Mx L ahead) Constricted, tapered maxillary arch (hourglass shape) Constricted mandibular arch (hourglass shape)
Other	—
Diagnosis	Angle Class II division 1 subdivision left Skeletal anterior open bite

severe skeletal open bite). Ashley also demonstrates dental compensations for her severe mandibular retrognathia (proclined mandibular incisors and upright maxillary incisors).

Q: In terms of her open bite, what other questions should you ask Ashley and her parents? What else should you check for? Why?

A: Ask Ashley and her parents if she is still growing. If she is still growing, then you need to consider this growth in forming her treatment plan and deciding when to initiate treatment. If she is still growing, use caution in doing anything irreversible (e.g., extracting teeth or surgery) until growth is complete and you are able to define your final treatment plan. If you proceeded with irreversible treatment and she was still growing, then she could grow out of your treatment. Ashley and her parents state that she reached menarche and completed growth years before. Next, show Ashley that her teeth are not touching in the front, and ask her when (and why) she developed this open bite. She thinks her front teeth have not touched for many years, but has no idea why they do not touch. Check for functional habits—tongue interpositional habit, thumb sucking, digit sucking, or lip biting. You do not detect any habits and she denies having any habits. Also, check for any temporary open bites due to permanent teeth erupting, ankylosis of permanent teeth that are not fully erupted, or lack of space for complete eruption of permanent teeth. Ashley does exhibit lack of space for the complete eruption of the maxillary right canine.

Q: What should you check for on Ashley's panoramic radiograph (hint: possible etiology of her open bite)?

A: Condylar degeneration—you need to confirm its absence. Degeneration of her condyles would result in downward and backward rotation of her mandible, creating the anterior open bite.

Q: Let's leave Ashley for a minute to examine an example of this concept. Krista is a 23-year-old woman who presents to you

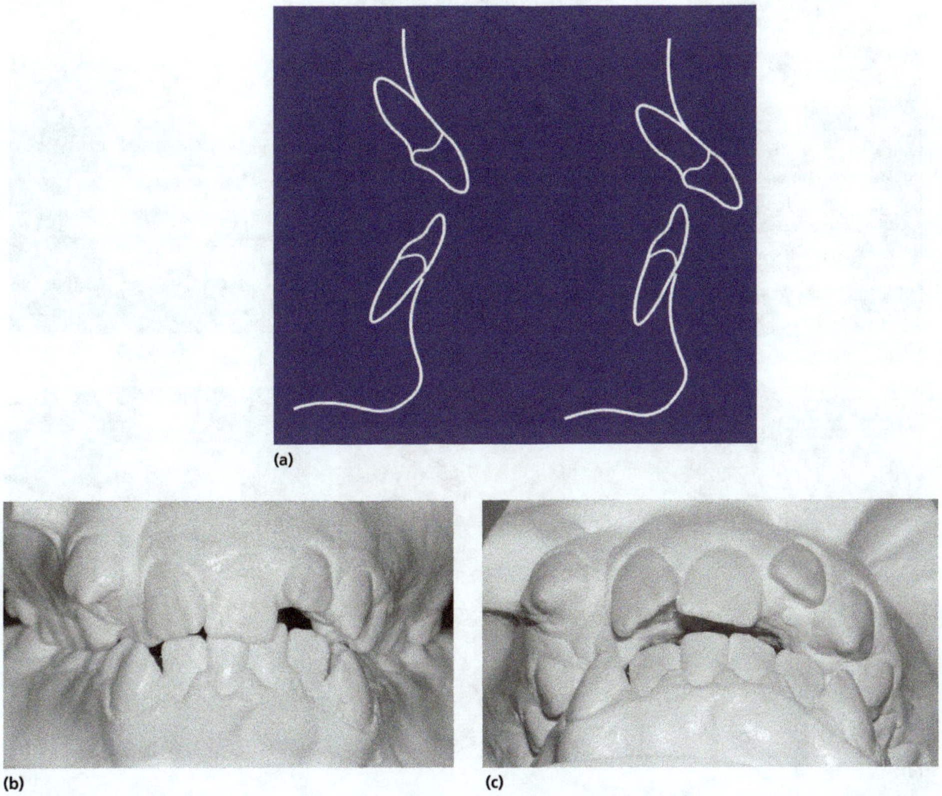

Figure 5.102 An anterior open bite exists when the mandibular anterior teeth do not touch the maxillary anterior teeth or the palate: (a, left) illustrates an anterior open bite, (a, right) illustrates an anterior open bite with "overlap"—the anterior teeth do not touch but appear to touch when viewed from the front, (b) illustrates Ashley's initial models viewed from the front, and (c) illustrates Ashley's models tipped up slightly. Ashley has an anterior open bite with overlap.

with an open bite (Figure 5.103a–d) and says that she did not have this open bite when she was growing up. She shows you a photograph from her teen years to prove this (Figure 5.103e). She says that she was in an automobile accident as a sophomore in high school, and she hit her chin on the steering wheel. In addition to her open bite, she complains of bilateral intermittent TMJ pain. Clinical examination reveals a maximum interincisal opening of 42 mm, a 2 mm CR—CO shift, and a 1.5 mm left lateral shift. She is without pain today and denies any medical problems. Figure 5.103f is her current panoramic image, and Figure 5.103g is a magnified image of her right condyle. What do you see?

A: Her right condylar head appears to be severely flattened.

Q: What question should you ask Krista about her bite immediately after the automobile accident?

A: Ask her if she remembers her bite being off immediately after the accident. If her bite had felt different, then she could have sustained a mandibular fracture. She says that she remembers her chin feeling sore, but her bite after the accident was normal.

Q: Condylar heads can have a variety of shapes. But with the Krista's history of trauma and resulting open bite, what do you suspect has happened here?

A: The trauma from the accident is probably at fault. The impact on her chin was transmitted to her mandibular condylar heads. Even without fracture, the blood supply to the condylar heads may have been interrupted resulting in bone death and resorption.

Q: What is your diagnosis for Krista?

A: Apertognathia (skeletal open bite) secondary to degenerative joint disease—avascular necrosis secondary to trauma [160]. This condition is relatively rare in the mandible, and is more frequently seen in hips (often requiring total hip replacement).

Q: Is there additional imaging you should recommend for Krista? Are there any other consultations you should request?

A: Yes, before considering any orthodontic treatment, you should have a CT scan made of her TM joints. These scans should be interpreted by a radiologist. In addition, you should rule out systemic etiologies. Referral to a rheumatologist would be appropriate.

Q: The radiologist confirms your diagnosis of condylar degeneration (both TMJs) most likely secondary to avascular necrosis. The rheumatologist rules out any systemic etiology for these degenerative changes. Krista is unhappy with her open bite and excess incisal show. She requests treatment for both concerns. Although we are not examining Krista's treatment in detail here, can you suggest treatment options specifically to correct her open bite and decrease her incisal display?

A: A maxillary LeFort I impaction osteotomy could correct her open bite and reduce her incisal display. A nonsurgical attempt could be made to intrude her entire maxillary dentition with TADs in order to close her open bite.

Q: What specific unknown do you face with Krista's condylar degeneration? How could you reduce this unknown?

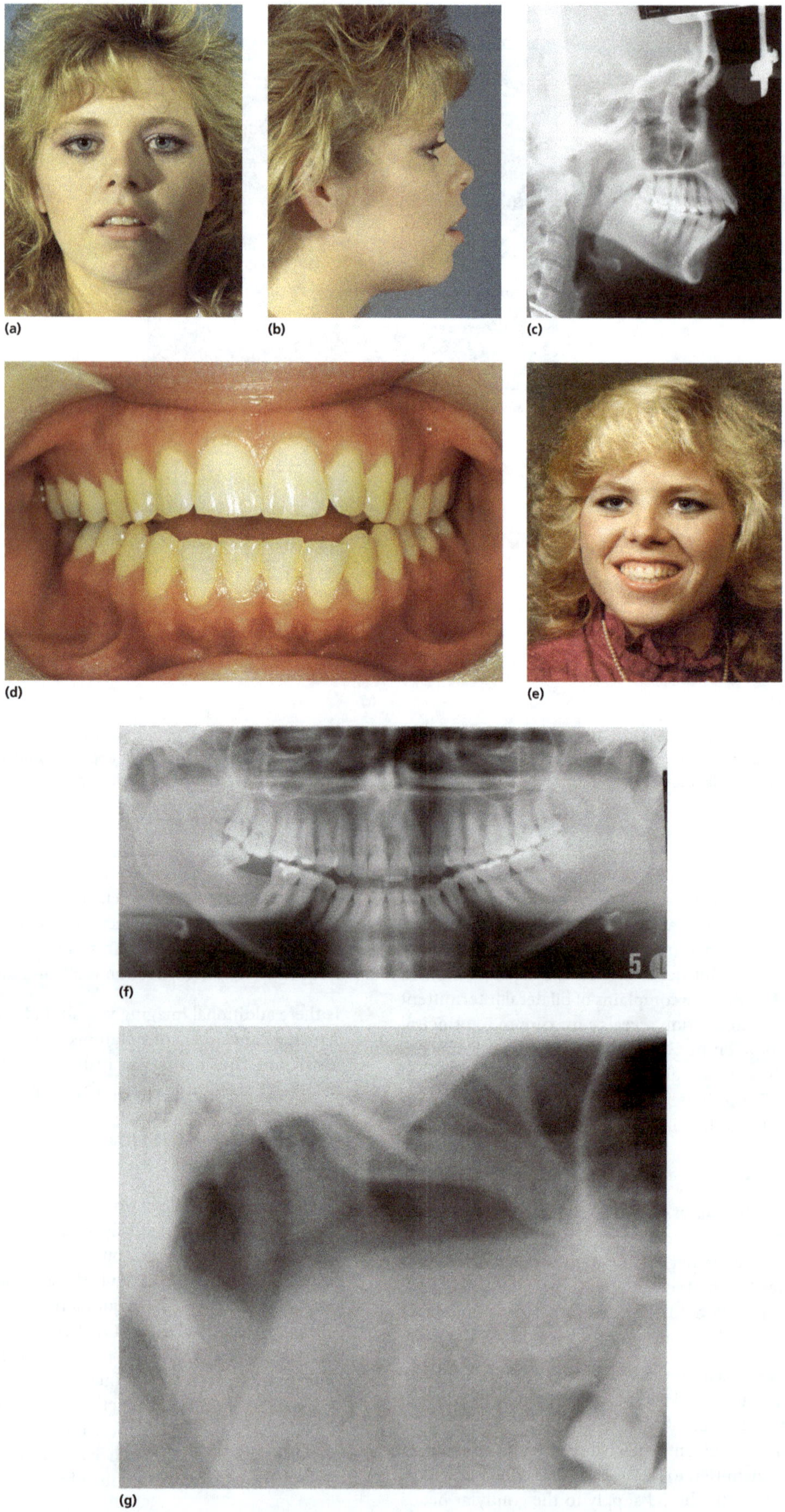

Figure 5.103 Records of Krista, who presents to you with an anterior open bite: (a, b) facial photographs, (c) lateral cephalograph, (d) intraoral photograph, (e) Krista's photograph taken in her junior year of high school showing the absence of an open bite, (f) pantomograph, and (g) magnified view of her right condyle from the pantomograph.

A: The major unknown you face is whether Krista's condylar degeneration is currently worsening or whether it will worsen with treatment. You should first ask Krista if her open bite is getting worse. She says she does not think so. You should then contact her general dentist to seek earlier panoramic images—to see what the condyles looked like before the accident and whether changes are occurring, recently. This was attempted, but historic images were unavailable. Whether you treat her surgically or nonsurgically, it would be wise to proceed slowly with treatment and monitor her condyles. Maybe first place braces, level and align arches, then evaluate her joints using another panoramic image in 9–12 months.

Q: With her TMJ history, do you feel comfortable with surgical treatment? Will her condylar degeneration worsen with surgery? Can you guarantee Krista that her condylar degeneration will not worsen?

A: A recent study of 18 patients with bilateral progressive condylar resorption who underwent orthognathic surgery [161] reported that four patients demonstrated condylar resorption with recurrence of open bite and retrognathism, four patients had a stable surgical result but currently have temporomandibular joint (TMJ) symptoms, and 10 patients had a stable surgical result (no change in postoperative occlusion or jaw position) without TMJ symptoms. Also, relapse occurred in patients having bimaxillary surgery with mandibular advancements greater than 5 mm. So, yes there is the chance that Krista could have a recurrence of condylar resorption with surgery. This is a risk she must be willing to take if a surgical option is taken.

Q: You discuss these risks with Krista, and she decides to proceed with surgery. In terms of the surgical procedure selected, the surgeon did something smart. To close the open bite, he had to impact the maxilla, but can you suggest what he decided about mandibular surgery?

A: He decided to avoid performing surgery on the proximal mandible (chin surgery only). By doing so, he avoided the possibility of diminishing blood supply to the proximal region, he avoided the possibility of torquing mandibular condyles with surgery, and (hopefully) he reduced the chances for a recurrence of condylar resorption.

Q: Krista had fixed appliances places, and her arches were leveled and aligned. She underwent a maxillary impaction osteotomy and genioplasty advancement (Figure 5.104a). She was debanded, and records were made 2 years later (Figure 5.104b–e). She continues to have occasional muscle soreness and her bite opened slightly in retention, but she is quite stable overall. She will continue to be monitored. Comparing her right condyle initially (Figure 5.103g) to her right condyle 2 years post deband (Figure 5.104e), what do you note?

A: Her right condyle appears stable. Condylar resorption has not re-occurred (at least as of this date).

Q: Let's return to Ashley's initial panoramic image (Figure 5.101i). Do you observe condylar degeneration or other pathology?

A: No. Ashley's condyles appear normal. A shape difference exists between her right and left condyles, and the necks of the condyles are long, but overt degeneration is not present. Furthermore, Ashley lacks any TMJ symptoms. However, you can always contact her family dentist to obtain historic panoramic images (to look for changes). This was not done.

Q: What else should you check for in terms of Ashely's open bite (hint: she exhibits mild adenoidal hypertrophy)?

A: Ashley's history of streptococcus infections should be obtained. If she is having multiple annual strep throats, having difficulty breathing, is an obligatory mouth breather, or is having episodes of sleep apnea, then she should be referred to an ortolaryngologist for an airway evaluation. However, you should inform Ashley and her parents that improving her airway will not guarantee a change in her facial growth pattern or guarantee stability of her orthodontic treatment. Last, an attempt should be made to have Ashley smile very broadly—to re-check her buccal corridors. This was not done.

Q: Is Ashley's open bite a dental open bite, a skeletal open bite, or a combination of both? What is the etiology of her open bite?

A: Ashley's open bite is a skeletal open bite due to maxillary vertical excess (VME: long soft tissue LAFH, ILG, long skeletal LAFH, steep MPA, maxillary first molar apicies erupted below palatal plane, palatal plane tipped down in posterior). She exhibits features of a classic skeletal open bite growth pattern: condyles growing posterior-superiorly instead of more vertically (Figure 5.105, curved red arrow), lack of posterior face height development, backward internal (true) mandibular rotation (curved blue arrows), a maxilla that has descended more than normal with a palatal plane which has rotated down posteriorly, and molars that have erupted more than normal (maxillary root apicies mildly erupted below palatal plane). As her mandible rotated downward and backward (yellow arrow), the mandibular plane angle steepened, the anterior face height increased, an ILG developed, and her anterior open bite resulted. Ashley lacks any habits that would have prevented her incisors from erupting. In fact, her mandibular incisors have supraerupted (Figure 5.101g, u) in an attempt to make contact with her maxillary incisors. *She does not have a functional habit or a dental open bite. Ashley is a skeletal open bite.*

Q: In what dimensions does Ashley exhibit apical base discrepancies? What are the *primary* problems in each dimension you must address?

A: Ashley has apical base (skeletal) discrepancies all three dimensions. See Table 5.11.

Q: What are the two general ways to close any anterior open bite? Which would you use to treat Ashley? Why?

A: Anterior open bites are closed by erupting anterior teeth (generally used for correcting dental open bites) and intruding posterior teeth (generally used for correcting skeletal open bites). *Erupting anterior teeth:* Ashley does not have a dental open bite. Her maxillary incisors are stepped up, but erupting them would only worsen her already excessive maxillary incisal display. Therefore, you should not erupt them (Figure 5.106a) unless you are planning to impact her maxilla surgically, intrude her maxillary dental arch with TADs, or accept the increased incisal display as a compromise when masking her skeletal open bite. Her mandibular incisors are already stepped up so you would not normally erupt them more (Figure 5.106a) unless you mask her skeletal open bite. Her maxillary incisors are upright so you would not wish to retract them/upright them further (Figure 5.106b) in order to rotate them around their apicies (erupting them). Her mandibular incisors are proclined. So, you could retract them/upright them (Figure 5.106b) which would tend to erupt them. However, they are already stepped up. You would not want to erupt them further unless you mask her skeletal open bite. *Intruding posterior teeth* (Figure 5.106c): intruding Ashley's mandibular posterior teeth with TADs, intruding her maxillary posterior teeth with TADs, or

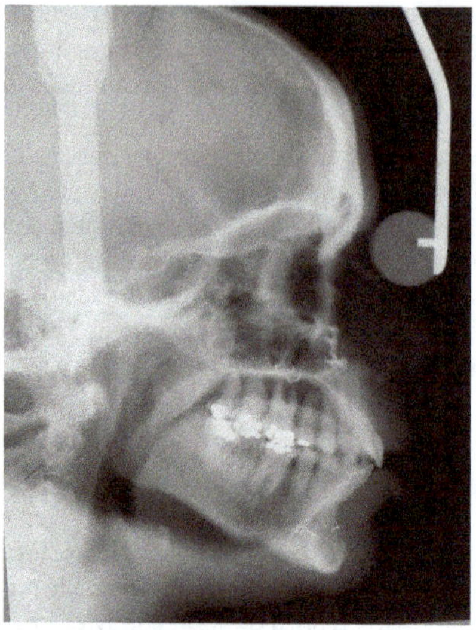

(a)

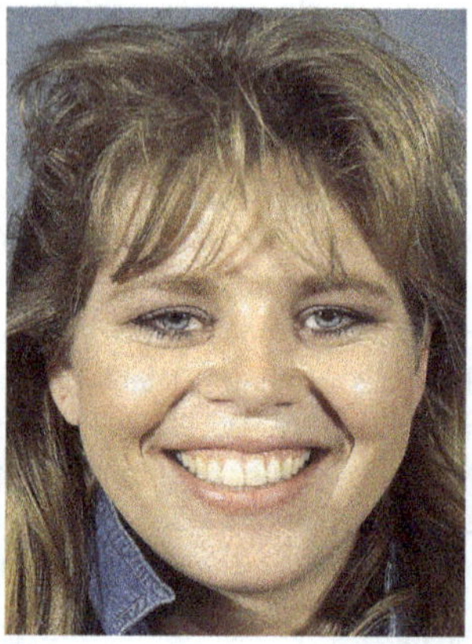

(b)

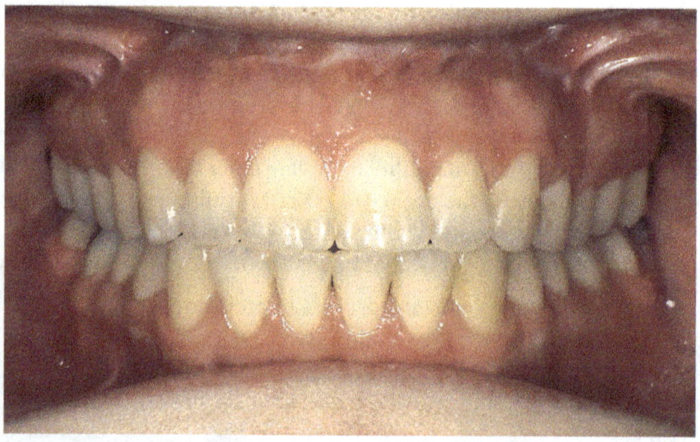

(c)

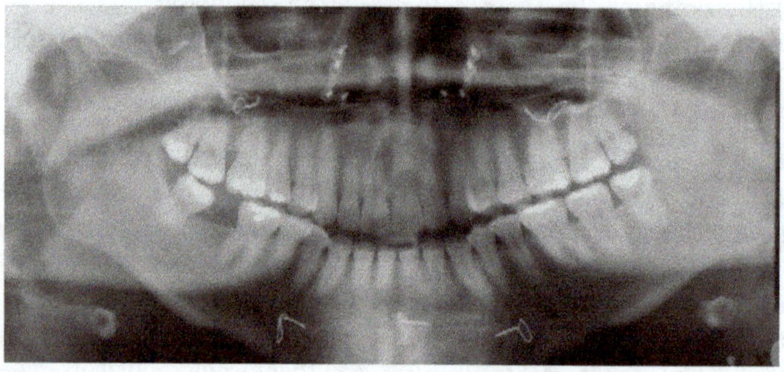

(d)

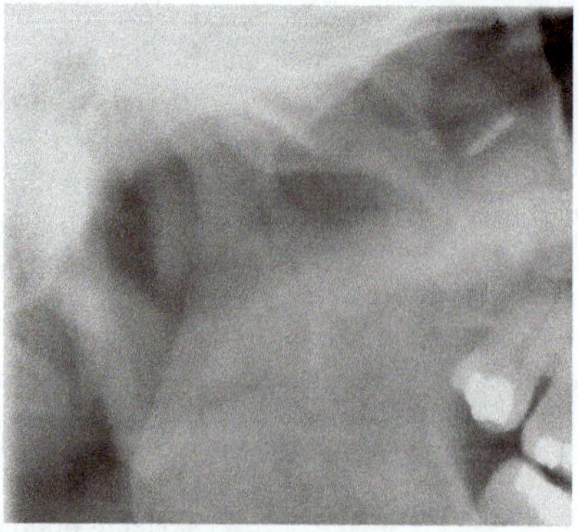

(e)

Figure 5.104 (a–e) Posttreatment records of Krista.

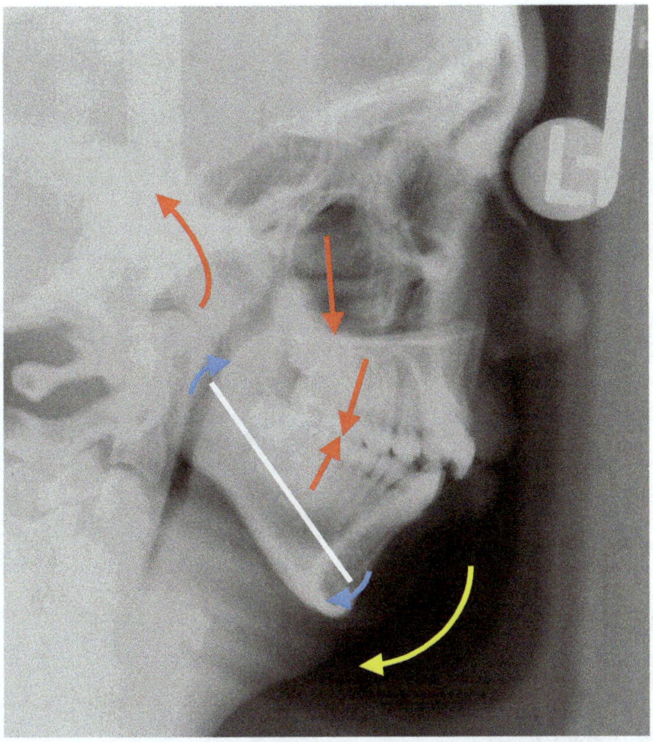

Figure 5.105 Ashley exhibits classic skeletal open bite growth features: condyles growing posterior-superiorly, lack of posterior face height development, backward mandibular internal (true) rotation, maxilla descending more than normal (palatal plane tipped down posteriorly), and molars erupting more than normal. As her mandible rotated CW downward and backward (yellow arrow), her mandibular plane steepened, her lower anterior face height increased, and an ILG and open bite resulted. Note: if Ashley's lower incisors had not supra-erupted (dental compensation for her skeletal open bite), then Ashley's anterior open bite would be much worse.

Table 5.11 Primary problems list for Ashley *(apical base/skeletal discrepancies italicized).*

AP	I II (2) II (5) II (5) *Maxillary skeletal retrusion* *Mandibular skeletal retrusion*
Vertical	*VME, skeletal open bite*
Transverse	*Maxillary transverse skeletal deficiency* with transverse dental compensations (maxillary second molar labial crown torque, mandibular first and second molar lingual crown torque) Note: If Ashley's posterior teeth were uprighted, then the crowns of the maxillary molars would tip lingually and the crowns of her mandibular molars would tip buccally—putting her in a posterior cross bite
Other	Blocked out maxillary right canine

"intruding" her maxillary posterior teeth with a LeFort I maxillary impaction osteotomy would be ideal and permit autorotation (CCW rotation) of the mandible around the condyles, reduction of her LLAFH, reduction of her incisal display, elimination of her ILG, and closure of her anterior open bite.

Q: What are your treatment goals?

A: To address Ashley's chief complaints, alleviate her crowding, achieve lip competence, and improve her chin projection. Additionally, it would be beneficial to reduce her incisal display, improve her transverse relationship/buccal overjet, position her maxillary permanent canines into a Class I relationship, obtain minimal overjet, and overcorrect her overbite. Although improving her maxillary skeletal retrusion could be considered a goal, if you cover Ashley's initial facial photos from the lower lip down—her midface appears quite attractive. So, moving her maxilla forward may not be a priority. In addition, if her maxilla were to be moved forward, care must be taken not to tip her nose up more as the anterior nasal spine comes forward.

Q: How would you address Ashley's anteroposterior apical base discrepancy?

A: *Orthopedics* (restrict maxillary AP growth, permit the mandible to continue growing, or accelerate mandibular growth). Since Ashley has completed growth, *orthopedics is not an option.* However, if one considers the use of TADs as orthopedic treatment (as opposed to masking or surgical treatment), then TADs could be used to intrude her posterior teeth—reducing her vertical dimension and improving her chin projection slightly through mandibular CCW rotation. But, the amount of rotation would be inadequate to correct her retrusive chin projection. Another approach would be to use TADs to reduce her vertical dimension and rotate her mandible forward plus include an advancement genioplasty to improve her chin projection.

Masking or camouflage (achieve a Class I canine relationship without addressing the underlying anteroposterior apical base discrepancy). This approach would not address her chief complaint ("jaw sits back"). However, if Ashley declined surgery, then teeth alignment could be a compromise which would improve her smile, and a genioplasty advancement could be used to improve her chin projection. Teeth could be moved into a canine Class I relationship using headgear, TADs, interarch Class II correctors, of various combinations of premolar extractions. But again, none of these treatments would address her chief complaint.

Surgery (mandibular advancement, maxillary impaction to advance her mandible through autorotation, and genioplasty advancement). Surgery could address her chief complaint in the AP direction.

Q: If a surgical option is selected, would you extract teeth?

A: To answer this question for the maxillary arch, you first need to decide if you are expanding the maxilla (RME, SARME). If you are expanding the maxilla (increasing arch perimeter), it would be advisable to re-evaluate the need for extractions *after* expansion. Mandibular extractions will be necessary in order to retract mandibular canines further Class II prior to a mandibular advancement osteotomy (which then restores the canines to a Class I relationship). Further, considering the 9 mm of mandibular anterior crowding and mandibular incisor proclination (FMIA = 46°), extraction in the mandibular arch would create space to upright the incisors.

Q: If you extract mandibular teeth prior to surgery, which teeth would you extract? Would you advise minimal anchorage or maximal anchorage during space closure? How would you achieve this anchorage?

A: Since only a mild mandibular dental arch asymmetry exists, you should extract symmetrically if you are going to extract. The mandibular first premolars should be extracted if a BSSO advancement is planned. Why? If you need to extract teeth, then generally extract teeth where the crowding exists (scratch where it itches). So, you should extract Ashley's mandibular first premolars instead of her second premolars. To maximize a mandibular advancement, the mandibular

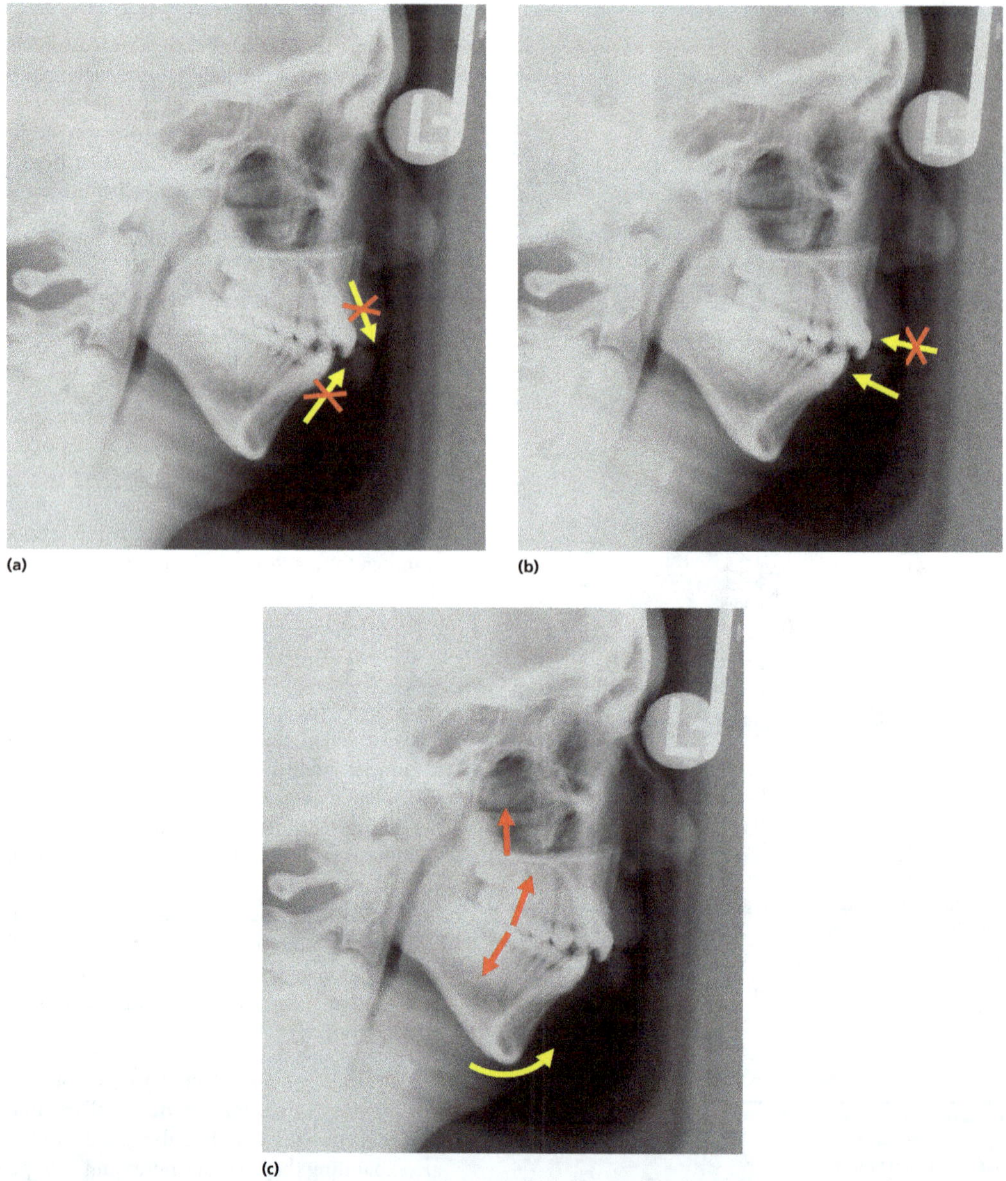

Figure 5.106 General ways to treat Ashley's anterior open bite: (a) Although Ashley's maxillary incisors are stepped up, unless you plan to impact her maxilla surgically, or intrude her maxillary teeth with TADs, erupting them will worsen her already excessive incisal display. Since her mandibular incisors are stepped up, it would not be ideal to erupt them more. (b) Since her maxillary incisors are upright, it would not be ideal to retract/upright them further in order to rotate them around their apicies (erupting them). You could retract/upright her proclined mandibular incisors which would tend to erupt them. However, her mandibular incisors are already stepped up, and you would not want to erupt them further unless you were masking her skeletal open bite. (c) Intruding Ashley's molars with TADs, or impacting her maxilla, would be ideal and permit autorotation of her mandible around the condyles, reduction of her LLAFH, elimination of her ILG, reduction of her incisal display, and closure of her anterior open bite (yellow arrow).

canines should be retracted through the entire first premolar extraction space—a movement requiring maximum posterior anchorage. That is, no reciprocal mesial movement of the mandibular second premolars or molars is desirable. The full extraction space should be used to retract the mandibular canines. TADs could be placed distal to the extraction site as anchorage. For instance, TADs could be placed between the mandibular first molars and second premolars. If inadequate room exists for the TADs, then space can first be opened between the teeth in order to make room for the TADs. Or, instead of using TADs, the patient could wear a headgear (J-hook headgear, Figure 5.107a–c) to the mandibular canines to retract them without any loss of mandibular posterior anchorage. In summary, Ashley's profile could benefit from a maximum mandibular advancement (up to 10 mm for high MPA patients like Ashley; 15 mm for flat MPA patients). Using TADs or headgear as anchorage will allow maximal retraction of mandibular canines through the extraction space and force the surgeon to maximally advance her mandible.

Q: How would you address Ashley's vertical apical base discrepancy?

A: *Orthopedics* (treatment that would reduce downward descent of the maxilla and reduce eruption of the maxillary and mandibular molars during growth). Since Ashley has completed growth,

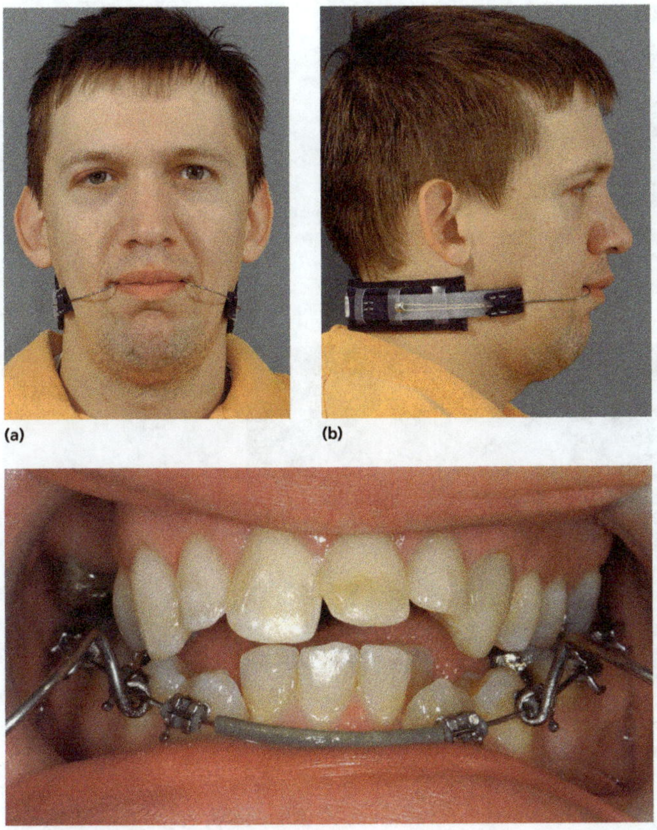

Figure 5.107 In Class II surgical patients, it is often desirable to maximally retract mandibular canines through first premolar extraction spaces. This movement forces the surgeon to maximally advance the mandible with a BSSO advancement osteotomy (bringing the mandibular canines forward into a Class I relationship, and maximally increasing chin projection). In order to achieve maximum mandibular canine retraction, TADs can be placed posteriorly as anchorage, or a J-hook cervical-pull headgear (a–c) can be worn to the canines.

orthopedics in the vertical dimension is not feasible. But again, one could consider the use of TADs to intrude teeth as orthopedics. Intrusion of posterior teeth with TADs could decrease Ashley's ILG and reduce her excess incisal display. The use of TADs could be coupled with an impaction genioplasty—to further reduce her LAFH and reduce her ILG.

Masking or camouflage (achieve open bite closure without addressing the underlying vertical apical base discrepancy). The lower incisors could be left overerupted (Figure 5.101u) by placing a curve of Spee in the mandibular archwire, and the maxillary incisors could be erupted during arch leveling (fixed appliances supported by vertical elastics). However, masking will not address Ashley's chief complaint of lip incompetence.

Surgery (maxillary impaction osteotomy) could be used in conjunction with a mandibular advancement and impaction genioplasty procedure to achieve an ideal result.

Q: How would you address Ashley's transverse apical base discrepancy?

A: *Orthopedics* (separating the hemi-maxillae at the midpalatal suture). RME—would result in both maxillary skeletal expansion and maxillary dental expansion. Figure 5.101l, n, and s illustrate just how narrow Ashley's maxilla is. If the maxilla is expanded, then excess posterior overjet is created to allow uprighting/elimination of lingual crown torque of the mandibular posterior teeth. Both arches can then be coordinated.

Masking or camouflage (correcting the minimal posterior overjet primarily by increasing molar transverse compensations (maxillary labial crown torque, mandibular lingual crown torque) and not by addressing the underlying transverse skeletal discrepancy). Ashley's maxilla is so narrow that achieving adequate transverse overjet with masking is not advised—it would result in excessive maxillary molar labial crown torque and excessive mandibular lingual crown torque.

Surgery

- SARME—would achieve adequate maxillary expansion. However, an attempt should first be made to achieve maxillary expansion with RME.
- Since a maxillary impaction surgery is planned anyway—a simultaneous multiple-piece maxillary osteotomy to expand the transverse would be reasonable. However, the magnitude of maxillary transverse expansion is limited with a multiple-piece maxillary osteotomy since you are stretching the palatal soft tissue quickly and may compromise the palatal blood supply if it is stretched too much (blanch the palatal soft tissue).

Q: What is a potential problem in attempting RME expansion in Ashley?

A: Her age. There is increased skeletal resistance to maxillary expansion at the maxillary bony articulations with increasing age [162, 163], and the *most marked effect of RME is before and during the pubertal growth spurt* [164]. In older patients, there is little orthopedic change [165], and expansion after pubertal growth spurt occurs mainly by dentoalveolar (not orthopedic) expansion [166]. At 16 years, 6 months old, Ashley's facial skeletal resistance may be too great to permit separation of her midpalatal suture with an RME appliance. However, you can attempt this approach, albeit slowly (0.25 mm per day, or 0.25 mm every other day when starting), and see if the midpalatal suture separates.

Q: How do you know if the midpalatal suture separates (splits)?

A: If a maxillary midline diastema forms during RME, or if an occlusal radiograph clearly shows a midpalatal split (Figure 5.108a, red arrows), then the suture has separated. If a midline diastema does not form, and if an occlusal radiograph does not clearly show a split, then only dental movement may be occurring. Compare the banded first molar on the right side of the image in Figure 5.108b, c. While the patient continued turning the screw, the midpalatal suture did not open. Instead, the molar on the right of the image was being driven buccally out of its socket. Clinically, the metal bar of the RME appliance will start impinging on the palatal soft tissue as the teeth, but not the hemi-maxillae, are moving buccally. Other signs that the midpalatal suture is not opening can include a sensation of lasting pressure from the screw, or pain.

Q: If the midpalatal suture does not split, what should you do?

A: This will depend on whether you have already achieved significant dental expansion of the maxillary molars with the expander. If only minimal expansion has occurred and you require much more, then you may consider surgical intervention (SARME or multiple-piece maxillary osteotomy). If significant dental expansion has already occurred, and the periodontium

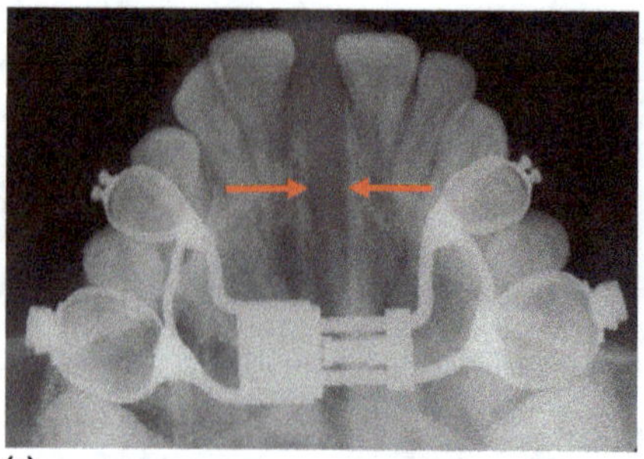

(a)

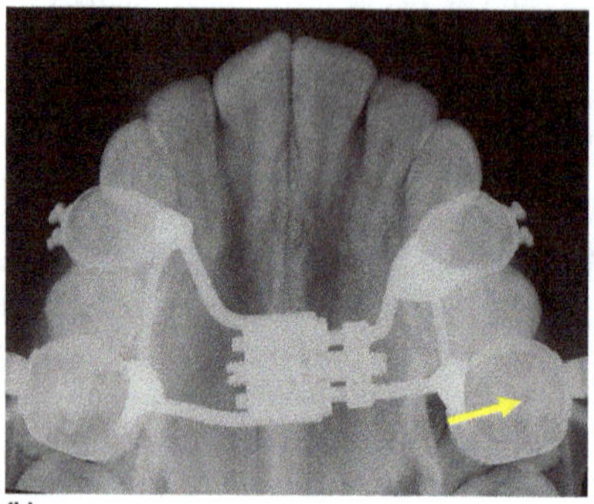

(b)

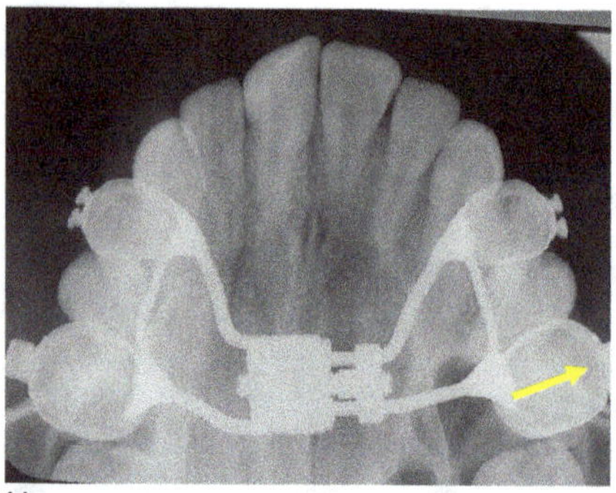

(c)

Figure 5.108 Effects of RME as viewed using occlusal radiographs: (a, red arrows) midpalatal suture split; (b, c) absence of midpalatal suture split as the screw is being opened, transverse expansion occurring only by first molar dental movement (yellow arrows).

appears robust, you must make the decision either to continue dental expansion *or* to stop and consider surgery.

Q: Assume that a surgical transverse correction is being considered. What general guidelines would you follow for choosing between a SARME or an MPMO to make the transverse correction?

A: Guidelines include the following:

- The *magnitude* of the transverse maxillary skeletal expansion needed is the most important factor you must consider. If the required maxillary skeletal expansion is 10 mm or more, than a SARME is indicated. Why? With a SARME, you are actually growing tissue as you expand. With an MPMO, you are stretching palatal tissue that could compromise the palatal blood supply.
- If the palatal vault is *low*, then a SARME may be indicated (again, there may be too much immediate stretching of the palatal soft tissue with an MPMO).
- If surgical expansion is the *only* dimension to be corrected with maxillary surgery, then a SARME is indicated. Why? There would be no reason to downfracture the maxilla to correct the transverse. But, if the maxilla will also be impacted, downgrafted, advanced, or set back, then an MPMO may be indicated.
- If a *very large step* exists between the posterior and anterior maxillary dentition, then an MPMO may be needed to move the maxillary segments independently.

Q: What unknowns do you face during Ashley's treatment? Are there any unknowns you need to eliminate before you define your final treatment plan?

A: The biggest unknown is whether Ashley's midpalatal suture will separate if you attempt RME. You need to address this before you can establish your final treatment plan. Also, cooperation, hygiene, and a hidden anteroposterior shift are possible unknowns.

Q: Ashley's maxillary anterior teeth are stepped up relative to her posterior teeth. How do you recommend treating this occlusal step (if she undergoes surgery)? Should you level this step with fixed appliances and archwires before surgery? Should you level it surgically (with an MPMO)?

A: Here is what we know: Ashley's maxillary anterior teeth are stepped up by 3–4 mm, except for her maxillary right canine which is blocked out (Figure 5.101t). Leveling anterior teeth stepped up by a few millimeters has been shown to be stable [60]. *Leaving* an anterior step in the occlusion prior to surgery would force you into an MPMO instead of a one-piece maxillary osteotomy. In terms of morbidity, it is generally better to minimize surgical segmentation of the maxilla. "The fewer the pieces, the fewer the problems." Considering the above, it is reasonable to level Ashley's maxillary arch prior to surgery.

Q: Based on everything, we have discussed thus far, what treatment options would you consider for Ashley? Suggest both a nonsurgical and a surgical treatment option. What specific treatment do you recommend?

A: To address Ashley's chief complaints, a surgical treatment plan must be considered. However, she was also presented with a nonsurgical option that would avoid surgical risks but would not address her complaint (retrusive jaw). The nonsurgical option started with an RME appliance and removable mandibular lingual arch (Wilson arch) in an *attempt* to expand the maxilla and upright the mandibular molars. This would be followed by re-evaluation for possible extraction of maxillary first premolars and mandibular second premolars. HPHG would be worn, or TADs placed, as needed to achieve a Class I molar and canine relationship. A TPA or expanded HG inner bow would maintain the maxillary transverse expansion. The arches would be leveled, aligned, and spaces closed. She would then be finished and retained. Ashley and her parents were informed that this treatment plan was a compromise.

The surgical treatment plan included an RME appliance (SARME if the RME failed) and removable mandibular lingual arch (Wilson arch) to upright the mandibular molars. This would be followed by re-evaluation for mandibular first premolar and wisdom teeth extractions, banding/bonding/leveling/aligning of the arches, space closure in the lower arch using maximum anchorage, LeFort I maxillary impaction osteotomy, mandibular BSSO advancement osteotomy, advancement genioplasty, finishing, and retention. After considering both options, Ashley and her parents chose the surgical option.

Q: What are the specific objectives of treatment for the maxilla, mandible, maxillary dentition, and mandibular dentition in all three planes of space?

A: Specific objectives of treatment for Ashley are as follows:

Maxilla

AP: Maintain anterior, protract posterior.

Vertical: Impact posterior, maintain anterior.

Transverse: Increase skeletal width.

Mandible

AP: Advance by surgical lengthening and advancement genioplasty.

Vertical: Decrease skeletal lower anterior facial height by autorotation and genioplasty.

Transverse: Maintain.

Maxillary dentition

AP: Protract molars and retract canines. Retract incisors.

Vertical: Maintain molars and incisors.

Intermolar width: Increase intermolar width.

Mandibular dentition

AP: Maintain molars. Retract canines and incisors.

Vertical: Eliminate reverse curve of Spee.

Intermolar/intercanine width: Increase intermolar by expansion. Increase intercanine widths by retraction.

Q: How did Ashley's treatment proceed?

A: An RME appliance was delivered, and Ashley was asked to turn it 1 turn/day for 14 days. She returned to the clinic at which time a midpalatal split was noted on a maxillary occlusal radiograph. Expansion continued at the same rate for another 14 days, and a Wilson arch was placed in the mandible. After the 11 mm screw of the RME appliance was opened completely, more expansion was deemed necessary and an impression for a new RME appliance was made. The new RME appliance was delivered (activation continuing), and the Wilson arch was activated to expand the mandibular intermolar width, upright the mandibular molars, and maintain coordination between the two arches. In addition, crossbite elastics were worn from the Wilson arch, bilaterally, to the buccal of the RME appliance to upright the mandibular molars more rapidly. Mandibular third molars and first premolars were extracted. TADs were placed between the mandibular second premolars and first molars. Mandibular canines were bonded, and their retraction begun. Expansion of the maxillary RME appliance was stopped when it was noted that the *roots of the maxillary first premolars were very prominent* in the buccal vestibule. The RME appliance was converted into a TPA. At this point, Ashley had attained 16 mm net maxillary expansion (Figure 5.109).

The mandibular canines were retracted through the entire mandibular first premolar extraction space using the TADs as anchorage (Figure 5.110).

Fixed appliances were placed on the remaining teeth of both arches. The arches were leveled/aligned and spaces

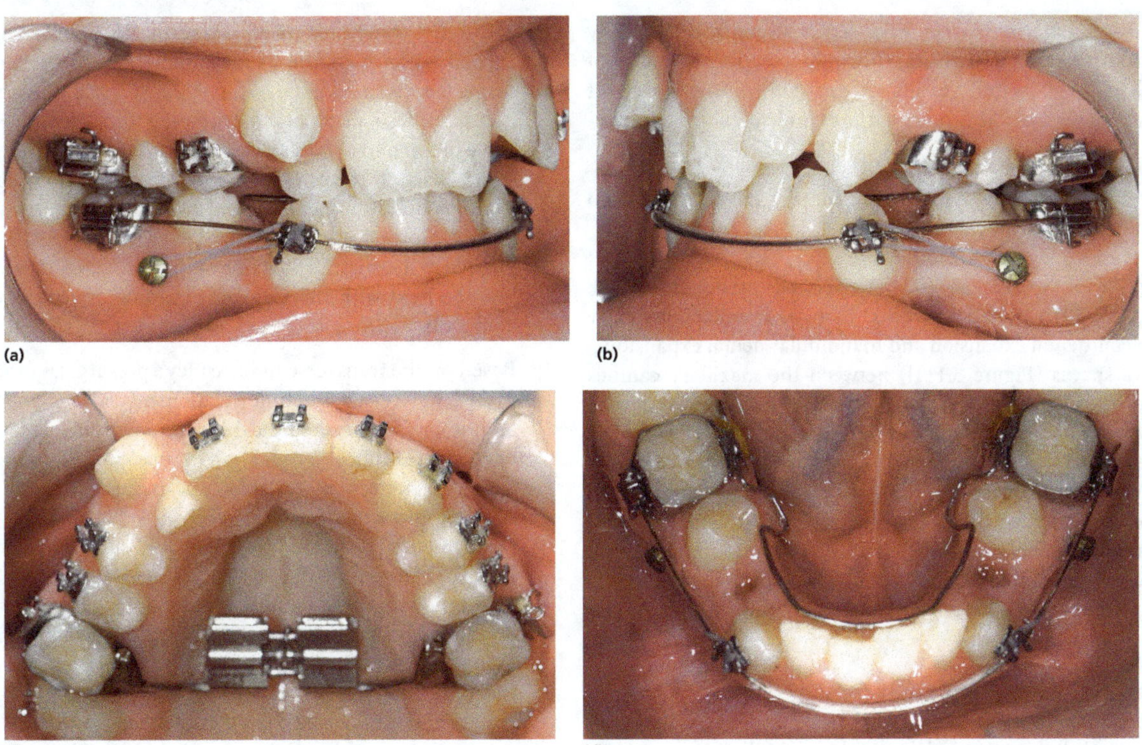

Figure 5.109 Progress records of Ashley: (a, b) expansion with an RME and retraction of the mandibular canines through the first premolar extraction sites using direct anchorage off TADs; (c) post expansion maxillary intermolar width was recorded at 55.8 mm, which represented a net intermolar expansion of 16 mm from the initial intermolar width of 39.8 mm; and (d) mandibular occlusal view showing removable Wilson arch.

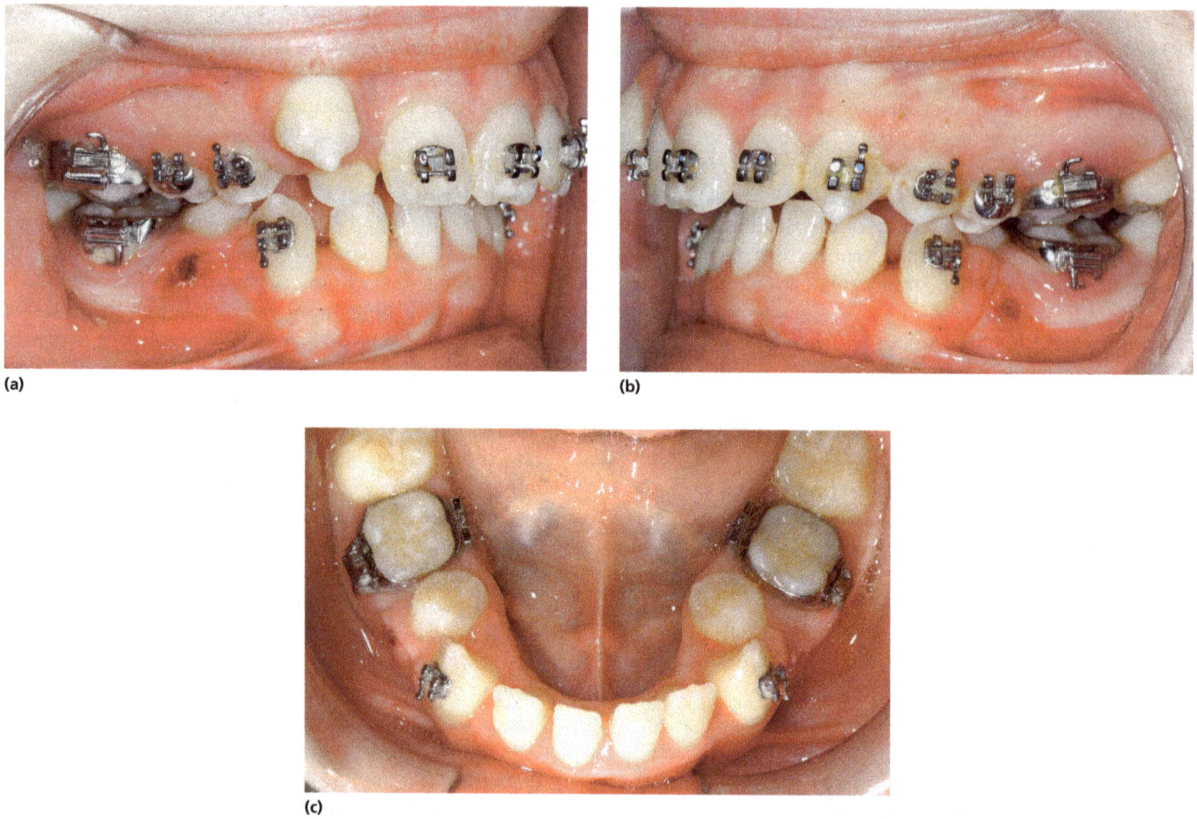

Figure 5.110 (a–c) Progress records of Ashley: mandibular canines were retracted through the entire first premolar extraction space. This is an example of maximum anchorage. That is, there was no reciprocal molar or premolar mesial movement during canine retraction using TADs as anchorage.

closed—except that spaces were left between the maxillary canines and lateral incisors (Iowa spaces, the purpose of which is to allow full seating of the canines into a perfect Class I relationship at surgery without interference from maxillary incisors).

Q: Figure 5.111 presents Ashley's pre-surgery records. What do you note?

A: Observations include the following:

- Significant expansion in both dental arches (compare Figure 5.101n, o with Figure 5.111l, m) as a result of maxillary skeletal/dental expansion and mandibular dental expansion.
- Iowa spaces (Figure 5.111l) between the maxillary canines and maxillary lateral incisors to allow full surgical canine Class I seating without incisor interference.
- Mandibular incisal uprighting and maxillary incisor proclination (Figure 5.111e). Ashley's facial appearance has worsened as these dental compensations were removed.
- Mandibular molars moved forward ~2 mm (Figure 5.111e). Did this occur during incisor retraction/space closure?
- There appears to have been a small amount of mandibular and maxillary growth.

Q: You believe that Ashley is ready for surgery. How should you proceed?

A: Presurgical diagnostic models should be made (Figure 5.112). Judge arch coordination when the models are hand articulated with canines Class I and in a best-fit transverse relationship. If additional transverse maxillary surgical expansion is needed, then duplicates of the models should be made and model surgery performed to (i) evaluate the occlusal fit with different multiple-piece maxillary osteotomies (e.g., two piece versus three piece) and (ii) determine the amount of additional expansion needed. If the canines cannot be seated into a Class I relationship because maxillary and mandibular incisors interfere, then the Iowa spaces should be increased in order to move the maxillary incisors further out of the way. A discussion should then be held with the surgeon regarding the optimal surgical approach.

Q: Based on the transverse fit of Ashley's presurgical models when placed in a Class I canine relationship, it was apparent that additional transverse surgical expansion was needed. Duplicates of her presurgical models were made and various model surgeries performed to assess the occlusal fit with different multiple-piece maxillary osteotomies. What are some multiple-piece maxillary osteotomies you would suggest to increase her maxillary transverse dimension?

A: The following three options were considered by sectioning duplicates of Ashley's maxillary model at the appropriate sites, repositioning the segments, and then bonding the segments together with wax to check for occlusal fit:

- A maxillary two-piece osteotomy to increase *both* the maxillary intercanine width and the posterior width (Figure 5.113). Note that the maxillary width widens more toward the posterior than the anterior because the maxillary central incisors are left

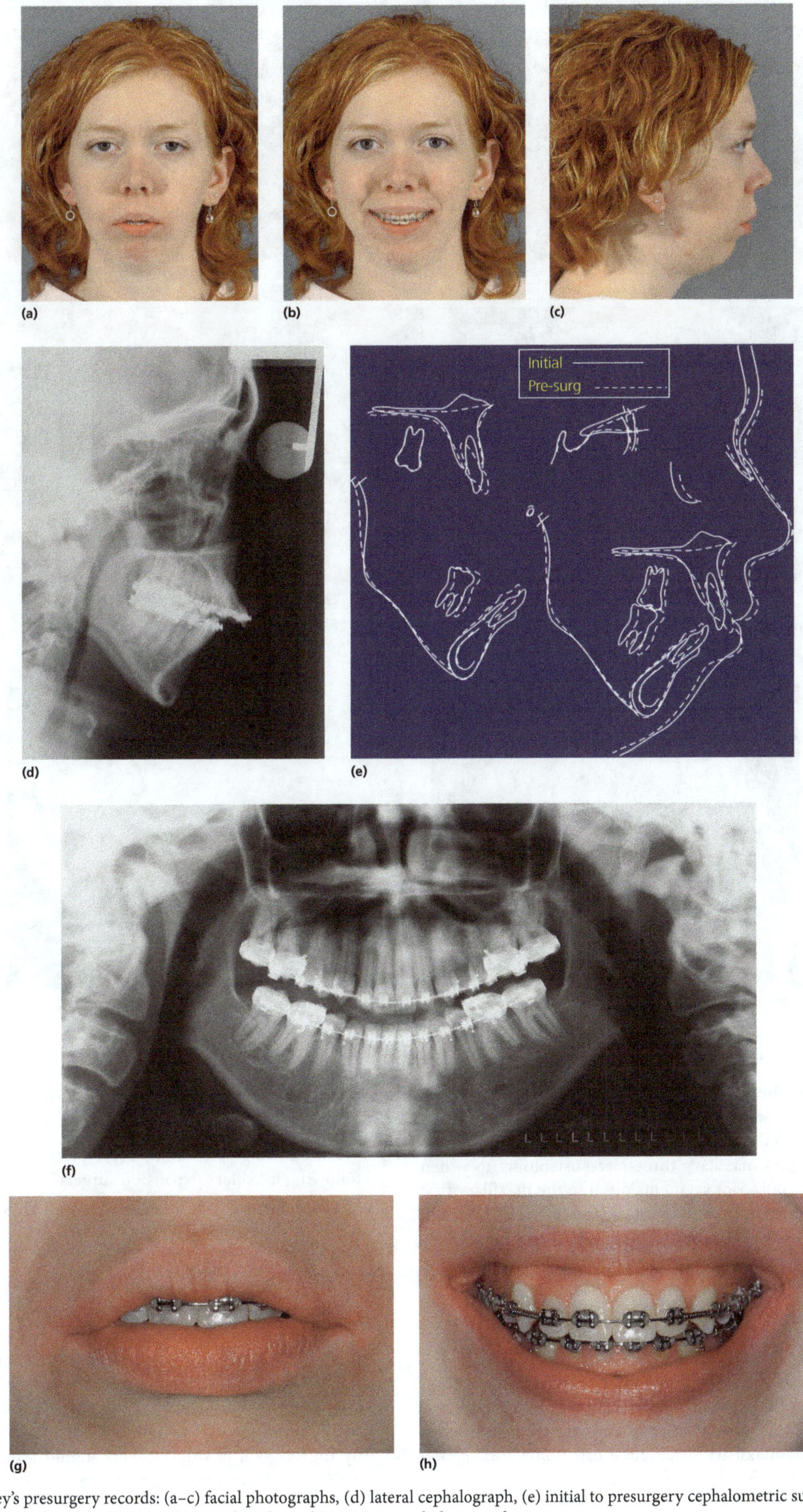

Figure 5.111 Ashley's presurgery records: (a–c) facial photographs, (d) lateral cephalograph, (e) initial to presurgery cephalometric superimposition, (f) pantomograph, (g) relaxed lip position, (h) posed smile, and (i–m) intraoral photographs.

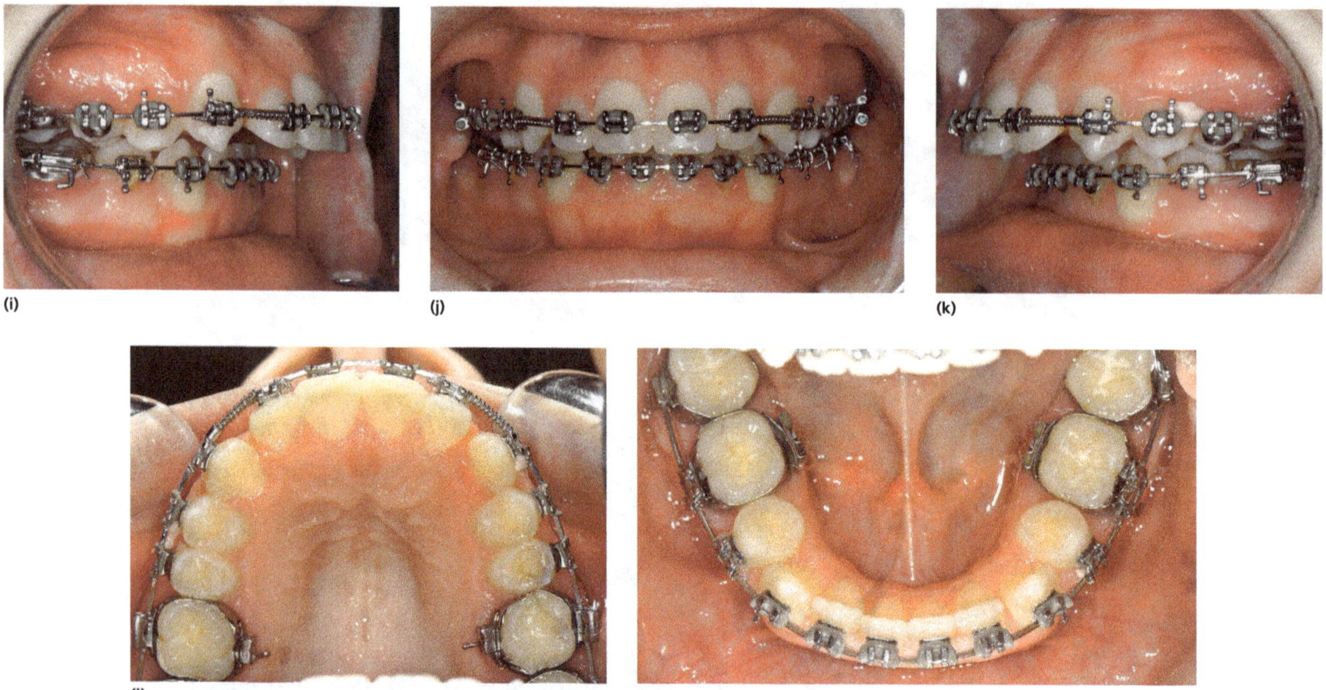

(i) (j) (k) (l) (m)

Figure 5.111 (Continued)

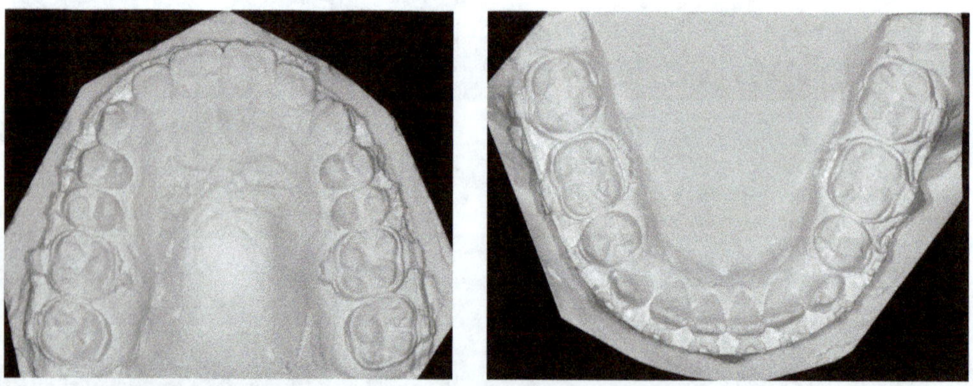

(a) (b)

Figure 5.112 (a–b) Occlusal views of Ashley's presurgical models.

in contact as the posterior arch is widened. The maxillary second molars would be left unopposed with this option because the mandibular first premolars were extracted.

- A nonextraction maxillary three-piece osteotomy to widen the maxillary posterior segments distal to the maxillary first premolars (since this is where the cuts are made). The width between the maxillary canines and between the maxillary first premolars does not change (Figure 5.114). Again, the maxillary second molars would be left unopposed with this nonextraction approach.
- A maxillary three-piece osteotomy including extraction of the maxillary second premolars to widen (and advance) the maxillary molar segments and place the maxillary second molars in occlusion with the mandibular second molars (Figure 5.115). It was concluded that the arches fit together best with this maxillary three-piece osteotomy. *This option was chosen as the best surgical option.*

Q: Is overexpansion generally recommended with an MPMO?
A: Yes, in anticipation of some transverse relapse.

Q: What chewing restrictions are typically given to the patient following maxillary expansion surgery?
A: For a SARME, generally there are no chewing restrictions. For a multiple-piece maxillary osteotomy, 2–6 weeks of chewing restrictions should be followed depending on the surgeon's philosophy.

Q: With multiple-piece maxillary osteotomies, the orthodontist must be concerned with transverse relapse because the palatal tissues are stretched during surgery. What protocol should be followed to help maintain the wider maxillary arch width following surgery?
A: A full-coverage occlusal splint (Figure 5.116) should be placed by the surgeon at surgery. This should remain in place for 6 weeks at which time it is removed and an immediate palatal

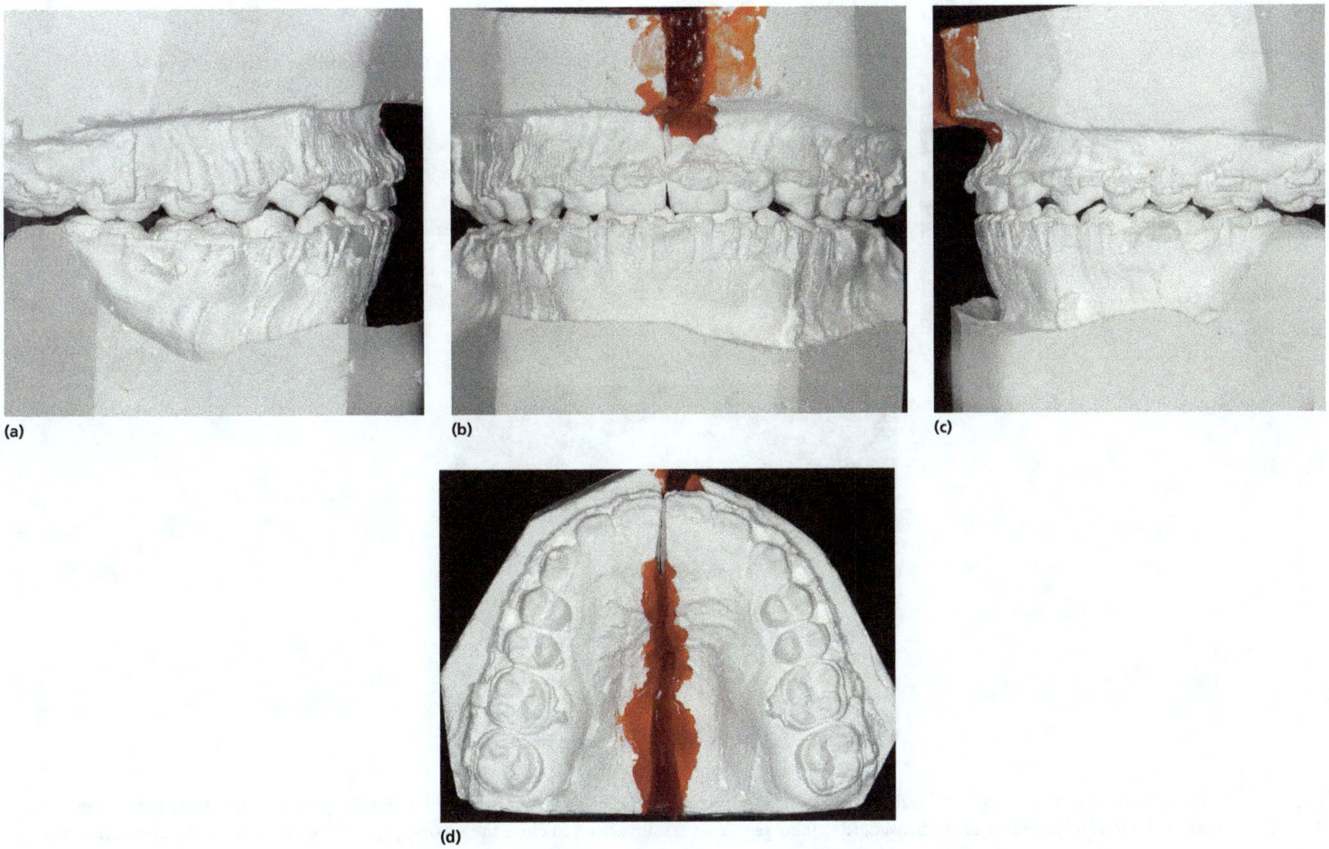

Figure 5.113 (a–d) Evaluation of Ashley's occlusal fit if a nonextraction maxillary two-piece osteotomy is performed.

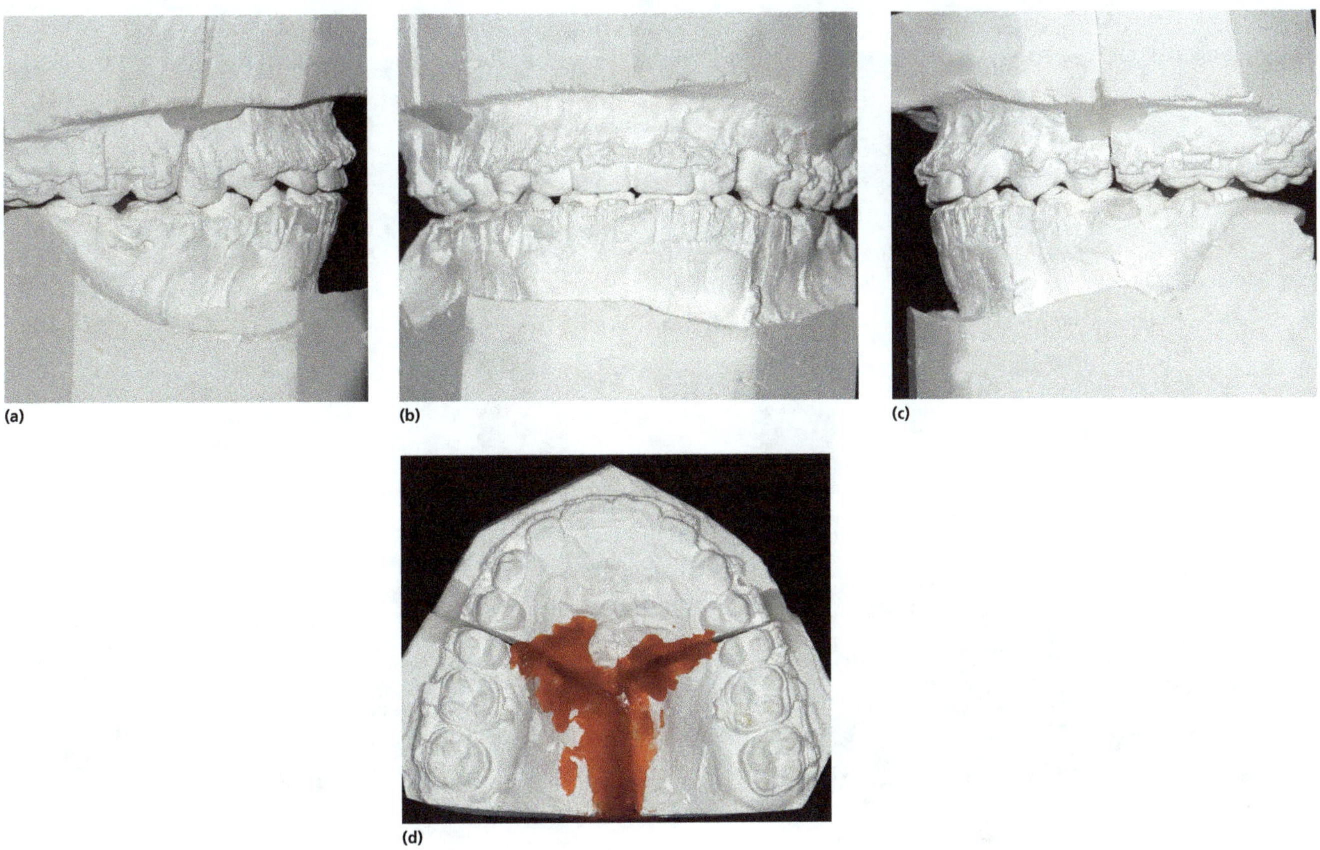

Figure 5.114 (a–d) Evaluation of Ashley's occlusal fit if a nonextraction maxillary three-piece osteotomy is performed. Only the maxillary width distal to the first premolars widens with this option (the maxillary intercanine width and inter-first-premolar widths remain unchanged).

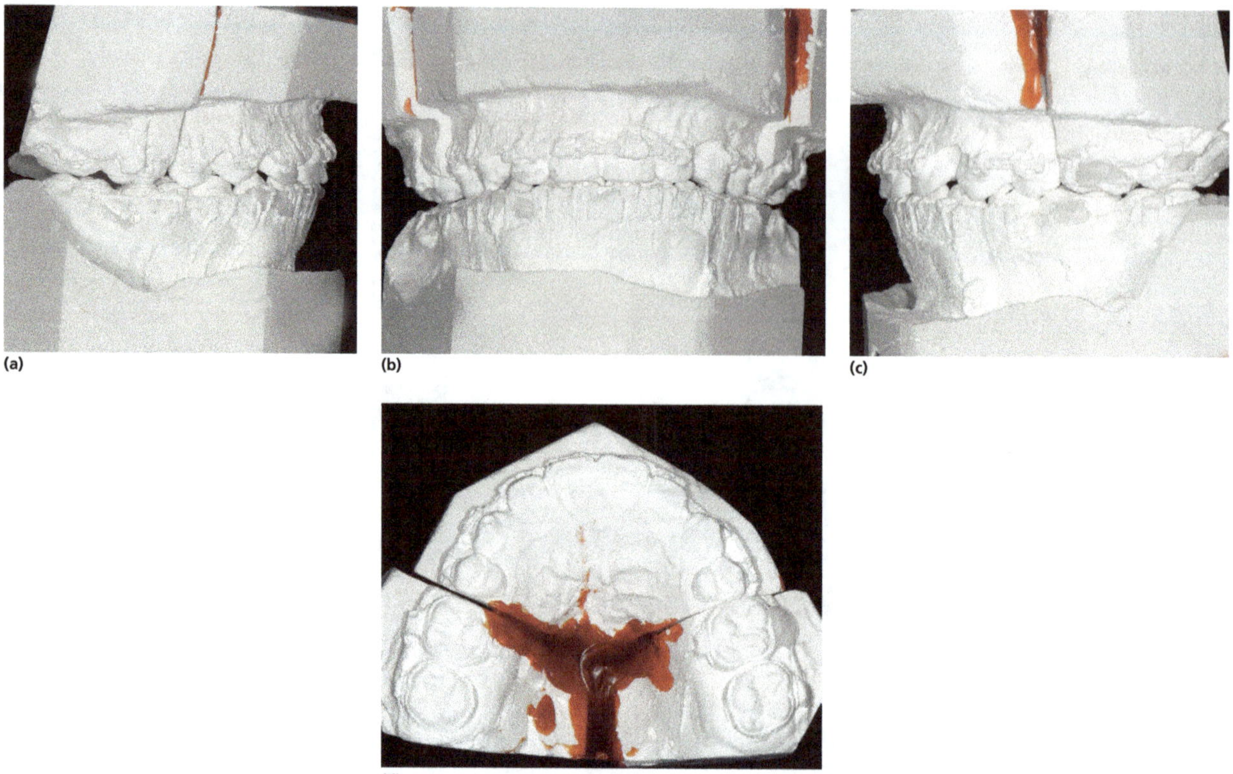

Figure 5.115 (a–d) Evaluation of Ashley's occlusal fit if her maxillary second premolars are extracted and a maxillary three-piece osteotomy is performed. Note that (i) only the intermolar widths are increased, (ii) molar segments are advanced to close the second premolar extraction space, and (iii) second molars are in occlusion. The occlusal fit of this option was the best.

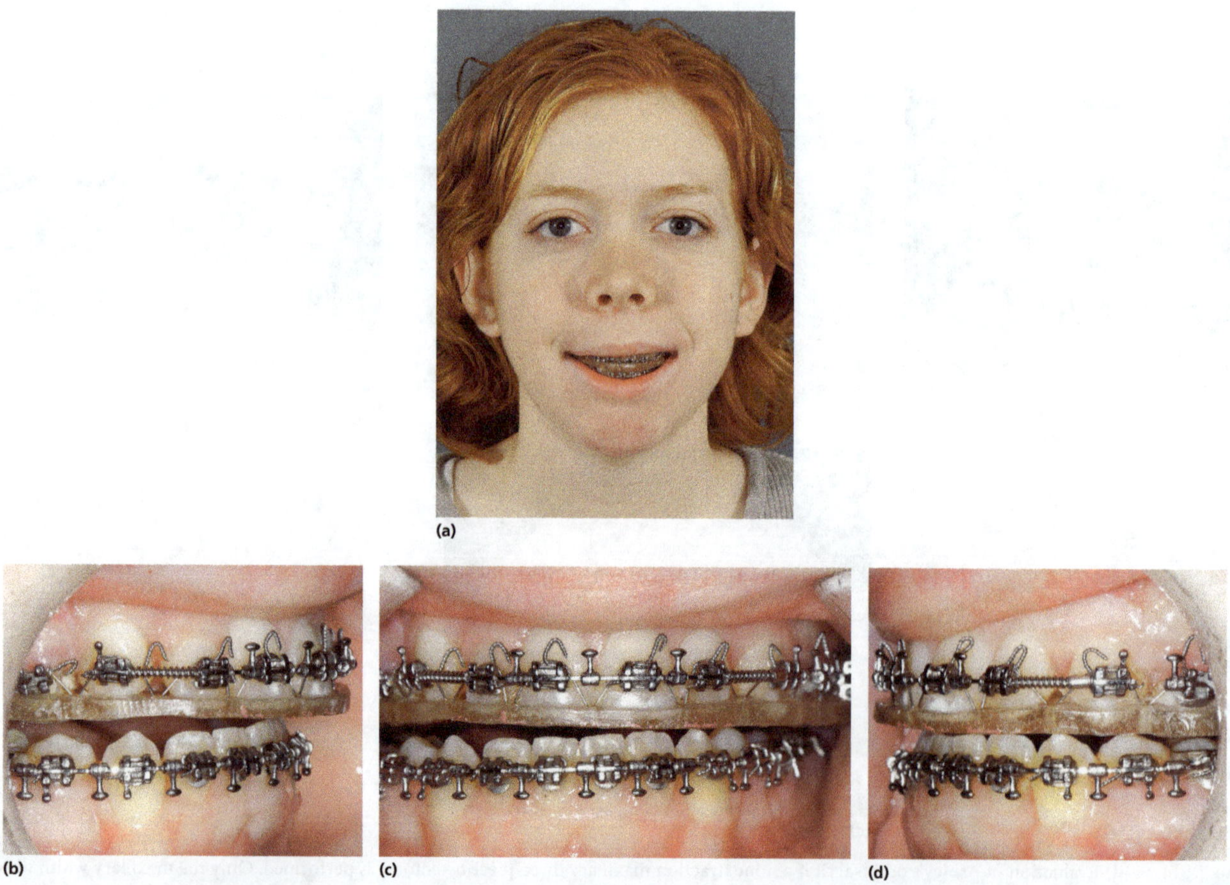

Figure 5.116 (a–d) One week postsurgery photographs.

splint fabricated, or TPA fitted, and worn. If the maxillary archwire was sectioned at surgery, then it should be replaced with a continuous wire at the 6-week appointment.

Q: Ashley's final surgery plan consisted of maxillary *first premolar* extractions, a maxillary three-piece LeFort I impaction/advancement osteotomy (posterior segments widened and moved anteriorly to close the extraction space), mandibular CCW autorotation, BSSO advancement, and genioplasty advancement. The night of her surgery, the surgeon called to state that the procedures went well. Note in Figure 5.116 that Ashley returned to the orthodontic clinic 1 week post surgery with her bite not properly seating. What questions should you ask the surgeons? What questions should you ask Ashley?

A: Ask the surgeon if he was able to get her occlusion properly seated in the operating room. The surgeon reports that her occlusion fit well at surgery. Then, ask Ashley whether she is wearing her guiding elastics. She was not wearing her guiding elastics and was asked to do so. By the next appointment (1 week later) Ashley's occlusion is perfectly seated in the splint. Four weeks later (6 weeks post surgery), the occlusal splint was removed, a maxillary impression made, and a palatal splint was immediately fabricated and delivered. This palatal splint was worn for the remainder of her treatment. A continuous archwire replaced the maxillary archwire sectioned during surgery.

Q: Finishing was completed. Ashley's final records are shown in Figure 5.117. What do you note?

A: Clearly, Ashley's smile has been improved dramatically. Her presurgery to final cephalometric radiographic superimposition (Figure 5.117f) reveals the surgical changes clearly.

- The maxilla was impacted at the posterior (differential impaction, not straight up). However, the anterior maxilla was also set back which is unfortunate since the patient initially had a retrusive maxilla. Why was the anterior maxilla set back? With extraction of the maxillary first premolars, the surgeon attempted to close the extraction spaces by bringing the posterior segments forward—but found that the tissue stretched too much—and had to set the anterior maxilla back to close the extraction site.
- The distal movement of the anterior maxilla (A-point) opened the NLA even more and retracted the maxillary lip slightly. This reduction of lip support does not benefit Ashley's profile esthetics.
- Soft tissue chin and B-point were brought forward significantly (Figure 5.117c)—but the profile was still retrusive. Why? Because the anterior maxilla was retracted during surgery—so the mandible could not be brought forward any more than it was. Further, to advance the mandible more, all mesial movement of the mandibular molars (Figure 5.111e) should have been prevented.
- LAFH was not shortened. Although the skeletal LAFH/TAFH decreased to 58% (Figure 5.117e), this was due to ANS descending (Figure 5.117f) and not to a true decrease in LAFH.
- The interlabial gap closed—apparently because the upper lip came down slightly.
- A Class I canine relationship was achieved (Figure 5.117h, j).
- Gingival height levels of the maxillary incisors are uneven.
- Canines are not coordinated (Figure 5.117i).
- Midlines are coincident.
- The mandibular right first premolar needs to erupt into occlusion.
- Inadequate lingual root torque of the maxillary right lateral incisor is noted (Figure 5.117k).
- Generalized root resorption/blunting (Figure 5.117g).
- Overbite is minimal (~10% OB).

Q: How was Ashley's open bite closed?

A: By impaction of her maxillary posterior and mandibular advancement (Figure 5.117f).

Q: If you could repeat Ashley's treatment, would you suggest any changes?

A: Yes. If RME was stopped because roots of the maxillary first premolars (anchorage teeth) were becoming buccally prominent, then *another RME appliance could have been fabricated without using the maxillary first premolars as anchorage* (maybe using the second premolars and first molars). This way, her maxilla should have been widened further with RME and a one-piece Le Fort I impaction osteotomy could be performed—instead of an MPMO.

Q: How would you retain this patient? What will you watch for?

A: Hawley retainers were placed. Small composite dots could be placed on the facial of the maxillary incisors to prevent apical movement (a clear retainer "snapping" in to place over the dots, or the Hawley labial bow snapping over the dots). Relapse toward an open bite and Class II relationship must be monitored. She should be followed for *at least* 4–6 months postsurgically to watch for relapse while she is still wearing orthodontic appliances ("active retention").

Q: If Ashley begins to relapse, how will you deal with it?

A: If Ashley begins to relapse to a mild-to-moderate Class II relationship, fixed appliances could be placed and Class II elastics, or a HPHG, could be worn (discuss HG force levels with the surgeon). If Ashley begins to relapse to a mild-to-moderate open bite, fixed orthodontic appliances could be placed and the bite closed with vertical elastics (and posterior enameloplasty). If she relapses to a severe Class II relationship or severe open bite, a second surgical procedure should be discussed.

Q: What are the "take-home" messages from this Ashley's treatment?

A: Take-home messages include the following:

- Ashley presented with a classic skeletal open bite due to VME (long soft tissue LAFH, ILG, long skeletal LAFH, steep MPA, maxillary first molar apicies erupted below palatal plane, and palatal plane tipped down in posterior) which resulted from condyles growing posterior-superiorly, lack of posterior face height development, backward mandibular internal (true) rotation, maxilla descending more than normal, and molars erupting more than normal. As her mandible rotated CW downward and backward, her mandibular plane steepened, her LAFH increased, and an ILG and open bite resulted. Ashley did not have a functional habit or a dental open bite.
- If Ashley's lower incisors had not supraerupted (dental compensation for her skeletal open bite), then Ashley's initial anterior open bite would have been *much* worse.
- In order to address her chief complaint, a surgical treatment option was chosen and consisted of a multiple-piece maxillary impaction osteotomy, a mandibular advancement osteotomy, and a genioplasty advancement osteotomy.
- Even with a girl as old as 16 years, you can still attempt to correct a transverse skeletal discrepancy with an RME

appliance. However, you must have a secondary plan (e.g., SARME or dental expansion) if you do not get a midpalatal split. Additional RME appliance expansion could have obviated the need for her *multiple-piece* maxillary osteotomy to gain extra arch width.

- Unlike maxillary expansion with a SARME, which is very stable, consider *overexpanding* with a multiple-piece maxillary osteotomy in anticipation of some relapse.
- To help maintain expansion with a MPMO, the surgeon should place a full coverage occlusal splint at the time of

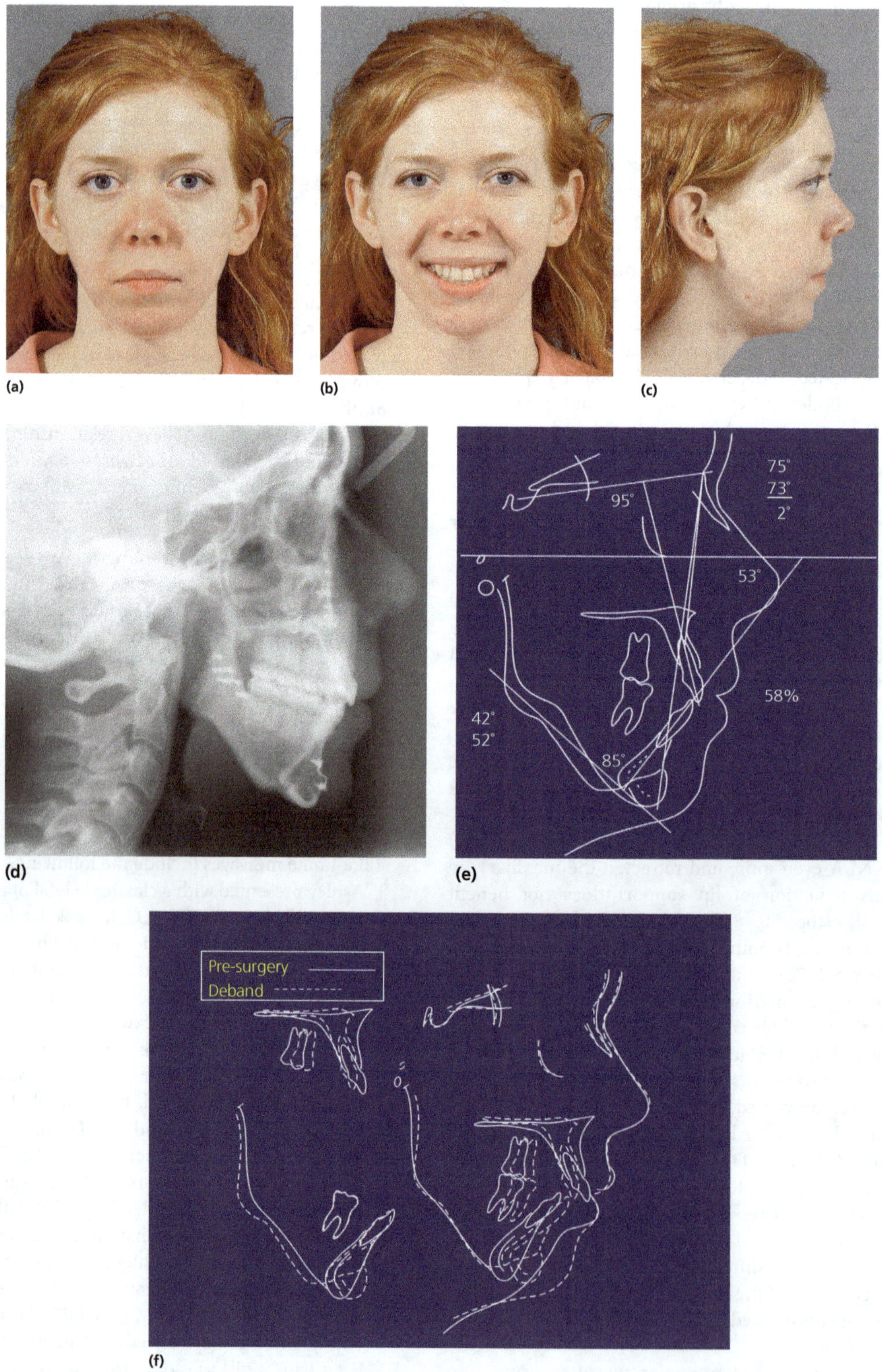

Figure 5.117 (a–l) Ashley's final records.

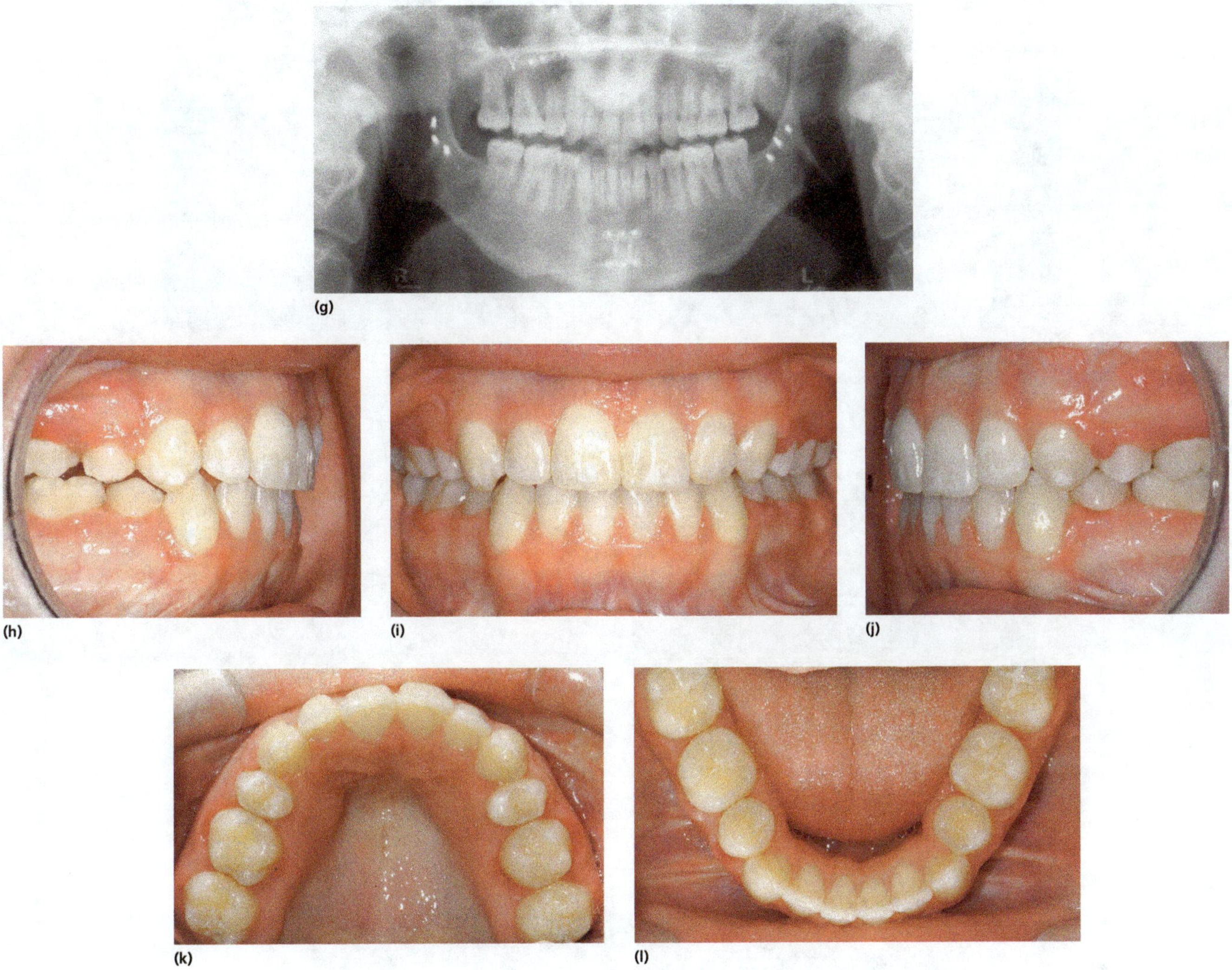

Figure 5.117 (Continued)

surgery. Six weeks post-surgery this should be replaced with an immediate palatal splint which is worn for the remainder of orthodontic treatment.

- Overbite at the end of Ashley's treatment was minimal (~10%). Ideally, her overbite should have been overcorrected to 20–40% OB (anticipating some relapse).
- Ashley's profile was still retrusive at the end of treatment because the anterior maxilla was retracted during surgery (the mandible could not be brought forward any more than it was). However, *TADs should have been left in place during mandibular incisor retraction* to prevent all mesial mandibular molar movement (Figure 5.111e). The surgeon would have then been forced to advance the mandible more.
- After you have defined your problem list, always ask yourself if there are any unknowns you should eliminate before establishing your final treatment plan. Our ability to obtain midpalatal suture separation, and correct the transverse skeletal discrepancy with an RME appliance, was the major unknown in Ashley's case.
- Exhaustively consider the costs/benefits of *all* treatment options. For Ashley, this included options of masking versus surgery, extraction versus nonextraction, and different multiple-piece maxillary osteotomies.
- The orthodontist should work closely with the surgeon in outlining the surgical treatment plan. Even then, unanticipated problems can arise in the operating room. The orthodontist and the surgeon are a team whose only goal is to provide the best possible care for the patient.

Case Alyson

Alyson is an 18-year, 1-month-old female who presents to you with the chief complaint, "I want my teeth straight and do not like the way my gums show when I smile." Her PMH and PDH are WRN. TMJ evaluation is WRN and CR=CO (Figure 5.118).

Q: List diagnostic findings/problems. What is your diagnosis?
A: See Table 5.12.

Q: Why does the patient have an "hourglass" contoured maxillary arch on the right side (Figure 5.118r)?
A: Posterior teeth erupt between the soft tissue trough created by the cheeks and tongue. The maxillary right molar and premolars

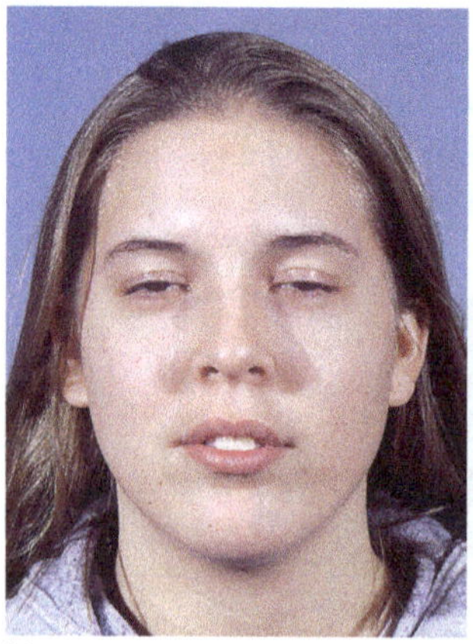
(a)

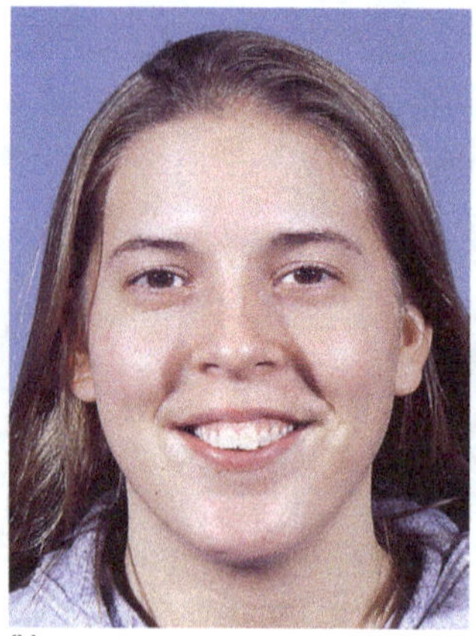
(b)

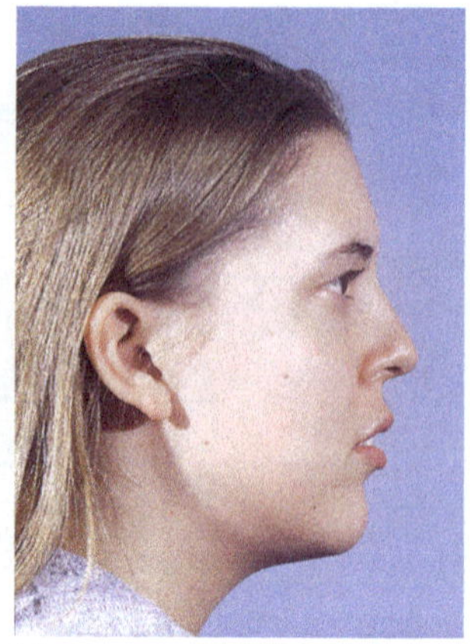
(c)

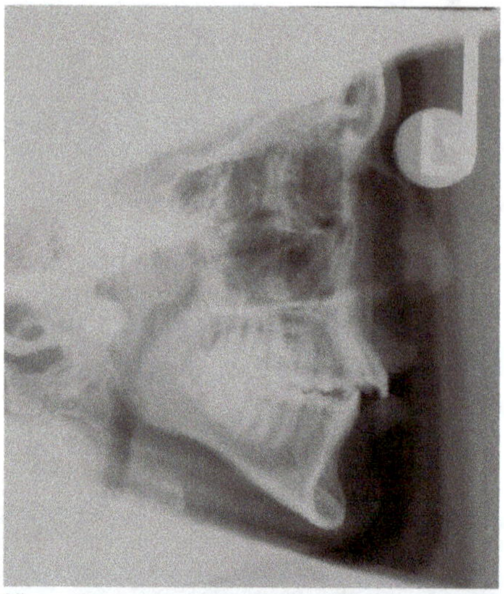
(d)

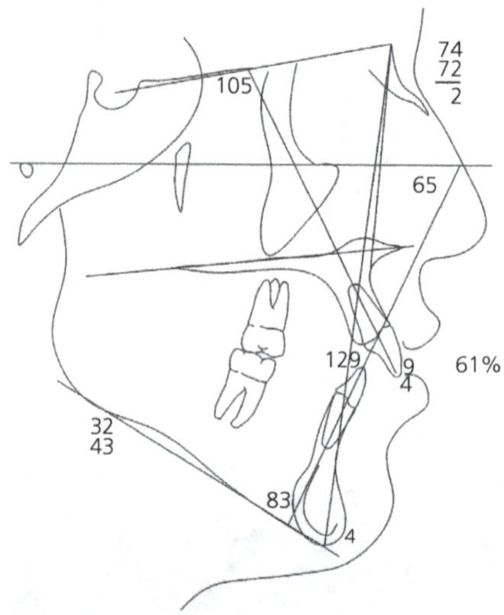

(e)

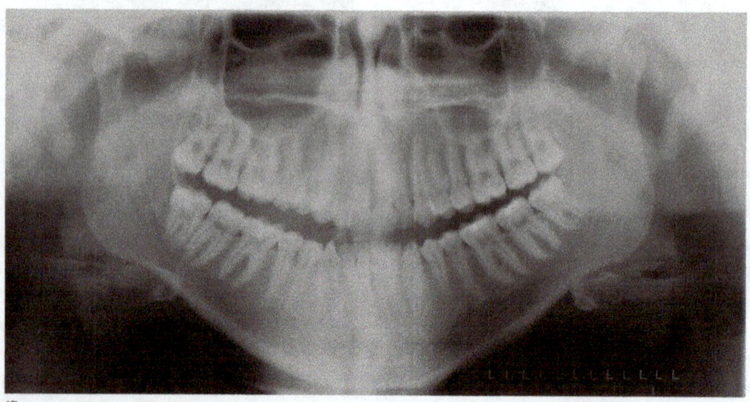
(f)

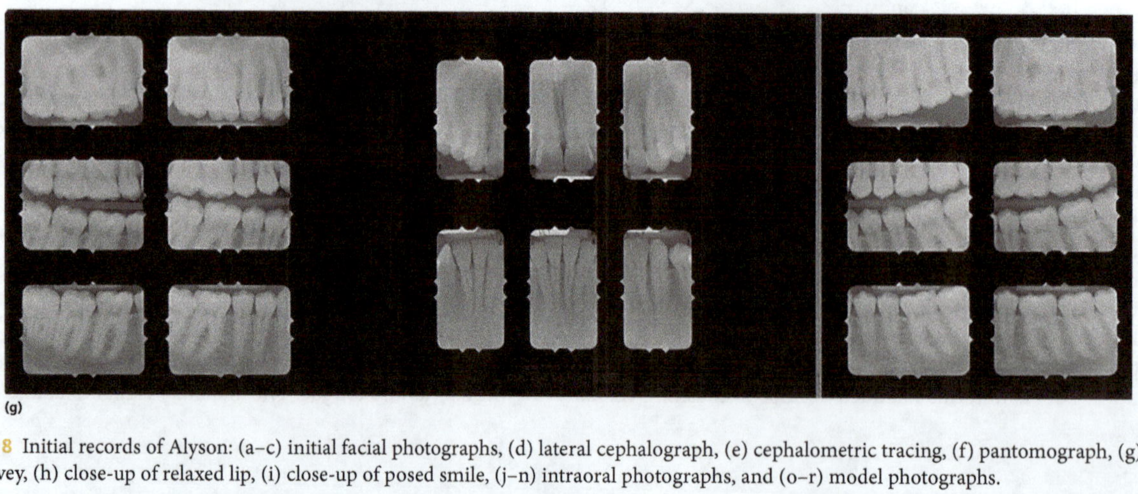
(g)

Figure 5.118 Initial records of Alyson: (a–c) initial facial photographs, (d) lateral cephalograph, (e) cephalometric tracing, (f) pantomograph, (g) complete mouth survey, (h) close-up of relaxed lip, (i) close-up of posed smile, (j–n) intraoral photographs, and (o–r) model photographs.

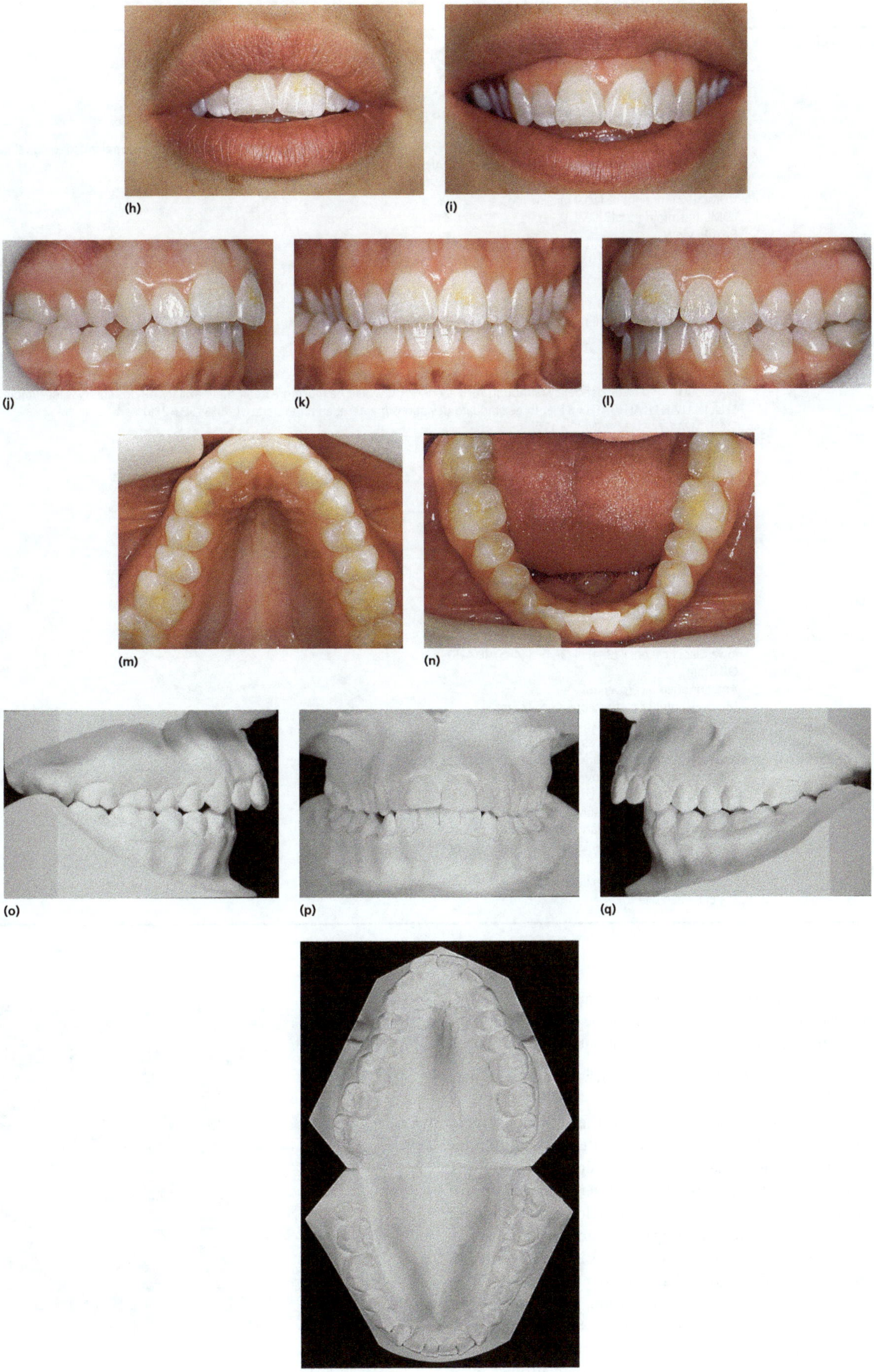

Figure 5.118 (Continued)

Table 5.12 Diagnostic findings and problem list for Alyson.

Full face and profile	**Frontal view**
	Soft tissue LLAFH (soft tissue Glabella-Subnasale < Subnasale-soft tissue Menton)
	ILG ~10 mm
	Upper lip length (philtrum length) 22 mm
	Exaggerated cupid's bow (commissure height exceeds philtrum length by >2–3 mm)
	Excessive incisal display at rest ~8 mm
	Excess gingival display in posed smile (maxillary lip vermillion border should be congruent with maxillary central incisor gingival margins)
	Buccal corridors do not appear especially wide, but Alyson may not be smiling
	Broadly in the posed smile photograph
	UDML 1–2 mm right of facial midline
	LDML 1–2 mm right of UDML
	Profile view
	Mildly convex profile
	Retrusive chin
	90° nasolabial angle
	Slightly upturned nose but lack of supratip break
	Protrusive/everted lower lip
	Slightly obtuse lip-chin-throat angle
Ceph analysis	**Skeletal**
	Maxillary skeletal AP deficiency (A-Point posterior to Nasion-perpendicular line)
	Mandibular AP skeletal deficiency (although ANB is only 2°, it would be much greater if the maxillary AP position was ideal/more forward)
	Skeletal LLAFH (LAFH/TAFH = 61%, three standard deviations greater than an average of 55%, SD = 2%)
	Steep MPA (FMA = 32°; SNMP = 43°)
	Short posterior face height
	VME (skeletal LLAFH; first molar apicies erupted below palatal plane, palatal plane tipped down in posterior)
	Effective bony Pogonion
	Mild adenoidal hypertrophy
	Mandibular incisors are supra-erupted
	Dental
	Maxillary incisor inclination WRN
	Ideal mandibular incisor inclination (FMIA = 65°)
	Open bite
Radiographs	Permanent dentition
	Third molars present
Intraoral photos and models	Angle Class II division 1 malocclusion
	Iowa Classification: II (3–4) II (3–4) II (4–5) II (4–5)
	OJ: 8 mm
	Anterior open bite (overlap)
	Maxillary anterior teeth stepped up ~2 mm
	Mandibular anterior teeth stepped up
	Right posterior lingual cross bite
	Intermolar widths: maxillary first molars 45.5 mm (between palatal cusps); mandibular first molars 51 mm (between central fossae)
	Mild maxillary anterior crowding (UTSALD = −2 mm)
	Mild mandibular anterior crowding (LTSALD = −2 mm)
	Dental arches are reasonably symmetric
	Anteriorly tapering maxillary arch w/hourglass shape on right
	Washboarding of mandibular anterior roots (Figure 5.118j–l)
Other	—
Diagnosis	Angle Class II division 1 malocclusion
	Skeletal open bite

erupted lingually, leaving Alyson in right lingual cross bite. This gives the maxillary arch an "hourglass" shape on the right. Such a constriction is not unusual in cases of unilateral cross bite.

Q: Are there additional photographs or other records you may wish to make?

A: With Alyson's chief complaint and her age, the option of surgery comes to mind. With any surgical candidate, you should take additional photographs that could be of value to you and the patient in deciding whether to pursue surgery. For example, if you had a skeletal deep bite patient (overclosed), you should have the patient open until their lips just touch to define where the soft tissue drape would ideally be positioned, vertically. Then, surgery would be directed at changing the facial skeleton to support that vertical soft tissue dimension. In Alyson's case, it could be useful to record 3/4 (45°, Figure 5.119) left and right facial views to examine malar (zygomatic) projection. That is, in a 45° facial view the malar eminence should project to or

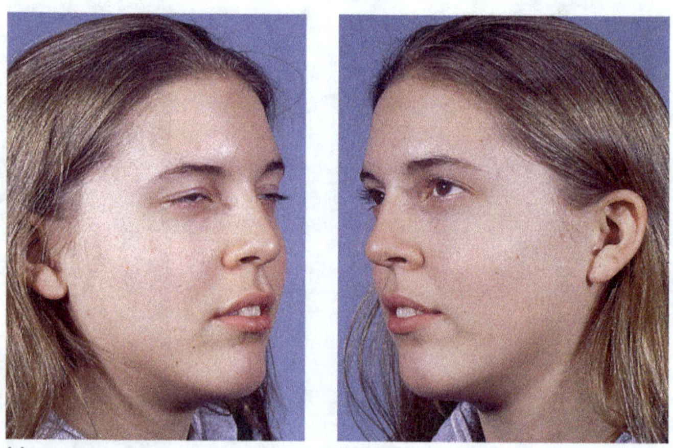

(a) (b)

Figure 5.119 (a, b) Right and left 3/4 facial views of Alyson (45° views).

beyond a line drawn vertically from the apex of the eye cornea. Lack of sufficient malar projection could be corrected with malar implants. Alyson appears to have adequate malar projection.

A frontal view with her holding a tongue blade in the posterior (Figure 5.120a) is helpful to check for an occlusal cant (tongue blade not parallel to the interpupillary line). In Alyson's case, the posteriorly placed tongue blade is parallel to her interpupillary line (i.e., she does not have an occlusal cant). Also, a view of her posturing forward into a Class I canine position (Figure 5.120b) is of value if you are considering a possible BSSO advancement or autorotation into a Class I canine relationship following maxillary impaction surgery.

Q: Are there other views of the models you should examine?

A: Yes. In addition to examining her molar AP position from the lingual (maxillary molar rotation can affect AP molar classification when viewed from the buccal), you should always separate the models to examine maxillary and mandibular posterior crown torque. Excessive maxillary posterior labial crown torque or excessive mandibular lingual crown torque can be compensations for an underlying maxillary transverse skeletal deficiency.

Q: In terms of Alyson's posterior crown torque (Figure 5.121), what do you observe?

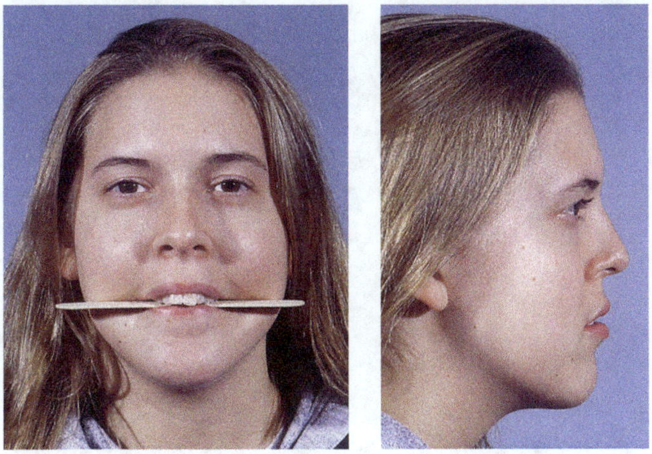

(a) (b)

Figure 5.120 (a) Evaluating Alyson for a posterior occlusal cant and (b) with her mandible postured forward into a Class I canine relationship.

A: Excess maxillary second molar labial crown torque and excess mandibular posterior lingual crown torque. Alyson has a transverse skeletal discrepancy with posterior transverse compensations masking that discrepancy. *If all her transverse compensations were removed (posterior teeth uprighted), then she could be in bilateral posterior cross bite.* Also note in Figure 5.121b a significant curve of Spee.

Q: Does Alyson have an open bite or overlap (OB when viewed from the front, Figure 5.118k, but lacking mandibular incisor contact)?

A: She has both. As soon as you tip her models up in the front (Figure 5.122a), you see that she has an open bite. A patient has "overlap" when there appears to be overbite as the dentition is viewed from the front, and yet the mandibular incisors are not actually touching the maxillary incisors or the palate (Figure 5.122b). This is true for Alyson. She has an open bite and overlap.

Q: Look at Alyson's cephalometric radiograph (Figure 5.118d). How has her mandibular incisor tooth eruption minimized her anterior open bite? What is this an example of?

A: Her mandibular incisors have undergone excessive eruption. Note the long, narrow alveolus that has resulted from this incisor eruption. If the mandibular incisors had not erupted excessively, then Alyson's anterior open bite would be *much* worse. This is an example of dental compensation for an underlying apical base discrepancy (excessive mandibular incisor eruption compensating for a severe skeletal open bite).

Q: What other questions should you ask Alyson about her open bite to complete a thorough history?

A: Other important questions include the following:

- Even though Alyson is over 18 years old, confirm that she has completed growth. Alyson states that she reached menarche and finished growing years ago.
- Since skeletal open bites can include a functional (dental open bite) component, if a functional habit is missed and/or not corrected then the open bite treatment can relapse later. Alyson denies any functional habits. While slowly separating her lips, you note that she does not have an anterior tongue positioning habit.
- Her open bite could have resulted from condylar degeneration—with the mandible rotating CW upward and backward. Check Alyson's panoramic film (Figure 5.118f) to confirm that degeneration of the mandibular condyles is not

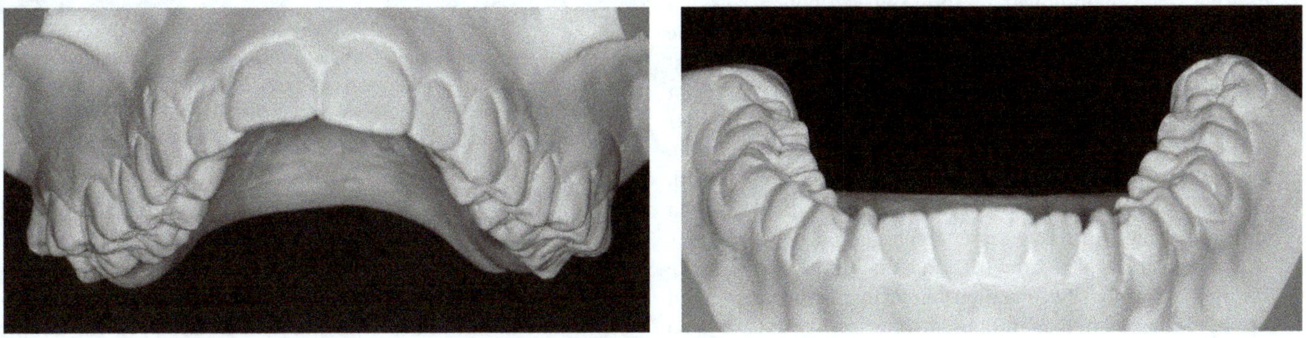

(a) (b)

Figure 5.121 (a, b) Separated model views to evaluate maxillary and mandibular posterior crown torque.

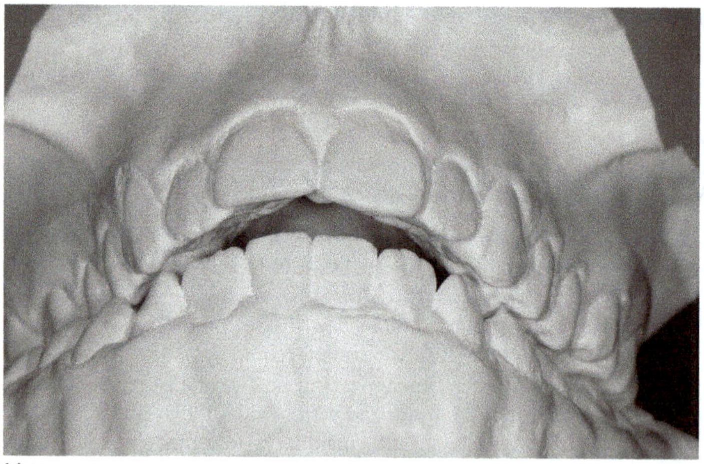

(a)

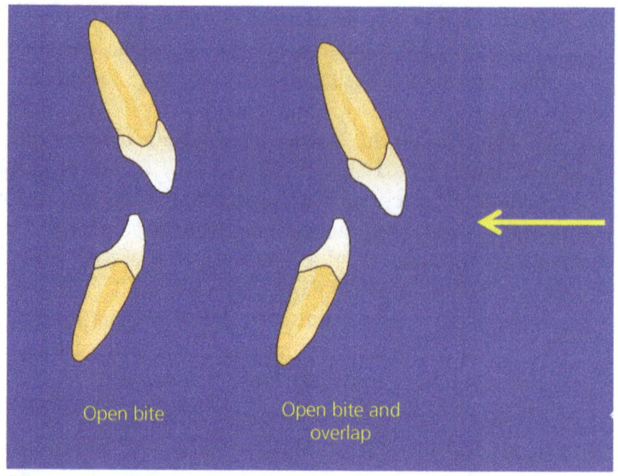

(b)

Figure 5.122 (a) As Alyson's articulated models are tipped up slightly, we see that she has an open bite (mandibular anterior teeth not in contact with maxillary anterior teeth or palate). (b) When viewed from the front (yellow arrow), open bites are present whether they can be seen directly or whether, like Alyson, they are not evident until the models are tipped up slightly. This latter relationship is termed "overlap."

evident—it is not. Further, she does not complain of any TMJ symptoms.

- Alyson's buccal corridors should be checked when she is smiling broadly. This was not done.
- Check for temporary open bites due permanent teeth still erupting, ankylosis of teeth that are not fully erupted, and permanent teeth that are not fully erupted due to a lack of space. Alyson does not appear to have these features.
- The mild adenoidal hypertrophy should be investigated. If Alyson has difficulty breathing, is an obligatory mouth breather, or has a history of sleep apnea, then her airway should be evaluated by otolaryngology. Alyson breathes nasally and does NOT report breathing difficulties when awake or asleep. Nor does she report recurrent episodes of pharyngitis.

Q: Is Alyson's open bite a skeletal open bite, a dental open bite, or a combination of both? What is the etiology of her open bite?

A: Alyson has a *skeletal open bite due to vertical maxillary excess (VME: soft tissue and skeletal LLAFH, excess maxillary growth in posterior/palatal plane tipped down in posterior, excess maxillary molar eruption)*. Alyson demonstrates a classic skeletal open bite growth pattern: condyles growing posterior-superiorly instead of more vertically (Figure 5.123, curved red arrow), lack of posterior face height development, backward internal (true) mandibular rotation (curved blue arrows), a maxilla that has descended more than normal/palatal plane that has rotated down posteriorly, and maxillary first molars that have erupted more than normal (maxillary first molar root apicies erupted below the palatal plane). As her mandible rotated downward and backward (yellow arrow), her mandibular plane angle steepened, her LAFH increased, she developed an ILG and excessive gingival display when smiling (facial soft tissue drape growth could not keep pace with vertical skeletal growth), and an anterior open bite resulted. Although her maxillary anterior teeth are stepped up by ~2 mm, her mandibular anterior teeth are also stepped up (not stepped down)—*Alyson lacks a functional habit and does not have a dental open bite.*

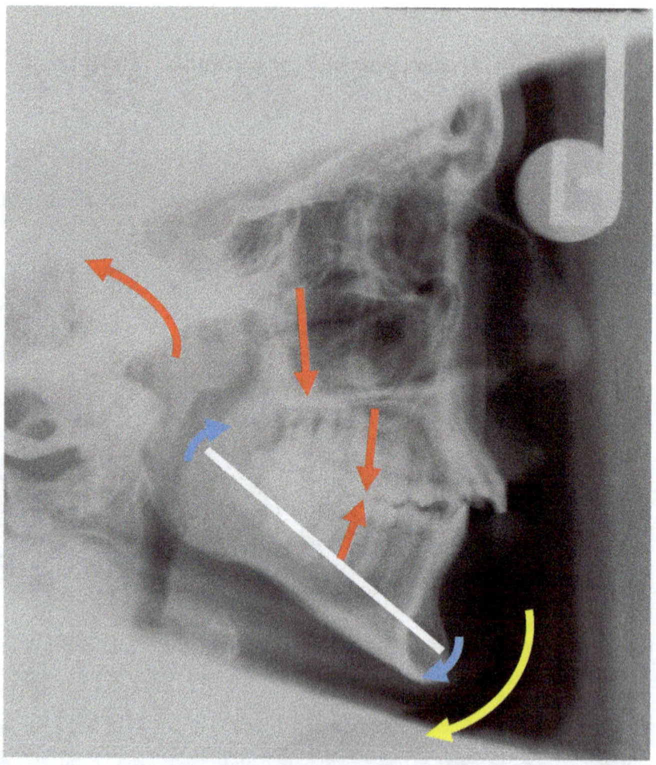

Figure 5.123 Alyson illustrates the classic growth features found in a skeletal open bite patient: condyles growing posterior-superiorly, lack of posterior face height development, backward mandibular internal (true) rotation, maxilla descending more than normal (palatal plane clearly rotated down posteriorly), and maxillary molars erupting more than normal (maxillary first molar apicies erupted well below her palatal plane). As her mandible rotated CW downward and backward (yellow arrow), her mandibular plane steepened, her LAFH increased, and an ILG and open bite resulted.

Q: Alyson demonstrates excessive incisal display when her lips are relaxed and excessive gingival display when smiling (Figure 5.118a, b). By contrast, Mohamed (Figure 5.124) displays

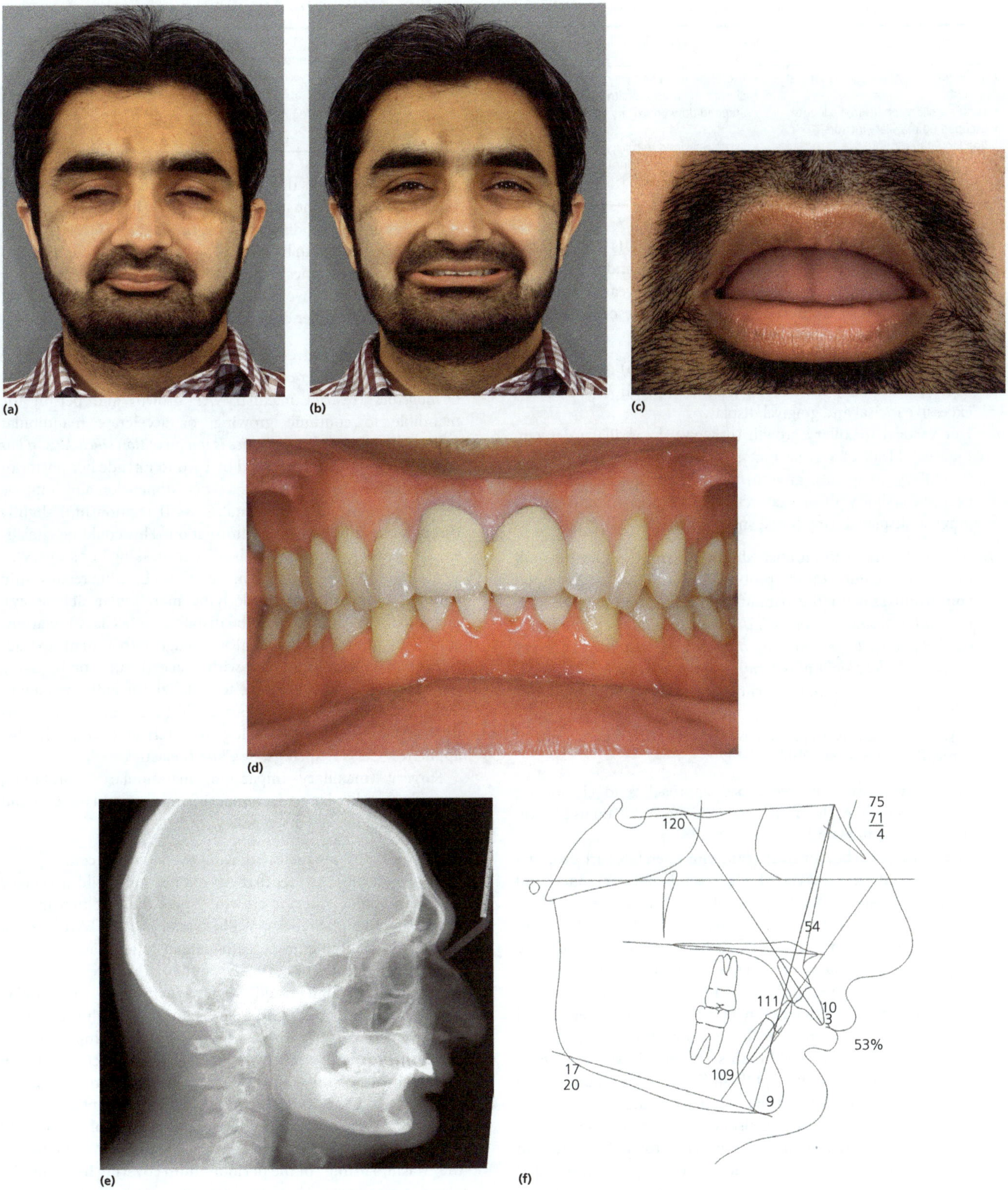

Figure 5.124 (a–f) Records of Mohamed, who exhibits inadequate incisal display.

inadequate incisal display when relaxed (Figure 5.124c) and inadequate incisal display when smiling (Figure 5.124b). Remember, ideal incisal display in a posed smile would find maxillary lip vermillion border at the level of the maxillary central incisor gingival margins. List the reasons why a patient can present with inadequate incisal display. List the reasons why a patient can present with excessive incisal display.

A: See Table 5.13.

Table 5.13 Possible reasons for inadequate or excessive incisal display.

Inadequate incisal display	Excess incisal display
• Inadequate maxillary corpus vertical growth • Long maxillary (philtrum) lip length • Stepped up maxillary incisors (inadequate eruption) • Worn or short incisor crowns • Hypoactivity of (smiling) facial muscles	• Excess maxillary vertical growth • Short maxillary lip (philtrum) length • Stepped down maxillary incisors (excess eruption) • Excessively long maxillary incisor crowns • Hyperactivity of (smiling) facial muscles • Delayed passive eruption (excess gingiva)

Q: Alyson has a 22 mm lip length (philtrum length). Is this a normal length? What is a normal lip length for women and men?

A: Yes, 22 mm is a normal lip length for an 18-year-old female. Lip lengths range from 17 to 23 mm for adolescent girls and 22–26 mm for adolescent boys [1].

Q: Alyson's teeth are stepped up (Figure 5.118k, p) *and* she has a normal (not short) maxillary lip length. So why does she exhibit excessive incisal and gingival display.

A: Her vertical maxillary growth (downward maxillary descent, Figure 5.118d, e) was so excessive that the soft tissue drape (maxillary lip vertical growth) has not kept pace. The result: excess maxillary display at rest (Figure 5.118a) and excess gingival display during posed smile (Figure 5.118b).

Q: Although the orthodontist should attempt to address all problems included on the problem list, and discuss potential compromises with the patient before beginning treatment, the *major problem(s) in each dimension (plus other problems, e.g., impacted teeth) must be the focus of treatment at every visit. Never lose sight of the major problem in each dimension.* What are Alyson's major (primary) problems you must stay focused on?

A: Alyson has significant apical base (skeletal) discrepancies in all three dimensions. See Table 5.14.

Q: There are really only two broad approaches to closing an anterior open bite. Describe them. Which would you use to you treat Alyson, and why?

A: The two approaches for closing anterior open bites are erupting anterior teeth (generally used to correct dental open bites) and intruding posterior teeth (generally used to correct skeletal open bites). *Erupting anterior teeth:* Alyson does not present with a dental open bite. Although her maxillary incisors are stepped up, you would not wish to erupt them to close her open bite (Figure 5.125a) as her incisal display would worsen, unless you planned to impact her maxilla and reduce her incisal display, or planned to settle for a compromised result with masking. Her mandibular incisors are already stepped up so you would not normally erupt them (Figure 5.125a) unless you were treating her skeletal open bite by masking it. Finally, her maxillary and mandibular incisors have normal angulations, so retracting/uprighting them (in order to rotate them around their apicies/erupt them) would not be recommended (Figure 5.125b). *Intruding posterior teeth* (Figure 5.125c): intruding Alyson's mandibular posterior teeth with TADs, intruding her maxillary posterior teeth with TADs, or intruding her maxillary posterior teeth with a LeFort I maxillary impaction osteotomy, would permit autorotation of the mandible around the condyles, reducing her LLAFH, reducing her incisal display, eliminating her ILG, and closing her anterior open bite. This would be the ideal approach in treating Alyson.

Table 5.14 Primary problems list for Alyson *(apical base/skeletal discrepancies italicized).*

AP	II (3–4) II (3–4) II (4–5) II (4–5) *Maxillary and mandibular skeletal retrusion*
Vertical	*Vertical maxillary excess, skeletal open bite*
Transverse	Unilateral right lingual cross bite—*maxillary transverse skeletal deficiency* with transverse dental compensations
Other	—

Q: What treatment goals do you recommend for Alyson?

A: Certainly, our goals must include addressing her chief complaint: reducing her gingival display (when smiling) and incisal display, straightening her teeth by correcting her cross bite, aligning and coordinating her arches, achieving a Class I canine relationship with over-corrected overbite (20–40% OB), and eliminating her overjet. Improving her chin projection would be ideal.

Q: How would you address Alyson's anteroposterior apical base discrepancy (consider orthopedics, masking, and surgery)?

A: *Orthopedics* (restrict maxillary AP growth and permit the mandible to continue growing, or accelerate mandibular growth). *Traditional orthopedics is not an option since Alyson has completed growth.* TADs could be used to intrude her posterior teeth which would reduce her vertical dimension and improve her chin projection (and dental Class II relationship) slightly through mandibular CCW autorotation. This could be considered orthopedic treatment (it is neither masking nor surgery).

Masking or camouflage (achieve a Class I canine relationship without addressing the underlying mandibular deficiency). Her maxillary canines could be distalized to a Class I relationship with intra-arch mechanics: headgear treatment, extraction of maxillary premolars with space closure, or by using maxillary TADs as anchorage to distalize the entire maxillary dentition. Her maxillary molars could be distalized and mandibular molars advanced using interarch mechanics: Herbst appliance, Class II springs, or Class II elastics.

Surgery (maxillary impaction, mandibular autorotation, possible mandibular advancement) Surgery would be ideal and could correct her AP discrepancy.

Q: If a surgical option is selected, would you extract teeth?

A: No. Considering the fact that Alyson has only mild maxillary and mandibular anterior crowding plus the fact that incisor angulation in both arches is WRN ($\underline{1}$ to SN = 105°; FMIA = 65°), there is no need to extract teeth—either to alleviate crowding or to upright incisors. If Alyson had a severely retrusive mandible/chin, one could suggest extracting mandibular premolars, retracting mandibular canines through the extraction space to worsen her Class II canine relationship, and then increasing chin projection by surgically advancing her jaw (bringing her canines surgically into a Class I relationship). But since her initial profile looks acceptable now (Figure 5.118c), this suggestion is not reasonable. The only factor that would lead one to consider mandibular extraction is the "washboarding" of the periodontium covering her mandibular anterior roots. That is, alignment of mandibular incisors could stress the mandibular anterior periodontium and cause recession. However, Alyson does have some attached keratinized attached tissue covering the mandibular anterior area—so, it is reasonable to simply monitor the mandibular anterior gingiva during leveling and aligning. If recession begins to occur, then a periodontist would need to graft the area. In summary, extractions are not necessary if a surgical option is chosen.

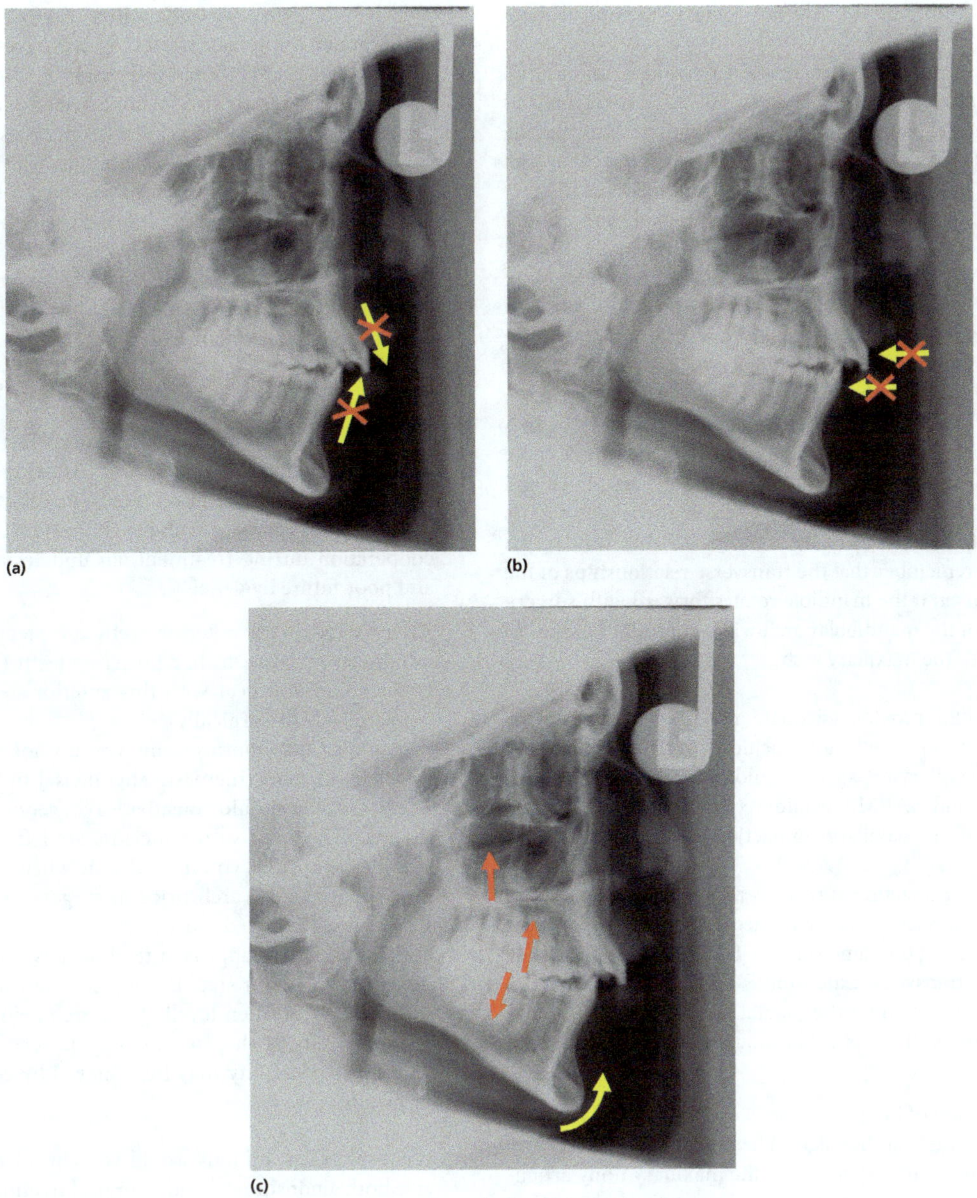

Figure 5.125 (a) Although Alyson's maxillary incisors are stepped up, unless you plan to impact her maxilla (or settle for a compromise by masking), you should not erupt them to close her open bite as you would worsen her incisal display. Since her mandibular incisors are already stepped up, it would not be ideal to erupt them more. (b) Since the angulation of her maxillary and mandibular incisors is WRN, you should not retract/upright them in order to rotate them around their apicies/erupt them. (c) Intruding Alyson's molars with TADs, or impacting her maxilla with surgery, would permit CCW autorotation of her mandible around the condyles, reducing her LLAFH, eliminating her ILG, reducing her incisal display, and closing her anterior open bite (yellow arrow).

Q: How would you address Alyson's vertical apical base discrepancy?

A: *Orthopedics* (treatment that would reduce downward descent of the maxilla and/or reduce eruption of the maxillary and mandibular molars during growth). Since Alyson has completed growth, traditional orthopedics is not an option. But again, one could consider the use of TADs to intrude teeth as orthopedics. Since the mandible is rotating around the condyles, for every millimeter of molar intrusion the anterior vertical will close somewhere around 2 mm.

Intrusion of her maxillary posterior *and* anterior teeth with TADs could reduce her LLAFH, interlabial gap, incisal display, and gingival display (when smiling). However, in order to achieve ideal incisal display (2–4 mm at rest), TAD intrusion of the maxillary arch would have to be 4+ mm.

Masking or camouflage (achieve anterior open bite closure without addressing the underlying vertical apical base discrepancy). The lower incisors could be left supra-erupted (Figure 5.121b) by maintaining a curve of Spee in the archwire. Erupting the (stepped up) maxillary incisors to close the open bite would not be advised—as the amount of incisal display would be increased. Masking will not address Alyson's chief complaint of excess incisal/gingival display.

Surgery (maxillary impaction osteotomy) could result in a normal LAFH, lip competence, and ideal incisal/gingival display.

Q: How would you address Alyson's transverse apical base discrepancy?

A: *Orthopedics* (separating hemi-maxillae at the midpalatal suture). RME would result in both maxillary skeletal expansion and maxillary dental expansion/buccal crown tipping. If the maxilla was expanded skeletally, then the resulting excess buccal overjet could be used to upright maxillary left second molars as they are brought lingually (labial crown torque eliminated) and upright mandibular posterior teeth as they are brought labially (lingual crown torque eliminated). The arches could be coordinated.

Masking or camouflage (correcting the posterior cross bite by increasing maxillary posterior labial crown torque and/or by increasing mandibular posterior lingual crown torque—and not by addressing the underlying transverse skeletal discrepancy). Since the only teeth in cross bite are the maxillary right first molar and right premolars (Figure 5.118o, q), and since these teeth are initially upright, the maxillary right first molar and premolars could be torqued labially to move them out of cross bite. Although increasing compensations in this way seems viable at first, remember that the transverse relationships of the arches will worsen if the mandible rotates forward with surgery (a wider part of the mandibular arch will be brought forward to coordinate with the maxillary arch).

Surgery

- SARME would provide adequate maxillary expansion to upright posterior teeth and achieve arch coordination. However, maxillary expansion could first be attempted with RME only, and SARME would require a second surgical procedure if a maxillary impaction osteotomy is later planned.
- If a maxillary impaction surgery is planned, then a simultaneous multiple-piece maxillary osteotomy could expand the transverse during the same surgery. However, the magnitude of maxillary transverse expansion is limited with an MPMO since you are stretching the palatal soft tissue quickly and may compromise the palatal blood supply if it is stretched too much.

Q: Is RME correction of her transverse likely? Why or why not?

A: Not likely, because of her age. There is increased skeletal resistance to maxillary expansion at the maxillary bony articulations with increasing age [162, 163]. The most marked effect of RME is before and during the *pubertal growth spurt* [164]. In older patients, there is little orthopedic change [165], and expansion after pubertal growth spurt occurs mainly by dentoalveolar (not orthopedic) expansion [166]. However, you can *attempt* to expand skeletally with an RME appliance at the rate of 0.25 mm per day, or 0.25 mm every other day when starting, and see if the midpalatal suture separates.

Q: If Alyson's midpalatal suture does not separate with an RME appliance, and you cannot gain enough transverse correction with only maxillary dental expansion, then how would you choose between expanding with a SARME or with an MPMO?

A: The major consideration is the *magnitude* of the transverse skeletal correction needed.

- If you need maxillary transverse skeletal expansion ≥10 mm, then a SARME is indicated (so you can actually grow palatal hard and soft tissue).
- If the only dimension you need to correct skeletally is the transverse dimension, then a SARME is indicated.
- If the palate is very low/flat, then a SARME may be indicated (too much immediate stretching of the palatal soft tissue may occur with an MPMO in this case).
- If the maxilla must also be impacted anyway, and if the magnitude of expansion needed is 8 mm or less, then an MPMO could be performed in conjunction with maxillary impaction—obviating the need for a separate (SARME) surgery.
- If a very large step (5–6+ mm) exists between the posterior and anterior dentition, then an MPMO may be necessary to align the maxillary segments independently with lessened possibility of relapse (which could occur if the anterior teeth were erupted during leveling).

Q: Are there *unknowns* that you should eliminate before you define Alyson's final treatment plan?

A: Yes. If you plan to attempt transverse correction using an RME appliance, then you should do this first—to see if a nonsurgical midpalatal suture separation is even possible. Other unknowns include the remote possibility of residual growth, Alyson's cooperation during treatment, an undetected CR—CO shift, and poor future hygiene.

Q: Alyson's maxillary anterior teeth are stepped up by a few millimeters relative to her posterior teeth (Figure 5.118o–q). How should you deal with this anterior step if you treat her nonsurgically or surgically?

A: If you treat her *nonsurgically*, you do not want to erupt her maxillary incisors (increasing her incisal and gingival display). Therefore, you should consider leaving compensating curve in the maxillary arch so the incisors are left stepped up. If you treat her *surgically*, you must decide whether you are going to level the maxillary arch prior to surgery or leave an anterior step to be corrected during surgery with an MPMO. The decision of which approach to choose is based on the *magnitude* of the anterior step. If it is only a few millimeters, which is the case here, then leveling her arch before surgery should be stable [60]. If the anterior step is very large (5–6+ mm), then greater stability may be achieved by correcting the step surgically.

Q: What treatment options would you consider for Alyson (provide both a nonsurgical and a surgical treatment option)? What treatment do you recommend?

A: An orthodontics only treatment plan was given but not recommended. It included extraction of maxillary first premolars, placement of fixed orthodontic appliances, and HPHG wear for posterior anchorage control during anterior tooth retraction (TADs could be used for anchorage instead). The right cross bite would be corrected with archwire coordination and cross bite elastics. Alyson's arches would be leveled and aligned, her maxillary canines retracted into a Class I relationship (molars Class II), and then her maxillary incisors retracted. A compensating curve would be left in the maxillary archwire to help prevent increased incisor display, and a curve of Spee would be left in the mandibular archwire. She would be finished and retained. The disadvantages of this approach are that it would not address her chief complaint, and you may not be able to fully correct her right cross bite. Further, as the maxillary incisors are retracted (Figure 5.126), the incisors will tend to rotate around their apicies, the bite will tend to deepen, and the incisal display could worsen (unless the deflected archwire/jaw musculature intrudes the maxillary incisors). It is Alyson's concern with excess gin-

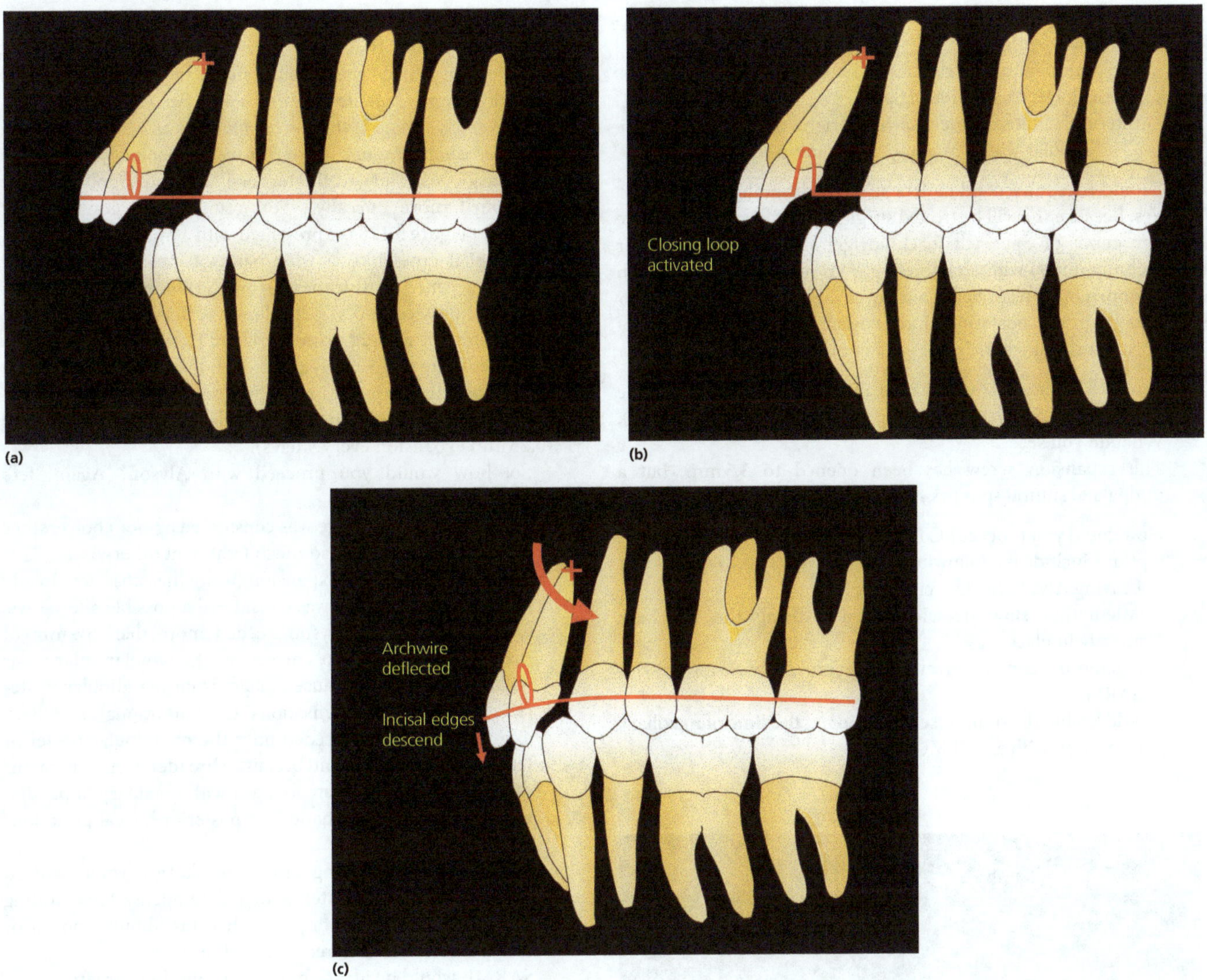

Figure 5.126 (a–c) As maxillary incisors are retracted, the incisors tend to rotate around their apicies, the bite tends to deepen, and incisal display tends to increase.

gival/incisal display which requires that a surgical option be entertained. With orthodontics alone, TADs could be used as anchorage to intrude the maxillary arch and reduce incisal display, but the initial incisal display at rest is large (~8 mm) and would require at least 4 mm of incisor intrusion to reduce to ideal (2–4 mm). It may be challenging to achieve this amount of intrusion with TADs.

A surgical treatment plan was given and recommended. It consisted of third molar removal and an attempt to achieve a midpalatal suture opening with an RME appliance. If a split did not occur, a SARME would be considered. Fixed orthodontic appliances would be placed, arches leveled and aligned (maxillary anterior step leveled), maxillary and mandibular posterior teeth uprighted (transverse compensations removed), and a one-piece maxillary impaction osteotomy with mandibular autorotation performed (the need for a mandibular advancement would be determined after the arches were leveled and aligned). Alyson would be finished with Class I molars and canines plus ideal overbite/overjet. The advantages of this plan are that it addresses the patient's chief (vertical) complaint and it corrects her transverse discrepancy. The disadvantages are the surgical risks. After considering both options, Alyson and her parents chose the surgical option.

Q: What are the specific objectives of treatment for the maxilla, mandible, maxillary dentition, and mandibular dentition in all three planes of space?

A: Specific objectives of treatment for Alyson are as follows:

Maxilla
- AP: Maintain.
- Vertical: Surgically impact posterior, maintain anterior.
- Transverse: Increase skeletal width.

Mandible
- AP: Advance by autorotation.
- Vertical: Decrease skeletal lower anterior facial height by autorotation.
- Transverse: Maintain.

Maxillary dentition
- AP: Maintain molars and canines. Upright incisors.
- Vertical: Maintain molars and incisors.

Intermolar width: Increase intermolar width.

Mandibular dentition

AP: Maintain molars canines and incisors.

Vertical: Decrease curve of Spee.

Intermolar/intercanine width: Upright molars to increase intermolar width. Maintain intercanine width.

Q: Should Alyson's second molars be banded/bonded?

A: Yes. Because she will be treated surgically, you *want* to eliminate her curve of Spee (tip back/upright/erupt her mandibular second molars) with arch leveling. This movement will worsen her open bite presurgically and force the surgeon to impact her maxilla in the posterior more. Postsurgically, if her curve of Spee returns, it will help to keep her bite closed down.

Q: An RME appliance was delivered and the screw was turned one turn per day for 2 weeks. A radiograph was made (Figure 5.127). What do you see?

A: The expansion screw has been opened to 3.5 mm, but a midpalatal sutural split has not resulted.

Q: How could you proceed? Consider all (at least 4) options.

A: Options include the following:

1 Leaving Alyson in right cross bite
2 Attempting slow dental expansion using the expander already in place
3 Attempting dental correction using cross-bite elastics
4 SARME
5 Addressing the transverse correction at the time of maxillary impaction with an MPMO

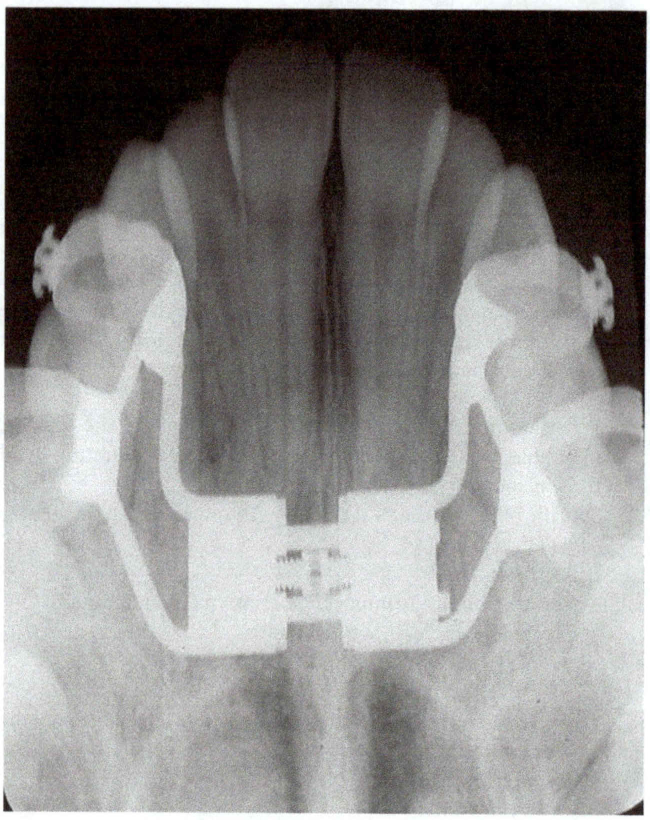

Figure 5.127 Maxillary occlusal radiograph of Alyson after 2 weeks of activating the RME screw 1 turn per day.

Slow dental expansion would be a viable alternative if the *magnitude* of the transverse posterior discrepancy was *mild (≤5 mm)*, if there was robust maxillary posterior buccal periodontium (*adequate bone and a wide band of attached keratinized gingiva*), and if there were *minimal or absent transverse posterior compensations* (posterior teeth reasonably upright or maxillary posterior teeth torqued lingually/roots already positioned more buccally). For example, the adult patient shown in Figure 5.128a–e presented with a mild bilateral posterior lingual cross bite, a wide band of attached keratinized gingiva, a generous thickness of buccal bone (Figure 5.128e, note thickness of buccal periodontium between red arrows), and reasonably upright posterior teeth. Her maxillary arch was expanded (Figure 5.128f–j) and cross bite corrected with 7 mm of slow dental expansion using a hyrax expansion screw appliance attached to the maxillary molars and first premolars (0.25 mm expansion every 4 days).

So, how would you proceed with Alyson? Again, let's consider our options:

1 Leaving her in cross bite was considered a poor choice, since she was going through so much treatment otherwise.
2 Slow maxillary dental expansion (using the expander already in place, Figure 5.127) was considered a possible alternative. On the one hand, Alyson needed more than 5½ mm of maxillary expansion to correct her first molar intermolar width discrepancy because of significant mandibular posterior transverse compensations (i.e., additional maxillary expansion would be needed once the mandibular posterior teeth were uprighted) and because a broader part of her mandibular arch would rotate forward with maxillary impaction surgery. On the other hand, her posterior buccal periodontium was robust.
3 Dental correction using cross-bite elastics would worsen Alyson's transverse posterior dental compensations (adding more lingual crown torque to her mandibular posterior teeth) and was considered a poor choice.
4 SARME would be ideal—but require another surgery.
5 Taking everything into consideration, a decision was made to correct her transverse discrepancy at the time of the LeFort I impaction osteotomy using an MPMO.

Fixed appliances were placed and the arches were leveled and aligned. Dental compensations were removed. Third molars were extracted, and spaces were placed between the maxillary lateral incisors and maxillary canines (Iowa spaces, to permit full seating of the posterior dentition during surgery without incisor interference).

Q: Figure 5.129 presents Alyson's presurgery records. Relaxed lip position is shown in Figure 5.129a, e, posed smiling is shown in Figure 5.129b, f, and exaggerated smiling is shown in Figure 5.129c, g.
What do you note?

A: Significant excess maxillary incisal and gingival display is evident. Figure 5.129e, f, and g underscores the importance of using incisal display *at rest* (following maxillary arch leveling) to determine the magnitude of surgical impaction and *not incisal/gingival display when smiling* (which is highly variable and dependent on musculature activity). Other features observed are as follows:

- Following arch leveling and aligning, an overt open bite is now present and extends to the premolars (Figure 5.129h–j).

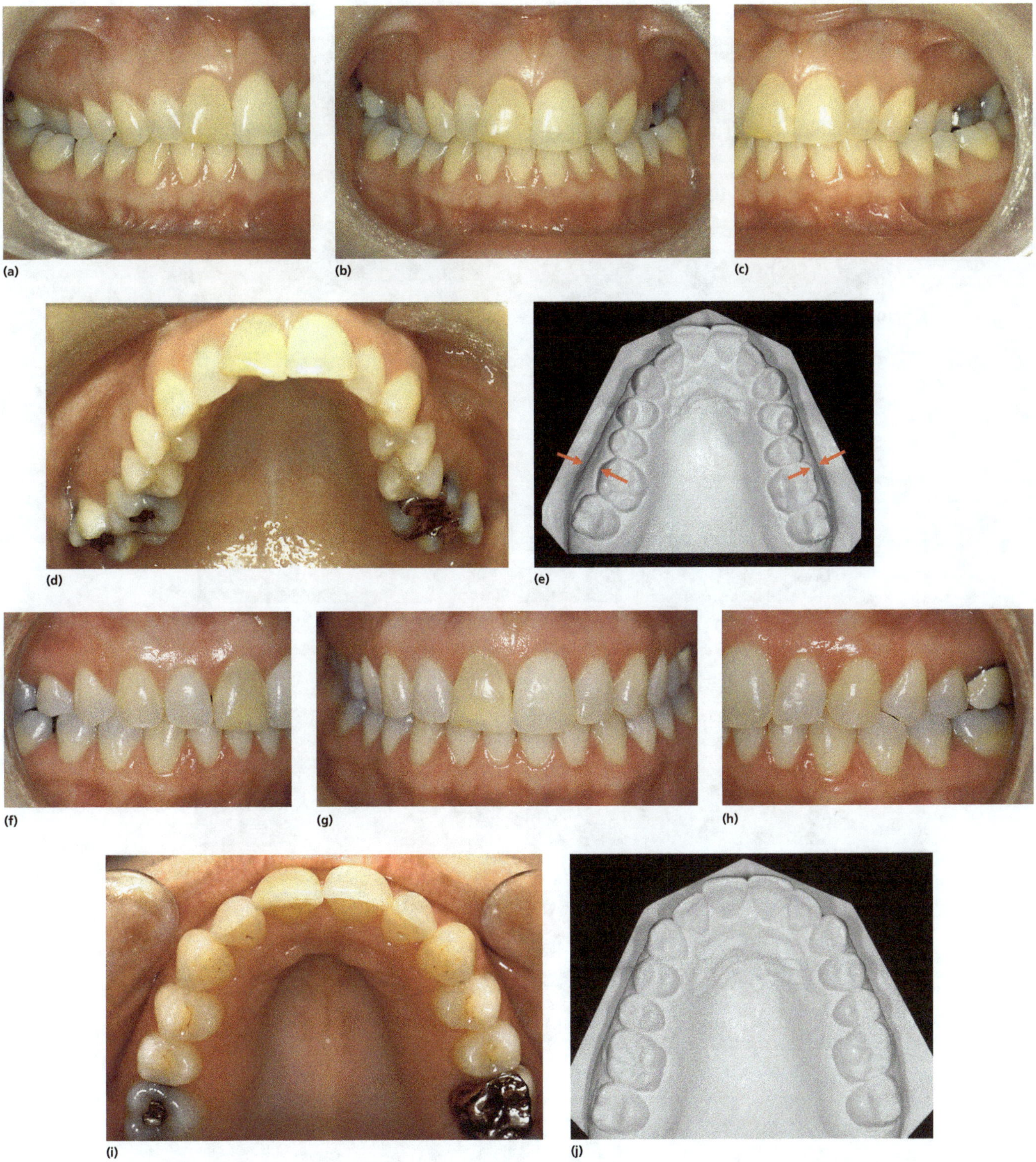

Figure 5.128 This adult patient was a good candidate for slow, dental, expansion: (a–c) mild bilateral posterior cross bite with wide band of attached keratinized gingiva, (d, e) reasonably upright posterior teeth and generous thickness of buccal bone. (f–j) Her maxillary arch was expanded by 0.25 mm, every 4 days, for a total of 7 mm.

Why? Mandibular posterior teeth were erupted with curve of Spee leveling—opening the bite.

- She is still Class II by about 4 mm (Figure 5.129h, j).
- Iowa spaces (Figure 5.129k) between the maxillary canines and maxillary lateral incisors are present to allow full canine Class I surgical seating without incisor interference.

Q: What other presurgical records should you make? How would use them?

A: A presurgical cephalometric radiograph should be taken and the final surgical predictions made using it. On the tracing, the maxilla is impacted (Figure 5.130, top left) to provide 4–5 mm of incisal display at rest (Figure 5.130, center). The posterior of

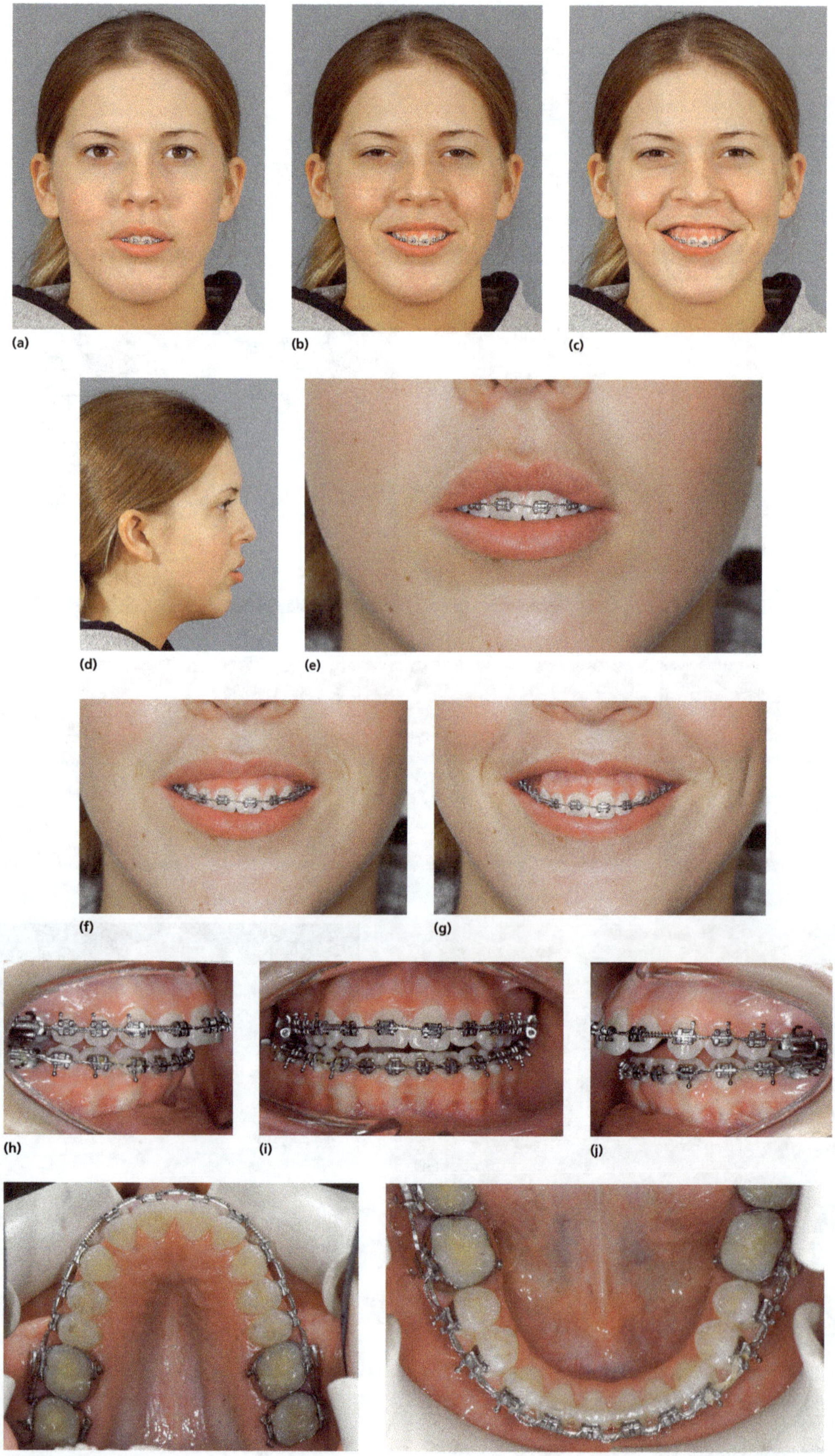

(a) (b) (c) (d) (e) (f) (g) (h) (i) (j) (k) (l)

Figure 5.129 (a–l) Presurgical records of Alyson.

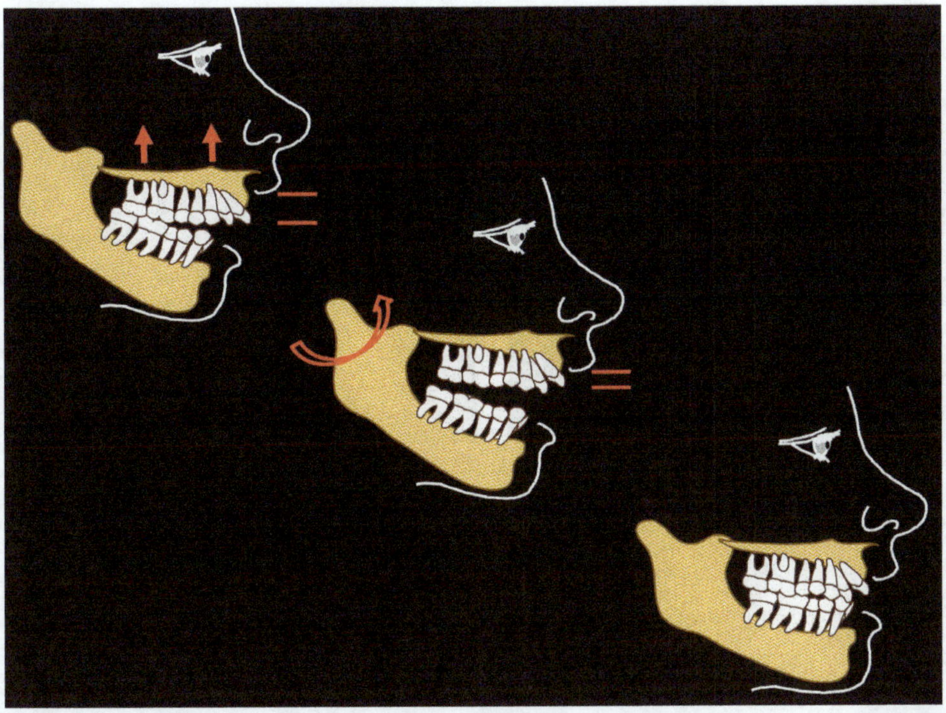

Figure 5.130 Use of a presurgical lateral cephalometric tracing for treatment planning maxillary surgery: the maxilla is impacted (top left) so that when the mandible autorotates forward and upward (center), the LAFH is reduced, 4–5 mm of maxillary incisal display at rest obtained, ILG reduced or eliminated, anterior open bite closed, and posterior teeth brought into occlusion (bottom right).

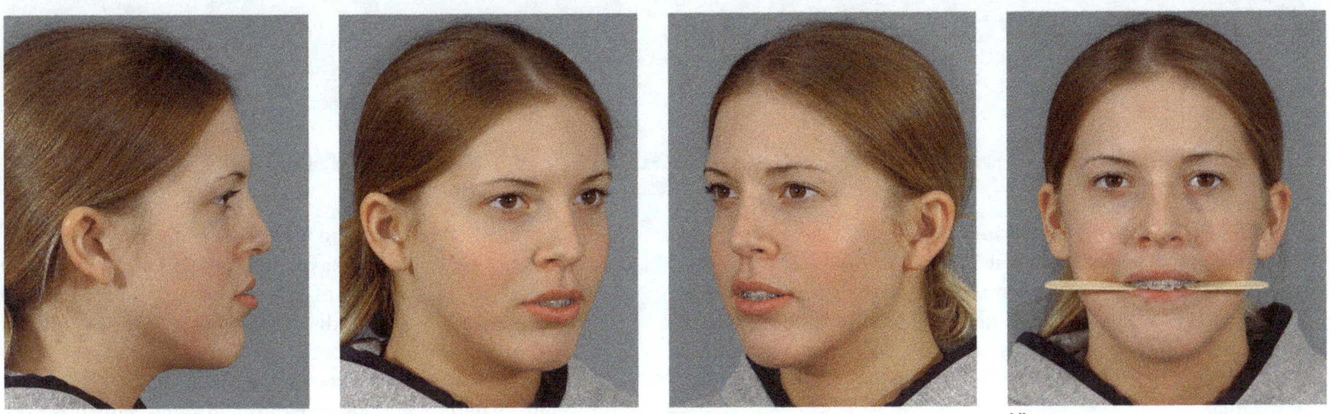

(a) (b) (c) (d)

Figure 5.131 Additional, presurgical photographs: (a) Alyson postured forward to a Class I canine relationship, (b, c) right and left ¾ (45°) facial views, (d) evaluation of maxillary right-to-left cant using a tongue blade. Note: even if these photographs were made initially, it is important to re-make them presurgically, since leveling and aligning the arches could have produced changes.

the maxilla is impacted enough so that the open bite is closed when the mandible is autorrotated CCW around the condyles (Figure 5.130 bottom right). You must evaluate whether a Class I canine relationship is achieved with this mandibular autorotation or whether a mandibular advancement (or setback) osteotomy will be necessary to achieve Class I canines. You must also evaluate whether the posterior maxilla must be impacted more (or less) than the anterior maxilla to achieve occlusal interdigitation.

A profile view of Alyson postured forward into a Class I canine relationship (Figure 5.131a) can give some idea of her postsurgical profile. As shown, her profile is relatively straight when she postured forward into a Class I canine relationship. Therefore, treating her nonextraction was probably a good choice (although her lower lip looks protruded). Left and right 45° facial photos (Figure 5.131b, c) can provide one final examination of her malar and maxillary projection, while biting on a tongue blade (Figure 5.131d) can help determine if an occlusal cant resulted during leveling which must be addressed during surgery. Finally, presurgery models should be made and evaluated when held in a Class I canine relationship (with best fit posterior transverse) to judge the anteroposterior and transverse occlusal coordination.

Q: Generally, in a young person like Alyson, is it better to overimpact her maxilla (resulting in less than 2 mm of incisal display at

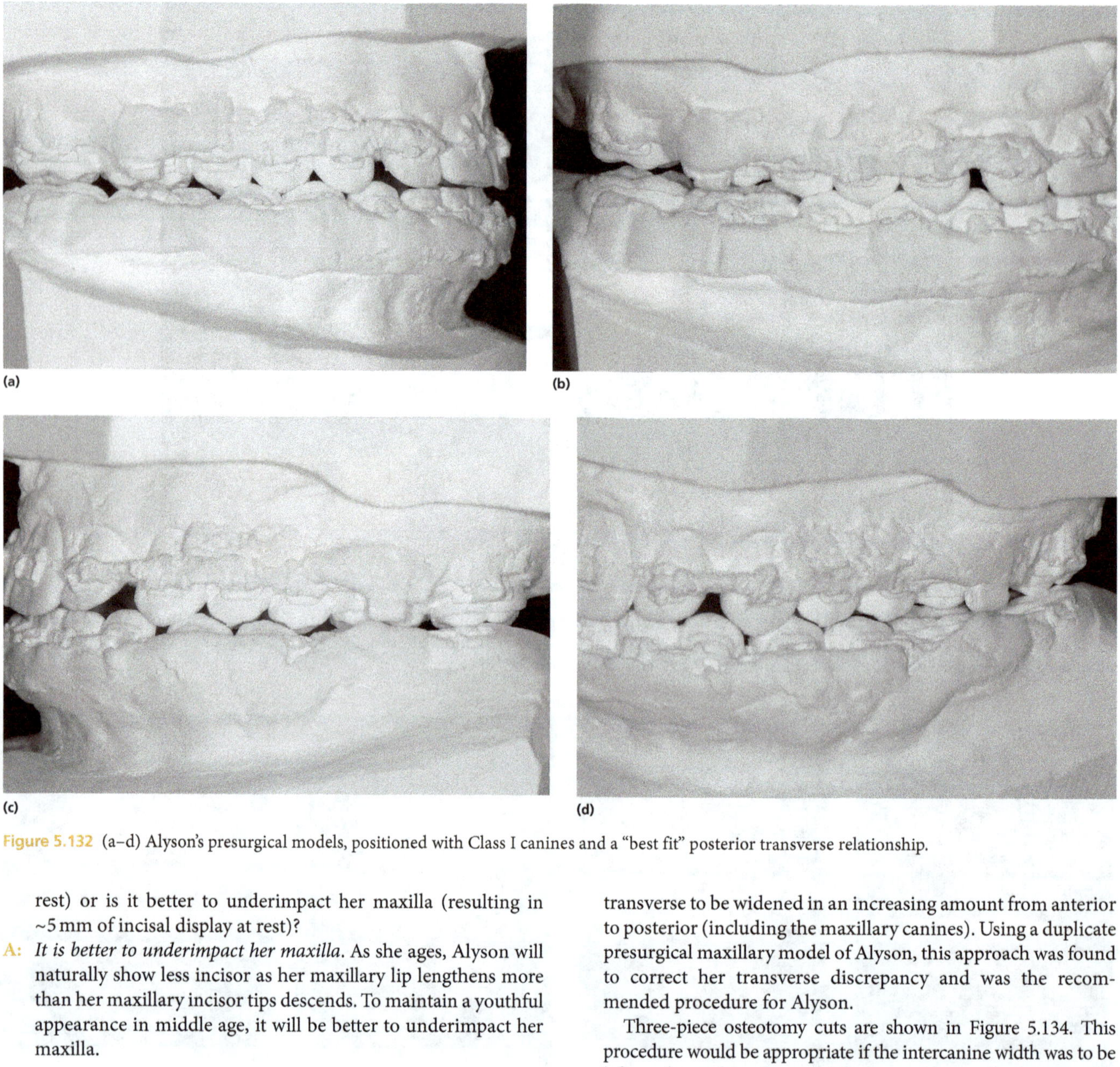

Figure 5.132 (a–d) Alyson's presurgical models, positioned with Class I canines and a "best fit" posterior transverse relationship.

rest) or is it better to underimpact her maxilla (resulting in ~5 mm of incisal display at rest)?

A: *It is better to underimpact her maxilla.* As she ages, Alyson will naturally show less incisor as her maxillary lip lengthens more than her maxillary incisor tips descends. To maintain a youthful appearance in middle age, it will be better to underimpact her maxilla.

Q: Look at Alyson's presurgery models when held in a Class I canine relationship with posterior transverse "best fit" (Figure 5.132). What do you note?

A: The left and right *anteroposterior* relationships (Figure 5.132a, c) look reasonable. But a transverse discrepancy, which *worsens from canine to second molar*, is seen bilaterally when looking down slightly on the models (Figure 5.132b, d).

Q: How will this transverse discrepancy affect your surgical recommendations?

A: Instead of performing a single-piece maxillary impaction osteotomy, a multiple-piece maxillary impaction osteotomy is indicated to widen the posterior maxilla.

Q: Would you recommend a two-piece or a three-piece maxillary impaction osteotomy?

A: A two-piece osteotomy is shown in Figure 5.133. A parasagittal cut, starting between the central incisors, allows the maxillary transverse to be widened in an increasing amount from anterior to posterior (including the maxillary canines). Using a duplicate presurgical maxillary model of Alyson, this approach was found to correct her transverse discrepancy and was the recommended procedure for Alyson.

Three-piece osteotomy cuts are shown in Figure 5.134. This procedure would be appropriate if the intercanine width was to be left unchanged, and you wished to widen only the posterior transverse (Figure 5.134b). Also, this procedure is appropriate if you had a large anterior step in the occlusion and wished to correct the step by vertically moving the anterior and posterior segments, independently (not by leveling the anterior step, presurgically).

Q: Should the surgeon consider overexpanding the maxilla with an MPMO?

A: Yes, the surgeon should consider overexpanding the maxilla.

Q: Using the presurgical records, a final surgical plan was established consisting of a Le Fort I two-piece differential impaction osteotomy (3 mm anterior impaction, 5 mm posterior impaction, 5 mm transverse maxillary expansion at the first molars, and mandibular autorotation). You receive a call the afternoon of the surgery. The surgeon states that intra-operative difficulties during Alyson's 9-hour surgery resulted in less maxillary expansion and less posterior impaction than was planned. There was excessive bleeding in the pterygoid plate

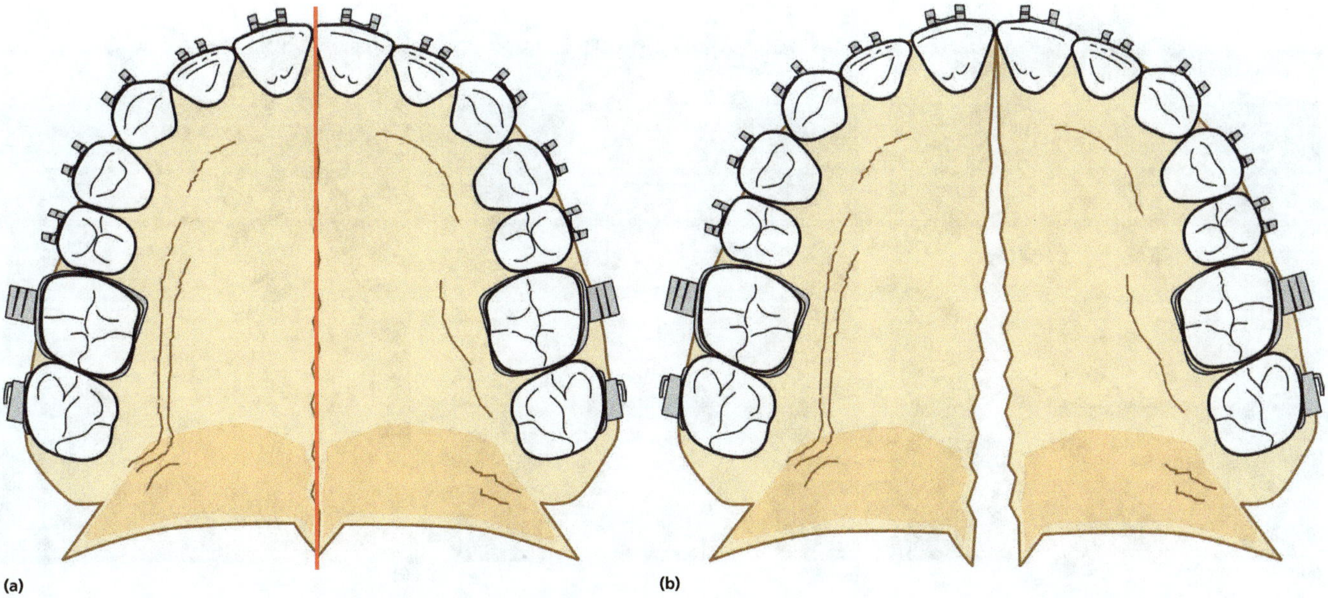

Figure 5.133 (a) The parasagittal cut and (b) transverse widening for a one-piece maxillary osteotomy. Note that the entire arch, from the canines posteriorly, is widened (increasingly).

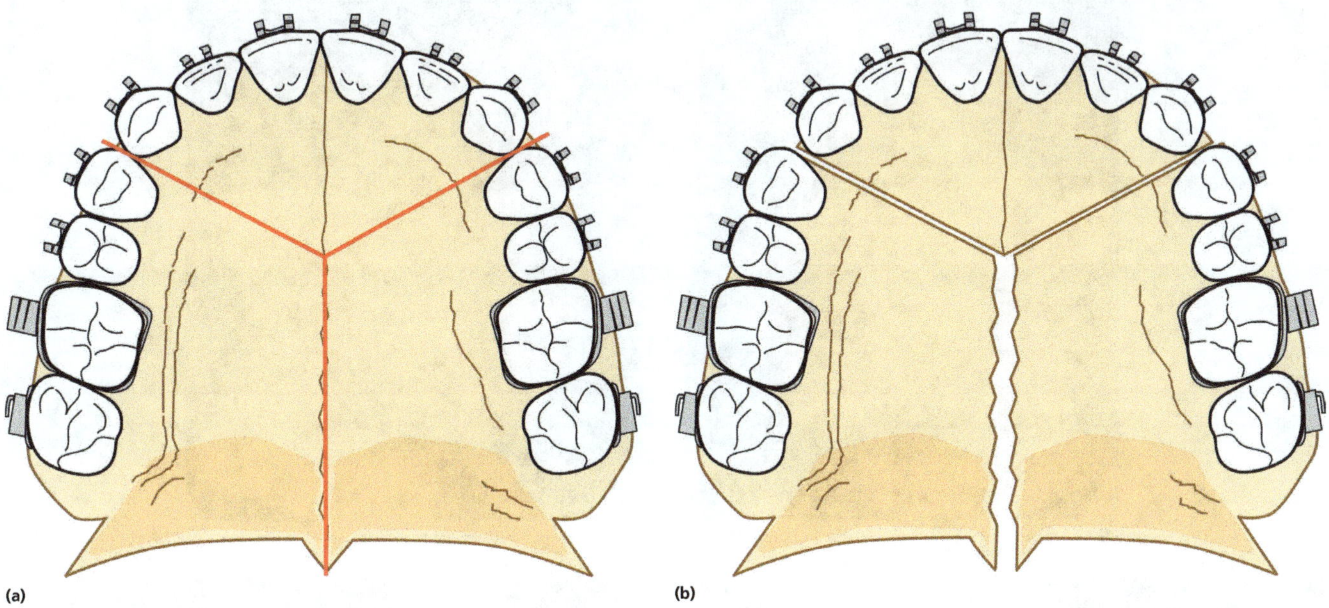

Figure 5.134 (a) The cuts and (b) posterior transverse widening for a three-piece maxillary osteotomy where the interpremolar and intermolar widths are to be increased, but the intercanine width is to be left unchanged.

region plus the occlusal splint broke and had to be reconstructed during surgery. Alyson returns to see you 10 days post surgery (Figure 5.135). What do you note?

A: As anticipated, Alyson presents with a less-than-ideal surgical result. Although minimal swelling is seen, she still has an interlabial gap. An occlusal splint is in place to hold the transverse correction, and she is wearing guiding elastics. A Class I molar relationship is observed on the right, and an end-on Class II (3–4 mm Class II) relationship is seen on the left. A deficient transverse width is also noted (not shown) which worsens posteriorly. A maxillary midline deviation of approximately 1.5 mm to the right is seen. Finally, note that the maxillary archwire was sectioned at the midline during surgery, as expected.

Q: Let's take a few moments to discuss guidelines for dealing with postsurgical problems such as we have here. What items would you consider as important in avoiding or dealing with postsurgery problems?

A: The following checklists (Tables 5.15, 5.16 and 5.17) are guidelines to avoid postsurgical problems.

Q: You dismiss Alyson and contact the surgeon. You describe the occlusal discrepancies you noted. How do you recommend proceeding?

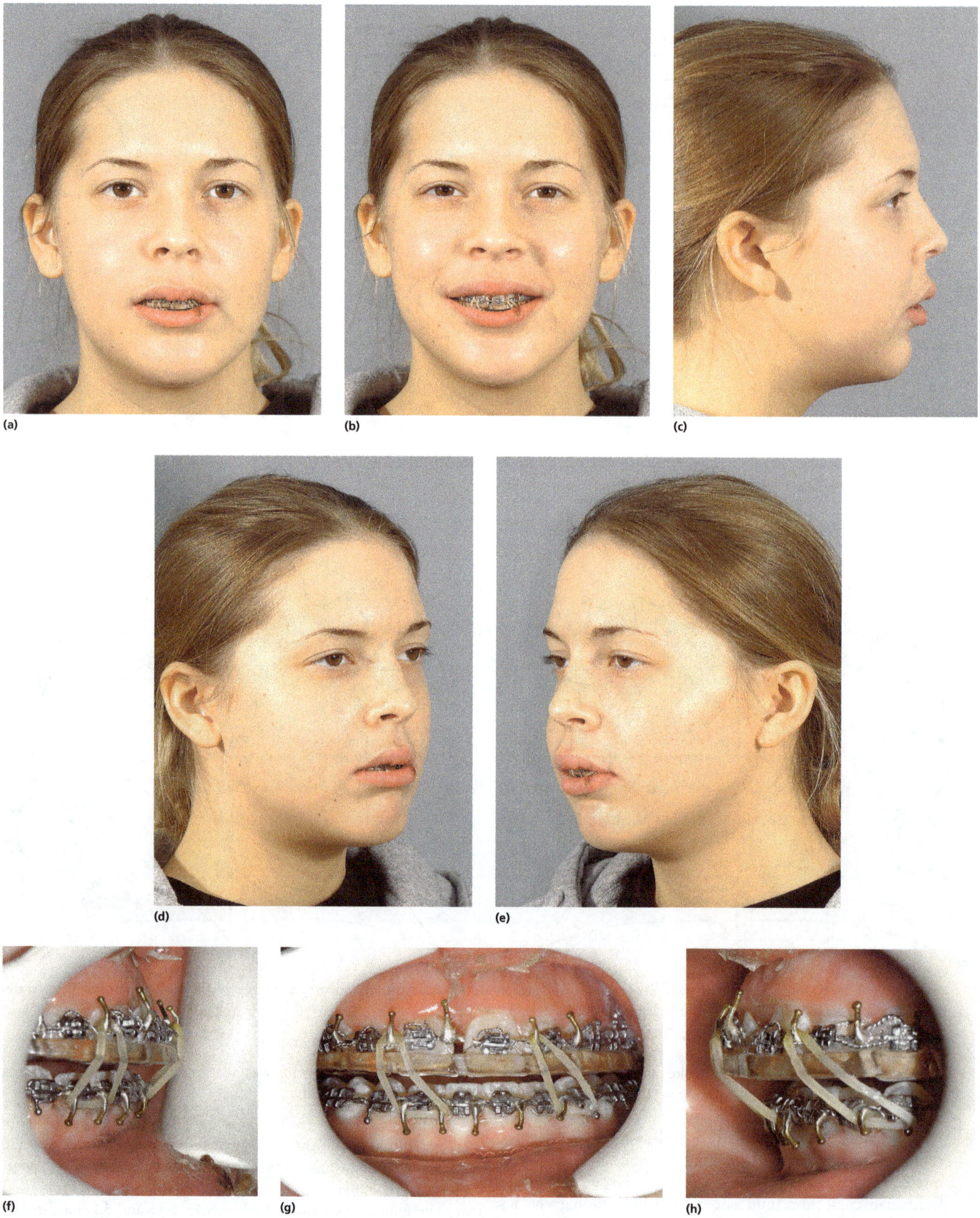

Figure 5.135 (a–h) Alyson at 10 days post surgery.

Table 5.15 Checklist to follow for surgical patients.

Presurgical tasks	◻ Verify relaxed lip incisal display *after leveling* to decide the magnitude of vertical anterior maxillary surgical incisor movement. ◻ Approve the articulated surgical occlusion (models mounted by the surgeon). ◻ Agree on proposed surgical movements and verify that surgical movements are within surgical limits. ◻ Schedule the patient to see you 1 week after the surgery date.
Postsurgical communication	◻ When should the surgeon contact the orthodontist? – Immediately after surgery (what was the surgical outcome?) – The surgeon should inform the orthodontist of problems (to better prepare for dealing with them) – **Q:** Was the bite seated during surgery? (If it was, then a later occlusal discrepancy could be due to edema/muscle spasms) ◻ Take care what you say in front of the patient. – Seek solutions to surgical problems the cause of which may have been indeterminate/unavoidable. – Put a positive spin on intervention—"surgery helped a lot, now we are completing treatment". ◻ Work together with the surgeon to discuss postsurgical treatment, including direction and magnitude of forces to be applied.
Postsurgical tasks	◻ See patient 1 week postoperatively (well within the first month window of accelerated bony remodeling/cellular activity/possible increased tooth movement) so that you can intercede effectively, as needed. ◻ Check for postsurgical occlusal discrepancies, including a repeatable bite at the 1 week postop appointment. ◻ Guiding elastics—guiding elastics help the patient learn to close into the new occlusion. This is necessary since the jaw muscular length and direction have been changed with surgery, edema, and muscle spasms may alter the correct closing position, proprioceptive sense may have been lost, and/or the patient may be numb. The focus of guiding elastics is on the muscles. Guiding elastics are *not* intended to move teeth. There is no specific length of time for wearing guiding elastics. Time of wear is a judgment call made between the surgeon and orthodontist ◻ Splints—an occlusal splint is worn by the patient for ~6 weeks following MPMOs to hold a transverse expansion. As soon as it is removed, a palatal splint is fabricated and worn for as long as possible through the completion of orthodontic treatment. If the maxillary archwire was sectioned at surgery, then it should be replaced with a continuous wire at the 6-week appointment

Table 5.16 Limits of orthognathic surgical movements.

Maxillary surgical limits	Downgraft	5–8 mm	Note: The maxilla cannot descend straight down due to changes in the occlusal plane angle as the mandible rotates down and back.
	Impaction	6–7 mm	In the posterior
		10 mm	In the anterior
	MPMO transverse expansion	8 mm	Limit depends on the height of the palate and posterior tooth torque; a low palate permits less expansion (soft tissue stretch); ideally, the presurgical posterior dentition should be without transverse compensations.
	Advancement	5–7 mm	Consider distraction osteogenesis if more maxillary advancement than this is required.
	Setback	5–6 mm	The limiting factor is running into the bony pterygoid plates. If you need a greater setback than this, consider extracting maxillary premolars so only the anterior segment is setback.
Mandibular surgical limits	Advancement	10 mm	In high MPA cases
		14–15 mm	In low MPA cases
			Note: Check for impingement of maxillary second molars on the ascending ramus during advancement. You may need to extract the maxillary second molars if maxillary second molar impingement occurs.
	Setback	10 mm	Be careful to avoid airway obstruction or of creating future sleep apnea problems.

Table 5.17 Guidelines for post-surgical biomechanics if occlusal discrepancies exist (i.e., not fully corrected or overcorrected).

General guidelines	• Use the same biomechanics that are used as for nonsurgical cases. • Discuss with your surgeon the level of forces, and direction of forces you intend to use • Try to stay with light forces—especially when beginning. • *Remember the direction of surgery*—do NOT immediately use mechanics that are opposite to the direction of the surgery. For example, if a mandibular advancement osteotomy overcorrected a Class II patient to a Class III relationship, do NOT begin pulling Class III elastics. You may eventually need to use Class III elastics, but give the patient some months to allow edema to be eliminated and muscular function to normalize before doing so.
Mild discrepancy	• Use standard orthodontic finishing treatment.
Moderate discrepancy	• Aggressive intercession may be required, or accept a compromise result.
Severe discrepancy	• Discuss with surgeon. • If you feel that the patient needs to go back into surgery, do it very soon so the patient has only one recovery period (if you wait a month before sending the patient to surgery, he/she will have two recovery periods.)

A: Alyson's treatment to this point was appropriate. Her discrepancy arose because of unanticipated problems during surgery. You stayed within reasonable limits for surgical movement, you checked her incisal display preoperatively, and you consulted with the surgeon regarding the cephalometric prediction. You approved the presurgical occlusion using articulated models, and Alyson wore her guiding elastics as recommended. The occlusal discrepancy on her left is moderate, and you should proceed with somewhat aggressive treatment to correct it. Considering the direction of the surgery (maxilla up), it would be reasonable to ask Alyson to wear an asymmetric left HPHG. Alyson was recalled at 14 days post op (Figure 5.136). Note that the edema has diminished but the left 3–4 mm Class II relationship is still evident. She was placed on an asymmetric left HPHG (Figure 5.136g) with light force, after conferring with the surgeon.

Q: At a follow-up appointment 3 weeks later (Figure 5.137), what do you note?

A: You see significant improvement in the anteroposterior relationship on her left (Figure 5.137). You did well.

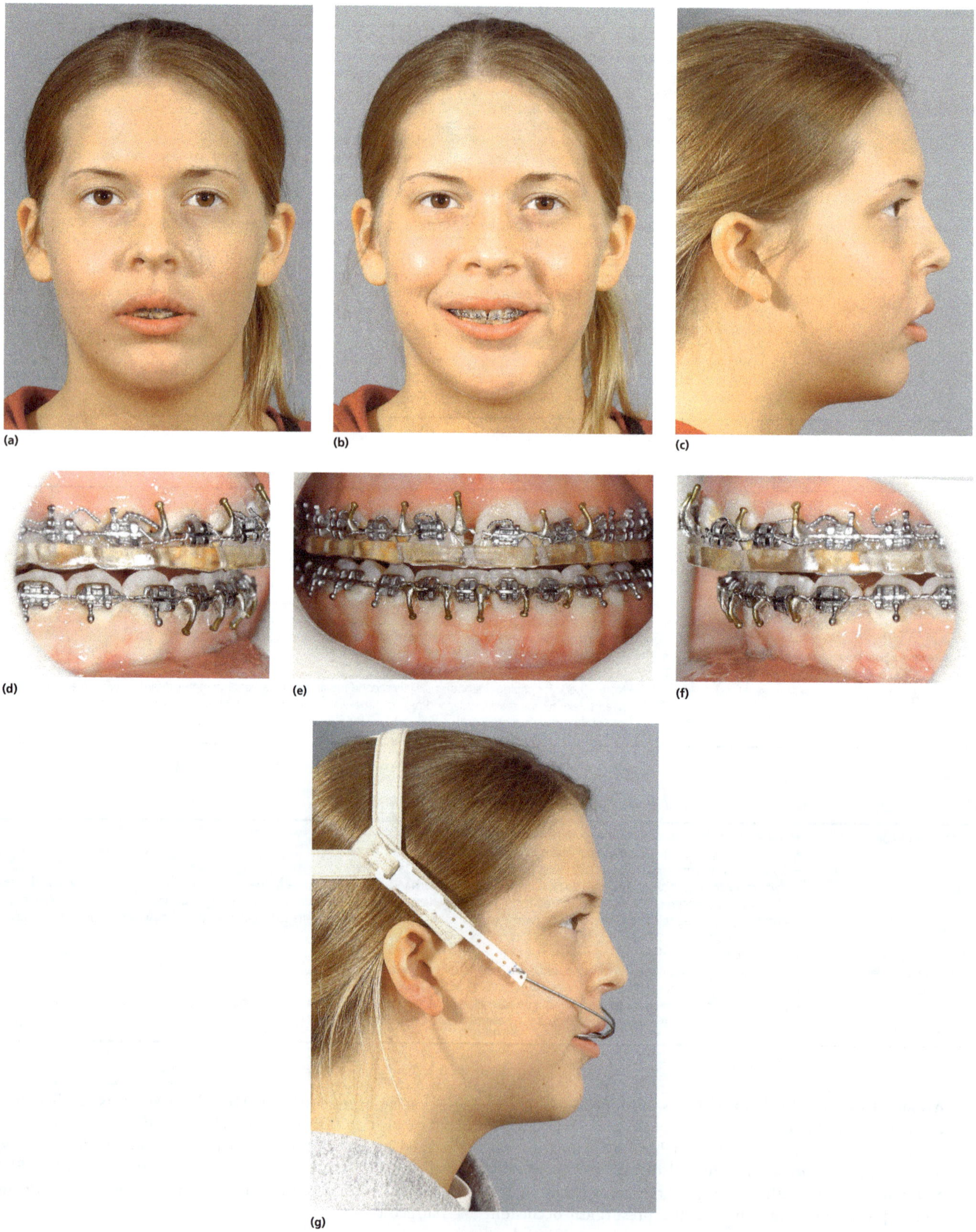

Figure 5.136 (a–g) Alyson at 14 days post surgery. After conferring with the surgeon, and based upon the direction of surgery (maxilla up) and postoperative occlusal discrepancies, Alyson was placed on an asymmetric left HPHG with light force.

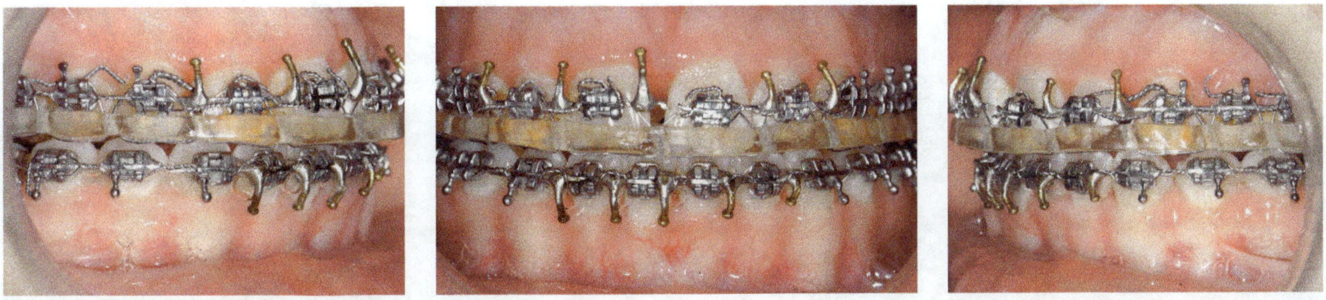

(a) (b) (c)

Figure 5.137 (a–c) Alyson at 5 weeks post surgery.

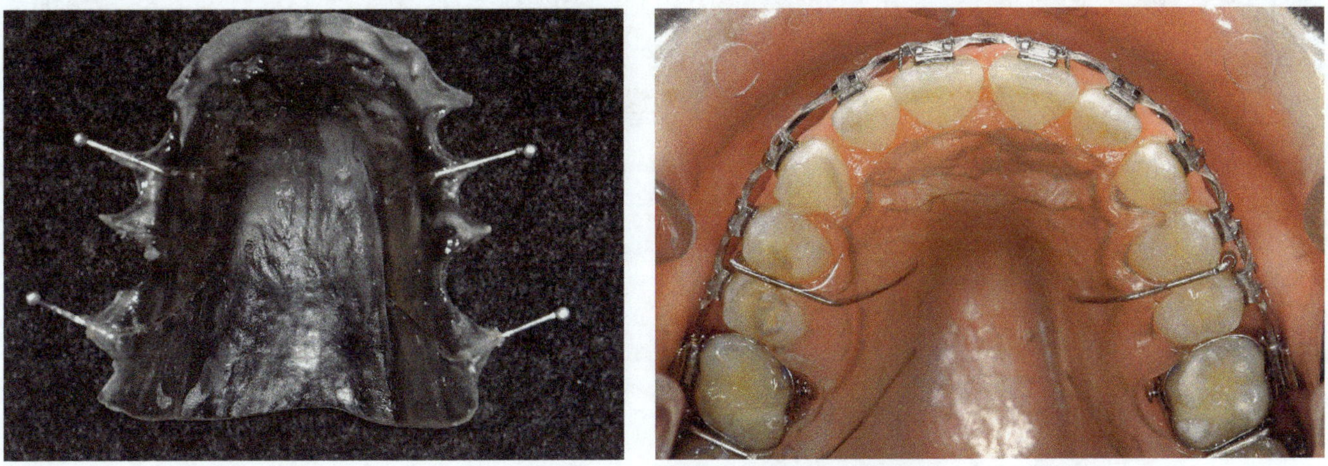

(a) (b)

Figure 5.138 (a, b) In order to minimize relapse of Alyson's maxillary surgical transverse expansion, a removable palatal splint should be fabricated and worn as soon as her occlusal splint is removed.

Q: As stated earlier, MPMO surgery resulted in less maxillary expansion then desired, and we are left with a few millimeters of residual maxillary transverse constriction on the left side. How do you proceed?

A: First, make sure that you *maintain* the transverse expansion that surgery provided. Remove the occlusal splint at 6 weeks, make a maxillary impression, and immediately prepare a removable palatal splint that Alyson should wear for as long as possible during the rest of treatment (Figure 5.138).

If the maxillary constriction was bilateral, then the maxillary archwire could be expanded (bilateral effect), an expanded 0.032 overlay archwire placed through the headgear tubes on the molar bands (bilateral effect), or bilateral cross-bite elastics worn. These treatments would also help insure stability of the MPMO expansion. Since Alyson's post-surgery transverse problem was primarily on the left, she was treated with a slightly expanded maxillary archwire plus cross-bite elastics on the left only (left elastic worn from maxillary first molar lingual to mandibular first molar buccal—to increase transverse OJ).

Q: With this approach to addressing the transverse postsurgical discrepancy, what changes do you anticipate in Alyson's left posterior transverse dental compensations?

A: Expect a worsening of left transverse compensations (buccal maxillary posterior crown torque and lingual mandibular posterior crown torque).

Q: The HPHG was continued and bilateral Class II elastics were worn. Iowa spaces were closed. Her orthodontic treatment was detailed and finished. Eight months of post surgical orthodontic intervention achieved the final result (Figure 5.139). What do you note?

A: A striking improvement in Alyson's appearance is seen by comparing Figures 5.118a–c to 5.139a–c. Her initial to final cephalometric radiographic superimposition (Figure 5.139f) illustrates the basis for these changes:

- A maxillary impaction osteotomy moved both ANS, PNS, and the maxillary dentition superiorly ~2–3 mm. This movement decreased incisal display and reduced LAFH as the mandible rotated CCW, bringing B-point upward and forward. Although the surgeon reported that problems in the pterygoid area prevented him from impacting the posterior maxilla as much as desired, open bite closure and excellent incisal display was achieved.
- Her maxilla *retracted* 2–3 mm, probably with postsurgery HPHG wear.
- Nasal shape was not altered.

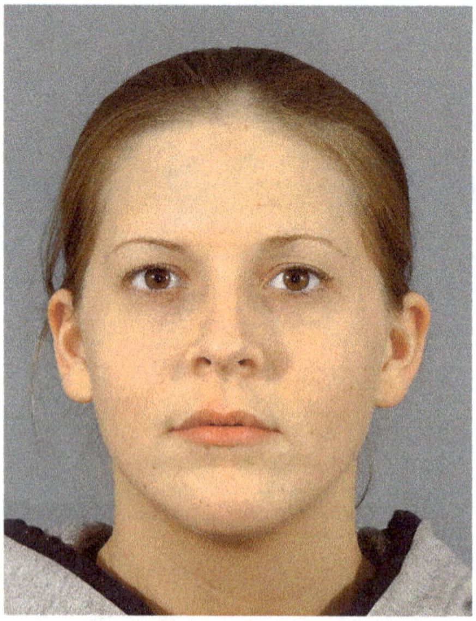
(a)

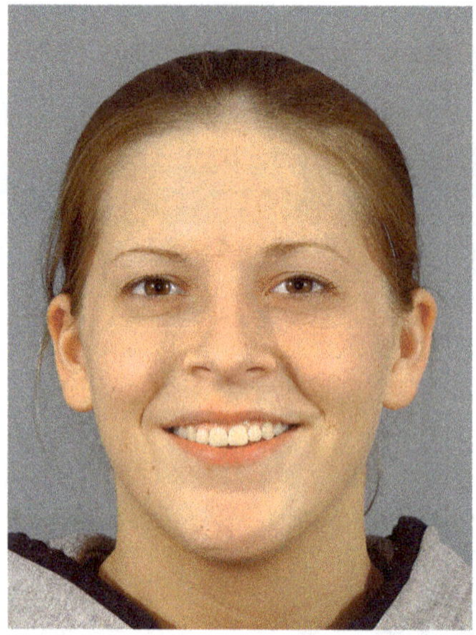
(b)

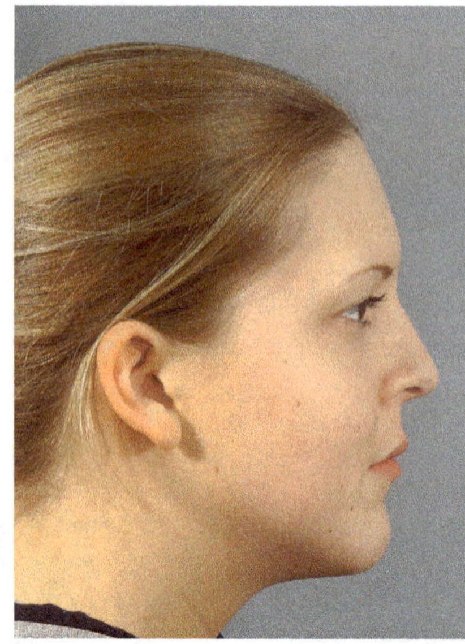
(c)

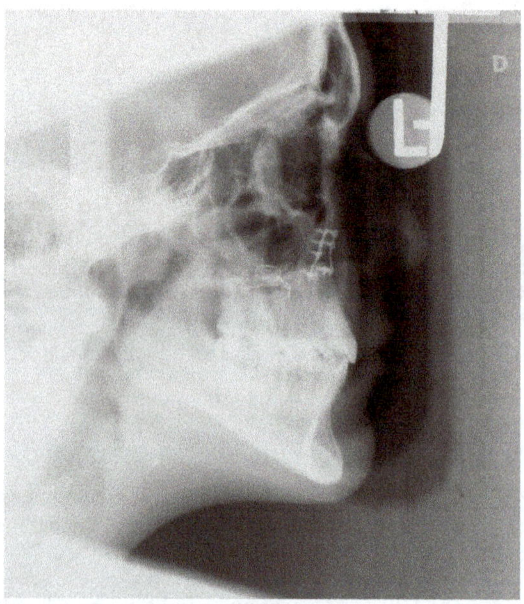
(d)

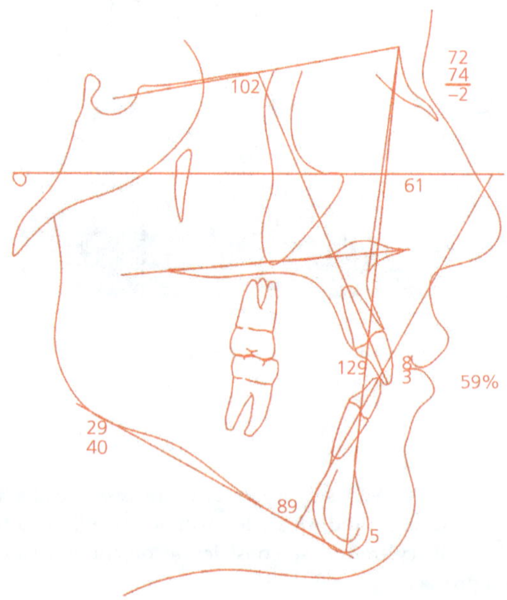

(e)

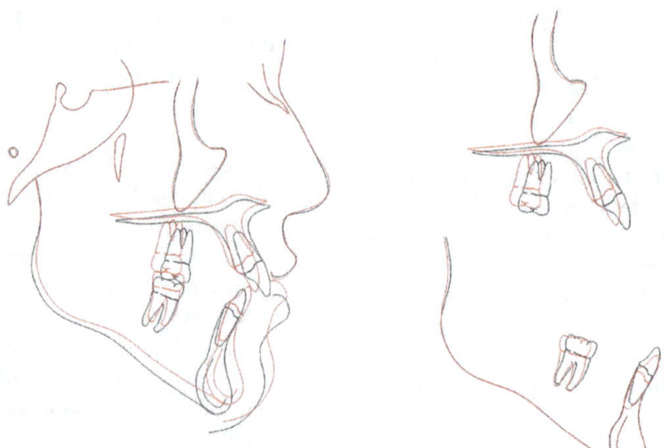
(f)

Figure 5.139 (a–n) Alyson's final records.

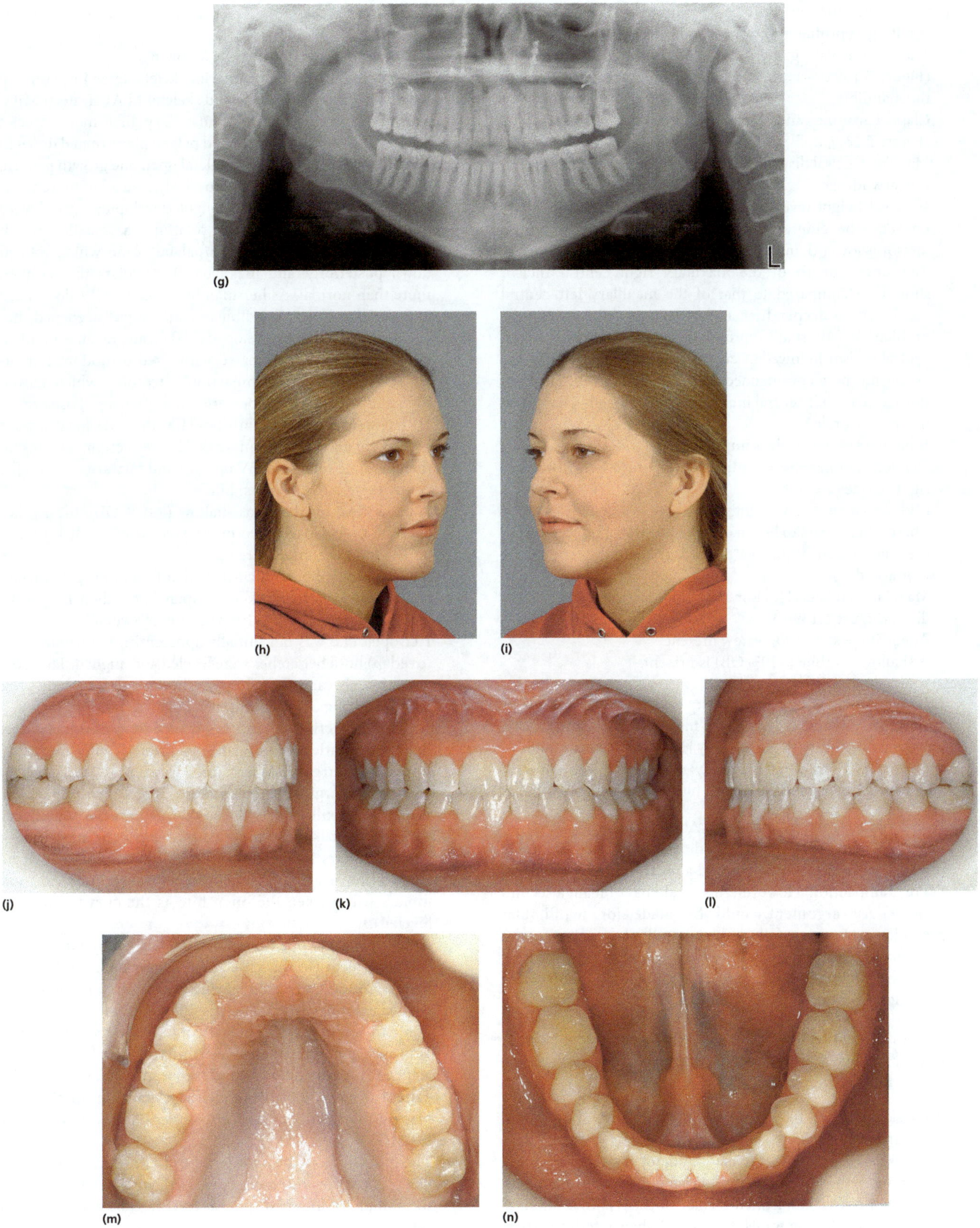

Figure 5.139 (Continued)

- Soft tissue chin and B-point were brought up and forward, resulting in profile improvement.
- The interlabial gap was reduced to a mere 1 mm (Figure 5.139a)—as the mandibular lip was carried up with the mandible.
- Class I canine and molar relationships were achieved (Figure 5.139j, l).
- Maxillary incisal display during a posed smile (Figure 5.139b) is nearly ideal.
- Gingival height levels of the maxillary incisors are slightly uneven—the gingival level of the maxillary right central incisor is lower than that of the maxillary left central incisor. The sulcus depth of the maxillary right central incisor should be compared to that of the maxillary left central incisor. If it is deeper, then a gingivectomy could correct the problem. An alternate approach, erupting the maxillary left central incisor followed by enameloplasty of the incisal edge, would not be recommended. Why? The gingival margin of the maxillary left central incisor is already ideally positioned in a posed smile.
- Broadness of her smile is improved.
- Her left canines are coordinated (Figure 5.139k), but her right canines are not.
- Midlines are not coincident.
- There still appears to be attached keratinized gingiva labial to the mandibular right central incisor—but this should be monitored.
- Maxillary left lateral incisor and canine are rotated out on the distal (Figure 5.139m).
- Adequate posterior OJ is now present.
- A shallow overbite (~10% OB) is present.

Q: How was Alyson's open bite closed?

A: As her maxilla moved up with the maxillary impaction osteotomy (and possibly with postsurgery HPHG wear), her mandible autorotated CCW around the condyles, moving B-point upward and forward, and closing the open bite.

Q: Would you suggest any changes to Alyson's surgery?

A: Probably not. A SARME would have provided an ideal transverse correction and allowed a more simple (one piece) LeFort I impaction. However, this would have meant a second surgery. An argument could be made for mandibular premolar extractions, followed by mandibular canine retraction, mandibular BSSO advancement, and resulting stronger chin projection. However, Alyson's profile is actually quite pleasing now.

Q: How would you retain this patient? What will you watch for?

A: Hawley retainers were placed. The possibility for surgical relapse must be monitored.

Q: If the skeletal open bite begins to return (relapse), how would you manage it?

A: The answer depends on the magnitude of the relapse. If it is very minor, then it could be left untreated or closed with posterior occlusal adjustment (enameloplasty). If is mild to moderate, and Alyson wants it corrected, then anterior vertical elastics could be worn between fixed appliances to erupt her anterior teeth (masking) or TADs could be used to intrude her posterior teeth (orthopedics?). If it is severe, then you need to consider another surgery.

Q: What are the "take-home" messages from treatment of this patient?

A: Take home-messages include the following:

- Alyson presented with an anterior skeletal open bite (vertical maxillary excess: soft tissue and skeletal LLAFH, steep MPA, short posterior face height, maxillary first molar apicies erupted below palatal plane, and palatal plane tipped down in posterior). She had a classic skeletal open bite growth pattern: condyles growing posterior-superiorly instead of more vertically, lack of posterior face height development, backward internal (true) mandibular rotation, a maxilla which descended more than normal/palatal plane which rotated down posteriorly, and maxillary first molars that erupted more than normal. As her mandible rotated CW downward and backward, her mandibular plane angle steepened, her LAFH increased, she developed an ILG, and an anterior open bite resulted. She was treated with fixed orthodontic appliances and a maxillary impaction osteotomy which moved PNS and the maxillary posterior dentition up. Postsurgical HPHG wear may have contributed to this maxillary upward movement and the 2–3 mm maxillary retraction. As a result, the mandible rotated CCW upward and forward (around the condyles), closing the open bite.
- Alyson's final overbite was shallow (~10% OB). Ideally, her overbite should have been overcorrected to 20–40% OB, in anticipation of some future relapse.
- If Alyson's mandibular incisors had not supra-erupted (dental compensation for her skeletal open bite), then her initial anterior open bite would have been *much* worse.
- Her open bite was not initially apparent in the frontal view (overlap) until her arches were leveled and aligned. Then, the open bite became apparent as her posterior teeth were erupted during curve of Spee leveling.
- It is good practice to band/bond second molars in skeletal open bite patients that will be treated with maxillary impaction surgery. Why? You want the open bite to worsen presurgically, to force the surgeon to impact the posterior maxilla more (Alyson's open bite worsened presurgically). It is good practice to *avoid* banding/bonding second molars in skeletal open bite patients that will be treated nonsurgically (since tipping back/erupting second molars will worsen the open bite as the curve of Spee is leveled).
- Anterior skeletal open bites are best treated by intrusion of posterior teeth (in this case surgical impaction of the maxilla). Masking (extrusion of anterior teeth) may not have yielded an esthetic, or stable, result for Alyson.
- You can attempt RME in patients of Alyson's initial age. However, you must have a secondary plan if you fail to achieve a midpalatal sutural separation (e.g., leave the patient in cross bite, RME dental expansion, masking by placing/increasing posterior compensations, SARME, or MPMO).
- The magnitude of the *anterior* upward movement of a maxillary impaction osteotomy is based, in large measure, on the amount of incisal display at rest after the maxillary arch is leveled.
- The surgical patient checklist provided with this case (and in the Appendix) can help reduce surgical-orthodontic problems. However, despite your and the surgeon's skill, unanticipated problems can arise during surgery. In Alyson's case, the

surgeon could neither impact nor widen the maxilla as much as was planned. The orthodontist must be prepared to intercede postsurgically to provide the patient with the best possible outcome.

References

1 Burstone CJ. Lip posture and its significance in treatment planning. *Am J Orthod.* 1967;**53**:262–84.

2 Schudy FF. The rotation of the mandible resulting from growth: its implications in orthodontic treatment. *Angle Orthod.* 1965;**35**:36–50.

3 Schudy FF. The control of vertical overbite in clinical orthodontics. *Angle Orthod.* 1968;**38**:19–39.

4 Bjork A, Skieller V. Facial development and tooth eruption. An implant study at the age of puberty. *Am J Orthod.* 1972;**62**:339–83.

5 Nemeth RB, Isaacson RJ. Vertical anterior relapse. *Am J Orthod.* 1974;**65**:565–85.

6 Bjork A, Skieller V. Normal and abnormal growth of the mandible. A synthesis of longitudinal cephalometric implant studies over a period of 25 years. *Eur J Orthod.* 1983;**5**:1–46.

7 Bjork A, Skieller V. Contrasting mandibular growth and facial development in long face syndrome, juvenile rheumatoid polyarthritis and mandibulofacial dysostosis. *J Craniofac Genet Dev Biol Suppl.* 1985;**1**:127–38.

8 Proffit WR. Later stages of development. In: Proffit WR, Fields HW, Sarver D. *Contemporary orthodontics.* 4th ed. St. Louis, MO: Mosby Elsevier; 2006. p. 107–29.

9 Cangialosi T. Skeletal morphologic features of anterior open bites. *Am J Orthod.* 1984;**85**:28–36.

10 Frush JO, Fisher RD. The dynesthetic interpretation of the dentogenic concept. *J Prosthet Dent.* 1958;**8**:558–81.

11 Buschang PH, Carrillo R, Russouw PE. Orthopedic correction of growing hyper-divergent, retrognathic patients with miniscrew implants. *J Oral Maxillofac Surg.* 2011;**69**:754–62.

12 Elder J, Tuenge R. Cephalometric and histologic changes produced by extraoral high-pull traction to the maxilla in Macaca mulatta. *Am J Orthod.* 1974;**66**:599–617.

13 Firouz M, Zernik J, Nanda R. Dental and orthopedic effects of high-pull headgear in treatment of Class II, division 1 malocclusion. *Am J Orthod Dentofacial Orthop.* 1992;**102**:197–205.

14 Baumrind S, Korn EL, Isaacson RJ, West EE, Molthen R. Quantitative analysis of the orthodontic and orthopedic effects of maxillary traction. *Am J Orthod.* 1983;**84**:384–98.

15 Kingsley NW. Die anomalien der zahnstellung und die defecte des gaumens (translated by LH Hollaender). Leipzig: A. Felix; 1881. Quoted by Bredy E, Baugut G, Hatle S. Der offene biB-eine historische betrachtung. *Fortschr Kieferorthop.* 1982;**43**:110–26.

16 Pearson LE. Vertical control in treatment of patients having backward-rotational growth tendencies. *Angle Orthod.* 1978;**48**:132–40.

17 Pearson LE. Vertical control in fully-banded orthodontic treatment. *Angle Orthod.* 1986;**56**:205–24.

18 Iscan HN, Dincer M, Gultan A, Meral O, Taner-Sarisoy L. Effects of vertical chin-cup therapy on the mandibular morphology in open-bite patients. *Am J Orthod Dentofacial Orthop.* 2002;**122**:506–11.

19 Deguchi T, Kuroda T, Minoshima Y, Graber TM. Craniofacial features of patients with Class III abnormalities: growth-related changes and effects of short-term and long-term chincup therapy. *Am J Orthod Dentofacial Orthop.* 2002;**121**:84–92.

20 Wendell PD, Nanda R, Sakamoto T, Nakamura S. The effects of chin cup therapy on the mandible: a longitudinal study. *Am J Orthod.* 1985;**87**:265–74.

21 Sugawara J, Asano T, Endo N, Mitani H. Long-term effects of chincup therapy on skeletal profile in mandibular prognathism. *Am J Orthod Dentofacial Orthop.* 1990;**98**:127–33.

22 Pancherz H. The Herbst appliance—its biologic effects and clinical use. *Am J Orthod.* 1985;**87**:1–20.

23 Schiavoni R, Grenga V, Macri V. Treatment of Class II high angle malocclusions with the Herbst appliance: a cephalometric investigation. *Am J Orthod Dentofacial Orthop.* 1992;**102**:393–409.

24 Dellinger EL. A clinical assessment of the Active Vertical Corrector—a non-surgical alternative for skeletal open bite treatment. *Am J Orthod.* 1986;**89**:428–36.

25 Barbre RE, Sinclair PM. A cephalometric evaluation of anterior openbite correction with the magnetic active vertical corrector. *Angle Orthod.* 1991;**61**:93–102.

26 Kiliaridis S, Egermark I, Thilander B. Anterior open bite treatment with magnets. *Eur J Orthod.* 1990;**12**:447–57.

27 Kuster R, Ingervall B. The effect of treatment of skeletal open bite with two types of bite-blocks. *Eur J Orthod.* 1992;**14**:489–99.

28 Gurton AU, Akin E, Karacay S. Initial intrusion of the molars in the treatment of anterior open bite malocclusions in growing patients. *Angle Orthod.* 2004;**74**:454–64.

29 DeBerardinis M, Stretesky T, Sinha P, Nanda RS. Evaluation of the vertical holding appliance in treatment of high-angle patients. *Am J Orthod Dentofacial Orthop.* 2000;**117**:700–5.

30 Villalobos FJ, Sinha PK, Nanda RS. Longitudinal assessment of vertical and sagittal control in the mandibular arch by the mandibular fixed lingual arch. *Am J Orthod Dentofacial Orthop.* 2000;**118**:366–70.

31 Umemori M, Sugawara J, Mitani H, Nagasaka H, Kawamura H. Skeletal anchorage system for open-bite correction. *Am J Orthod Dentofacial Orthop.* 1999; **115**:166–74.

32 Sherwood KH, Burch JG, Thompson WJ. Closing anterior open bites by intruding molars with titanium miniplate anchorage. *Am J Orthod Dentofacial Orthop.* 2002;**122**:593–600.

33 Kuroda S, Katayama A, Takano-Yamamoto T. Severe anterior open-bite case treated using titanium screw anchorage. *Angle Orthod.* 2004;**74**:558–67.

34 Kuroda S, Sakai Y, Tamamura N, Deguchi T, Takano-Yamamoto T. Treatment of severe anterior open bite with skeletal anchorage in adults: comparison with orthognathic surgery outcomes. *Am J Orthod Dentofacial Orthop.* 2007; **132**:599–605.

35 Southard TE, Franciscus RG, Fridrich KL, Nieves MA, Keller JC, Holton NE, et al. Restricting facial bone growth with skeletal fixation: a preliminary study. *Am J Orthod Dentofacial Orthop.* 2006;**130**:218–23.

36 Ingervall B, Bitsanis E. A pilot study of the effect of masticatory muscle training on facial growth in long-face children. *Eur J Orthod.* 1987;**9**:15–23.

37 English JD. Early treatment of skeletal open bite malocclusions. *Am J Orthod Dentofacial Orthop.* 2002;**121**:563–5.

38 Parks LR, Buschang PH, Alexander RA, Dechow P, Rossouw PE. Masticatory exercises as an adjunctive treatment for hyperdivergent patients. *Angle Orthod.* 2007;**77**:457–62.

39 Lee H, Park Y. Treatment and posttreatment changes following intrusion of max-illary posterior teeth with miniscrew implants for open bite correction. *Korean J Orthod.* 2008;**38**:31–40.

40 Sugawara J, Baik UB, Umemori M, Takahashi I, Nagasaka H, Kawamura H, et al. Treatment and posttreatment dentoalveolar changes following intrusion of man-dibular molars with application of a skeletal anchorage system (SAS) for open bite correction. *Int J Adult Orthodon Orthognath Surg.* 2002;**17**:243–53.

41 Sheffler NR, Proffitt WR, Phillips C. Outcomes and stability inf patients with ante-rior open bite and long anterior face height treated with temporary anchorage devices and maxillary intrusion splint. *Am J Orthod Dentofac Orthop.* 2014;**146**:594–602.

42 Lew KK. Changes in lip contour following treatment of maxillary protrusion with esthetic orthodontic appliances. *J Esthet Dent.* 1992;**4**:16–23.

43 Sarver DM, Johnston MW. Skeletal changes in vertical and anterior displacement of the maxilla with bonded rapid palatal expansion appliances. *Am J Orthod Dentofacial Orthop.* 1989;**95**:462–86.

44 Chang JY, McNamara JA Jr, Herberger TA. A longitudinal study of skeletal side effects induced by rapid maxillary expansion. *Am J Orthod Dentofacial Orthop.* 1997;**112**:330–7.

45 Lineberger MW, McNamara JA, Baccetti T, Herberger T, Franchi L. Effects of rapid maxillary expansion in hyperdivergent patients. *Am J Orthod Dentofacial Orthop.* 2012;**142**:60–9.

46 Al-Nimri KS. Vertical changes in Class II division 1 malocclusion after premolar extractions. *Angle Orthod.* 2006;**76**:52–8.

47 Gkantidis N, Halazonetis DJ, Alexandropoulos E, Haralabakis NB. Treatment strategies for patients with hyperdivergent Class II division 1 malocclusions: is vertical dimension affected? *Am J Orthod Dentofacial Orthop.* 2011;**140**:346–55.

48 Kim YH, Han UK. The versatility and effectiveness of the multiloop edgewise archwire (MEAW) in treatment of various malocclusions. *World J Orthod.* 2001;**2**:208–18.

49 Renfroe EW. *Edgewise.* Philadelphia, PA: Lea & Febiger; 1975.

50 Strang RHW, Thompson WM. *A textbook of orthodontia.* Philadelphia, PA: Lea & Febiger; 1958.

51 Alexander RG. Countdown to retention. *J Clin Orthod.* 1987;**21**:526–7.

52 Steffen JM, Haltom FT. Five-cent tooth positioner. *J Clin Orthod.* 1987;**21**:528–9.

53 Kim YH. Anterior openbite and its treatment with multiloop edgewise archwire. *Angle Orthod.* 1987;**57**:290–321.

54 Jarabak JR, Fizzell JA. *Technique and treatment with the light-wire appliances; light differential forces in clinical orthodontics.* St. Louis, MO: C.V. Mosby; 1963.

55 Thurow RC. *Technique and treatment with the edgewise appliance*. St. Louis, MO: C.V. Mosby; 1962.

56 Pearson LE. Treatment of Class II backward rotating malocclusion. In: Nanda R, editor. *Biomechanics in clinical orthodontics*. Philadelphia, PA: W. B. Saunders; 1997. p. 281–93.

57 Mojdehi M, Buschang PH, English JD, Wolford LM. Postsurgical growth changes in the mandible of adolescents with vertical maxillary excess growth pattern. *Am J Orthod Dentofacial Orthop*. 2001;**119**:106–16.

58 Rosenberg A, Muradin MS, van der Bilt A. Nasolabial esthetics after Le Fort I osteotomy and V-Y closure: a statistical evaluation. *Int J Adult Orthodon Orthognath Surg*. 2002;**17**:29–39.

59 Fontes AM, Joondeph DR, Bloomquist DS, Greenlee GM, Wallen TR, Huang GJ. Long-term stability of anterior open-bite closure with bilateral sagittal split osteotomy. *Am J Orthod Dentofacial Orthop*. 2012;**142**:792–800.

60 Lo FM, Shapiro PA. Effect of presurgical incisor extrusion on stability of anterior open bite malocclusion treated with orthognathic surgery. *Int J Adult Orthodon Orthognath Surg*. 1998;**13**:23–34.

61 Fridrich KL, Casko JS. Genioplasty strategies for anterior facial vertical dysplasias. *Int J Adult Orthodon Orthognath Surg*. 1997;**12**:35–41.

62 Proffit WR. Section II: the development of orthodontic problems. In: Proffit WR, editor. *Contemporary orthodontics*. 3rd ed. St. Louis, MO: C.V. Mosby; 2000. p. 100–1.

63 Bell WH, Proffit WR, White RP. *Surgical correction of dentofacial deformities*. Philadelphia, PA: W. B. Saunders; 1980.

64 Edwards CB, Marshall SD, Qian F, Southard KA, Franciscus RG, Southard TE. Longitudinal study of facial skeletal growth completion in 3 dimensions. *Am J Orthod Dentofacial Orthop*. 2007;**132**:762–8.

65 Greenlee GM, Huang GJ, Chen SS, Chen J, Koepsell T, Hujoel P. Stability of treatment for anterior open-bite malocclusion: a meta-analysis. *Am J Orthod Dentofacial Orthop*. 2011;**139**:154–69.

66 Janson G, Crepaidi MV, Freitas KM, de Freitas MR, Janson W. Stability of anterior open-bite treatment with occlusal adjustment. *Am J Orthod Dentofacial Orthop*. 2010;**138**:14e1–7; discussion 14–5.

67 Espeland L, Dowling PA, Mobarak KA, Stenvik A. Three-year stability of open-bite correction by 1-piece maxillary osteotomy. *Am J Orthod Dentofacial Orthop*. 2008;**134**:60–6.

68 Proffit WR, Turvey TA, Phillips C. Orthognathic surgery: a hierarchy of stability. *Int J Adult Orthodon Orthognath Surg*. 1996;**11**:191–204.

69 Teittinen M, Tuovinen V, Tammela L, Schatzie M, Peltomaki T. Long-term stability of anterior open bite closure corrected by surgical-orthodontic treatment. *Eur J Orthod*. 2012;**34**:238–43.

70 Solano-Hernandez B, Antonarakis GS, Scolozzi P, Kiliaridis S. Combined orthodontic and orthognathic surgical treatment for the correction of skeletal anterior openbite malocclusion: a systematic review on vertical stability. *J Oral Maxillofac Surg*. 2013;**71**:98–109.

71 Ericson S, Kurol J. Early treatment of palatally erupting maxillary canines by extraction of the primary canines. *Eur J Orthod*. 1988;**10**:283–95.

72 Power SM, Short MB. An investigation into the response of palatally displaced canines to the removal of deciduous canines and an assessment of factors contributing to favourable eruption. *Br J Orthod*. 1993;**20**:215–23.

73 Leonardi M, Armi P, Franchi L, Baccetti T. Two interceptive approaches to palatally displaced canines: a prospective longitudinal study. *Angle Orthod*. 2004;**74**:581–6.

74 Baccetti T, Mucedero M, Leonardi M, Cozza P. Interceptive treatment of palatal impaction of maxillary canines with rapid maxillary expansion: a randomized clinical trial. *Am J Orthod Dentofacial Orthop*. 2009;**139**:657–61.

75 Bonetti G, Zanarini M, Incerti Parenti S, Marini I, Gatto MR. Preventive treatment of ectopically erupting maxillary permanent canines by extraction of deciduous canines and first molars: a randomized clinical trial. *Am J Orthod Dentofacial Orthop*. 2011;**139**:316–23.

76 Pinto AS, Buschang PH, Throckmorton GS, Chen P. Morphological and positional asymmetries of young children with functional unilateral posterior crossbite. *Am J Orthod Dentofacial Orthop*. 2001;**120**:513–20.

77 Pirttiniemi P, Kantomaa T, Lahtela P. Relationship between craniofacial and condyle path asymmetry in unilateral cross-bite patients. *Eur J Orthod*. 1990;**12**:408–13.

78 Myers DR, Barenie JT, Bell RA, Williamson EH. Condylar position in children with functional posterior crossbites: before and after crossbite correction. *Pediatr Dent*. 1980;**2**:190–4.

79 Yoshikane TT. Characteristics of functional posterior crossbites in the deciduous and mixed dentitions [thesis]. Los Angeles: University of California, School of Dentistry; 1989.

80 Hesse KL, Artun J, Joondeph DR, Kennedy DB. Changes in condylar position and occlusion associated with maxillary expansion for correction of functional unilateral posterior crossbite. *Am J Orthod Dentofacial Orthop*. 1997;**111**:410–8.

81 O'Byrn BL, Sadowsky C, Schneider B, BeGole EA. An evaluation of mandibular asymmetry in adults with unilateral posterior crossbite. *Am J Orthod Dentofacial Orthop*. 1995;**107**:394–400.

82 Harrison JE, O'Brien KD, Worthington HV. Orthodontic treatment for prominent upper front teeth in children. *Cochrane Database Syst Rev*. 2007:CD003452.

83 Proffit WR, Tulloch JF. Preadolescent Class II problems: treat now or wait? *Am J Orthod Dentofacial Orthop*. 2002;**121**:560–2.

84 Tulloch JF, Proffit WR, Phillips C. Outcomes in a 2-phase randomized clinical trial of early Class II treatment. *Am J Orthod Dentofacial Orthop*. 2004;**125**:657–67.

85 Ghafari J, Shofer FS, Jacobsson-Hunt U, Markowitz DL, Laster LL. Headgear versus function regulator in the early treatment of Class II division 1 malocclusion: a randomized clinical trial. *Am J Orthod Dentofacial Orthop*. 1998;**113**:51–61.

86 Keeling SD, Wheeler TT, King GJ, Garvan CW, Cohen DA, Cabassa S, et al. Anteroposterior skeletal and dental changes after early Class II treatment with bionators and headgear. *Am J Orthod Dentofacial Orthop*. 1998;**113**:40–50.

87 Dolce C, McGorray SP, Brazeau L, King GJ, Wheeler TT. Timing of Class II treatment: skeletal changes comparing 1-phase and 2-phase treatment. *Am J Orthod Dentofacial Orthop*. 2007;**132**:481–9.

88 Kim JH, Viana MA, Graber TM, Omerza FF, BeGole EA. The effectiveness of protraction face mask therapy: a meta-analysis. *Am J Orthod Dentofacial Orthop*. 1999;**115**:675–85.

89 Jager A, Braumann B, Kim C, Wahner S. Skeletal and dental effects of maxillary protraction in patients with angle class III malocclusion. *J Orofac Orthop*. 2001;**62**:275–84.

90 Wells AP, Sarver DM, Proffit WR. Long-term efficacy of reverse pull headgear therapy. *Angle Orthod*. 2006;**76**:915–22.

91 Turley PK. Managing the developing Class III malocclusion with palatal expansion and facemask therapy. *Am J Orthod Dentofacial Orthop*. 2002;**122**:349–52.

92 Tulloch JFC, Phillips C, Proffit WR. Early versus late treatment of Class II malocclusion: preliminary results from the UNC clinical trial. In: McNamara JA Jr, editor. *Orthodontic treatment: outcome and effectiveness*. Craniofacial growth series. Ann Arbor: Center for Growth and Development, University of Michigan; 1995. p. 113–38.

93 Ballard CF, Gwynne-Evans E. Discussion of the mouth breather. *Proc R Soc Med Sect Paediatr*. 1958;**51**:279–85.

94 Hartgerink DV, Vig PS. Lower anterior face height and lip incompetence do not predict nasal airway obstruction. *Angle Orthod*. 1989;**59**:17–23.

95 Trask GM, Shapiro GG, Shapiro PA. The effects of perennial allergic rhinitis on dental and skeletal development: a comparison of sibling pairs. *Am J Orthod Dentofacial Orthop*. 1987;**92**:286–93.

96 Justus R. Correction of anterior open bite with spurs: long-term stability. *World J Orthod*. 2001;**2**:219–31.

97 Proffit WR, Mason RM. Myofunctional therapy for tongue-thrusting: background and recommendations. *J Am Dent Assoc*. 1975;**90**:403–11.

98 O'Brien K. Is early treatment for Class II malocclusions effective? Results from a randomized controlled trial. *Am J Orthod Dentofacial Orthop*. 2006;**129**:S64–5.

99 O'Brien K, Wright J, Conboy F, Appelbe P, Davies L, Connolly I, et al. Early treatment for Class II division 1 malocclusion with the Twin-block appliance: a multi-center, randomized, controlled trial. *Am J Orthod Dentofacial Orthop*. 2009;**135**:573–9.

100 LaHaye MB, Buschang PH, Alexander RG, Boley JC. Orthodontic treatment changes of chin position in Class II division 1 patients. *Am J Orthod Dentofacial Orthop*. 2006;**130**:732–41.

101 Kirjavainen M, Kirjavainen T, Hurmerinta K, Haavikko K. Orthopedic cervical headgear with an expanded inner bow in Class II correction. *Angle Orthod*. 2000;**70**:317–25.

102 Jakobsson SO. Cephalometric evaluation of treatment effect on Class II, division 1 malocclusions. *Am J Orthod*. 1967;**53**:446–57.

103 Tulloch JF, Phillips C, Koch G, Proffit WR. The effect of early intervention on skeletal pattern in Class II malocclusion: a randomized clinical trial. *Am J Orthod Dentofacial Orthop*. 1997;**111**:391–400.

104 Wheeler TT, McGorray SP, Dolce C, Taylor MG, King GJ. Effectiveness of early treatment of Class II malocclusion. *Am J Orthod Dentofacial Orthop*. 2002;**121**:9–17.

105 Almeida-Pedrin RR, Almeida MR, Almeida RR, Pinzan A, Ferreira FP. Treatment effects of headgear biteplane and bionator appliances. *Am J Orthod Dentofacial Orthop*. 2007;**132**:191–8.

106 Thurman MM, King GJ, Ramsay DS, Wheeler TT, Phillips C. The effect of an anterior biteplate on dental and skeletal Class II correction using headgears: a cephalometric study. *Orthod Craniofac Res*. 2011;**14**:213–21.

107 Baccetti T, Franchi L, Stahl F. Comparison of 2 comprehensive Class II treatment protocols including the bonded Herbst and headgear appliances: a double-blind study of consecutively treated patients at puberty. *Am J Orthod Dentofacial Orthop*. 2009;**135**:698.e1–10; discussion 698–9.

108 Franchi L, Alvetro L, Giuntini V, Masucci C, Defraia E, Baccetti T. Effectiveness of comprehensive fixed appliance treatment used with the Forsus Fatigue Resistant Device in Class II patients. *Angle Orthod*. 2011;**81**:678–83.

109 Heinig N, Göz G. Clinical application and effects of the Forsus spring. A study of a new Herbst hybrid. *J Orofac Orthop*. 2001;**62**:436–50.

110 Janson G, Sathler R, Fernandes TM, Branco NC, Freitas MR. Correction of Class II malocclusion with Class II elastics: a systematic review. *Am J Orthod Dentofacial Orthop*. 2013;**143**:383–92.

111 Mann KR, Marshall SD, Qian F, Southard KA, Southard TE. Effect of maxillary anteroposterior position on profile esthetics in headgear-treated patients. *Am J Orthod Dentofacial Orthop*. 2011;**139**:228–34.

112 Tanner JM. *Growth at adolescence*. 2nd ed. Oxford, England: Blackwell Scientific Publications; 1962. Figure 6, p. 16.

113 Schendel SA, Eisenfeld J, Bell WH, Epker BN, Mishelevich DJ. The long-face syndrome: vertical maxillary excess. *Am J Orthod*. 1976;**70**:398–408.

114 Vig PS, Hall DJ. The inadequacy of cephalometric radiographs for airway assessment. *Am J Orthod*. 1980;**77**:230–3.

115 Schwab RJ. Upper airway imaging. *Clin Chest Med*. 1998;**19**:33–54.

116 Krouse J, Lund V, Fokkens W, Meltzer EO. Diagnostic strategies in nasal congestion. *Int J Gen Med*. 2010;**3**:59–67.

117 Vig KW. Nasal obstruction and facial growth: the strength of evidence for clinical assumptions. *Am J Orthod Dentofacial Orthop*. 1998;**113**:603–11.

118 Linder-Aronson S. Respiratory function in relation to facial morphology and the dentition. *Angle Orthod*. 1979:**6**:59–71.

119 McNamara JA. Influence of respiratory pattern on craniofacial growth. *Angle Orthod*. 1981;**51**:269–300.

120 Fields HW, Warren DW, Black K, Phillips CL. Relationship between vertical dentofacial morphology and respiration in adolescents. *Am J Orthod Dentofacial Orthop*. 1991;**99**:147–54.

121 Souki BQ, Pimenta GB, Souki MQ, Franco LP, Becker HM, Pinto JA. Prevalence of malocclusion among mouth breathing children: do expectations meet reality? *Int J Pediatr Otorhinolaryngol*. 2009;**73**:767–73.

122 Franco LP, Souki Q, Pereira TB, Meyge de Brito G, Goncalves Becker HM, Pinto JA. Is the growth pattern in mouth breathers comparable with the counterclockwise mandibular rotation of nasal breathers? *Am J Orthod Dentofacial Orthop*. 2013;**144**:341–8.

123 Petraccone Caixeta AC, Andrade I Jr, Bahia Junqueira Pereira T, Franco LP, Becker HM, Souki BQ. Dental arch dimensional changes after adenotonsillectomy in prepubertal children. *Am J Orthod Dentofacial Orthop*. 2014; **145**:461–8.

124 Iwasaki T, Saitoh I, Takemoto Y, Inada E, Kakuno E, Kanomi R, et al. Tongue posture improvement and pharyngeal airway enlargement as secondary effects of rapid maxillary expansion: a cone-beam computed tomography study. *Am J Orthod Dentofacial Orthop*. 2013;**143**:235–45.

125 Baratieri C, Alves M Jr, de Souza MM, de Souza Araujo MT, Maia LC. Does rapid maxillary expansion have long-term effects on airway dimensions and breathing? *Am J Orthod Dentofacial Orthop*. 2011;**140**:146–56.

126 Bluestone CD. Current indications for tonsillectomy and adenoidectomy. *Ann Otol Rhinol Laryngol Suppl*. 1992;**155**:58–64.

127 Mahony D, Karsten A, Linder-Aronson S. Effects of adenoidectomy and changed mode of breathing on incisor and molar dentoalveolar heights and anterior face heights. *Aust Orthod J*. 2004;**20**:93–8.

128 Miles PG. Effects of adenoidectomy and changed mode of breathing [comments on the Mahony article]. *Aust Orthod J*. 2005;**21**:65–6.

129 Coatoam GW, Behrents RG, Bissada NF. The width of keratinized gingiva during orthodontic treatment: its significance and impact on periodontal status. *J Periodontol*. 1981;**52**:307–13.

130 Karlsen AT. Association between facial height development and mandibular growth rotation in low and high MP-SN angle faces: a longitudinal study. *Angle Orthod*. 1997;**67**:102–10.

131 Hansen K, Koutsonas TG, Pancherz H. Long-term effects of Herbst treatment on the mandibular incisor segment: a cephalometric and biometric investigation. *Am J Orthod Dentofacial Orthop*. 1997;**112**:92–103.

132 Marshall WA, Tanner JM. Puberty. In: Falkner F, Tanner JM, editors. *Human growth*. Vol **2**. 2nd ed. New York, NY: Plenum Publishing; 1986. p. 171–209.

133 Barrett AA, Baccetti T, McNamara JA Jr. Treatment effects of the light-force chincup. *Am J Orthod Dentofacial Orthop*. 2010;**138**:468–76.

134 Rudee DA. Proportional profile changes concurrent with orthodontic therapy. *Am J Orthod*. 1964;**50**:421–34.

135 Morgenthaler TI, Kagramanov V, Hanak V, Decker PA. Complex sleep apnea syndrome: is it a unique clinical syndrome? *Sleep*. 2006;**29**:1203–9.

136 Jacobson RL, Schendel SA. Treating obstructive sleep apnea: the case for surgery. *Am J Orthod Dentofacial Orthop*. 2012;**142**:435, 437, 439, 441–2.

137 El-Ad B, Lavie, P. Effect of sleep apnea on cognition and mood. *Int Rev Psychiatry*. 2005;**17**:277–82.

138 Aloia MS, Sweet LH, Jerskey BA, Zimmerman M, Arnedt JT, Millman RP. Treatment effects on brain activity during a working memory task in obstructive sleep apnea. *J Sleep Res*. 2009;**18**:404–10.

139 Neill AM, Angus SM, Sajkov D, McEvoy RD. Effects of sleep posture on upper airway stability in patients with obstructive sleep apnea. *Am J Respir Crit Care Med*. 1997;**155**:199–204.

140 Xiheng G, Chen W, Hongyu Z, Weimin K, Li A, Li L, et al. The study of the influence of sleep position on sleep apnea [Internet]. Dublin, OH: Cardinal Health; 2003. Available from: http://www.withoutsnoring.com/of-03-249.html (cited August 8, 2014).

141 Loord H, Hultcrantz E. Positioner—a method for preventing sleep apnea. *Acta Otolaryngol*. 2007;**127**:861–8.

142 Szollosi I, Roebuck T, Thompson B, Naughton MT. Lateral sleeping position reduces severity of central sleep apnea/Cheyne-Stokes respiration. *Sleep*. 2006;**29**:1045–51.

143 Vennelle M, White S, Riha RL, Mackay TW, Engleman HM, Douglas NJ. Randomized controlled trial of variable-pressure versus fixed-pressure continuous positive airway pressure (CPAP) treatment for patients with obstructive sleep apnea/hypopnea syndrome (OSAHS). *Sleep*. 2010;**33**:267–71.

144 Steward DL. Effectiveness of multilevel (tongue and palate) radiofrequency tissue ablation for patients with obstructive sleep apnea syndrome. *Laryngoscope*. 2004;**114**:2073–84.

145 Ahrens A, McGrath C, Hagg U. A systematic review of the efficacy of oral appliance design in the management of obstructive sleep apnea. *Eur J Orthod*. 2011;**33**:318–24.

146 Almeida FF, Lowe AA, Otsuka R, Fastlicht S, Farbood M, Tsuiki S. Long-term sequellae of oral appliance therapy in obstructive sleep apnea patients: part 2. Study-model analysis. *Am J Orthod Dentofacial Orthop*. 2006;**129**:205–13.

147 Pirklbauer K, Russmueller G, Stiebellehner L, Nell C, Sinko K, Millesi G, et al. Maxillomandibular advancement for treatment of obstructive sleep apnea syndrome: a systematic review. *J Oral Maxillofac Surg*. 2011;**69**:e165–76.

148 Jung RE, Pjetursson BE, Glauser R, Zembic A, Zwahlen M, Lang NP. A systematic review of the 5-year survival and complication rates of implant-supported single crowns. *Clin Oral Implants Res*. 2008;**19**:119–30.

149 Dueled E. Gotfredsen K, Trab Damsgaard M, Hede B. Professional and patient-based evaluation of oral rehabilitation in patients with tooth agenesis. *Clin Oral Implants Res*. 2009;**20**:729–36.

150 Engeseth L. Mutilating dental traumas: outcome of treatment involving orthodontics, transplantation, implants, and prosthodontics [thesis]. Oslo, Norway: University of Oslo; 2009. p. 1–45.

151 Zachrisson BU, Rosa M, Toreskog S. Authors' response to letters to the editor. *Am J Orthod Dentofacial Orthop*. 2011;**140**:138–9.

152 Chang M, Wennstrom JL, Odman P, Andersson B. Implant supported single-tooth replacements compared to contralateral natural teeth. Crown and soft tissue dimensions. *Clin Oral Implants Res*. 1999;**10**:185–94.

153 Thilander B, Odman J, Lekholm U. Orthodontic aspects of the use of oral implants in adolescents: a 10-year follow-up study. *Eur J Orthod*. 2001;**23**:715–31.

154 Bernard JP, Schatz JP, Christou P, Belser U, Killaridis S. Long-term vertical changes of the anterior maxillary teeth adjacent to single implants in young and mature adults. A retrospective study. *J Clin Periodontol*. 2004;**31**:1024–8.

155 Jemt T. Single implants in the anterior maxilla after 15 years of follow-up: comparison with central implants in the edentulous maxilla. *Int J Prosthodont*. 2008;**21**:400–8.

156 Nordquist GG, McNeill RW. Orthodontic vs restorative treatment of the congenitally absent lateral incisor—long-term periodontal and occlusal evaluation. *J Periodontol*. 1975;**46**:139–43.

157 Robertsson S, Mohlin B. The congenitally missing upper lateral incisor. A retrospective study of orthodontic space closure versus restorative treatment. *Eur J Orthod*. 2000;**22**:697–710.

158 Kinzer GA, Kokich VO Jr. Managing congenitally missing lateral incisors. Part II: tooth-supported restorations. *J Esthet Restor Dent*. 2005;**17**:76–84.

159 Kokich VO Jr, Kinzer GA, Janakievski J. Congenitally missing maxillary lateral incisors: restorative replacement. Counterpoint. *Am J Orthod Dentofacial Orthop*. 2011;**139**:435, 437, 439 passim.

160 Lafforgue, P. Pathophysiology and natural history of avascular necrosis of bone. *Joint Bone Spine*. 2006;**73**:500–7.

161 Huang YL, Pogrel MA, Kaban LB. Diagnosis and management of condylar resorption. *J Oral Maxillofac Surg.* 1997;**55**:114–9; discussion 119–20.
162 Betts NJ, Vanarsdall RL, Barber HD, Higgins-Barber K, Fonseca RJ. Diagnosis and treatment of transverse maxillary deficiency. *Int J Adult Orthodon Orthognath Surg.* 1995;**10**:75–96.
163 Shetty V, Caridad JM, Caputo AA, Chaconas SJ. Biomechanical rationale for surgical-orthodontic expansion of the adult maxilla. *J Oral Maxillofac Surg.* 1994;**52**:742–9; discussion 750–1.
164 Krebs A. Midpalatal suture expansion studies by the implant method over a seven-year period. *Rep Congr Eur Orthod Soc.* 1964;**40**:131–42.
165 Wertz R, Dreskin M. Midpalatal suture opening: a normative study. *Am J Orthod.* 1977;**71**:367–81.
166 Baccetti T, Franchi L, Cameron CG, McNamara JA Jr. Treatment timing for rapid maxillary expansion. *Angle Orthod.* 2001;**71**:343–50.

CHAPTER 6

Posterior Open Bites

Introduction

Jay is a 15-year-old male (Figure 6.1) who presents with the chief complaint "My back teeth don't touch and it makes it hard to chew." PMH is noncontributory, PDH is routine, and TMJs are asymptomatic, CR = CO.

Q: What are Jay's diagnostic findings and problems in the vertical dimension?

A: He has a bilateral posterior open bite. His anterior teeth and the distal of his maxillary first molars are in occlusion, but his canines, premolars, and the mesial of his first molars are not in occlusion. Although Jay appears to have a long LAFH in the frontal view (Figure 6.1a, soft tissue Glabella–Subnasale < Subnasale–soft tissue Menton), he appears to have a normal LAFH in the profile view (Figure 6.1c) and his lips are competent. His skeletal LAFH is slightly greater than normal (LAFH/TAFH = 57%), but his MPA is WRN (FMA = 27°; SNMP = 32°). So overall, Jay is *NORMAL vertically, but he has a bilateral posterior open bite.*

Q: Why correct posterior open bites?

A: Posterior open bites can adversely affect the ability to chew, and anterior teeth may undergo excessive wear without the occlusal support of posterior teeth.

Q: What do you suspect is the cause of Jay's bilateral posterior open bite?

A: The fact that the right and left openings have a classic "football" shape should lead you to suspect that an interpositional tongue posture habit is preventing the posterior teeth from erupting. Of course, tongue interposition could be an adaptation to the open bite, not the cause.

Q: In addition to an interpositional tongue posture habit preventing tooth eruption, can you list at least 6 other potential causes of posterior open bites?

A: Other potential causes of posterior open bites include the following:

- Digit interposition habits.
- Temporary posterior open bite occurring after normal exfoliation of primary molars but before permanent teeth have time to erupt into occlusion with the opposing dentition.
- Ankylosis of teeth, which prevents their complete eruption into occlusion (note that in Figure 6.1f–i, the right maxillary second primary molar lacks a successor and appears to be ankylosed—a step in the level of the alveolar process bone crest height exists between the second primary molar and adjacent permanent teeth indicating the second primary molar has stopped erupting).
- Class III growth resulting in an edge-to-edge incisor relationship could potentially create a posterior open bite (Figure 6.2a–f), especially if a tongue interpositional habit is acquired as a result.
- Lack of space for complete tooth eruption (teeth blocked out).
- Systemic factors found in patients with certain syndromes, such as cleidocranial dysplasia, ectodermal dysplasia, Gardner syndrome, and Apert syndrome.
- Primary failure of eruption.
- Some treatments for sleep apnea may create posterior open bites [1].
- A very constricted maxilla (no room for the tongue).

Q: *Anterior* open bites can be treated in only one of two ways: eruption of anterior teeth (generally done in cases of dental anterior open bites where normal eruption of anterior teeth has been impeded by a habit) or intrusion of posterior teeth (generally done in cases of skeletal anterior open bites). However, *posterior* open bites can be corrected in only one way. How?

A: By erupting posterior teeth until they are in occlusion (Figure 6.3). Orthodontic eruption of posterior teeth could include using fixed appliances with posterior vertical elastics or leveling a curve of Spee. Surgical eruption of posterior teeth could include a segmental maxillary downgraft osteotomy or distraction osteogenesis [2, 3]. Of course, prosthodontic treatment (buildups, crowns, implant replacement with elongated crowns, or overlay removable partial dentures) can also close posterior open bites.

Q: What is primary failure of eruption?

A: The term "primary failure of eruption" was originated by Proffit and Vig [4] and refers to a tooth not erupting due to a disturbance in its eruption mechanism.

Q: What signs have been used to describe primary failure of eruption (PFE)? List at least six.

A: The following signs are characteristic of primary failure of eruption [4–8]:

- First molars are always involved and present with supracrestal appearance and no apparent barrier to eruption (100% for genetically confirmed PFE).
- Posterior teeth are more frequently affected.
- If a tooth in a more anterior position is affected, teeth more posterior are usually affected as well (i.e., when the premolars are affected, molars are also likely to be affected).
- Both primary and permanent teeth can be affected.

Orthodontics in the Vertical Dimension: A Case-Based Review, First Edition. Thomas E. Southard, Steven D. Marshall and Laura L. Bonner.

- The condition is often bilateral (50/50 for PFE patients versus 80/20 unilateral/bilateral for ankylosis).
- Teeth in both arches are often affected (91% of those with genetically confirmed PFE).
- Affected teeth resorb the alveolar bone above the crown, may erupt into initial occlusion, and then cease to erupt further, or may fail to erupt entirely.
- Involved teeth may be displaced back and forth with manual pressure (indicating that they are not, initially, ankylosed). However, involved teeth tend to become ankylosed as soon as orthodontic eruptive forces are applied.
- If a small area of ankylosis is broken by manipulating the ankylosed tooth, it might be possible to move the tooth for a short time, but re-ankylosis is inevitable.
- Other concurrent skeletal (Class III malocclusion for 63% of genetically confirmed PFE patients) and dental (tooth agenesis, microdontia of maxillary lateral incisors, anomalous root morphology) anomalies may be present.

Q: A patient presents to you with a posterior open bite of the right first molars. You suspect that the posterior open bite resulted from either primary failure of eruption or ankylosis of the maxillary first molar. What is a key distinguishing feature between primary failure of eruption and ankylosis?

A: In primary failure of eruption, more distal teeth to the one involved will also be affected. In ankylosis, more distal teeth will erupt normally [8]. In other words, if primary failure of eruption has prevented the first molar from erupting, then a series of radiographs will also show the second molar not erupting. If ankyloses has prevented the first molar from erupting, then a series of radiographs will show the second molar erupting.

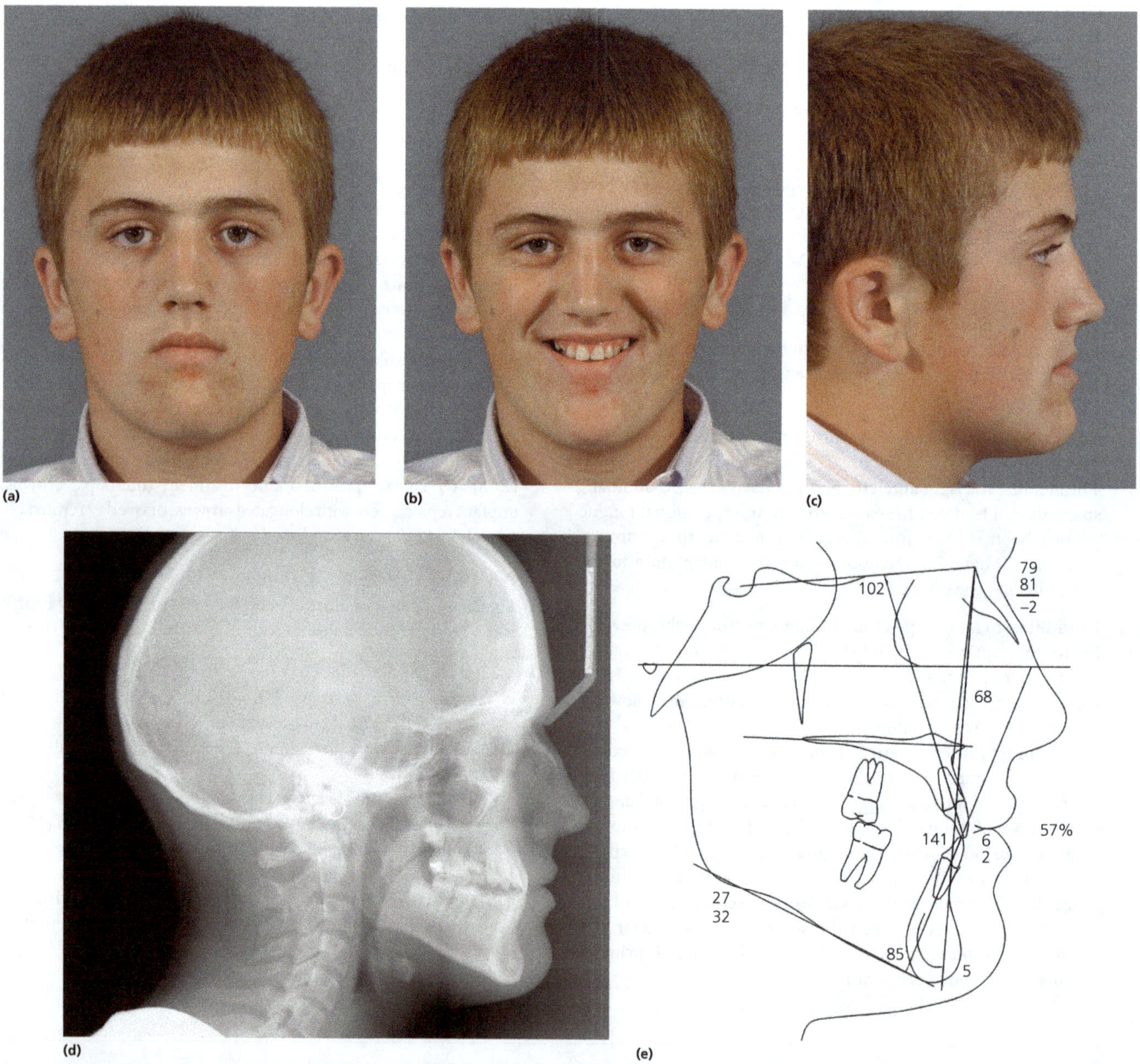

Figure 6.1 Initial records of Jay: (a–c) initial facial photographs, (d) lateral cephalograph, (e) cephalometric tracing,

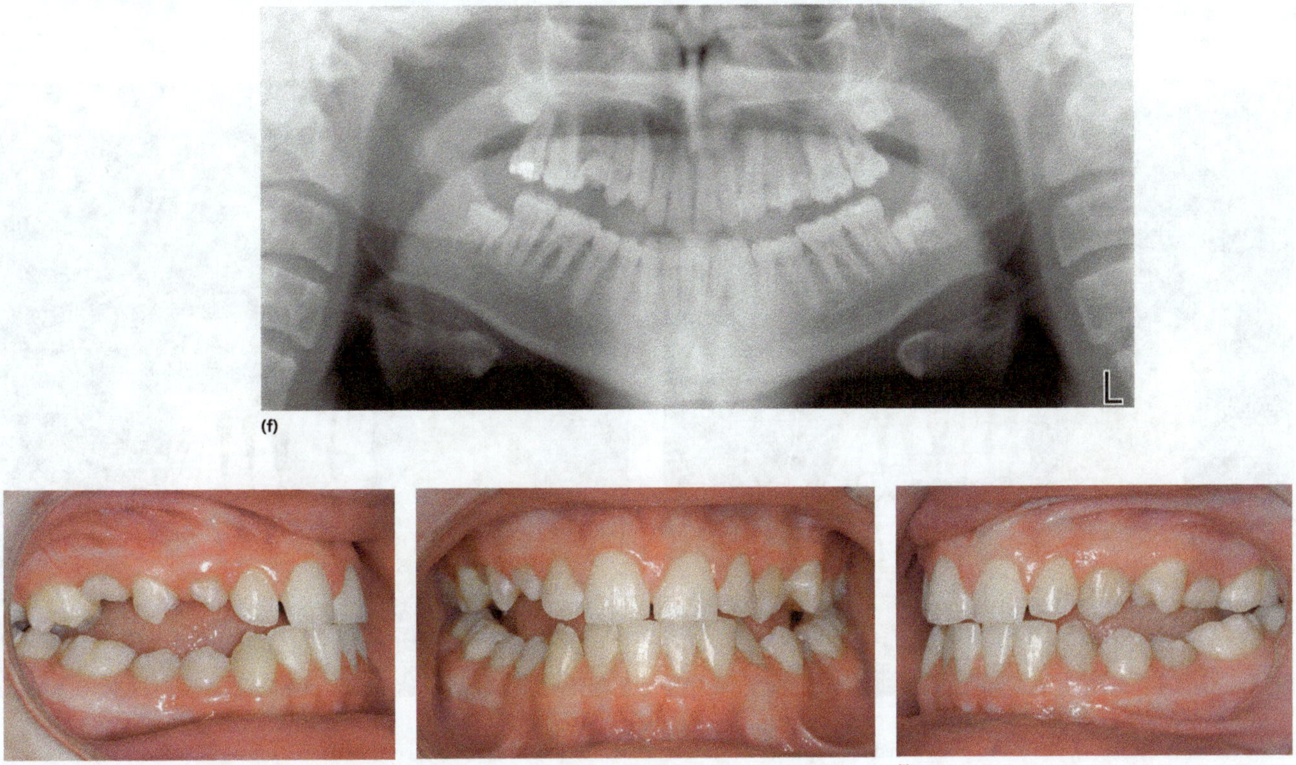

(f)

(g) (h) (i)

Figure 6.1 (Continued) (f) pantomograph, and (g–i) intraoral photographs.

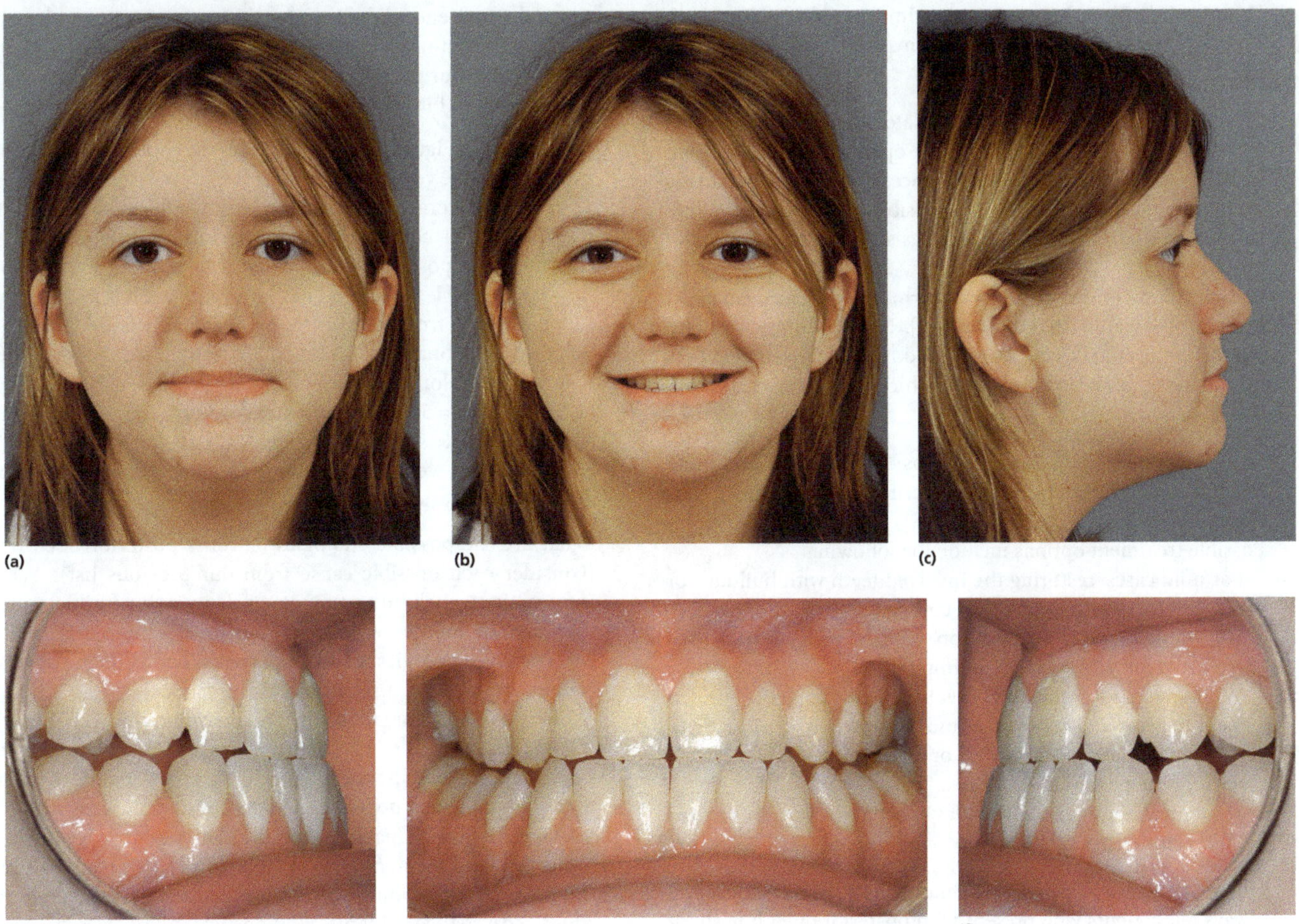

(a) (b) (c)

(d) (e) (f)

Figure 6.2 (a–f) Bilateral posterior open bite potentially due to rapid Class III growth with resulting edge-to-edge incisor contact and tongue habit.

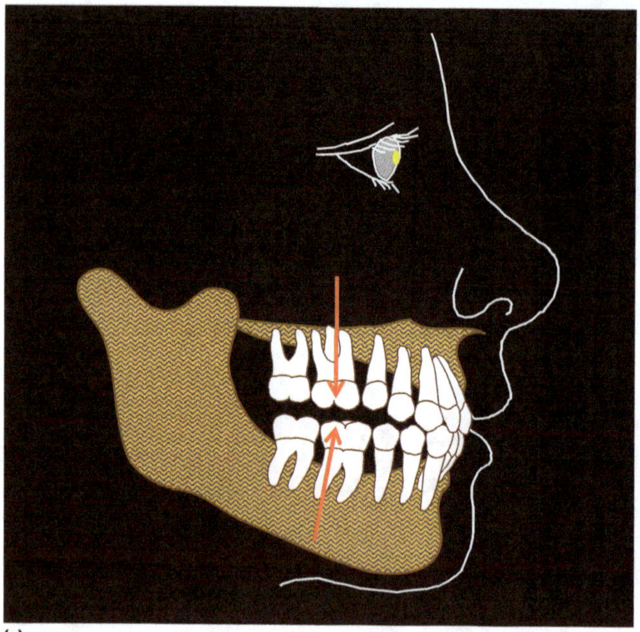
(a)

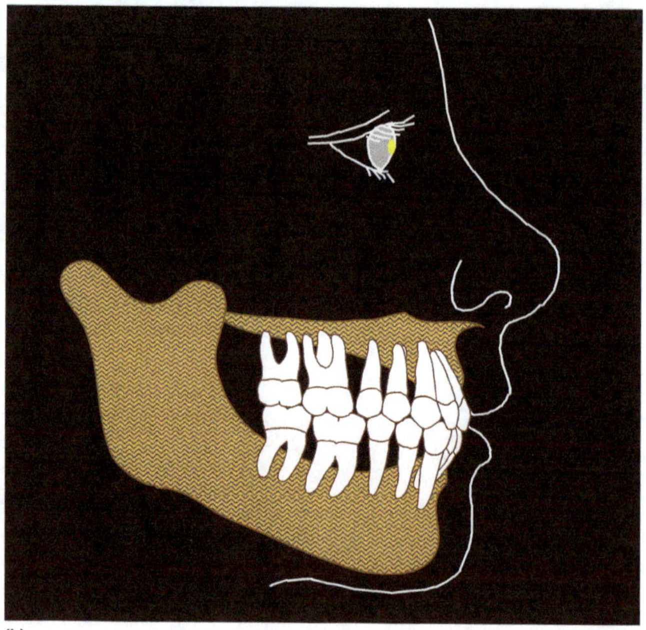
(b)

Figure 6.3 (a, b) Posterior open bites are corrected by erupting posterior teeth with orthodontics or surgery. Prostheses (e.g. overlay dentures) can also be used.

Q: Does Jay (Figure 6.1) present with primary failure of eruption?

A: Probably not. If the premolars were involved, the molars would usually be involved.

Q: A patient presents to you with a unilateral posterior open bite. In addition to the possibility of the open bite resulting from isolated ankylosis, severe lack of space, or a tongue posturing problem, you also consider the possibility of primary failure to erupt. What is the underlying basis for primary failure of eruption?

A: Pedigree and clinical findings confirm that primary failure of eruption is an inherited disorder [9]. Nonsyndromic primary failure of eruption has an autosomal-dominant genetic mode of inheritance [5]. The mechanism by which this prevents eruption is unknown.

Q: What are possible treatment options for posterior open bite resulting from primary failure of eruption? Suggest at least three.

A: Possible treatment options include the following:

- For mild cases, restoring the involved teeth with buildups or crowns after vertical growth is complete [10].
- For moderate cases, extraction of the involved teeth and replacement with bone grafts/implants.
- With first and second molar involvement, leaving the affected teeth in place and accept a premolar occlusion.
- A segmental osteotomy [4, 11] or distraction osteogenesis [2] to close the posterior open bite.
- A removable prosthetic (overlay) partial denture to provide posterior occlusion [12].

Q: How difficult are posterior open bites to treat? What should you always tell patients who present with posterior open bite about your ability to close, and maintain closure of, posterior open bites?

A: Clinical experience demonstrates that posterior open bite can be one of the, if not *the*, most difficult orthodontic problem to correct. Tell your patients that you may not be able to close their posterior open bite or to keep it closed.

Q: Look at Tom (Figure 6.4). What are his diagnostic findings and problems in the vertical dimension (Figure 6.4)?

A: Tom has a bilateral posterior open bite, which extends from his maxillary right central incisor posteriorly and from his left first premolar posteriorly (note: *his second molars occlude; you might just be able to see this in* Figure 6.4h). He has a soft tissue LLAFH in the frontal view (Figure 6.4a, soft tissue Glabella–Subnasale < Subnasale–soft tissue Menton), his lips are competent, his cephalometric skeletal LAFH is greater than normal (LAFH/TAFH = 58%, over one standard deviation greater than average of 55%, sd = 2%), but his MPA is WRN (FMA = 22°, SNMP = 27°). Overall, Tom is mildly long vertically, and he has a bilateral posterior open bite.

Q: What are the possible etiologies of Tom's posterior open bite (consider each possible cause from our previous list)? What information is helpful to support or deny each possible cause? Of these possibilities, which do you believe is the cause?

A: The possible etiologies for Tom's posterior open bite include the following:

- Interpositional tongue habit. To determine this, ask Tom to close his eyes and relax. Then, as you ask him to open his eyes (to distract his attention), quickly/gently separate his lips (Figure 6.5). *Tom does have an interpositional tongue habit.*
- Class III growth pattern resulting in edge-to-edge incisor contact and posterior open bite (and possible resulting tongue interposition habit). To determine this, ask Tom if he noticed a change in his bite relationship while he was growing. He denies noticing any such change. Additionally, look for wear facets on molars, premolars, and canines indicating

these teeth had prior occlusal contact in function or parafunction before he grew Class III. On inspection, no such attrition is noted on premolars and canines.

- Digit sucking or other habits. Tom denies any such habits.
- Ankylosis of teeth. Check to see if the posterior teeth appear immobile upon palpation. They do not.
- Systemic factors. Tom states that he is in perfect health.
- Primary failure of eruption. Since teeth more distal to the ones involved in the posterior open bite are not affected (i.e., his second molars occlude), primary failure of eruption is probably not the cause.

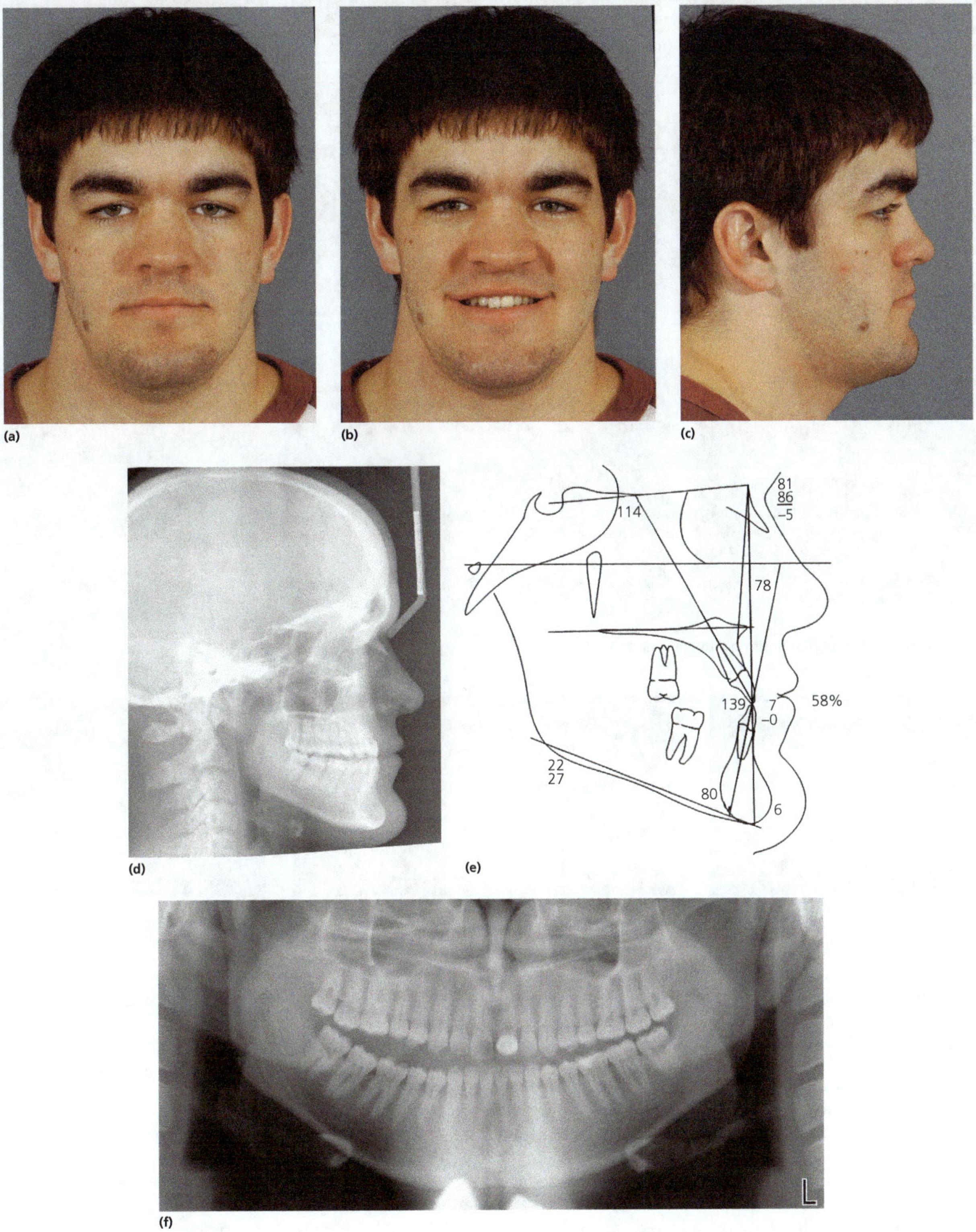

Figure 6.4 (a–k) Initial records of Tom.

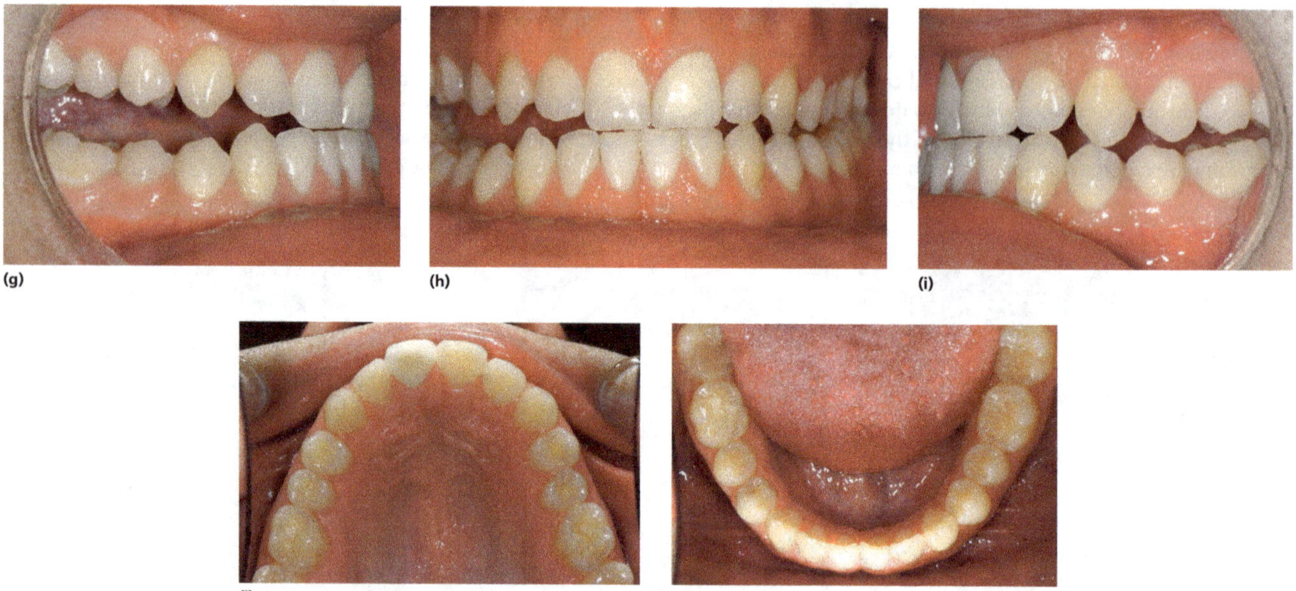

(g) (h) (i) (j) (k)

Figure 6.4 (Continued)

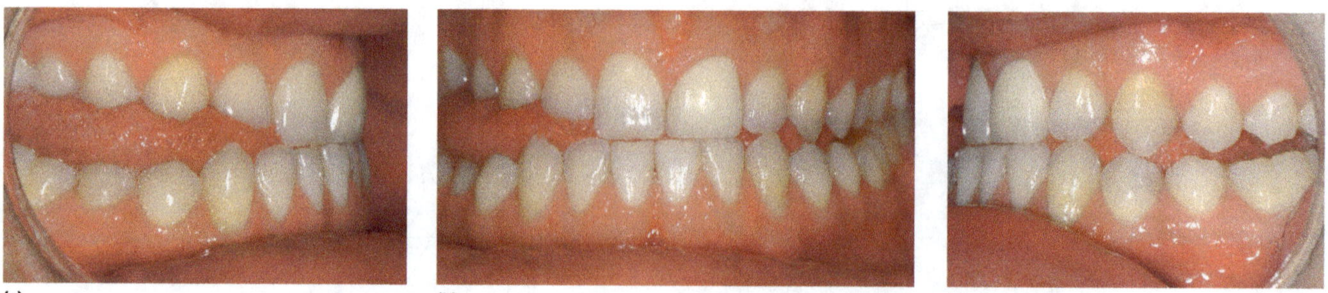

(a) (b) (c)

Figure 6.5 (a–c) Tom has an interpositional tongue habit.

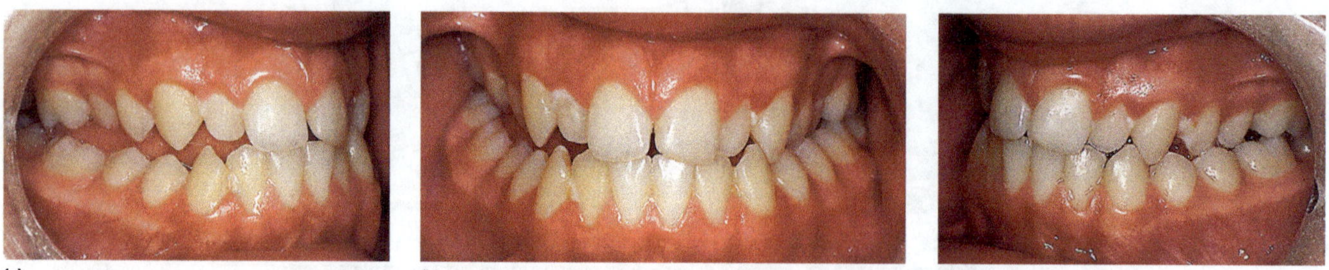

(a) (b) (c)

Figure 6.6 (a–c) A unilateral right posterior open bite due to an interpositional tongue habit.

In summary, *the most likely cause of Tom's bilateral posterior open bite is his interpositional tongue habit.* This may have developed as he grew Class III.

Q: A unilateral right posterior open bite, due to an interpositional tongue habit, is shown in Figure 6.6. Can you list four appliances or techniques to help correct an interpositional tongue habit?

A: Appliances or techniques to help correct an interpositional tongue habit include the following:

1 Loops to block the tongue soldered to an LLHA (Figure 6.7a, b)
2 Loops to block the tongue included as part of a removable retainer (Figure 6.7c)
3 Wearing a tooth positioner
4 Vertical "criss-cross" elastics worn between fixed appliances in each arch (Figure 6.7d, e).

Q: What was the error made in fabricating the LLHA in Figure 6.7a?

A: The loops were placed unilaterally. Blocking a tongue unilaterally can compel the tongue to seek the contralateral side (creating a new open bite). A better design is the appliance in Figure 6.7c with bilateral loops. (However, a problem with any removable appliances is that the patient may simply choose to not wear it.)

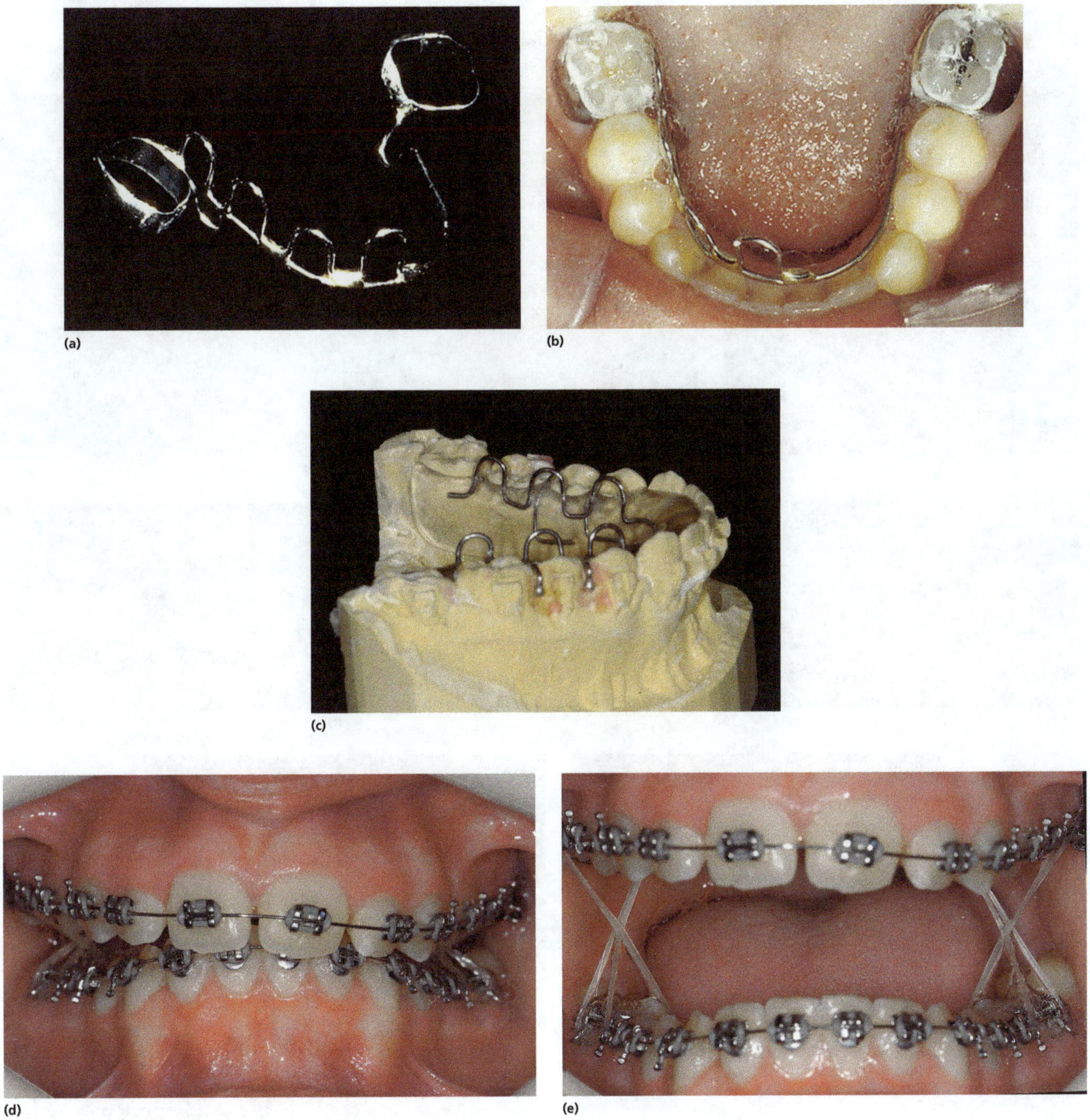

Figure 6.7 Techniques to help close posterior open bites by blocking the tongue: (a–c) loops soldered to an LLHA or embedded in a mandibular Hawley retainer and (d, e) vertical "criss-cross" elastics.

Q: What are the advantages of using vertical "*criss-cross*" elastics shown in Figure 6.7e?

A: With criss-cross elastics, the tongue is kept out of the posterior open bite when the elastics are worn, the vertical component of force from the elastics erupts the posterior teeth to close the open bite, the elastics may be easier for the patient to insert than vertical buccal elastics, and criss-cross forces eliminate transverse effects that would normally occur, if vertical elastics were only worn on the buccal.

Q: Grace is an adolescent patient with a history of bilateral posterior open bite due to an interpositional tongue habit (Figure 6.8). What are your options for attempting to close her posterior open bite?

A: A removable retainer fabricated with bilateral loops to keep the tongue out of the open-bite space (Figure 6.9). Other options include bilateral vertical loops soldered to an LLHA, a tooth positioner, or fixed appliances with vertical criss-cross elastics.

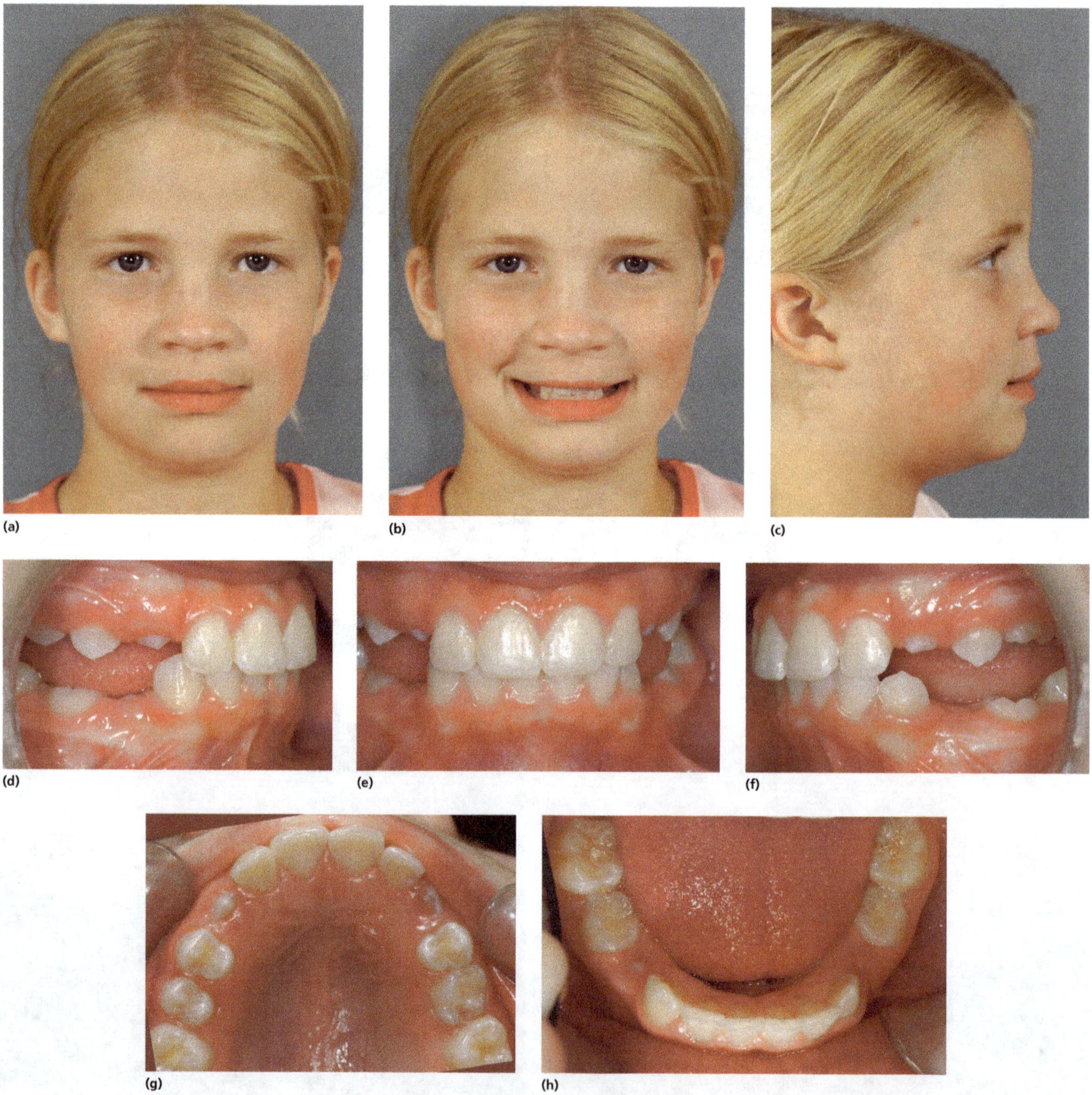

Figure 6.8 (a–h) Initial records of Grace who presented with a bilateral posterior open bite due to an interpositional tongue habit.

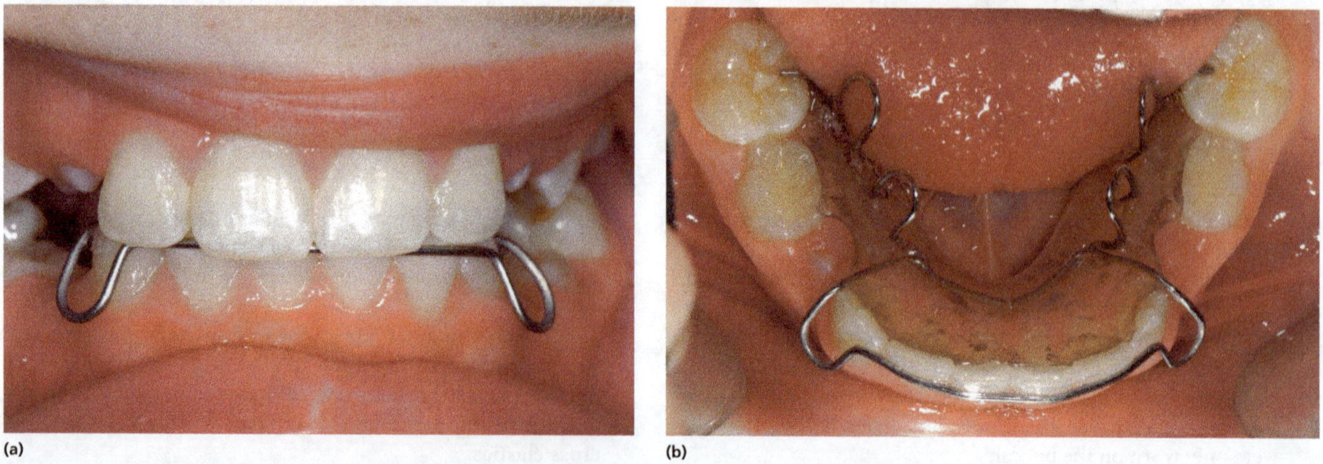

Figure 6.9 (a, b) Grace was placed in a mandibular Hawley retainer with bilateral loops to block her tongue.

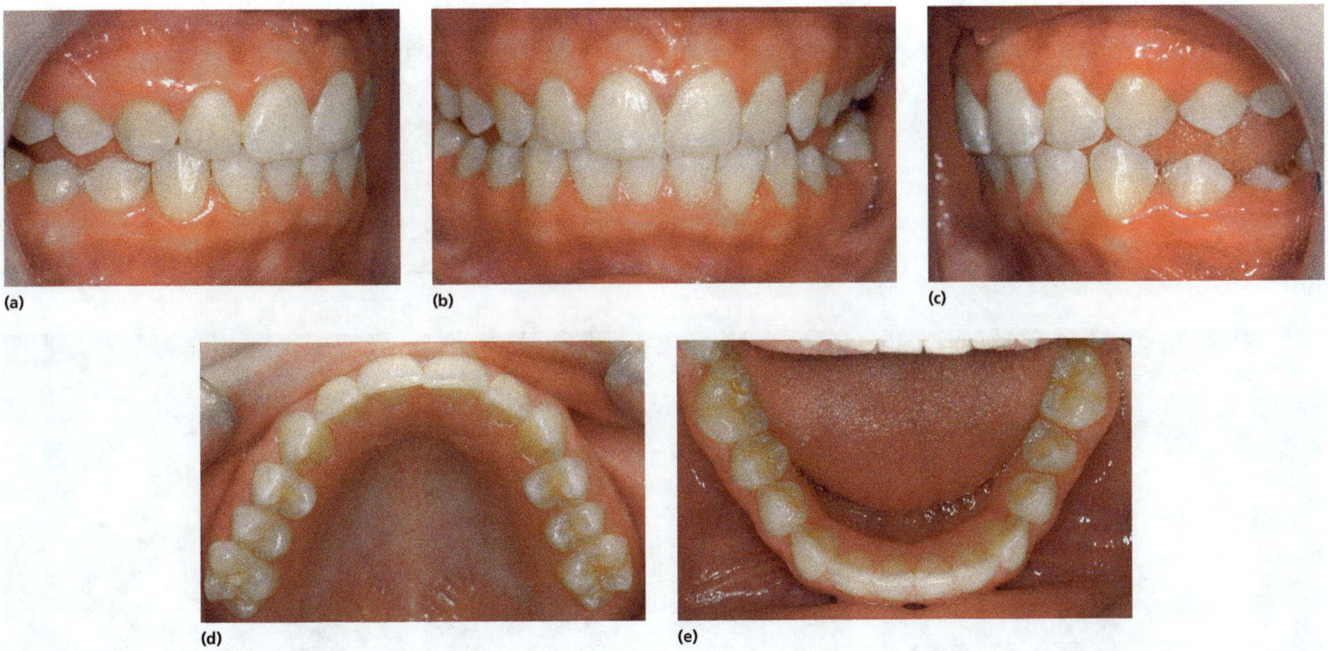

Figure 6.10 (a–e) Grace wore a retainer with posterior loops, but it was ineffective in retraining her tongue or closing her posterior open bite.

Q: Grace stated she was compliant in wearing the retainer with loops for months. But, her posterior open bite did not improve because her tongue would find a way around the loops (Figure 6.10, note posterior interpositional tongue habit still present). What do you recommend now?

A: Although fixed appliances with vertical criss-cross elastics could be used, the orthodontist chose a simpler solution because Grace was compliant. A tooth positioner was fabricated to block her tongue (Figure 6.11a–c). She wore this religiously and successfully closed her posterior open bite (Figure 6.11d–k). No other treatment was provided. She continued to wear the positioner as a retainer for 6 months, and was then placed in Hawley retainers.

Q: Figure 6.12 show Grace 6 years later. Her posterior open bite is still closed. What principle does this case illustrate (hint: habit correction)?

A: If the interpositional tongue habit causing a posterior open bite can be eliminated, then correction of the open bite, and long-term stability of the correction, can be achieved.

Q: Using fixed orthodontic appliances and vertical elastics, you successfully close a unilateral left posterior open bite in a patient with an interpositional tongue habit. The patient is debanded and placed in retainers. A year later, the patient presents with relapse of the unilateral left posterior open bite. Do you have any suggestions for correcting this relapse without using full fixed appliances again?

A: You could attempt to correct the posterior open bite with a tooth positioner. This was done without improvement. You could place bilateral lingual loops in the patient's maxillary or mandibular retainers to keep the tongue out of the open-bite space. This was attempted without improvement. Finally, you could place facial buttons on the left posterior teeth and run vertical elastics (Figure 6.13a–d). In this patient, once the bite was closed, the elastics were continued for 4 additional months. The elastics were then discontinued, but the buttons were left on the teeth until it could be verified that the open bite remained closed. Note: the retainers (Figure 6.13d) are worn *with* the vertical elastics to prevent the left posterior teeth from "rolling" lingually. This approach proved to be immediately successful (Figure 6.13e), and successful long-term. Figure 6.13f shows the same patient some years later with successful maintenance of the posterior open bite closure. Why? The habit was corrected.

Q: You suspect that the right posterior open bite in an adolescent patient (Figure 6.14) may be an example of primary failure of eruption. The maxillary right permanent first molar has not erupted into occlusion, while the maxillary left permanent first molar has erupted into occlusion. What should you do to help determine if you are right about the etiology?

A: First, try to check the radiographic history of tooth eruption for this patient. An unsuccessful attempt was made to obtain earlier dental radiographs, to determine if the maxillary right second molar was erupting. A decision was made to recall the patient in 1 year. At that time, additional radiographs were made.

Q: Dental radiographs were made 1 year later (Figure 6.15)? What do you see? What does this mean?

A: The *maxillary right second molar has continued to erupt* over the maxillary right first permanent molar. This means that this is probably *not* a case of primary failure of eruption. If both molars were failing to erupt, then it could likely be a case of primary failure of eruption. The maxillary right first molar is simply ankylosed.

Q: Knowing this, what options do you have? How should you proceed?

A: You could attempt to break the ankylosis by luxating the maxillary right first molar and by immediately placing vertical elastic force on the tooth to bring it into the arch. Instead, a decision was made to extract the ankylosed maxillary right first molar, place the patient in fixed appliances, and use a vertical elastic (Figure 6.16a) to bring the maxillary right second molar forward and into occlusion (Figure 6.16b–l). Note that the maxillary right third molar is continuing to erupt.

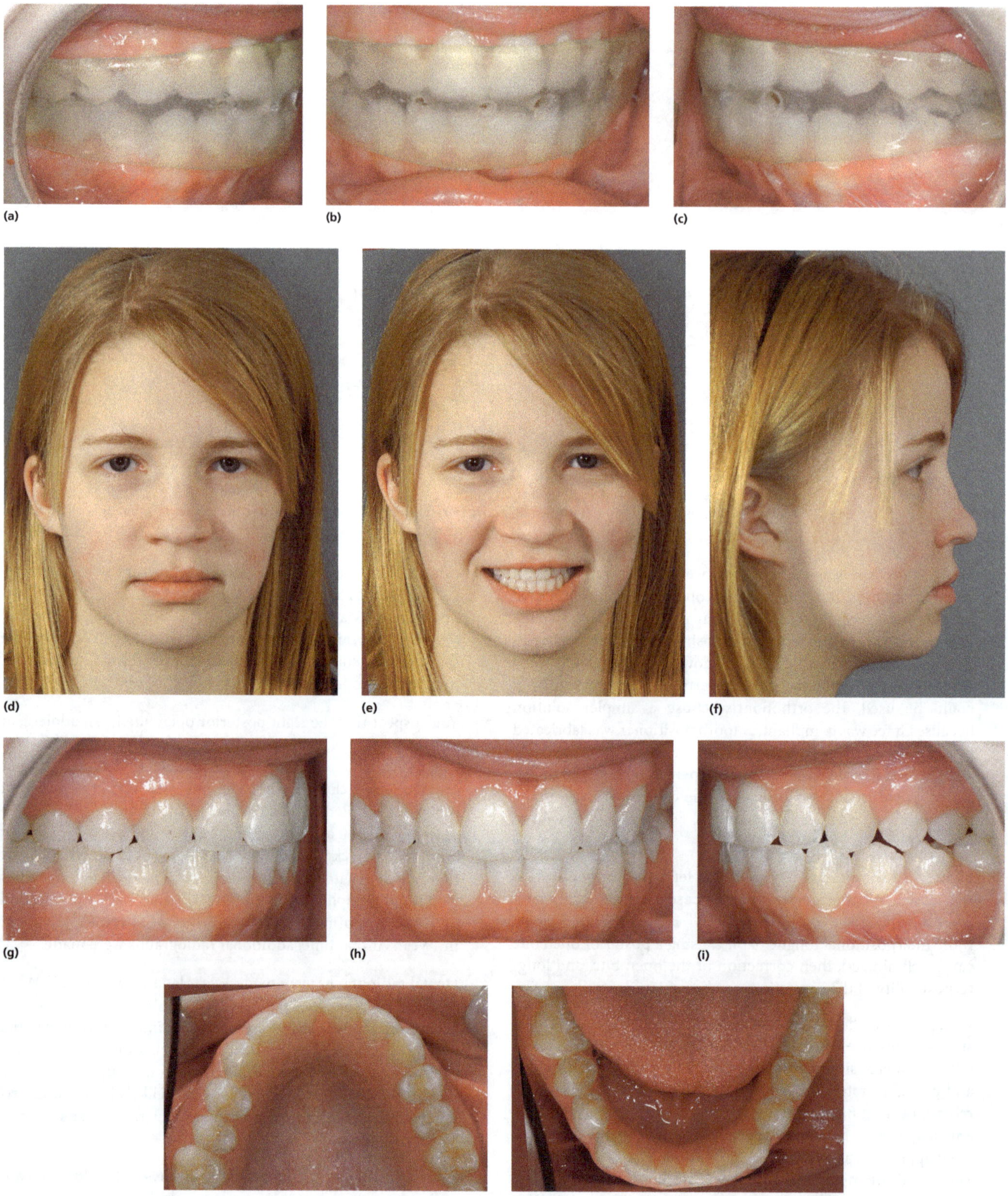

Figure 6.11 (a–c) Grace was next placed in a tooth positioner which (d–k) corrected her tongue habit and permitted her posterior teeth to erupt, closing her open bite. No other treatment was provided.

Q: An adolescent patient with a unilateral right posterior open bite presents to your associate (Figure 6.17), and your associate asks for your treatment advice. How do you recommend he proceed?

A: You advise him to seek historical dental radiographs to help detail the eruption history of these teeth. Such radiographs are found to be unavailable. You next advise him to wait 6 months and then re-evaluate eruption. After 4 months, he takes a

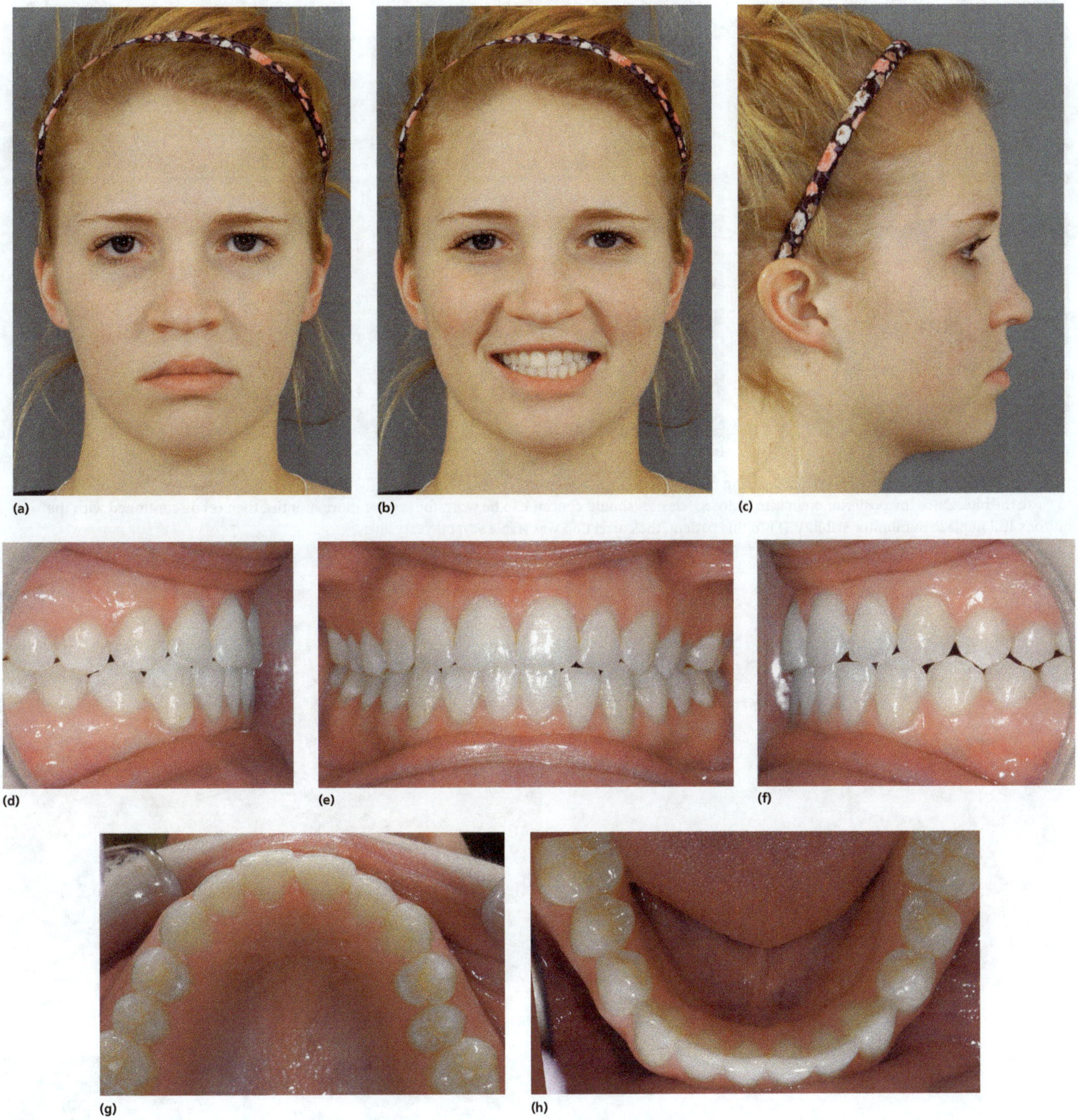

Figure 6.12 (a–h) Grace 6 years later. She has worn Hawley retainers for over 5 years, and her posterior open bite is still closed. The tooth positioner was effective in correcting her posterior tongue interposition habit.

complete mouth series of dental radiographs (Figure 6.18a) and is disappointed that the maxillary right first molar has not erupted. Without speaking to you, he concludes that the maxillary right first molar cannot erupt because it is blocked out by the maxillary right second premolar. He places the patient in fixed orthodontic appliances (Figure 6.18b–d), opens space for the maxillary right first molar, and attempts to erupt the maxillary right first molar and premolars using vertical elastics. He is unsuccessful erupting the maxillary right first molar. He concludes that this is a case of primary failure of eruption, aligns the arches, and debands the patient (Figure 6.18e–g).

Q: You see the same patient during a retention visit, and then discuss this patient with your associate. (i) Was the maxillary right first molar "blocked out" by the maxillary right second premolar? (ii) Was this a case of primary failure of eruption? (iii) Did your associate treat the patient appropriately?

A:

1 When you compare Figures 6.17c and 6.18a, it is tempting to conclude that the maxillary right first permanent molar is being blocked from erupting by the maxillary right second premolar. But this is not the case. Remember, the maxillary right first molar probably erupted long before the maxillary

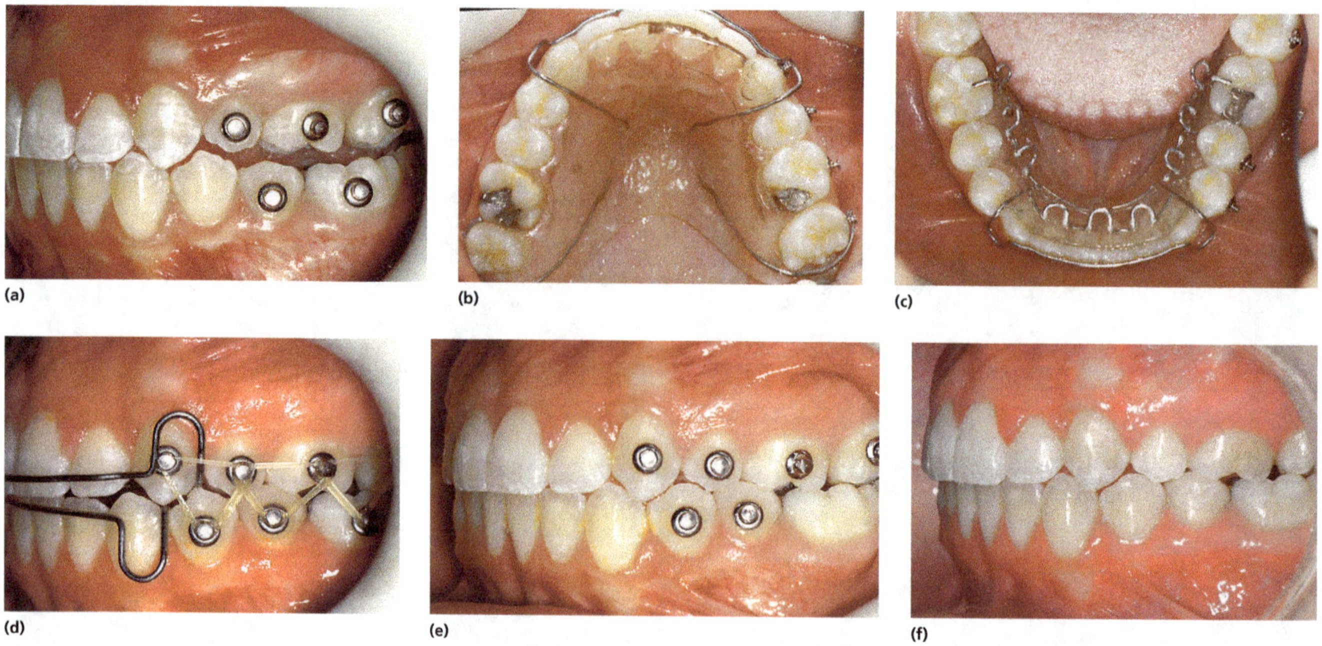

Figure 6.13 If a posterior open bite returns during retention, then (a–c) buttons can be bonded labially, and (d) vertical elastics worn with the retainers in to close the bite. Once the posterior open bite is closed, elastics should continue to be worn for several more months, then (e) discontinued with the buttons still in place to monitor stability. (f) In this patient, the correction was stable several years later.

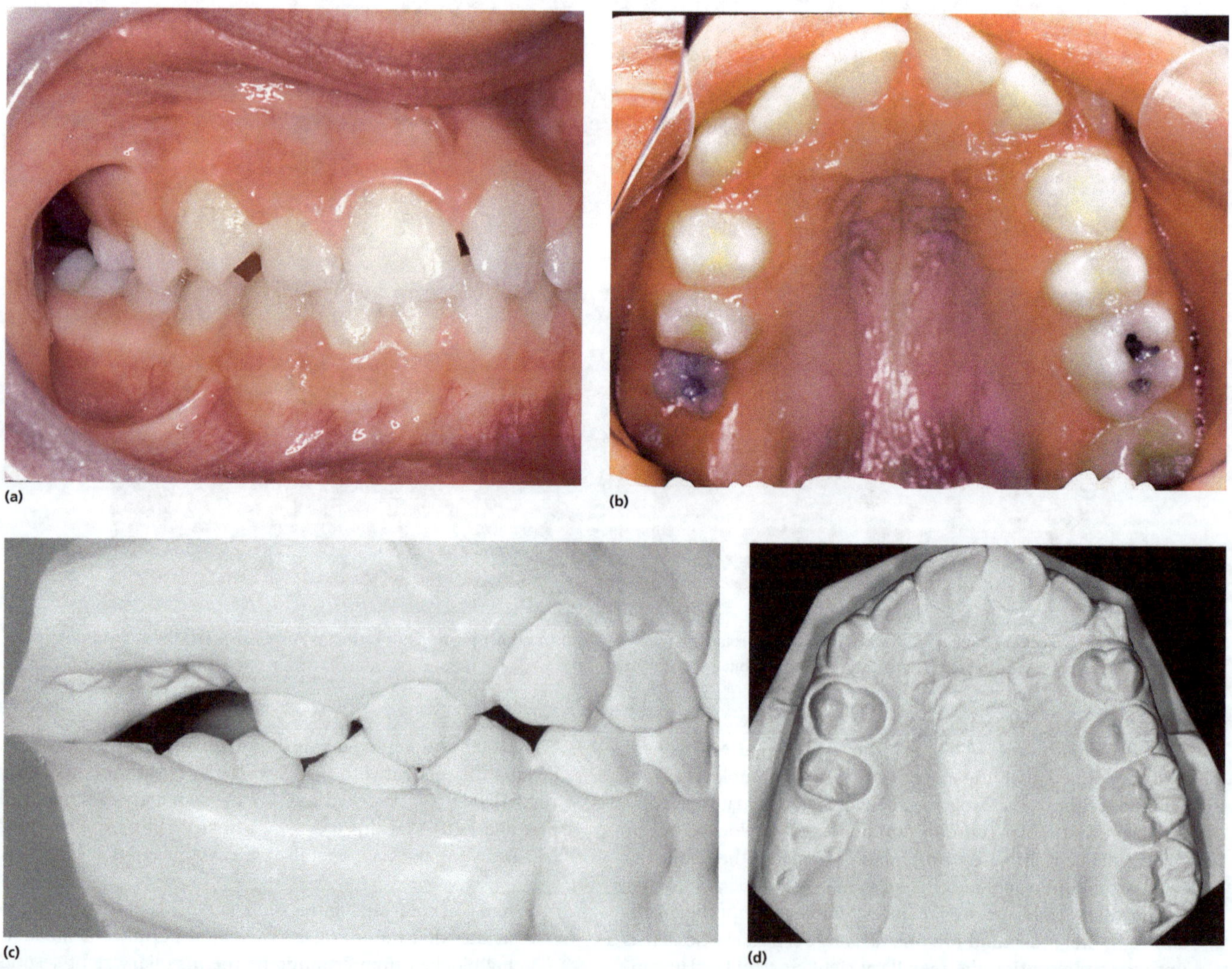

Figure 6.14 (a–e) Adolescent patient presenting with a right posterior (molar) open bite.

right second premolar erupted. Even in cases of maxillary first molar ectopic eruption under a maxillary right primary second molar, the maxillary right permanent first molar should not become blocked out under the second premolar when the primary second molar exfoliates.

2 Comparing Figure 6.17c with 6.18a (taken several months later), it appears that the maxillary second molar is continuing to erupt. Therefore, *this is a case of maxillary first molar ankylosis and not primary failure of eruption.*

3 Instead of running the vertical elastic from the mandibular teeth to the ankylosed maxillary first molar (Figure 6.18b), which would only erupt the mandibular teeth, your associate should have bypassed the maxillary first molar (not bonded it) and run a vertical elastic from the mandibular teeth to

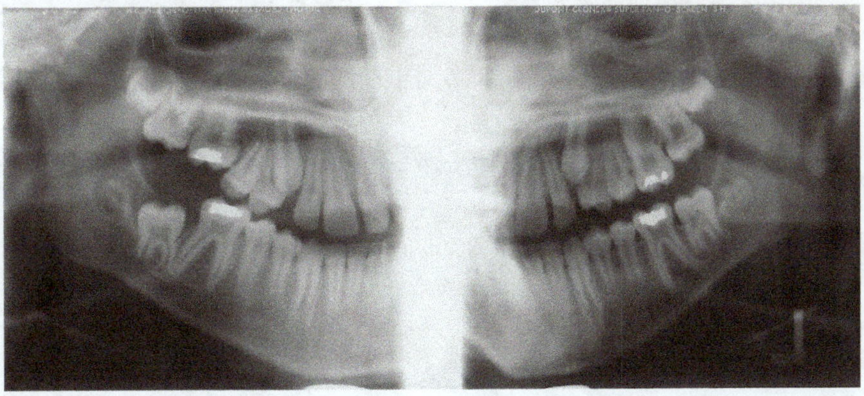

(e)

Figure 6.14 (Continued)

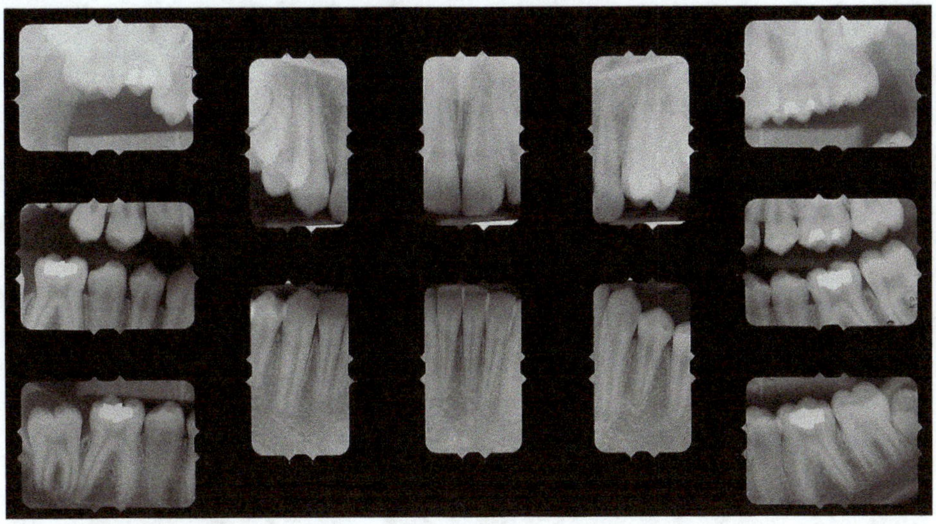

Figure 6.15 Dental radiographs of the patient in Figure 6.14 made 1 year later.

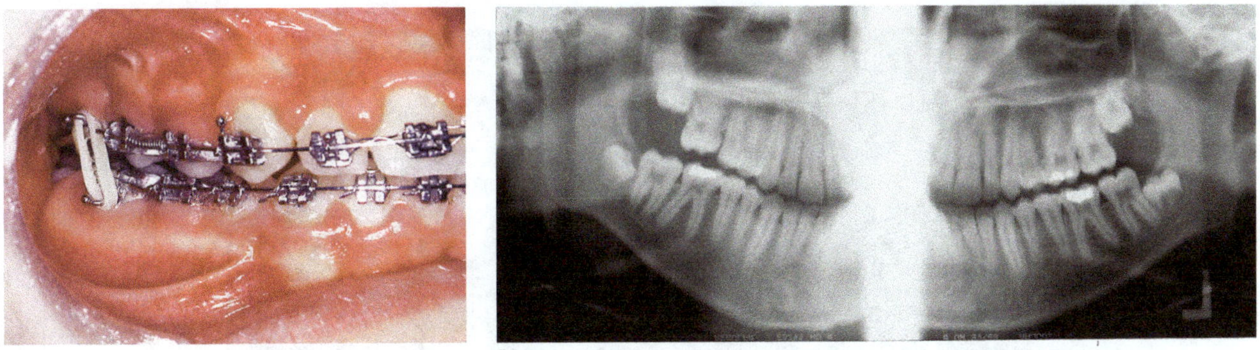

(a) (b)

Figure 6.16 Treatment of the patient in Figures 6.14 and 6.15: (a–f) The ankylosed maxillary right first molar was extracted. Fixed appliances were placed, and vertical elastics used to erupt the right second molar forward into occlusion. Eruption of the maxillary right third molar will be followed.

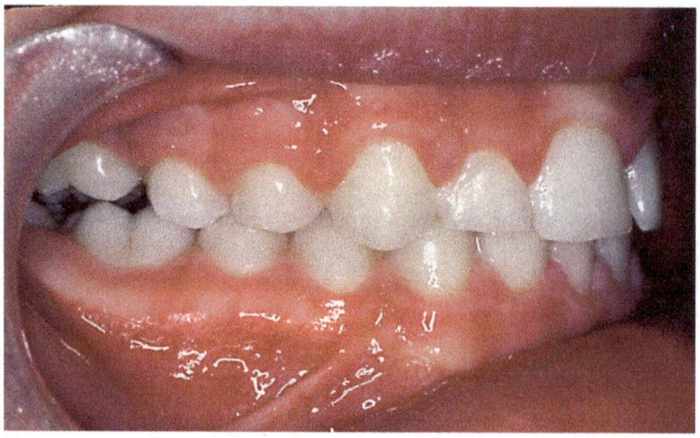

(c)

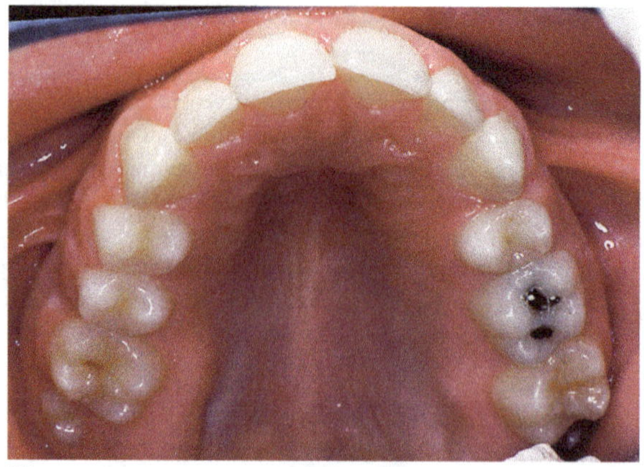

(d)

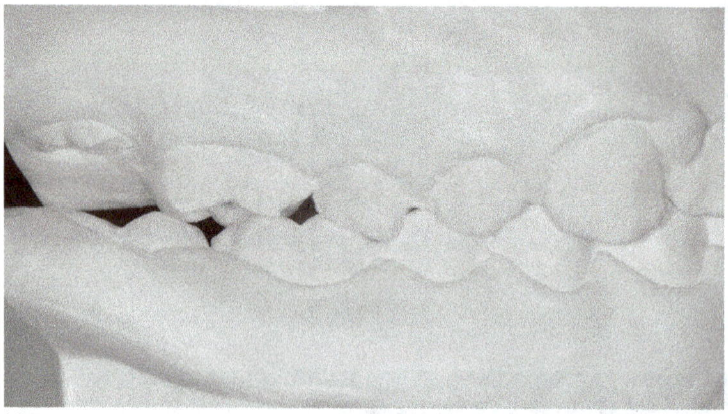

(e)

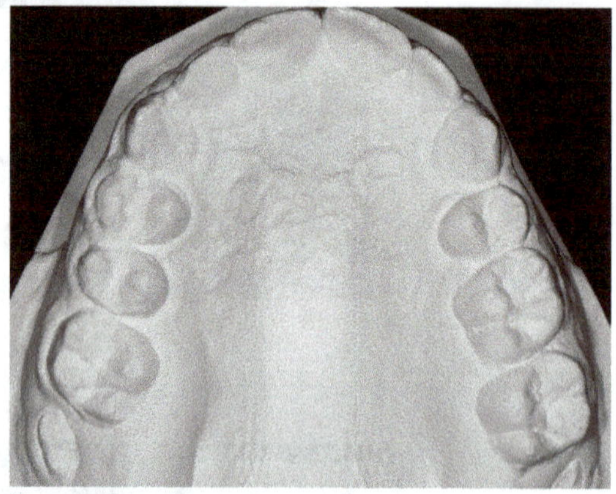

(f)

Figure 6.16 (Continued)

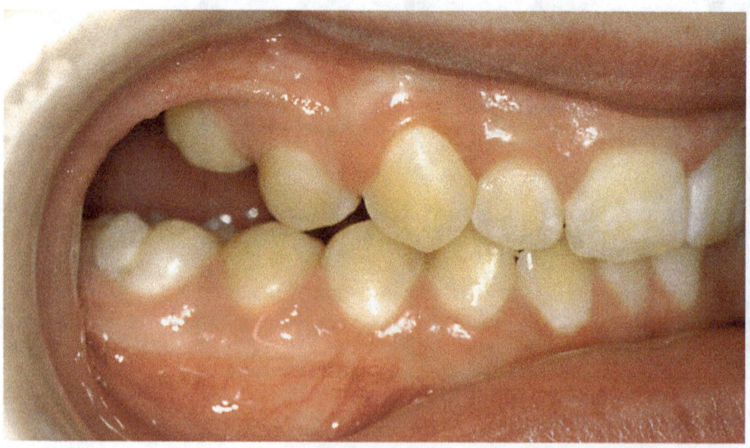

(a)

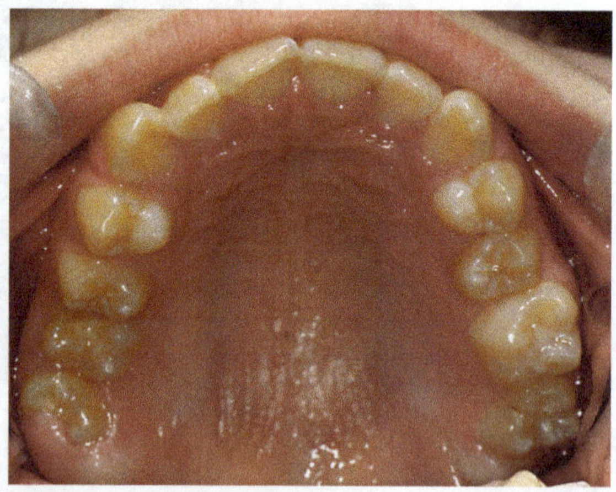

(b)

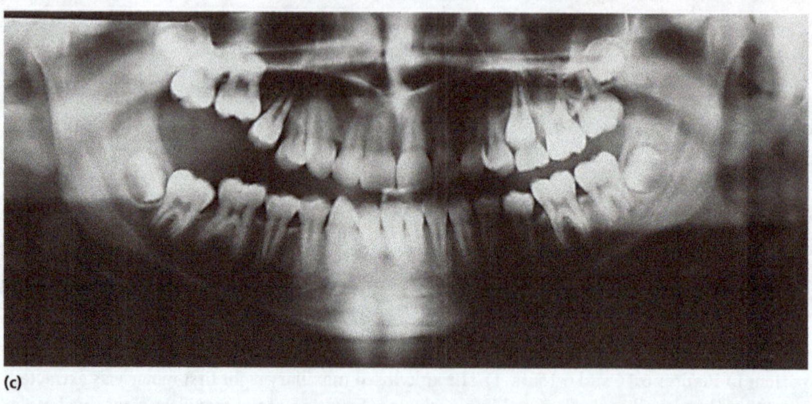

(c)

Figure 6.17 (a–c) An adolescent patient with a unilateral right posterior open bite.

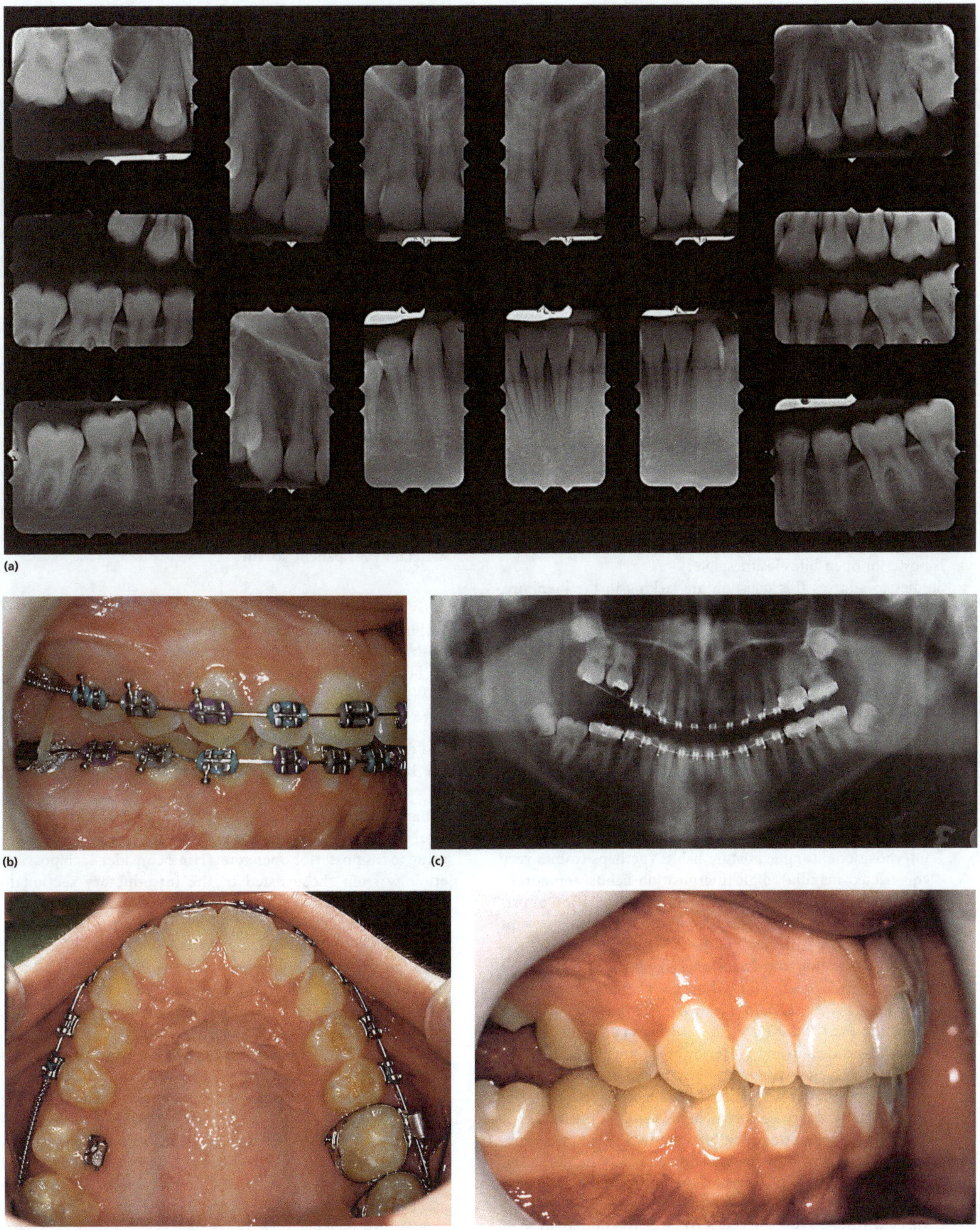

(a) (b) (c) (d) (e)

Figure 6.18 Treatment of the patient shown in Figure 6.17: (a–d) Progress records and (e–g) deband records of the same adolescent patient.

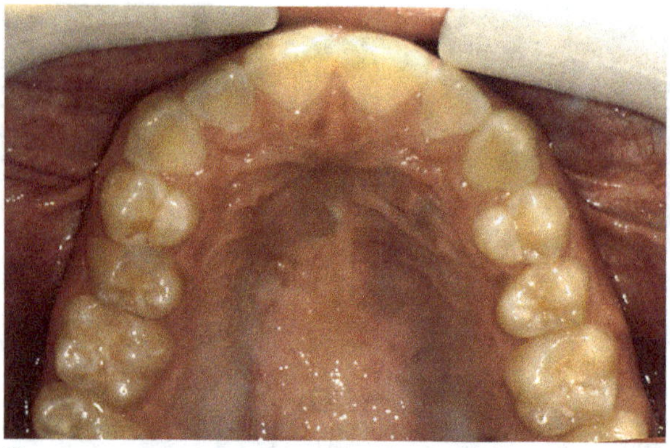

(f)

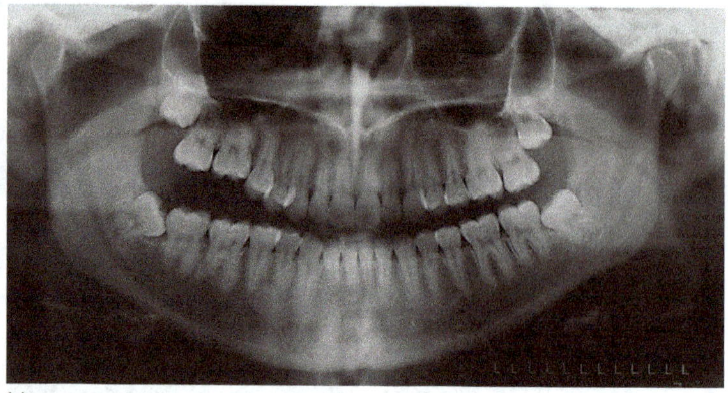

(g)

Figure 6.18 (Continued)

only the maxillary right second molar and premolars (erupting them). Of course, the maxillary right first molar would have been left unerupted in a far more apical position (along with a significant bony crest height step). Other options would have been to attempt luxation/forced eruption of the ankylosed maxillary right first molar, or to extract the maxillary right first molar and substitute the maxillary right second molar for it.

Q: Is posterior open-bite closure stable?

A: Studies to address this question are lacking in the literature. Clinical experience suggests that elimination of the tongue interposition habit is the key to stability for cases caused by the tongue habit. The adage, "posterior open bite closure and maintenance of closure may be the most challenging problem confronting the orthodontist" is an indication of the difficulty maintaining stability of a treated posterior open bite.

Q: In summary, what are your "take-home messages" regarding etiology, identifying, treating, and retaining posterior open-bite patients?

A: Take-home messages include the following:

- Posterior open bites result from a range of causes, including interpositional tongue posture habits (perhaps from a very constricted maxilla), digit interposition habits; temporary posterior open bites as a result of normal exfoliation of primary molars, but before permanent teeth have time to erupt into occlusion; ankylosis of teeth, which prevents their complete eruption into occlusion; lack of space for complete tooth eruption (teeth blocked out); systemic factors found in patients with certain syndromes; primary failure of eruption; and Class III growth resulting in an edge-to-edge incisor relationship and posterior open bite.
- The hallmark of a posterior open bite is occlusal contact of anterior teeth but lack of occlusal contact of posterior teeth. The patient is otherwise normal in the vertical dimension.
- Treatment of posterior open bites consists of erupting posterior teeth until they are in occlusion. If a habit caused the open bite, the habit must be eliminated. Orthodontic eruption of posterior teeth could include using fixed appliances with posterior vertical elastics or leveling a curve of Spee with archwires. Surgical eruption could include a segmental maxillary downgraft osteotomy or distraction osteogenesis. Of course, prosthodontic treatment (buildups, crowns, implant replacement with elongated crowns, or overlay RPDs) can close posterior open bite, and these treatments can also be viewed as another form of posterior tooth eruption.
- Closure of posterior open bite, and retention of closure of posterior open bite, can be one of the most difficult problems an orthodontist can face. Tell your patient that you may not be able to close, or to keep closed, a posterior open bite. Tell them to expect relapse and the possible need for retreatment. Retain your patient, for life.

Case Mark

Mark (Figure 6.19) is a 10-year, 2-month-old boy who presents to you with the CC, "I would like to have straight teeth and not have spaces between my teeth." PMH includes seasonal allergies and ADHD (Rx: Adderall), PDH WRN. TMJ and periodontal evaluations are WRN. CR = CO.

Q: List diagnostic findings/problems. What is your diagnosis?

A: See Table 6.1

Q: What are *all* possible etiologies of Mark's posterior open bite? List them and judge whether each could be contributing to his posterior open bite. (Hint: consider each possible etiology from those listed in the introductory section to Chapter 6.)

A: Possible posterior open bite etiologies include the following:

- Interpositional tongue habit: Mark has a "football" shape to his posterior open bite, especially on his left. Have Mark relax while you talk to his parents, then ask Mark to open his eyes (to distract him) as you quickly/gently separate his lips and check for an interpositional tongue habit. This was not done, but *a tongue habit could be contributing to his open bite.*
- Digit interposition habits: no inquiry was made regarding possible digit habits with Mark. This should have been done but was overlooked. *A digit habit could be contributing.*
- Temporary posterior open bites occurring while permanent teeth are erupting: yes, *transient eruption of posterior teeth could be playing a role in Mark's posterior open bite, especially in the first premolar area.*
- Ankylosis of teeth which prevents their complete eruption into occlusion: yes, it looks like the *maxillary left second primary molar could be ankylosed, and at least partially, contributing to the left posterior open bite.*

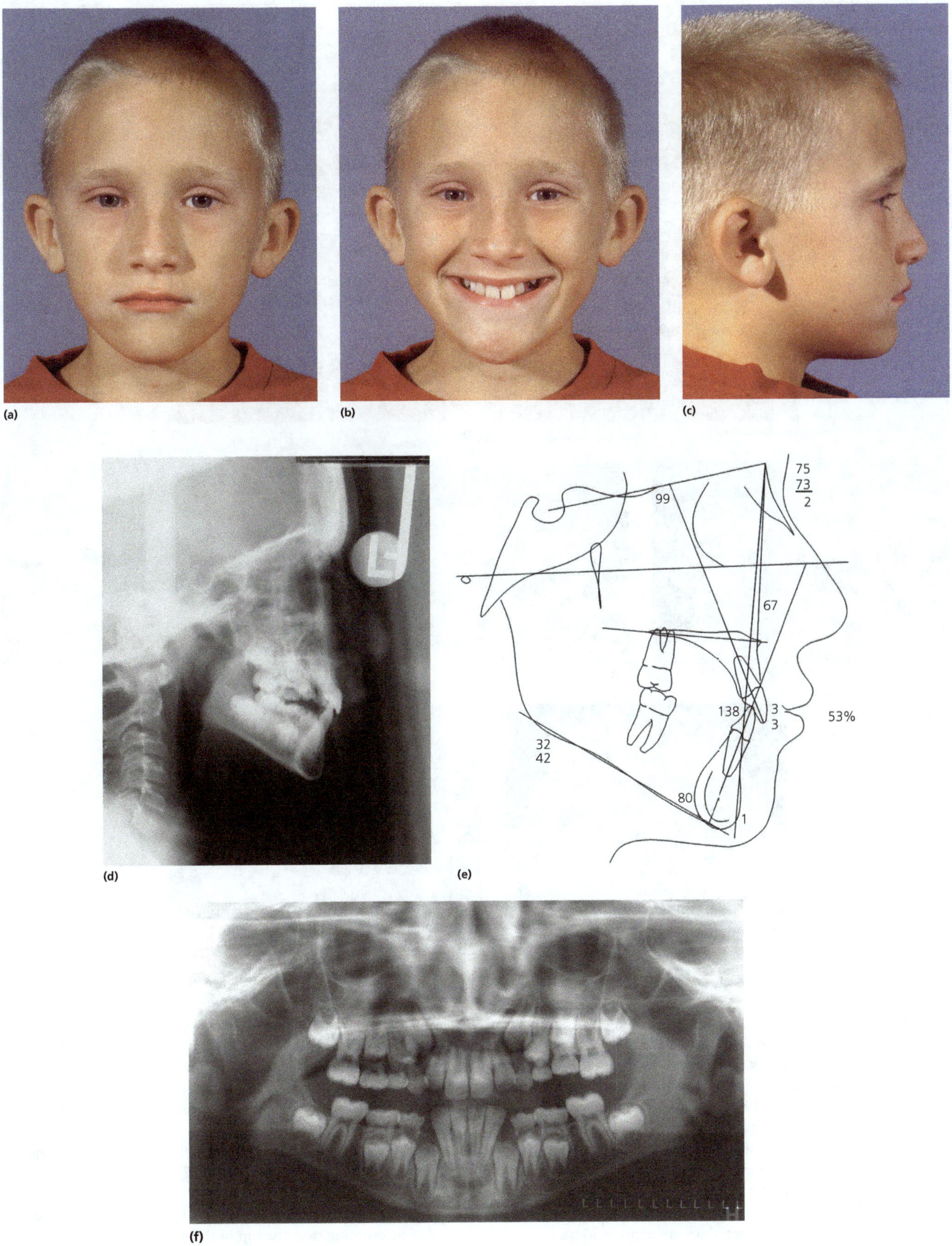

Figure 6.19 Initial records of Mark: (a–c) initial facial photographs, (d) lateral cephalograph, (e) cephalometric tracing, (f) pantomograph, (g–k) intraoral photographs, and (l–p) model photographs.

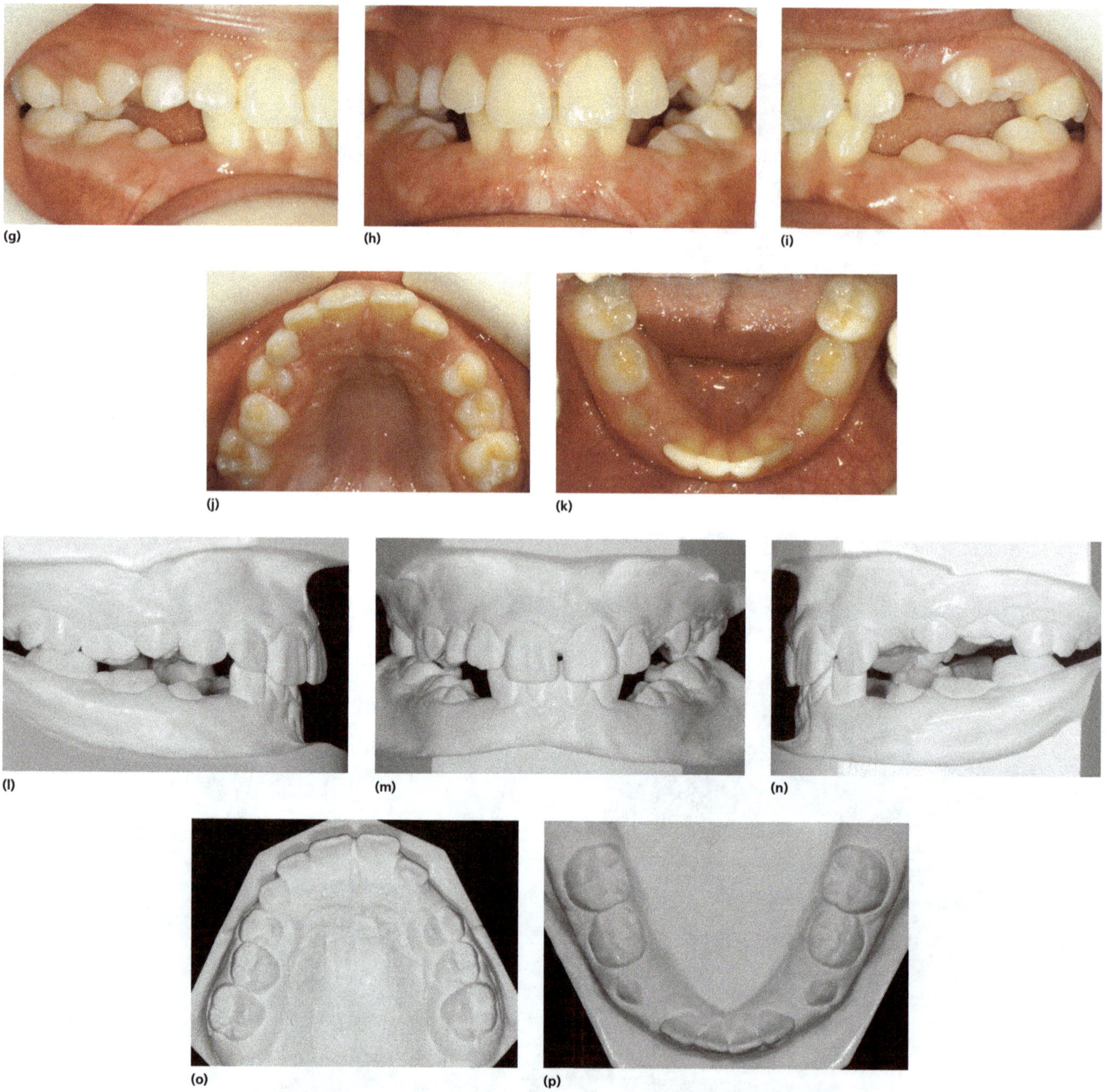

Figure 6.19 (Continued)

- Rapid excessive mandibular growth resulting in an edge to edge incisor relationship and bilateral posterior open bite: does not apply to Mark.
- Lack of space for complete tooth eruption (teeth blocked out): *lack of space for the mandibular canines could be contributing to the open bite at those locations.*
- Systemic factors: does not apply to Mark.
- Primary failure of eruption: since Mark's first molars are in occlusion, this does not appear to be a case of primary failure of eruption.
- Treatments for sleep apnea: does not apply to Mark.

In summary, at this stage of dental development, an interpositional tongue habit, digit habit, transient eruption of his first premolars, and ankylosis of his maxillary left second primary molar are factors that could contribute to Mark's posterior open bite. But, the precise reason(s) for the posterior open bite remains unknown. The open bite may be transient, closing with normal eruption of the permanent canines and premolars.

Q: What are your options for dealing with the (possibly) ankylosed maxillary left primary second molar?

A: Options include the following:

- Since the maxillary left permanent first molar does not appear to be erupting over the top of the maxillary left primary second molar (Figure 6.19f, n), you could simply monitor eruption of the maxillary left second premolar. Eruption of

Table 6.1 Diagnostic findings and problem list for Mark.

Full face and profile	**Frontal view** Symmetric Vertical proportions appear normal (soft tissue Glabella—Subnasale = Subnasale—soft tissue Menton) Adequate incisal display in posed smile, but the maxillary incisors are stepped down Relative to the occlusal plane Lip competence UDML: WRN **Profile view** Slightly convex/retrusive profile and chin NLA WRN Mildly everted lower lip
Ceph analysis	**Skeletal** Maxillary anteroposterior position mildly retrusive (A-point slightly behind Nasion-perpendicular line) ANB angle of 2° is WRN (but it would be greater, maybe 4°, if the maxillary AP position was ideal/more forward) Maxillary molar root apicies positioned *above* the palatal plane Steep MPA (FMA = 32°; SNMP = 42°) LAFH WRN (LAFH/TAFH = 53%) **Dental** Upright maxillary incisors ($\underline{1}$ to SN = 99°) Mandibular incisor angulation WRN (FMIA = 67°)
Radiographs	Mandibular primary second molar occlusal surfaces are stepped *below* the occlusal plane of the mandibular permanent first molars, but alveolar process bone crest height appears normal. That is, short primary second molar clinical crown height caused this occlusal surface step, not primary second molar ankylosis. Maxillary left primary second molar alveolar bone crest height appears stepped up compared to the maxillary left permanent first molar (ankylosed primary molar?)
Intraoral photos and models	Angle Class I Iowa Classification: I X X I OJ: 3 mm OB: 60% Maxillary incisors stepped down with respect to maxillary posterior teeth Bilateral posterior open bite Late mixed dentition (panoramic image made before models and photos) Inadequate room for mandibular permanent canines (excluding Leeway space) LDML: 1.5 mm right of UDML
Other	—
Diagnosis	Angle Class I malocclusion bilateral posterior open bite

the second premolar may be delayed by 6 months in the case of an ankylosed primary second molar, but the bone should be normal after the maxillary left second premolar erupts [13–15].

- If the maxillary left permanent first molar begins to erupt over the maxillary left primary second molar (potentially blocking eruption of the second premolar), then you may need to tip the maxillary left permanent first molar distally (and maintain it there).
- Another option is to extract the maxillary left primary second molar and place a space maintainer (e.g., Nance button) to maintain the anteroposterior position of the maxillary left permanent first molar. However, since the root of the maxillary left second premolar (Figure 6.19f) does not yet appear to be 1/2–2/3 developed, this approach could actually slow its eruption as bone heals over it.

Q: What are your options for dealing with the inadequate space for the (blocked out) permanent mandibular canines?

A: Options include the following:

- Doing nothing (no immediate treatment). However, when the mandibular primary second molars eventually exfoliate, a portion of the mandibular leeway space will be lost by mesial drift of the mandibular permanent first molars, which could potentially drift into a Class III relationship [16]. It would be better to maintain the leeway space (entirely) for eruption of the mandibular permanent canines and also to maintain the Class I molar relationship.
- Placement of an LLHA. Estimates of mandibular leeway space range from 3.4 mm [17] to 5 mm total for the total arch, depending on the size of the second premolar successors [18]. An average of 4 mm total arch leeway space is estimated to exist in the maxillary arch [18]. Depending on the mesial-distal width of the mandibular second premolars, 76% [19, 20] of mixed-dentition patients can be treated to satisfactory mandibular anterior alignment through the placement of an LLHA; 84% if 2 mm or less of initial crowding is permitted [20]. Because Mark's mandibular incisors are in an excellent cephalometric inclination (FMIA = 67°, Figure 6.19e) with excellent alignment, nonextraction treatment of the lower arch (LLHA placement) makes sense.
- Extraction of a mandibular incisor. Since Mark's maxillary lateral incisors are not small, excess incisor and canine OJ will be present later, if a lower incisor is extracted.
- Extraction of posterior teeth (e.g., first premolars). This would not be reasonable since Mark's anterior crowding is minimal, you have 3–4 mm of mandibular arch leeway space to work with, and his maxillary and mandibular incisors are upright.

Q: What are Mark's primary problems you observe in each dimension and other major problems?

A: See Table 6.2

Q: What are your treatment goals?

A: Achieve eruption of all permanent teeth into a fully seated Class I occlusion with ideal overbite and overjet.

Q: What unknowns exist? Does Mark have any unknowns that you should eliminate before you define your final treatment plan or do something irreversible?

Table 6.2 Primary problems list for Mark.

AP	—
Vertical	Bilateral (probably transient) posterior open bite
Transverse	—
Other	—

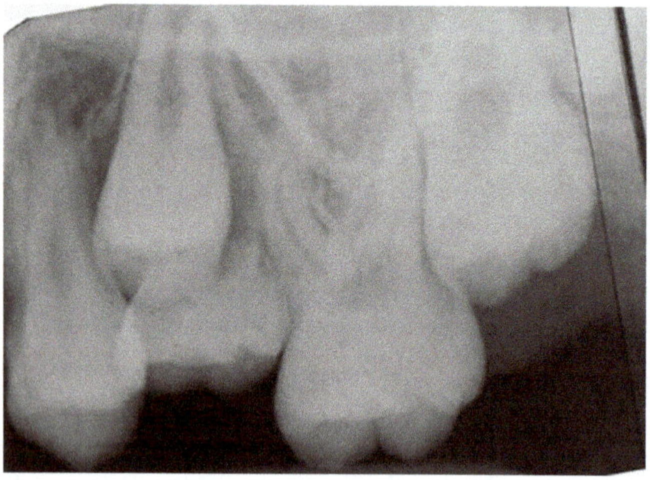

Figure 6.20 One year later—a periapical radiograph of Mark's maxillary left primary second molar and erupting permanent second premolar.

A: *The precise etiology of his posterior open bite is a major unknown.* Additional unknowns include Mark's growth and compliance, an undetected CR–CO shift, and future development of his dentition. You should definitely try to determine the cause of his posterior open bite before doing anything irreversible. If habits causing the posterior open bite are detected, every effort should be made to correct the habits.

Q: What treatment do you recommend for Mark at this time, or do you just want to monitor him? What do you recommend doing?

A: A decision was made to monitor his posterior open bite for 1 year. An LLHA was placed and eruption of permanent teeth monitored. Placing an LLHA was smart. But, he was not checked for a tongue interposition/digit habit. This was a mistake.

Q: One year later, Mark was recalled. It was noted that his maxillary left primary second molar was not showing normal vertical drift and a periapical radiograph was made (Figure 6.20). What do you see?

A: The maxillary left second premolar is resorbing the maxillary left primary second molar root properly, but the maxillary left permanent first molar is *tipping mesially over the primary tooth* (potentially blocking eruption of the maxillary left second premolar).

Q: How would you deal with this situation (mesial tipping of the first molar over the primary tooth)?

A: By regaining the space that was lost if you feel the maxillary left second premolar will be blocked from erupting. Mark was placed on an asymmetric left headgear to upright/distalize the maxillary left permanent first molar and create space for the maxillary left second premolar to erupt.

Six months later, normal tooth eruption was judged to be occurring. The LLHA was removed. Fixed appliances were placed, arches were leveled and aligned, headgear discontinued, and a panoramic image was made (Figure 6.21).

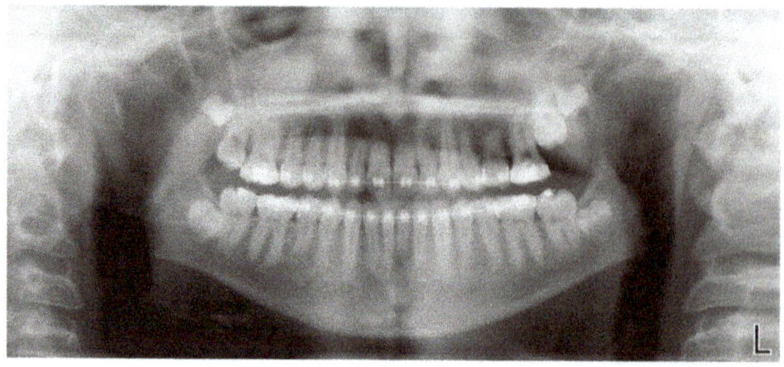

Figure 6.21 Mark's progress panoramic image following leveling and aligning of his dental arches.

A posterior open bite was then noted on Mark's left side, and he was asked to wear left posterior vertical elastics to close it. The posterior open bite was thought to be improved with elastic wear. Mark was debanded after 2 years in full appliances (Figure 6.22) and placed in Hawley retainers. Note a mild (molar) posterior open bit appears on his lateral cephalometric radiograph (Figure 6.22c), but is not seen on study models (Figure 6.22g, i). Also note the slight Class III molar relationship on his right (Figure 6.22g).

Q: Let's compare the maxillary right and left second molars as seen in Figures 6.19f and 6.21. What difference do you note?

A: Both second molars began at about the same level and developmental stage (Figure 6.19f). However, the maxillary right second molar now appears to be erupting normally while the left is delayed (Figure 6.21).

Q: What could be happening to the maxillary left second molar? What could this be an example of?

A: The maxillary left second molar could be ankylosed or an example of primary failure of eruption.

Q: How do you handle the unerupted maxillary left second molar?

A: Option include the following:

- Since Mark is stable now, you could simply monitor eruption of the maxillary left second. It will probably not erupt, but it may erupt. Monitoring it reduces your unknowns.
- If you think it is ankylosed, then you could surgically expose it, luxate it to break the bony union, and then try to erupt it immediately (before it ankyloses again).
- If you think this is an example of primary failure of eruption, then you could consider (i) extracting it and replacing it with a bone graft/implant (heroic), (ii) leaving it unerupted and accepting a first molar occlusion, and (iii) treating it with a segmental osteotomy or distraction osteogenesis to close the posterior open bite (heroic).
- After discussions with Mark and his parents, a decision was made to monitor the maxillary left second molar's eruption.

Q: Three years later Mark presents for a retention check (Figure 6.23). What are the primary problems in each dimension and other major problems at this retention check?

A: See Table 6.3

Q: Examine the cephalometric superimposition of deband and 3 years post deband (Figure 6.23f). How did the Class III dental relationship develop?

A: Mandibular growth. B-point has grown forward much more than A-point. Considering the intraoral Class III relationship, is his

LDML deviation to the left due to more right mandibular growth then left mandibular growth, or is it due slippage of anterior tooth contacts? It could be due to either, or possibly both.

Q: Remember that you previously considered future growth an unknown? What is a major unknown(s) now?

A: *Future growth is still a major unknown.* The Class III relationship could worsen. Another unknown is the cause of the left maxillary posterior teeth not erupting.

Q: What options do you have for dealing with Mark's Class III relationship?

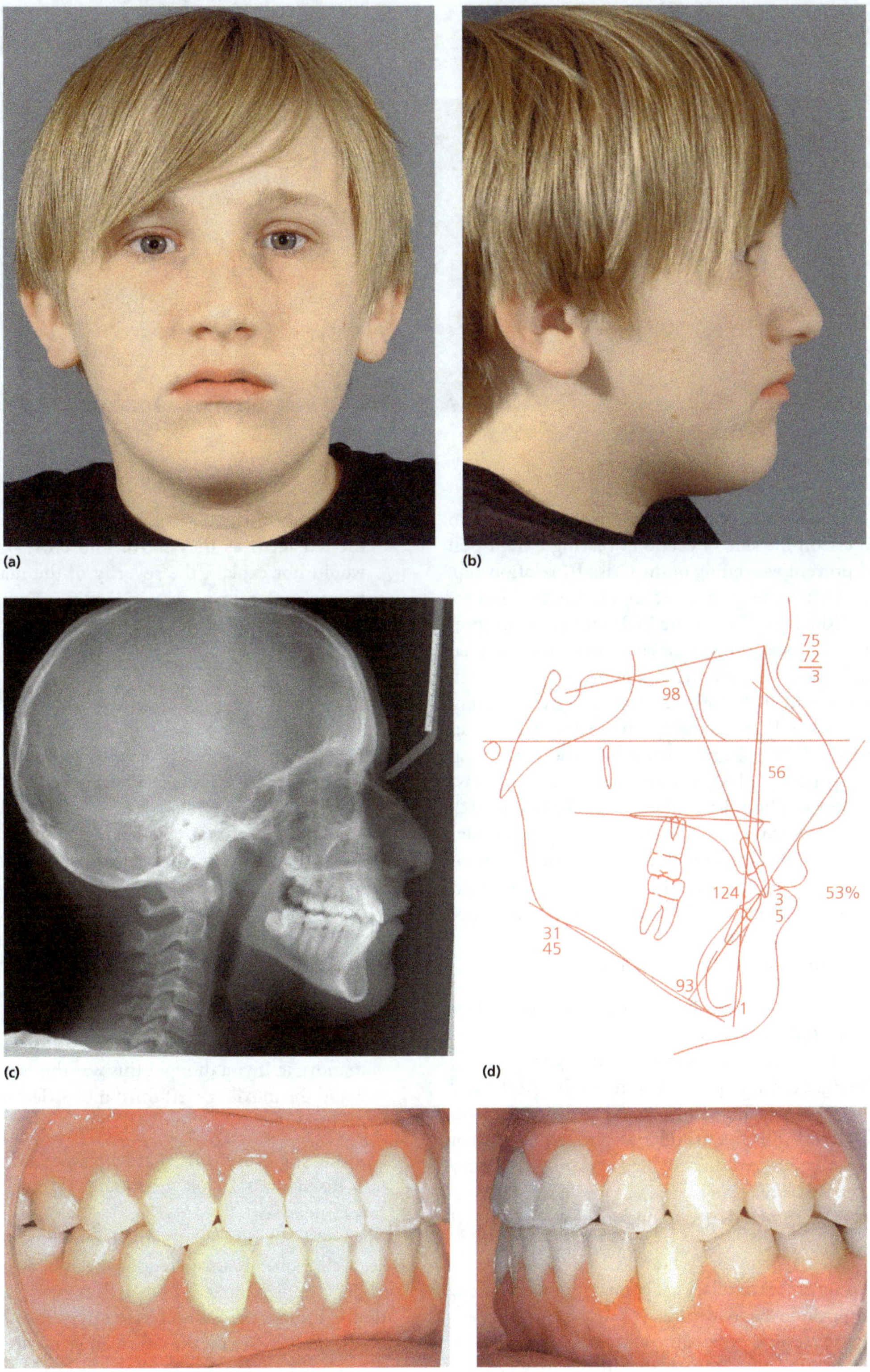

Figure 6.22 (a–k) Deband records of Mark.

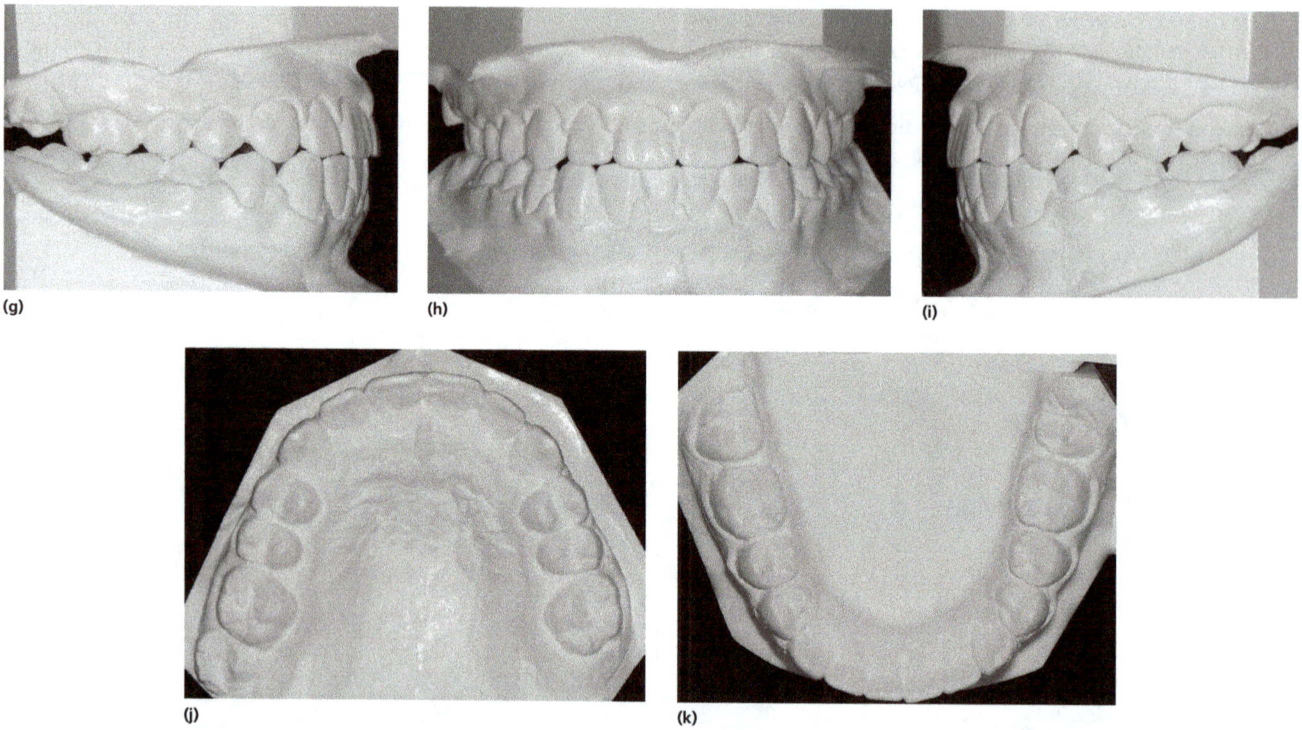

Figure 6.22 (Continued)

A: The problem is that we do not know if Mark will continue to grow more. To err on the side of caution, wearing a high-pull chin cup could prevent worsening of the Class III relationship, if Mark would be willing to wear it. He should wear it until we are sure he is finished growing. If the high-pull chin cup prevented forward mandibular growth; and if his maxilla continued to grow forward, then his Class III relationship may correct. Even if he just wore the high-pull chin cup enough to prevent worsening of his Class III relationship, then Class III elastics could make the final AP 1–2 mm correction. Another option would be to place buccal TADs (or miniplates) to permit Class III elastic wear between both jaws all day long. This approach could selectively slow down or prevent further mandibular growth and enhance forward growth of the maxilla. A poor solution would be to extract mandibular premolars at this time. Why? Irreversible treatments should be postponed until major unknowns, such as growth, are reduced. Further, a 1–2 mm Class III relationship is too small to warrant extraction.

Q: How did the open bite at the maxillary lateral incisors occur?
A: Possible reasons include the following:

- The maxillary right lateral incisor was initially stepped up relative to the right central incisor (Figure 6.19h). At deband (Figure 6.22h), the maxillary right lateral incisor edge was approximately even with the maxillary right central incisor edge. So, eruption of the right lateral incisor during maxillary arch leveling could be relapsing.
- The amount of anterior OB is decreasing as the right Class III worsens.

Q: How did the step-up of the maxillary left second premolar occur?
A: Possible reasons include the following:

- The maxillary left second premolar could be ankylosed.
- An interpositional tongue habit, or other habit, may be contributing. This was never evaluated.
- Asymmetric right mandibular growth could be discluding the left teeth as they move into cross bite. But, this effect would not explain the severity of the maxillary left second premolar step-up as seen in Figure 6.23j

Q: Compare the maxillary left second molar vertical position in Figures 6.21 and 6.23g. What do you note?
A: It appears that the maxillary left second molar has not erupted any more.

Q: What treatment options would you *now* consider for the unerupted maxillary left second molar?
A: Options include the following:

- You could continue to annually monitor the maxillary left second and third molars with a panoramic image. As long as they are not pathologically involved or creating periodontal problems, you could just leave them alone.
- If you thought the maxillary left second molar was simply ankylosed, then you could expose it, luxate it to break the ankylosis, and immediately attempt to erupt it. Or, you could extract it.
- If you thought the maxillary left second molar was an example of failure of eruption, then it would ankylose if you attempted to move it. If you thought this was the case, you could extract it and the maxillary left third molar (leaving a left first molar occlusion).

Q: Considering everything that has happened thus far, and all of our discussions, what treatment (if any) would you now recommend?
A: Mark was offered, and accepted, retreatment. His maxillary left second molar (considered to be ankylosed), and all third molars, were extracted. Both arches were placed in fixed orthodontic appliances, the arches were leveled/aligned, and vertical elastics were worn on the left side to close the open bite. Neither the current Class III relationship, nor the potential worsening Class III relationship, were addressed.

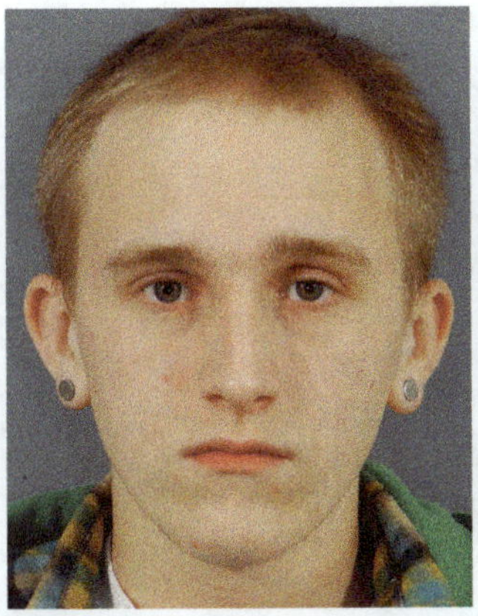

(a)

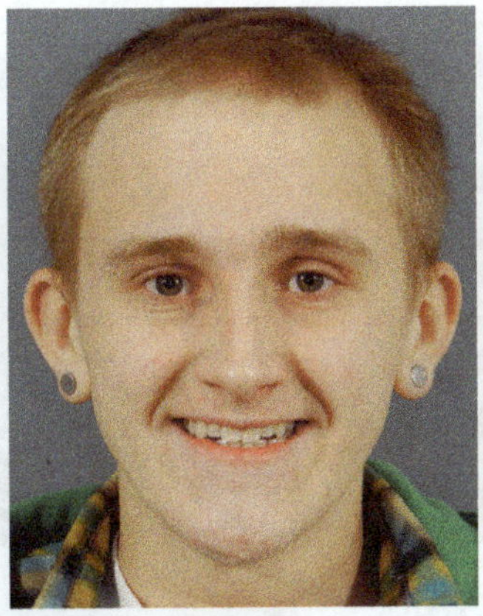

(b)

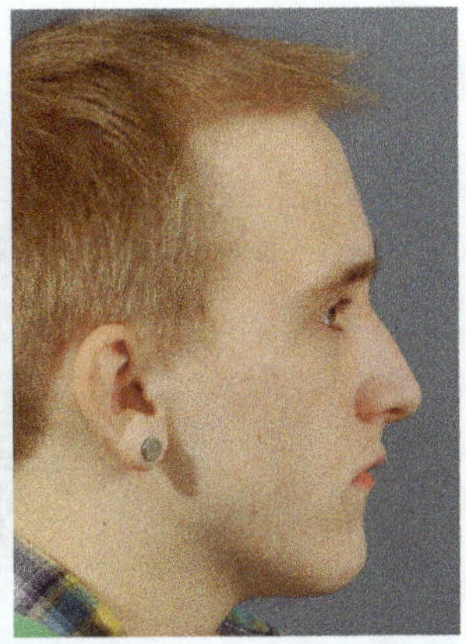

(c)

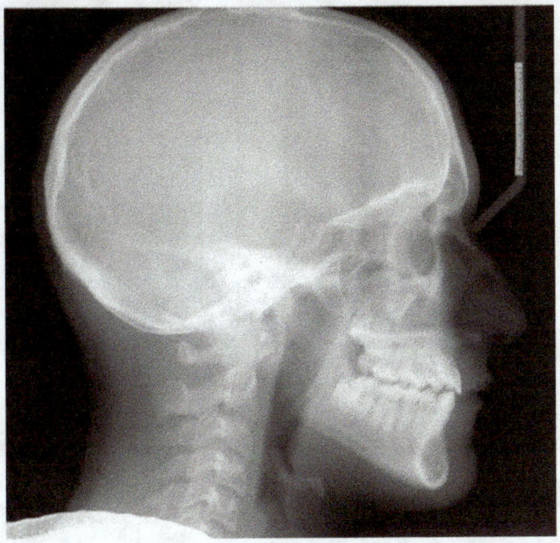

(d)

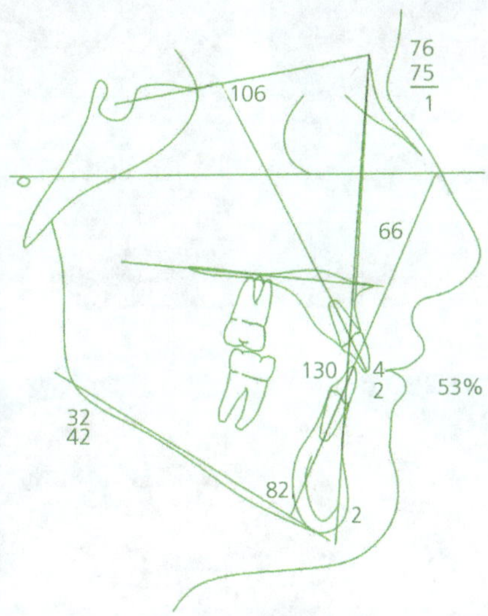

(e)

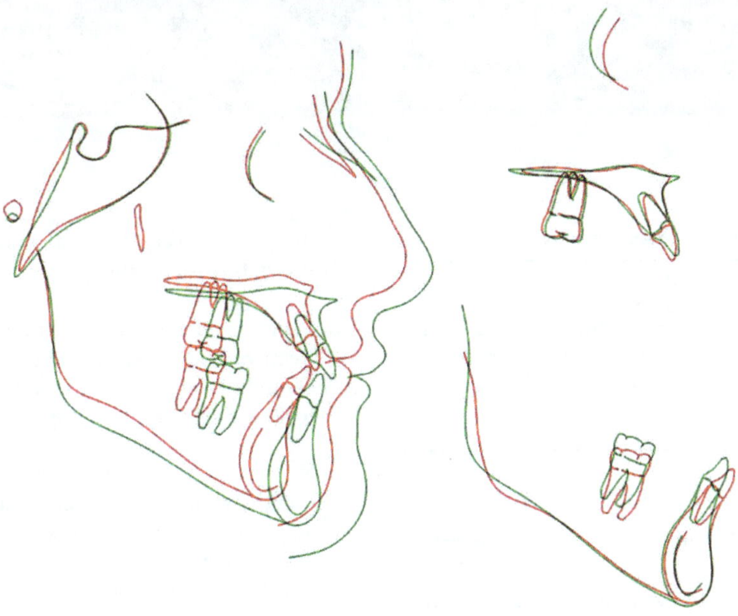

(f)

Figure 6.23 (a–l) Three-year retention records of Mark.

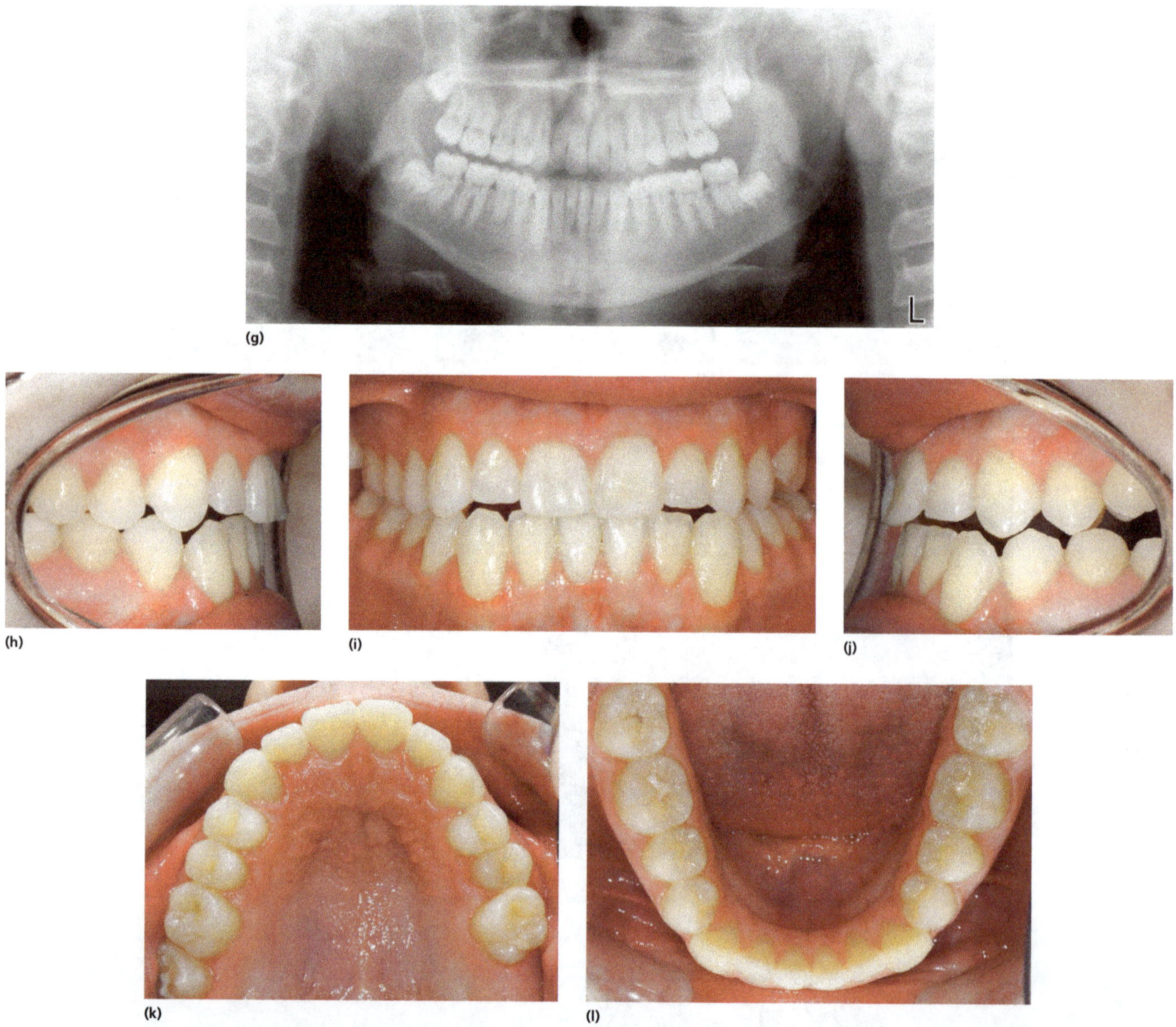

Figure 6.23 (Continued)

Table 6.3 Primary problems list for Mark after 3 Years in retention.

AP	Mild Class III (1–2) mm canine relationship
Vertical	Anterior open bite (lateral incisors)
	Left posterior open bite (maxillary left second premolar stepped up, maxillary left second molar unerupted)
Transverse	Cross-bite left canines
	LDML deviates left
Other	—

Q: Progress photos are shown 8 months into treatment (Figure 6.24). What has happened?

A: The left posterior open bite has worsened and a right-to-left cant of the maxillary arch has developed—despite Mark wearing left vertical elastics.

Q: Why has this happened?

A: The maxillary left (stepped up) second premolar is very likely ankylosed, and its inclusion in the arch has resulted in intrusion of the other left maxillary posterior teeth and in the right-to-left cant.

Q: How do you now recommend proceeding?

A: Remove the maxillary left second premolar bracket and continue with left anterior and posterior vertical elastics to try to close the left posterior open bite.

Q: Mark is very compliant in wearing his vertical elastics. Three months later, you re-evaluate his occlusion (Figure 6.25). What do you see? Mark's parents ask you what is happening—what do you tell them?

A: The left posterior open bite is not closing, and the Class III relationship is not improving.

Tell Mark and his parents that late mandibular growth could be occurring, along with the possibility of a tongue interposition habit, ankylosis of the maxillary left second premolar and first molar, and the possibility of primary failure of eruption.

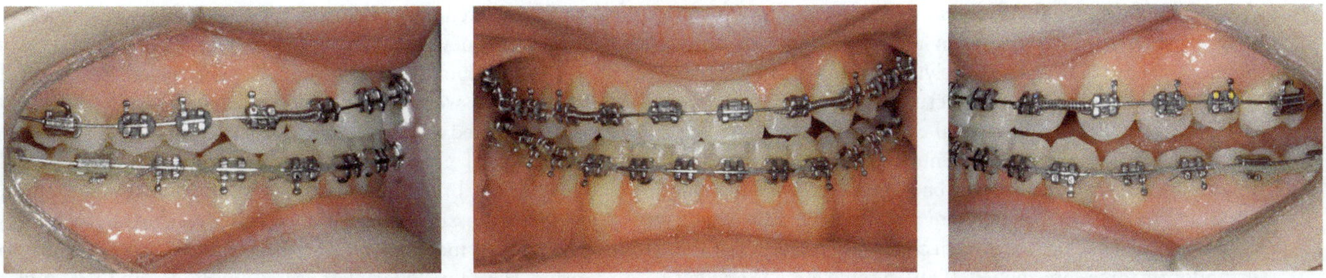

(a) (b) (c)

Figure 6.24 (a–c) Second treatment progress photos of Mark.

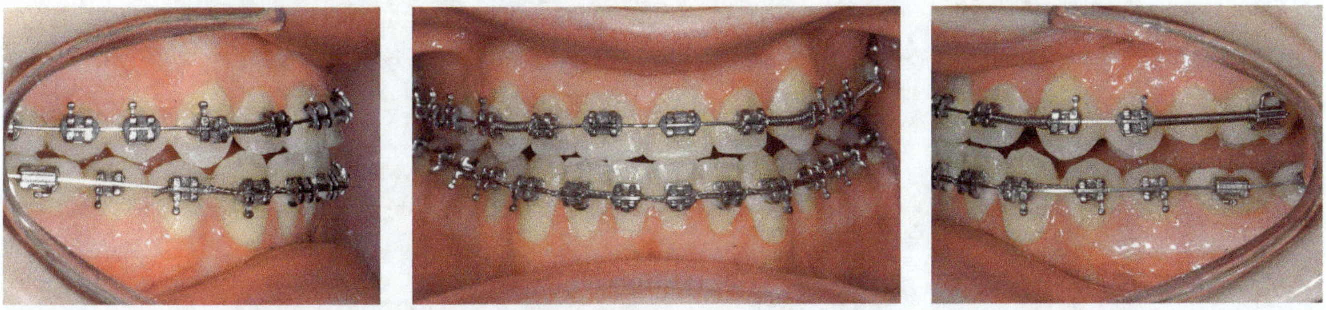

(a) (b) (c)

Figure 6.25 (a–c) Progress photos 3 months after removing the maxillary left second premolar bracket.

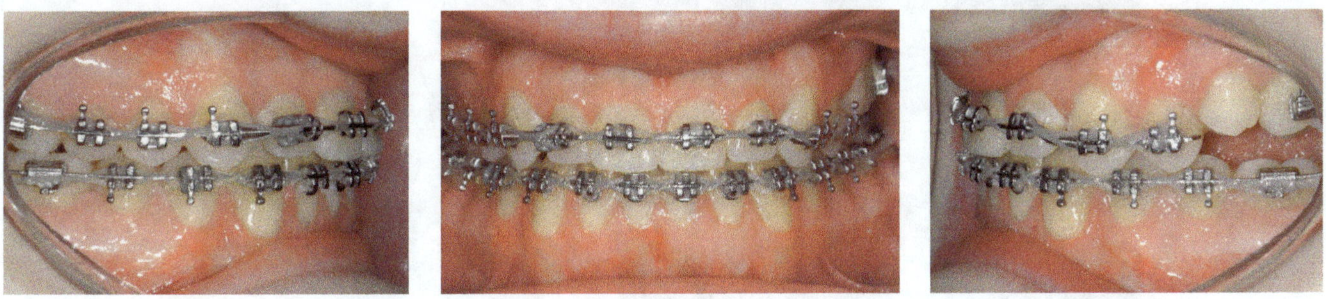

(a) (b) (c)

Figure 6.26 (a–c) Mark's occlusion several months after the maxillary archwire was sectioned distal to the maxillary left first premolar (freeing the remaining maxillary arch from the ankylosed maxillary left second premolar and first molar). Class III elastics and anterior vertical elastics were worn, prn.

Q: Let's step back for a moment to look at the big picture. What do you now believe is the most likely cause of Mark's left posterior open bite—a tongue habit or primary failure of eruption?

A: *Since Mark is complying with left anterior and posterior vertical elastic wear (elastics would tend to keep his tongue lingual), the most likely cause of the left posterior open bite is primary failure of eruption.*

Q: What do you do? How would you proceed?

A: A discussion was held with Mark and his parents. They elected to correct his Class III relationship and to attempt closure of Mark's left posterior open bite to, and including, only the maxillary first premolar. The maxillary archwire was sectioned distal to the maxillary left first premolar to free the rest of the maxillary arch from the ankylosed maxillary left second premolar and first molar. Mark was placed on Class III elastics on the right (elastics worn from the maxillary right first molar to the mandibular right canine). On the left side, a Class III elastic was worn from the maxillary left first premolar to the mandibular left canine. Anterior vertical elastics were worn bilaterally.

Q: Within a few months Mark's occlusion has improved dramatically (Figure 6.26), and he was soon debanded (Figure 6.27). Is Mark an example of primary failure of eruption?

A: *Mark is very likely an example of primary failure of eruption.* Let's look at how primary failure of eruption facts each relate to Mark.

- First molars are always involved: in this case, the maxillary left first molar was affected.
- Posterior teeth are more frequently affected: Mark's maxillary left second premolar, first molar, and second molar were affected.
- If a tooth in a further anterior position is affected, then more posterior teeth are usually affected as well: all teeth on Mark's maxillary left side distal to the maxillary left first premolar were affected.
- The condition is bilateral for 50% of PFE patients: in Mark's case, the condition was unilateral.

- Affected teeth resorb the alveolar bone above the crown and may erupt into initial occlusion and then cease to erupt further, or may fail to erupt entirely: Mark's maxillary left second premolar and first molar erupted into occlusion but ceased to erupt later with vertical elastic pull. The maxillary left second molar never erupted into occlusion.
- Involved teeth may be displaced back and forth with manual pressure (indicating that they are not, initially, ankylosed). However, involved teeth tend to become ankylosed as soon as orthodontic forces are applied. If an eruptive force is applied to the affected teeth, then the force will cause them to ankylose. It was never noted whether mobility of Mark's maxillary second premolar and first molar was checked. But, even if these teeth were initially mobile, they became ankylosed when erupted forces were applied.
- In a case of primary failure of eruption, if a small area of ankylosis is broken by manipulating the ankylosed tooth, it might be possible to move the tooth for a short time, but re-ankylosis is inevitable. It was wise to discontinue attempts to bring Mark's maxillary left second premolar and first molar

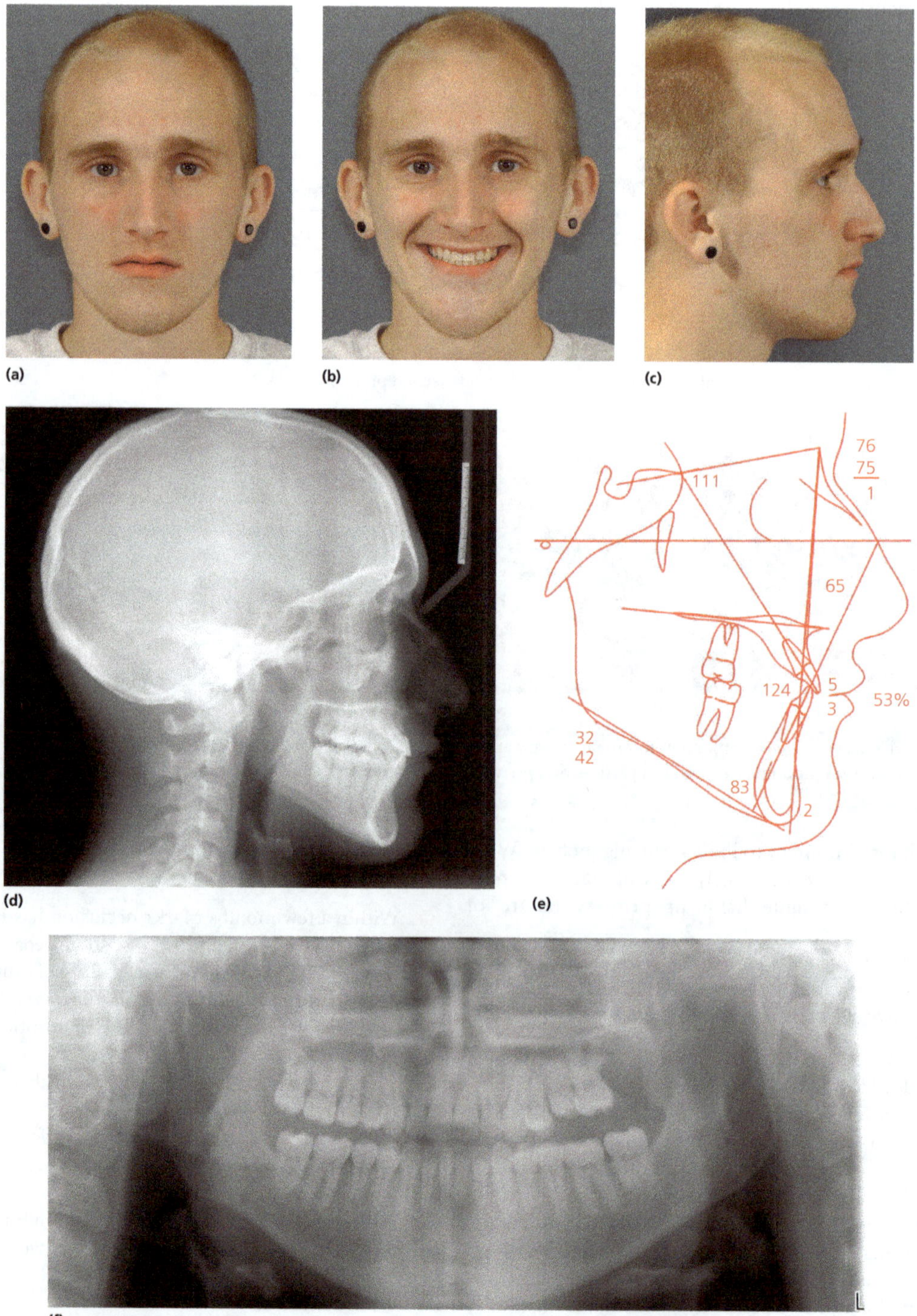

Figure 6.27 (a–k) Second treatment deband records of Mark.

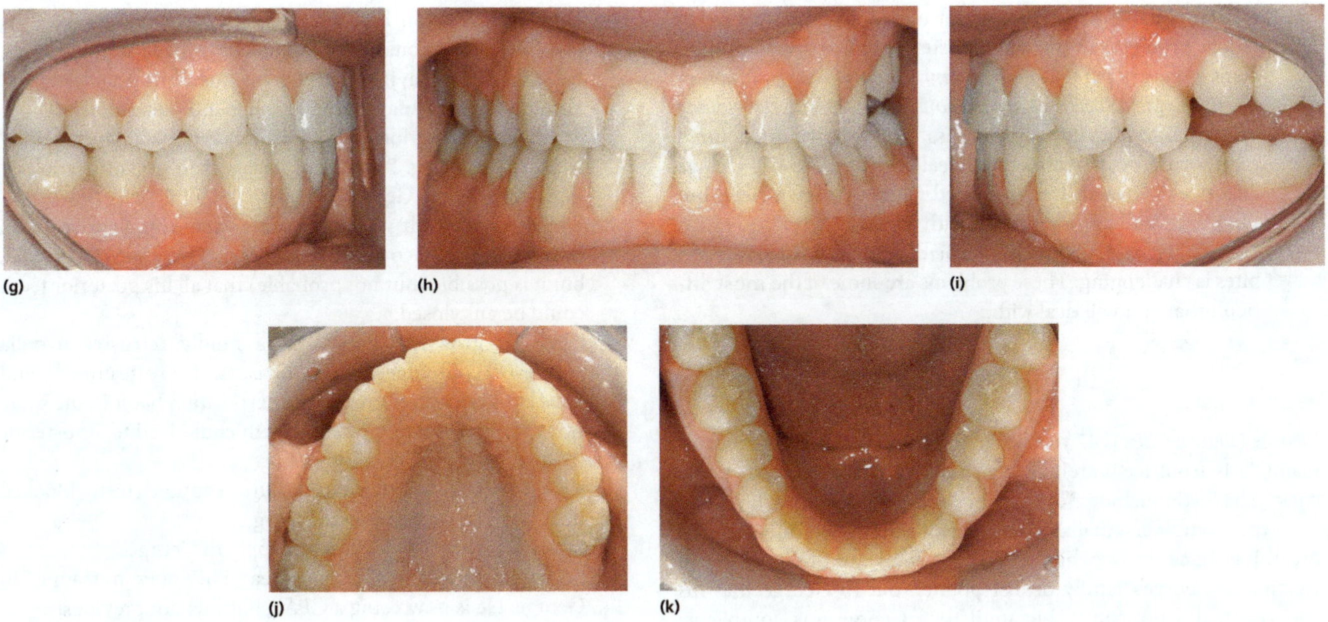

Figure 6.27 (Continued)

into occlusion, orthodontically. Freeing these teeth from the rest of the arch allowed the left open bite to be closed anterior to them.

- Other concurrent skeletal and dental anomalies may be present: Mark was Class III.

Q: What are your future options for Mark's ankylosed maxillary left second premolar and first molar?

A: Let's consider each of the possible options:

- Restoring the involved teeth with buildups or crowns after vertical growth is complete would not be reasonable for Mark because of the large left open-bite magnitude.
- Extraction of the involved teeth and replacement with bone grafts/implants would be reasonable, especially if Mark desires more chewing surface on his left side.
- Leaving the affected teeth in place and accepting a first premolar occlusion would be reasonable if Mark is satisfied with his present left occlusion.
- Performing a segmental osteotomy or distraction osteogenesis to close the left posterior open bite is a possible (heroic) treatment.
- Fabrication of a removable prosthetic (overlay) partial denture to provide greater left occlusion: this is a reasonable alternative, although not likely accepted by a young man.

Of these options, Mark chose to wear Hawley retainers and to maintain the left first premolar occlusion with a posterior open bite.

Q: What features of Mark's development were continually ignored throughout treatment?

A: Features include the following:

- Mark's Class III growth potential. Once this was detected at his 3-year retention check, it should have been addressed. Correcting his Class III relationship with elastics without knowing whether his growth was complete was a gamble. Even at this time, it would be prudent to consider placing Mark on a high-pull chin cup (and monitoring his AP) until you are sure growth is complete.
- A possible tongue or digit habit as an etiologic factor in his posterior open bite. This was not even considered until the second round of orthodontic treatment.

Q: What are your "take-home messages" for Mark?

A: Take-home messages include the following:

- Mark presented with a Class I molar occlusion, normal transverse relationship, normal anterior vertical relationship, and a bilateral posterior open bite. As a 10-year-old, the posterior open bite was assumed to be transient, resulting from his transitional dentition. The possibility that it could be due to a tongue interposition habit, or a digit habit, was completely ignored. The possibility that it could be due to primary failure of eruption was rightfully discounted because his first permanent molars were in occlusion.
- One difficulty in identifying cases of primary failure of eruption (which Mark most likely was) is that affected teeth may erupt into initial occlusion and then cease to erupt further.
- Placement of an LLHA to provide leeway space for Mark's erupting mandibular canines, and monitoring tooth eruption/development, was a good decision. When he returned a year later, the maxillary left first molar was found to be tipping mesially over the ankylosed maxillary left primary second molar. The decision to regain space by distalizing the maxillary left first molar with a headgear was good. The first sign that something unexpected was happening was after fixed appliances were placed and a mild left posterior open bite developed. Although this was initially closed with vertical elastics, 3 years following deband, the open bite reappeared. The continued worsening of this left posterior open bite with retreatment led to the suspicion that Mark exhibited primary failure of eruption. Successful treatment by *not* including the affected (ankylosed) teeth and accepting a left first premolar occlusion was reasonable.
- Teeth affected by primary failure of eruption may initially appear mobile, but will ankylose if subjected to orthodontic forces.

- Even in a patient with a posterior open bite, you must never ignore problems in the anteroposterior or transverse dimensions. *At every patient appointment, examine every patient in all three facial/occlusal dimensions and act on developing problems.* Mark's developing class III relationship required monitoring post-treatment to deal with the growth change effectively. Growth was identified as an unknown here, but not monitored closely or dealt with appropriately.
- Correcting and maintaining correction of posterior open bites is challenging. These problems are some of the most difficult that you will deal with.

Case George

George (Figure 6.28) is 47 years old and presents with the chief complaint, "My front teeth are wearing, and I have missing teeth in the back." His PMH includes "occasional chest pain upon exertion, and my wife complains that I snore when sleeping and even stop breathing once in a while." PDH includes routine restorative treatment. George's family dentist pointed out to George that his back teeth did not touch, but until then George was completely unaware that his back teeth were supposed to touch. TMJs: occasional bilateral "popping," but no pain. CR=CO. Periodontal status is WRN.

Q: List diagnostic findings/problems. What is your diagnosis?
A: See Table 6.4

Q: You query George further about his medical complaints. He says he occasionally feels a dull pain across the center of his chest upon exertion which is relieved by rest. He says that less exertion is required to cause the pain in cold weather. What problems do you suspect?
A: The chest pain upon exertion could be angina pectoris (myocardial eschemia), which should be addressed immediately, along with his sleep apnea.

Q: How do you proceed with these medical symptoms?
A: Refer George to an internist immediately for evaluation of both conditions. The internist reports back that George's occasional chest pain is angina pectoris and will be treated. George was referred to a sleep clinic and an otolaryngologist. Sleep apnea was confirmed. George underwent a polysomnography test, an uvulopalatoplasty, and now wears a CPAP every night. He is compliant with wearing the CPAP.

Q: In terms of George's posterior open bite, what should you check for? What questions should you ask George?
A: You should check for a tongue interposition habit. Have George close his eyes. Then, as you ask him to open his eyes (to distract him), gently retract his lips and check for a tongue habit. This was *not* done. Also, ask George if he has any habits (digit sucking, etc.) that would cause his posterior open bite. This was not done.

Q: What are *all* the possible etiologies of George's posterior open bite? List them and judge whether you think each could be contributing to his open bite.
A: Possible posterior open-bite etiologies include the following:

- Interpositional tongue habit. Even though George was not examined for a tongue posture habit, *key signs of this etiology are his mandibular posterior teeth crowns being "rolled" labially (torqued labially), his mandibular anterior spacing, and his broad mandibular arch—all features probably caused by excess tongue pressure.*
- Digit interposition habits. No inquiry was made regarding possible digit habits. This should have been done. A digit habit could be playing a role in his open bite but would not account for the labial torque of the mandibular molars.
- Temporary posterior open bites occurring while permanent teeth are erupting. Because of his age, this potential etiology does not apply to George.
- Ankylosis of teeth which prevents their complete eruption into occlusion. George's tooth mobility was never checked, but it is possible (but not probable) that all his posterior teeth could be ankylosed.
- Class III growth. George has a mildly retrusive maxilla (ANB=0°) and edge-to-edge incisors. These features could have led to a posterior tongue interposition habit in the same way that excess mandibular growth could lead to a posterior tongue interposition habit.
- Lack of space for complete tooth eruption (teeth blocked out). This does not apply to George.
- Systemic factors. This does not apply to George.
- Some treatments for sleep apnea. This does not apply to George. He is now using a CPAP, but was not previously.
- Primary failure of eruption. Let's examine each characteristic of primary failure of eruption and decide whether each could apply to George:
  1. First molars are always involved. George only has the mandibular right first molar, and it appears erupted with the other mandibular right posterior teeth.
  2. Posterior teeth are more frequently affected. *Yes, this would apply to George.*
  3. If a tooth in a more anterior position is affected, teeth more posterior are usually affected as well. *Yes.*
  4. Both primary and permanent teeth can be affected. *Yes.*
  5. The condition is bilateral. *Yes*, this is true for George.
  6. Teeth in both arches are often affected. *Yes*, George's open bite is bilateral.
  7. Affected teeth resorb the alveolar bone above the crown, and may erupt into initial occlusion and then cease to erupt further, or may fail to erupt entirely. *Yes.*
  8. Involved teeth may be displaced back and forth with manual pressure (indicating that they are not, initially, ankylosed). However, involved teeth tend to become ankylosed as soon as orthodontic eruptive forces are applied. This is *unknown for George.*
  9. If a small area of ankylosis is broken by manipulating the ankylosed tooth, it might be possible to move it for a short time, but re-ankylosis is inevitable. *Unknown.*
  10. Other concurrent skeletal and dental anomalies may be present. Excluding tooth loss, George has no other obvious skeletal or dental anomalies.

Q: In summary, what do you suspect is the most likely cause of George's bilateral posterior open bite?
A: *A tongue-positioning habit is the most likely cause of George's posterior open bite.* Yes, there is the possibility that he is an example of primary failure of eruption. And yes, there is the possibility that all his posterior teeth are ankylosed. But, the most probable cause of his open bite is tongue interpositioning habit (as a way for George to maintain a patent airway?).

Q: Considering the fact that the tongue has created a very broad mandibular arch and torqued the mandibular posterior teeth labially, what could this be a case of? How would you test for it?

A: George could be an example of macroglossia or psuedomacroglossia. Although there are no *objective* diagnostic criteria to diagnose macroglossia, the possible diagnostic criteria observed in George include excessive labial/buccal tip of teeth, and sleep apnea. Crenations of teeth on the tongue border (scalloping) is another possible criteria but was not observed. George's tongue could be of normal size but still appear enlarged (psuedomacroglossia) due to habitual posturing, hypertrophied tonsils/adenoidal tissue, low palatal vault, small arches which decrease oral cavity volume (doubtful, since George has such a broad mandibular arch), severe mandibular deficiency (not in George's case), and tumors, cysts, and so on.

Q: Since George could be an example of macroglossia or psuedomacroglossia, would you recommend a partial glossectomy before treating George orthodontically?

A: No. Although case reports of true macroglossia have been reported purporting the value of partial glossectomy [21, 22],

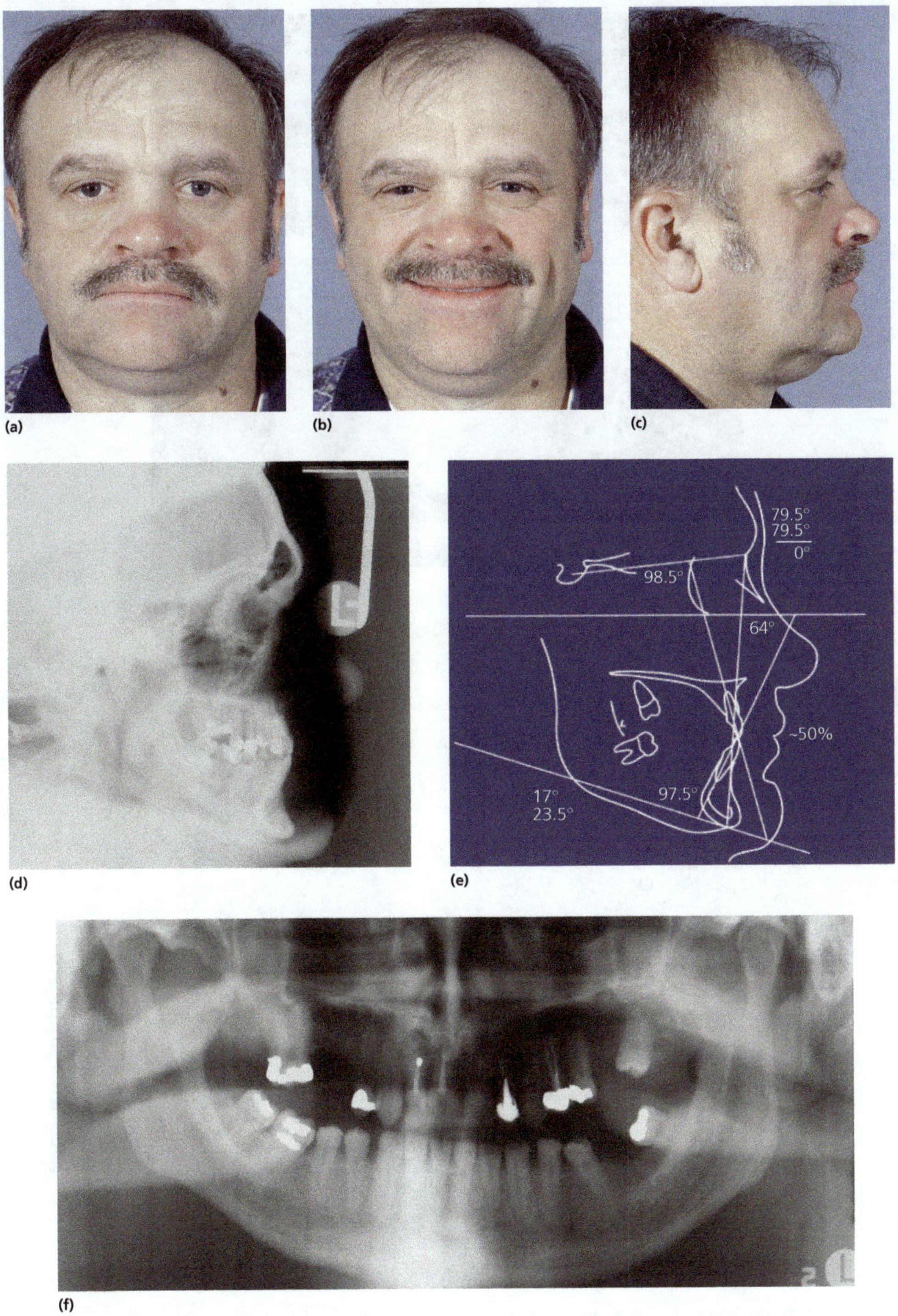

Figure 6.28 Initial records of George: (a–c) initial facial photographs, (d) lateral cephalograph, (e) cephalometric tracing, (f) pantomograph,

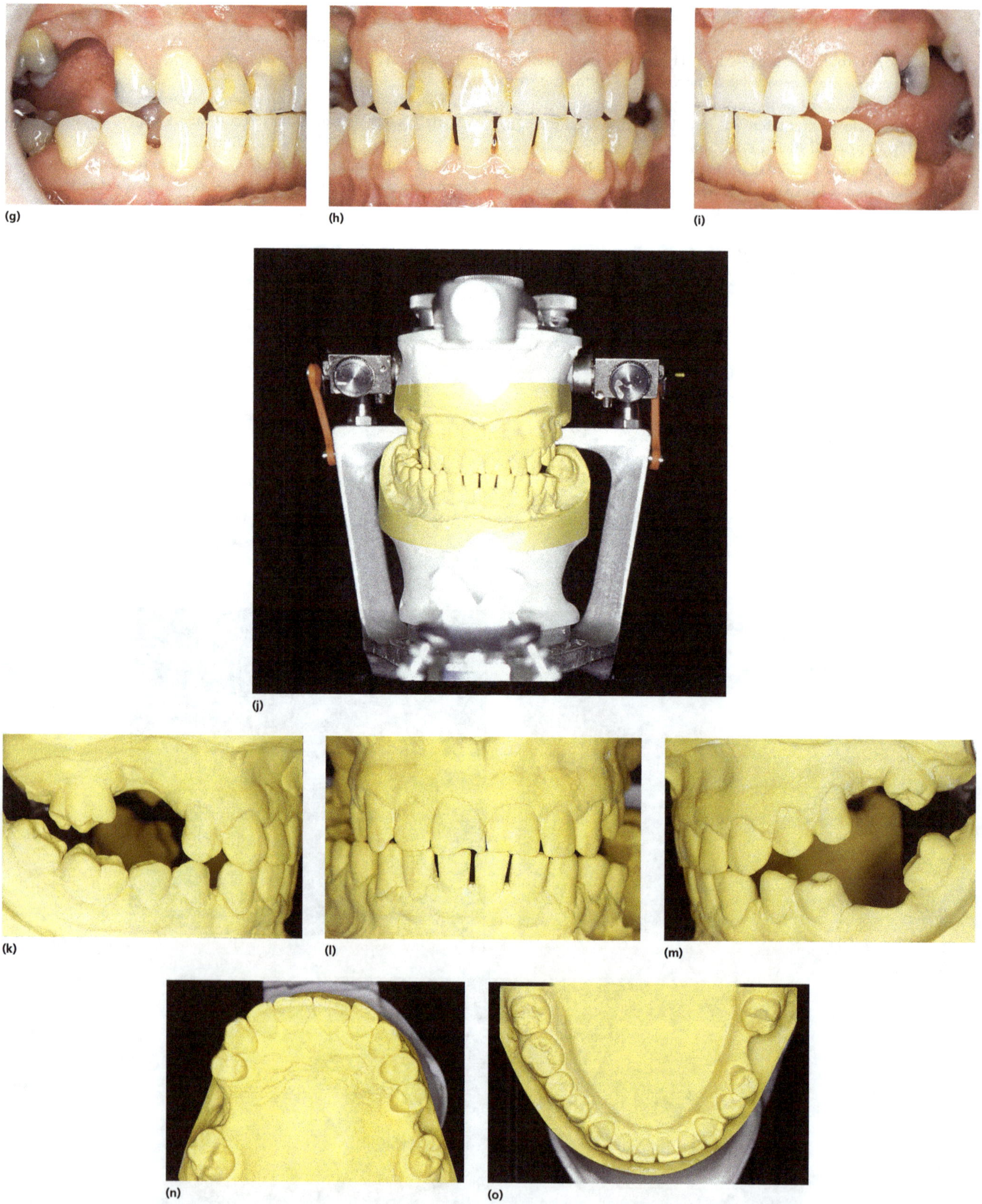

Figure 6.28 (Continued) (g–i) intraoral photographs, (j) models mounted on an articulator, and (k–o) model photographs.

it is considered of little or no value by some surgeons (In a conversation with two colleagues from the University of Iowa College of Dentistry, Department of Oral and Maxillofacial Surgery (Fridrich KL and Burton RG 2010), oral communication, October 25.) A partial glossectomy would be of no value in treating a case of psuedomacroglossia.

Table 6.4 Diagnostic findings and problem list for George.

Full face and profile	**Frontal view**
	Right-to-left cant of lips and lower border of mandible
	Soft tissue LAFH appears WRN (although he appears overclosed)
	Broad alar base width
	Minimal incisal display at rest (not shown here, can be seen in lateral cephalometric radiograph)
	Less than ideal central incisor display when smiling (maxillary central incisor gingival margins above upper lip vermillion margin)
	UDML 2–3 mm L of facial midline (not easily seen here)
	Profile view
	Relatively straight profile
	NLA covered by mustache (although it appears acute in the lateral cephalometric radiograph)
	Strong chin projection
	Cervicomental lipomatosis (redundant submental tissue)
	Obtuse lip–chin–throat angle
Ceph analysis	**Skeletal**
	Maxillary AP position is slightly retrusive (A-point behind Nasion perpendicular)
	Mandibular AP position is WRN (ANB = 0°, but maxilla is retrusive)
	Short skeletal LAFH (LAFH/TAFH = 50%, over two standard deviations less than normal of 55%, sd = 2%)
	Flat MPA (FMA = 17°; SNMP = 23.5°)
	Strong bony and soft tissue Pogonion
	Uneven right and left mandibular borders (lower border of mandible cant)
	Dental
	Upright maxillary incisors (maxillary incisor to SN = 98.5°)
	Mandibular incisor inclination WRN (FMIA = 64°)
	Posterior open bite evident at molars
Radiographs	Missing teeth #s 1, 3, 4, 14, 15, 18, 19, and 30
	Endodontic treatment teeth #s 8, 9, 10, and 12
	Retained root tip tooth #4
	Maxillary right condylar head appears flattened
Intraoral photos and models	Angle Class II division 2 subdivision right
	Iowa Classification: X II(4) I X (mounted models)
	OJ: 0 mm
	OB: 0%
	Bilateral posterior open bite
	Bilateral posterior lingual cross bite
	Bilateral mandibular posterior *labial* crown torque
	Mandibular anterior spacing
	3 mm curve of Spee
	LDML ~2 mm to right of UDML
	Maxillary and mandibular arches relatively symmetric
	Right-to-left occlusal cant
	Very broad mandibular arch
	Very thin and chipped enamel of maxillary incisors
Other	—
Diagnosis	Angle Class II division 2 subdivision right
	Bilateral posterior open bite and bilateral lingual cross bite

Q: Looking ahead to dealing with the bilateral posterior open bite, how might closure of the posterior open bite affect George's sleep apnea?

A: If George must hold his tongue forward to maintain a patent airway, then closing the posterior open bite could force his tongue lingual and back, obstructing his airway and worsening his sleep apnea. George's otolaryngologist was consulted. He felt that closure of the open bite would not worsen George's sleep apnea. Your highest priority in treating George should be *not to compromise George's airway* or worsen his sleep apnea. Even with orthodontic treatment approval from the otolaryngologist, it is important for you to monitor George's breathing/sleeping as treatment progresses. Periodically, ask George how he is doing with the CPAP and whether he exhibits hypersomnia (excess daytime sleepiness). Better yet, talk to his wife.

Q: Considering the magnitude of George's bilateral posterior *cross bite*, his sleep apnea, and his tongue interposition habit, do you have any thoughts about whether you should correct his posterior cross bite or leave it?

A: It may be prudent to leave George in posterior cross bite in order to avoid restricting his tongue space. His canines, however, could be ideally positioned.

Table 6.5 Primary problems list for George.

AP	X II (4) I X skeletal relationships WRN
Vertical	Bilateral posterior open bite
Transverse	Bilateral posterior lingual cross bite
Other	Missing teeth #s 1, 3, 4, 14, 15, 18, 19, and 30

Q: Are you concerned with the finding of occasional bilateral TMJ "popping"? Does it warrant treatment?

A: George does not exhibit TMJ pain. Asymptomatic disc displacement alone does not warrant treatment [23], and progression of a TM click to a more serious, nonreducing disk, is uncommon [24].

Q: What are your treatment goals?

A: Attempting to close (and maintain closure of) his posterior open bite, aligning and coordinating his arches, and achieving a Class I canine relationship with ideal overbite (10–20%) and overjet.

Q: Always stay focused on the patient's primary problems in each dimension (plus other major problems). What are George's primary problems?

A: George's primary problems are shown in Table 6.5

Q: How would you address George's vertical apical base discrepancy?
A: Trick question. There is no vertical *apical base* discrepancy. The jaws are in a good vertical orientation (Figure 6.28e). As a matter of fact, there is really not a significant apical base discrepancy in any dimension. George's posterior cross bite is impressive, but much of that cross bite is due to the labial "rolling out" of mandibular molars from tongue pressure.

Q: Rephrasing the question: how would you address George's posterior open bite? Suggest at least three techniques.
A: Possible techniques include the following:

- Assuming that a tongue interposition habit is causing George's open bite (not ankylosis or primary failure of eruption), then simply leveling the curve of Spee could erupt mesially tipped mandibular molars as they are uprighted/tipped distally. This could help close the posterior open bite.
- Posterior vertical elastics (criss-cross elastics) could be worn between fixed appliances in both arches to close the posterior open bite.
- Segmental osteotomies, or segmental distraction osteogenesis, could achieve posterior bite closure.
- Depending on how much the posterior open bite closed with the aforementioned techniques, the posterior teeth could be restored with buildups, implants, or crowns to close any residual posterior open bite. A removable prosthetic (overlay) partial denture could be used to provide posterior occlusion.

Q: An attempt to keep George's tongue out of the posterior open bite could be made using a tooth positioner, mandibular retainer with bilateral posterior loops, or an LLHA with soldered bilateral posterior loops. Would this be a good idea in George's particular case?
A: You could see how George tolerates wearing a tooth positioner or removable mandibular Hawley retainer with posterior loops. If he is able to wear those at night, then you could watch to see if his posterior open bite improves as teeth erupt. An LLHA with soldered posterior loops would *not* be a good idea, since he could not remove it if his breathing suffered.

Q: What should you tell George about the prognosis for closing (and maintaining closure of) his posterior open bite?
A: Tell him that there is no guarantee that the posterior open bite can be closed or that it will remain closed, especially if his tongue habit is not corrected. Even if surgery is used to close the open bite, muscle (tongue) may win over teeth and bone. There is one possibility of guaranteeing posterior open-bite closure. If the bite could be closed using osseointegrated implants (and crowns), then the bite should stay permanently closed.

Q: How could George's right Class II (4 mm) canine relationship be corrected?
A: If anterior overjet can be created by closing mandibular spaces, then the right Class II canine relationship could be corrected using Class II elastics, other interarch Class II correctors (e.g., Jasper Jumpers and Forsus), or reciprocal space closure between the maxillary right canine and maxillary right molar.

Q: Are there *unknowns* that you should eliminate before you establish George's final treatment plan?
A: The effect of treatment on his sleep apnea and your ability to close the posterior open bite are the two major unknowns. As just stated, you could begin treatment by putting George in a tooth positioner or mandibular retainer with posterior loops to see how he tolerates a new tongue position (this was not done). Other unknowns include cooperation, an undetected shift, and hygiene.

Q: Would you consider treating George nonextraction? With extraction of anterior teeth? With extraction of posterior teeth?
A: Considering the fact that George has so many missing teeth already, significant spacing in both arches, upright maxillary incisors, and reasonable inclination of his mandibular incisors, attempting nonextraction treatment is recommended.

Q: What treatment options would you consider for George? Suggest both a surgical and nonsurgical option.
A: After establishing his problem list, treatment goals, identifying the major problem in each dimension (plus other problems), identifying unknowns, and considering non-extraction/extraction approaches, the following options were considered:

- Orthodontic/prosthodontic treatment only:
  - Obtain an endodontic evaluation to assess previous RCT.
  - Consult with prosthodontics.
  - Band/bond dental arches, level and align arches, upright molars/reduce posterior open-bite (mesially tipped molars should erupt as they are uprighted/tipped distally).
  - Close mandibular anterior spaces and create OJ.
  - Correct right Class II canine relationship by reciprocal maxillary space closure.
  - Leave in posterior cross bite.
  - Refer to prosthodontics—overlay removable partial denture and fixed partial dentures to complete posterior open-bite closure.
- Orthodontic/surgical/prosthodontic treatment:
  - Obtain an endodontic evaluation to assess previous RCT.
  - Consult with oral surgery and prosthodontics.
  - Band/bond dental arches and level and align arches.
  - Close mandibular anterior spaces and create OJ.
  - Perform a three-piece Le Fort I maxillary osteotomy—correct midlines, inferiorly reposition maxillary left and right segments to close the posterior open-bite.
  - Leave in posterior cross bite.
  - Prosthodontic treatment, prn.

Q: Considering everything we have discussed thus far, what treatment do you recommend?
A: George elected to attempt nonsurgical treatment.

Q: What are the specific objectives of treatment for the maxilla, mandible, maxillary dentition, and mandibular dentition in all three planes of space?
A: Specific objectives of treatment for George are as follows:

Maxilla
AP: Maintain.
Vertical: Maintain.
Transverse: Maintain.

Mandible
AP: Maintain.
Vertical: Maintain.
Transverse: Maintain.

Maxillary dentition
AP: Maintain molars (upright and protract). Maintain canines and incisors.
Vertical: Erupt molars. Maintain canines and incisors.
Intermolar width: Maintain intermolar width.

Mandibular dentition

AP: Upright molars (distalize crowns). Retract canines and incisors.

Vertical: Erupt molars. Maintain incisors

Intermolar/intercanine width: Maintain intermolar and intercanine widths.

Q: How did George's treatment proceed?

A: Fixed appliances were placed in both arches. The arches were leveled to 0.017 × 0.025 stainless steel archwires at which time a mandibular 0.036 stainless steel "overlay" wire was placed to constrict the mandibular arch (Figure 6.29). This was done to attempt correction of his posterior cross bite (contradicting our earlier plan to leave him in cross bite and leave room for his tongue). Why? George, and his wife, reported that orthodontic treatment was not affecting his breathing or sleeping. His sleep apnea was well controlled with the CPAP.

Spaces were closed in the mandibular anterior. The mandibular archwire was increased to 0.019 × 0.025″ stainless steel (Figure 6.30, note overlay wire in Figure 6.30e).

Because the right canine Class II relationship had appeared to improve, Class II elastics were worn on the right to make the AP correction. Cross-bite elastics were worn on the left. All mandibular spaces were closed except for the mandibular left first molar edentulous area. Vertical elastics were worn minimally, only for a few months at the end of treatment on the left posterior. George was debanded and placed in a tooth positioner, to maintain the occlusion and keep his tongue away from the teeth, and later in vacuum-formed (temporary) retainers.

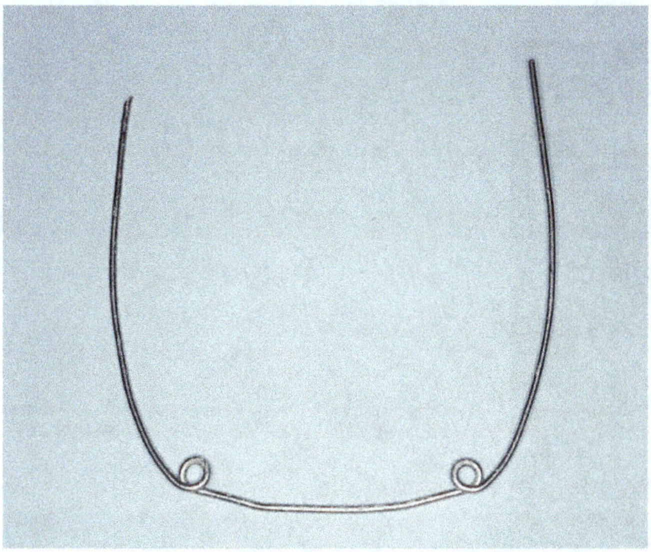

Figure 6.29 Constricted 0.036 stainless steel overlay wire to reduce George's mandibular posterior labial crown torque and constrict the arch.

Q: Once goals were achieved with George's treatment, what principle was violated?

A: George should have been maintained in fixed appliances, in "active retention" for months before debanding, to monitor stability/help insure stability. He was not.

Q: Deband records are shown in Figure 6.31. What do you observe?

A: George's deband records show:

- There was no change in his facial, smile, or profile esthetics (Figure 6.28a–c vs. Figure 6.31a–c).
- As his mesially tipped molars were uprighted and tipped distally (Figure 6.31f), they erupted. Surprisingly, this orthodontic movement alone nearly closed the posterior open bite on the right and completely closed the posterior open bite on the left (Figure 6.31m, o). Remember, vertical elastics were never used on the right and were only used on the left for a short while at the end of treatment.
- Mandibular incisor edges were retracted.
- Right canines are still Class II by 1–2 mm.
- Midlines are not coincident by 1 mm.

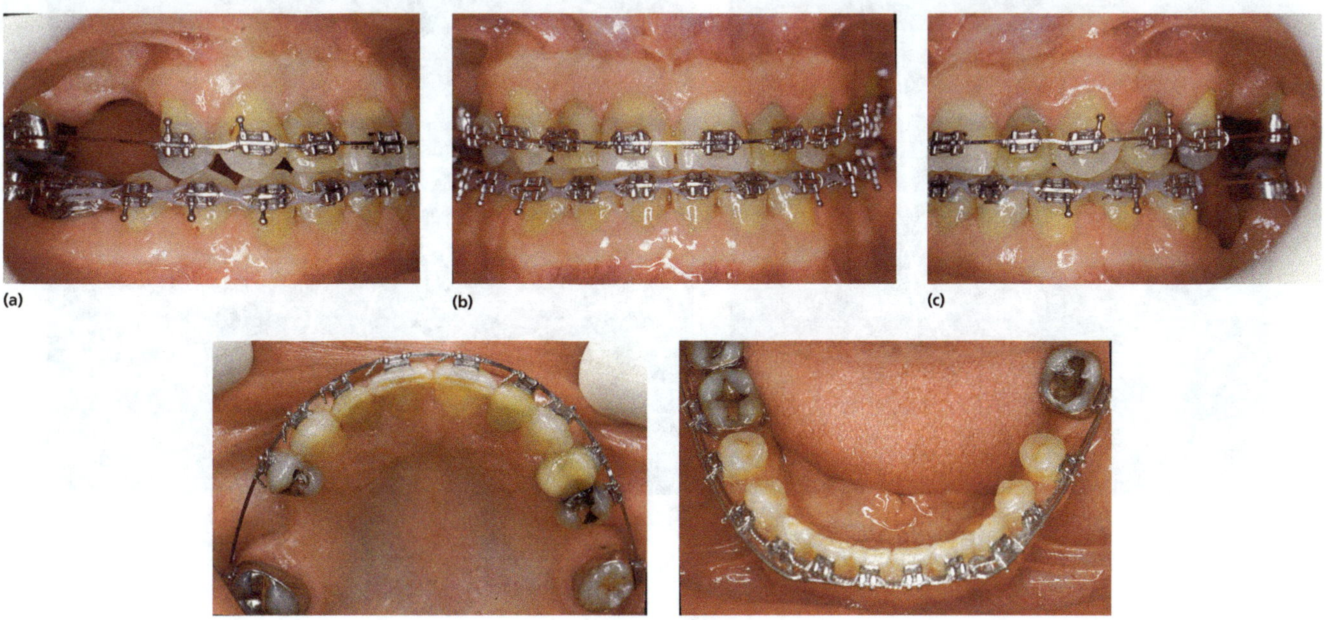

(a) (b) (c) (d) (e)

Figure 6.30 (a–e) George's progress records.

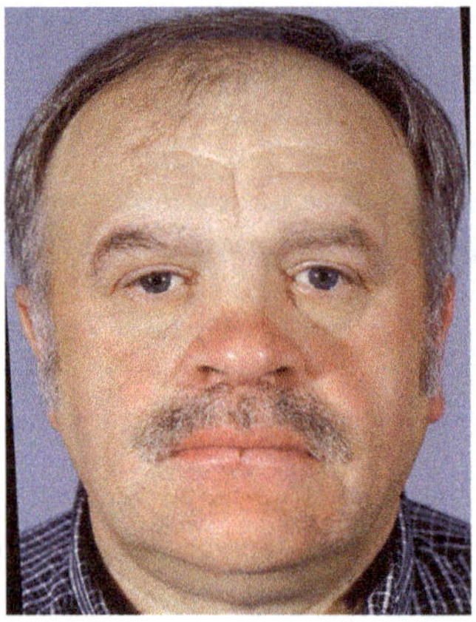
(a)

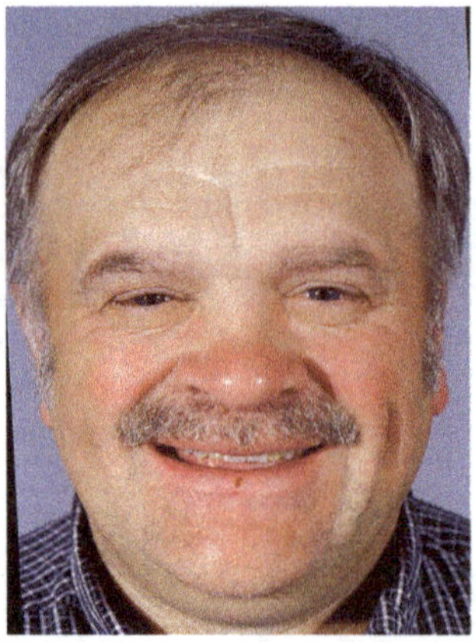
(b)

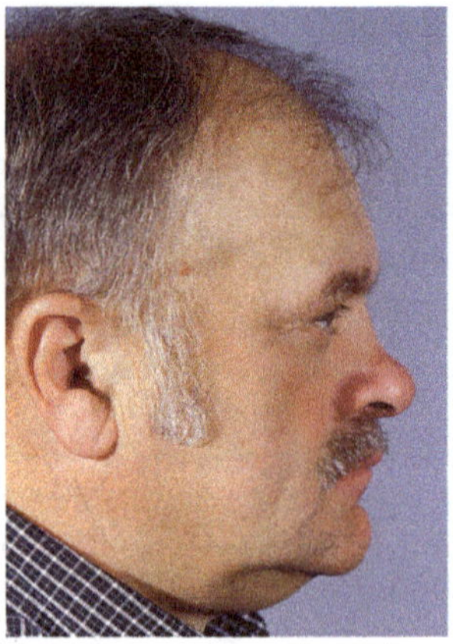
(c)

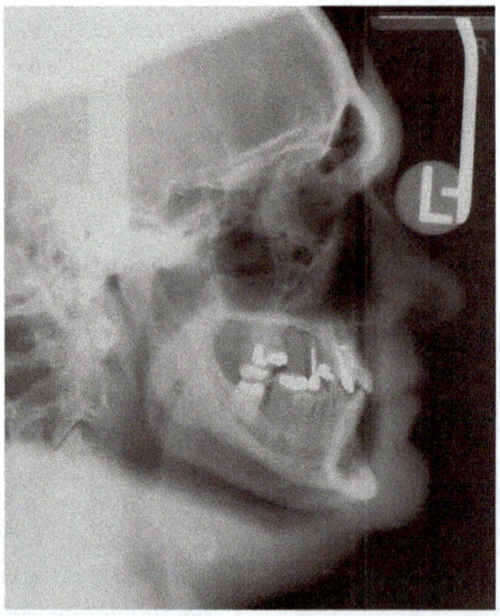
(d)

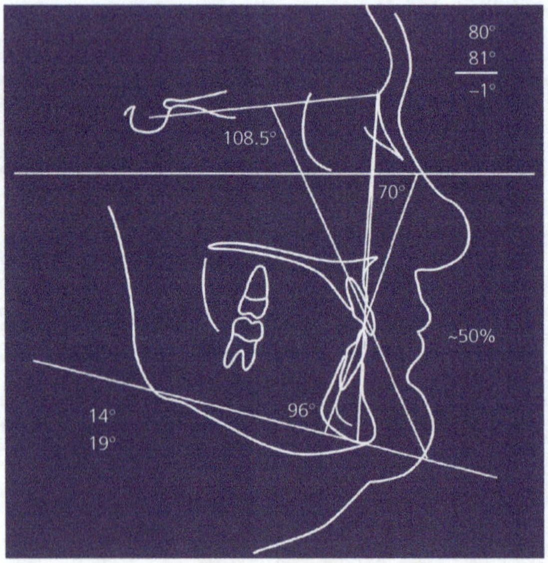

(e)

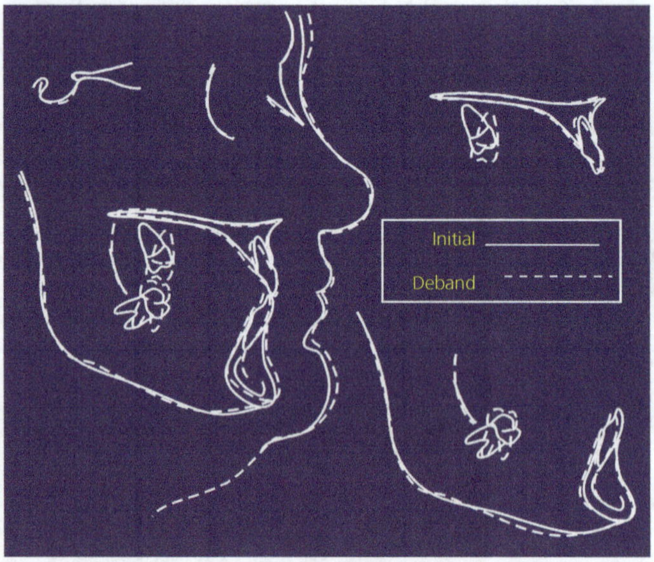

(f)

Figure 6.31 (a–q) George's deband records.

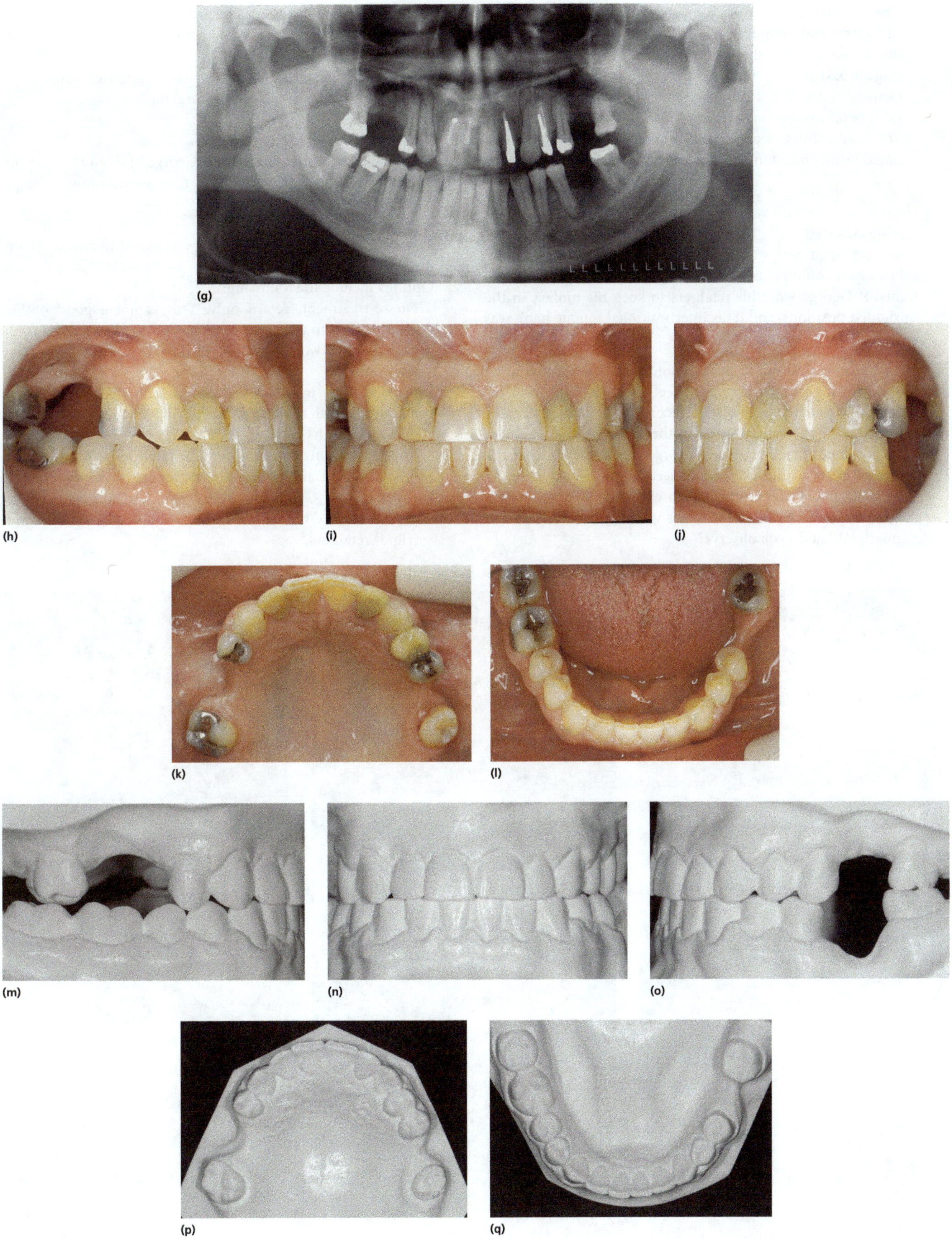

Figure 6.31 (Continued)

- The bilateral cross bite has been corrected.
- Maxillary and mandibular left canines exhibit too much distal root tip, and the roots of many teeth are nonparallel (Figure 6.31g).
- Generalized root blunting is seen throughout the dentition (Figure 6.31g).
- Tooth 20 exhibits a periapical radiolucency—this was evaluated by an endodontist who recommended monitoring.

Q: Considering how successful George's posterior open bite closure was, what do you now think your chances are of maintaining closure?

A: Since his open bite was closed (surprisingly) by uprighting molars, you could assume that this correction would be maintained if George wore his retainers to keep his molars in the uprighted positions, and if his interpositional tongue habit was corrected by the open-bite closure.

Q: Next, George underwent prosthodontic treatment, including crowns for his maxillary anterior teeth and an FPD from his mandibular left first premolar to second molar. New vacuum-formed retainers were fabricated as the occlusion changed with each prosthetic treatment, and George was asked to wear the retainers all the time except when eating or when drinking something hot. George returned to clinic some months later (Figure 6.32) stating that he wore his vacuum-formed retainers regularly. What do you observe?

A: Observations include the following:
- Unfortunately, his bilateral posterior open bite *and* cross bite have returned.
- Space has opened distal to the mandibular right canine and distal to the mandibular left central incisor.

Q: Why did this relapse happen?

A: This is speculation, but either George did NOT wear his vacuum-formed retainers all the time or his tongue simply overpowered these retainers.

Q: What are your options now? What additional treatment, if any, do you recommend?

A: Options include the following:
- No re-treatment, retain only. This is not a good option. George went to the expense of the left FPD so that he could chew, and he would still like to be able to chew. He cannot chew now.
- Place George in Hawley retainers with bilateral posterior loops in one arch to try to correct his tongue habit. Monitor posterior tooth eruption.
- Re-treat with fixed orthodontic appliances. Close the mandibular spaces, and close the posterior open bites with vertical elastics. Hold George in "active retention" for an extensive period of time before debanding. Retain him with Hawley (rigid) retainers.

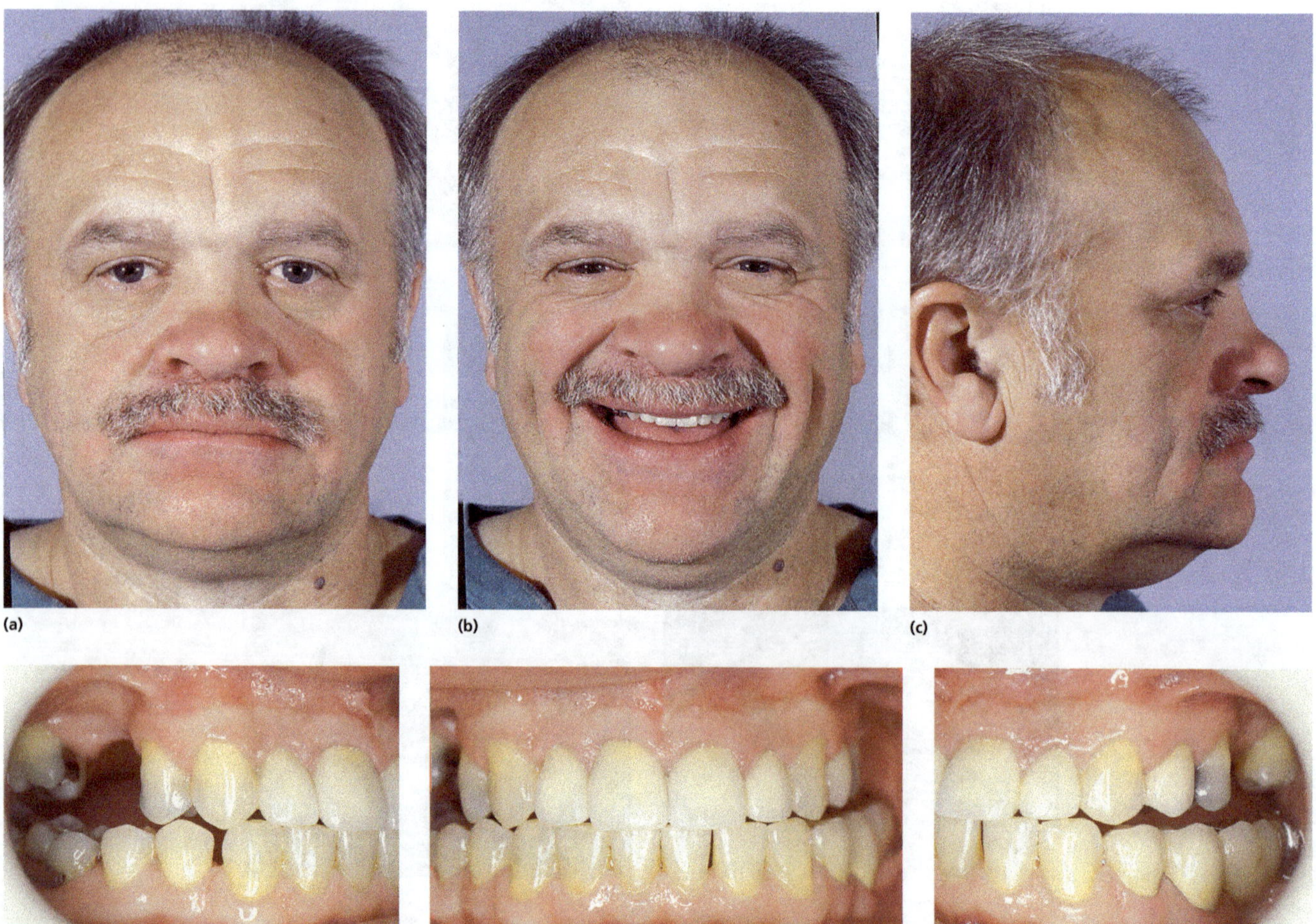

(a) (b) (c) (d) (e) (f)

Figure 6.32 (a–n) Records of George following prosthodontic treatment. George stated that he had been wearing his vacuum-formed retainers, regularly.

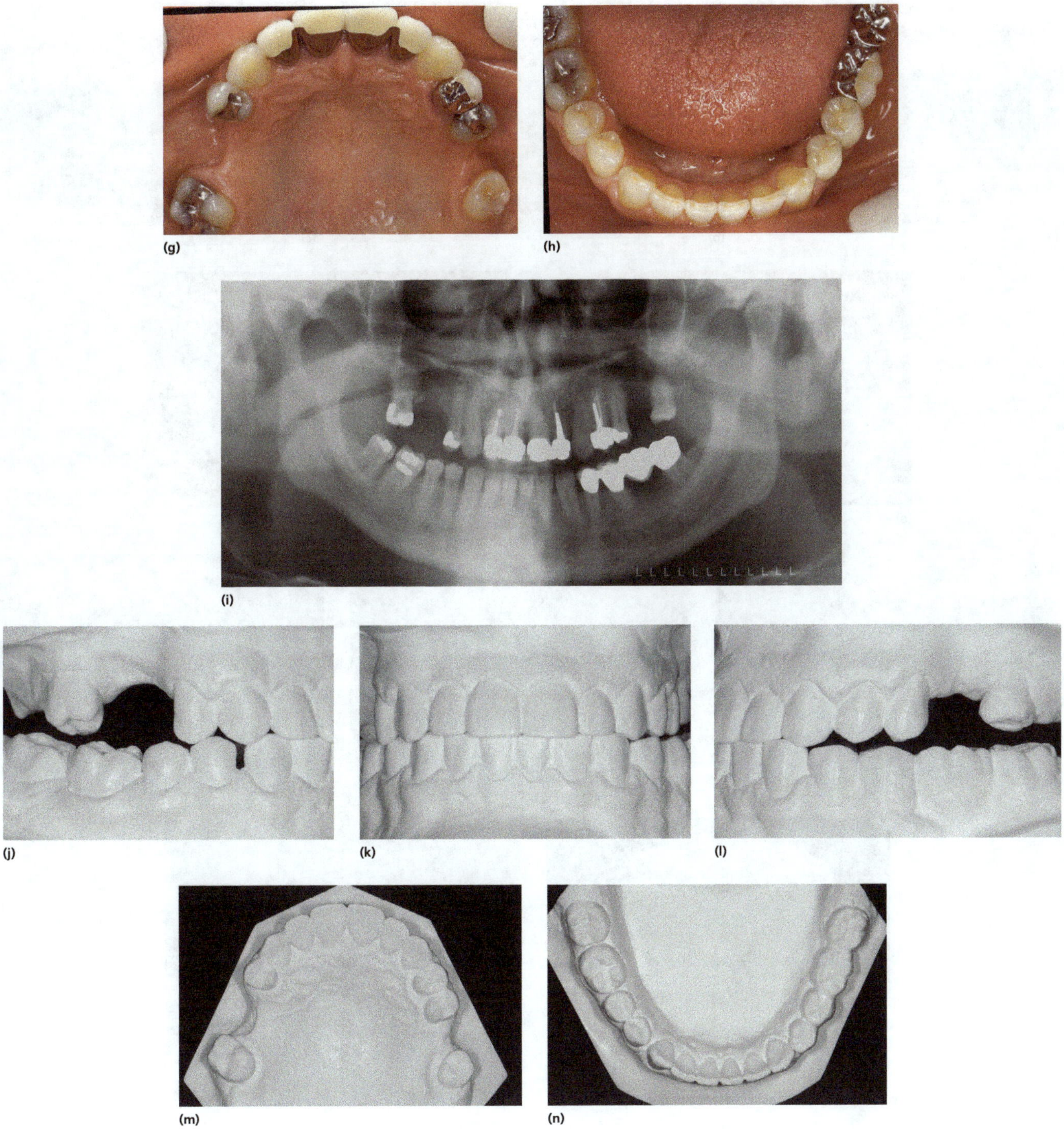

Figure 6.32 (Continued)

- Re-treat with a surgical procedure. This is not a good option. Treatment could relapse all over again unless better retention compliance (with relatively rigid retainers) is achieved.
- Place an overlay maxillary RPD so that George can chew but allow the tongue to fill the current transverse space (this was the option that George selected, Figure 6.33).

Q: George has been subsequently followed for years, and his occlusion appears stable. What are your take-home pearls from this case?

A: Take-home pearls include the following:

- George presented with a bilateral posterior open bite caused by an interpositional tongue habit. Although this habit was never confirmed clinically, key signs of it included his mandibular posterior teeth crowns being "rolled" labially (torqued labially), mandibular anterior spacing, and a very broad mandibular arch. His significant posterior lingual cross bite was also caused by his tongue—pushing his mandibular posterior teeth labially. Both conditions were successfully treated by uprighting/distal tipping his molars (erupting them) and tipping his mandibular molars lingually using a constricted overlay archwire and fixed appliances. This treatment later relapsed either from poor retainer compliance or excessive tongue force. Final transverse stability was achieved by permitting the tongue to occupy a large enough space. Final

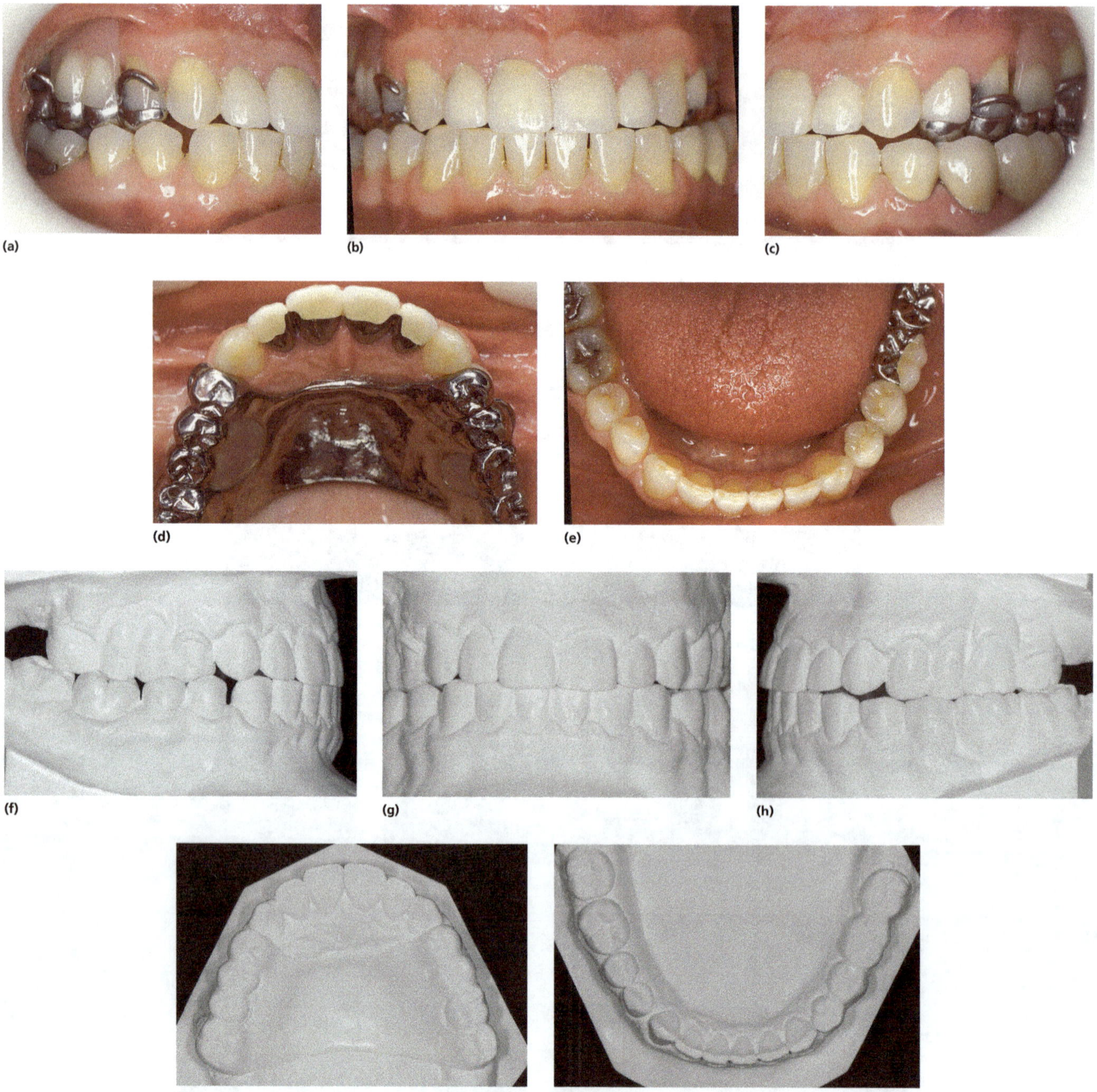

(a) (b) (c) (d) (e) (f) (g) (h) (i) (j)

Figure 6.33 (a–j) Final records of George with overlay maxillary RPD.

posterior occlusal function was achieved using an overlay removable partial denture.

- Any time you are faced with a posterior open bite, consider *all* possible etiologies of the open bite before defining your treatment plan. These etiologies include the following:
  - Interpositional tongue habit
  - Digit habit
  - Temporary posterior open bites occurring while permanent teeth are erupting
  - Ankylosis of teeth
  - Class III growth with development of a tongue posturing habit
  - Lack of space for complete tooth eruption
  - Systemic factors
  - Primary failure of eruption
  - Some treatments for obstructive sleep apnea
- Initially, there existed the possibility that George was an example of primary failure of eruption or posterior teeth ankylosis. However, both of these possibilities were proved wrong by the fact that his posterior teeth moved during treatment.
- Posterior open bites are corrected by erupting posterior teeth with fixed appliances and archwires (uprighting mesially tipped posterior teeth), posterior vertical elastics, surgery, or prosthodontics.
- George's posterior tongue interposition habit was never corrected. A better treatment would have begun by attempting to modify his habit (wearing a tooth positioner or

removable mandibular Hawley retainer with posterior loops to block the tongue). If George was able to wear those at night (or day and night), then you could monitor to see if his posterior open bite improved with tooth eruption alone. A major, unanswered, question still remains—why does George have this habit?

- Regarding his transverse relationship, heavy (e.g., 0.032″ stainless steel) overlay wires can be very effective in generating *bilateral* forces to constrict or expand dental arches. Such overlay wires do not generate unilateral forces. If you require *unilateral* orthodontic transverse expansion or constriction, consider "stepping-in" or "stepping-out" the archwire for single teeth or consider cross-bite elastics for multiple teeth.
- Should we have left George in posterior cross bite in order to avoid restricting his tongue space (no overlay wire) as we originally considered? Yes, if I had to treat George again, I would probably leave him in posterior lingual cross bite (canines properly coordinated) to provide adequate tongue space.
- Initial closure of George's posterior open bite was remarkably successful. However, in retrospect, George should have been maintained in fixed appliances, in "active retention," for (many) months before debanding. This would have given us a chance to monitor the stability of his correction. Additionally, instead of being placed in (flexible) vacuum-formed retainers, it may have been prudent to immediately place George in *rigid* removable Hawley retainers the *same day he was debanded.* Unlike the flexible light vacuum-formed retainers, if George wore the rigid retainers, then relapse may have been far less. Ultimately, guaranteed stability may only come from placement of posterior implants connected to posterior teeth and from correction of his tongue habit.
- Posterior open bites can be very, very difficult problems to correct and to maintain corrected.
- Your first priority with George was to monitor him to confirm that his airway was never compromised during treatment.

Case Kreslyn

Kreslyn (Figure 6.34) is a 15-year, 4-month-old who presents and with the chief complaint, "I was referred for treatment by my dentist." PMH includes Gordon Syndrome (Rx: hydrochlorothiazide), and PDH is WRN. Periodontal tissues are WRN. TMJs: Anterior disc displacement (ADD) with reduction, no pain. CR—CO shift of 1 mm forward and left.

Q: List diagnostic findings/problems. What is your diagnosis?

A: See Table 6.6

Q: We failed to obtain one critical piece of information thus far. What is it?

A: Kreslyn's chief complaint. She told us that her family dentist referred her for treatment, but we do not know Kreslyn's concerns (if any). What does she want? What do her parents want? Further discussions of her condition led to the understanding that Kreslyn wants a nice smile and to be able to chew food. *Determine what your patient's desires are*, not just the referring doctor's.

Q: Kreslyn's face is reasonably symmetric. And yet she is Class III (molar) on the right and Class II (molar) on the left. How do you explain this?

A: She has a dental asymmetry with her maxillary left posterior ahead of her maxillary right posterior by 2–3 mm.

Q: What is Gordon Syndrome?

A: It is a rare familial autosomal-dominant syndrome characterized by a mutation in the chloride channel in the distal renal tubule, which results in enhanced chloride resorption. It is also characterized by hyperkalemia, normal glomerular filtration, and hypertension. Clinical findings include short stature, muscle weakness, intellectual impairment, impaired growth, dental abnormalities, and severe hypertension by the third decade. Correction of physiologic abnormalities is achieved with thiazide diuretics.

Q: Kreslyn appears mandibular prognathic in the frontal view (Figure 6.34a). However, her mandible is relatively normal (Figure 6.34d, e). Why?

A: Kreslyn's mandible *is* relatively prognathic, relative to a deficient maxilla, that is. Class III patients with excessive mandibular AP growth, deficient maxillary AP growth, or a combination of both can all appear to be mandibular prognathic. Cephalometric analysis can eliminate confusion regarding maxillary and mandibular absolute AP positions. Try covering Kreslyn's maxillary area with your fingers in Figure 6.34a–c. You will notice that her mandibular projection appears reasonably referenced to the rest of her face. Clues of maxillary deficiency in Kreslyn's case include her flat paranasal areas, inferior sclera show, and deep paranasal folds when smiling. However, these clues are not present in every patient with maxillary AP hypoplasia. Why? The facial soft tissue drape tends to mask underlying skeletal imbalances. For example, if the soft tissue is thick, then it can mask underlying skeletal deficiencies; if it is thin, then it can mask excesses. On the other hand, if the soft tissue is thick, then it can exaggerate excesses; or if the soft tissue is thin, then it can exaggerate deficiencies.

Q: List possible etiologies of Kreslyn's posterior open bite. Specifically, list etiologies that you feel *could* be implicated in her posterior open bite, and list etiologies that you feel *could not* be implicated.

A: Etiologies that could be implicated include the following:

- Interpositional tongue habit (with associated constricted maxilla).
- Ankylosis of primary posterior teeth preventing their complete eruption. You would expect to see continued eruption of permanent teeth and (radiographically) a vertical alveolar crest step between ankylosed primary teeth and adjacent erupting permanent teeth. We *do* see such alveolar crest steps (indicating ankylosis, Figure 6.34f) in the maxillary right primary second molar, maxillary left primary second molar, and mandibular right primary second molar, but not in the mandibular left primary second molar.
- Class III growth resulting in an edge-to-edge incisor relationship, especially if a tongue interpositional habit is acquired as a result.

Etiologies not implicated include the following:

- Digit habit. Kreslyn denies any such habit.
- Temporary posterior open bites seen soon after loss of the primary molars and before complete emergence of the permanent tooth. Not a probable cause of Kreslyn's posterior open bite because Kreslyn lacks permanent successors for her primary teeth
- Lack of space for complete tooth eruption (teeth blocked out). Not a probable cause. Her maxillary primary second molars, and mandibular right primary second molar, are

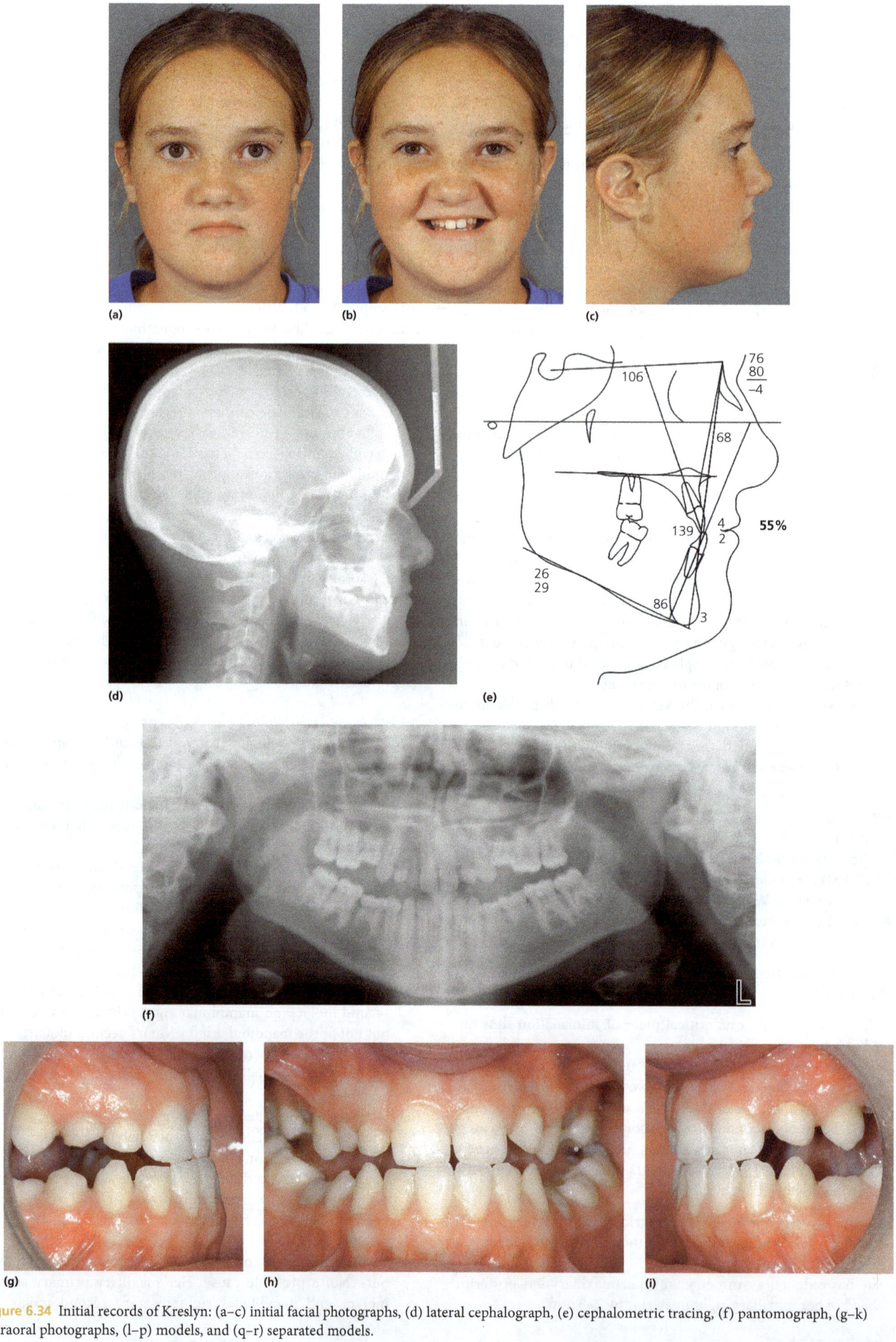

Figure 6.34 Initial records of Kreslyn: (a–c) initial facial photographs, (d) lateral cephalograph, (e) cephalometric tracing, (f) pantomograph, (g–k) intraoral photographs, (l–p) models, and (q–r) separated models.

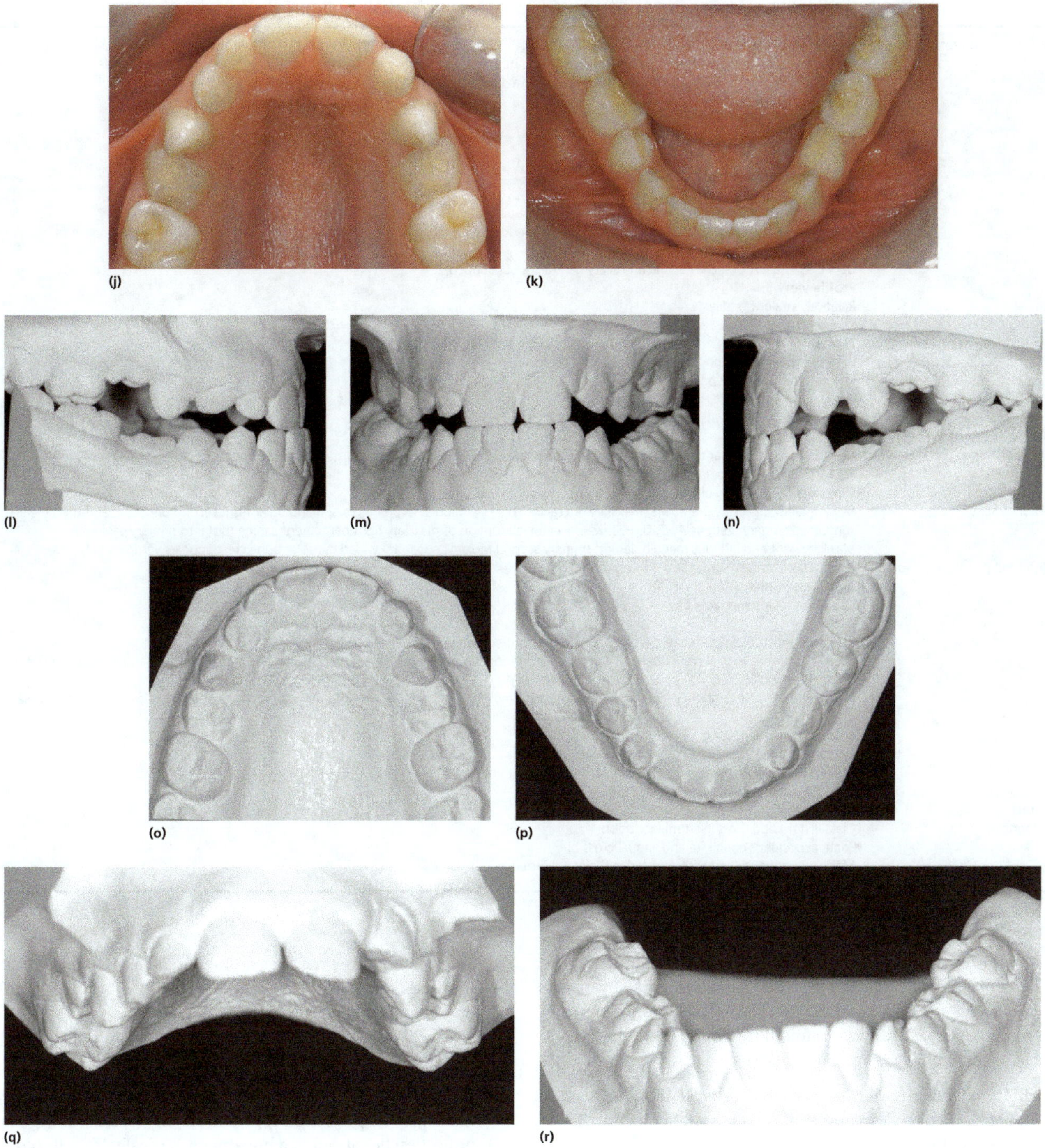

Figure 6.34 (Continued)

blocked out because they are ankylosed with the permanent molars erupting up and over them.

- Systemic factors found in patients with certain syndromes, such as cleidocranial dysplasia, ectodermal dysplasia, Gardner syndrome, and Apert syndrome. Not a probable cause because Gordon syndrome does not present with a feature of posterior open bite.
- Primary failure of eruption. Not a probable cause because if a tooth in a further anterior position is affected, more posterior teeth are usually affected as well. In Kreslyn's case, the more posterior permanent teeth appear to be erupting normally. Also, Kreslyn's posterior open bite is symmetric (primary failure of eruption is usually asymmetric).
- Some treatments for sleep apnea (Kreslyn is not being treated for sleep apnea).

Q: Every time, *every time* you meet with a patient for a case presentation (or a treatment appointment), you should first check what?

A: Check the patient's bite once again to look for a shift. If you cannot confirm centric relation position, then your entire treatment plan (or your last treatment decision) could have been based on an inaccurate jaw relationship. If you are unsure of the

Table 6.6 Diagnostic findings and problem list for Kreslyn.

Full face and profile	**Frontal view**
	Reasonably symmetric (chin pointed deviated approximately 1 mm to left)
	Soft tissue LAFH WRN (and yet she has a mildly overclosed appearance)
	Prognathic appearance
	Inferior sclera show
	Lip competence
	Flat paranasal areas
	Deep paranasal folds when smiling
	Large buccal corridors (constricted maxilla)
	Right-to-left cant of maxillary arch (compared to interpupillary line, Figure 6.34b)
	~0.5 mm incisal display at rest less than ideal central incisor display when smiling (maxillary central incisor gingival margins apical to maxillary lip vermillion margin)
	UDML ~1 mm left of facial midline (maxillary central incisors tipped)
	Profile view
	Relatively straight profile
	Obtuse NLA
Ceph analysis	**Skeletal**
	Retrusive maxillary AP position (A-Point behind Nasion-perpendicular line)
	Normal mandibular AP position
	Skeletal LAFH WRN (LAFH/TAFH=55%)
	Slight discrepancy between left and right mandibular borders
	Dental
	Maxillary incisors appear to have normal inclination (although $\underline{1}$ to SN = 106°, this large angle could be due to a high Sella position)
	Ideal mandibular incisor inclination (FMIA = 68°)
	Bilateral posterior open bite evident
Radiographs	Missing teeth: maxillary premolars, maxillary lateral incisors, mandibular left premolars, mandibular right second premolar, and third molars retained primary teeth #s A, C, D, H, J, K, L, T ectopic eruption of maxillary right permanent canine (distal to primary canine)
	Maxillary right and left plus mandibular left primary second molars appear ankylosed (alveolar bone crest appears vertically deficient)
Intraoral photos and models	Angle Class III molar right, Class II molar left
	Iowa Classification: III (1–2) III (8) III (6) II (2–3)
	OJ: ~−1 mm, anterior cross bite
	OB: 0%
	Maxillary central incisors are stepped down relative to molars bilateral posterior open bite
	Bilateral posterior lingual cross bite with transverse posterior compensations (maxillary posterior labial crown torque and mandibular posterior lingual crown torque)
	Maxillary transverse deficiency (maxillary first molar intermolar palatal cusp width = 34 mm; mandibular first molar intermolar central fossa width = 40 mm)
	Maxillary anterior spacing
	Dental asymmetry maxillary left posterior ahead 2–3 mm
	Maxillary and mandibular midlines approximately coincident
	Robust mandibular anterior periodontium
Other	Poor hygiene
Diagnosis	Class III right and Class II left malocclusion
	Bilateral posterior open bite and lingual cross bite
	Maxillary transverse and anteroposterior skeletal deficiency

presence of a shift at the case presentation, then do whatever you need to do to help you detect (eliminate) the shift before finalizing a treatment plan (e.g., RME, level and align arches, and biteplate). Kreslyn was found to have a 1 mm forward and left shift at her case presentation.

Q: In terms of her posterior open bite, what else should you check for at Kreslyn's case presentation? In terms of her incisal display, what else should you check for?

A: Check for a tongue interposition habit as a cause of her posterior open bite. Kreslyn was asked to remain perfectly still and to close her eyes. She was then asked to open her eyes (to distract her), while her lips were gently and quickly retracted. A tongue interposition habit was detected (Figure 6.35a–c). Therefore, we conclude that *Kreslyn's posterior open bite is due to a combination of tongue habit, ankylosis of primary maxillary molars, and ankylosis of the mandibular right primary molar.* Also, you should examine the amount of incisal display she exhibits when relaxed (Figure 6.35d) and in posed smile (Figure 6.35e). Note the near absence of incisal display when relaxed, despite the fact that the maxillary central incisors are stepped down relative to the posterior teeth (Figure 6.34h, m). She exhibits less than ideal incisal display in posed smile (border of maxillary lip hangs below the maxillary central incisal gingival margin).

Q: Figure 6.36 shows 45° facial views that, in some cases of severe midface deficiency, may demonstrate deficient zygomatic (malar) process projection. However, in these views Kreslyn's malar process projection appears adequate (soft tissue zygomatic projection lies ahead of a line drawn vertically from the corneal apex). Are there other facial views you should photograph?

A: One view that may be helpful, but was not made, is a view with Kreslyn separating her teeth *just wide enough to have her lips barely touching*—to demonstrate elimination of the possible soft tissue overclosure. In other words, with the inadequate incisal display Kreslyn exhibits when relaxed (even with her maxillary incisors being stepped down), we would have expected her soft tissue drape to reflect a need for increased vertical skeletal length. If she can open (with her lips just touching) and eliminate a mildly overclosed appearance, then this observation could help us decide to down graft her anterior maxilla slightly if we also decide to surgically advance her deficient maxilla.

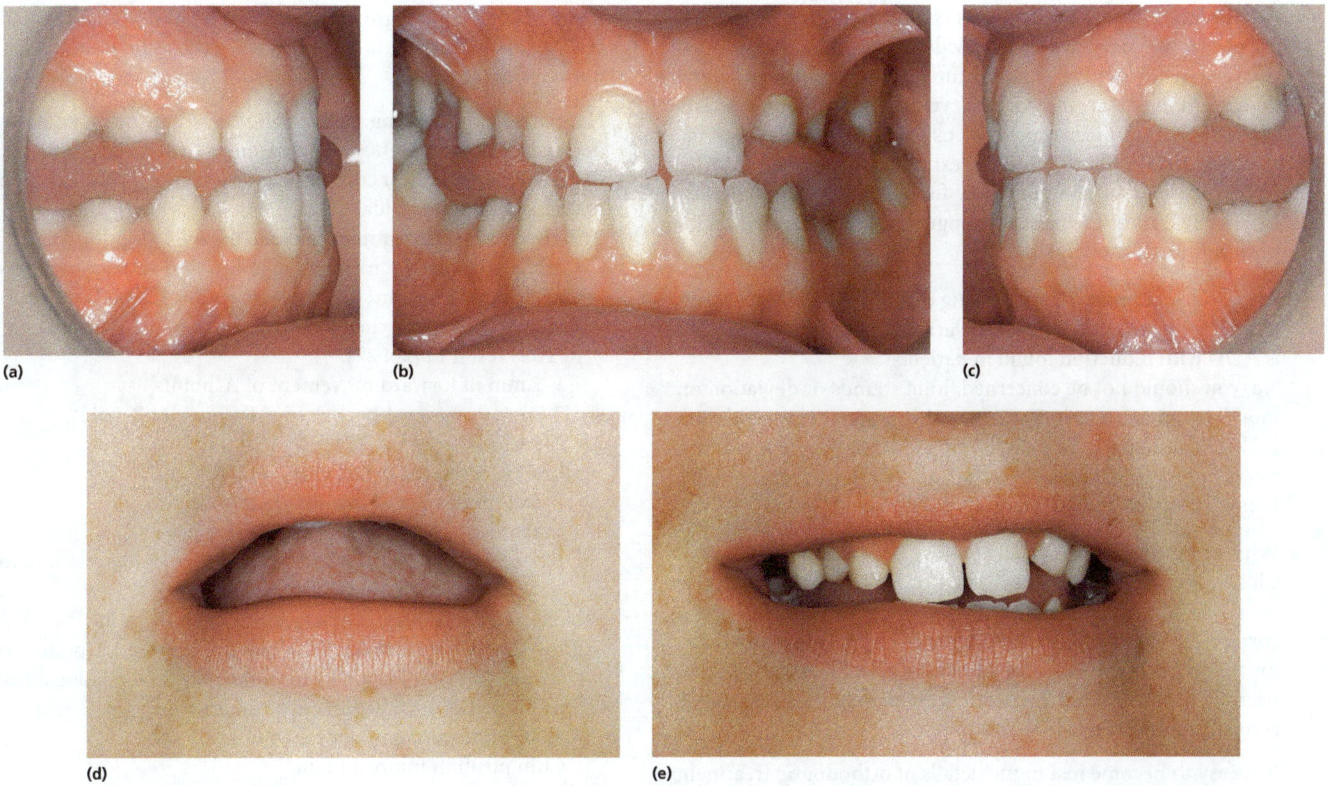

Figure 6.35 Additional records of Kreslyn: (a–c) posterior interpositional tongue habit, (d) approximately 0.5 mm incisal display when relaxed, and (e) posed smile.

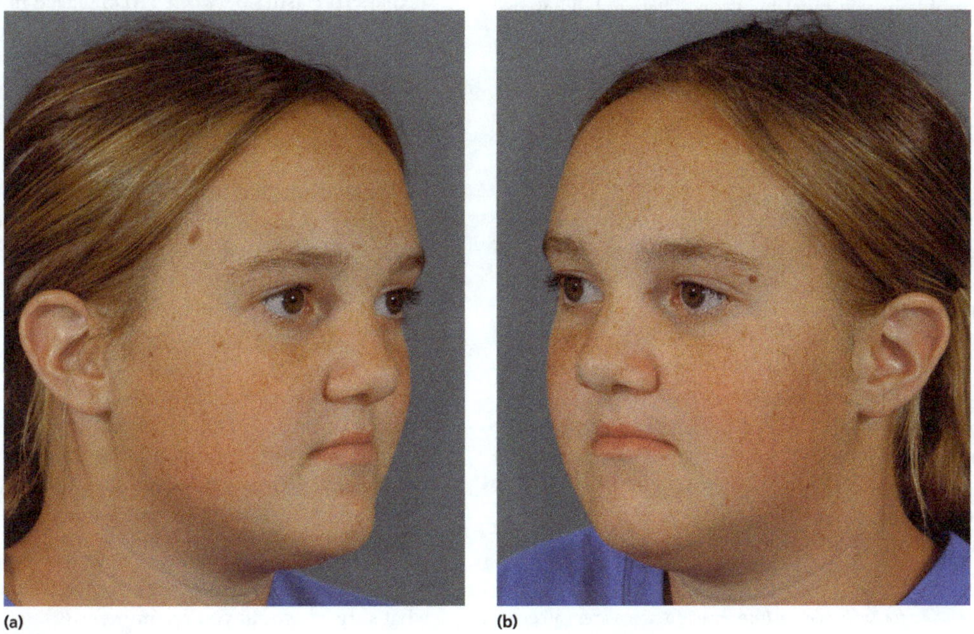

Figure 6.36 (a) Right and (b) left 45° facial views.

Q: Kreslyn's parents ask you how her interpositional tongue habit developed. Can you answer with certainty or offer speculation as to how it developed?

A: The development of her interpositional tongue habit cannot be established with certainty. A probable explanation is that, with a narrow maxilla and ankylosed primary molars, the tongue developed a habit of resting between the dental arches instead of the tongue resting against the constricted palate. A posterior open bite would develop, and worsen, as the tongue prevented permanent canines and premolars from erupting into occlusion.

Additionally, since the tongue was not habitually resting against the palate, the maxillary skeletal width may not have developed adequately, furthering the need for the tongue to seek lateral interposition as it grew (a vicious cycle). Although possible, it is improbable that macroglossia or psuedomacroglossia was the cause. Why? The lower molars exhibit *lingual* crown torque (transverse dental compensation for a narrow maxilla)—*not* labial crown torque (due to the tongue pushing the mandibular posterior teeth laterally).

Q: Are you concerned with the finding of anteriorly displaced disk (ADD) with reduction? Does it warrant treatment? How often is ADD with reduction found in patients?

A: No, you should not be concerned. Joint sounds or deviation on mouth opening occur in 50% of a healthy nonpatient population [25]. Asymptomatic disc displacement *alone* does not warrant treatment [23]. Progression of a TM click to a more serious, nonreducing disk, is uncommon [24].

Q: What are your treatment goals?

A: Close (and maintain closure of) Kreslyn's bilateral posterior open bite, improve her smile esthetics (increase incisal display), correct her bilateral posterior lingual cross bite, align and coordinate arches, achieve a Class I canine relationship with ideal overbite (10–20%) and overjet, and prepare her for restorative reconstruction, as needed.

Q: It is easy to become lost in the details of orthodontic treatment and to lose sight of the major problems that must be addressed. Every time, *every time*, you examine a patient in treatment you should assess the primary problem in each dimension (plus any other major problem, e.g., impacted teeth, spacing, and hygiene). These are the problems you must focus on. That said, what are Kreslyn's primary problems?

A: See Table 6.7

Q: Poor hygiene was identified as a *primary* problem. Why?

A: By causing dental and periodontal destruction, inadequate hygiene can force early patient debanding before treatment is complete. Poor hygiene is always a primary problem.

Q: Of the three general approaches to treating Kreslyn's Class III apical base discrepancy (orthopedics, masking/camouflage, or surgery), would you recommend orthopedics?

A: No. Although you could attempt orthopedic treatment using RPHG, high-pull chin cup, or Class III elastics worn between maxillary and mandibular TADs, at 15 years 4 months of age, it would be unusual for Kreslyn to have enough growth potential remaining to permit full orthopedic correction. Of course, you could ask Kreslyn and her parents whether she is still growing. If she is still growing, you could consider orthopedic treatment. They were asked—her parents stated that Kreslyn stopped growing over a year ago and that she had reached menarche years before that. Orthopedic treatment is not reasonable.

Table 6.7 Primary problems list for Kreslyn *(apical base/skeletal discrepancies italicized)*

AP	III (1–2) III (8) III (6) II (2–3) *maxillary skeletal retrusion*
Vertical	Bilateral posterior open bite resulting from lateral tongue interposition and ankylosed primary molars, inadequate incisal display
Transverse	Bilateral posterior lingual cross bite *maxillary skeletal transverse deficiency*
Other	Missing teeth #s 4, 5, 7, 10, 12, 13, 20, 21, 29 and third molars Maxillary dental arch asymmetry—left posterior ahead of right posterior Poor hygiene

Q: Hypothetically speaking, if Kreslyn was still growing and you decided to attempt orthopedic treatment—what is the effect of RPHGs, high-pull chin cups, or Class III elastics worn between maxillary and mandibular TADs?

A: The effects of each treatment include the following:

- RPHGs advance the maxilla (A-point) and restrict mandibular (B-point) forward growth—correcting Class III relationships. Specifically, when coupled with an RME appliance, RPHGs result in [26, 27]:
  - 1–2 mm of forward movement of A-point.
  - 2.5 mm downward/backward movement of B-point.
  - MPA increasing by 1.5°.
  - LAFH increasing by 2.9 mm.
  - Labial movement of maxillary incisors.
  - Lingual movement of mandibular incisors.
  - *Overcorrection* of the Class III with RPHG use is key to treatment with this appliance.
- High-pull chin cups restrict mandibular (B-point) forward growth and, simultaneously, allow the maxilla (A-point) to continue growing forward, correcting Class III relationships: Specifically, high-pull chin cups result in [28]:
  - ANB improvement (compared to controls).
  - Chin position improvement.
  - Inhibition of mandibular ramal and body length growth.
  - Backward rotation of mandible.
  - Closure of gonial angle.
  - MPA (FMA) flattened compared to controls.
- Class III elastics between TADS placed in the infrazygomatic and anterior mandibular regions advance the maxilla (4 mm) and restrict mandibular growth (2 mm) [29]. Remember, none of these three treatments normalizes growth. *Once the Class III correction is made, orthopedically, it must be held until growth is complete.*

Q: Of the three general approaches to treating Kreslyn's Class III apical base discrepancy, could she be treated with *masking*? If yes, how would you do it?

A: Yes, Kreslyn could be treated to a satisfactory dental result with masking (leaving her maxillary skeletal AP deficiency uncorrected). Maxillary primary anterior teeth could be extracted. Then, using her ankylosed maxillary primary molars as anchorage, Kreslyn could be placed in fixed appliances and her maxillary permanent canines advanced with springs to a Class I relationship with her mandibular canines and the maxillary permanent central incisors advanced out of cross bite. Prosthodontic treatment would follow.

Q: Of the three general approaches to treating Kreslyn's Class III apical base discrepancy, would you recommend *surgery*? If yes, what surgery would you recommend?

A: A maxillary advancement osteotomy could provide a satisfactory dental and skeletal result. Simultaneously downgrafting her anterior maxilla could improve her incisal display (and reduce her overclosed appearance) but would also rotate her mandible down and back (possibly necessitating a mandibular surgical procedure).

Q: If you decided to include a maxillary anterior down graft, when would your make the decision to include it?

A: After fixed appliances were placed and the maxillary arch was leveled and aligned. Then you could evaluate Kreslyn's incisal display when relaxed.

Q: Since she could be treated with either masking or surgery (but not orthopedics), how do you determine which option to pursue?

A: A complete discussion of Kreslyn's findings and problems should be held at the case presentation. If potential benefits of improved facial balance (decrease of paranasal flatness and paranasal folds, reduced prognathic appearance) outweighs the risks, then surgery would be the appropriate treatment choice. This discussion was held. Kreslyn and her parents chose the surgical treatment option.

Q: How would you address Kreslyn's vertical apical base discrepancy?

A: Trick question. Her soft tissue LAFH and skeletal LAFH are both WRN. Her incisal display could be improved with an anterior maxillary down graft osteotomy, but this will lengthen her LAFH and possibly create an interlabial gap.

Q: Let's rephrase this question. How would you address Kreslyn's posterior open bite?

A: We are fortunate that Kreslyn's permanent molars are in occlusion. Since permanent successors for the primary molars are missing, prosthetic replacement of the missing premolars immediately comes to mind. Removable partial dentures could be fabricated to close the posterior open bite. However, the ideal solution would be implants and crowns. Why? Osseointegrated implants/crowns could provide posterior bite closure and maintain *stable* closure (the tongue cannot move them). Her permanent canines could be erupted during leveling (with vertical elastics, prn). Of course, if the resting tongue interposition habit is not resolved, the posterior open bite at the canines could return. Or worse, the tongue could seek a new resting position and force the permanent molars apart.

Q: What should you tell Kreslyn about the prognosis for closing (and maintaining closure of) her posterior open bite?

A: Tell her that there is generally no guarantee that posterior open bites can be closed or kept closed. Muscle (tongue interposition habit) can win over tooth and bone, even if the open bite is closed with surgery. However, in her case the use of osseointegrated implants (plus crowns) could, theoretically, prevent the open bite from returning at all implant locations.

Q: Discuss the three general approaches to treating Kreslyn's *transverse* apical base discrepancy (6 mm first molar intermolar transverse maxillary deficiency, significant maxillary labial crown torque, significant mandibular lingual crown torque). What are the advantages and disadvantages of each? What do you recommend?

A: Advantages and disadvantages include the following:

- Orthopedics, using an RME appliance, could be attempted. However, at 15 years, 4 months of age (and well past her pubertal growth spurt), Kreslyn's skeletal resistance to separation of the midpalatal suture (especially skeletal resistance from the zygomatic buttress) could prevent sutural separation. Before you attempt sutural expansion with an RME appliance, you need to inform Kreslyn and her parents that surgical widening may be necessary, if the RME is unsuccessful.
- Masking the transverse discrepancy is possible (increasing transverse compensations—increasing maxillary posterior labial crown torque and increasing mandibular lingual crown torque). But, it is not ideal and not recommended. The increased compensations would be significant. Further, as illustrated in Figure 6.34o, there is simply not enough bone *buccal* to the maxillary first molars to permit maxillary intermolar widening via buccal root translation through bone.
- Surgery (SARME) would be effective in widening the maxillary apical base. However, surgery (multiple piece maxillary osteotomy at the time of a maxillary advancement osteotomy) may be heroic in terms of the magnitude of expansion needed (6 mm first molar intermolar transverse maxillary deficiency, plus additional widening if maxillary and mandibular transverse compensations are eliminated).
- *Recommendation: attempt RME. If a maxillary sutural split is not achieved, then widen the maxilla with a SARME.*

Q: If you attempt maxillary sutural expansion with an RME appliance, which teeth would you attach the RME appliance to?

A: You could band the maxillary first molars and canines and attach the RME appliance to these teeth. Or, you could band the maxillary first molars and extend a heavy wire (0.036″ or 0.045″ stainless steel wire) forward from the RME appliance along the lingual surfaces of the ankylosed maxillary primary second molars—then *bond* the lingual surfaces of the primary molars to the heavy wire (without banding them).

Q: If you attempt maxillary sutural expansion with an RME appliance, then how/when do you know that the midpalatal suture is *not* splitting?

A: The most obvious sign is failure for a maxillary midline diastema to form within a few days to a week of opening the RME appliance (at an expansion rate of 0.25–0.50 mm per day). Other signs include absence of a midpalatal split when viewed on an occlusal radiograph, pain, pressure that does not quickly dissipate after the screw is turned, and impingement of the RME wires into the lateral walls of the palate (indicating buccal molar expansion through bone without buccal skeletal expansion).

Q: Are there unknowns that you should eliminate *before* you define Kreslyn's final treatment plan? Especially, are there unknowns that should be eliminated before you do something irreversible (e.g., extract teeth and perform surgery)?

A: Yes. You should attempt RME. You do not know whether you will need to plan for surgical expansion until you attempt this first. Kreslyn's ability to correct her tongue interposition habit is an unknown. Growth is no longer an unknown since her parents stated that Kreslyn stopped growing over a year ago. Other unknowns include cooperation, an undetected shift, hygiene, and the final position of her maxillary incisors following leveling of the upper arch.

Q: Should you treat Kreslyn nonextraction, with extraction of anterior teeth, or with extraction of posterior teeth?

A: Nonextraction. With good anterior dental alignment in both arches, absence of many permanent teeth, maxillary anterior spacing, and normal incisor angulation in both arches (incisors not proclined), nonextraction treatment would be the most reasonable approach.

Q: What consultations should you have before deciding on a final treatment plan?

A: You should have consultations with the oral surgeon and prosthodontist before beginning.

Q: Considering everything we have discussed, what treatment options would you consider for Kreslyn? What treatment do you recommend?

A: After establishing her chief complaint, problem list and treatment goals, identifying the primary problems in each dimension (plus other), identifying unknowns, and deciding to treat her nonextraction, only a surgical treatment option was considered and recommended:

1. Attempt RME—the surgeon later recommended MPMO for transverse expansion during maxillary advancement osteotomy, if the RME is unsuccessful.
2. Retain primary teeth until implant grafting (because Kreslyn has completed growth, we are not concerned that her ankylosed molar alveolar crest defects will worsen).
3. Band/bond dental arches and level and align arches.
4. Close mandibular anterior spaces and create OJ.
5. All space distribution and tooth positioning are determined by the prosthodontist and surgeon (for implant placement).
6. Maxillary Le Fort I advancement osteotomy with possible anterior down grafting (possible need for mandibular surgery—depending on mandibular rotation during maxillary surgery).
7. Extraction of Kreslyn's retained primary teeth.
8. After healing, iliac bone grafts in preparation for dental implants.
9. Orthodontic finishing.
10. Final prosthodontic approval before orthodontic deband.
11. Prosthodontic reconstruction.

Q: What are the specific objectives of treatment for the maxilla, mandible, maxillary dentition, and mandibular dentition in all three planes of space?

A: Specific objectives of treatment for Kreslyn are as follows:

Maxilla

AP: Surgical advancement.
Vertical: Maintain.
Transverse: Increase skeletal transverse width

Mandible

AP: Advance chin position by autorotation.
Vertical: Decrease skeletal lower anterior facial height by autorotation.
Transverse: Maintain.

Maxillary dentition

AP: Maintain molars, left canine and incisors. Protract right canine.
Vertical: Maintain molars and canines. Maintain incisors.
Intermolar width: Increase intermolar width.

Mandibular dentition

AP: Maintain molars and canines. Retract incisors.
Vertical: Maintain molars. Maintain incisors.
Intermolar/intercanine width. Maintain intermolar and intercanine widths.

Q: How did Kreslyn's treatment progress?

A: An RME appliance, banded to the maxillary first molars *and* canines, was fabricated. Maxillary expansion (1 turn per day, 0.25 mm per day) was attempted and successful—a midline diastema was seen within the first week. Continued expansion was checked every two weeks. When her maxillary first molar lingual cusps were nearly edge-to-edge with her mandibular buccal cusps (to permit removal of transverse compensations), further expansion was discontinued and held. After 4 months, the RME appliance was replaced with a TPA. Lingual torque was placed in the TPA to decrease the maxillary first molar buccal compensations. A decision was made to extract the ankylosed maxillary primary second molars. Fixed 0.022 slot edgewise appliances were placed, the arches were leveled and aligned, and the archwires increased to 0.019×0.025 inch stainless steel. Discussions were held regularly with the surgeon and prosthodontist. Models of the arches were made every 2–3 months to check for transverse and anteroposterior arch coordination in preparation for surgery. Spaces were adjusted for maxillary and mandibular implants. Following surgery, Kreslyn's canines would be Class I while her first molars would be Class II. Presurgical records were made (Figure 6.37), and we followed the "Checklist for Surgical Patients" found in the Appendix to minimize postsurgical problems. A Le Fort I maxillary advancement osteotomy/anterior down graft was completed.

Postsurgically, space distribution adjustments were continued until the prosthodontist was satisfied. After 4 months, Kreslyn's remaining primary teeth were extracted. Following healing of the extraction sites, interiliac crest bone was harvested and grafting/augmentation of the maxillary and mandibular edentulous ridges was completed (maxillary premolar sites, maxillary lateral incisor sites, and mandibular premolar sites). Maxillary and mandibular implants were placed 4 months after grafting. Archwires were left in place for 3 months following implant placement, at which time Kreslyn was debanded and placed in temporary retainers. (Space was blocked out between the implants and the vacuum-formed retainers to avoid pressure from being placed on the implants.) Hawley retainers were delivered following the completion of prosthodontic treatment.

Q: Deband records are presented in Figure 6.38, and records made after placement of provisional crowns were fabricated are presented in Figure 6.39.
Final records, after completion of prosthodontic treatment, are shown in Figure 6.40. (Note that Figures 6.40a, c, and e are *initial* images, included for comparison.) What do you observe?

A: Observations of her records include the following:

- A dramatic improvement in her smile.
- Her overclosed appearance has been eliminated.
- Paranasally, her face is fuller, but she still exhibits deep paranasal grooves when smiling.
- Increased fullness to her upper lip (Figure 6.40b versus 6.40a).
- Less prominent appearance to her chin in the frontal view.
- Kreslyn exhibits a much broader maxillary arch (Figure 6.40c versus 6.40d) and smaller buccal corridors.
- Maxillary right-to-left occlusal cant is still present (compared to interpupillary line).
- Maxillary midline is right of the facial midline by approximately 2 mm.

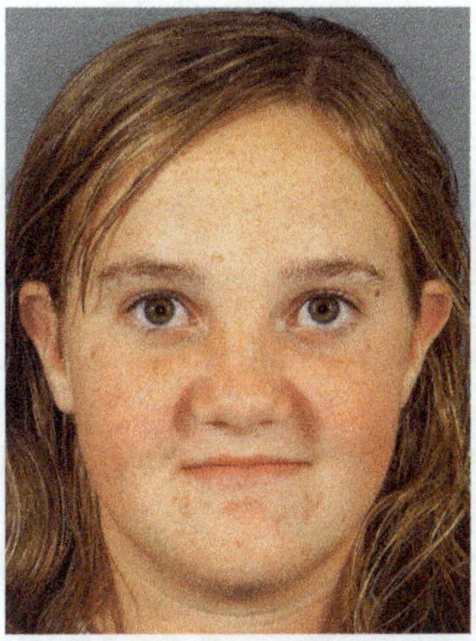
(a)

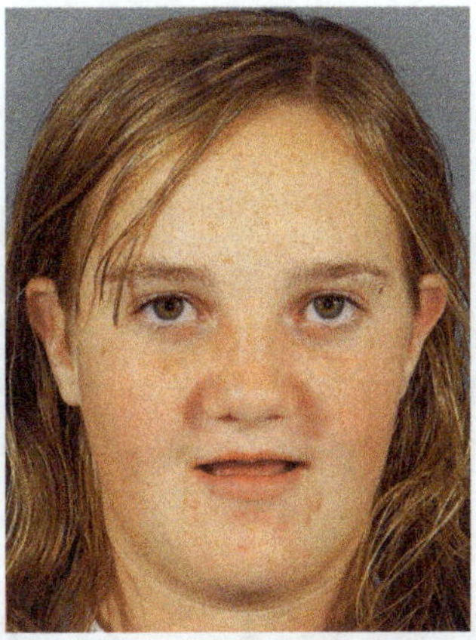
(b)

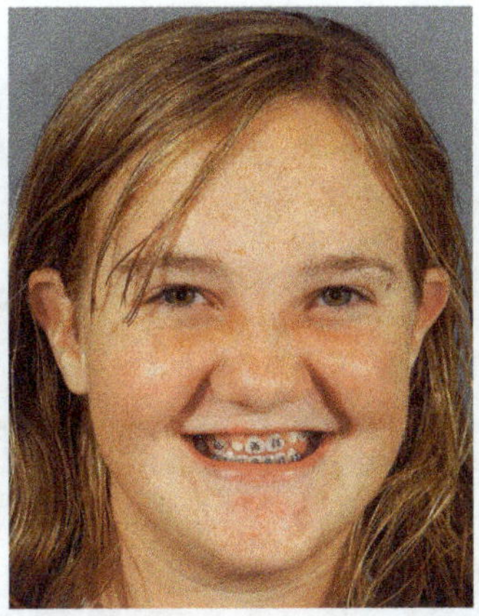
(c)

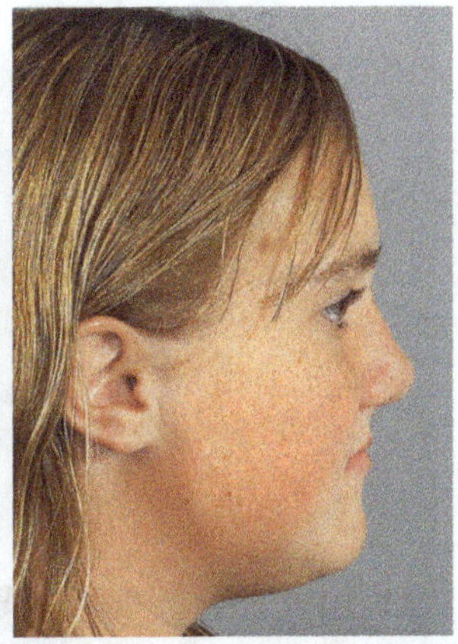
(d)

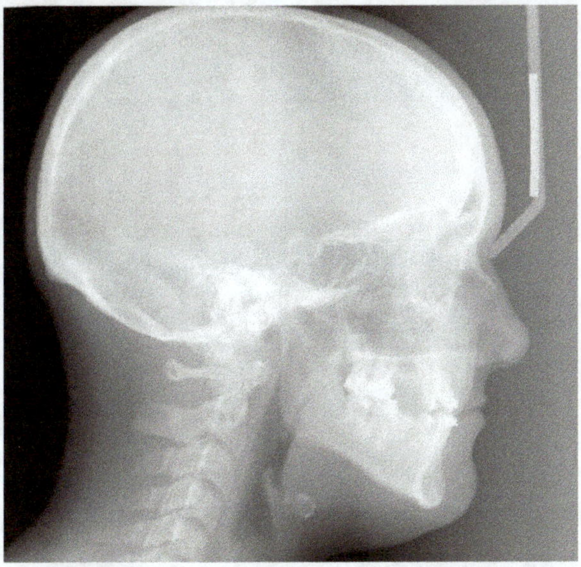
(e)

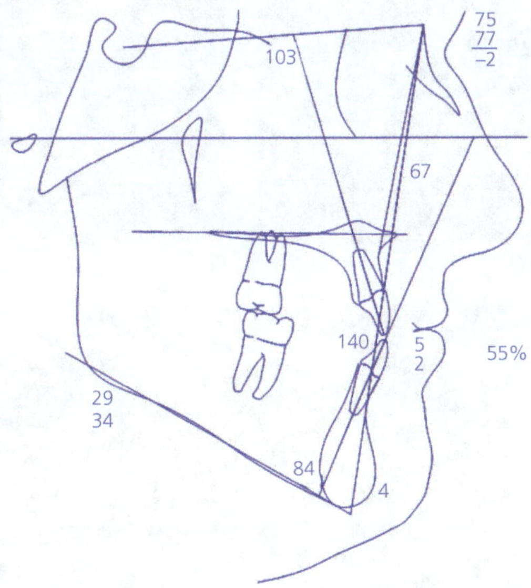

(f)

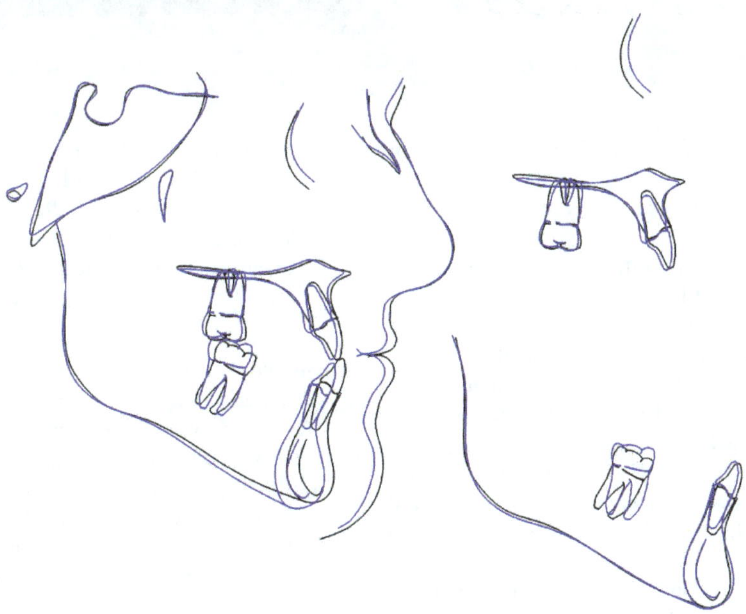
(g)

Figure 6.37 (a–m) Presurgical records of Kreslyn.

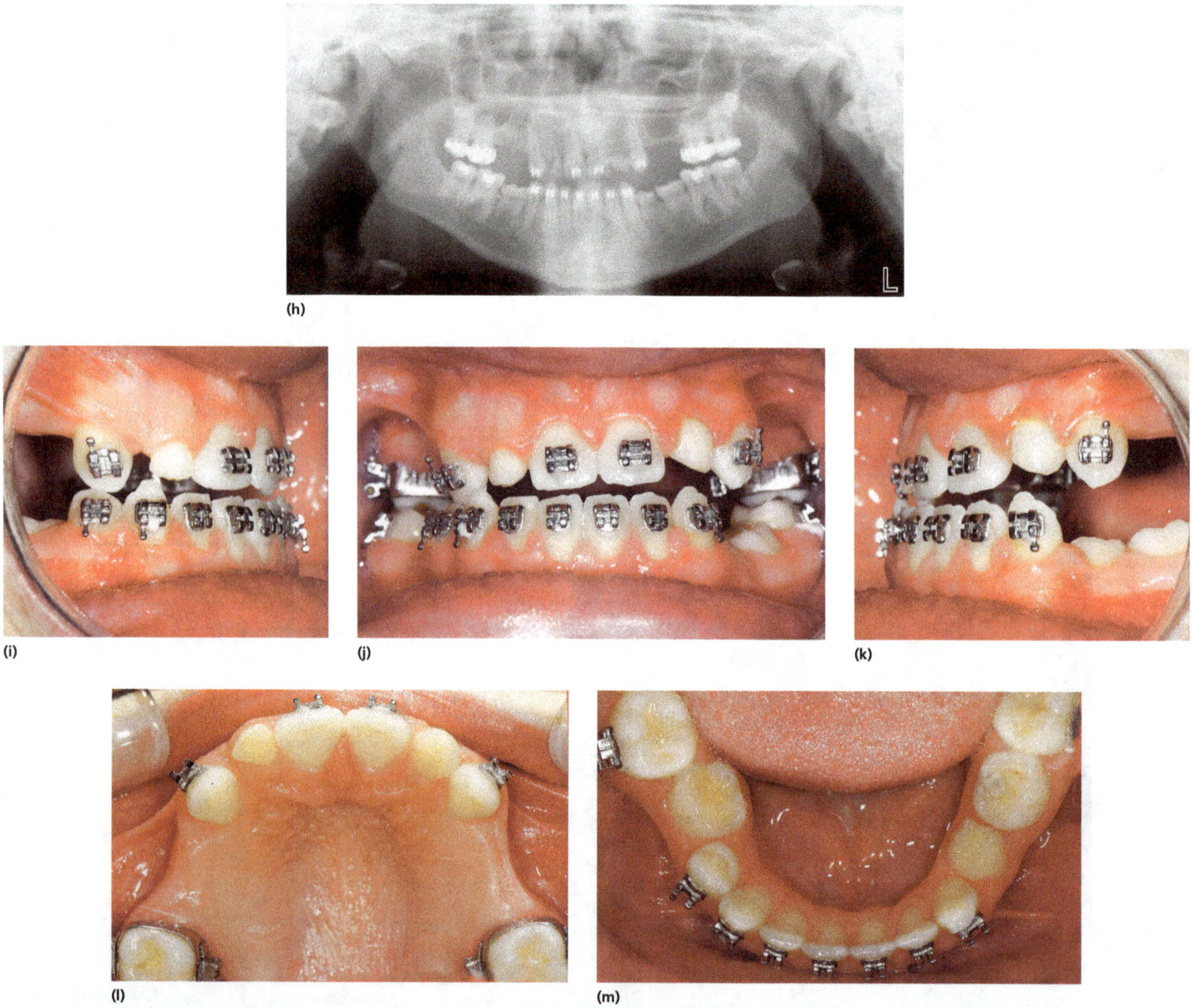

Figure 6.37 (Continued)

- She now has a convex profile (retrusive chin) compared to an initially straight profile.
- Even with the maxillary advancement, the maxilla is still retrusive (Figure 6.40h).
- Overall cephalometric superimposition (Figure 6.40i) shows that the maxilla was brought forward and down in the anterior (increasing her incisal display), and up in the posterior, rotating the mandible down and back. The maxillary lip has descended, and the nasolabial angle has opened up. Mandibular molars have erupted, and maxillary molars have moved distally and erupted.
- Right occlusal AP relationship is Class III by approximately 2 mm, midlines are not coincident, left occlusal AP relationship is Class I, and OB is approximately 10% (Figure 6.40k–m).
- Maxillary right lateral incisor gingival margin is more apical than the maxillary right canine or central incisor gingival margins (instead, the relationship should be "high-low-high").
- Bilateral posterior open bite was closed.
- Transverse dental compensations (maxillary buccal crown torque and mandibular lingual crown torque) are still present in the molars (Figure 6.39i, j).
- The mesiodistal widths of some posterior crowns were exaggerated in order to fill edentulous spaces.
- Maxillary canines are rotated (distal surfaces rotated to the labial).

Q: Should her maxillary right-to-left occlusal cant have been eliminated? Can you suggest why this was *not* done?

A: Yes, to achieve an ideal result, the left side of her maxilla should have been down grafted slightly more—to align the right-to-left occlusal plane with her interpupillary line (Figure 6.40d). However, in order to maintain her occlusion with this movement, a concomitant mandibular osteotomy would have been necessary. Kreslyn and parents declined mandibular surgery.

Q: What is the millimeter threshold for a right-to-left occlusal cant before lay persons notice it?

A: Right-to-left cants greater than or equal to 3 mm must usually exist for lay persons to notice it [30].

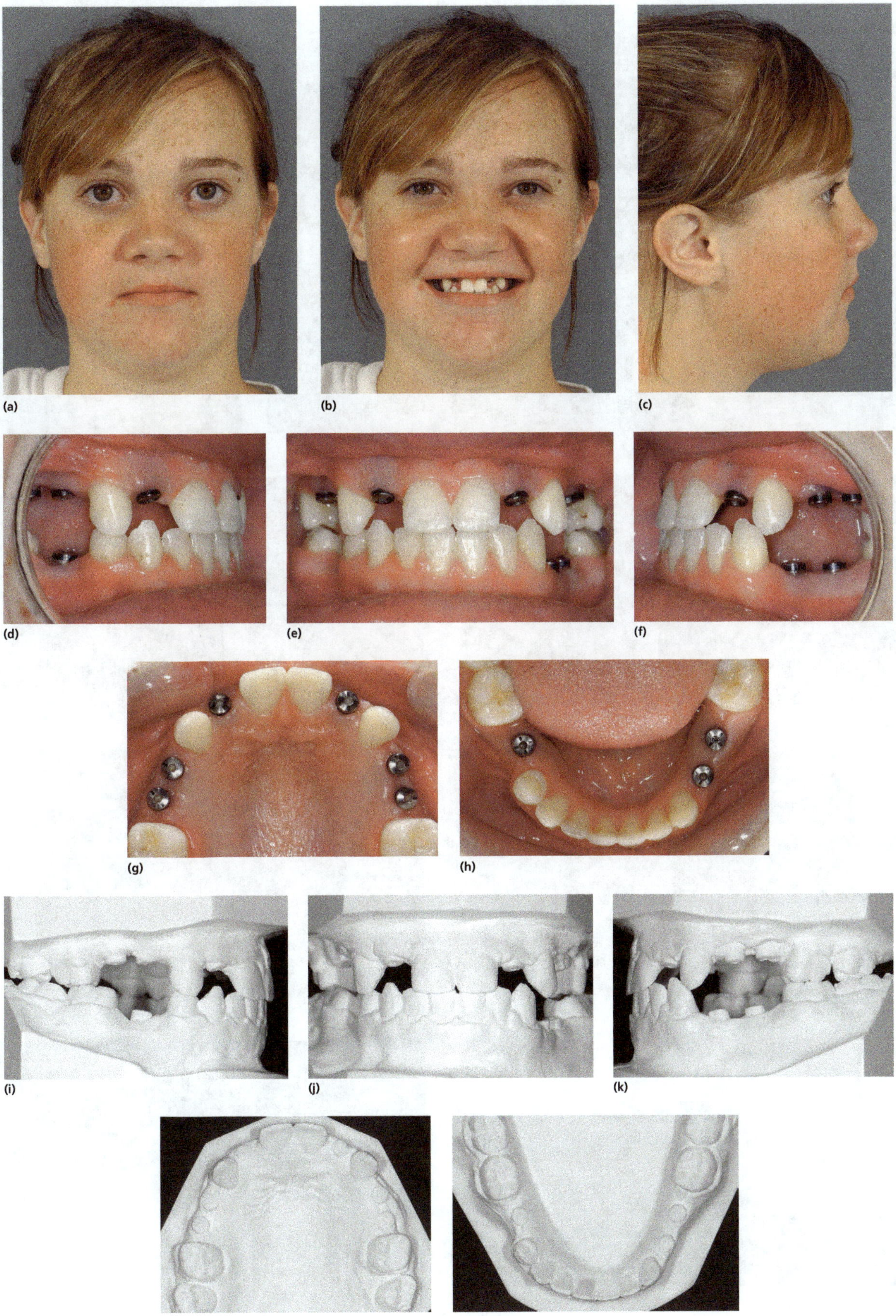

(a) (b) (c) (d) (e) (f) (g) (h) (i) (j) (k) (l) (m)

Figure 6.38 (a–m) Deband records of Kreslyn.

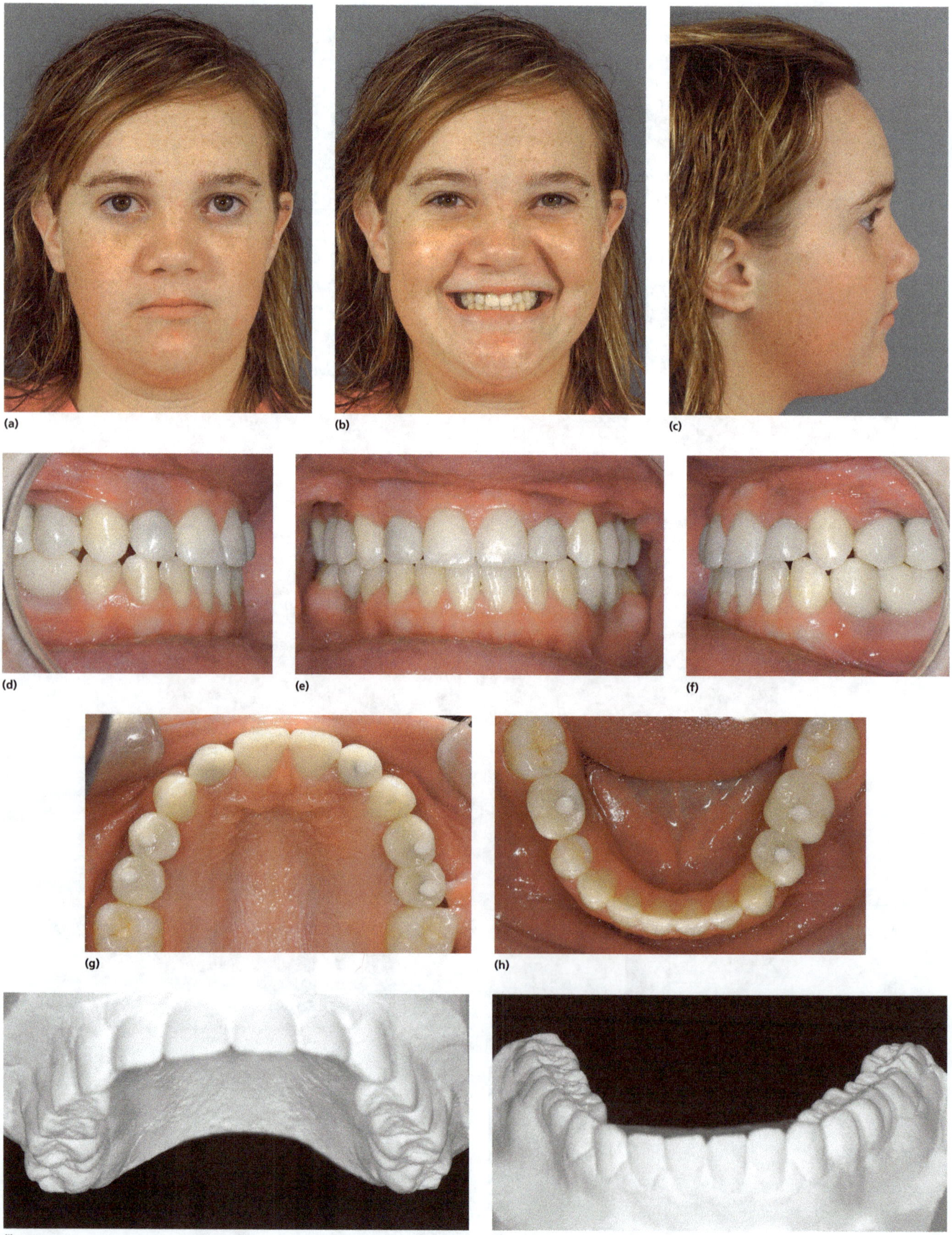

Figure 6.39 (a–j) Kreslyn after placement of provisional restorations.

Q: List other, nonsurgical, treatments which can improve right-to-left occlusal cants.

A: Selective intrusion of individual anterior teeth, enameloplasty of anterior teeth, or anterior veneers can correct very mild right-to-left cants. TADs can be used as anchorage to intrude multiple anterior teeth and eliminate cants (with vertical elastics used to erupt teeth in the opposing arch).

Q: Try to predict Kreslyn's long-term retention success.

A: Since her posterior open bite was closed using implants and crowns, maintenance of the open bite closure could be successful. The danger is that her tongue habit was never corrected. Thwarted by the implants, her tongue could see to create an open bite somewhere elsewhere in her mouth. Finally, Kreslyn needs to wear retainers at night, for life, in order to maintain her tooth alignment attained with treatment.

Q: Kreslyn returns 4 years later. (Figure 6.41, Figure 6.41c is her profile view from 4 years earlier at deband.) She is wearing her maxillary and mandibular Hawley retainers faithfully. What has happened to her posterior occlusion?

A: Long-term maintenance of her closed bilateral posterior open bite has been achieved. No other open bites have developed. Also, note that her profile esthetics have improved as her nasal tip has descended (Figure 6.41d, current profile view).

Q: What are your take-home pearls from this patient?

A: Take-home pearls include the following:

- Kreslyn presented with a Class III malocclusion secondary to maxillary anteroposterior deficiency, posterior cross bite secondary to maxillary transverse deficiency, normal vertical skeletal proportions but inadequate incisal display, and a bilateral posterior open bite. Her posterior open bite was due a tongue interposition habit, constricted maxilla, plus ankylosis of primary molars. Kreslyn's maxillary anteroposterior deficiency was treated with a Le Fort I maxillary advancement osteotomy, her maxillary transverse deficiency was treated with RME, her inadequate incisal display was treated by anteriorly downgrafting the maxilla, and her bilateral posterior open bite was treated using osseointegrated implants and crowns to replace congenitally missing teeth.
- When a patient presents with a posterior open bite, the orthodontist must consider all possible etiologies, including: interpositional tongue or digit habit, ankylosis of primary or permanent posterior teeth, temporary posterior open bites seen soon after loss of the primary molars, lack of space for complete tooth eruption (teeth blocked out), systemic factors found in patients with certain syndromes, and primary failure of eruption. *Successful treatment is based on etiology.*
- First principle: posterior open bites can be very, very difficult problems to correct and to maintain corrected.
- Posterior open bites are corrected by erupting posterior teeth—correcting habits, using fixed appliances with archwires or vertical elastics to upright/erupt posterior teeth, or using surgery/prosthodontics to attain posterior occlusal interdigitation.
- Muscle (tongue interposition) wins over tooth and bone. Not correcting Kreslyn's tongue habit was a stability gamble. Orthodontic/surgical posterior open bite correction can fail, and the posterior open bite can return, if a tongue interposition habit is not corrected. The tongue loses against osseointegrated implants. Implants can be the heroes in posterior open bite correction stability.
- In spite of the fact that Kreslyn's tongue interposition habit was never addressed, long-term (4 year) stability of her posterior bite was achieved. Why? Her posterior open bite was closed with dental implants. Also, RME expansion/uprighting lingually inclined mandibular molars possibly made room for the tongue, and the tongue was possibly retrained to remain lingual to the dentition with open-bite closure.

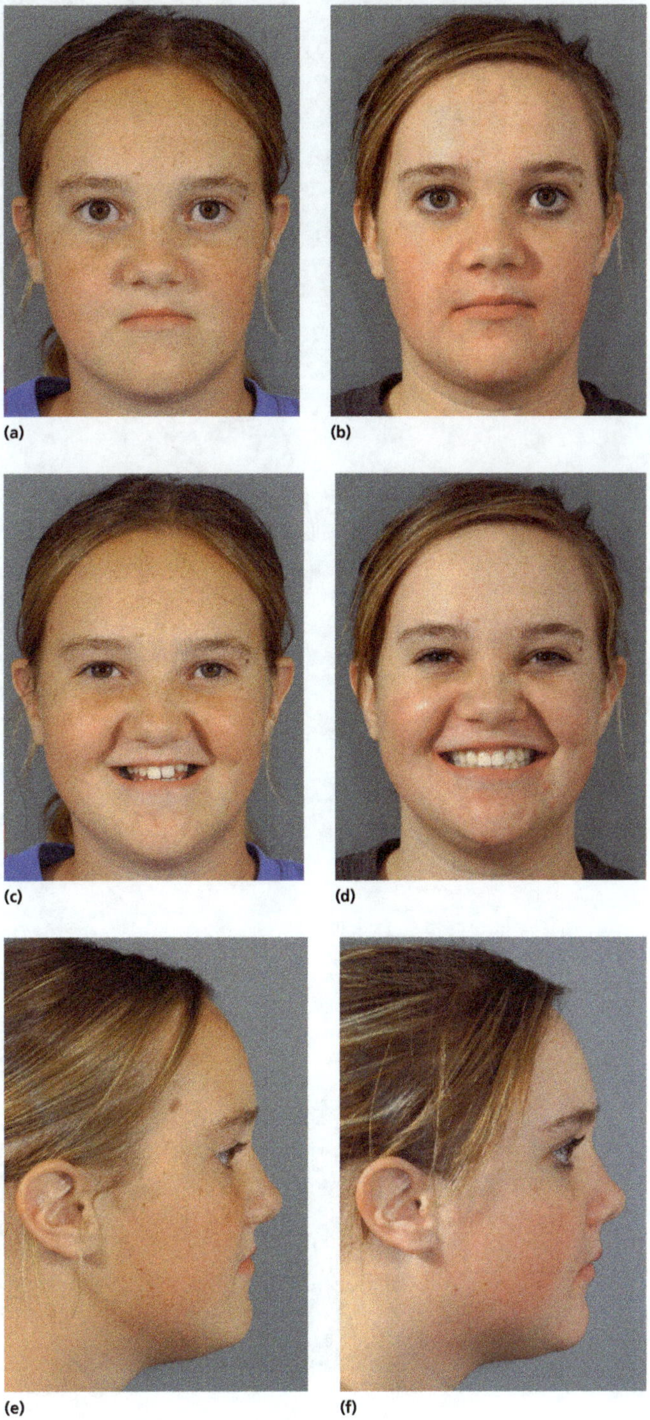

Figure 6.40 Final records of Kreslyn: (a, c, and e) initial facial photographs; (b, d, and f) final facial photographs; (g–t) final records.

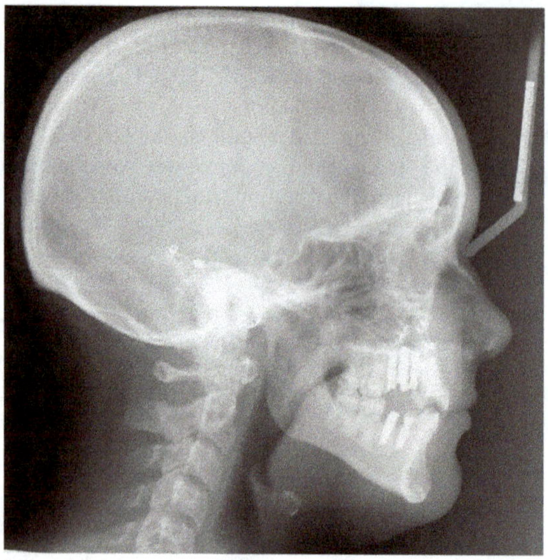

(g)

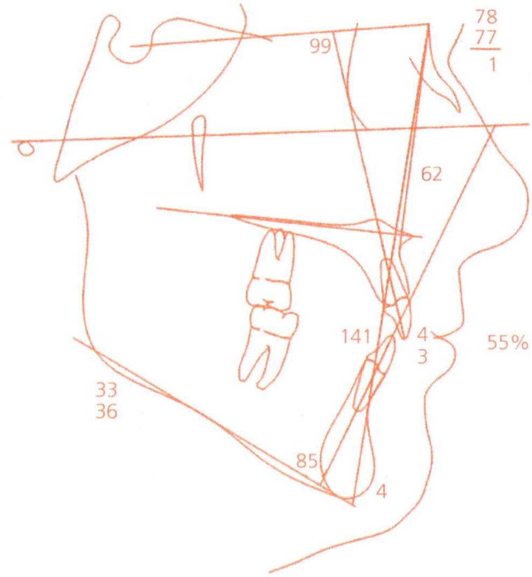

(h)

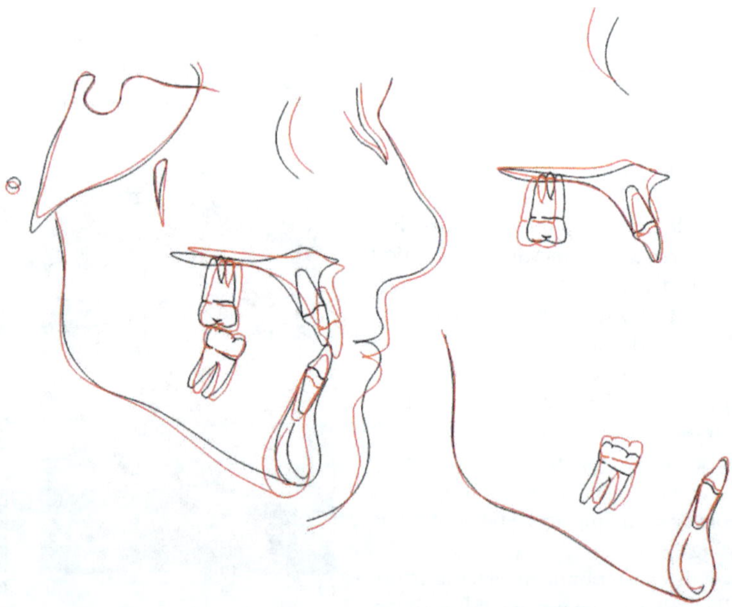

(i)

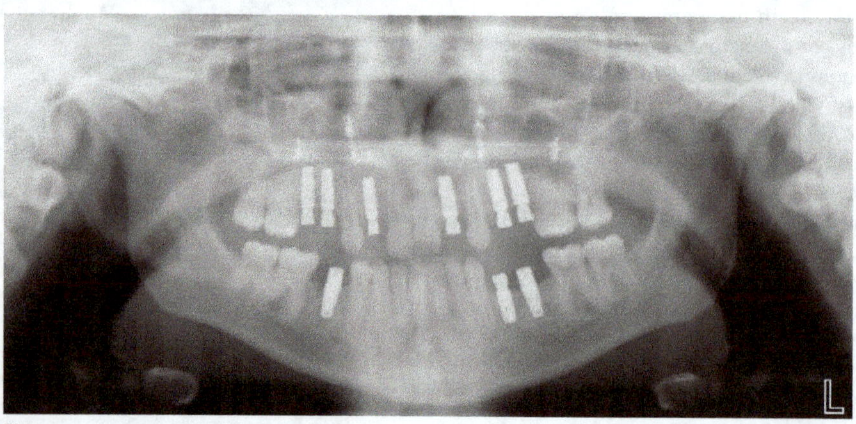

(j)

Figure 6.40 (Continued)

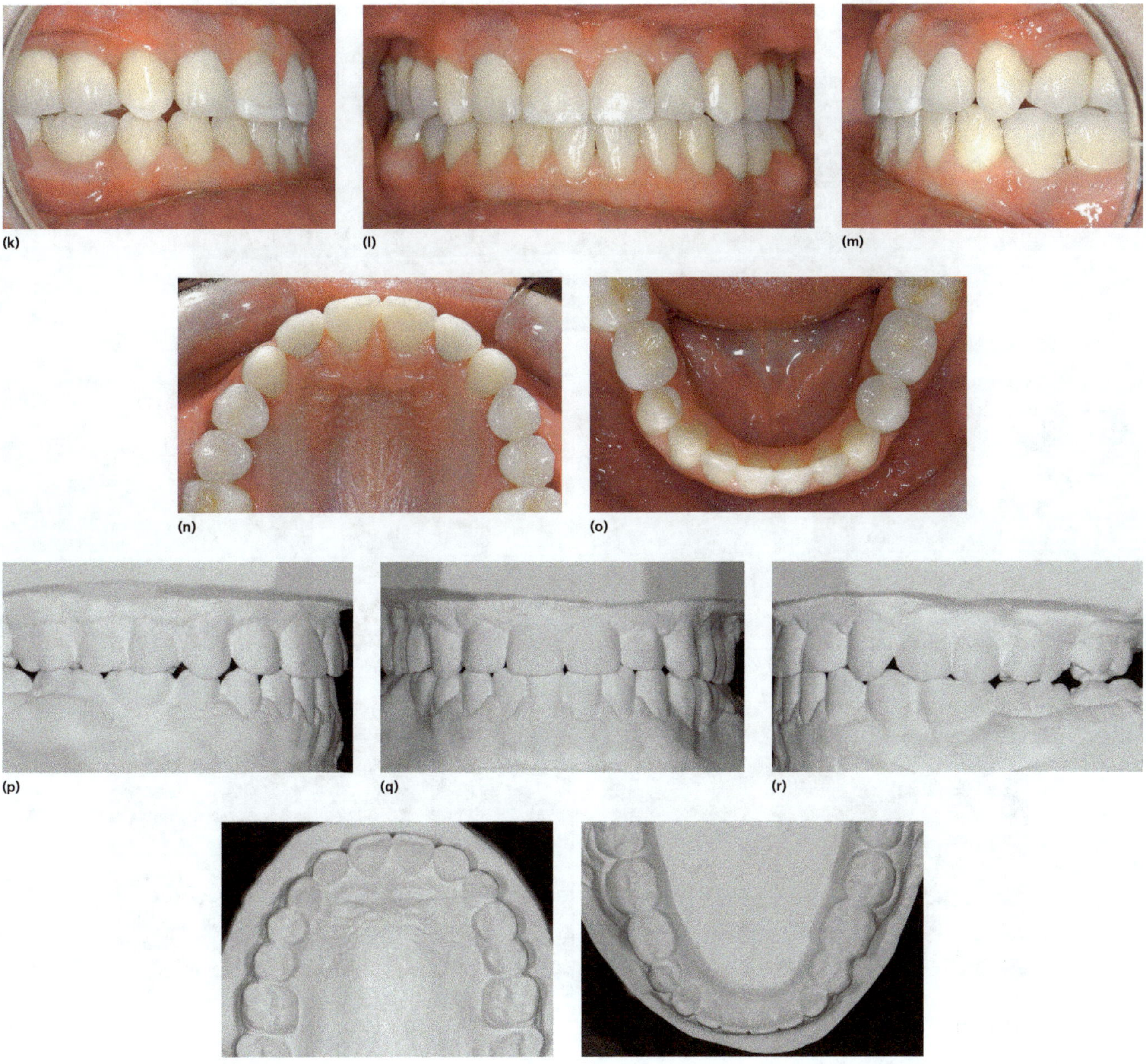

(k) (l) (m) (n) (o) (p) (q) (r) (s) (t)

Figure 6.40 (Continued)

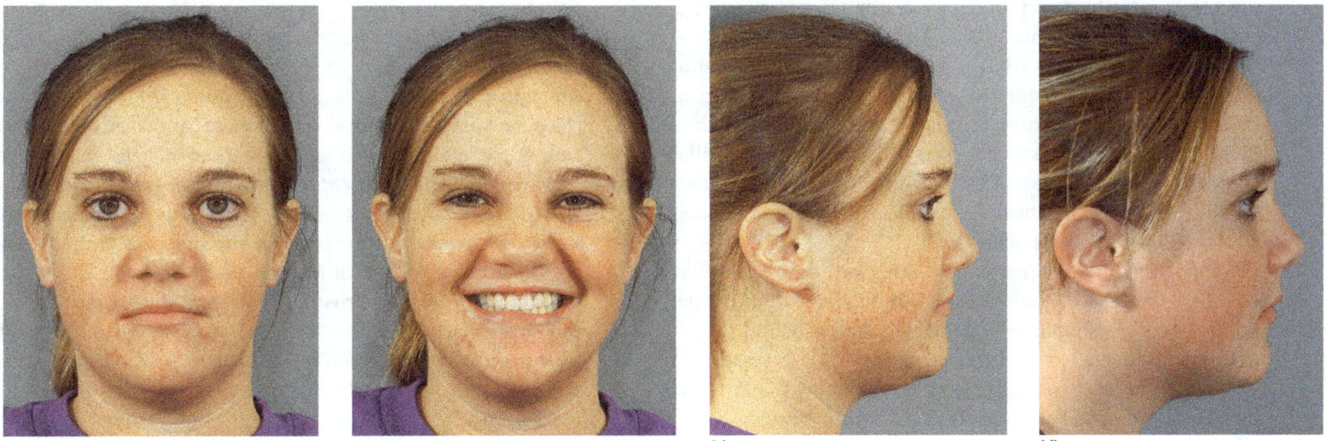

(a) (b) (c) (d)

Figure 6.41 (a–j) Four-year retention records of Kreslyn. (d) Deband profile view for comparison.

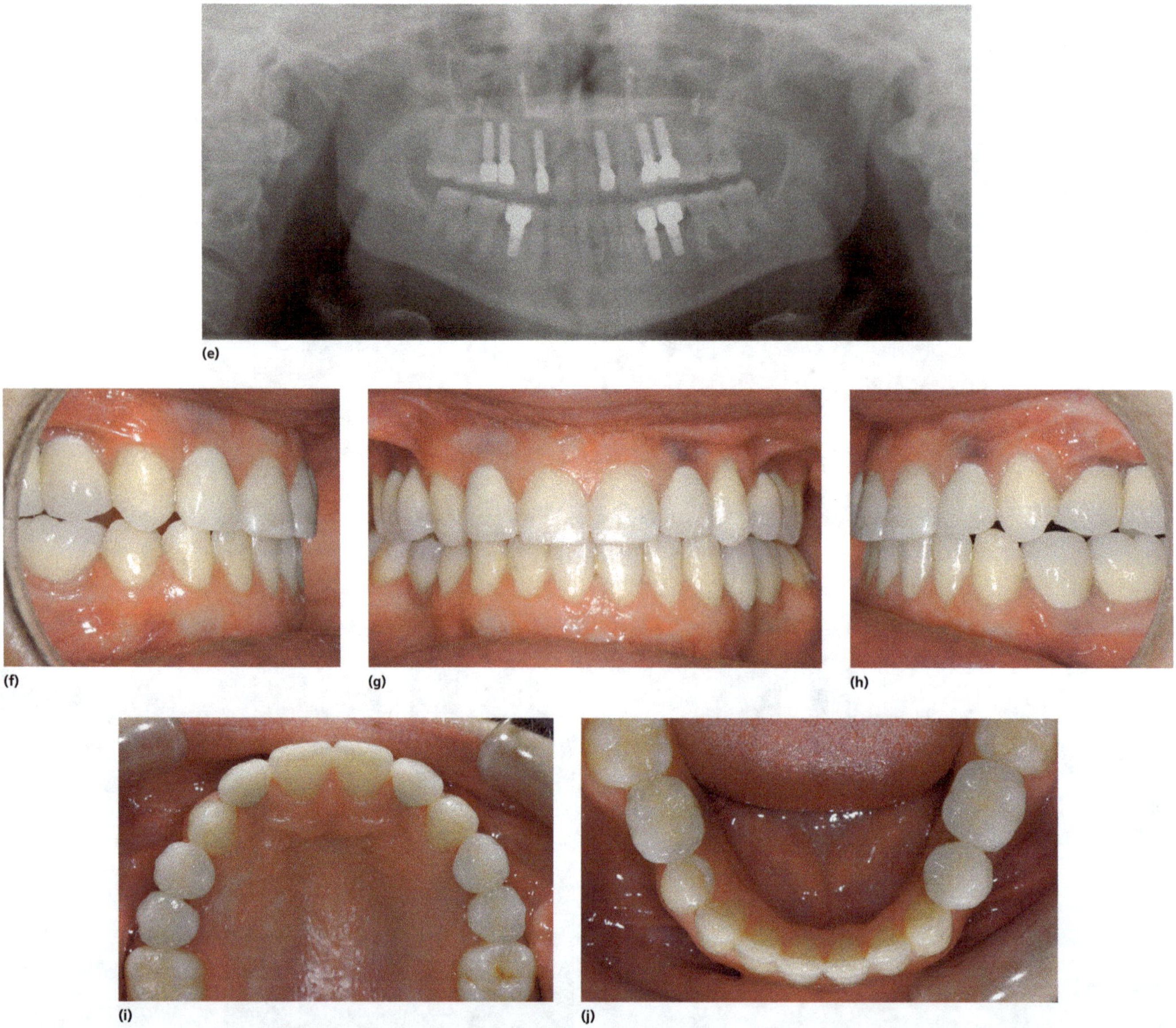

Figure 6.41 (Continued)

- Whenever attempting RME in an older child, be prepared. Have an alternate plan ready if you fail to achieve a midpalatal suture opening. This could include leaving the patient in posterior cross bite, improving posterior OJ by increasing posterior dental compensations, SARME, or MPMO.
- Kreslyn's posterior cross bite was successfully treated with RME. If we had not achieved a midpalatal split with RME, then we had initially considered expanding the maxilla with a SARME. However, our surgeon later believed that the maxilla could be adequately expanded with an MPMO (since the maxilla would be "relatively" expanded as it was surgically advanced relative to the mandible).
- *Large buccal corridors (constricted maxillae) do affect smile esthetics.* Contrast Figure 6.40c with Figure 6.40d. Large buccal corridors should be included in your problem list.
- Kreslyn's right-to-left occlusal cant was not addressed. It could have been corrected when the maxilla was anteriorly down grafted, but changing the cant would have necessitated a mandibular surgery to rotate the mandibular occlusal plane to match the maxillary occlusal plane. Kreslyn and her parents declined mandibular surgery. An advancement genioplasty could have improved Kreslyn's final profile esthetics.
- In any maxillary down graft surgery, care must be taken NOT to increase the LAFH to the point where an ILG is created.
- Archwires were left in place for 3 months following implant placement at which time Kreslyn was debanded and placed in temporary retainers. This was a potential mistake. Whenever possible, *leave the patient in orthodontic appliances until immediately before final prosthetic restoration placement*. That is, take archwires out for implant surgery, and immediately put the archwires back in to hold everything in place. Take the archwires out for prosthodontic provisional placement, and immediately put the archwires back in to make final adjustments. We have seen too many preprosthodontic cases compromised because teeth/roots shifted between deband and final prosthetic placement, even when patients faithfully wear their retainers.

- Communication is the key to successful multidisciplinary treatment. The prosthodontist tells the orthodontist where he/she wants the teeth/jaws moved. The orthodontist tells the prosthodontist if this can be done, and then does his/her best to achieve that movement. Discuss the case often. Strive for ideal treatment or discuss compromises. Form a team with family practice dentists, oral surgeons, periodontists, prosthodontists, and endodontists. Check your ego at the front door. You are here to serve. You work for the patient and all other doctors on your team.

References

1 Perez CV, de Leeuw R, Okeson JP, Carlson CR, Li HF, Bush HM, et al. The incidence and prevalence of temporomandibular disorders and posterior open bite in patients receiving mandibular advancement device therapy for obstructive sleep apnea. *Sleep Breath.* 2013;**17**:323–32.

2 Kater WM, Kawa D, Schafer D, Toll D. Treatment of posterior open bite using distraction osteogenesis. *J Clin Orthod.* 2004;**38**:501–4.

3 Shirota T, Hishida M, Yamaguchi T, Kurabayashi H, Maki K, Shintani S. Posterior maxillary segmental distraction for the treatment of severe lateral open bite caused by primary failure of tooth eruption: a case report. *J Oral Maxillofac Surg Med Pathol.* 2013;**25**:39–42.

4 Proffit WR, Vig KW. Primary failure of eruption: a possible cause of posterior open-bite. *Am J Orthod.* 1981;**80**:173–90.

5 Stellzig-Eisenhauer A, Decker E, Meyer-Marcotty P, Rau C, Fiebig BS, Kress W, et al. Primary failure of eruption (PFE)—clinical and molecular genetics analysis. *J Orofacial Orthopedics.* 2010;**71**:6–16.

6 Ahmad S, Bister D, Cobourne MT. The clinical features and aetiological basis of primary eruption failure. *Eur J Orthod.* 2006;**28**:535–40.

7 Rhoads SG, Hendricks HM, Frazier-Bowers SA. Establishing the diagnostic criteria for eruption disorders based on genetic and clinical data. *Am J Orthod Dentofacial Orthop.* 2013;**144**:194–202.

8 Frazier-Bowers SA, Koehler KE, Ackerman JL, Proffit WR. Primary failure of eruption: further characterization of a rare eruption disorder. *Am J Orthod Dentofacial Orthop.* 2007;**131**:578.e1–e11.

9 Frazier-Bowers SA, Simmons D, Wright JT, Proffit WR, Ackerman JL. Primary failure of eruption and PTH1R: the importance of a genetic diagnosis for orthodontic treatment planning. *Am J Orthod Dentofacial Orthop.* 2010;**137**:160e1–7; discussion 160–1.

10 Yatani H, Watanabe EK, Kaneshima T, Yamashita A, Suzuki K. Etched-porcelain resin bonded onlay technique for posterior teeth. *J Esthet Dent* 1998;**10**:325–32.

11 Piattelli A, Eleuterio A. Primary failure of eruption. *Acta Stomatol Belg* 1991;**88**:127–30.

12 Siegel SC, O'Connell A. Oral rehabilitation of a child with primary failure of tooth eruption. *J Prosthodont.* 1999;**8**:201–7.

13 Kurol J. Early treatment of tooth-eruption disturbances. *Am J Orthod Dentofacial Orthop.* 2002;**121**:588–91.

14 Kurol J, Koch G. The effect of extraction of infraoccluded deciduous molars: a longitudinal study. *Am J Orthod.* 1985:**87**:46–55.

15 Kurol J, Thilander B. Infraocclusion of primary molars and the effect on occlusal development, a longitudinal study. *Eur J Orthod.* 1984;**6**:277–93.

16 Rebellato J, Lindauer SJ, Rubenstein LK, Isaacson RJ, Davidovitch M, Vroom K. Lower arch perimeter preservation using the lingual arch. *Am J Orthod Dentofacial Orthop.* 1997;**112**:449–56.

17 Nance HN. The limitations of orthodontic treatment: mixed dentition diagnosis and treatment. *Am J Orthod Oral Surg.* 1947;**33**:177–223.

18 Moyers RE. *Standards of Human Occlusal Development.* Ann Arbor, MI: Center for Human Growth and Development, the University of Michigan; 1976. p. 371.

19 Dugoni SA, Lee JS, Varela J, Dugoni AA. Early mixed dentition treatment: postretention evaluation of stability and relapse. *Angle Orthod* 1995;**65**:311–20.

20 Brennan MM, Gianelly AA. The use of the lingual arch in the mixed dentition to resolve incisor crowding. *Am J Orthod Dentofacial Orthop.* 2000;**117**:81–5.

21 Miyawaki S, Oya S, Noguchi H, Takano-Yamamoto T. Long-term changes in dentoskeletal pattern in a case with Beckwith-Wiedemann syndrome following tongue reduction and orthodontic treatment. *Angle Orthod.* 2000;**70**:326–31.

22 Hotokezaka H, Matsuo T, Nakagawa M, Mizuno A, Kobayashi K. Severe dental open bite malocclusion with tongue reduction after orthodontic treatment. *Angle Orthod.* 2001;**71**:228–36.

23 Greene CS, Laskin DM. Long-term status of TMJ clicking in patients with myofascial pain and dysfunction. *J Am Dent Assoc.* 1988;**117**:461–5.

24 Pullinger AG, Seligman DA. TMJ osteoarthritis: A differentiation of diagnostic subgroups by symptom history and demographics. *J Craniomandib Disord.* 1987;1:251–6.

25 Huber MA, Hall EH. A comparison of the signs of temporomandibular joint dysfunction and occlusal discrepancies in a symptom-free population of men and women. *Oral Surg Oral Med Oral Pathol.* 1990;**70**:180–3.

26 Ngan P, Hagg U, Yiu C, Merwin D, Wei SH. Treatment response to maxillary expansion and protraction. *Eur J Orthod.* 1996;**18**:151–68.

27 Ngan P. Early timely treatment of Class III malocclusions. *Sem Orthod.* 2005;**11**:140–5.

28 Deguchi T, Kuroda T, Minoshima Y, Graber TM. Craniofacial features of patients with Class III abnormalities: growth-related changes and effects of short-term and long-term chincup therapy. *Am J Orthod Dentofacial Orthop.* 2002;**121**:84–92.

29 De Clerck H, Cevidanes L, Baccetti T. Dentofacial effects of bone-anchored maxillary protraction: a controlled study of consecutively treated Class III patients. *Am J Orthod Dentofacial Orthop.* 2010;**138**:577–81.

30 Kokich VO Jr, Kiyak HA, Shapiro PA. Comparing the perception of dentists and lay people to altered dental esthetics. *J Esthet Dent.* 1999:**11**;311–24.

Appendix

Cephalometrics Primer

There are many cephalometric analyses. In this section we present a straightforward analysis which has served us well.

Q: Lateral cephalometric radiographs provide valuable anteroposterior and vertical relationship information. What are the five most important relationships measured from lateral cephalometric radiographs?

A: The five most important relationships are (Figure A.1):

1. maxillary anteroposterior skeletal position
2. mandibular anteroposterior skeletal position
3. vertical skeletal relationships
4. maxillary incisor angulation
5. mandibular incisor angulation

Q: When taking a patient's lateral cephalometric radiograph, the lips should be relaxed. What do you notice when comparing the cephalometric radiograph to the profile photograph of the patient shown in Figure A.2?

A: An interlabial gap (ILG) is present on the radiographic profile but absent on the photographic profile. The presence of an ILG could be very important for treatment planning in the vertical dimension, and should be recorded in both the cephalometric radiograph and facial photographs. *Always verify that the patient's soft tissue in the profile photograph matches the soft tissue on the lateral cephalometric radiograph.*

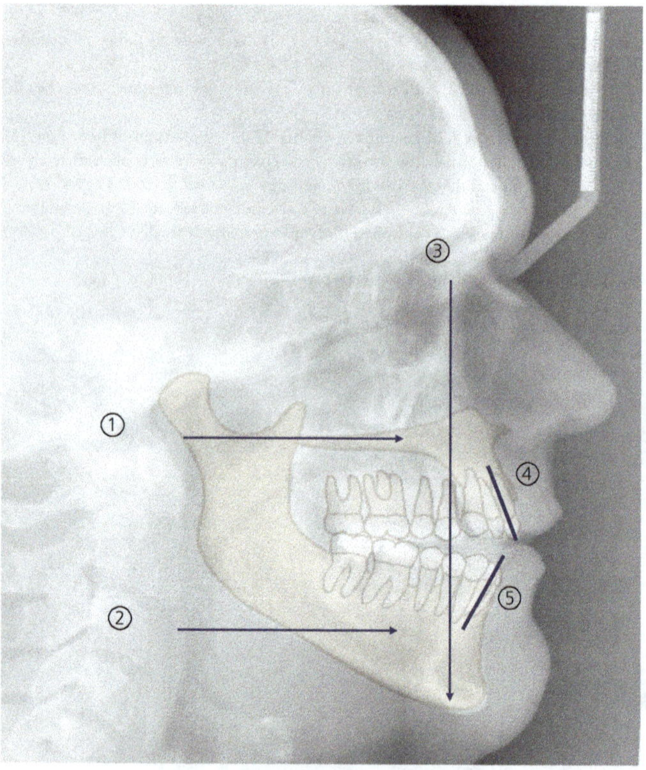

Figure A.1 Five important relationships determined from a cephalometric radiograph. Numbers 1–5 refer to definitions in the text.

Q: How do you judge *ideal* maxillary AP position on a cephalometric radiograph?

A: On the lateral cephalometric tracing, draw Frankfort Horizontal (FH) between *anatomic* Porion and Orbitale (Figure A.3a, b). Next, draw a line downward from Nasion (N) passing perpendicular to FH (Figure A.3c, d). An *ideal maxillary AP position is one in which A-Point lies on the Nasion perpendicular line* [1, 2]. Another way of saying this is that a line drawn from Nasion to A-Point (N-A line) makes a 90° angle with FH (i.e. angle FH-NA = 90°).

Q: If A-Point lies *nearly* on Nasion perpendicular, but not exactly on Nasion perpendicular, should the maxilla be classified as either AP deficient or AP excessive, but not normal?

A: Not necessarily. A *range of normal* exists in cephalometric analysis. If a patient presents with a cephalometric measurement that is close to normal, but not precisely normal, that measurement may still be considered to fall "within the range of normal" or WRN. In other words, if A-Point sits slightly behind or slightly ahead of Nasion perpendicular, than the maxillary AP position may still be considered WRN. Or, if the posterior-inferior angle formed by the N-A line and FH (NA-FH angle) is, say 89° or 91°, then the maxillary AP position may still be considered WRN.

Q: How would you describe the maxillary AP position in the cephalometric tracing shown in Figure A.4a? Figure A.4b?

A: The maxillary AP position is very deficient (retrusive) in Figure A.4a. The maxillary AP position is very excessive (protrusive) in Figure A.4b.

Q: How would you describe the maxillary AP position in the cephalometric radiograph and tracing shown in Figure A.5?

A: In this patient, A-Point lies ahead of Nasion-perpendicular (NA-FH angle is 93°). This patient presents with maxillary AP excess (protrusion).

Orthodontics in the Vertical Dimension: A Case-Based Review, First Edition. Thomas E. Southard, Steven D. Marshall and Laura L. Bonner.

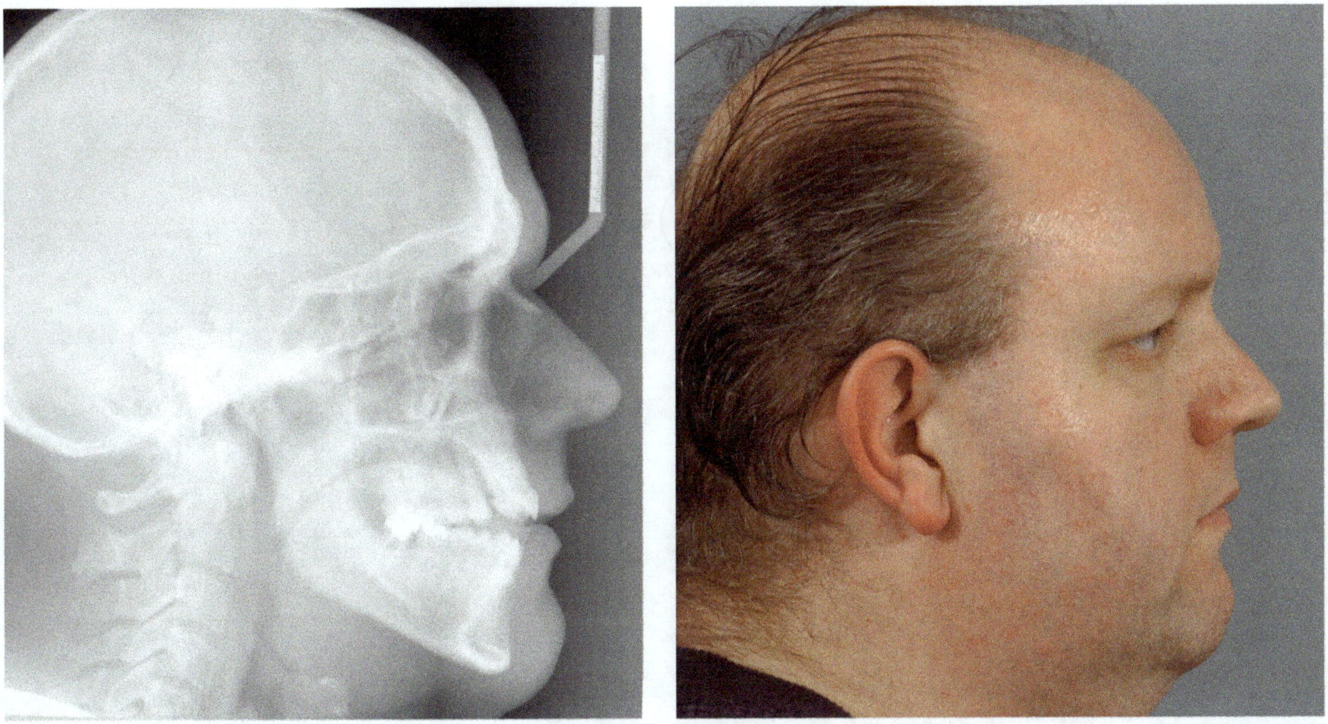

(a) (b)

Figure A.2 (a) Cephalometric radiograph and (b) profile photograph depicting inconsistency in recording the patient's inter-labial gap (ILG).

Q: How would you describe the maxillary AP position in the cephalometric radiograph and tracing shown in Figure A.6?

A: A-Point lies behind Nasion perpendicular (NA-FH angle is 85°). This patient presents with maxillary AP deficiency (retrusion).

Q: How do you judge *ideal* mandibular AP position on a cephalometric radiograph—if maxillary AP is WRN?

A: *If maxillary AP position is WRN, then simply use the ANB angle.* As shown in Figure A.7a, when maxillary AP is WRN the line N-A lies coincident with Nasion perpendicular. In this case, an ideal mandibular AP position will be found when a 2° or 3° angle is formed between lines N-A and N-B (Figure A.7b, c), that is ANB = 2° or 3°.

Q: How would you describe the mandibular AP position in the cephalometric tracing shown in Figure A.8a, b? Figure A.8c, d?

A: The mandibular AP position is deficient (retrusive) in Figure A.8a, b. The mandibular AP position is excessive (protrusive) in Figure A.8c, d.

Q: How do you judge mandibular AP position when the maxillary AP position is *not* WRN? For example, how do you judge the mandibular AP position in Figure A.9?

A: Judging the mandibular AP position when the maxillary AP position is not WRN includes:

- Just as you did when judging maxillary skeletal AP position, *relate the mandible to Nasion perpendicular.* Measure (estimate) the angle formed between Nasion perpendibular and the N-B line. What is the logic of doing this? This angle would be the ANB angle if the maxilla was WRN (that is, if the N-A line was coincident with Nasion perpendicular).
- *If you measure the angle formed between Nasion perpendicular and the N-B line to be 2° or 3°, then the mandibular AP position is WRN. Otherwise, it is deficient or excessive.* For instance, in Figure A.9a, b the angle formed between Nasion perpendicular and the N-B line is 8°. Clearly, both the mandible and the maxilla are deficient. Most seasoned orthodontists would draw this same conclusion without actually measuring angles. Likewise, in Figure A.9c, d the angle formed between Nasion perpendicular and the N-B line is -2°. The mandibular AP is excessive (maxilla is deficient).
- As an alternative, you can often use logic to judge mandibular AP position. For instance, if you measure an ANB angle to be 3°, and the maxilla is AP deficient, then logic would dictate that the mandible must also be deficient.

Q: How would you judge the mandibular AP position for the patient shown in Figure A.10?

A: Mandibular skeletal AP retrusion

Q: How would you judge the mandibular AP position for the patient shown in Figure A.11?

A: Mandibular AP skeletal protrusion

Q: How would you describe the maxillary and mandibular AP positions for the patient shown in Figure A.12?

A: Maxillary *and* mandibular AP skeletal retrusion (deficiency)

Q: How would you describe the maxillary and mandibular AP positions for the patient shown in Figure A.13?

A: Maxillary AP skeletal retrusion (deficiency) and mandibular AP skeletal WRN

Q: Instead of using Nasion-perpendicular to judge maxillary and mandibular AP positions, why not use SNA and SNB angles?

A: *SNA and SNB angles are too dependent upon the vertical position of Sella* to be of value in judging maxillary and mandibular skeletal AP positions. For instance, normal values

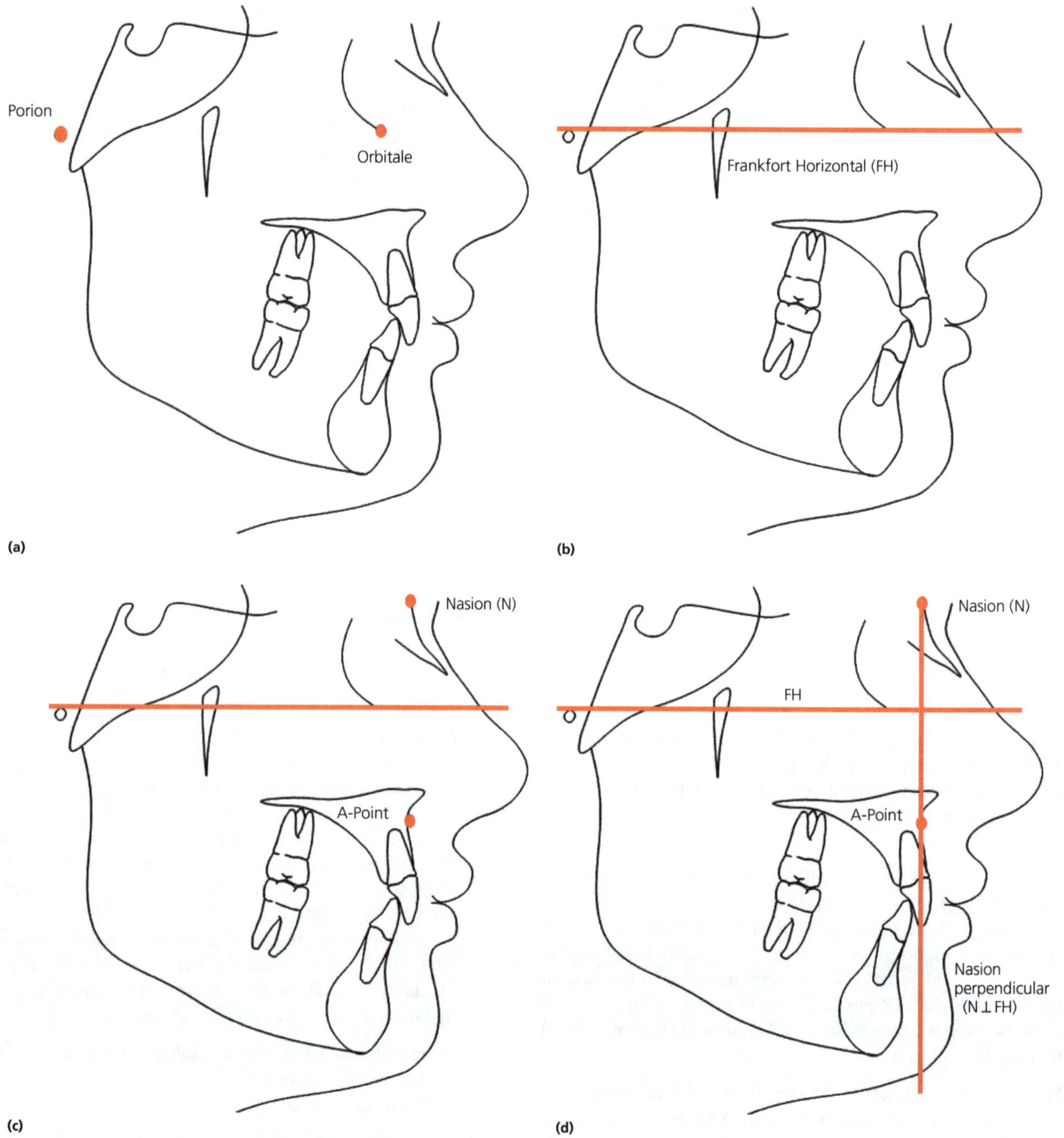

Figure A.3 Construction of FH and a vertical line beginning at Nasion (N) perpendicular to FH. (a, b) Construction of FH and (c, d) a vertical line beginning at Nasion (N) perpendicular to FH. For this subject, A-Point lies on Nasion perpendicular exemplifying an ideal maxillary AP position.

for SNA and SNB angles are 82° and 80°, respectively. But in Figure A.14a (patient with normal maxilla and mandible but "high Sella") SNA and SNB angles are 85° and 83°—incorrectly suggesting maxillary and mandibular AP skeletal protrusion. Then, in Figure A.14b (same patient, but low sella) SNA and SNB angles are 77° and 74°—suggesting maxillary and mandibular skeletal retrusion. The use of SNA and SNB angles can be misleading.

Of course, you could argue that adjustments can be made to SNA and SNB to compensate for Sella being high or low. The normal angular difference between SN and FH is 7°(normal SN-MP = 32° and normal FMA = 25°, a difference of 7°). So, for the "high Sella" in Figure A.14a, where the angular difference between SN and FH is 4° (SN-MP = 27° and FMA = 23°), you could reduce SNA and SNB by 3°, making them 82° and 79°, respectfully (indicating normal maxillary and mandibular AP positions). Conversely, for the "low Sella" in Figure A.14b, where the angular difference between SN and FH is 12° (SN-MP = 35° and FMA = 23°) you could increase SNA and SNB by 5°, again making them 82° and 79°, respectfully.

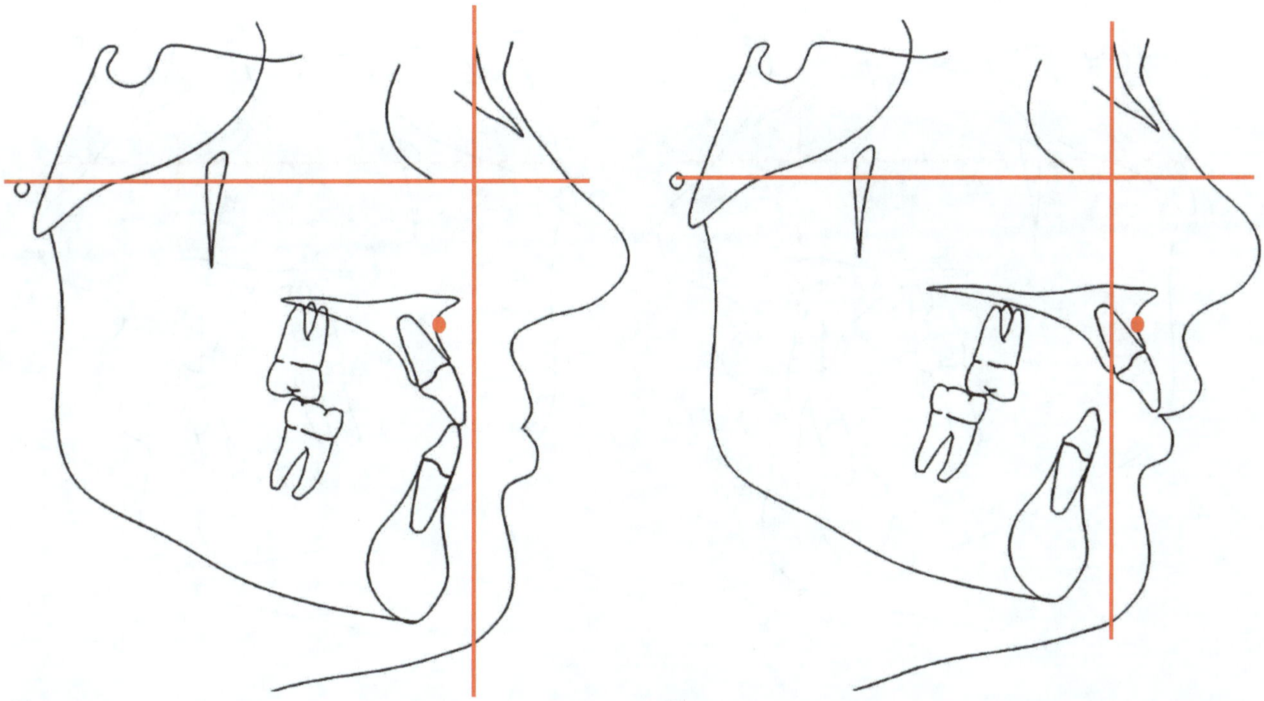

(a) (c)

Figure A.4 (a) Cephalometric tracing where A-Point lies considerably behind Nasion perpendicular, and the maxillary AP position is deficient/retrusive. (b) Cephalometric tracing where A-Point lies considerably ahead of Nasion perpendicular, and the maxillary AP position is excessive/protrusive.

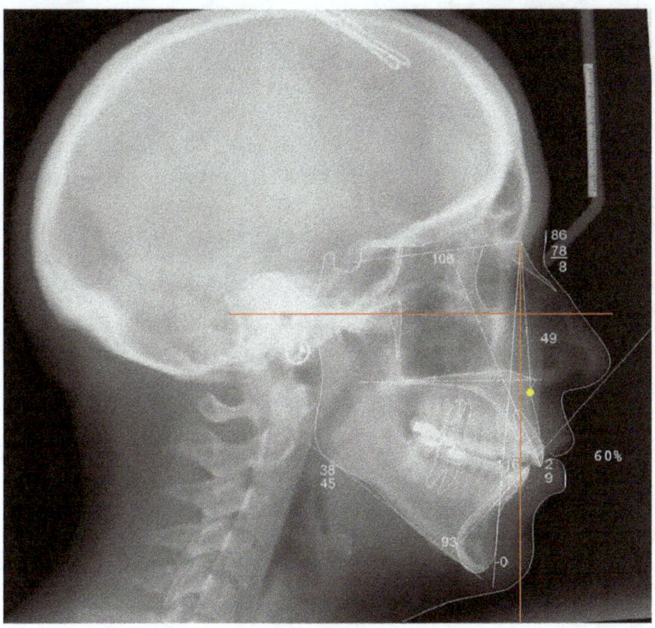

Figure A.5 Cephalometric radiograph and tracing where A-Point (yellow dot) lies ahead of Nasion perpendicular (NA-FH angle is 93°). This patient presents with maxillary AP excess (protrusion).

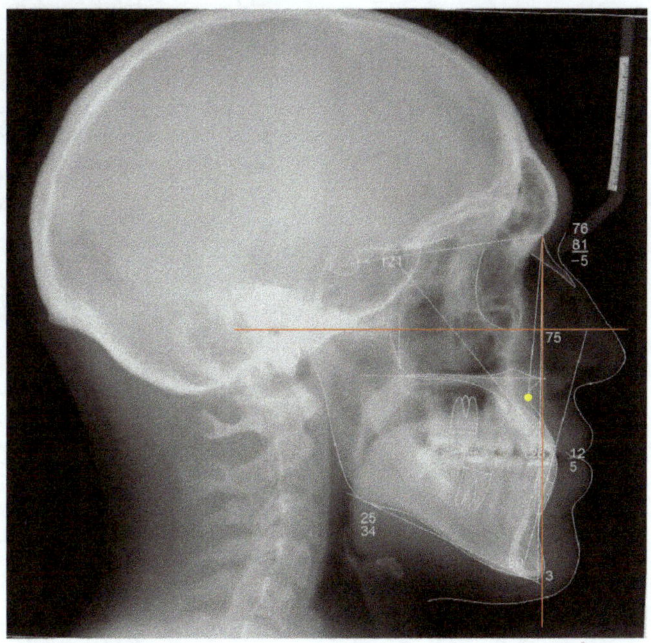

Figure A.6 Cephalometric radiograph and tracing where A-Point (yellow dot) lies behind Nasion perpendicular (NA-FH angle is 85°). This patient presents with maxillary AP deficiency (retrusion).

Q: How do you judge vertical skeletal relationships from a cephalometric radiograph?

A: There are a number of measurements that can help make this assessment:

- *Ratio of the lower anterior facial height to total anterior facial height*: measures the portion of the total height of the face contributed by the basal and alveolar portions of the jaws (Figure A.15). The average LAFH/TAFH ratio is 55% with a 2% standard deviation [3].
- *Steepness or flatness of the mandibular plane*: measured as an angle between MP and FH (FMA) or S-N line (SN-MP angle). These angular measurements are depicted in Figure A.16. Ideally, FMA = 25° and SN-MP = 32°. Angle SN-MP values >

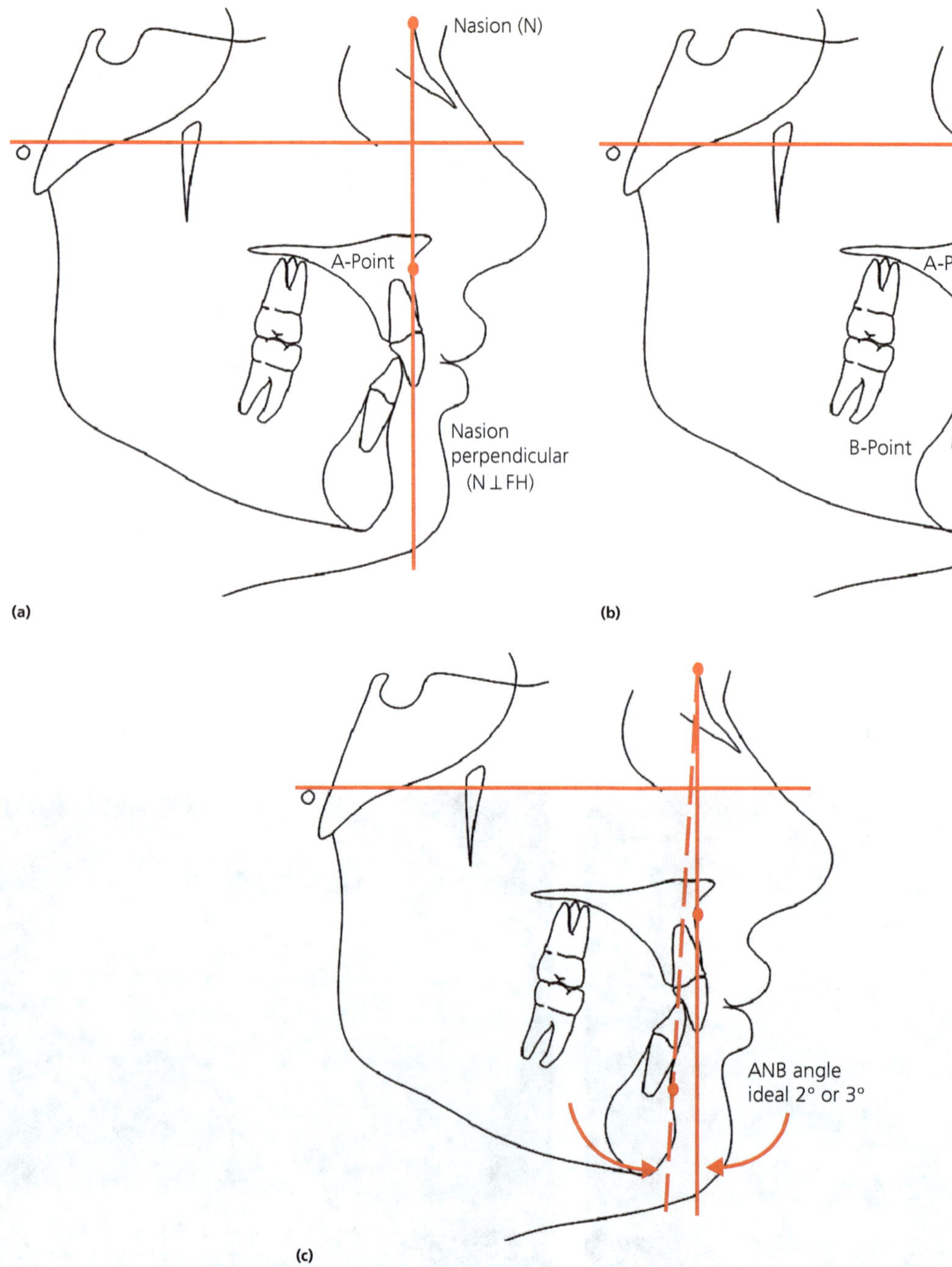

Figure A.7 (a) When the maxillary AP position is WRN, (b, c) an ideal mandibular AP position exists when ANB = 2° or 3°.

32° (FMA values > 25°) indicate increasing facial hyperdivergence while angle SN-MP values below 32° (FMA values < 25°) indicate contracting facial hypodivergence.

- Ratio of Posterior Facial Height (PFH) to Anterior Facial Height (AFH): the most common description of the PFH/AFH ratio is the quotient (Sella to Gonion distance)/(Nasion to Menton distance) as shown in Figure A.17 [4]. A ratio of 0.59 to 0.63 is WRN. A ratio less than 0.59 indicates a hyperdivergent pattern tending toward skeletal open bite. A ratio greater than 0.63 indicates a hypodivergent pattern tending toward skeletal deep bite. Because the ratio is mathematically related to the angle SN-MP, we choose the SN-MP angle and FMA to describe the vertical relationship of the jaws -instead of PFH/AFH.

Q: Evaluate the patient's vertical relationships in Figure A.18.
A: This patient's vertical relationship is normal and nearly ideal (LAFH/TAFH = 55%, FMA = 26°, SN-MP angle = 32°).

Q: Evaluate the patient's vertical relationship in Figure A.19.
A: She has a long lower anterior facial height (LLAFH), LAFH/TAFH = 60% and a very steep MPA (FMA = 38°, SN-MP angle = 45°).

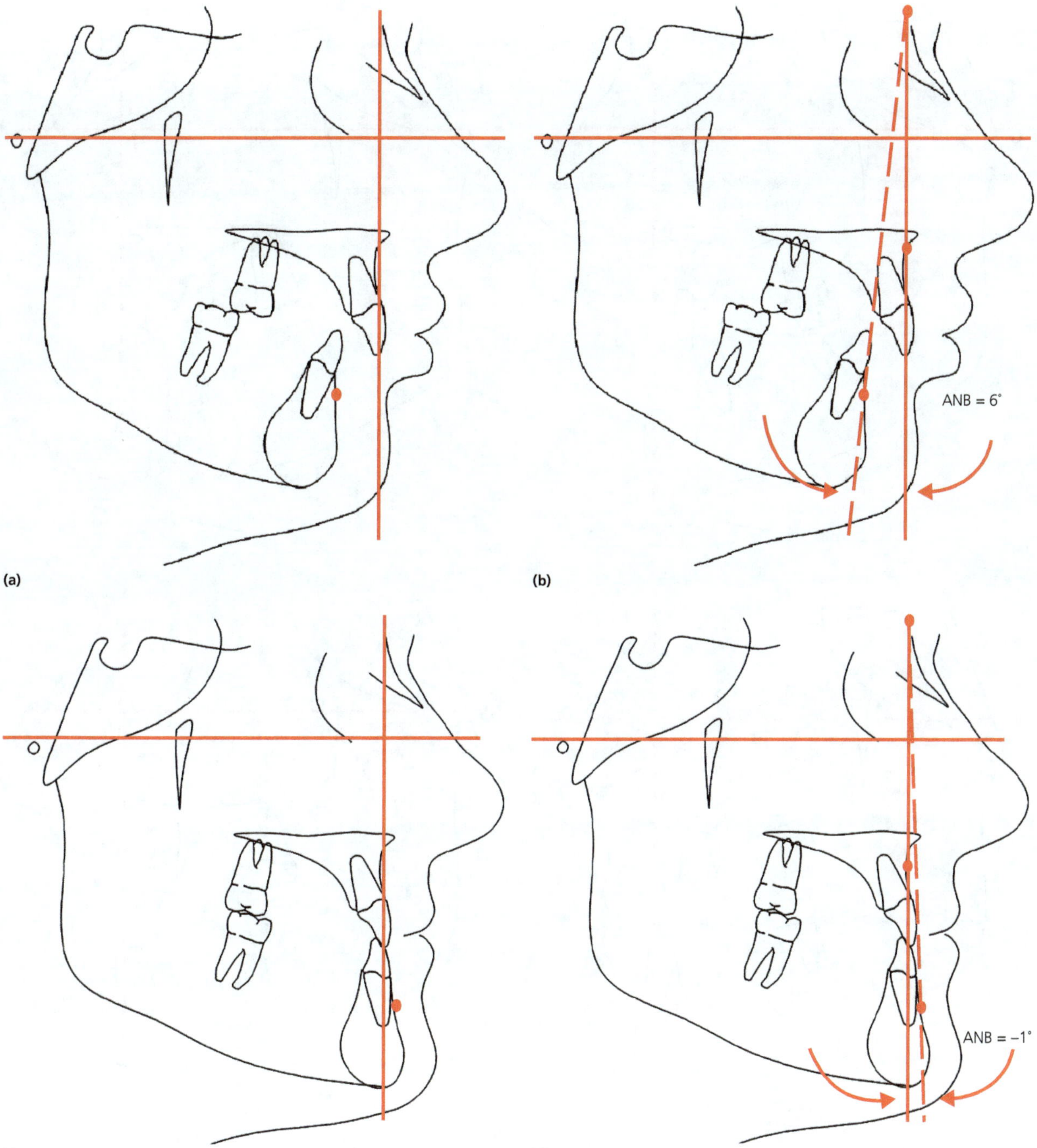

Figure A.8 Cephalometric tracings where the maxillary AP position is WRN: (a, b) mandibular AP deficiency (retrusion); (c, d) mandibular AP excess (protrusion).

Q: Evaluate the patient's vertical relationship in Figure A.20.

A: She has a short LAFH (LAFH/TAFH = 50%) and a very flat MPA (FMA = 15°, SN-MP angle = 20°).

Q: How do you judge maxillary incisor angulation?

A: Maxillary incisor angulation is judged *using the angle formed by the axis if the maxillary central incisors and the Sella—Nasion line (1-SN angle)*. This angle should lie within the range of 101–104°. 1-SN angles greater than 104° indicate proclined maxillary incisors. 1-SN angles less than 104° indicate retroclined (upright) maxillary incisors. Also, *the long axis of the maxillary incisor should project close to, or through, the distal contour of the orbit* (Figure A.21). This position can vary with maxillary incisor inclination, but also with forward or backward maxillary skeletal AP position.

Q: How do you judge mandibular incisor angulation?

A: Mandibular incisor angulation is judged *using the angle formed by the axis of the mandibular central incisors and Frankfort Horizontal, termed the Frankfort Mandibular Incisor Angle (FMIA)*. This angle should lie within the range of 65–68° (Figure A.21). FMIAs greater than 68° indicate retroclined

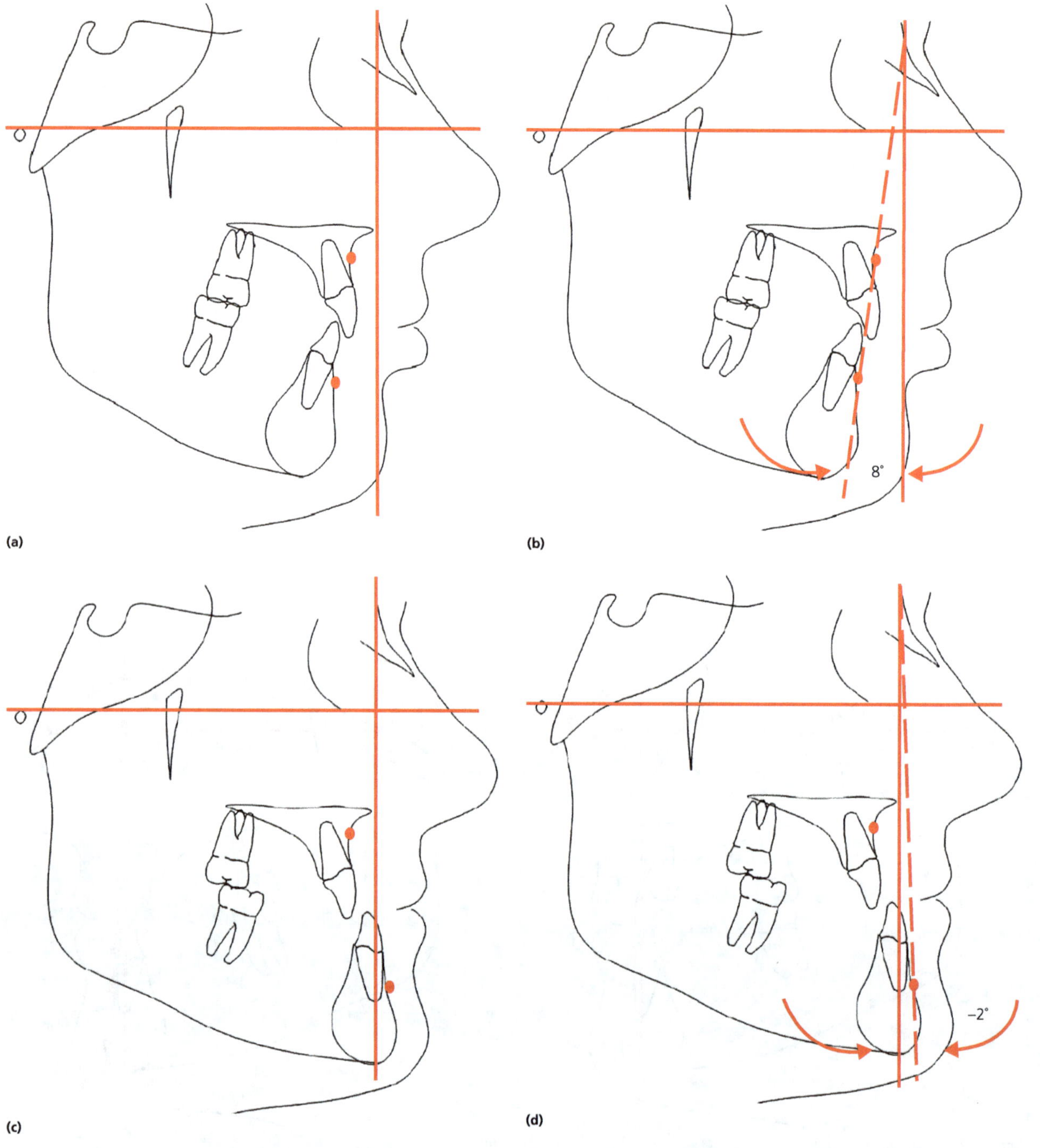

Figure A.9 Judging mandibular AP position when the maxillary AP position is not WRN: (a, b) Using the angle formed between Nasion perpendicular and the N-B line (8°), the mandible is judged to be deficient. (c, d) Using the same simple measurement, this mandible is judged to be excessive.

(upright) mandibular incisors. FMIAs less than 65° indicate proclined mandibular incisors.

Q: We recommend using FMIA to judge lower incisor angulation. If instead, you use the angle formed by the intersection of the mandibular central incisor axis and the mandibular plane (incisor mandibular plane angle, IMPA) to judge lower incisor angulation, you must be careful. Why?

A: Imagine that the lower incisors are fixed in the mandible. Mandibular incisor proclination varies with the steepness of the MPA—which is reflected in changes in FMIA but *not* in IMPA. That is, as the mandibular plane is rotated upward and forward, the mandibular incisors are increasingly uprighted with respect to the face. This will be reflected in increasing values of FMIA while IMPA remains fixed. Conversely, as the mandibular plane is rotated downward and backward, the mandibular incisors are increasingly proclined with respect to the face. This will be reflected in decreasing values of FMIA while IMPA remains fixed. We recommend using FMIA, not IMPA, to judge mandibular incisor proclination.

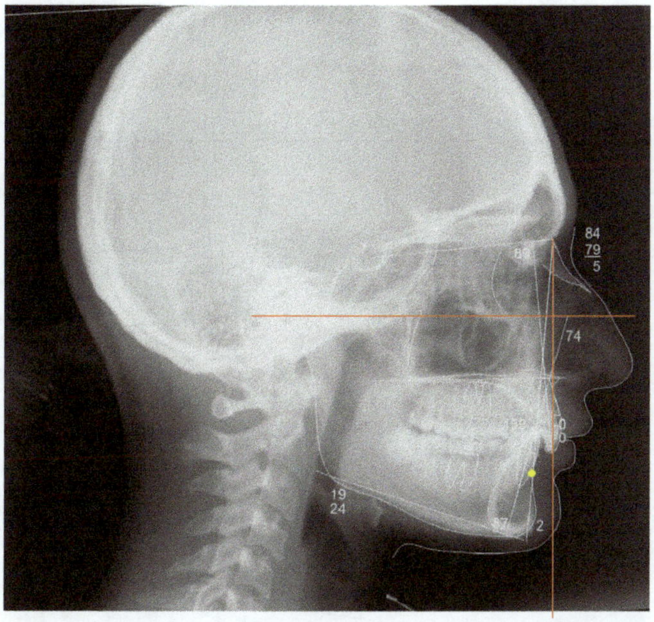

Figure A.10 Cephalometric radiograph and tracing where the maxilla is WRN (A-Point lies on Nasion-perpendicular), but the ANB angle is 5° (B-Point is indicated in yellow). The diagnosis is mandibular skeletal AP retrusion (deficiency).

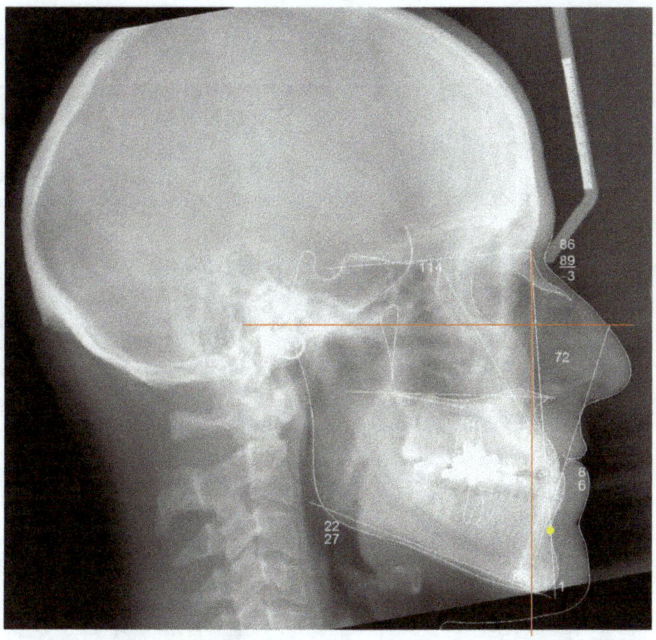

Figure A.11 Cephalometric radiograph and tracing where the maxilla is WRN (A-Point lies on Nasion-perpendicular), but ANB = −3° (B-Point is indicated in yellow). The diagnosis is mandibular AP skeletal protrusion (excess).

Q: Judge maxillary and mandibular incisor angulations in Figure A.5.
A: Proclined maxillary incisors, proclined mandibular incisors.

Q: Judge maxillary and mandibular incisor angulation in Figure A.6.
A: Proclined maxillary and upright mandibular incisors.

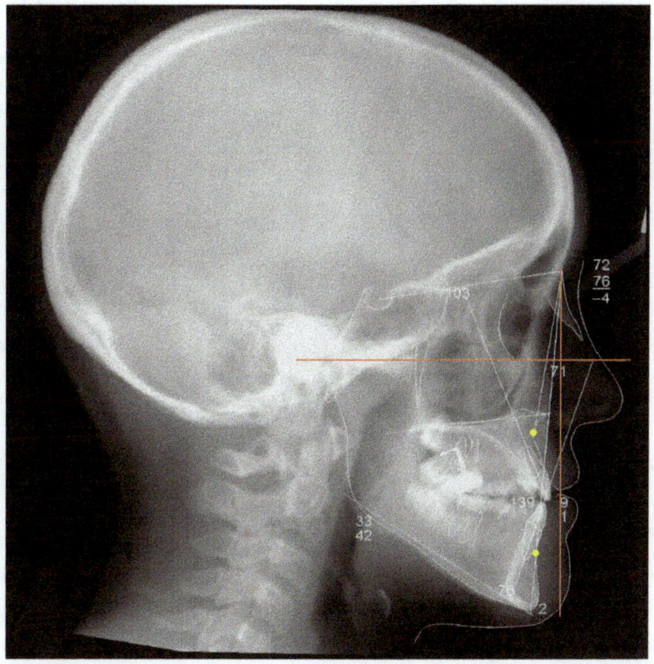

Figure A.12 Cephalometric radiograph and tracing showing an AP deficient maxilla (A-Point is quite distal to Nasion-perpendicular) and an AP deficient mandible (the angle formed by Nasion perpendicular and the N-B line exceeds 4°). A-Point and B-Point are indicated in yellow.

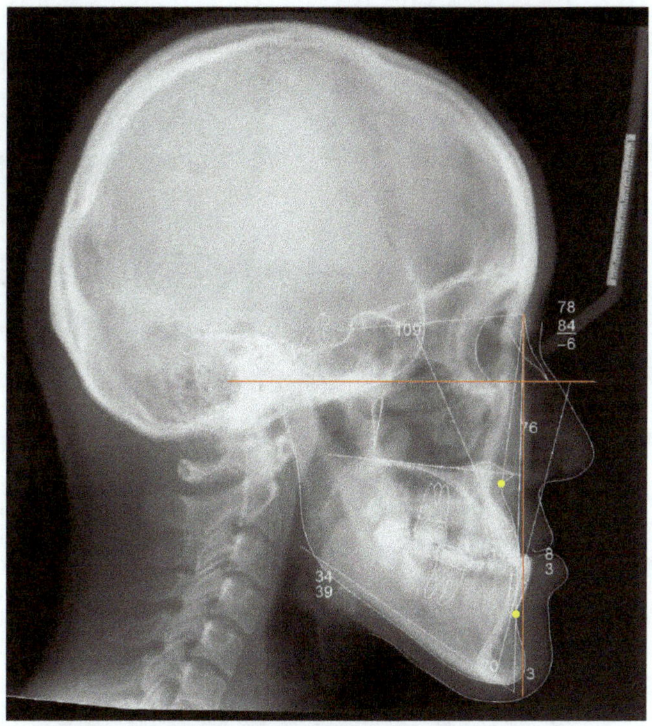

Figure A.13 Cephalometric radiograph and tracing showing an AP deficient maxilla (A-Point is quite distal to Nasion-perpendicular) and a mandible WRN (the angle formed by Nasion perpendicular and the N-B line is 2°). A-Point and B-Point are indicated in yellow.

Q: Judge maxillary and mandibular incisor angulation in Figure A.10.
A: Upright maxillary and mandibular incisors.

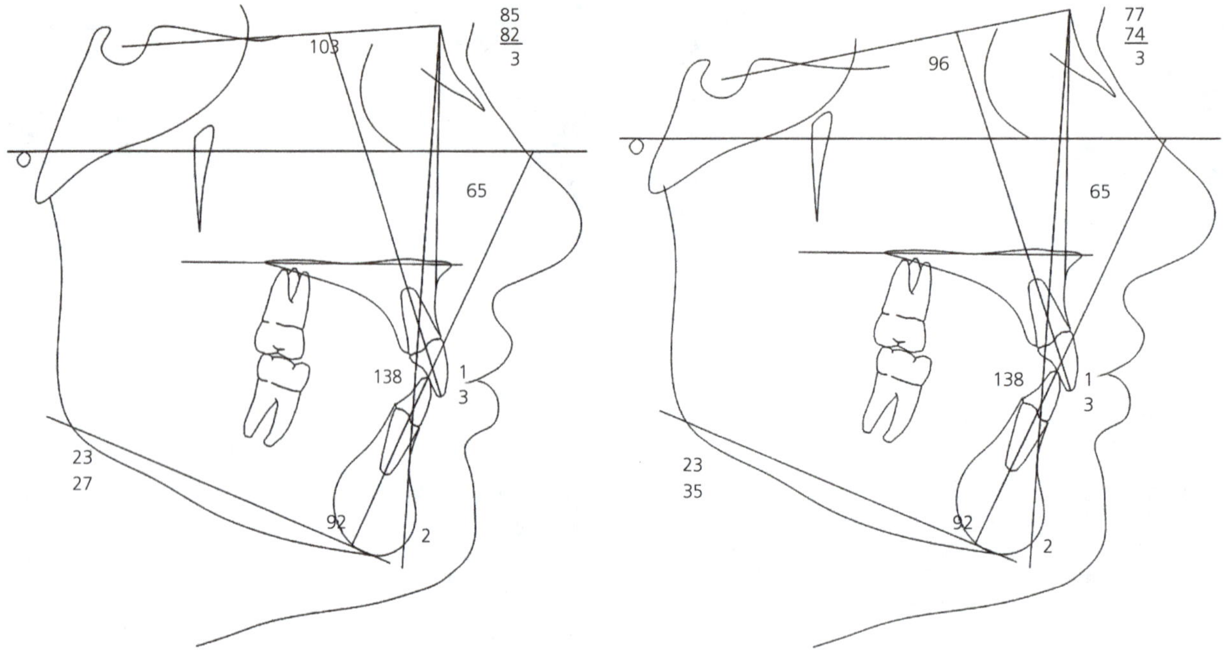

(a) (b)

Figure A.14 Effect of Sella vertical position on $\underline{1}$-SN, SNA, and SNB. (a) A "high" Sella results in larger values of $\underline{1}$-SN, SNA, and SNB and (b) a "low" Sella results in smaller values. Note also that the ANB angle is independent of Sella vertical position.

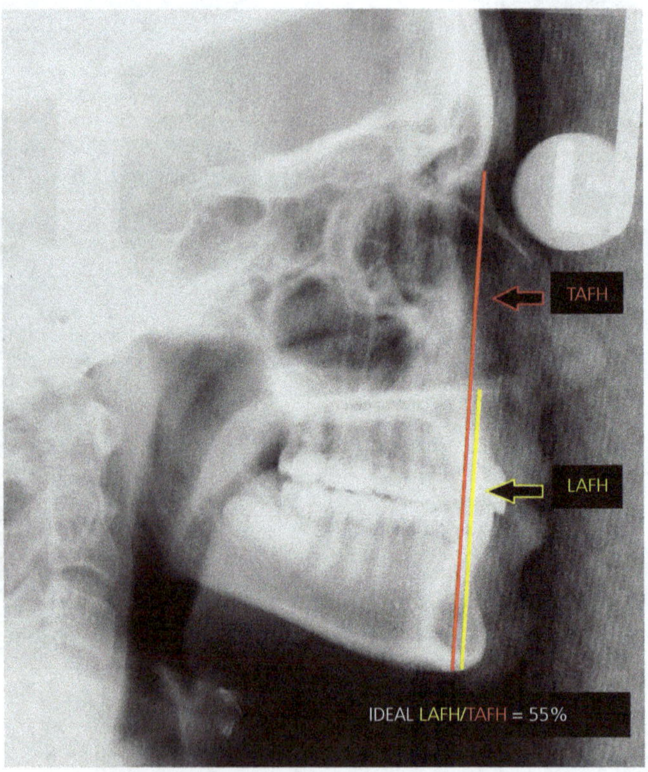

Figure A.15 Cephalometric radiograph showing the measurement of TAFH (distance from Nasion to Menton) and LAFH (distance along a parallel line from Menton to the projection of anterior nasal spine perpendicular to the Nasion-Menton line). The linear distances are combined into a percentage ratio LAFH/TAFH.

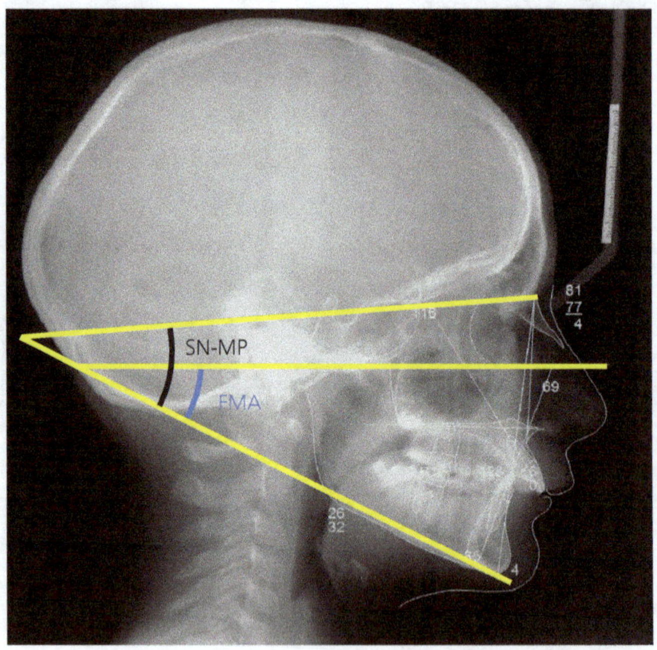

Figure A.16 Depiction of the angles formed by the Frankfort Horizontal and the Mandibular plane (FMA) and by the Sella-Nasion line and the Mandibular plane (SN-MP).

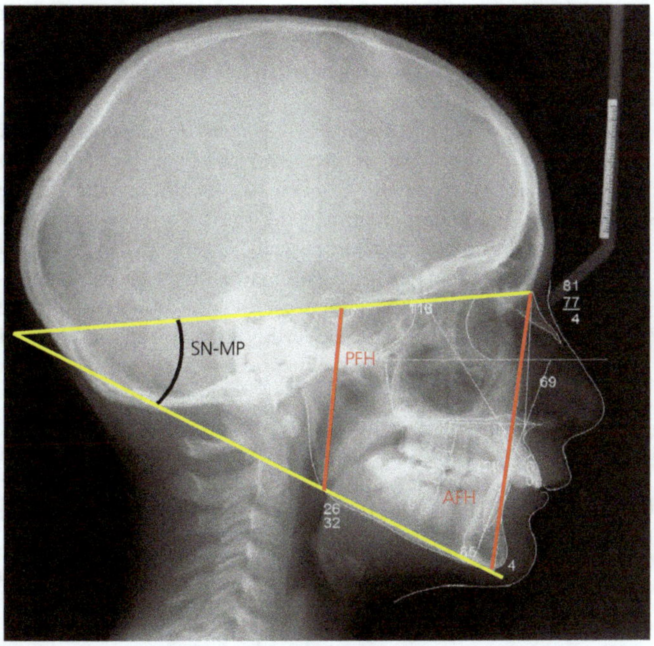

Figure A.17 Measurement of Posterior Facial Height (PFH) and Anterior Facial Height (AFH). For any individual, the ratio PFH/AFH is a mathematical relationship that defines the individual's SN-MP angle.

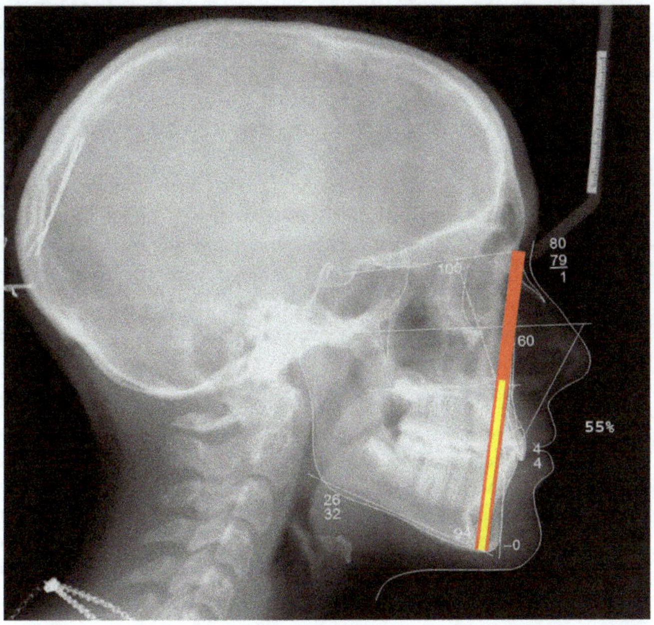

Figure A.18 Cephalometric radiograph and tracing illustrating a LAFH/TAFH (yellow/red) ratio of 55%, SN-MP angle = 32°, and FMA = 26°.

Q: Judge maxillary and mandibular incisor angulations in Figure A.12.

A: Normally inclined maxillary incisors, upright mandibular incisors.

Q: Judge maxillary and mandibular incisor angulations in Figure A.13.

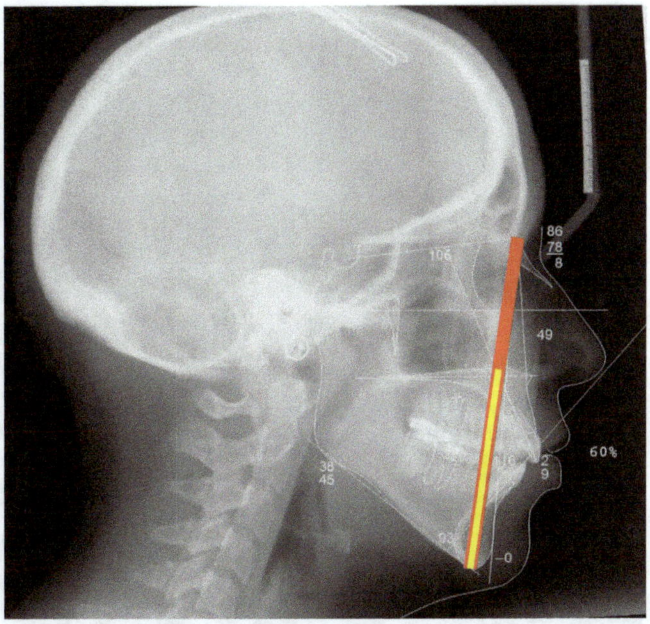

Figure A.19 Cephalometric radiograph and tracing illustrating a LAFH/TAFH (yellow/red) ratio of 60%, SN-MP angle = 45°, and FMA = 38°

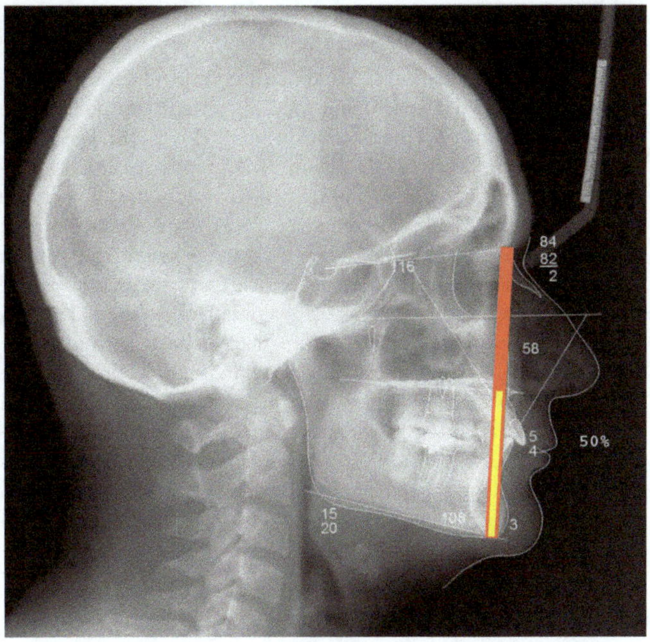

Figure A.20 Cephalometric radiograph and tracing illustrating a LAFH/TAFH (yellow/red) ratio of 50%, SN-MP = 20°, and FMA = 15°.

A: Proclined maxillary incisors, upright mandibular incisors.

Q: This Cephalometrics Primer described an analysis using anatomic landmarks to define reference points and lines. However, there are other approaches to lateral cephalometric analysis. What is "natural head position" and what is the advantage of using natural head position in cephalometric analysis?

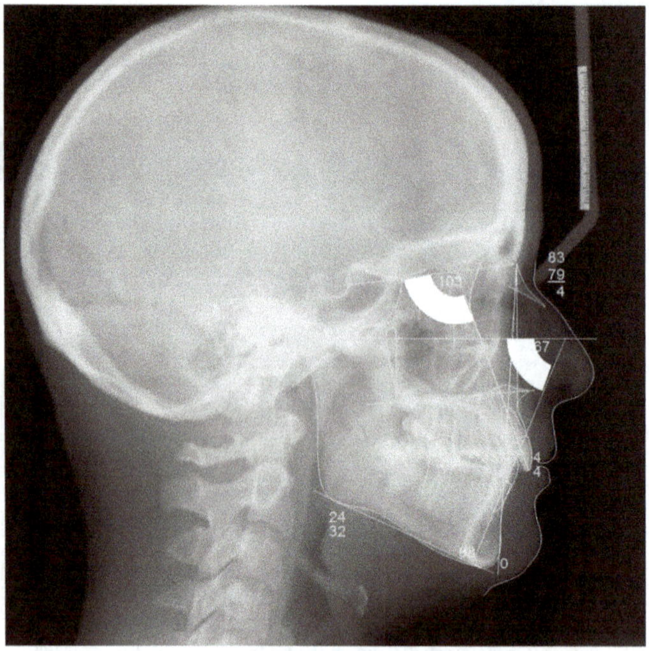

Figure A.21 Cephalometric radiograph and tracing illustrating normal maxillary and mandibular incisor relationships (1-SN = 103°, a line through the long axis of the maxillary central incisors projects through the distal of the orbits, and FMIA = 67°).

A: Natural head position is a standardized reproducible orientation of the head in space while focusing on a distant point at eye level [5]. This concept was introduced by Downs [6], Bjerin [7], Morrees, and Kean [8]. To obtain photographs or lateral cephalometric radiographs in natural head position, the subjects are typically seated in a relaxed state with the head unsupported and their eyes looking into their own image in a mirror [8]. An extracranial vertical line (true vertical) is used as a reference while interpreting lateral cephalometric radiographs and clinical photographs obtained in natural head position. The advantage of using natural head position is that it eliminates the biological variability inherent to anatomic reference points and lines. It is important to distinguish between natural head position and natural head posture. While natural head position is fixed and standardized for all individuals, the natural head posture is a functional or postural position of the head for each individual [5].

Q: What is estimated natural head position?

A: In scenarios when clinical photographs and lateral cephalometric radiographs are not obtained in the patient's natural head position, an "estimated natural head position" can be used. The photographs and lateral cephalometric can be "rotated" to the patient's natural head position [9, 10]. This is, however, subject to the judgment of the clinician.

Q: Can you offer any "take home pearls" regarding cephalometric analysis?

A: Take home pearls include:

- *Interpret cephalometric measurements in view of clinical impressions.* Your cephalometric skeletal analysis should always reflect what you observed clinically. For example, if you conclude (cephalometrically) that a patient has a mandibular AP skeletal deficiency, then this conclusion should be reflected in a retrusive (convex) photographic profile.
- *Never treat patients to satisfy cephalometric norms.* Deviation in cephalometric values away from average values can help compose your patient problem list, but these values alone should not dictate treatment decisions. For example, if you determine that (cephalometrically) a patient has proclined mandibular incisors, then you may decide to leave the incisors proclined if the patient's profile is attractive and the mandibular incisors are reasonably aligned. You must take all factors into consideration when treatment planning, not just cephalometric values.
- All cephalometric analyses have their weaknesses. The weakness of the aforementioned analysis is that it relies on Nasion. If Nasion is shifted far backward or far forward for a particular patient, then the analysis we presented could result in misleading conclusions. After all is said and done, base your final judgments of maxillary AP, mandibular AP, and vertical skeletal relationships on clear thinking and clinical impressions.

Iowa AP Classification Primer

The occlusion depicted in Figure A.22 illustrates a nearly ideal AP dental relationship and interdigitation of posterior teeth, what Edward H. Angle would call Class I "normal" occlusion [11]. Even the distobuccal cusp of the upper first permanent molar occludes with the mesiobuccal cusp of the lower second molar, as suggested by Andrews [12]. When you state that this patient has a "Class I occlusion," every orthodontist knows exactly what you mean and can visualize it.

The Angle classification scheme [13] describes malocclusion based largely on the variation of permanent first molar inter-arch anteroposterior relationships (variation from the maxillary first molar mesiobuccal cusp tip being aligned with the mandibular first molar buccal groove). Angle reasoned that the maxillary first molars were the most dependable reference from which to judge the position of other teeth:

> So important is the influence of these teeth in the building of the dental apparatus that we believe Nature exercises the greatest care in locating them, especially the upper first molars—which we call the keys to occlusion—and so places them that the rest of the dental apparatus may be completed normally; ...the first permanent upper molar furnishes more nearly than any other tooth or point in the anatomy an exact scientific basis from which to reason on malocclusion. [13]

Expanding upon the three *bilateral* molar AP relationship categories (Class I, Class II, and Class III), Angle conceived of a seven category classification system by adding subcategories for incisor inclination and unilateral inter-arch molar AP discrepancies:

- Class I
- Class II division 1
- Class II division 1 subdivision
- Class II division 2
- Class II division 2 subdivision
- Class III
- Class III subdivision

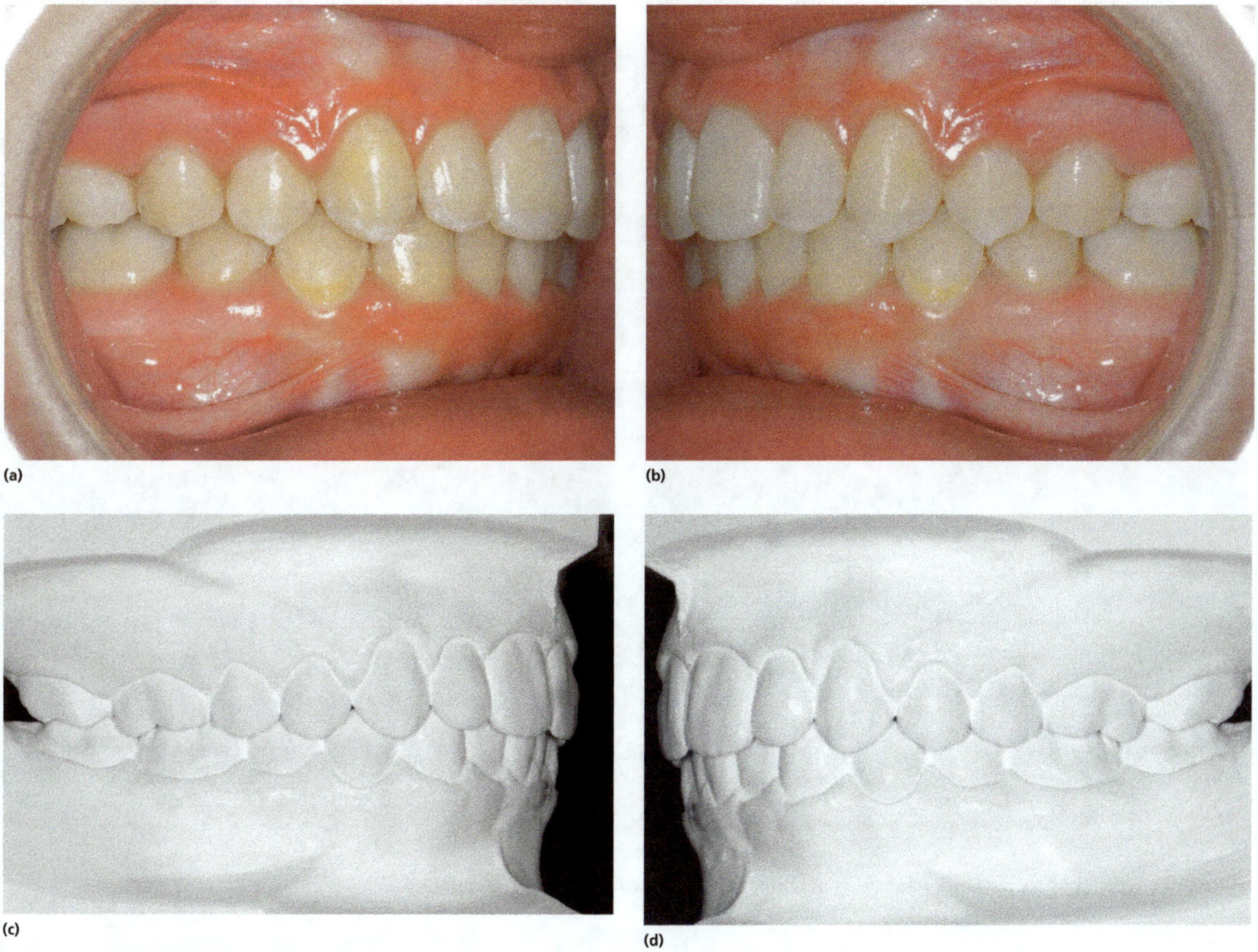

Figure A.22 (a–d) A patient with ideal Class I occlusion.

Although widely used today, Angle's classification scheme suffers from weaknesses:

- It constrains the diagnosis of inter-arch AP dental relationships to discrete categories. However, variation of inter-arch AP dental relationships is *continuous*, not discrete.
- *It does not permit the orthodontist to clearly visualize the magnitude of the AP discrepancy.* In other words, a Class II malocclusion with a 4 mm discrepancy is classified the same as a Class II malocclusion with a 10 mm discrepancy.
- It does not classify inter-arch canine relationships. And yet, canines are just as much keys of the dental arches as first molars are.
- It cannot classify malocclusions that are Class II molar on one side and Class III molar on the other.

Consider the patient shown in Figure A.23. According to Angle's system, this patient would be classified as Class I malocclusion (with a 2 mm molar AP discrepancy, the mesiobuccal cusps of the maxillary first molars are not beyond one-half of the mesial cusp of the mandibular molars). This classification gives no indication of the severity of the AP inter-arch discrepancy, or even that there is a discrepancy. Simply put, with a diagnosis of Class I you cannot infer whether the AP inter-arch discrepancy is non-existent, mild (perhaps amenable to correction with elastics), or severe (perhaps requiring orthognathic surgery for correction). Further, Angle's classification ignores canine relationships—which are at least as important as molar AP relationships in order to obtain maximum intercuspation.

To address these shortcomings, faculty at the University of Iowa (including ourselves and Dr. Robert Staley) developed a simple modification of the Angle classification system. This modification, which we call the Iowa Classification, is used throughout this text and consists of describing the patient's right molar, right canine, left canine, and left molar relationships in terms of millimeter deviation from Class I. The Iowa Classification system permits ready communication and visualization of the patient's AP relationship.

For example, the patient shown in Figure A.23 is re-classified in Figure A.24 according to the Iowa Classification as follows: Beginning with the right-side inter-arch first molar relationship, the AP discrepancy is measured to be Class II by 2 mm. The right-side inter-arch canine AP discrepancy is then measured to be Class II by 4 mm. The left-side inter-arch canine discrepancy is then measured to be Class II by 5 mm. And finally, the left-side inter-arch

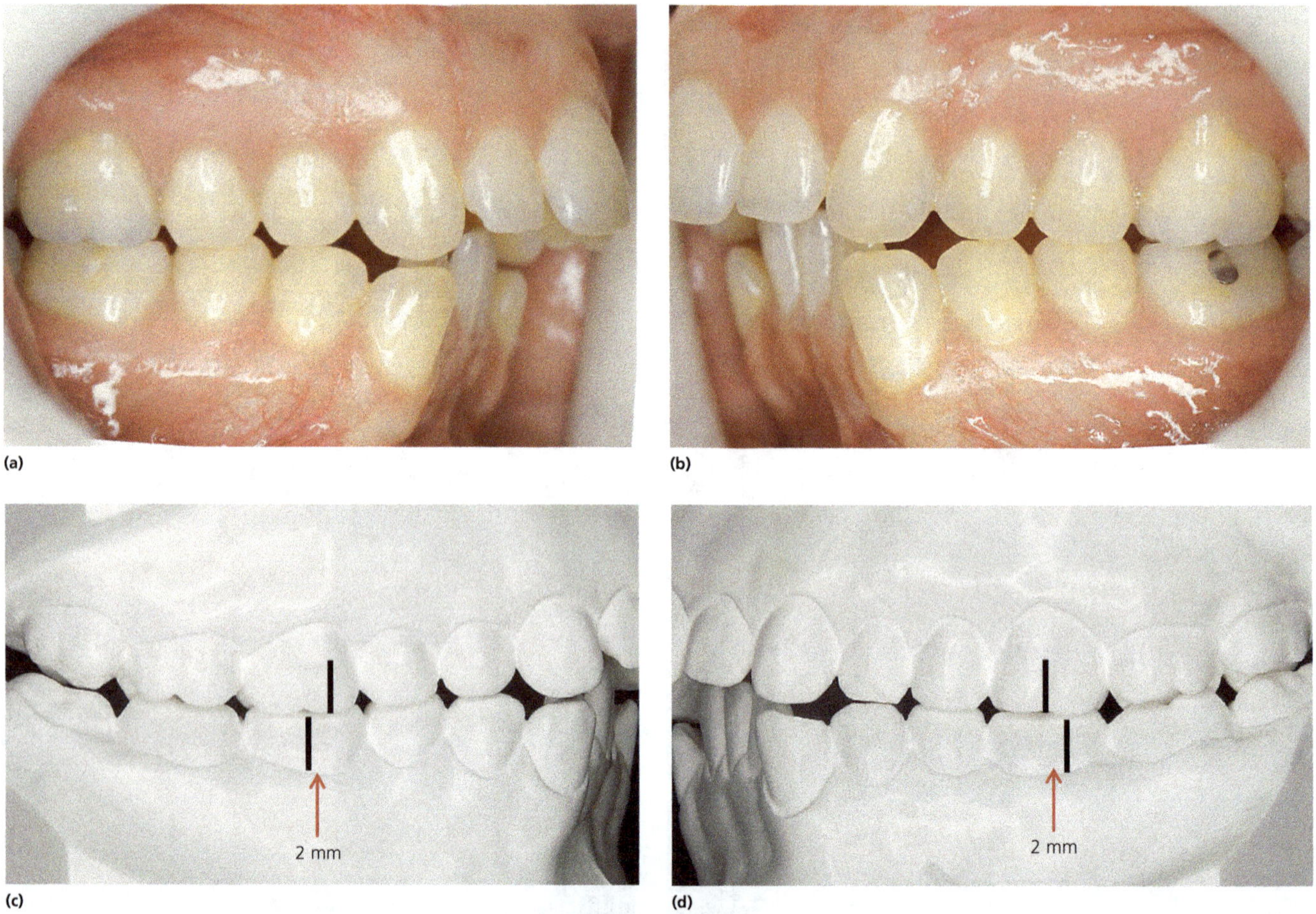

Figure A.23 Patient with a Class I malocclusion according to the Angle system.

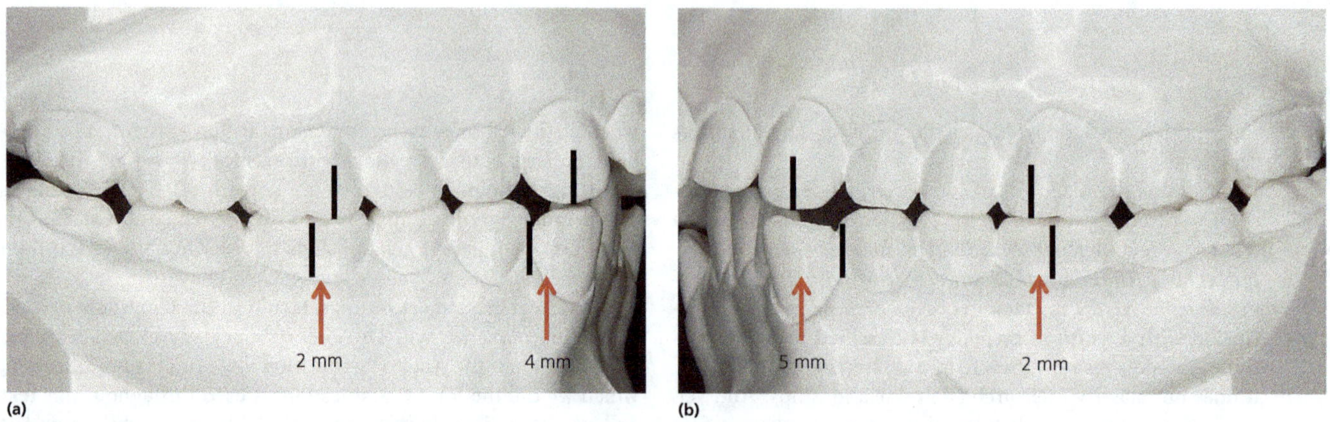

Figure A.24 The Iowa Classification measurements for the patient in Figure A.23. The shorthand notation for this classification is II(2) II(4) II(5) II(2).

first molar AP discrepancy is measured to be 2 mm. The shorthand notation of the Iowa Classification for this patient is:

Right-side II (2 mm) II (4 mm) II (5 mm) II (2 mm) Left-side, or simply,

II(2) II(4) II(5) II(2) ; read as "Class II by 2, 4, 5, 2 mm"

Q: Classify the patient shown in Figure A.25.
A: III(3) III(3) III(3) III(3)

Q: Classify the subdivision patient shown in Figure A.26.
A: II(3) II(3) I I

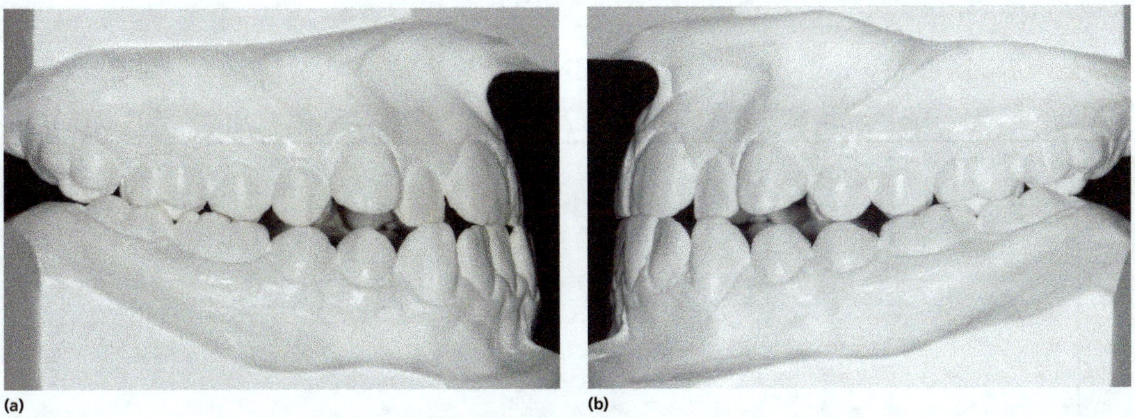

Figure A.25 (a, b) Patient who is Class III, bilaterally, by 3 mm at molars and canines.

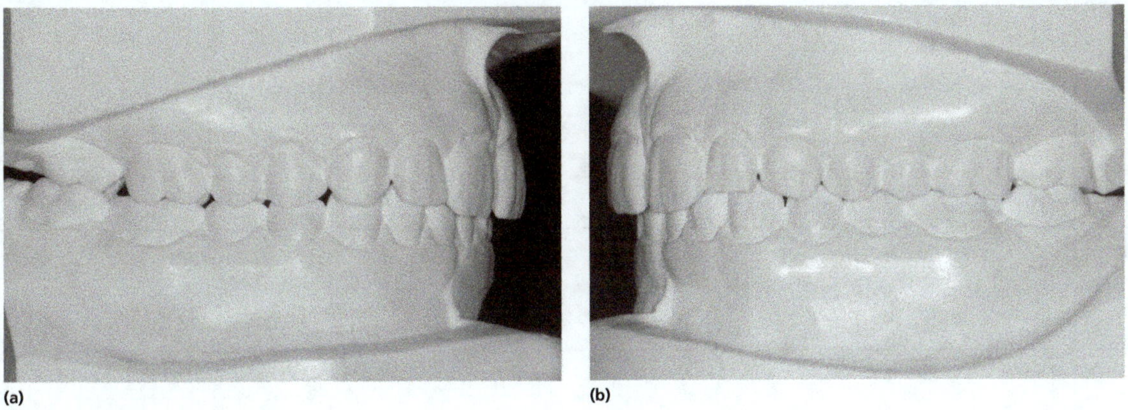

Figure A.26 (a, b) Subdivision patient.

Tables for Reference

Table A.1 Template: Diagnostic findings and problems list.

Full face and profile	FRONTAL VIEW PROFILE VIEW
Ceph analysis	SKELETAL DENTAL
Radiographs	
Intraoral photos and models	
Other	
Diagnosis	

Table A.2 Template: Primary problems list.

AP	
Vertical	
Transverse	
Other	

Table A.3 Checklist to follow for surgical patients.

Pre-surgical tasks	☐ Verify relaxed lip incisal display *after leveling* to decide the magnitude of vertical maxillary surgical incisor movement ☐ Approve the articulated surgical occlusion (models mounted by the surgeon) ☐ Agree on proposed surgical movements and verify that surgical movements are within surgical limits ☐ Schedule the patient to see you 1 week after the surgery date
Post-surgical communication	☐ When should the surgeon contact the orthodontist? – immediately after surgery (what was the surgical outcome?) – the surgeon should inform the orthodontist of problems (to better prepare for dealing with them) – **Q:** was the bite seated during surgery? (if it was, than a later occlusal discrepancy could be due to edema/muscle spasms) ☐ take care what you say in front of the patient – seek solutions to surgical problems the cause of which may have been indeterminate / unavoidable – put a positive spin on intervention—"surgery helped a lot, now we are completing treatment" ☐ Work together with the surgeon to discuss post-surgical treatment, including direction and magnitude of forces to be applied
Post-surgical tasks	☐ See patient 1 week post-operatively (well within the first month window of accelerated bony remodeling/cellular activity/possible increased tooth movement) so that you can intercede effectively, as needed. ☐ Check for post-surgical occlusal discrepancies, including a repeatable bite at the 1 week post-op appointment ☐ Guiding elastics—guiding elastics help the patient learn to close into the new occlusion. This is necessary since the jaw muscular length and direction have been changed with surgery, edema and muscle spasms may alter the correct closing position, proprioceptive sense may have been lost, and/or the patient may be numb. The focus of guiding elastics is on the muscles. Guiding elastics are *not* intended to move teeth. There is no specific length of time for wearing guiding elastics. Time of wear is a judgment call made between the surgeon and orthodontist. ☐ Splints—an occlusal splint is worn by the patient for approximately 6 weeks following MPMOs to hold a transverse expansion. As soon as it is removed, a palatal splint is fabricated and worn for as long as possible through the completion of orthodontic treatment. If the maxillary archwire was sectioned at surgery, then it should be replaced with a continuous wire at the 6 week appointment.

Table A.4 Limits of orthognathic surgical movements.

Maxillary surgical limits	Downgraft	5–8 mm	Note: The maxilla cannot descend straight down due to changes in the occlusal plane angle as the mandible rotates down and back
	Iimpaction	6–7 mm 10 mm	In the posterior In the anterior
	MPMO transverse expansion	8 mm	Limit depends on the height of the palate and posterior tooth torque; a low palate permits less expansion (soft tissue stretch); ideally, the pre-surgical posterior dentition should be without transverse compensations
	Advancement	5–7 mm	Consider distraction osteogenesis if more maxillary advancement then this is required
	Setback	5–6 mm	The limiting factor is running into the bony pterygoid plates. If you need greater setback than this, consider extracting maxillary premolars so only the anterior segment is setback
Mandibular surgical limits	Advancement	10 mm 14–15 mm	In high MPA cases In low MPA cases Note: check for impingement of maxillary 2nd molars on the ascending ramus during advancement. You may need to extract the maxillary 2nd molars if maxillary 2nd molar impingement occurs
	Setback	10 mm	Be careful to avoid airway obstruction or of creating future sleep apnea problems

Personal communication with Drs. Kirk Fridrich and Steve Fletcher, University of Iowa College of Dentistry Department of Oral and Maxillofacial Surgery, September 16, 2013.

Table A.5 Guidelines for post-surgical biomechanics if occlusal discrepancies exist (i.e., not fully corrected or overcorrected).

General guidelines	• Use the same biomechanics that are used as for non-surgical cases • Discuss with your surgeon the level of forces, and direction of forces, you intend to use • Try to stay with light forces—especially when beginning • *Remember the direction of surgery*—do NOT immediately use mechanics that are opposite to the direction of the surgery. For example, if a mandibular advancement osteotomy overcorrected a Class II patient to a Class III relationship, do NOT begin pulling Class III elastics. You may eventually need use Class III elastics, but give the patient some months to allow edema to be eliminated and muscular function to normalize before doing so.
Mild discrepancy	• Use standard orthodontic finishing treatment
Moderate discrepancy	• Aggressive intercession may be required, or accept a compromise result
Severe discrepancy	• Discuss with surgeon • If you feel that the patient needs to go back into surgery, do it very soon so the patient has only 1 recovery period (if you wait a month before sending the patient back to surgery, he/she will have two recovery periods.)

Abbreviations

ANB angle formed by A-Point—Nasion—B-Point
ADD anteriorly displaced disk
AP anteroposterior
BSSO bilateral sagittal split osteotomy
CC chief complaint
CO centric occlusion
CPHG cervical pull headgear
CR centric relation
CW clockwise
CCW counter-clockwise
FH Frankfort horizontal
FMA angle formed by Frankfort horizontal to mandibular plane
FMIA angle formed by Frankfort horizontal to mandibular incisor
HPHG highpull headgear
ILG interlabial gap
IMPA angle formed by lower incisor to mandibular plane
IPR interproximal reduction

LLAFH	long lower anterior facial height (soft tissue clinically or skeletal cephalometrically)
LAFH	lower anterior facial height (soft tissue clinically or skeletal cephalometrically)
LDML	lower dental midline
LLHA	lower lingual holding arch
LTSALD	lower tooth size arch length discrepancy
Mn	mandibular
MPMO	multiple piece maxillary osteotomy
MP	mandibular plane
MPA	mandibular plane angle
Mx	maxillary
NLA	nasolabial angle
OB	overbite
OJ	overjet
PDH	past dental history
PFE	primary failure of eruption
PMH	past medical history
RME	rapid maxillary expansion
SARME	surgically assisted rapid maxillary expansion
SN	Sella-Nasion
SNA	angle formed by Sella—Nasion—A-Point
SNB	angle formed by Sella—Nasion—B-Point
SNMP	angle formed by Sella—Nasion to mandibular plane
TAD	temporary anchorage device
TAFH	total anterior facial height (skeletal cephalometrically)
TMJ	temporomandibular joint
UDML	upper dental midline
UTSALD	upper tooth size arch length discrepancy
U1	maxillary central incisor
L1	manidbular central incisor
WRN	within the range of normal

Appendix References

1 Riedel R. *A cephalometric roentgenographic study of the relation of the maxilla and associated parts to the cranial base in normal and malocclusion of the teeth [master's thesis]*. Evanston, IL: Northwestern University;1948.

2 McNamara JA Jr. A method of cephalometric evaluation. *Am J Orthod.* 1984;**86**:449–69.

3 Wylie W, Johnson E. Rapid evaluation of facial dysplasia in the vertical plane. *Angle Orthod.* 1952;**22**:165–82.

4 Siriwat PP, Jarabak JR. Malocclusion and facial morphology is there a relationship? An epidemiologic study. *Angle Orthod.* 1985;**55**:127–38.

5 Moorees CFA. Natural head position: the key to cephalometry. In: Jacobson A, Jacobson RL, editors. *Radiographic cephalometry: from basics to 3-D imaging.* 2nd ed. Chicago, IL: Quintessence; 2006. pp. 153–60.

6 Downs WB. Analysis of the dentofacial profile. *Angle Orthod.* 1956;**4**:191–212.

7 Bjerin R. A comparison between the Frankfort Horizontal and the sella turcica-nasion line as reference planes in cephalometric analysis. *Acta Odontol Scand.* 1957;**15**:1–12.

8 Moorrees CFA, Kean MR. Natural head position, a basic consideration in the interpretation of cephalometric radiographs. *Am J of Phys Anthropol.* 1958;**16**:213–34.

9 Jiang J, Xu T, Lin J. The relationship between estimated and registered natural head position. *Angle Orthod.* 2007;**77**:1019–24.

10 Moorrees CF. Natural head position—a revival. *Am J Orthod Dentofacial Orthop.* 1994;**105**:512–3.

11 Angle EH. Classification of malocclusion. *Dent Cosmos.* 1899;**41**:248–64, 350–7.

12 Andrews L. The six keys to normal occlusion. *Am J Orthod Dentofacial Orthop.* 1972;**62**:296–309.

13 Angle EH. *Treatment of malocclusion of the teeth: Angle's system.* Philadelphia, PA: SS White Dental Manufacturing Company; 1907.

Index

Page numbers in *italics* refer to illustrations.

Orthodontics in the Vertical Dimension: A Case-Based Review, First Edition. Thomas E. Southard, Steven D. Marshall and Laura L. Bonner.

www.ingramcontent.com/pod-product-compliance
Lightning Source LLC
LaVergne TN
LVHW062155200926
848484LV00007B/1915